NINTH EDITION

An Introduction to
HUMAN DISEASE

Pathology and Pathophysiology Correlations

LEONARD V. CROWLEY, MD

Biology Department
Century College
University of Minnesota Medical Center, Fairview
Minneapolis, Minnesota

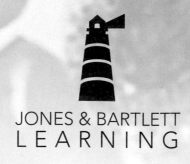

JONES & BARTLETT
LEARNING

World Headquarters
Jones & Bartlett Learning
5 Wall Street
Burlington, MA 01803
978-443-5000
info@jblearning.com
www.jblearning.com

Jones & Bartlett Learning books and products are available through most bookstores and online booksellers. To contact Jones & Bartlett Learning directly, call 800-832-0034, fax 978-443-8000, or visit our website, www.jblearning.com.

Substantial discounts on bulk quantities of Jones & Bartlett Learning publications are available to corporations, professional associations, and other qualified organizations. For details and specific discount information, contact the special sales department at Jones & Bartlett Learning via the above contact information or send an email to specialsales@jblearning.com.

Production Credits

Chief Executive Officer: Ty Field
President: James Homer
SVP, Editor-in-Chief: Michael Johnson
SVP, Chief Marketing Officer: Alison M. Pendergast
Publisher: Cathleen Sether
Executive Editor: Shoshanna Goldberg
Associate Acquisitions Editor: Megan R. Turner
Editorial Assistant: Agnes Burt
Editorial Assistant: Sean Coombs

Production Editor: Amanda Clerkin
Rights & Photo Researcher: Sarah Cebulski
Marketing Manager: Jody Yeskey
V.P., Manufacturing and Inventory Control: Therese Connell
Composition: Circle Graphics, Inc.
Cover Design: Kristin E. Parker
Cover Image: Courtesy of Leonard V. Crowley
Printing and Binding: Courier Kendallville
Cover Printing: Courier Kendallville

To order this product, use ISBN: 978-1-4496-6559-3

Library of Congress Cataloging-in-Publication Data
Crowley, Leonard V., 1926-
    An introduction to human disease : pathology and pathophysiology correlations / Leonard V. Crowley. — 9th ed.
        p. ; cm.
    Includes bibliographical references and index.
    ISBN 978-1-4496-3240-3
    I. Title.
    [DNLM: 1. Disease. 2. Pathology. QZ 4]

    616.07—dc23

                                                    2011050945

6048
Printed in the United States of America
16 15 14 13 12   10 9 8 7 6 5 4 3 2 1

In Memoriam

Dr. Leonard Crowley passed away on February 5, 2012. We honor his memory as a dedicated practitioner, educator, and author.

Dedication

To my wife, who was very helpful and understanding.

Reviewers

The author wishes to thank...

Christine K. Bieszczad, PhD
Colby-Sawyer College

Carol J. Bunge, RN, MHA
University of Southern Indiana

L. Fleming Fallon, Jr., MD, DrPH
Bowling Green State University

Julie A Fisher, PhD, RN
Professor, Nursing
Wesley College

Jennifer Green-Williams, RHIT, RMA, EMT-I
Neosho County Community College

Jill-Renae Gulczinski, MS, PA-C
Kettering College Physician Assistant Program
Kettering College of Medical Arts

Seema Jejurikar
Bellvue College

Julia Lapp, PhD, RD, CDN
Department of Health Promotion and Physical
Education
Ithaca College

Lisa Ochs, MSN, RN
Burlington County College

Emmanuel Osunkoya, MD, MPH
Chicago State University

Shallee T. Page, PhD, MA
University of Maine at Machias

Sara S. Plaspohl, DrPH, CIM, CIP
Armstrong Atlantic State University

Peter C. Sayles
North Country Community College

Shonna Snyder
Gardner Webb University

Julie Vining Smith, PhD
William Carey University

Brief Contents

Contents

14   THE HEMATOPOIETIC AND LYMPHATIC SYSTEMS   341

21 THE LIVER AND THE BILIARY SYSTEM   553

22 THE PANCREAS AND DIABETES MELLITUS   590

26 THE NERVOUS SYSTEM 698

Preface

THERE HAVE BEEN MANY NEW DEVELOPMENTS AND ADVANCES in medicine since the last edition of this book. This edition has many rewritten sections to incorporate new concepts and treatment methods. I have rearranged the location of the material in some chapters, added material on some new diseases that have become more important in medical practice, added some new tables to existing chapters, and updated the annotated list of references. I have expanded the annotations, which can be used to supplement the text material. I have concentrated primarily on references in the *New England Journal of Medicine* and the *Journal of the American Medical Association* because they are the most likely journals to be available in the libraries used by students. The same basic organization of the book has been retained as described in the "About the Book" section, because the format seems to be popular with students. The student workbook has been rearranged in some areas to conform to the textbook chapters, and also was upgraded by adding questions dealing with the new material.

New material has been added to almost every chapter, and many new references have been added.

- Chapter 1 contains additional material on the applications and limitations of PET scans.
- Chapter 2 describes the role of microRNA and how it regulates gene functions.
- Chapter 5 contains new material on lupus erythematosus and scleroderma and also includes two new photographs.
- Chapter 6 has expanded material on herpes zoster (shingles) and the vaccine to prevent it.
- Chapter 7 deals with *Pneumocystis jiroveci*, which now is classified as a fungus.
- Chapter 8 contains updated material on HIV, including recommendations for early treatment to prevent damage to the immune system and to help prevent the spread of HIV to contacts.
- Chapter 9 explains that prenatal tests for Down syndrome now are offered to all women, not just older women. The tests are described, along with their applications and limitations.
- Chapter 10 describes new, less-aggressive treatment of Hodgkin disease and other neoplastic diseases affecting the bone marrow to reduce the risk of later therapy-related complications.
- Chapters 11 and 12 explain how new anticoagulant drugs offer treatment advantages over Warfarin. The d-dimer test helps diagnose a pulmonary embolism.
- Chapter 13 contains an expanded section on artificial heart valves, with several new photographs, and describes new methods of valve replacement. Treatment of acute coronary syndromes is updated, along with case studies.
- Chapter 14 provides a new section on oxygen transport by hemoglobin, along with an expanded section on problems related to sickle cell trait. Immunosuppression of the bone marrow before marrow transplant is less aggressive and yields better results.
- Chapter 15 contains an augmented chest CT screening test for lung carcinoma that permits earlier detection and improves survival but is more expensive and also yields false-positive results.
- Chapter 16 contains updated material on the harmful effects of estrogen-progestin on breast cancer risk, and risk-reduction surgery for *BRCA*-positive women is discussed.
- Chapter 17 discusses the role of PAP smears and tests for HPV infection. A new postcoital contraceptive is available.
- Chapter 18 provides additional material on twin-to-twin transfusion.

- Chapters 19 and 20 describe the risks and benefits of kidney transplantation, with emphasis on new approaches that reduce the need for continuous immunosuppression. Treatment of prostatic carcinoma on young and elderly men is described. Nephrectomy is not always necessary when treating kidney carcinoma.
- Chapter 21 describes non-alcohol–related fatty liver and cirrhosis. New treatment for hepatitis C improves results.
- Chapter 22 contains expanded sections on diabetes, prediabetes, and treatment.
- Chapter 23 contains additional sections on GI tract foreign bodies, with case studies and photographs. The section on eating disorders has been updated and expanded. Gluten enteropathy is considered, and new photographs have been added.
- Chapter 26 contains additional material on prenatal intrauterine treatment of meningomyelocele.
- Chapter 27 provides and expanded section on osteogenesis imperfecta, and a new photograph has been added. A new section on pectus excavatum with two photographs and its effect on cardiopulmonary function has been added, along with new material on Marfan syndrome and its relationship to pectus excavatum.

Although the book has undergone considerable updating and rewriting, I have attempted to retain the same basic format and orientation of the earlier editions, emphasizing the major structural and functional changes of disease and the basic principles of treatment in a straightforward, user-friendly manner. Normal structure and function are interrelated and so also are the structural derangements associated with disease (pathology) and the accompanying disturbances in organ function (pathophysiology). Moreover, if one has a clear concept of the structural derangements associated with disease, one also has a better grasp of the relevant pathophysiology and can usually also deduce the clinical manifestations of various diseases and understand how treatment can influence the course of a disease.

I would like to thank the many persons teaching human disease courses who provided the publisher and me with helpful suggestions and editorial comments that helped to improve this edition. Special thanks also go to the staff at Jones & Bartlett Learning for their enthusiasm, help, and encouragement during the preparation of this edition.

About the Book

PURPOSE AND SCOPE OF THE BOOK

This book is based on courses given for many years to students in nursing and other health professions. It is designed to provide a solid foundation on which students can build for the remainder of their professional careers. A fundamental knowledge of disease requires a clear conception of both the structural and the functional changes caused by disease in tissues and organs, as a basis for understanding the clinical manifestations and principles of treatment. Consequently, to facilitate learning, many illustrations of the salient features of the more important diseases have been included. Photographs of x-ray films, angiograms, and CT scans also are used where appropriate because such studies are widely used by health professionals to diagnose disease and evaluate response to therapy. A number of brief case studies have been included so that students can more easily relate the clinical manifestations, diagnosis, and treatment of a specific disease to an individual patient.

ORGANIZATION

The book is organized into two main sections. The first section, comprising the first 12 chapters, deals with general concepts and with diseases affecting the body as a whole. The second section, which includes the remaining 15 chapters, considers the various organ systems and their diseases.

In the first section, Chapter 1 discusses manifestations of disease, classification, diagnosis, and principles of treatment. Chapter 2 considers the organization and basic function of cells and tissues in health and disease. Chapter 3 deals with genes, chromosomes, cell division, and chromosome analysis, as well as the HLA system and its relation to disease. Chapters 4 and 5 consider the body's defenses, the inflammatory reaction and the immune system, and their disorders. Chapters 6 and 7 are concerned with the various pathogenic microorganisms and parasites and the diseases they cause. This material is followed by a discussion of the transmission and control of communicable diseases in Chapter 8 and includes discussion of the clinically important sexually transmitted diseases. Chapter 9 considers congenital and hereditary diseases, and Chapter 10 deals with tumors. Chapter 11 describes the coagulation of the blood and conditions in which the blood does not clot normally. Chapter 12 considers conditions in which the blood clots too readily and its attendant complications—thrombosis and embolism.

In the second section, the individual organ systems and their diseases are considered in a systematic manner, with emphasis on the more common and important diseases. Basic pathologic physiology, pathology, and principles of diagnosis and treatment are discussed. Newer diagnostic procedures and methods of treatment are emphasized. Chapter 13 describes diseases of the cardiovascular system and includes an extensive discussion of coronary heart disease, one of the most prevalent diseases in the developed nations of the world. Diseases of the hematopoietic and lymphatic systems are considered together in Chapter 14, followed by diseases of the respiratory system in Chapter 15. Chapters 16, 17, and 18 should be considered as a unit: diseases of the breast, the female reproductive system, prenatal development, and diseases associated with pregnancy. Chapter 19, diseases of the urinary system, and Chapter 20, which is concerned with the male reproductive system, are also best considered as a unit. Chapter 21 describes derangements of the liver and biliary system. This is followed in Chapter 22 by diseases of the pancreas, including diabetes mellitus. The upper and lower intestinal tracts and their diseases follow in Chapter 23. Chapter 24 departs from the organ system approach and considers disturbances of fluid, electrolyte, and acid–base balance. The material is introduced here rather than in the first section because it is more easily understood and related to specific organ system diseases when considered after Chapters 19 through 23. The final three chapters deal, respectively, with diseases of the endocrine glands, nervous system, and musculoskeletal system.

STUDY AIDS AND SPECIAL FEATURES

Various learning and study aids are included to enhance the usefulness of the book. Learning objectives, review questions, and a detailed outline summary are provided for each chapter. Literature for further study is listed at the end of each chapter, and a listing of general references is included at the end of the book. These additional sources should prove useful to students who wish to pursue a subject in greater detail. A glossary with a pronunciation guide is appended to the end of the text. This may prove useful to students who have not already had a course in medical terminology and can serve as a convenient reference for other students who wish a quick review of a particular term. Words appearing in the glossary are set in boldface type in the text and set off in the margin for easy reference.

ACKNOWLEDGMENTS

Many people helped with the book in various ways, and I would like to acknowledge their assistance. Several colleagues at Minneapolis and Saint Paul Hospitals, with which I have been associated, and in the Department of Laboratory Medicine and Pathology at the University of Minnesota made suggestions and comments. Colleagues in the Department of Family Practice and Community Health at the University of Minnesota and at the West Side Community Health Center in St. Paul also provided helpful comments. Several of the concepts and clinical cases used in the book were based on these clinical contacts and activities.

Resource Preview

INSTRUCTOR'S MEDIA CD

ISBN 978-1-4496-6552-4

Preparing for class has never been easier. This impressive resource will not only save you time but also afford you more flexibility than ever before.

Included on the Media CD are:

- PowerPoint Presentations: Provide a compelling way to make presentations that are educational and engaging to your students. The slides can be modified and edited to fit your specific classroom needs.
- Full-Color Image Bank: Using photographs and illustrations from the text, you can incorporate graphics into your PowerPoint presentations or present a specific image for further discussion.

go.jblearning.com/crowley9e

This fully integrated website allows students and instructors to become active participants in the learning process. The *Human Disease* website incorporates:

- Anatomy and Physiology Review with interactive figure labeling exercises.
- Animated flashcards and crossword puzzles for quizzing and reviewing key terms.
- Interactive glossary, allowing students to search by term, chapter, or to browse alphabetically.
- Web links directing students to additional resources on the Internet.

CHAPTER 1

General Concepts of Disease: Principles of Diagnosis

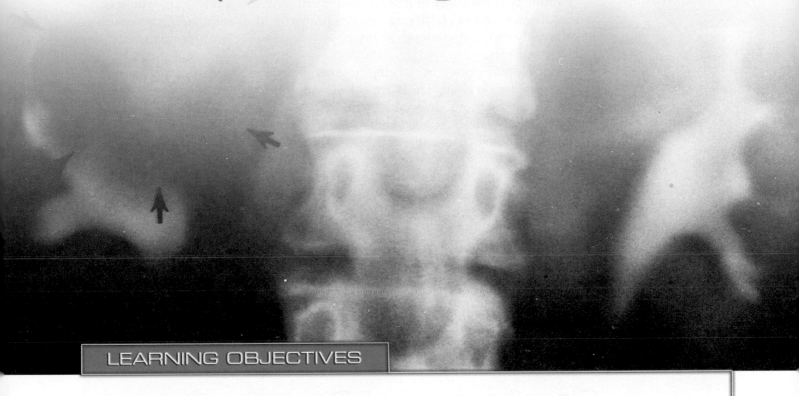

LEARNING OBJECTIVES

1 Define the common terms used to describe disease, such as lesions, organic and functional disease, symptomatic and asymptomatic disease, etiology, and pathogenesis.

2 List the major categories of human disease.

3 Explain the approach that a practitioner uses to make a diagnosis and decide on a patient's treatment.

4 Describe the various types of diagnostic tests and procedures that can help the practitioner make a diagnosis and decide on proper treatment.

Characteristics of Disease

Any disturbance of structure or function of the body may be regarded as **disease**. A disease is often associated with well-defined, characteristic structural changes called **lesions** that are present in various organs and tissues. One can recognize lesions by examining the diseased tissue with the naked eye, which is called a gross examination, or with the aid of a microscope, which is called a histologic examination. Sometimes histologic examinations are supplemented by specialized studies that evaluate the properties of the cell membranes and the proteins within the cells. A disease associated with structural changes is called an **organic disease**.

Disease
Any disturbance of the structure or function of the body.

Lesion (lē'shun)
Any structural abnormality or pathologic change.

Organic disease
A disease associated with structural changes in the affected tissue or organ.

Functional disease
A disease that is not associated with any recognizable structural changes in the body.

Pathology
The study of the structural and functional changes in the body caused by disease.

In contrast, a **functional disease** is one in which no morphologic abnormalities (*morphe* = structure or shape) can be identified even though body functions may be profoundly disturbed. However, as we develop new methods for studying cells, we can sometimes identify previously unrecognized abnormalities that disturb cell functions. Consequently, many of the traditional distinctions between organic and functional disease are no longer as sharply defined as in the past.

Pathology is the study of disease, and a pathologist is a physician who specializes in diagnosing and classifying diseases primarily by examining the morphology of cells and tissues. A clinician is any physician or other health practitioner who cares for patients.

A disease may cause various subjective manifestations, such as weakness or pain, in an affected individual: These are called symptoms. A disease may also produce objective manifestations, detectable by the clinician, which are called signs or physical findings. In many diseases, the quantity of blood cells in the circulation may change and so may the biochemical constituents in the body fluids. These alterations are reflected as abnormal laboratory test results.

A disease that causes the affected individual no discomfort or disability is called an asymptomatic disease or illness. A disease is often asymptomatic in its early stages. If the disease is not treated, however, it may progress to the stage where it causes subjective symptoms and abnormal physical findings. Therefore, the distinction between asymptomatic and symptomatic disease is one of degree, depending primarily on the extent of the disease.

Etiology
(ē-tē-ol′ō-jē)
The cause, especially the cause of a disease.

Pathogenesis
(path-ō-jen′e-sis)
Manner in which a disease develops.

The term **etiology** means cause. A disease of unknown etiology is one for which the cause is not yet known. Unfortunately, many diseases fall into this category. If the cause of a disease is known, the agent responsible is called the etiologic agent. The term **pathogenesis** refers to the manner by which a disease develops, and a pathogen is any microorganism, such as a bacterium or virus, that can cause disease.

Classifications of Disease

Diseases tend to fall into several large categories, although the diseases in a specific category are not necessarily closely related. Rather, the lesions produced by the various diseases in a category are morphologically similar or have a similar pathogenesis. Diseases are conveniently classified in the following large groups:

1. Congenital and hereditary diseases
2. Inflammatory diseases
3. Degenerative diseases
4. Metabolic diseases
5. Neoplastic diseases

CONGENITAL AND HEREDITARY DISEASES

Congenital and hereditary diseases are the result of developmental disturbances. They may be caused by genetic abnormalities, abnormalities in the numbers and distribution of chromosomes, intrauterine injury as a result of various agents, or an interaction of genetic and environmental factors. Hemophilia—the well-known hereditary disease in which blood does not clot properly—and congenital heart disease induced by the German measles virus are examples of diseases in this category.

INFLAMMATORY DISEASES

Inflammatory diseases are those in which the body reacts to an injurious agent by means of inflammation. Many of the diseases characterized by inflammation, such as a sore throat or pneumonia, are caused by bacteria or other microbiologic agents. Others, such as "hay fever," are a manifestation of an allergic reaction or a hypersensitivity state in the patient. Some diseases in this category appear to be caused by antibodies formed against the patient's own tissues, as occurs in some uncommon diseases classified as autoimmune diseases. The etiology of still other inflammatory diseases has not been determined.

DEGENERATIVE DISEASES

In degenerative diseases, the primary abnormality is degeneration of various parts of the body. In some cases, this may be a manifestation of the aging process. In many cases, however, the degenerative lesions are more advanced or occur sooner than would be expected if they were age related and are distinctly abnormal. Certain types of arthritis and "hardening of the arteries" (arteriosclerosis) are common examples of degenerative diseases.

METABOLIC DISEASES

The chief abnormality seen in metabolic diseases is a disturbance in some important metabolic process in the body. For example, the cells may not be utilizing glucose normally, or the thyroid gland may not properly regulate the rate of cell metabolism. Diabetes, disturbances of endocrine glands, and disturbances of fluid and electrolyte balance are common examples of metabolic diseases.

NEOPLASTIC DISEASES

Neoplastic diseases are characterized by abnormal cell growth that leads to the formation of various types of benign and malignant tumors.

Health and Disease: A Continuum

Health and disease may be considered two extremes of a continuum. At one extreme is severe, life-threatening, disabling illness with its corresponding major effect on the physical and emotional well-being of the patient. At the other extreme is ideal good health, which may be defined as a state of complete physical and mental well-being. The healthy person is emotionally and physically capable of leading a full, happy, and productive life that is free of anxiety, turmoil, and physical disabilities that limit activities. Between these two extremes are many gradations of health and disease, ranging from mild or short-term illness that limits activities to some extent to moderate good health that falls short of the ideal state. The midpoint in this continuum may be considered a "neutral" position in which one is neither ill nor in ideal good health. In this continuum, most of us are somewhere between midposition and the ideal state.

The goal of traditional medicine is to cure or ameliorate disease. This is accomplished by various means, ranging from administering an antibiotic to cure an infection to very complex "high-technology" treatments such as kidney transplants and heart surgery. The advances of modern medicine have done much to relieve suffering and advance human welfare, but modern medicine does not guarantee good health. Health is more than an absence of disease; it is a condition in which body and mind function efficiently and harmoniously as an integrated unit. Consequently, we must take an active part in achieving good health by assuming some responsibility for our own physical and emotional well-being. This means practicing such common sense measures as eating properly, exercising moderately, and avoiding harmful excesses such as overeating, smoking, heavy drinking, or using drugs, which can disrupt physical or emotional well-being. Taking responsibility for one's health also requires using one's mind constructively, expressing emotions, and feeling good about oneself. Positive mental attitudes are essential for good health because negative feelings may be reflected in disturbed bodily functions that are manifested as disease.

Principles of Diagnosis

Diagnosis
The determination of the nature and cause of a patient's illness.

Prognosis
The probable outcome of a disease or a disorder; the outlook for recovery.

The determination of the nature and cause of a patient's illness by a physician or other health practitioner is called a **diagnosis**. It is based on the practitioner's evaluation of the patient's subjective symptoms, the physical findings, and the results of various laboratory tests, together with other appropriate diagnostic procedures. When the practitioner has reached a diagnosis, he or she can then offer a **prognosis**: an opinion concerning the eventual outcome of the disease. Then a course of treatment is instituted.

THE HISTORY

The clinical history is a very important part of the evaluation. It consists of several parts:

1. The history of the patient's current illness
2. The past medical history
3. The family history
4. The social history
5. The review of systems

The history of the present illness elicits details concerning the severity, time of onset, and character of the patient's symptoms. Many diseases have characteristic symptoms. The patient's description of the oppressive substernal pain of a heart attack or the pain and urinary disturbances associated with a bladder infection, for example, may provide very helpful information that suggests the correct diagnosis. The past medical history provides details of the patient's general health and previous illnesses. These data may shed light on the patient's current problems as well. The family history provides information about the health of the patient's parents and other family members. Some diseases, such as diabetes and some types of heart disease, tend to run in families. The social history deals with the patient's occupation, habits, alcohol and tobacco consumption, and similar data. This information may also relate to the patient's general health and current problems. The review of systems inquires as to the presence of symptoms other than those disclosed in the history of the present illness; such symptoms might suggest disease affecting other parts of the body. For example, the practitioner inquires about such symptoms as pain or burning on urination, which suggest an abnormality of the urinary tract and coughing, shortness of breath, or chest pain, which may indicate disease of the respiratory system. In this way, possible dysfunctions of other organ systems are evaluated by systematic inquiry.

THE PHYSICAL EXAMINATION

The physical examination is a systematic examination of the patient. The practitioner places particular emphasis on the part of the body affected by the illness, such as the ears, throat, chest, and lungs in the case of a respiratory infection. Any abnormalities detected on the physical examination are correlated with the clinical history. At this point, the practitioner begins to consider the various diseases or conditions that would fit with the clinical findings. Sometimes, more than one possible diagnosis need to be considered. In a differential diagnosis, the practitioner considers a number of diseases that are characterized by the patient's symptoms. For example, if a patient complains of shortness of breath and abnormalities are detected when the lungs are examined with a stethoscope, the practitioner may consider both chronic lung disease and chronic heart failure in the differential diagnosis.

Often, the practitioner can narrow the list of diagnostic possibilities and arrive at a correct diagnosis by using selected laboratory tests or other specialized diagnostic procedures. In difficult cases, the clinician may also wish to obtain the opinion of a medical consultant who is a physician with special training and experience in the type of medical problem presented by the patient.

When dealing with patients who have long-standing chronic diseases such as chronic heart, kidney, or lung disease, or some types of cancer, the physician may be assisted by a disease-management team composed of a group of persons with special skills that are useful in the care and treatment of patients with these diseases. The management team may include persons who can explain to patients the nature of their disease, the goals of treatment, and how patients can contribute to their own care. Other health care team members such as dieticians, nurse clinicians, physician assistants, respiratory therapists, physiotherapists, and pharmacists can bring their own special skills to help physicians care for patients with chronic illnesses who require long-term care and who have special needs. Often, the team approach to management of patients with chronic diseases reduces the long-term cost of medical care, improves the patients' satisfaction with the quality of their medical care, and contributes to a more favorable response to treatment.

TREATMENT

After the diagnosis has been established, a course of treatment is initiated. There are two different types of treatment: specific treatment and symptomatic treatment.

A specific treatment is one that exerts a highly specific and favorable effect on the basic cause of the disease. For example, an antibiotic may be given to a patient who has an infection that is responsive to the antibiotic, or insulin may be given to a patient with diabetes. Symptomatic treatment, as the name implies, makes the patient more comfortable by alleviating symptoms but does not influence the course of the underlying disease. Examples are the treatment of fever, pain, and cough by means of appropriate medications. Unfortunately, there are no specific treatments for some diseases. Consequently, the clinician must be content with treating the manifestations of the disease, without being able to influence its ultimate course.

Screening Tests for Disease

PURPOSE AND REQUIREMENTS FOR EFFECTIVE SCREENING

Many diseases that respond to treatment are asymptomatic initially. If untreated, however, the disease often progresses slowly, causing gradual but progressive organ damage until eventually the person is seriously ill with far advanced organ damage caused by the disease. Unfortunately, treatment of late-stage disease is often much less effective and may not be able to restore the function of the organs that have been damaged. Had the disease been identified and treated in its early asymptomatic stage, the disease-related organ damage could have been prevented or minimized, and the affected person would have been spared the discomfort, disability, and shortened survival associated with late-stage disease.

A successful screening program should fulfill the following requirements:

1. A significant number of persons in the group being screened must be at risk for the disease.
2. A relatively inexpensive noninvasive test that does not yield an excessively high number of false-positive or false-negative results must be available to screen for the disease.
3. Early identification and treatment of the disease will favorably influence the health or welfare of the person with the disease.

GROUPS SUITABLE FOR SCREENING

Screening tests should target a group of persons in whom there is a relatively high frequency of disease, and tests should also target the age group in whom the disease is likely to be present. If the disease, for example, has its onset in middle age, then screening adolescents and children in the target group would not be productive.

SUITABLE SCREENING TESTS

Screening a group of persons for a disease in its early asymptomatic stage requires some type of test that can identify some characteristic manifestation of the disease, such as high blood sugar in the case of diabetes or the presence of blood in the stool in the case of a colon tumor. A test used for screening should be reasonably inexpensive and should have few false-positive results (test is positive when no disease is present) and few false-negative results (test is negative when disease is present). If the test produced a large number of false-positive results in the group being screened, many persons with false-positive test results would have to undergo more extensive and sometimes invasive testing, as well as a comprehensive medical evaluation, only to find that the test result was a "false alarm" and that they did not have the disease. On the other hand, less sensitive screening tests would yield an excess of false-negative tests, and many persons who actually had the disease would not be detected.

BENEFITS OF SCREENING

Screening test results should provide some benefit to the person being screened. Generally, there is no point in screening for a disease if no treatment is available to arrest the progression of the disease.

Examples of widely used cost-effective screening tests for disease include urine tests to detect glucose in the urine as a screening test for diabetes, tests to detect blood in the stools to screen for colon tumors, Papanicolaou smears (Pap tests) to screen for abnormalities in the epithelium of the uterine cervix that predispose to cancer, and breast x-ray examinations (mammograms) to screen for very early breast cancer at a stage when it can be treated most effectively.

SCREENING FOR GENETIC DISEASE

Screening tests can also be used to screen for carriers of some genetic diseases that are transmitted from parent to child as either dominant or recessive traits. When many persons in a population carry a recessive gene that can be detected by relatively simple screening tests, identifying carriers allows the affected persons to make decisions regarding future childbearing or management of a future pregnancy. One high-incidence recessive gene for which screening is available is the sickle hemoglobin gene, which occurs in about 8% of the black population. A child born to two carriers of the sickle hemoglobin gene who receives the sickle hemoglobin gene from each parent will develop a severe anemia called sickle cell anemia. The sickle hemoglobin gene and its clinical manifestations are considered in the hematopoietic and lymphatic systems discussion. Other examples of genetic diseases for which screening is available are described in the discussion on congenital and hereditary diseases.

Diagnostic Tests and Procedures

A wide array of diagnostic tests and procedures are available to help the practitioner diagnose and treat the patient properly. They fall into two classifications: invasive procedures and noninvasive procedures. Invasive procedures are so-named because the patient's body is actually "invaded" in some way in order to obtain diagnostic information. Such procedures involve introducing needles, catheters, or other instruments into the patient's body. Noninvasive procedures are those that entail no risk or minimal risk or discomfort to the patient, such as a chest x-ray or an examination of the urine.

Many diagnostic procedures entail some degree of risk or discomfort to the patient. The risk is greater with invasive procedures, but even some noninvasive procedures are not completely harmless. A chest x-ray, for example, exposes the patient to radiation. Even a relatively simple procedure such as the collection of a blood sample for a laboratory test may be complicated by bleeding around the vein or by formation of a blood clot in the vein at the site of puncture. Therefore, with any diagnostic procedure, the practitioner must balance the possible disadvantages to the patient against the benefits that may be derived from the information obtained by the procedure. Patients also must be fully informed about the possible risks and benefits so that they can make informed decisions as to whether or not to consent to the procedure. It would be unwise to perform a potentially risky diagnostic procedure if the information gained would not contribute significantly to the diagnosis or would not greatly influence the course of treatment. The physician would be much more likely to employ a diagnostic procedure that could provide much useful information at little or no risk to the patient.

Diagnostic tests and procedures can be classified in several major categories:

1. Clinical laboratory tests
2. Tests that measure the electrical activity of the body
3. Tests using radioisotopes (also called radionuclides)
4. Endoscopy
5. Ultrasound procedures
6. X-ray examinations
7. Magnetic resonance imaging (MRI)
8. Positron emission tomography (PET scans)
9. Cytologic and histologic examination of cells and tissues removed from the patient

CLINICAL LABORATORY TESTS

Clinical laboratory tests have many uses. They can be used to determine the concentration of various constituents in the blood and urine, which are frequently altered by disease. For example, the concentration of a substance in the blood called urea is elevated if the kidneys are not functioning properly because this constituent is normally excreted by the kidneys. The concentrations of hemoglobin and the quantity of red cells are reduced in patients with anemia. One also can determine the concentration (activity) of enzymes in the blood. Sometimes, the enzyme level is elevated because (a) enzymes are leaking from diseased or injured organs, (b) enzyme synthesis is increased as a result of disease, or (c) excretion of enzymes is impaired because disease has caused blockage of normal excretory pathways.

Clinical laboratory tests are also used to evaluate the functions of organs. Clearance tests measure the rate at which a substance such as urea or creatinine is removed from blood and excreted in the urine. This provides a measure of renal (kidney) function. Pulmonary function tests measure the rate at which air moves in and out of the lungs. Determinations of the concentration of oxygen and carbon dioxide in the blood also can indicate pulmonary function by evaluating how efficiently the lungs can oxygenate the blood and eliminate carbon dioxide, and a simple device applied to the finger can calculate rapidly the amount of oxygen carried by hemoglobin as another measure of pulmonary function. Tests that measure the uptake and excretion of various substances by the liver are used as a measure of liver function. One also can detect substances that are likely to be produced by tumors growing within the body and measure their concentration. Serial analyses of these substances can be used to monitor the response of certain tumors to treatment. Microbiologic tests detect the presence of disease-producing organisms in urine, blood, and feces. They also determine the responsiveness of the organisms to antibiotics. Serologic tests detect and measure the presence of antibodies as an indication of response to infectious agents.

TESTS OF ELECTRICAL ACTIVITY

Several different tests measure the electrical impulses associated with various bodily functions and activities. These include the electrocardiogram (ECG), the electroencephalogram (EEG), and the electromyogram (EMG). The most widely used of these tests is the ECG. Electrodes attached to the arms, legs, and chest are used to measure the serial changes in the electrical activity of the heart during the various phases of the cardiac cycle. The ECG also identifies disturbances in the heart rate or rhythm and identifies abnormal conduction of impulses through the heart. Heart muscle injury, such as occurs after a heart attack, also can be recognized by means of characteristic abnormalities in the cardiogram. The EEG measures the electrical activity of the brain, often called brain waves, by means of small electrodes attached to different areas in the scalp. Brain tumors, strokes, and many other abnormalities of cerebral structure or function may cause altered brain wave patterns that are detected by this examination. The EMG measures the electrical activity of skeletal muscle during contraction and at rest. Abnormal electrical activity is often encountered in various inflammatory or degenerative diseases involving the skeletal muscles. The test is performed by inserting a needle into the muscle that is being studied. The speed at which a nerve conducts impulses also can be measured by means of electrodes taped to the surface of the skin over the nerve being tested. Abnormal conduction of nerve impulses, encountered in some diseases, can be identified by such studies.

RADIOISOTOPE (RADIONUCLIDE) STUDIES

The function of various organs can be evaluated by administering a substance labeled with a radioactive material called a radioisotope. Specially designed radiation detectors then measure the uptake and excretion of the labeled substance. For example, in certain types of anemia, one measures the absorption and excretion of radioisotope-labeled vitamin B_{12}, which is a vitamin required for normal blood formation. The ability of the thyroid gland to concentrate and utilize radioactive iodine is used as a measure of thyroid function and also can be used to detect tumors within the thyroid gland. One may administer a radioactive material that is filtered out or concentrated in a tissue or organ and then measure the radioactivity by radiation detectors applied to the exterior of the body and connected to a computer. For example, specially processed albumin labeled with a radioisotope may be administered intravenously as a measure of pulmonary blood flow. The material is filtered out and retained in the lungs as the blood flows through them. If blood flow to a part of the lung is inadequate for any reason, less radioactivity is recorded in that area. This technique is frequently used to detect the presence of blood clots in the lung that impede blood flow to parts of the lung. Phosphorus-containing isotopes are concentrated in the skeletal system. If there are deposits of tumor in bone, the isotopes are concentrated around the tumor deposits and can be easily identified (FIGURE 1-1). Radioactive materials injected intravenously also can be used to evaluate blood flow to heart muscle and to identify areas of damaged heart muscle.

ENDOSCOPY AND LAPAROSCOPY

An **endoscopy**, or endoscopic examination (*endo* = within + *skopeo* = examine), is an examination of the interior of the body by means of various types of rigid or flexible tubular instruments that are named according to the part of the body they are designed to examine. These instruments have a system of lenses for viewing and a light source to illuminate the region being examined. An esophagoscope, for example, is used to examine the interior of the esophagus; a gastroscope to examine the stomach; and a bronchoscope to examine the trachea and major bronchi. An instrument for viewing the interior of the bladder is called a cystoscope. A sigmoidoscope is a rigid tube used to examine the rectum and the sigmoid colon, and a colonoscope is a flexible tube that can be used to examine the entire length of the colon. An instrument called a **laparoscope** is used to visualize the abdominal and pelvic organs, and the procedure is called laparoscopy, which can be used not only to examine abdominal and pelvic organs but also to perform various surgical procedures, such as removal of the gallbladder (cholecystectomy), appendix (appendectomy), ovary (oophorectomy), and other surgical procedures that formerly were removed through much larger abdominal incisions. To perform a laparoscopic procedure, the peritoneal cavity is inflated first with carbon dioxide, which separates the organs within the peritoneal cavity so that they can be visualized more easily. Then the laparoscope is inserted through a small incision in the abdominal wall, often in or near the umbilicus. If a surgical procedure is to be performed, such as an appendectomy or cholecystectomy, one or two additional small incisions are needed in order to insert the instruments used to perform the surgical procedure and remove the organ from the abdominal cavity.

ULTRASOUND

Ultrasound is a technique for mapping the echoes produced by high-frequency sound waves transmitted into the body. Echoes are reflected wherever there is a change in the density of the tissue. The reflected waves are recorded on sensitive detectors, and images are produced. This method is widely used to study the uterus during pregnancy because it does not require the use of potentially harmful radiation and poses no risk to the fetus (FIGURE 1-2). The technique can be used to determine the

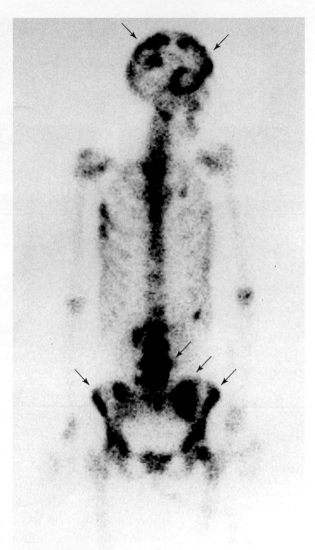

FIGURE 1-1 Radioisotope bone scan of head, chest, and pelvis. Dark areas (*arrows*) indicate the concentration of radioisotope around tumor deposits in bone.

Endoscopy
(en-däs′kō-pē)
An examination of the interior of the body by means of various lighted tubular instruments.

Laparoscope
(lap′-ă-rō-skōp)
A long tubular telescope-like instrument passed through the abdominal wall to examine structures within the peritoneal cavity.

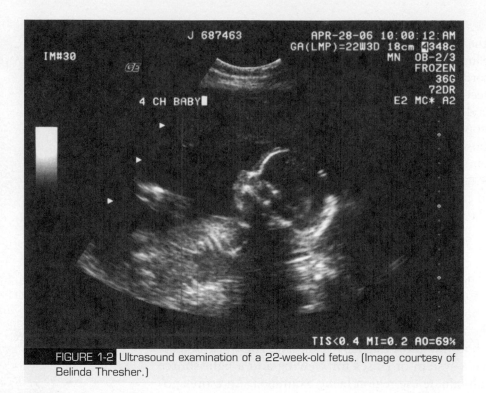

FIGURE 1-2 Ultrasound examination of a 22-week-old fetus. (Image courtesy of Belinda Thresher.)

position of the placenta and the fetus within the uterus; it also can identify some fetal abnormalities and detect twin pregnancies. Ultrasound is also often used to examine the cardiovascular system. When used for this purpose, the procedure is usually called an **echocardiogram**. The prefix term "echo" refers to the reflected sound waves. An echocardiogram can detect the structure and function of the heart valves. The procedure can detect valve abnormalities and identify blood clots that sometimes form on the heart valves in association with infection of the valve as well as determining abnormal communications between adjacent cardiac chambers. Abnormal blood flow patterns—characteristic of congenital or acquired valvular heart disease—can also be detected. An ultrasound examination can distinguish a significant heart murmur caused by a valve or chamber abnormality from a murmur caused by turbulent blood flow within a structurally normal heart, which is clinically significant. In many cases, ultrasound has replaced some radiology procedures because ultrasound avoids radiation, is not an invasive procedure, and is usually less expensive. Ultrasound can determine the thickness of the ventricular walls and septum and the size of the ventricular chambers during systole and diastole. It can also identify gallstones in the gallbladder and abnormalities in the prostate suspicious for prostate cancer. The technique has many other applications in medicine.

X-RAY EXAMINATION

X-ray examinations are conducted in many ways, but the basic principle is the same for all types of x-ray studies. X-rays are passed through the part of the body to be examined, and the rays leaving the body expose an x-ray film. The extent to which the rays are absorbed by the tissues as they pass through the body depends on the density of the tissues. Tissues of low density, such as the air-filled lungs, transmit most of the rays, and thus, the film exposed to x-rays passing through them appears black. Tissues of high density, such as bone, absorb most of the rays; the film remains unexposed and appears white. Tissues of intermediate densities appear as varying shades of gray. The x-ray image produced on the film is called a radiograph or **roentgenogram**. The same basic principle is used to obtain x-ray films of the

Echocardiogram
An examination of the heart by means of an ultrasound procedure.

Roentgenogram
(rent'gen-ō-gram)
A photograph taken with x-rays.

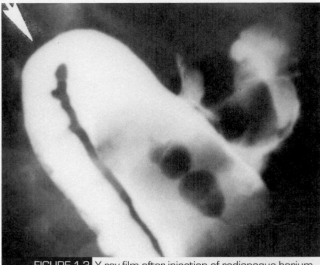

FIGURE 1-3 X-ray film after injection of radiopaque barium sulfate suspension into colon (barium enema), illustrating narrowed area (*arrow*) that impedes passage of bowel contents.

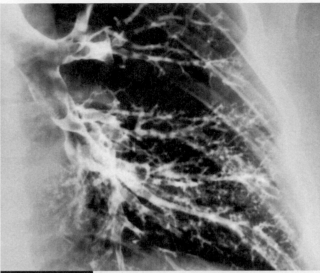

FIGURE 1-4 Bronchogram illustrating normal branching of bronchi and bronchioles that are normal in caliber and appearance.

breast. This procedure is called **mammogram**. The applications and limitations of the mammogram procedure are considered in diseases of the breast.

Although the linings of internal organs such as the intestinal tract, urinary tract, bronchi, fallopian tubes, and biliary tract have little contrast, they can be examined by administering a dense radiopaque substance called contrast medium. It coats and adheres to the lining of the structure being examined and enhances its visibility. To examine the interior of the gastrointestinal tract, for example, one gives the patient a suspension of barium sulfate to swallow or administers it as an enema. The opaque barium coats the lining of the intestinal tract, and an abnormality in the lining shows on the film as an irregularity in the column of barium (FIGURE 1-3). The lining of the bronchi can be visualized by instilling a radiopaque oil into the bronchi. The oil forms a thin film on the bronchial mucosa and delineates the contours of the bronchi. This procedure is called a bronchogram (FIGURE 1-4).

One uses the same principle to visualize the urinary tract. A radiopaque substance is injected into a vein and is excreted in the urine as the blood flows through the kidney, outlining the contour of the urinary tract. This is called an intravenous pyelogram (IVP) (FIGURE 1-5). Another method is to introduce the dye directly into both ureters through tubes that are inserted into both ureters by means of a cystoscope introduced into the bladder. This procedure is called a retrograde pyelogram. To visualize the gallbladder, the patient ingests tablets of radiopaque material that is absorbed into the circulation, excreted by the liver in the bile, and concentrated in the gallbladder. Gallstones can be identified because they occupy space in the gallbladder and cause irregularities in the radiopaque material concentrated there (FIGURE 1-6).

One can also use contrast material to study the flow of blood in large arteries and to identify areas of narrowing or obstruction. This procedure is called an **arteriogram** or **angiogram** (*angio* = blood vessel). A small flexible catheter is inserted into a large artery in the arm or leg and advanced into the aorta until it is positioned at the opening of the artery that is to be examined. Radiopaque material is then injected through the catheter. It mixes with the blood, and its flow through the vessel is followed by means of a series of x-ray films. If the vessel is narrowed by disease, the film will show areas in which the column of opaque material is narrowed. A complete obstruction of the vessel appears as an interruption of the column. Arteriography

Mammogram
(mam′ō-gram)
An x-ray of the breast, used to detect tumors and other abnormalities within the breast.

Arteriogram
(är-tēr′ē-ō-gram)
An x-ray technique for studying the caliber of blood vessels by injection of radiopaque material into the vessel.

Angiogram
(an′jē-ō-gram)
Same as arteriogram.

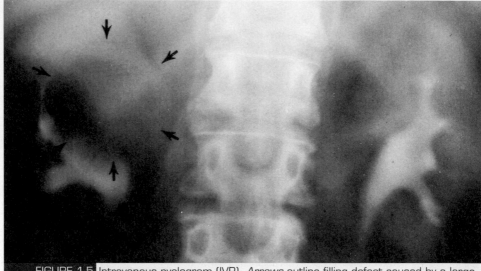

FIGURE 1-5 Intravenous pyelogram (IVP). *Arrows* outline filling defect caused by a large cyst in kidney that distorts renal pelvis and calyces. The opposite kidney appears normal.

Cardiac catheterization
A specialized technique to determine the blood flow through the chambers of the heart and to detect abnormal communications between cardiac chambers.

....

Computed tomographic (CT) scan
(tō-mo-graf'ik)
An x-ray technique producing detailed cross-sectional images of the body by means of x-ray tube and detectors connected to a computer. Sometimes called a CAT scan.

is often used to detect narrowing or obstruction of the coronary arteries or of the carotid arteries in the neck, which carry blood to the brain (FIGURE 1-7). Obstruction of the pulmonary arteries by blood clots also can be identified by arteriography. In this case, the catheter used to inject the radiopague material is inserted into a large vein in the arm, threaded up the vein and through the right side of the heart, and positioned in the pulmonary artery.

This same basic method can be used to study the flow of blood through the heart and can detect abnormal communications between cardiac chambers. This type of study is called **cardiac catheterization.**

Computed Tomographic Scans

A **computed tomographic scan** (**CT scan**) is performed by a highly sophisticated x-ray machine that produces images of the body in cross section by rotating the x-ray tube around the patient at various levels. The x-ray tube is mounted on a movable frame opposite an array of sensitive radiation detectors that encircle the

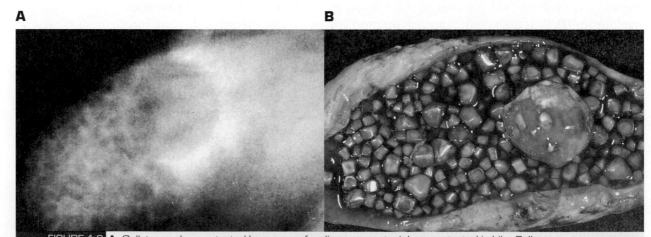

FIGURE 1-6 **A**, Gallstones demonstrated by means of radiopaque material concentrated in bile. Gallstones occupy space and appear as radiolucent (dark) areas within radiopaque (white) bile. Note the large radiolucent area, indicating a large gallstone, surrounded by smaller radiolucent areas, representing multiple smaller stones. **B**, Opened gallbladder removed surgically from the same patient. Compare appearance and location of stones with x-ray appearance.

patient. As the x-ray tube moves around the patient, the radiation detectors record the amount of radiation passing through the body (FIGURE 1-8). In computerized scanning, the amount of radiation absorbed is not read directly on an x-ray film. Instead, the data from the radiation detectors are fed into a computer, which reconstructs the data into an image that reproduces the patient's anatomy as a cross-section picture. The image is displayed on a television monitor and can be recorded on film (FIGURE 1-9). As with conventional x-rays, dense substances are white, and less dense substances appear darker in proportion to the amount of radiation they transmit. The individual organs appear sharply separated from one another because the various parts of the body are separated by planes of fat, which have very low density. These separations increase contrast between adjacent organs. Abnormalities of internal organs that cannot be identified by means of standard x-ray examinations can often be discovered with CT scans. FIGURE 1-10 shows a renal cyst located by CT scan.

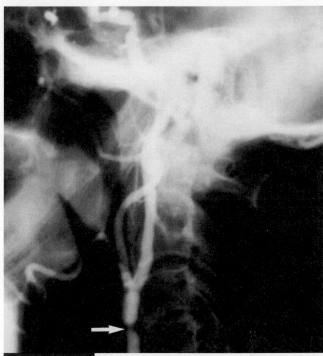

FIGURE 1-7 Narrowing of carotid artery in neck (*arrow*) demonstrated by carotid angiogram.

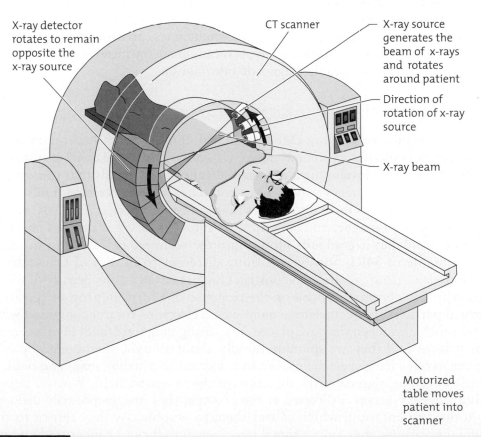

X-ray detector rotates to remain opposite the x-ray source

CT scanner

X-ray source generates the beam of x-rays and rotates around patient

Direction of rotation of x-ray source

X-ray beam

Motorized table moves patient into scanner

FIGURE 1-8 Computed tomographic (CT) scan. The patient lies on a table that is gradually advanced into the scanner. X-ray tube mounted in scanner rotates around patient, and radiation detectors also rotate so that detectors remain opposite the x-ray source. Data from radiation detectors generate computer-reconstructed images of the patient's body at multiple levels.

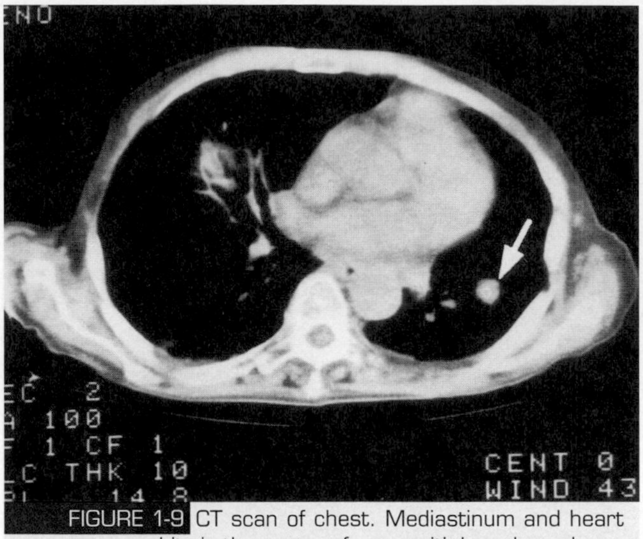

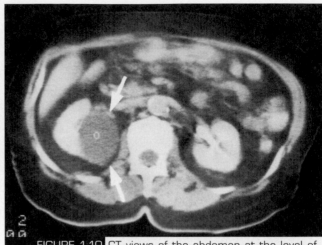

FIGURE 1-9 CT scan of chest. Mediastinum and heart appear white in the center of scan, with less-dense lungs on either side. The *arrow* indicates a lung tumor, which appears as white nodule in lung.

FIGURE 1-10 CT views of the abdomen at the level of kidneys, illustrating a fluid-filled cyst in the kidney (*arrow*). The cyst appears less dense than surrounding renal tissue. The opposite kidney (*right* side of photograph) appears normal.

Use of CT has increased greatly in recent years and provides much useful information. Much of the increased use has been for screening asymptomatic persons for unsuspected lung or colon tumors and for some screening studies in children. However, CT delivers a much greater dose of radiation than a standard x-ray examination, such as a chest x-ray, and some physicians are concerned that repeated CT examinations may deliver a significant and possibly excessive amount of radiation to the patient. Ultrasound examination, which sometimes can provide the same information without any radiation exposure, is recommended whenever it can substitute for CT to provide comparable diagnostic information.

MAGNETIC RESONANCE IMAGING

Magnetic resonance imaging (MRI)
A diagnostic procedure that yields computer-generated images based on the movement of hydrogen atoms in tissues subjected to a strong magnetic field.

Magnetic resonance imaging (MRI) produces computer-constructed images of various organs and tissues somewhat like CT scans. The device consists of a strong magnet capable of developing a powerful magnetic field; coils that can transmit and receive radiofrequency waves; and a computer, which receives impulses from the scanner and forms them into images that can be interpreted. The MRI scanner with the enclosed magnet and coils appears similar to a CT scanner. The patient lies on a table that is gradually moved into the scanner, as is done in CT scans. The principle of MRI, however, is quite different from that of CT scanning, which uses ionizing radiation to construct images based on the density of tissues. MRI scans, in contrast, depend on the response of hydrogen protons (positively charged particles in the nucleus around which electrons rotate) contained within water molecules when they are placed in a strong magnetic field. Hydrogen protons behave as if they are spinning rapidly about an axis, surrounded by orbiting negatively charged electrons. When subjected to a strong magnetic field, the protons become aligned in the direction of the magnetic field. When a pulse of radiofrequency waves is directed at the protons, they are temporarily dislodged from their orientation, which causes them to wobble. As they return to their original positions, they emit a signal (resonance) that can be measured and used to produce the computer-constructed images. Body tissues, which have a high water content, are a rich source of protons capable of excitation. The intensity of the signals produced is related to the varying water content of body tissues and

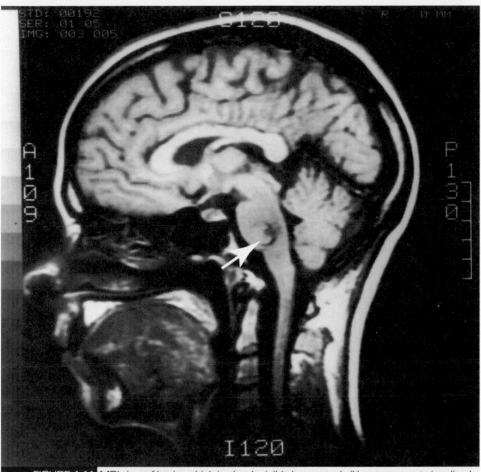

FIGURE 1-11 MRI view of brain, which is clearly visible because skull bones are not visualized by MRI. The white line surrounding the brain represents scalp tissue. The *arrow* indicates a malformation composed of blood vessels within the brain stem.

to the strength and duration of the radiofrequency pulse. Because an MRI does not use ionizing radiation, the patient does not receive radiation exposure. An MRI does expose the patient to strong magnetic fields and radiowaves, but this appears relatively safe on the basis of current knowledge.

Applications

An MRI detects many of the same types of abnormalities detected by a CT, and a CT is superior to an MRI for many applications. An MRI, however, offers distinct advantages over CT in special situations, as, for example, when attempting to detect abnormalities in tissues surrounded by bone, such as lesions in the spinal cord, orbits or near the base of the skull (FIGURE 1-11). In these locations, bone interferes with scanning because of its density, but it does not produce an image in MRI because the water content of bone is low. MRI also provides a sharp contrast between gray and white matter within the brain and spinal cord, which differ in their water content. For this reason, the technique is useful for demonstrating areas where myelin sheaths of nerve fibers have been damaged, as in a neurologic disease called multiple sclerosis (described in the discussion on the nervous system). MRI may also be superior to mammography for detecting breast carcinoma in a selected group of women who have a higher than normal risk of breast carcinoma (described in the discussion about breast disease). Further improvements in equipment will undoubtedly increase the usefulness of this diagnostic procedure.

POSITRON EMISSION TOMOGRAPHY

Related to radioisotope studies but much more complex and sophisticated is one of the newest of the diagnostic imaging tests called positron emission tomography (PET), or simply PET scans. Positrons are unique subatomic particles that have the same mass as electrons but carry a positive charge. They are formed when atoms such as carbon, oxygen, or nitrogen are bombarded in a cyclotron with high-energy particles, which breaks down the atomic nuclei and releases the positrons along with other subatomic particles. The positrons escaping from the nuclei collide with negatively charged electrons circling the nuclei, producing radiation that can be detected and measured by means of sensitive radiation detectors.

One uses PET scans to study body functions by injecting into the subject a biochemical compound, such as glucose, that is labeled with a positron-emitting isotope and then assessing the distribution and metabolism of the compound by measuring the radiation produced within the body by the isotope-labeled compound. The radiation output, measured by sensitive radiation detectors, is fed into a computer that constructs computer-generated images similar to those obtained with CT scans. Such studies provide information on the metabolic activities of the organ or tissue being studied, the site within an organ where the compound is being metabolized, and the blood flow to the organ being studied.

Although originally developed for research studies, PET scans have moved from the research laboratory into medical practice. A major application is to assess biochemical functions within the brain. One can detect and measure changes in brain functions associated with various neurologic diseases such as strokes, brain tumors, Alzheimer disease, Parkinson disease, and some hereditary degenerative diseases of the nervous system. The method has also been used to some extent to evaluate changes in blood flow and metabolism in heart muscle after a heart attack. PET scans following intravenous infusion of a labeled glucose compound have also been used to distinguish a benign from a malignant tumor growing within the body, based on the greater glucose uptake and metabolic activity within a malignant tumor, in contrast to the much lower labeled glucose uptake in a benign tumor. This same approach is also used to identify deposits of malignant tumor that have spread throughout the body by demonstrating the increased glucose uptake within the tumor deposits. When PET scans are used to determine how widely a malignant tumor has spread throughout the body, the initial PET scan is often followed by a follow-up scan after a course of treatment in order to evaluate the response to treatment. Because a PET scan is usually performed along with a CT scan, repeated PET–CT scans subject the patient to significant amounts of radiation. In addition, when a PET scan is used to aid in tumor diagnosis and to evaluate response to treatment, false-positive results may be obtained. Areas of inflammation are also associated with increased glucose uptake, which may be very difficult to distinguish from a tumor.

Although PET scans provide useful information, there are some drawbacks to their widespread application. They are very expensive procedures and may not be widely available. Because positron-emitting isotopes must be produced in a cyclotron, the isotopes produced have a very short duration of activity (half-life), and one must have facilities for incorporating the isotope into the biochemical compound required for the PET scan procedure.

CYTOLOGIC AND HISTOLOGIC EXAMINATIONS

Cells covering the surfaces of the body are continually cast off and replaced by new cells. Abnormal cells can often be identified in the fluids or secretions that come in

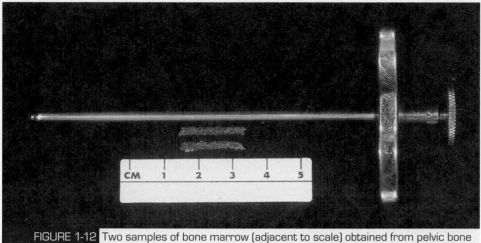

FIGURE 1-12 Two samples of bone marrow (adjacent to scale) obtained from pelvic bone by means of a specially designed needle, shown in the upper part of the photograph.

contact with the epithelial surface. This type of examination is called a Papanicolaou smear, or simply **Pap smear**, after the physician who developed the procedure. It is widely used as a screening test for recognizing early cancer of the uterus and can be used to detect cancers in other locations as well. The Pap smear is discussed in the section on neoplasms.

Diseased tissues have abnormal structural and cellular patterns that can be recognized by the pathologist. Consequently, it is often possible to determine the cause of a patient's disease by histologic examination of a small sample of tissue removed from the affected tissue or organ. This procedure is called a **biopsy**. Samples of tissue can be obtained from any part of the body. Gastroscopes, bronchoscopes, and other instruments used for endoscopic examination, for example, are constructed so that specimens for biopsy can be obtained while the internal organs are being examined. Biopsy specimens can also be taken directly from internal organs such as the liver or kidney by inserting a thin needle through the skin directly into the organ. Samples of bone marrow are obtained in this way, and bone-marrow biopsy is often performed to diagnose blood disease (FIGURE 1-12).

Pap smear
A study of cells from various sources, commonly used as a screening test for cancer.

Biopsy
(bī′op-sē)
Removal of a small sample of tissue for examination and diagnosis by a pathologist.

QUESTIONS FOR REVIEW

1. What are the five major categories of disease?
2. What are the definitions of the following terms: *etiology, symptom of disease, sign of disease, diagnosis,* and *prognosis*?
3. How does an organic disease differ from a functional disease?
4. What principal factors does the physician evaluate in arriving at a diagnosis?
5. What is the difference between specific and symptomatic treatment?
6. What are the major categories of diagnostic tests and procedures that can help the practitioner make a diagnosis? Give some examples.
7. What is the difference between an invasive and a noninvasive procedure?
8. What are the basic concepts on which the following procedures are based: Pap smear, x-ray examinations, ultrasound, electrocardiogram, and CT scans?

SUPPLEMENTARY READINGS

Baerlocher, M. O., and Detsky, A. S. 2010. Discussing radiation risks associated with CT scans in patients. *Journal of the American Medical Association* 304:2170–71.
  ▶ Use of CT has doubled every 2 years since the 1980s, as have concerns about the associated radiation risks and radiation-related cancers. Most patients are not informed of radiation risks associated with CT scans, and many patients with cardiovascular disease have multiple CT examinations. Physicians should explain to patients the reason for the procedures, the expected benefits, and the radiation-related risks and should obtain an informed consent for the procedure.

Brenner, D. J., and Hall, E. J. 2007. Computed tomography—an increasing source of radiation exposure. *New England Journal of Medicine* 357:2277–84.
  ▶ CT has revolutionized diagnostic radiology, and its use has increased greatly in recent years. It is used now for screening procedures on healthy patients to identify unsuspected colon or lung tumors and for total body screening; its use has also increased in pediatric patients. CT delivers a much greater radiation exposure than a standard x-ray examination, such as a chest x-ray. Too many CT exams are being performed and many may not be justified by medical need. In order to reduce radiation exposure to the patient, ultrasound examinations or MRI should substitute for CT whenever possible.

Dinan, M. A., Curtis, L. H., Hammill, B. G., et al. 2010. Changes in the use and costs of diagnostic imaging among Medicare beneficiaries with cancer, 1999–2006. *Journal of the American Medical Association* 303:1625–31.
  ▶ Imaging costs among Medicare patients with cancer increased from 1999 to 2006, which outpaced the rate of increase in the total costs among Medicare beneficiaries with cancer. In each cancer type, the number of PET scans increased at a mean annual rate of 35.9–53.6%. Patients with lung cancer or lymphoma had the largest increase in PET use.

Einstein, A. J., Weiner, S. D., Bernheim, A., et al. 2010. Multiple testing, cumulative radiation dose, and clinical indications in patients undergoing myocardial perfusion imaging. *Journal of the American Medical Association* 304:2137–44.
  ▶ The US Food and Drug Administration proposes reducing unnecessary radiation exposure. CT scans associated with perfusion of coronary arteries account for a large proportion of the radiation exposures. Many patients with suspected coronary artery disease have multiple tests, which lead to very high cumulative doses of radiation. Ways to reduce unnecessary repeat testing are described.

Figley, N. M., ed. 1983. Diagnostic imaging and related sciences. *American Journal of Roentgenology* (special section: NMR) 141:1101–353.
  ▶ A detailed reference on the various applications and limitations of nuclear magnetic resonance in medical diagnosis.

Guttmacher, A. E., Collins, F. S., and Carmona, R. H. 2004. The family history: More important than ever. *New England Journal of Medicine* 351:2333–6.
  ▶ We do patients a disservice if we fail to realize the value of the family history in pinpointing some of the more common diseases that have a hereditary or genetic component. A government-sponsored website is available that allows people to collect, organize, and maintain their family history in their own computers (www.hhs.gov/familyhistory). Patients are encouraged to bring their family history to their healthcare provider for further discussion, evaluation, and use.

Jacobson, H. G. 1987. Fundamentals of magnetic resonance imaging. Council on Scientific Affairs. *Journal of the American Medical Association* 258:3417–23.

▶ Describes principles and applications of this powerful diagnostic tool.

Juweid, M. E., and Cheson, B. D. 2006. Positron-emission tomography and assessment of cancer therapy. *New England Journal of Medicine* 354:496–507.

▶ A comprehensive, well-illustrated article dealing with the applications and limitations of PET scans used for the evaluation and treatment of malignant tumors.

Khoury, M. J., McCabe, L., and McCabe, E. R. 2003. Population screening in the age of genomic medicine. *New England Journal of Medicine* 348:50–8.

▶ Newborn infants are routinely screened for several inherited diseases so that early diagnosis can allow prompt treatment, thereby preventing the long-term adverse effects caused by the disease. Screening of adults for selected diseases can also provide benefits to the affected persons.

Matchar, D. B. 1990. Decision making in the face of uncertainty: The case of carotid endarterectomy. *Mayo Clinic Proceedings* 65:756–60.

▶ Excellent discussion of risks and benefits of therapeutic procedures, as well as biases. The wish to do everything possible for the patient must not lead to misguided actions.

McNutt, R. A. 2004. Shared medical decision making: Problems, process, progress. *Journal of the American Medical Association* 292:2516–8.

▶ Decisions about options for treatment of a disease should be a joint effort on the part of both the physician and the patient, and the patient needs to understand that every decision is influenced by uncertainty and risk. The physician can explain the possible risks and benefits of various methods of treatment, but the patient must make the final decision.

OUTLINE SUMMARY

Characteristics of Disease

DISTURBANCE OF STRUCTURE OR FUNCTION

Lesions: structural changes identified by gross or microscopic examination.

Symptoms: subjective manifestations.

Signs: objective findings.

Terminology:

Asymptomatic disease: not associated with symptoms or discomfort.

Symptomatic disease: associated with symptoms and abnormal physical findings.

Etiology: cause of disease.

Pathogenesis: manner in which disease develops.

Classifications of Disease

Congenital and hereditary disease: caused by genetic or chromosomal abnormality, intrauterine injury, or interaction of genetic and environmental factors.

Inflammatory disease: associated with inflammation.

Degenerative disease: associated with degeneration of tissues or organs.

Metabolic disease: associated with disturbed metabolic processes.

Neoplastic disease: characterized by various benign and malignant tumors.

Health and Disease: A Continuum

BASIC CONCEPTS

Health and disease are two extremes of a continuous spectrum.

Good health is more than absence of disease.

Modern medicine can cure disease but cannot guarantee good health.

Each individual must assume responsibility for achieving good health.

Principles of Diagnosis

DIAGNOSIS

Clinical history: information obtained from patient.

Physical examination: objective findings obtained by clinician.

Differential diagnosis: consideration of possible diseases that could be responsible for clinical manifestations.

TREATMENT

Specific treatment: produces specific curative effect.
Symptomatic treatment: alleviates symptoms but does not alter course of disease.

Screening Tests for Disease

Purpose is to detect early asymptomatic disease amenable to treatment, thereby preventing or minimizing late-stage organ damage.
Requirements for effective screening:
Significant population at risk for disease.
Inexpensive noninvasive test available to detect the disease.
Early identification and treatment favorably influences outcome.
Screening for genetic disease useful in selected cases.

Diagnostic Tests and Procedures

CATEGORIES OF DIAGNOSTIC PROCEDURES

Invasive procedure: "invades" patient's body to obtain diagnostic information.
Noninvasive procedure: not associated with significant risk or discomfort.

TYPES OF PROCEDURES

Clinical laboratory tests: chemical, serologic, microbiologic tests on blood and body fluids.

Tests that measure electrical activity: ECG, EEG, EMG.
Radioisotope studies: determine uptake and excretion of radioactive materials.
Endoscopy: examines interior of body with specially designed instruments.
Ultrasound: high-frequency sound waves directed into the body creates echoes based on differing densities of body organs. Used to evaluate body structure and functions.
X-ray examination: *x-rays absorbed in proportion to density of tissue.*
X-rays using contrast media: outline structures that cannot be visualized on standard films.
CT scans: x-rays transmitted to the computer produce cross-section views through various levels of the body.
MRI: detects same type of abnormalities as CT, but based on movement of protons in magnetic field; has advantages over CT in special situations.
PET scans: measure metabolism of biochemical compounds labeled with positron-emitting isotopes as measure of organ function.
Very expensive procedure; applications and limitations still being explored.
Major current application is assessment of brain functions in health and disease.
Cytologic and histologic examinations: smears and biopsy samples taken from patient's body have characteristic patterns that permit recognition of disease.

http://health.jbpub.com/humandisease/9e

Human Disease Online is a great source for supplementary human disease information for both students and instructors. Visit this website to find a variety of useful tools for learning, thinking, and teaching.

CHAPTER 2

Cells and Tissues: Their Structure and Function in Health and Disease

LEARNING OBJECTIVES

1 Make a sketch of the general structure of a typical cell.

2 Explain how cells are organized to form tissues. Diagram the fundamental structure of the four basic types of tissues.

3 Explain how tissues are organized to form organ systems.

4 Write a general description of the three germ layers and their derivatives.

5 Describe how cells utilize the genetic code within DNA chains to convey genetic information to daughter cells during cell division.

6 Explain the process by which the DNA in the nucleus directs the synthesis of enzymes and other proteins in the cytoplasm.

7 Illustrate how materials move in and out of cells. List five processes by which cells adapt to changing conditions.

8 Explain three ways in which an aging cell becomes increasingly vulnerable to injury.

Organization of Cells

The cell is the basic structural and functional unit of the body. Groups of similar cells arranged to perform a common function form **tissues**. Tissues in turn are grouped together in different proportions to form **organs**, and groups of organs functioning together form **organ systems**. Finally, the various organ systems are integrated to form a functioning organism. Dysfunction at any of these levels of organization can cause disease.

Tissue *A group of similar cells joined to perform a specific function.*

Organs *A group of different tissues organized to perform a specific function.*

Organ systems *A group of organs that function together as a unit, such as the various organs of the gastrointestinal tract.*

The Cell

Cells having different functions differ somewhat in structure, but all have certain features in common (FIGURE 2-1). Each cell consists of a nucleus surrounded by the cytoplasm. The nucleus, which contains the genetic information stored in the cell, directs the metabolic functions of the cell, and structures in the cytoplasm carry out these directions. Within the cytoplasm are numerous small structures called **organelles**, which play an important part in the functions of the cell. The cytoplasm also contains filaments of structural protein that form the framework (cytoskeleton) of the cell. Some cells also contain filaments of contractile protein. The cytoplasm, nucleus, and organelles are surrounded by membranes composed of lipid and protein molecules, which separate these structures from one another.

THE NUCLEUS

The nucleus contains two different types of nucleic acid combined with protein. **Deoxyribonucleic acid (DNA)** is contained in the chromosomes, which are long and thin in the nondividing cell and cannot be identified as distinct structures. Instead, they appear as a network of granules called nuclear chromatin. **Ribonucleic acid (RNA)** is contained in spherical intranuclear structures called nucleoli (singular, nucleolus). The nucleus is separated from the cytoplasm by a double-layered nuclear membrane. Small pores in the nuclear membrane permit the nucleus and cytoplasm to communicate.

THE CYTOPLASM

The cytoplasm of the cell consists of a mass of protoplasm surrounded by a cell membrane, which acts selectively to allow some materials to pass into and out of the cell while it restricts the passage of others. It contains various organelles and may also contain products that accumulate within the cell, such as glycogen and fat. The most important organelles are the mitochondria, endoplasmic reticulum, Golgi apparatus, lysosomes, centrioles, and the tubules and filaments comprising the cytoskeleton of the cell. Some diseases are associated with characteristic abnormalities in cytoplasmic

Organelle
A small structure present in the cytoplasm of the cell, such as a mitochondrion.

Deoxyribonucleic acid (DNA)
The nucleic acid present in the chromosomes of the nuclei of cells that carries genetic information.

Ribonucleic acid (RNA)
A type of nucleic acid contained in the nucleoli of cells. A component of messenger, transfer, and ribosomal RNA.

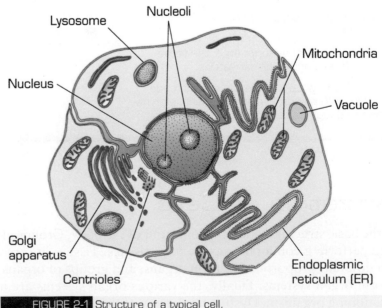

FIGURE 2-1 Structure of a typical cell.

organelles. The functions of the organelles are described in the following section and summarized in TABLE 2-1.

Mitochondria are sausage-shaped structures that contain enzymes capable of converting food materials into energy by oxidizing them. The cell uses this energy to manufacture a high-energy compound called **adenosine triphosphate (ATP)**, the fuel that powers the chemical reactions in the cell.

The **endoplasmic reticulum** is an interconnected network of tubular channels enclosed by membranes. This network communicates with both the nuclear membrane and the cell membrane. Rough endoplasmic reticulum (RER) has numerous small nucleoprotein particles called **ribosomes** attached to the external surfaces of its membranes. Its name derives from the knobby appearance that the attached ribosomes give the membranes, and its function is to synthesize protein that will be secreted by the cell. The attached ribosomes synthesize protein molecules that accumulate within the tubules of the RER and are eventually secreted. Digestive enzymes and antibody proteins, for example, are produced in this way. The second type of endoplasmic reticulum lacks ribosomes and is called the smooth endoplasmic reticulum (SER). Its membranes contain enzymes that synthesize lipids and some other substances.

The **Golgi apparatus** consists of groups of flattened membranelike sacs located near the nucleus. These sacs are connected with the tubules of the RER. The proteins produced by the ribosomes attached to the RER pass through the RER tubules into the Golgi apparatus, where large carbohydrate molecules are synthesized and

Mitochondria
(mīt-o-kon′drē-uh)
Rod-shaped structures in the cell capable of converting foods into energy to power the cell.

Adenosine triphosphate (ATP)
A high-energy phosphate compound that liberates energy to power numerous cellular metabolic processes.

Endoplasmic reticulum
A mass of hollow tubular channels within the cytoplasm of the cell, frequently bordered by ribosomes.

Ribosome
A small cytoplasmic organelle that serves as the site of protein synthesis. Ribosomes are usually attached to the endoplasmic reticulum but may be free in the cytoplasm.

Golgi apparatus
(gol′jē)
A group of membrane-lined sacs found in the cytoplasm of the cell near the nucleus.

TABLE 2-1

Major cell organelles and their functions

Organelle	Function
Mitochondria	Convert food materials into energy to make adenosine triphosphate (ATP) used to power the chemical reactions in the cell
Rough endoplasmic reticulum (RER)	Tubular ribosome-containing channels that synthesize protein to be secreted by cells
Smooth endoplasmic reticulum (SER)	Tubular channels containing enzymes that synthesize lipids and some other compounds within the cells
Golgi apparatus	Flat sacs located near nucleus attach carbohydrate molecules to the proteins synthesized by RER
Lysosomes	Spherical organelles in cytoplasm containing digestive enzymes that break down worn-out cell organelles and material brought into cell by phagocytosis
Centrioles	Short cylinders that form the mitotic spindle that separates chromosomes during cell division
Cytoskeleton	Protein tubules and filaments that form structural framework of cells and promote cell functions such as motility and phagocytosis

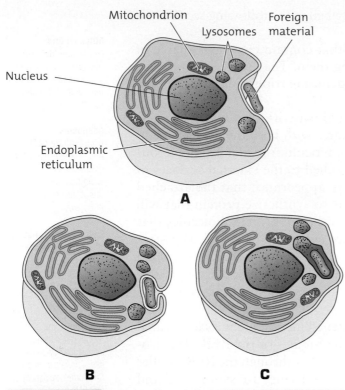

Nucleus

Mitochondrion

Lysosomes

Foreign material

Endoplasmic reticulum

A

B   **C**

FIGURE 2-2 Digestion of engulfed material by lysosomes. **A,** Extensions of cytoplasm from phagocytic cell begin to surround particulate material. **B,** Cytoplasmic extensions engulf material and form phagocytic vacuole containing the engulfed material. **C,** Lysosome and phagocytic vacuole merge, and enzymes from lysosome digest the engulfed material.

combined with the proteins. Then they are formed into secretory granules and eventually discharged from the cell.

Lysosomes (*lysis* = dissolving + *soma* = body) are cytoplasmic organelles made by the Golgi apparatus that are filled with potent digestive enzymes. They function as the "digestive system" of the cell. Lysosomes break down material brought into the cell by phagocytosis; they also degrade worn-out intracellular components such as mitochondria and other organelles, making the breakdown products available to be recycled or excreted from the cells. When particulate material is ingested by **phagocytosis**, the particle becomes enclosed within a membrane-lined vacuole called a phagocytic vacuole. A lysosome then merges with the phagocytic vacuole, and their cell membranes fuse, allowing the digestive enzymes contained in the lysosome to flow into the phagocytic vacuole and digest the engulfed material. Digestion is accomplished entirely within the phagocytic vacuole, which prevents digestive enzymes from leaking into the cytoplasm of the cell and causing injury to the cell (FIGURE 2-2). The same type of digestive process is involved when worn-out components are broken down within cells. Unfortunately, in some diseases, the lysosomal enzymes are unable to function properly, and incompletely digested material accumulates within lysosomes, disrupting cell functions.

Closely related to lysosomes are smaller structures called **peroxisomes**, which contain enzymes that break down various potentially toxic intracellular molecules. The name of this organelle (*peroxi* = peroxide + *soma* = body) comes from hydrogen peroxide (H_2O_2), a potentially toxic by-product of enzyme action that is promptly decomposed by one of the enzymes in the peroxisome.

Centrioles are short cylindrical structures located adjacent to the nucleus. In cell division, they move to opposite poles of the cell and form the mitotic spindle. The spindle fibers attach to the chromosomes and cause them to separate in the course of cell division.

The **cytoskeleton** of the cell consists of three different types of protein tubules and filaments that form the structural framework of the cell and also are responsible for cell movements, such as phagocytosis. Microtubules are the largest cytoskeletal components, and microfilaments are the smallest. Intermediate filaments are small tough protein filaments that reinforce the interior of the cell, hold the organelles in proper position within the cell, and along with the other cytoskeletal structures are responsible for the characteristic shape of each specific type of cell. There are five different types of intermediate filaments that can be identified in cells by specific histologic techniques. Each type of intermediate filament is characteristic of a specific type of cell.

Identification and characterization of intermediate filaments in cells often provide both diagnostic and prognostic information. In some diseases, such as the degenerative disease of the nervous system called Alzheimer disease (described in the discussion on

Lysosome
A small cytoplasmic vacuole containing digestive enzymes.

Phagocytosis
(fag-o-sī-tō′sis)
Ingestion of particulate of foreign material by cells.

Peroxisome
(per-ok′-si-sōm)
A cytoplasmic organelle containing various enzymes, including those that decompose potentially toxic hydrogen peroxide.

Centrioles
Short cylindrical structures located adjacent to the nucleus that participate in the formation of spindle fibers during cell division.

Cytoskeleton
(sigh′-toe-skeleton)
Protein tubules and filaments that form the structural framework of cells.

the nervous system), the intermediate filaments exhibit characteristic abnormalities that establish the diagnosis of the disease. Identification of the type of intermediate filaments in cells is also useful in the diagnosis of tumors (described in neoplastic disease discussion). Sometimes, when a pathologist is examining a biopsy of a malignant tumor, the tumor cells may be so immature and abnormal that it may be very difficult to determine the type of cell that gave rise to the tumor. Identifying a specific type of intermediate filament in the tumor cells helps determine the type of cell from which the tumor arose, which allows the pathologist to make a more precise diagnosis and provide a more reliable prognosis.

Tissues

A tissue is a group of similar cells joined together to perform a specific function. Tissues are classified into four major groups:

1. Epithelium
2. Connective and supporting tissues
3. Muscle tissue
4. Nerve tissue

EPITHELIUM

Epithelium consists of groups of cells closely joined together (FIGURE 2-3). Epithelial cells cover the exterior of the body and line the interior body surfaces that communicate with the outside, such as the gastrointestinal tract, urinary tract, and vagina. Epithelium

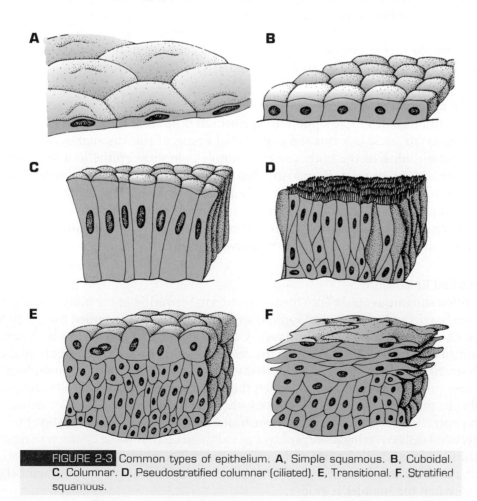

FIGURE 2-3 Common types of epithelium. **A**, Simple squamous. **B**, Cuboidal. **C**, Columnar. **D**, Pseudostratified columnar (ciliated). **E**, Transitional. **F**, Stratified squamous.

forms glands such as the thyroid and pancreas and also makes up the functional cells (often called **parenchymal cells** or **parenchyma**) of organs that have excretory or secretory functions, such as the liver and the kidneys. The individual cells may be flat and platelike (squamous cells), cube-shaped (cuboidal cells), or tall and narrow (columnar cells). Many columnar epithelial cells have become specialized to absorb or secrete, and some contain hairlike processes called cilia. Epithelial cells may be arranged in a single layer (simple epithelium) or may be several layers thick (stratified epithelium).

Endothelium and Mesothelium

The interiors of the heart, blood vessels, and lymphatic vessels are lined by a layer of simple squamous epithelium called **endothelium** (*endo* = within). A similar type of epithelium lining the pleural, pericardial, and peritoneal cavities is called **mesothelium** (*meso* = middle). Although these linings are classified as types of epithelium, they arise along with the connective tissues from the embryonic germ layer called the **mesoderm** and are therefore much more closely related to connective tissue than to other types of epithelium. Consequently, they are considered separately and are given distinct names. Moreover, tumors arising from endothelium or mesothelium behave more like tumors originating from connective tissue. They are classified with the connective tissue tumors rather than with tumors arising from surface, glandular, or parenchymal epithelium. This subject is considered in the discussion on neoplastic disease.

The Structure of Epithelium

Epithelial cells are supported by a thin basement membrane. The cells are firmly joined to each other, and the deeper layers of epithelium are firmly anchored to the basement membrane so that the epithelial cells remain relatively fixed in position. There are no blood vessels in epithelium. The cells are nourished by diffusion of material from capillaries located in the underlying connective tissue.

Simple Epithelium

The distribution of simple squamous epithelium is limited. It forms the lining of the pulmonary air sacs. It forms the endothelial lining of the vascular system and the mesothelial lining of the body cavities. Simple columnar epithelium lines most of the gastrointestinal tract. Pseudostratified columnar epithelium is a type of simple columnar epithelium in which the cells are so tightly packed together that their nuclei appear to lie at different levels. This gives an appearance of stratification. Pseudostratified epithelium is often ciliated. This type of epithelium lines most of the respiratory tract and is present in a few other areas.

Stratified Epithelium

Stratified squamous epithelium forms the external covering of the body and also lines the oral cavity, esophagus, and vagina. Stratified epithelium is named for the appearance of the most superficial cell layer. Consequently, this epithelium is designated "stratified squamous" even though the deeper layers are composed of cuboidal cells. The stratified squamous epithelium that forms the top layer of the skin undergoes a process called keratinization, in which the top layers of squamous cells accumulate a fibrous protein called **keratin** (FIGURE 2-4). This fibrous protein forms a dense layer that protects the underlying cells. Transitional epithelium consists of a layer of large superficial cells covering a deeper layer of cuboidal cells. It is the characteristic lining of the bladder and other parts of the urinary tract. The superficial cells of transitional epithelium become flattened when the bladder is distended and resume their original shape when the bladder is empty.

A   B

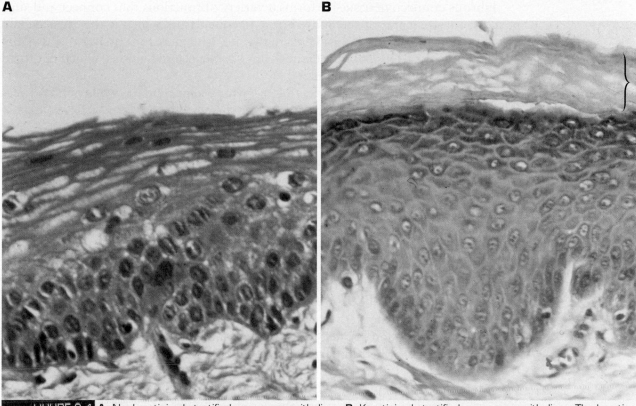

FIGURE 2-4 **A**, Nonkeratinized stratified squamous epithelium. **B**, Keratinized stratified squamous epithelium. The keratin layer (*bracket*) forms a dense acellular covering that protects the underlying epithelial cells (original magnification × 400).

Functions of Epithelium

Epithelium performs many different functions. All types of epithelium perform a protective function. Columnar epithelium, such as that lining the intestinal tract, is specialized to absorb and secrete. Other types of epithelium form glands that secrete mucus, sweat, oil, enzymes, hormones, or other products. Glands, such as the pancreas, that discharge their secretions through a duct onto an epithelial surface are called **exocrine glands** (*exo* = out). **Endocrine glands** (*endo* = within), such as the thyroid and adrenals, discharge their secretions directly into the bloodstream.

CONNECTIVE AND SUPPORTING TISSUES

Connective and supporting tissues consist of relatively small numbers of cells incorporated in a large amount of extracellular material called **matrix** in which are embedded various types of fibers. The proportions of cells, fibers, and matrix vary greatly in different types of connective tissue. Connective tissue fibers are of three types. Collagen fibers are long, flexible fibers composed of a protein called collagen. They are strong but do not stretch. Elastic fibers are composed of a protein called elastin. They are not as strong as collagen but stretch readily and return to their former shape when the stretching force is released. Reticulin fibers are very similar to collagen but are quite thin and delicate.

Connective and supporting tissues include various types of loose and dense fibrous tissue, elastic tissue, reticular tissue, adipose tissue, cartilage, and bone. Hematopoietic (blood-forming) tissue and lymphatic (lymphocyte-forming) tissue also are classified as types of connective tissue, primarily because, like other types of connective tissue, they originate from the mesoderm.

Exocrine glands
A gland that discharges its secretions through a duct onto a mucosal surface, in contrast to an endocrine gland that delivers its secretions directly into the bloodstream.

Endocrine glands
A gland that discharges its secretions directly into the bloodstream, in contrast to an exocrine gland that discharges its secretion through a duct onto a mucosal surface.

Matrix (mā'trix)
Material in which connective tissue cells are embedded.

Fibrous connective tissue performs a variety of functions that connect and support the various parts of the body. Loose fibrous tissue, which is the most widely distributed, forms the tissue just beneath the skin (subcutaneous tissue) and also fills in around organs. Dense fibrous tissue forms ligaments and tendons, which reinforce joints and attach muscles to bone.

Elastic tissue forms membranes that are wrapped around the walls of blood vessels and are responsible for the characteristic distensibility of large arteries. Elastic membranes also form part of the walls of the trachea and bronchi.

Reticular tissue is a special type of connective tissue characterized by a fine meshwork of reticulin fibers that form the supporting framework of various organs such as the liver, spleen, and lymph nodes.

Adipose tissue is a variety of loose fibrous tissue containing large numbers of fat cells. Fat is a stored form of energy and also functions as padding and insulation.

Cartilage is a type of supporting tissue in which the cells are dispersed in a dense matrix. There are three types of cartilage. Hyaline cartilage is the most common. It is blue and translucent and contains only a few fine collagen fibers suspended in the abundant matrix. Hyaline cartilage covers the ends of bones where they form movable joints, forms the greater part of the laryngeal and tracheal cartilages, and connects the ribs to the sternum. Elastic cartilage contains yellow elastic fibers in the matrix and is found in only few locations, such as the cartilaginous portions of the ears. The elastic fibers impart a flexibility to the cartilage that is lacking in other types of cartilage. Fibrocartilage contains many dense collagen bundles embedded in the matrix. It is found in areas where cartilage is subjected to marked weight-bearing stresses. It forms the disks between the vertebral bodies and some of the cartilages in the knee joints; it is also present in few other locations.

Bone is a highly specialized, rigid supporting tissue in which the matrix containing the bone-forming cells is impregnated with calcium salts.

MUSCLE TISSUE

Muscle cells contain filaments of specialized intracellular contractile proteins called actin and myosin. These are arranged in parallel bundles. During contraction of a muscle fiber, actin filaments slide inward on the myosin filaments, somewhat like pistons, causing the fiber to shorten. There are three types of muscle fibers. Smooth muscle is located primarily in the walls of hollow internal organs such as the gastrointestinal tract, biliary tract, and reproductive tract, and in the walls of the blood vessels where the muscle regulates the caliber of the vessels to control blood flow to the tissues; and in the skin where they attach to hair follicles and control elevation of the hairs. Smooth muscle functions automatically and is not under conscious control. Striated muscle moves the skeleton and is under voluntary control. Cardiac muscle is found only in the heart. It resembles striated muscle but has some features common to both smooth and voluntary muscle.

NERVE TISSUE

Nerve tissue is composed of nerve cells called **neurons,** which transmit nerve impulses, and supporting cells called **neuroglia.** Neuroglial cells are more numerous than neurons. They are of three different types. **Astrocytes** are long, star-shaped cells having numerous highly branched processes that interlace to form a meshwork. Astrocytes form the structural framework of the central nervous system in the way that the connective tissue fibers form the framework of internal organs. **Oligodendroglia** are small cells with scanty cytoplasm that surround individual nerve cells in the central nervous system. **Microglia** are phagocytic cells comparable to the macrophages found in other tissues.

Neuron (nū′ron)
A nerve cell, including the nerve cell body and its processes.

Neuroglia
(noo-rog′-lē-ah)
Supporting cells of tissue of the nervous system.

Astrocyte
A large stellate cell having highly branched processes. Forms the structural framework of the nervous system. One of the neuroglial cells.

Oligodendroglia
(ol′ig-ō-den-drog′li-ah)
One type of neuroglia that surrounds nerve fibers within the central nervous system.

Microglia
(mī-krog′-lē-ă)
Phagocytic cells of the nervous system comparable to macrophages in other tissues.

Organs and Organ Systems

An **organ** is a group of different tissues that is integrated to perform a specific function. Generally, one tissue performs the primary function characteristic of the organ, and the other tissues perform a supporting function, such as providing the vascular and connective tissue framework for the organ. The functional cells of an organ are often called the **parenchymal cells,** and the total mass of functional tissue is called the **parenchyma.** The supporting framework of the organ is called the **stroma.** In the liver, for example, the parenchymal cells are formed by cords of epithelial cells that perform the many metabolic functions characteristic of the liver, such as the synthesis of protein and the excretion of bile. The cord cells are supported by a framework of connective tissue fibers. Numerous thin-walled blood vessels are interspersed between the cell cords, and the entire liver is surrounded by a capsule composed of dense fibrous tissue.

An organ system is a group of organs that is organized to perform complementary functions, such as the reproductive system, the respiratory system, and the digestive system. Finally, the various organ systems are integrated into a functioning individual.

The Germ Layers and Their Derivatives

The highly complex structure of the entire body evolves from a single cell, the fertilized ovum, by a complex process that includes periods of cell multiplication, differentiation, and organization to form organs and organ systems. (Prenatal development is considered in the discussion on prenatal development and diseases associated with pregnancy.) As the fertilized ovum grows, its cells differentiate into two groups. The peripheral group of cells is called the **trophoblast.** This forms the placenta and other structures that will support and nourish the embryo. The inner group of cells is called the **inner cell mass.** These are the cells that will give rise to the embryo, and they soon become arranged into three distinct layers called the **germ layers.** Each layer will form certain specialized tissues and organs (FIGURE 2-5). The outer layer,

Organ
A group of different tissues organized to perform a specific function.

Parenchymal cell
(par-en'ki-mul)
The functional cell of an organ or tissue.

Parenchyma
(par-en'ki-muh)
The functional cells of an organ, as contrasted with the connective and supporting tissue that forms its framework.

Stroma (strō'muh)
The tissue that forms the framework of an organ.

Trophoblast
Cell derived from the fertilized ovum that gives rise to the fetal membranes and contributes to the formation of the placenta.

Inner cell mass
A group of cells that are derived from the fertilized ovum and are destined to form the embryo.

Germ layers
The three layers of cells derived from the inner cell mass, each layer destined to form specific organs and tissues in the embryo.

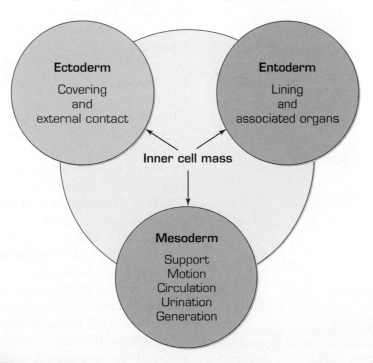

FIGURE 2-5 Derivatives of the germ layers (simplified scheme).

Ectoderm (ek'tō-derm)
The outer germ layer in the embryo that gives rise to specific organs and tissues.

Entoderm (en'tō-derm)
The inner germ layer of the embryo that gives rise to specific organs and tissues.

Mesoderm
(me'zō-derm)
The middle germ layer of the embryo, which gives rise to specific organs and tissues.

Genetic code
(jen-et'ik kōd)
The information carried by the codons of DNA molecules in chromosomes.

Base
A solution containing an excess of hydroxyl ions and having a pH greater than 7.0.

called the **ectoderm** (*ecto* = outer + *derm* = skin), forms the external covering of the body and the various organs that bring the individual into contact with the external environment: the nervous system, eyes, and ears. The inner layer, called the **entoderm** (*ento* = within), forms the internal "lining": the epithelium of the pharynx, the respiratory tract, the gastrointestinal tract and the organs closely associated with it (the liver, biliary tract, and pancreas), and some parts of the urogenital tract. The **mesoderm** (*meso* = middle) is the layer of cells sandwiched between the other two layers. From these cells are derived the various supporting tissues (connective tissues, cartilage, and bone), muscle, the circulatory system (heart, blood, and blood vessels), and major portions of the urogenital system. Each normal cell in the body is part of a community of cells and is integrated with its neighbors so that it functions along with other cells to meet the body's needs.

Cell Function and the Genetic Code

The chromosomes contain a series of messages called the **genetic code**. It is this code that regulates the various functions of the cell. The genetic code is contained within the structure of DNA and is transmitted to each newly formed cell in cell division.

THE STRUCTURE OF DNA

The chromosomes are composed of DNA combined with protein. The basic structural unit of DNA, called a nucleotide, consists of a phosphate group linked to a five-carbon sugar, deoxyribose, which in turn is joined to a nitrogen-containing compound called a **base** (FIGURE 2-6A). There are two different types of DNA bases: a purine base, which contains a fused double ring of carbon and nitrogen atoms, and a pyrimidine base, which contains only a single ring. There are four different bases in DNA: the purine bases adenine and guanine and the pyrimidine bases thymine and cytosine. Consequently, there are four different nucleotides in DNA, each containing a different base (FIGURE 2-6B). The nucleotides are joined together in long chains, with the nitrogen bases projecting at right angles from the long axes of the chains. A DNA molecule consists of two strands of DNA that are held together by weak chemical attractions between the bases of the adjacent chains. The chemical structure of the bases is such that only adenine can pair with thymine and only guanine can pair with cytosine. Bases that pair in this way are called complementary bases, and there are 3 billion pairs of complementary bases (base pairs) in the human genome. The DNA chains are twisted into a double spiral somewhat like a spiral staircase, with the sugar and phosphate groups forming the two railings and the complementary base pairs forming the steps (FIGURE 2-7A, B, AND C).

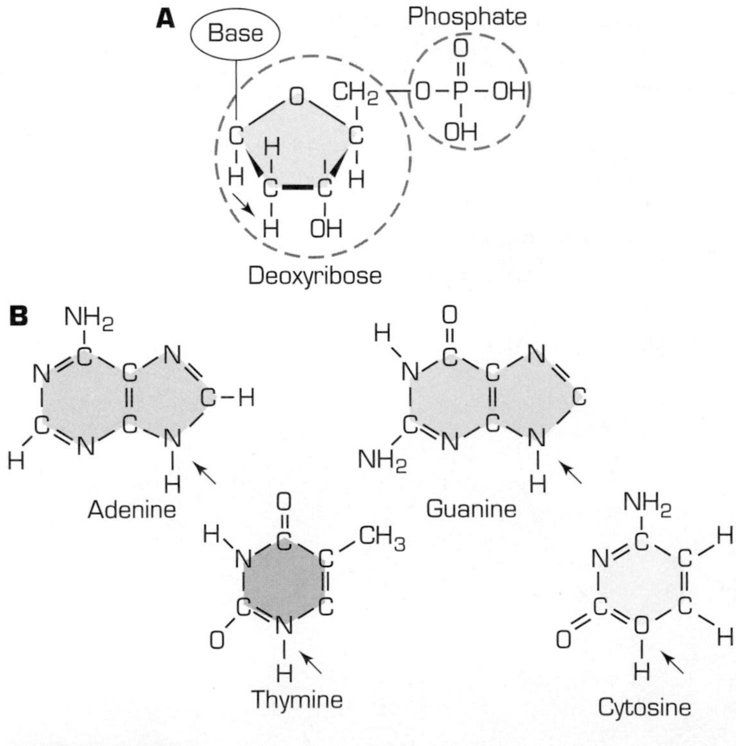

FIGURE 2-6 General structure of DNA nucleotide. **A,** Deoxyribose is identical with ribose except for the absence of an oxygen atom (site of missing oxygen indicated by *arrow*). **B,** Structure of the bases. The *arrows* indicate sites at which bases are joined to deoxyribose.

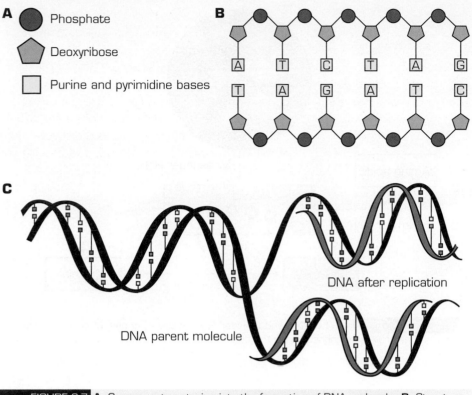

FIGURE 2-7 **A**, Components entering into the formation of DNA molecule. **B**, Structure of double stranded DNA. **C**, Duplication (replication) of DNA molecule.

DUPLICATION (REPLICATION) OF DNA

As a cell prepares to divide, the double strands of DNA duplicate themselves. The two chains separate, and each chain serves as the model for the synthesis of a new chain (FIGURE 2-7C). Because adenine always pairs with thymine and guanine with cytosine, the arrangement of the nucleotides in the original chains determines how the nucleotides will reassemble to form the new chains. The process of duplication forms two double strands, each containing one of the original strands plus a newly formed strand. In this way, each of the two daughter cells produced by cell division receives an exact duplicate of the genetic information possessed by the chromosomes of the parent cell.

THE GENETIC CODE

The DNA in the nucleus "tells the cell what to do" by directing the synthesis of enzymes and other proteins by the ribosomes located in the cytoplasm. The "instructions" are carried by messenger RNA (mRNA), so named because it carries the message encoded in the DNA to the ribosomes in the cytoplasm. mRNA is quite similar to DNA but consists of only a single rather than a double strand. It also differs by containing the five-carbon sugar ribose instead of deoxyribose and a base called uracil instead of thymine. During synthesis of mRNA, the DNA chains partially separate, and the DNA serves as the model on which the mRNA is assembled. Therefore, the information transported on the mRNA strand is an exact copy of the genetic information possessed by the nuclear DNA.

The mRNA strand leaves the nucleus through the pores in the nuclear membrane and becomes attached to the ribosomes in the cytoplasm, which are small nucleoprotein particles where enzymes and other proteins are constructed from individual amino acids. The combination of amino acids required to assemble the protein is

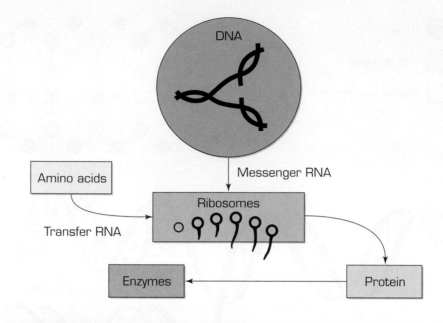

FIGURE 2-8 Role of mRNA and transfer RNA in the synthesis of enzymes and other proteins by ribosomes in the cytoplasm.

determined by the information contained in the mRNA strand. The amino acids are transported to the ribosomes by means of another type of RNA called transfer RNA (tRNA), so named because it "picks up" the required amino acids from the cytoplasm and transfers them to the ribosomes where they are assembled in proper order, as specified by the mRNA (FIGURE 2-8).

Recently, another type of RNA has been described, which does not function like messenger, ribosomal, and transfer RNA. It is called **microRNA** (miRNA) because it is a smaller molecule than other RNA molecules, and its unique function is to regulate the activity of individual genes. About 1,000 different miRNA molecules have been described, each regulating the activity of a specific gene that it controls. This subject is considered in the section dealing with the human genome and its functions.

MicroRNA
Small RNA molecules that regulate the activity of individual genes.

Movement of Materials Into and Out of Cells

In order for the cell to function properly, oxygen and nutrients must enter the cell, and waste products must be eliminated. Materials entering and leaving the cell must cross the cell membrane, which limits the passage of some molecules and is freely permeable to others. Materials cross the cell membrane in three ways:

1. Diffusion and osmosis
2. Active transport
3. Phagocytosis and pinocytosis

DIFFUSION AND OSMOSIS

Diffusion is the movement of dissolved particles (solute) from a more concentrated to a more dilute solution. Osmosis is the movement of water molecules from a dilute solution to a more concentrated solution (FIGURE 2-9). Both are passive processes that

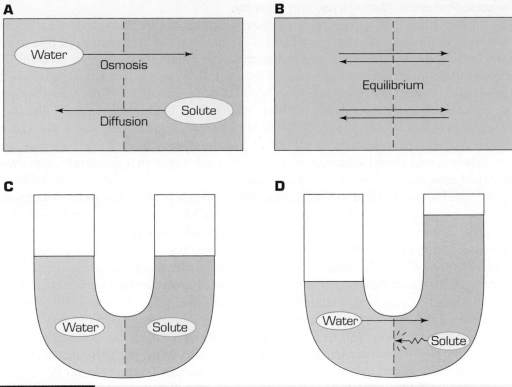

FIGURE 2-9 **A**, Processes of osmosis and diffusion across a porous membrane indicated by *dashed line*. **B**, At equilibrium, the concentrations of water and solute molecules are equal on both sides of membrane. **C**, The left compartment of U tube contains water. The right compartment contains solute impermeable to membrane. **D**, Water molecules diffuse freely across membrane, but solute molecules are unable to diffuse. The volume of solute increased by diffusion of water molecules into the solute. The volume of water in left limb of the U tube falls as water moves into the solute in the right limb of the U tube.

do not require the cell to expend energy. If the membrane is freely permeable to both water and solute particles (FIGURE 2-9A, B), the solute particles diffuse from the higher solute concentration on the right side of the membrane into the lower solute concentration on the left side. At the same time, water molecules diffuse in the opposite direction, from the more dilute solution on the right side of the membrane into the more concentrated solution on the left side. At equilibrium, the concentrations of solute particles and water molecules are the same on both sides of the membrane. Solute and water molecules continue to move in both directions across the membrane after equilibrium is attained, but the movements are equal in both directions, which does not change in the equilibrium volume and concentration of the solutions on the two sides of the membrane.

The situation is quite different if the membrane is not permeable to the solute particles in the solution on one side of the membrane (FIGURE 2-9C, D). Water molecules move by osmosis from the left side of the membrane into the more concentrated solution on the right side (containing fewer water molecules). Because diffusion of solute is restricted by the membrane but movement of water molecules across the membrane is not, the volume of the solution on the right side of the membrane increases, and its solute concentration falls as the water molecules move by osmosis across the membrane. Eventually, the solutions on both sides of the membrane have the same concentration of water molecules, but their volumes are quite different.

Osmotic Pressure, Osmolarity, and Tonicity

The "water-attracting" property of a solution, which can be measured, is called its osmotic activity or osmotic pressure and is related to the concentration of dissolved particles in the solution. The more concentrated the solution, the higher its osmotic pressure. The quantitative expression of the osmotic pressure of a solution is called **osmolarity**. Osmolarity reflects the number of dissolved particles in the solution, not the molecular weight or valence of the particles. For a substance such as glucose, which does not dissociate in solution, 1 mole (the molecular weight of the substance in grams) dissolved in water to a volume of 1 liter has an osmolarity of 1 osmole per liter (abbreviated Osm/L). However, 1 mole of a substance that dissociates into two univalent ions (such as sodium chloride) has an osmolarity of 2 Osm/L. One mole of a salt containing a divalent ion such as calcium chloride ($CaCl_2$) has an osmolarity of 3 Osm/L because the salt dissociates into three particles: one calcium and two chloride ions. The osmolarity of body fluids is usually expressed in milliosmoles per liter (mOsm/L) because body fluids contain low concentrations of dissolved particles (1 Osm = 1,000 mOsm). Movement of water and solute between the extracellular fluid (interstitial fluid and fluid components of blood and lymph) and the intracellular fluid (fluid within the cells) is regulated by the cell membrane, which is permeable to water and some solutes but relatively impermeable to others. The osmolarity of extracellular fluids varies from about 280 to 295 mOsm/L, and the intracellular osmolarity is the same, as the two fluid compartments are in equilibrium. Most of the solutes in the extracellular fluid that contribute to its osmolarity are sodium (Na^+), chloride (Cl^-), and bicarbonate (HCO_3^-) ions. In contrast, the major intracellular ions are potassium (K^+) and phosphate (PO_4^{-3}). The sodium–potassium ion differences on the two sides of the cell membrane, which are essential for normal cell functions, are controlled by the cell.

The term tonicity, which is sometimes used to refer to the osmotic effects produced by a solution, is not quite the same as osmolarity. For practical purposes, however, we can consider that an **isotonic solution** (*iso* = equal) is osmotically equivalent to the patient's own body fluids and can safely be administered intravenously to patients. Generally, only isotonic solutions are used for intravenous administration. A **hypertonic solution** (*hyper* = above) is more concentrated. Cells exposed to a hypertonic solution shrink because water moves by osmosis from the cells into the hypertonic fluid. In contrast, a **hypotonic solution** (*hypo* = below) is a dilute solution, and cells exposed to a hypotonic solution swell as water moves by osmosis from the hypotonic fluid into the cells where the osmolarity is higher. The osmotic flow of water into cells, such as red cells, may be so great that the cell membranes of the overdistended cells may rupture, causing the cells to collapse and the hemoglobin to leak from the cells.

Osmotic Pressure Differences Between Cells and Extracellular Fluids

If the osmolarity of the extracellular fluid (ECF) is higher than that within the cells, water flows by osmosis from the cell into the ECF, causing the cell to shrink. Conversely, if the osmolarity of the ECF is lower than that of the cells, water moves by osmosis into the cells, causing the cells to swell. Normally, the osmotic pressures within the cell and in the ECF are equal; therefore, the shape and water content of the cells do not change. In disease, the osmolarity of the ECF may be abnormally low or high, which will lead to secondary changes in the water content of the cells and will impair their function. For example, a person with severe uncontrolled diabetes may have a very high blood glucose concentration that increases the ECF osmolarity because the glucose is unable to enter the cell. Consequently, the cells shrink because water moves by osmosis from the cells into the extracellular fluid. Conversely, cells swell in patients with kidney disease who consume excess water

Osmolarity
A measure of the osmotic pressure exerted by a solution.

Isotonic solution
A solution having essentially the same osmolarity as body fluids so that cells neither shrink nor swell when exposed to the solution.

Hypertonic solution
A solution having a greater osmolarity than body fluids, which causes cells to shrink in such a solution because water moves by osmosis from the cells into the hypertonic solution.

Hypotonic solution
A solution having a lower osmolarity than body fluids, causing cells in the solution to swell because water moves by osmosis from the hypotonic solution into the cells.

because the diseased kidneys are unable to excrete the water efficiently. The excess water dilutes the ECF, which lowers its osmolarity, and water moves by osmosis from the diluted body fluids into the cells.

ACTIVE TRANSPORT

Active transport is the transfer of a substance across the cell membrane from a region of low concentration to one of higher concentration. The process requires the cell to expend energy because the substance must move against a concentration gradient. Many metabolic processes depend on active transport of ions or molecules. For example, in order for the cell to function normally, the intracellular potassium concentration must be higher than the concentration in the ECF, and the intracellular sodium concentration must be much lower. This is accomplished by a mechanism that actively transports potassium into the cell and simultaneously moves sodium out.

PHAGOCYTOSIS AND PINOCYTOSIS

Phagocytosis is the ingestion of particles that are too large to pass across the cell membrane. The cytoplasm flows around the particle, and the cytoplasmic processes fuse, engulfing the particle within a vacuole in the cytoplasm of the cell. A similar process called **pinocytosis** consists of the ingestion of fluid rather than solid material.

Phagocytosis
(fag-o-sī-tō′sis)
Ingestion of particulate of foreign material by cells.

Pinocytosis
(pīn′o-sī-tō′sis)
Liquid absorption by cells in which a segment of cell membrane forms small pockets and engulfs the liquid. Similar to phagocytosis, except that liquids rather than particulate material are ingested.

Adaptations of Cells to Changing Conditions

Cells respond to changing conditions in various ways. Common adaptive mechanisms are:

1. Atrophy
2. Hypertrophy and hyperplasia
3. Metaplasia
4. Dysplasia
5. Increased enzyme synthesis

In many instances, the adaptation enables the cells to function more efficiently. Sometimes, however, the adaptive change may be detrimental to the cell, as occurs in dysplasia.

ATROPHY

Atrophy is a reduction in the size of cells in response to diminished function, inadequate hormonal stimulation, or reduced blood supply. The cell decreases in size in order to "get by" under the less favorable conditions. For example, skeletal muscles are reduced in size when an extremity is immobilized in a cast for long periods, and the breasts and genital organs shrink after menopause as a result of inadequate estrogen stimulation. A kidney becomes smaller if its blood supply becomes insufficient because of narrowing of the renal artery.

HYPERTROPHY AND HYPERPLASIA

If cells are required to do more work, they may increase either their size or their number in order to accomplish their task. **Hypertrophy** is an increase in the size of

Hypertrophy
An enlargement or overgrowth of an organ caused by an increase in size of its constituent cells.

individual cells without an actual increase in their numbers. The large muscles of a weight lifter, for example, result from hypertrophy of individual muscle fibers. The number of fibers is not increased. Similarly, the heart of a person with high blood pressure often enlarges as a result of hypertrophy of the individual cardiac muscle fibers. This occurs because the heart must work harder in order to pump blood at a higher than normal pressure.

Hyperplasia
(hī-per-plā′sē̄-uh)
An increase in the number of cells.

Hyperplasia is an increase in the size of a tissue or organ caused by an increase in the number of cells. Hyperplasia occurs in response to increased demand. For example, the glandular tissue of the breast becomes hyperplastic during pregnancy in preparation for lactation. Endocrine glands such as the thyroid may enlarge in order to increase their output of hormones.

METAPLASIA

Metaplasia
(met-uh-plā′sē-yuh)
A change from one type of cell to a more resistant cell type.

Metaplasia is a change from one type of cell to another type that is better able to tolerate some adverse environmental condition. For example, if the lining of the bladder is chronically irritated and inflamed, the normal transitional epithelial lining may assume the characteristic structure of a thick layer of squamous epithelium. The metaplastic epithelium is more resistant to irritation and is better able to protect the bladder wall in the presence of chronic infection.

DYSPLASIA

Dysplasia
(dis-plā′sē-yuh)
Abnormal maturation of cells.

Dysplasia (*dys* = bad + *plasia* = formation) is a condition in which the development and maturation of cells are disturbed and abnormal. The individual cells vary in size and shape, and their relationship to one another is also abnormal (FIGURE 2-10). Dysplasia of epithelial cells may result from chronic irritation or inflammation. In some cases,

A **B**

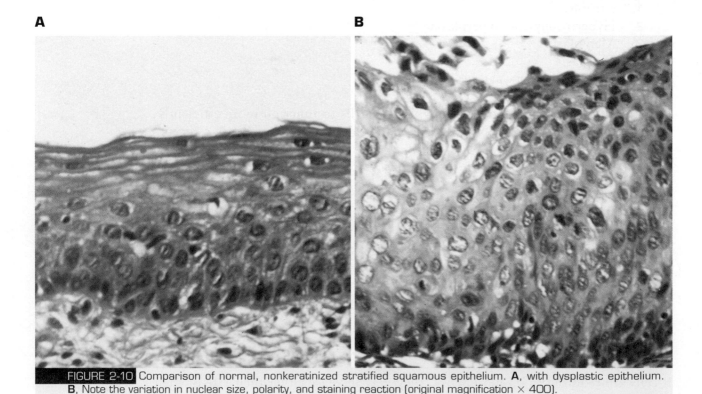

FIGURE 2-10 Comparison of normal, nonkeratinized stratified squamous epithelium. **A**, with dysplastic epithelium. **B**, Note the variation in nuclear size, polarity, and staining reaction (original magnification × 400).

dysplasia may progress to formation of a tumor; this is called **neoplasia**. The epithelium covering the uterine cervix is a common site of dysplasia, and cervical epithelial dysplasia sometimes progresses to cervical cancer. This subject is discussed in the female reproductive system.

INCREASED ENZYME SYNTHESIS

Increased synthesis of enzymes is another adaptive change that occurs in cells. Sometimes, cells are called on to inactivate or detoxify drugs or chemicals by means of the enzymes present in the smooth endoplasmic reticulum (SER). If increased demands are placed on the cells, they respond by synthesizing more SER enzymes so that drugs or chemicals can be processed more efficiently. After the cells increase their ability to handle such chemicals or drugs, they can rapidly eliminate other substances that are handled by means of the same enzyme systems. A person accustomed to heavy consumption of alcohol, for example, is able to metabolize the alcohol more efficiently because of this adaptive change. Such an individual may also metabolize and eliminate other drugs at a greatly accelerated rate. Consequently, if a physician administers a medication that is metabolized by the same enzyme systems, the usual therapeutic doses of the medications may be ineffective.

Cell Injury, Cell Death, and Cell Necrosis

CELL INJURY

An injured cell may exhibit various morphologic abnormalities. The two most common changes are cell swelling and fatty change.

Cell Swelling

A normally functioning cell actively transports potassium into the cell and moves sodium out. This process requires the cell to expend energy. If the cell is injured and unable to function normally, the transport mechanism begins to fail. Sodium diffuses into the cell, and water moves into the cell along with the sodium, causing the cell to swell. If the swelling continues, fluid-filled vacuoles may accumulate within the cell, and eventually, it may rupture.

Fatty Change

If the enzyme systems that metabolize fat are impaired, leading to accumulation of fat droplets within the cytoplasm, fatty change may occur. This condition is a common manifestation of liver cell injury because liver cells are actively involved in fat metabolism.

CELL DEATH AND CELL NECROSIS

A cell dies if it has been irreparably damaged. Several hours after the cell dies, various structural changes begin to take place within the nucleus and cytoplasm. Lysosomal enzymes are released and begin to digest the cell. The nucleus shrinks and either dissolves or breaks into fragments. Sometimes, calcium is deposited in the dead cells and tissues. These structural changes are termed cell **necrosis**. All necrotic cells are dead, but a dead cell is not necessarily necrotic because

Neoplasia
(nē-ō-plā′se-yuh)
The pathologic process that results in the formation and growth of a tumor.

Necrosis (nek-rō′sis)
Structural changes associated with cell death.

A   B

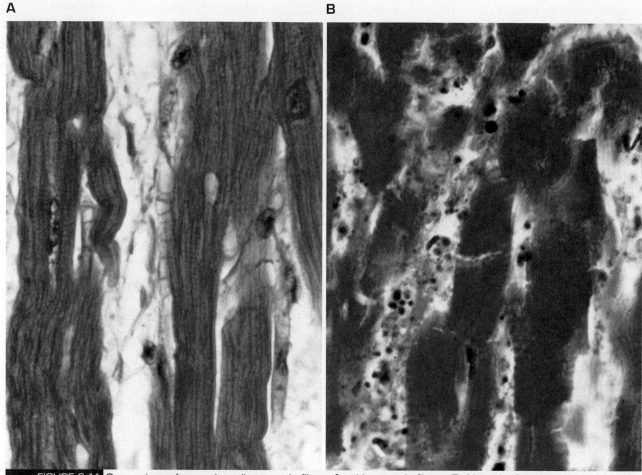

FIGURE 2-11 Comparison of normal cardiac muscle fibers **A**, with necrotic fibers. **B**, Note the fragmentation of fibers, the loss of nuclear staining, and the fragmented bits of nuclear debris (original magnification × 400).

the structural changes that characterize cell death take several hours to develop. Necrotic cells are easily recognized on histologic examination because they appear quite different from normal cells in both their structural and their staining characteristics (FIGURE 2-11).

PROGRAMMED CELL DEATH: APOPTOSIS

Not all cell death results from cell injury. All normal cells have a predetermined life span and are programmed to die after a specific period of time. The number of functional cells in all our body tissues is determined by a balance between proliferation of new cells and death of older "worn-out" cells. The older cells die because they are genetically programmed to "shut down" when they have reached the end of their predetermined life span. This form of programmed self-destruction is called **apoptosis.** The rates of cell proliferation and cell death vary in different body tissues. If the genes that regulate apoptosis become deranged and cease to function properly, cells may continue to proliferate instead of dying as they should. Excessive numbers of cells may accumulate in organs or tissues, which disrupts their functions and leads to disease. Some tumors appear to result from failure of the normal mechanisms regulating apoptosis.

Apoptosis
(ah-pop-toe′-sis,
or ah-po-toe′-sis)
*Programmed cell death
that occurs after a cell has
lived its normal life span.*

Aging and the Cell

All organisms grow old and eventually die, and each species has a predetermined life span. Although human life expectancy has increased over the years, the increase is chiefly because early deaths from infectious diseases, accidents, and other conditions have been greatly reduced. The causes of aging are not well understood but appear to reside in the cell. Although each type of cell has a definite life span, under normal circumstances, cell longevity is also influenced by environmental factors. The life span of an individual in turn reflects the survival of the various populations of cells that together form the individual.

Many investigators believe that aging of cells is genetically programmed and is an inherent property of the cell itself. Examples can be seen in the graying of the hair, which is the result of an eventual failure of the hair cells to produce pigment, and in menopause, which is a predetermined failure of reproductive function. Aging changes in the brain appear to be caused by the wearing out and eventual death of neurons, which are not capable of cell division. The degenerative changes in the walls of arteries, called arteriosclerosis, are thought to be caused partially by a gradual failure of the endothelial cells lining the blood vessels to prevent fatty substances from seeping into the arterial walls. The common type of arthritis seen in older persons begins as an aging change in the cartilage covering the ends of the bones.

As a cell ages, many of its enzyme systems become less active, and the cell becomes less efficient in carrying out its functions. The cell also becomes more susceptible to harmful environmental influences that may shorten its life. For example, the life span of a red cell is 4 months, and therefore the red cells circulating in the bloodstream vary greatly in age, ranging from newly produced cells to those nearing the end of their life span. Each red cell contains enzyme systems that generate its energy, enable it to perform its varied metabolic functions, and maintain the hemoglobin in a condition suitable for transporting oxygen. As the red cell ages and its enzyme systems gradually decline, the cell is less able to protect itself from injury than is a young, "vigorous" cell. If the red cells are exposed to harmful drugs or antibodies that damage the cell membranes, it is the older cells that bear the brunt of the damage and die. The younger cells are able to survive and continue to function.

An example of aging change in cells that affects the organism as a whole can be seen in the lymphocytes of which our immune system is composed. These cells help eliminate pathogenic organisms and also eliminate any of our own cells that become abnormal and have the potential of forming tumors. The cells of the immune system become less efficient as they age. Consequently, the aging individual becomes more susceptible to various infectious diseases, which can shorten the life span. The aging immune system also becomes less able to eliminate abnormal cells that arise sporadically within the body. This may predispose to the formation of malignant tumors, which occur with increasing frequency in older persons.

Aging of cells may also be caused by damage to cellular DNA, RNA, and cytoplasmic organelles that occurs at a pace more rapid than the cell's ability to repair itself. According to this concept, these components become damaged by radiation or other environmental factors or by accumulation of metabolic products within cells. Eventually, the cells begin to malfunction. Some cells can repair the damage and continue to function. Others cannot and die. The more efficient the repair process within the cell, the more likely the cell is to survive.

In summary, cells have a finite life span. However, the less they are exposed to harmful environmental influences and the more efficient they are in repairing their own malfunctions, the greater their chances for survival to a "ripe old age."

QUESTIONS FOR REVIEW

1. How does the nucleus direct the activities of the cell? What is the genetic code, and what is its role in directing the functions of the cell?
2. What are the functions of the following organelles: rough endoplasmic reticulum, ribosomes, lysosomes, and centrosomes?
3. How is epithelium classified, and what are its functions? Why are mesothelium and endothelium considered separately from other types of epithelium?
4. What are the germ layers, and what are their functions?
5. What is the difference between atrophy and hypertrophy, between metaplasia and dysplasia, and between cell death and cell necrosis?
6. What morphologic abnormalities are manifested by an injured cell? Why do they develop?
7. What factors cause a cell to age?

SUPPLEMENTARY READINGS

Guyton, A. C., and Hall, J. E. 2006. *Textbook of medical physiology.* 11th ed. Philadelphia: Elsevier Saunders.

▶ Good sections on cell biology.

Hetts, S. W. 1998. To die or not to die: An overview of apoptosis and its role in disease. *Journal of the American Medical Association* 279:300–7.

▶ A review of programmed cell death and how derangement of the process can lead to various diseases.

Levine, A. J. 1995. The genetic origins of neoplasia (Editorial). *Journal of the American Medical Association* 273:592.

▶ Mutations in three groups of genes contribute to the origins and progression of neoplasms: oncogenes, tumor suppressor genes, and DNA repair genes. Mutations that convert proto-oncogenes into oncogenes include amplifications, translocations, and point mutations, and they act as dominant mutations. Mutations of tumor suppressor genes are the basis of inherited predisposition to cancer and are inherited in the heterozygous state. A random mutation of the remaining normally functioning allele leads to loss of regulator function that results in malignancy. DNA repair genes correct errors in DNA duplication, and loss of gene function increases the mutation rate.

OUTLINE SUMMARY

Organization of Cells

Basic structural and functional unit.
Forms tissues, organs, and organ systems.

The Cell

COMPOSITION

Nucleus: contains genetic information and directs activities.
Cytoplasm: carries out metabolic activities directed by nucleus.

Mitochondria: oxidize food to form ATP, energy source of cell.
Endoplasmic reticulum: two types of hollow tubes in cytoplasm. RER has ribosomes and synthesizes protein. SER has enzymes and synthesizes lipids and other materials.
Golgi apparatus: functions with endoplasmic reticulum to synthesize and package secretory granules, which are eventually discharged.
Lysosomes: vacuoles containing digestive enzymes.
Centrioles: short cylinders that form mitotic spindle during cell division.

Tissues

EPITHELIUM
Structure:
Forms coverings and linings.
Simple: one layer thick.
Stratified: multiple layers.
Endothelium and mesothelium: separate category.
Forms parenchymal cells of excretory or secretory organs.
Function:
Protection.
Absorption.
Secretion.
Forms glands: exocrine and endocrine.

CONNECTIVE AND SUPPORTING TISSUES
Structure and function:
Fibrous connective tissue: connection and support.
Elastic tissue: stretches. Wrapped around blood vessels.
Reticular tissue: framework of liver, spleen, lymph nodes.
Adipose tissue: energy storage, padding, insulation.
Cartilage and bone: support.

MUSCLE TISSUE
Structure and function:
Smooth: in walls of hollow organs and blood vessels. Regulatory.
Striated: moves skeleton under voluntary control.
Cardiac: found only in heart. Properties intermediate between smooth and skeletal muscle.

NERVE TISSUE
Structure and function:
Impulse transmission.
Composed of nerve cells and supporting cells: neuroglia.

Organs and Organ Systems

ORGANS
A group of different tissues integrated to perform a specific function.
Composed of parenchymal (functional) cells and stromal (supporting) cells.

ORGAN SYSTEMS
A group of organs that perform related functions; for example, reproductive system.

The Germ Layers and Their Derivatives

FUNCTION
Embryonic cell layers that give rise to specific tissues and organs.
Ectoderm: external coverings, nervous system, eyes, ears.
Entoderm: lining of body and associated organs.
Mesoderm: supporting tissue, muscle, circulatory system, urogenital system.

Cell Function and the Genetic Code

FUNCTION
DNA composed of chains of nucleotides containing genetic information.
In cell division, original chain serves as model for building new chain.

GENETIC CODE
Nucleus directs activities of cytoplasm by means of mRNA, which attaches to ribosomes and directs protein synthesis.
Transfer RNA brings amino acids to ribosomes for assembly as specified by nucleotides in mRNA.
MicroRNA: a unique RNA that regulates the activity of individual genes.

Movement of Materials Into and Out of Cells

DIFFUSION AND OSMOSIS
Diffusion: movement of solute from concentrated to dilute solution.
Osmosis: movement of water from dilute to more concentrated solution.
Osmotic pressure: a measure of concentration.
Depends on number of dissolved particles.
Tonicity often used interchangeably with osmolarity.

ACTIVE TRANSPORT
Transfer of materials against a concentration gradient.
Necessary to maintain proper concentration of intracellular and extracellular ions.

PHAGOCYTOSIS AND PINOCYTOSIS
Phagocytosis: ingestion of particulate material.
Pinocytosis: ingestion of water.

Adaptations of Cells to Changing Conditions

NATURE OF ADAPTATIONS
Atrophy: reduction in size in response to unfavorable conditions.
Hypertrophy: increase in cell size for more efficient function.
Hyperplasia: increase in number of cells to increase functional capabilities.
Metaplasia: change from one type of cell to a more resistant type.
Dysplasia: disturbed development. May proceed to neoplasia.
Increased enzyme synthesis: adaptation in order to inactivate or detoxify materials more efficiently.

Cell Injury, Cell Death, and Cell Necrosis

CELL INJURY

Cell swelling: mechanism for transporting sodium out of cell begins to fail when cell is injured. Sodium diffuses into cell along with water, causing cell to swell.

Fatty change: fat metabolism impaired; fat accumulates in cell.

CELL DEATH AND NECROSIS

Cell death follows irreparable injury.

Structural changes that follow called cell necrosis.

PROGRAMMED CELL DEATH: APOPTOSIS

Cells have predetermined life span and are genetically programmed to die eventually.

If regulatory mechanisms fail, cells continue to proliferate. Accumulation of excessive numbers of cells disrupts organ functions.

Some tumors result from failure of regulatory mechanisms controlling cell longevity.

Aging and the Cell

BASIC CONCEPTS

Cells and organisms have predetermined life span.

Harmful environmental factors damage DNA, RNA, and organelles. This shortens life span.

Cells are capable of repairing damage. The more efficient the repair process, the greater the likelihood of cell survival.

---

http://health.jbpub.com/humandisease/9e

Human Disease Online is a great source for supplementary human disease information for both students and instructors. Visit this website to find a variety of useful tools for learning, thinking, and teaching.

Chromosomes, Genes, and Cell Division

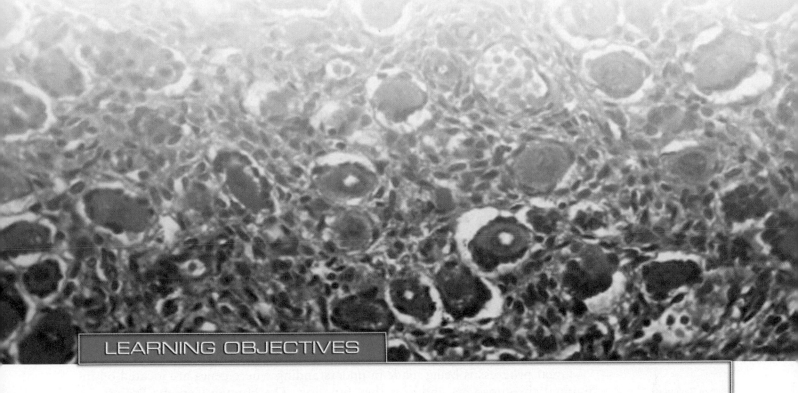

1 Describe how chromosomes are studied. Explain how a karyotype is determined.

2 Compare mitosis and meiosis.

3 Compare spermatogenesis and oogenesis. Explain the implications of abnormal chromosome separations in the course of meiosis in older women.

4 Describe the inheritance pattern of genes and define dominant, recessive, codominant, and sex-linked inheritance.

5 Describe the HLA system, and explain its application to organ transplantation and its relationship to disease susceptibility.

6 Describe the applications and limitations of gene therapy.

Chromosomes

The activities of cells are controlled by the chromosomes present in the nucleus. In the somatic cells (cells other than those giving rise to eggs and sperm), chromosomes exist in pairs. One member of each pair is derived from the male parent and one member from the female parent. Except for the sex chromosomes, both members of the pair are similar in size, shape, and appearance and are called **homologous chromosomes**. In human beings, the normal chromosome component is 22 pairs of **autosomes** (the general term for chromosomes other than the sex chromosomes) and one pair of **sex chromosomes**.

Homologous chromosomes
A matched pair of chromosomes, one derived from each parent.

Autosome (aw′tō-sōm)
A chromosome other than a sex chromosome.

Sex chromosomes
The X and Y chromosomes that determine genetic sex.

Genome (jee′nōm)
The total of all the genes contained in a cell's chromosomes.

Gene product
A protein or enzyme specified (coded) by a gene.

Exon
The part of a chromosomal DNA chain that codes for a specific protein or enzyme.

Intron
A noncoding part of a chromosomal DNA chain.

Human Genome Project (jee′-nōm)
An international collaboration of scientists who mapped the nucleotide sequence of the entire human genome.

As described in the discussion on cells and tissues: their structure and function in health and disease, the chromosomes are composed of double coils of deoxyribonucleic acid (DNA) combined with protein. The genes, which are the basic units of inheritance, are segments of the DNA chains that determine some property of the cell. Genes are sometimes described as being arranged along the chromosome like beads on a string.

The total of all the genes contained in a cell's chromosomes is called its **genome** and is the same in all cells; however, not all genes are expressed (active) in all cells, and not all genes are active all the time. Some genes code for specific enzymes or other proteins that the cell needs in order to function, and others act as regulators to control the activities of neighboring genes. An enzyme or other protein specified by a gene, which is transcribed into messenger RNA and translated through transfer RNA and cytoplasmic ribosomes into protein, is called the **gene product**.

There are about 20,000 genes in the human genome arranged on 23 pairs of chromosomes containing over 3 billion pairs of DNA bases. Each pair consists of adenine paired with thymine or guanine paired with cytosine. Actually, only a very small percentage of the total DNA in the human genome consists of genes that direct the synthesis of enzymes or other proteins specified by messenger RNA. We do not know much about the functions of the remaining DNA, which is interspersed between the genes. The parts of the DNA chains that code for specific proteins are called **exons**, and the parts of the DNA chains interspersed between the exons are called **introns**. When parts of the DNA chains are translated into messenger RNA in order to make a gene product in the cytoplasm, both the genes (exons) and the noncoding parts of the DNA chains (introns) are transcribed, but the introns are removed from the messenger RNA before it leaves the nucleus. Only the coding sequences that specify the protein to be constructed are delivered to the ribosomes by the messenger RNA.

The genes that are expressed in a given cell determine both its structure and its functions, which is why a liver cell, for example, has a different structure from that of a blood cell and functions differently as well.

Great progress is being made in understanding where genes are located on individual chromosomes and how they function. The **Human Genome Project**, an international collaboration of many scientists working together, has constructed a "road map" of our entire genome by determining the locations of the individual genes on each of our chromosomes, which is an enormous scientific achievement. Genomics is the study of gene structure, and attempts to correlate the structure of the genes with the effects of the genes (gene expression) in the individual.

REGULATION OF GENE FUNCTION BY MICRORNA

A major undertaking in recent years has been attempting to understand the role of the microRNA (miRNA) molecules that regulate the expression of genes. Usually, miRNAs act by inhibiting or blocking the action of messenger RNA, thereby preventing synthesis of the protein (gene product) directed by messenger RNA, which in turn blocks the function of the gene.

MiRNAs are produced by many cells in the body, which affect how the organs function. Each miRNA recognizes a distinct set of messenger RNAs that code for specific gene products. Some miRNAs may completely change the characteristics and functions of the cells under their control; many play a role in cell growth, differentiation, and cell death. Dysfunction of miRNA has been described in many diseases, although sometimes, it is uncertain whether the miRNA dysfunction caused the disease or occurred as a result of the disease. The disease may have resulted either from failure of the cell to produce a required miRNA or from malfunction of the miRNA that had been produced. Some investigators believe that failure of brain neurons to produce miRNA may be responsible for some neurologic diseases. Many investigations are also underway dealing with the role of miRNAs on the growth of cancer cells and their role in diseases resulting from dysfunction of cells in specific organs. Perhaps, as investigators learn more about miRNA malfunctions and dysfunctions, physicians may be able to apply new concepts about miRNA to the control of cancer, Alzheimer disease, heart disease and other health-related problems.

SINGLE NUCLEOTIDE POLYMORPHISMS

Although we have been very successful in mapping the genome, much work remains. The sequence of base pairs in the human genome is almost (over 99%) identical in everybody. However, there are minor variations in many of the nucleotides contained in the individual genes of different individuals. These variations are called single nucleotide polymorphisms, usually abbreviated as SNPs and pronounced "snips." The single nucleotide variation may affect how the gene functions, such as how rapidly a cell enzyme inactivates a drug or environmental toxin or repairs damage to cell DNA. SNPs may also explain why some persons respond differently to various foods, antibiotics, or other drugs. Differences in the ability to detoxify potential carcinogens may influence susceptibility to some cancers, which may explain why inhaled carcinogens in tobacco smoke cause lung cancer in some persons but not in others. Many studies are underway analyzing multiple genes in individuals within specific groups having risk factors for some disease or condition (constructing a "gene profile"). Studies of this type attempt to define a specific profile that can predict a favorable response to a specific drug, can determine genetic susceptibility to certain cancers, or can predict susceptibility to some chronic diseases such as diabetes or Alzheimer disease.

Eventually, as the human genome gives up its secrets, we will be able to understand how variations in the structure of the same gene leads to different effects on body functions in health and disease. Hopefully, we may be able to apply this information to provide more effective medical care and perhaps prevent or favorably influence the course of some diseases.

SEX CHROMOSOMES

Genetic sex is determined by the composition of X and Y chromosomes. The cells of a normal female contain two X chromosomes, and those of a normal male contain one X and one Y chromosome. The small Y chromosome consists almost entirely of genes concerned with male sexual differentiation. In contrast, the large X chromosome contains a large number of genes that direct many important cell activities.

X Chromosome Inactivation: The Lyon Hypothesis

Because the cells of the female contain two X chromosomes, they would be expected to contain much more genetic material than those of the male, whose cells contain only one X chromosome. Female cells, however, function as though they contained only genetic material equivalent to that of a single X chromosome. The reason for this paradoxical behavior is that one of the X chromosomes is inactivated and nonfunctional. In the female, the genetic activity of both X chromosomes is only essential during the first week of embryonic development. Thereafter, one of the X chromosomes in each of the developing cells is inactivated. With only rare exceptions, the inactivation occurs in a random manner, as illustrated in FIGURE 3-1. After the initial inactivation of an X chromosome has occurred, the same paternal- or maternal-derived X chromosome will also be inactivated in all descendants of the precursor cell. The inactivated X chromosome appears as a small, dense mass of chromatin attached to the nuclear membrane of somatic cells. This structure can

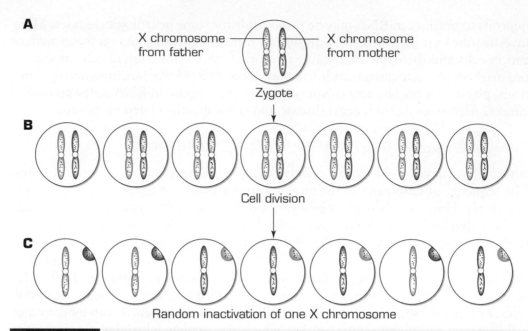

FIGURE 3-1 Concept of random inactivation of X chromosome. **A**, Fertilized egg (zygote) contains two functionally active X chromosomes, and both are necessary during early development. **B**, Cell divisions of the zygote give rise to many daughter cells, each containing two active X chromosomes. **C**, One of the X chromosomes in each cell (either X chromosome derived from the mother or the father) is inactivated in a random manner, giving rise to two cell populations with respect to the X chromosome. The descendants of each of these cells also contain the same inactivated X chromosome.

Barr body
The inactivated X chromosome that is applied to the nuclear membrane in the female. Sex chromatin body.

be identified in the cells of a normal female and is called a sex chromatin body or **Barr body** after the man who first described it (FIGURE 3-2A).

Because the X chromosome inactivation is random, the inactivated X is of paternal origin in some cells and of maternal origin in others, and the percentages of inactivated paternal- and maternal-derived X chromosomes are not necessarily equal. Consequently, the genes on the X chromosome that function in a woman's cell will depend on which X chromosome is active in the cell, as the other X chromosome is inactivated and nonfunctional. According to this concept, called the Lyon hypothesis after the woman who first described it, a female is composed of a mixture of two types of cells with respect to the active X chromosome. This hypothesis has explained some of the pecu-

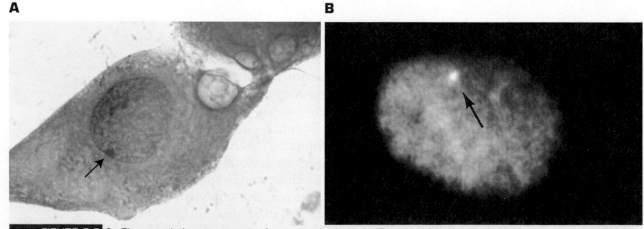

FIGURE 3-2 **A**, Characteristic appearance of sex chromatin body (Barr body) in the nucleus of a squamous epithelial cell. **B**, Fluorescent Y chromosome (*arrow*) in nucleus of intact cell.

liarities of the behavior of genes carried on the X chromosome in males and females, as described in later sections dealing with X-linked genetic diseases.

Identification of Sex Chromosomes in Intact Cells

An inactivated X chromosome in an intact cell of a normal female can be identified as a sex chromatin body attached to the nuclear membrane of the cell (FIGURE 3-2A). It is also possible to identify the Y chromosome in the cells of a normal male. The Y chromosome stains intensely with certain fluorescent dyes as a bright fluorescent spot within the nucleus of the intact cell when a suitably stained preparation is examined microscopically under ultraviolet light (FIGURE 3-2B).

A combination of staining and ultraviolet light makes it possible to determine the X and Y chromosome composition of intact cells. The cells of the normal male possess the fluorescent spot but lack the sex chromatin body, and the cells of the normal female contain the sex chromatin body but lack the fluorescent spot. Cells for examination are usually obtained by scraping the mucosa of the cheek gently with a tongue depressor and preparing slides from this material. However, cells obtained from any convenient site may be used for examination.

Cell Division

There are two types of cell division: **Mitosis** is characteristic of somatic cells. **Meiosis** is a specialized type of cell division that occurs during the development of the eggs (ova) and sperm, a process called **gametogenesis**. In mitosis, each of the two new cells (called the **daughter cells**) resulting from the cell division receives the same number of chromosomes that were present in the precursor cell (called the parent cell). In meiosis, the number of chromosomes is reduced so that the daughter cells receive only half of the chromosomes possessed by the parent cell.

MITOSIS

Mitosis is characteristic of somatic cells, but not all mature cells are able to divide. Some mature cells, such as skeletal and cardiac muscle cells and nerve cells, do not divide. Others, such as connective tissue cells and liver cells, divide as needed to replace lost or damaged cells or to heal an injury. Yet others divide continually, such as those lining the testicular tubules that produce sperm cells and those in the bone marrow that continually replace the circulating cells in the bloodstream. Regardless of the frequency of cell division, the rate of cell division is controlled closely to match the body's needs, and excess cells are not normally produced.

Many factors regulate cell growth and cell division. Often the stimulus that induces a cell to divide does not originate within the cell itself but comes from other cells. Various soluble growth-promoting substances called **growth factors** are secreted by neighboring cells and bind to receptors on the cell membrane of the target cell, which activates the receptors. The activated receptors in turn transmit biochemical signals to the "machinery" inside the cell, which induces the cell to divide. Genes within the cell also play an important role. Some promote cell growth by directing the production of the receptors on the cell surface to which the growth factors can attach. Other genes generate inhibitory signals that suppress cell growth and division. Depending on the signals, either the cell is induced to grow and divide or its growth is inhibited. These intracellular communications allow normal cells to divide often enough to accomplish their functions and replenish cell losses from injury or normal aging but restrain excessive proliferation. Moreover, normal cells cannot continue to divide indefinitely. They are programmed to undergo a limited number of cell divisions, and then they die.

Mitosis
The type of cell division of most cells in which chromosomes are duplicated in the daughter cells and are identical with those in the parent cell. The characteristic cell division found in all cells in the body except for the gametes.

Meiosis (mī-o′sis)
A special type of cell division occurring in gametes (ova and sperm), in which the number of chromosomes is reduced by one-half in the ovum and sperm.

Gametogenesis
(gam′ē-to-gen′esis)
The development of mature eggs and sperm from precursor cells.

Daughter cell
A cell resulting from division of a single cell (called the parent cell).

Growth factor
A soluble growth promoting substance produced by cells that attaches to receptors on the cell membrane of other cells, which activates the receptors and initiates events leading to growth or division of the target cells.

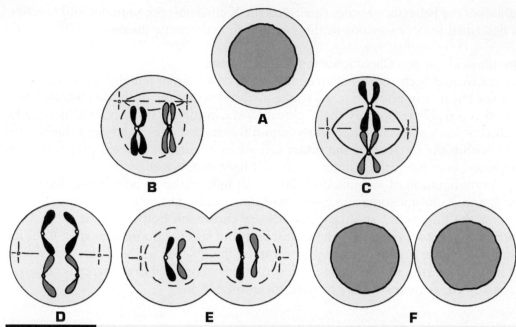

FIGURE 3-3 Stages of mitosis. The behavior of only one pair of homologous chromosomes is shown. **A**, Prior to cell division. **B**, Prophase. **C**, Metaphase. **D**, Anaphase. **E**, Telophase. **F**, Daughter cells resulting from mitosis, each identical to the parent cell.

Chromatid (krō′mä-tid)
One of two newly formed chromosomes held together by the centromere.

Before a cell begins mitosis, its DNA chains are duplicated to form new chromosome material. Each chromosome and its newly duplicated counterpart lie side by side. The two members of the pair are called **chromatids**. Mitosis is the process by which chromatids separate. (The use of the terms chromosomes and chromatids may at times be confusing. Each chromosome duplicates itself before beginning cell division. Because there are normally 46 chromosomes in each somatic cell, just prior to cell division, there are actually the equivalent of 92 chromosomes in the cell (i.e., 46 × 2). When the chromosomes shorten in the course of cell division, each chromosome can be seen to actually consist of two separate chromosomes that are still partially joined where the spindle fibers attach. The term chromatids is applied to the still-joined chromosomes at this stage. As soon as they separate, they are again called chromosomes.)

Mitosis is divided into four stages (FIGURE 3-3): prophase, metaphase, anaphase, and telophase.

Prophase

Each chromosome thickens and shortens. The centrioles migrate to opposite poles of the cell and form the mitotic spindle, which consists of small fibers radiating in all directions from the centrioles. Some of these spindle fibers attach to the chromatids. The nuclear membrane breaks down toward the end of prophase.

Metaphase

Centromere
The structure that joins each pair of chromatids formed by chromosome duplication.

The chromosomes line up in the center of the cell. At this stage, the chromatids are partially separated but still remain joined at a constricted area called the **centromere**, which is the site where the spindle fibers are attached.

Anaphase

The chromatids constituting each chromosome separate to form individual chromosomes, which are pulled to opposite poles of the cell by the spindle fibers.

Telophase

The nuclear membranes of the two daughter cells reform and the cytoplasm divides, forming two daughter cells. Each is an exact duplicate of the parent cell.

MEIOSIS

Meiotic cell division reduces the number of chromosomes by half and also leads to some intermixing of genetic material between homologous chromosomes. The process entails two separate divisions called the first and second meiotic divisions (FIGURE 3-4).

First Meiotic Division

As in mitosis, each chromosome duplicates itself before beginning cell division, forming two chromatids. During prophase, each homologous pair of chromosomes come to lie side by side over their entire length. This association is called a **synapse**. At this stage, there is frequently some interchange of segments between homologous chromosomes, which is called a **crossover**. The pairing of homologous chromosomes and the interchange of genetic material during prophase is the characteristic feature of meiosis. In the female, the two X chromosomes synapse in the same way as autosomes, but in the male, the X and Y chromosomes synapse end to end and do not exchange segments.

In metaphase, the paired chromosomes become arranged in a plane within the middle of the cell. During anaphase, the homologous chromosomes separate and

Synapse (sin′aps)
Pairing of homologous chromosomes in meiosis.

Crossover
Interchange of genetic material between homologous chromosomes during synapse and meiosis.

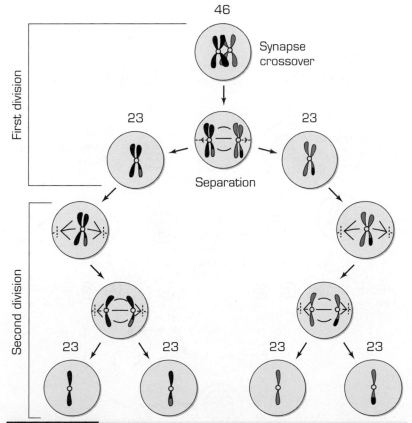

FIGURE 3-4 Stages of meiosis. The behavior of only one pair of homologous chromosomes is indicated. In the first meiotic division, each daughter cell receives only one member of each homologous pair, and the chromosomes are not exact duplicates of those in the parent cell. The second meiotic division is like a mitotic division, but each cell contains only 23 chromosomes.

move to opposite poles of the cell. Each chromosome consists of two chromatids, but they do not separate at this stage. In telophase, two new daughter cells are formed. Each daughter cell contains only one member of each homologous pair of chromosomes; consequently, the chromosomes in each daughter cell are reduced by half. The chromosomes in the daughter cells are also somewhat different from those in the parent cell because of the interchange of genetic material during synapse.

Second Meiotic Division

The second meiotic division is similar to a mitotic division. The two chromatids composing each chromosome separate and two new daughter cells are formed, each containing half of the normal number of chromosomes.

Gametogenesis

Gonad (gō'nad)
A general term referring to either the ovary or the testis.

Gametes
Reproductive cells, eggs, and sperm, each containing 23 chromosomes, which unite during fertilization to form a zygote containing 46 chromosomes.

The testes and ovaries, called **gonads**, contain precursor cells called germ cells, which are capable of developing into mature sperm or ova. The mature germ cells are called **gametes**, and the process by which they are formed is **gametogenesis**. The development of sperm (spermatogenesis) and of ova (oogenesis) is similar in many respects (FIGURE 3-5).

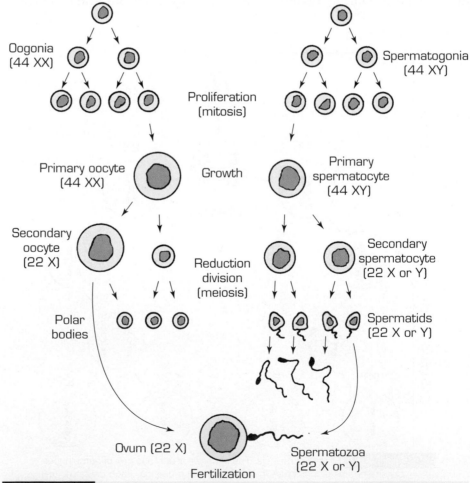

FIGURE 3-5 Sequence of events in gametogenesis. The numbers and letters in parentheses refer to the chromosomes in the cell. Numbers indicate autosomes; letters designate sex chromosomes.

SPERMATOGENESIS

The precursor cells in the testicular tubules are called *spermatogonia* (singular term, spermatogonium). Each contains a full complement of 46 chromosomes. Spermatogonia divide by mitosis to form primary spermatocytes, which, like the precursor cells, contain 46 chromosomes. The primary spermatocytes then divide by meiosis. In the first meiotic division, each primary spermatocyte forms two secondary spermatocytes, each containing 23 chromosomes. Each secondary spermatocyte completes the second meiotic division and forms two **spermatids**, also containing 23 chromosomes, and the spermatids mature into sperm. The entire process of spermatogenesis takes about 2 months, and sperm are being produced continually.

Spermatids
Germ cells in a late stage of sperm development just before complete maturation to form mature sperm.

OOGENESIS

The precursors of the ova are called *oogonia* (singular term, oogonium). Each contains 46 chromosomes. Oogonia divide repeatedly in the fetal ovaries before birth, forming primary oocytes, which contain 46 chromosomes. The oocytes then become surrounded by a single layer of cells called **granulosa cells** or follicular cells, forming structures called primary follicles (FIGURE 3-6). The primary oocytes in the follicles begin the prophase of the first meiotic division during fetal life but do not carry the division through to completion. A very large number of primary follicles are formed, but many of them degenerate during infancy and childhood. However, about a half million of the primary follicles persist into adolescence, and the loss continues throughout the woman's reproductive years. During each reproductive cycle, several oocytes begin to mature; however, usually only one is ovulated, and the others degenerate. Nevertheless, there is still a great excess of oocytes. Even if one egg were released over a reproductive span of 40 years, only 480 eggs would be ovulated, and only a few, if any, would ever be fertilized. At menopause, only a few thousand oocytes remain, and the decline continues until, eventually, there are no oocytes left in the ovaries of a postmenopausal woman.

Granulosa cells
(gran-u-lō′suh)
Cells lining the ovarian follicles.

The ovaries with their contained primary follicles remain inactive until puberty. Then cyclic ovulation begins under the influence of the pituitary gonadotrophic hormones, follicle-stimulating hormone (FSH), and luteinizing hormone (LH). During each menstrual cycle, a number of primary follicles begin to grow, but normally only one follicle comes to full maturity and is ovulated. When the oocyte is discharged,

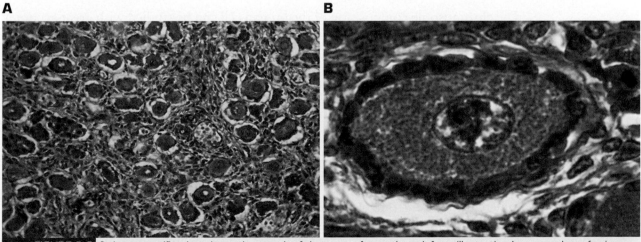

A   **B**

FIGURE 3-6 **A**, Low-magnification photomicrograph of the ovary of a newborn infant, illustrating large number of primary follicles distributed throughout the ovary (original magnification × 100). **B**, High-magnification photomicrograph illustrating a primary follicle composed of a central oocyte surrounded by a collar of granulosa cells (original magnification × 400).

it completes its first meiotic division and gives rise to two daughter cells, which are unequal in size. One daughter cell, which receives half of the chromosomes (one member of each homologous pair) and almost all of the cytoplasm, is called a secondary oocyte (23 chromosomes). The other daughter cell, which receives the remaining 23 chromosomes but almost none of the cytoplasm, is called the first **polar body** and is discarded. The newly formed secondary oocyte promptly begins its second meiotic division, which will lead to the formation of the mature ovum and a second polar body, each containing 23 chromosomes. The meiotic division is not completed, however, unless the ovum is fertilized.

Polar body
Structure extruded during the meiosis of the oocyte. Contains discarded chromosomes and a small amount of cytoplasm.

COMPARISON OF SPERMATOGENESIS AND OOGENESIS

Spermatogenesis and oogenesis have many similarities, but there are two major differences.

First, four spermatozoa are produced from each precursor cell in spermatogenesis, but only one ovum is formed from each precursor cell in oogenesis. The other three "daughter cells" derived from the meiotic divisions are discarded as polar bodies.

Second, spermatogenesis occurs continually and is carried through to completion in about 2 months. Consequently, seminal fluid always contains relatively "fresh" sperm. In contrast, the oocytes are not produced continually. All of the oocytes present in the ovary were formed before birth and have remained in a prolonged prophase of the first meiotic division from fetal life until they are ovulated. This may be why congenital abnormalities that result from abnormal separation of chromosomes in the course of gametogenesis are more frequent in older women. The ova released late in a woman's reproductive life have been held in prophase for as long as 45 years before they finally resume meiosis at the time of ovulation. These ova have been exposed for many years to potentially harmful radiation, chemicals, or other injurious agents, and this predisposes them to abnormal separation of chromosomes when cell division is resumed. If the chromosomes do not separate normally in meiosis, an ovum may end up with either an excess or a deficiency of chromosomes. If the abnormal ovum is fertilized, a fetus that has an abnormal number of chromosomes may be conceived. This subject is considered in the discussion on congenital and hereditary diseases.

Chromosome Analysis

The chromosome composition of the human cell can be studied with great accuracy by culturing cells in a suitable medium. The presence of abnormalities in chromosome number or structure also can be detected in this way. Usually, human blood is used as a source of cells for these studies; the blood lymphocytes can be induced to undergo mitotic division. Certain chemicals are added to stop the mitotic division after the chromosomes have become separate and distinct, and consequently, many cells arrested in mitosis accumulate in the culture medium. Additional methods are employed to cause swelling of the cells, which are then prepared, and the chromosomes can be examined. FIGURE 3-7 illustrates the appearance of a swollen cell arrested in mitosis with the chromosomes well separated. A normal dividing cell arrested in mitosis contains 46 chromosomes, each consisting of two chromatids joined at their centromeres. Chromosomes are classified according to their size, the location of the centromere, the relative lengths of the chromatids that extend outward from the centromere (called the arms of the chromosome), and the pattern of light and dark bands along the chromosome. Each chromosome has its own unique structure. The separated chromosomes from a single cell are photographed, and

A

B

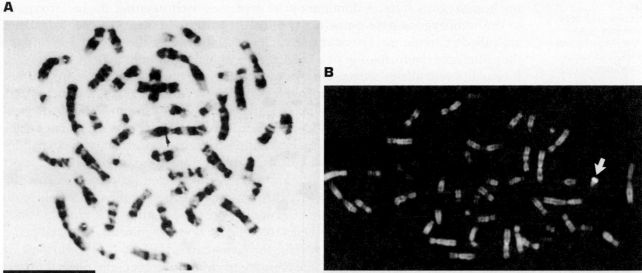

FIGURE 3-7 The appearance of chromosomes from a single cell arrested in mitosis, illustrating the banded pattern that facilitates the identification of individual chromosomes. The two chromatids composing each chromosome lie side by side. **A**, Giemsa stain (photograph courtesy of Dr. Jorge Yunis). **B**, Fluorescent stain. The *arrow* indicates intensely stained Y chromosome (photograph courtesy of Patricia Crowley-Larsen).

the individual chromosomes in the photograph are arranged in a standard pattern called a **karyotype**. FIGURE 3-8 illustrates the karyotype of a female, as indicated by the paired X chromosomes, with Y chromosome absent. The karyotype illustrated is not normal; there is an extra chromosome 21. (Chromosomal abnormalities are considered in the discussion on congenital and hereditary diseases.)

Karyotype
(ka̅ r′-e̅-o̅-type)
An arrangement of chromosomes from a single cell arrangement in pairs in descending order according to size of the chromosomes and the positions of the centromeres.

Genes and Inheritance

A gene is a section of the DNA chain that determines some property of the cell. Each gene occupies a specific site on the chromosome; this site is called the **locus** of the gene. Chromosomes exist in pairs except in the ova and sperm. Consequently, genes are also paired, and the members of each pair are located at corresponding gene loci on homologous chromosomes. Alternate forms of a gene that can occupy the same locus are called **alleles**, and any one chromosome can carry only one allele at a given locus. An individual is homozygous for a gene if both alleles are the same and **heterozygous** if the alleles are different.

Genes are responsible for inherited traits, but the effects that they produce (called the expression of the gene) vary with different genes. A **recessive gene** is one that produces an effect only in

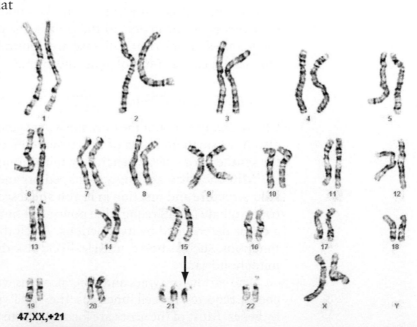

47,XX,+21

FIGURE 3-8 Karyotype of female. There is an extra chromosome 21 (*arrow*) characteristic of Down syndrome (photograph courtesy of Patricia Crowley-Larsen).

Locus
The position of a gene on a chromosome. Different forms (alleles) of the same gene are always found at the same locus on a chromosome.

Allele (äh'lēl)
One of several related genes that may occupy the same locus on a homologous chromosome.

Heterozygous
(het'er-o-zī'gus)
Having two different alleles at given gene loci on the homologous pair of chromosomes.

Recessive gene
A gene that expresses a trait only when present in the homozygous state.

Dominant gene
A gene that expresses a trait in the heterozygous state.

Sex-linked gene
Gene present on the X chromosome.

Hemizygous
A term applied to genes located on the X chromosome in the male.

the homozygous state. A **dominant gene** expresses itself in either the heterozygous or the homozygous state. Sometimes both alleles of a pair are expressed. Such alleles are called codominant. For example, each of the alleles that direct hemoglobin synthesis induces the formation of a specific type of hemoglobin in the red blood cells. If two different alleles are present, two different types of hemoglobin are produced.

Genes carried on sex chromosomes are called **sex-linked genes**, and the effects that they produce are called sex-linked traits. The small Y chromosome carries few genes other than those that direct male sex differentiation, but the much larger X chromosome carries many genes in addition to those concerned with sexual development. For practical purposes, only X-linked traits are recognized, and most are recessive. The female carrier of a recessive X-linked trait is normal because the effect of the defective allele on one X chromosome is offset by the normal allele on the other X chromosome. The male, however, possesses only one X chromosome. Consequently, he can be neither heterozygous nor homozygous for X-linked genes and is called **hemizygous** (*hemi* = half) for genes carried on the X chromosome. If the male receives an X chromosome containing a defective gene, the normal offsetting allele possessed by the female carrier is lacking, and the defective X-linked gene functions like a dominant gene when paired with the Y chromosome.

GENE IMPRINTING

Genes occur in pairs on homologous chromosomes, and each parent contributes one gene to the pair. In the case of identical genes, it had been assumed that a specific gene contributed by the mother functioned the same as the identical gene contributed by the father, but sometimes, it does matter which parent contributed a specific gene. Even when the mother and father contribute identical genes, the genes may have different effects because the genes have been modified in the parents during spermatogenesis or oogenesis. This modification process, which is called gene imprinting, probably involves addition of methyl groups to the DNA molecules of the gene. The imprinting does not change the basic structure of the gene, only the way the gene is expressed in the offspring. Sometimes, a gene from the female parent is imprinted differently from the same gene in a male parent, which modifies the expression (behavior) of the gene in the offspring. In a few hereditary diseases, the manifestations of the disease are determined by which parent contributed the abnormal gene, a result of gene imprinting.

MITOCHONDRIAL GENES AND INHERITANCE

Chromosomes are not the only site where genes are located in the cell. Mitochondria also have small amounts of DNA that contain some of the genes that are required for synthesis of energy-generating mitochondrial proteins.

Mitochondria are sausage-shaped organelles (described in the cells and tissues: their structure and function in health and disease chapter) that generate the adenosine triphosphate (ATP) required to power cell functions. The number of mitochondria in a cell is determined by its functions. A cell that needs lots of energy to carry out its functions, such as nerve, muscle, liver, or kidney cell, may contain several thousand mitochondria.

The various enzymes and other proteins within the mitochondria that produce the energy required for cell functions (the "ATP-generating machinery") are determined by genes. Most of the genes are located within the chromosomes in the cell nuclei, and they are inherited like other genes as described previously. Mitochondrial genes also code for some of the ATP-generating components, and they are inherited differently than genes on chromosomes. As mitochondria wear out, other mitochondria divide to replace them, and mutations may occur as the mitochondrial DNA duplicates (replicates) by a rather simple process to produce new mitochondria. Because there are several mitochondrial DNA molecules in each mitochondrion and several thousand mitochondria in an active cell, a cell may contain a mixture of normal mitochondria and mitochondria containing mutated DNA. Mitochondrial DNA mutations may not affect cell function unless there are such a large number of mitochondrial DNA mutations that the energy-generating capability of the cells is impaired.

A number of rare diseases have been described that result from inherited abnormalities of mitochondrial DNA, and the severity of the disease manifestations is related in part to the number of mutated mitochondria. Hereditary diseases caused by mitochondrial gene mutations are inherited differently than are hereditary diseases caused by mutations of genes carried on chromosomes because mitochondria are not transmitted from parents to child like chromosomes. The human ovum contains a very large number of mitochondria, but sperm contain very few. Consequently, transmission of abnormal mitochondrial DNA from parents to child is almost invariably from the mother. Paternal transmission is extremely rare.

Genes of the Histocompatibility (HLA) Complex

Successful transplantation of organs from one person to another requires that the antigens present on the cells of the organ donor resemble as closely as possible those of the recipient. (Organ transplantation is considered in the discussion on immunity, hypersensitivity, allergy, and autoimmune diseases.) The antigens present on cells are determined by a cluster of genes on chromosome 6. This group of genes, which was first identified in laboratory animals in connection with transplantation experiments, is called the **major histocompatibility complex** (MHC). In humans, these cell surface proteins (antigens) were first identified on peripheral blood leukocytes. Consequently, they were named **human leukocyte antigens** (HLA antigens), and the human major histocompatibility complex is often called the **HLA system**. Often, the designations HLA complex and HLA antigens and MHC complex and MHC antigens are used interchangeably. They refer to the unique, genetically determined cell-surface antigens that we possess to set us apart from other persons. They are our self-antigens.

Although the HLA surface proteins are often called HLA antigens, their antigenicity actually depends on whether they are one's own proteins or the HLA proteins of another person. The HLA proteins on a person's own cells (called self-antigens) are unique for the person possessing them and are recognized by the immune system as being part of that person, not as being foreign; they are, however, foreign proteins (non–self-antigens) in another person in whom they are antigenic and incite an immune response.

Originally, MHC proteins were considered of interest only with respect to organ transplantation because transplantation of cells containing MHC proteins different from those of the transplant recipient was followed by rejection of the transplant unless the immune system was suppressed. However, we know now that they have a much larger role, in that they take part in generating immune responses to foreign antigens of all types. The interaction of the HLA antigens with the various cells of the immune system is considered in the discussion on immunity, hypersensitivity, allergy, and autoimmune diseases.

The HLA complex consists of four separate but closely linked gene loci designated HLA-A, HLA-B, HLA-C, and HLA-D, and there are additional subdivisions within

Major histocompatibility complex (his-tō′com-pat-i-bil′i-tē) *A group of genes on chromosome 6 that determine the antigens on the surface of cells.*

Human leukocyte antigens *Unique histocompatibility antigens (self-antigens) on the surface of cells. Also called major histocompatibility complex (MHC) antigens.*

HLA system *The genes of the histocompatibility complex and the antigens that they determine on the surface of cells.*

the HLA-D locus. There are more than 1200 different allelic genes that can occupy the gene loci within the HLA system. Each gene locus has multiple alleles. Each allele is designated by a specific letter to designate the locus and a number to indicate the allele, such as HLA-B27. A set of HLA genes on one chromosome is called a **haplotype** and is transmitted as a unit. Because chromosomes are paired, each person has two haplotypes, each consisting of four HLA genes. The two haplotypes together determine a total of eight HLA proteins on the cell. Because of the large number of alleles in the HLA system, the chances of two persons who are not identical twins having the same HLA proteins on their cells is very remote. When performing HLA typing of proposed donors for an organ transplant, one attempts to match the major antigens of the donor as closely as possible with those of the recipient. It is impossible to get a perfect match because of the huge number of HLA alleles, but the more closely the HLA antigens match, the better the chances that the graft will survive.

The surface proteins within the HLA system fall into two major groups, designated MHC Class I proteins and MHC Class II proteins. The Class I proteins are determined by the HLA-A, HLA-B, and HLA-C genes and are present on virtually all nucleated cells and on blood platelets, which are small cytoplasmic fragments of large nucleated bone marrow cells called megakaryocytes (described in the hematopoietic and lymphatic systems). Class I proteins are not found on the surface of mature red blood cells, however, because these cells lack nuclei. Class II proteins are determined by the HLA-D genes and are found on only a few types of cells—those that play very important roles in the immune response: phagocytic cells called macrophages, along with related cells having functions similar to those of macrophages, and some types of lymphocytes (described in the discussion on immunity, hypersensitivity, allergy, and autoimmune diseases).

FIGURE 3-9 illustrates the inheritance of HLA haplotypes. Each child receives one of two possible haplotypes from each parent. Consequently, a child has only one haplotype in common with each parent. Because of the way in which chromosomes are transmitted from parent to child, the child has any one of four different

Haplotype
(hap'lō-tīp)
A set of HLA genes on one chromosome that is transmitted as a set.

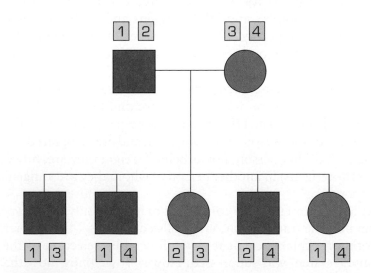

FIGURE 3-9 The possible distribution of HLA haplotypes illustrated in a family of five children. Each haplotype consists of four separate linked HLA genes and is arbitrarily designated by an arabic numeral. The four possible combinations of haplotypes are illustrated in the first four children. In this example, the haplotype of the fifth child is the same as that of the second child.

combinations of HLA haplotypes, as shown in the illustration by the haplotypes of the first four children. There is a one in four probability that two children will both possess the same pair of haplotypes. In this example, each of the first four children has a different combination of HLA haplotypes. The fifth child, however, has the same haplotypes as the second child, indicating that organ transplantation between these two children would have a much better chance for success than would transplantation between individuals having different haplotypes.

HLA TYPES AND SUSCEPTIBILITY TO DISEASE

Certain HLA types appear to predispose to specific diseases. The most striking example of such an association is between HLA-B27 and a particular type of arthritis of the spine and the sacroiliac joints. HLA-B27 is present in about 5% of the random white population but is found in about 90% of persons affected with this type of arthritis, indicating that a B27-positive individual is much more likely to develop this disease than is a person of a different HLA type. However, the presence of the B27 type indicates only a predisposition to the disease. It does not mean that any given individual will invariably be affected because no more than about 25% of B27-positive persons ever develop this type of arthritis. Predisposition to other diseases also has been associated with this HLA type.

Similar associations exist between certain HLA-D types and specific diseases, which are considered in other chapters. The diseases include a type of diabetes, prone to develop in children and young adults, called type 1 diabetes (discussion on pancreas and diabetes mellitus) and a type of arthritis called **rheumatoid arthritis** (discussion on musculoskeletal system).

The reason for the association of specific diseases with HLA types seems to be related to the relation of the HLA gene complex to genes controlling the immune response. The genes that regulate immunity are closely associated with the HLA genes. Individuals having certain specific HLA types also appear to possess genes that are less capable of regulating their immune responses when subjected to antigenic stimulation. Consequently, they seem prone to develop abnormal immune responses that are directed against their own cells and tissues. This type of abnormal reaction leads to cell and tissue injury or dysfunction, which causes various diseases classified as **autoimmune diseases** (discussion on immunity, hypersensitivity, allergy, and autoimmune diseases). In contrast, persons of a different HLA type have immune response genes that regulate responses to antigenic stimulation in a more normal manner.

Genes and Recombinant DNA Technology (Genetic Engineering)

Genes direct the synthesis of gene products—that is, enzymes or other proteins that play a role in the activities of the cells that make the proteins. Cells make many important biologic products, such as insulin, growth hormone, proteins that regulate the immune responses, and proteins that activate the body's clot-dissolving mechanisms. Many of these proteins are used in clinical medicine: insulin to treat diabetes; growth hormone, which allows a child with a growth hormone deficiency to grow normally; and proteins to unplug blocked coronary arteries of patients with heart attacks. Recent advances in DNA technology have led to the development of methods for large-scale production of these and many other important biologic products. The technology that paved the way for these advances has been called by various names: **recombinant DNA technology** (because genes from two different sources are being recombined in a single organism), **genetic engineering** (because genes are being

Rheumatoid arthritis
(rōōm′uh-toyd)
A systemic disease primarily affecting the synovium with major manifestations in the small joints.

Autoimmune disease
A disease associated with formation of cell-mediated or humoral immunity against the subject's own cells or tissue components.

Recombinant DNA technology
Methods for combining a gene from one organism, such as a gene specifying insulin synthesis, with genes from another organism, such as a bacterium.

Genetic engineering
Same as recombinant DNA technology.

Gene splicing
Same as recombinant DNA technology.

Plasmid (plas'-mid)
A small, circular DNA molecule separate from the main bacterial chromosome.

manipulated), or **gene splicing** (because a piece of genetic material is being cut open and another piece of genetic material is being spliced into it).

Whatever name one uses for it, the process requires the insertion of a gene that encodes a desired product, such as insulin, into a bacterium or yeast. If a bacterium is used, the gene is inserted into a small circular DNA segment within the bacterium, called a **plasmid**, which is distinct from the main bacterial chromosome. The circular plasmid is opened by means of an enzyme that "cuts" the plasmid DNA so that the desired gene can be inserted between the cut ends of the plasmid. After the gene has been inserted, the bacterial plasmid contains not only its own genes but also the new gene, which directs the synthesis of the desired protein. The bacterial–foreign gene combination (recombinant DNA) is now carried along by the bacterium as it divides repeatedly to produce a large population of bacterial cells, each producing large quantities of the desired protein that can be purified and used for various purposes.

Other applications of DNA technology in biology and medicine are based on these same principles. DNA technology has been a source of insight into the molecular basis of genetic diseases by increasing our understanding of normal gene structure and function; it has application in the prenatal diagnosis of genetic diseases by identifying abnormal genes and gene products in fetal cells. When the structure of a normal gene that specifies a gene product is known, it is possible to identify a mutation of the gene in fetal cell DNA obtained from amnionic fluid cells. The prenatal diagnosis of genetic diseases by DNA analysis of fetal cells is considered in the discussion on congenital and hereditary diseases.

Gene Therapy

One of the most exciting advances in DNA technology—gene therapy—is an extension of the principles of recombinant DNA technology. In recombinant DNA technology, a gene is inserted into a bacterial or yeast cell to make a protein. In gene therapy, a normal gene is inserted into a defective cell lacking an enzyme or structural protein that the cell needs in order to function effectively, and the inserted gene compensates for the missing or dysfunctional gene.

For the successful application of gene therapy, several goals must be achieved:

1. One must identify and select the correct gene to insert into the cell.
2. One must choose the proper cell to receive the gene.
3. One must select an efficient means of getting the gene into the cell.
4. One must ensure that the newly inserted gene can function effectively long enough within the cell to make the therapy worthwhile and doesn't disrupt other important cell functions.

The identification of the gene for insertion involves the same approaches used in recombinant DNA technology. The agent (vector) used to introduce the gene into the selected cell is usually a virus, although sometimes the gene can be coupled to a lipid or other material that is taken into the cell by endocytosis. Gene therapy targets somatic cells, not the germ cells that produce eggs and sperm, and gene therapy directed at germ cells is not considered either feasible or desirable.

Although gene therapy appears promising, there are risks related to possible disruption of cell functions caused by the inserted genes, as was demonstrated when a gene inserted into a lymphocyte-producing stem cell disrupted the function of other genes regulating cell growth and differentiation and caused lymphocytic leukemia in the person receiving the inserted gene. Other unexpected, serious complications have also followed gene therapy trials, making investigators extremely cautious about undertaking gene therapy projects.

Gene therapy has great potential, but it also has limitations. The correct gene must be inserted into the correct cell to substitute for a dysfunctional gene, but the inserted gene must not disrupt the activities of other cellular genes that regulate other cell functions. Gene therapy shows great promise as a powerful tool for fighting against disease, but much work remains to be done before gene therapy can be applied widely in clinical medicine.

QUESTIONS FOR REVIEW

1. What is meant by the following terms: *homologous chromosomes, autosomes, sex chromosome, Barr body, gene, gametogenesis,* and *centrosome?*
2. How does the process of mitosis compare with meiosis?
3. What are the differences between spermatogenesis and oogenesis?
4. What is a chromosome karyotype? How is it obtained? How is it used?
5. What is the MHC? What is its function? What is its relationship to disease susceptibility?
6. What is a haplotype? How are haplotypes inherited by children from their parents? What are the chances that two children will have the same haplotype?

SUPPLEMENTARY READINGS

Attia, J., Ioannidis, J. P., Thakkinstian, A., et al. 2009. How to use an article about genetic association: A: Background concepts. *Journal of the American Medical Association* 301:74–81.
  ▶ A review of the types of DNA variations, including SNPs, insertions, and deletions, and how they affect protein function. Describes genomewide association studies, in which thousands of genetic variants are tested for association with disease, such as coronary artery disease, diabetes, and breast cancer.
  ▶ Differences in gene structure that occur in less than 1% of the population are called mutations. Those that occur more frequently are called SNPs. Some affect the structure of a protein produced by the gene; others affect gene function, although they do not affect the protein made by the gene. More than 12 million SNPs have been identified. Many genomewide association studies attempt to establish whether specific SNPs are associated with a specific disease, which may be difficult to accomplish because often, SNP under consideration is associated with other SNPs that may have no effect on the disease association being studied.

Bamshad, M. 2005. Genetic influences on health: Does race matter? *Journal of the American Medical Association* 294:937–46.
  ▶ Many diseases and responses to therapeutic drugs are sometimes influenced by gene variants that vary in frequency or are completely different among racial groups.

Dong, L. M., Potter, J. D., White, E., et al. 2008. Genetic susceptibility to cancer: The role of polymorphisms in candidate genes. *Journal of the American Medical Association* 209:2423–36.
  ▶ Many of the nucleotide polymorphisms responsible for genetic variations have been identified, which have contributed to understanding their function and their role in influencing susceptibility to cancer. In many cases, variations in some of the enzymes

that metabolize potential carcinogens may account for differences in susceptibility to various cancers.

Falls, J. G., Pulford, D. J., Wylie, A. A., et al. 1999. Genomic imprinting: Implications for human disease. *American Journal of Pathology* 154:635–47.

▶ A review article dealing with how genes are imprinted, the characteristics of imprinted genes, diseases related to imprinted genes, and how imprinted genes may play a role in human cancer by inactivating tumor suppressor gene functions.

Feero, W. G., Guttmacher, A. E., and Collins, F. S. 2010. Genomic medicine— An updated primer. *New England Journal of Medicine* 362:2001–11.

▶ A very good summary of the clinical applications of genomic medicine illustrated by genetic studies performed on woman with a breast cancer, indicating how a gene expression profile performed on the excised tumor helps determine what additional treatment she should receive to reduce her risk of a recurrence of the tumor. The article also illustrates the complex interaction of genes with SNPs and miRNAs that influence the expression of a gene. A glossary of genomic terms also is provided.

Lupski, J. R. 2007. Structural variations in the human genome. *New England Journal of Medicine* 356:1169–71.

▶ Many mutations result from a change in a single nucleotide, which changes the sequence of nucleotides that codes for the gene, resulting in the synthesis of a different protein that may function differently than the protein that it replaces, as is the case in the sickle cell gene mutation. However, some mutations are not caused by single nucleotide mutation, but instead result from large deletions, duplications, or inversions of large gene segments.

Manolio, T. A. 2010. Genomewide association studies and assessment of risk of disease. *New England Journal of Medicine* 363:166–76.

▶ Many conditions are caused by SNPs. Only 12% of SNPs are located in the protein-coding regions of genes. The rest are located in the regions between the genes or in the parts of the DNA that are not transcribed (the introns). Genomewide association studies attempt to relate the inheritance of groups of SNPs to specific traits.

Migeon, B. R. 2006. The role of X inactivation and cellular mosaicism in women's health and sex-specific diseases. *Journal of the American Medical Association* 295:1428–33.

▶ X chromosome inactivation in females equalizes gene expression in males and females. Females are mosaics for genes on the X chromosome, which ameliorates the harmful effects of an X-linked mutation. Diseases caused by X chromsome mutations are always more severe in males. The greater frequency of autoimmune diseases in females may be related to the mosaic cell populations resulting from X chromosome inactivation.

Viel, K. R., Ameri, A., Abshire, T. C., et al. 2009. Inhibitors of factor VIII in black patients with hemophilia. *New England Journal of Medicine* 360:1618–27.

▶ This article illustrates how SNPs may have far-reaching effects on treatment. Factor VIII protein (antihemophilic factor) used to treat patients with hemophilia is prepared by recombinant DNA technology or from human blood plasma (described in Abnormalities of Blood Coagulation). Some treated patients develop inhibitors (antibodies) against factor VIII protein, which reduces its effectiveness and complicates treatment. The problem occurs more frequently in black than in white patients.

▶ The authors demonstrated six minor variations in the factor VIII protein (antihemophilic globulin) related to polymorphism (SNPs) of the gene coding for the protein, which they designated H1 through H6. The factor VIII administered to hemophilia patients contains the H1 and H2 protein, which is also contained in the factor VIII protein made by white patients. In contrast, the gene for factor VIII in blacks coded for proteins H3, H4, and H5. Consequently, factor VIII polymorphism caused reduced responsiveness to the administered factor VIII in blacks because they formed anti-factor VIII antibodies directed against H1 and H2 proteins lacking in their own factor VIII. This report demonstrates how SNPs may affect the biologic response to treatment in some persons but not in others.

OUTLINE SUMMARY

Chromosomes

STRUCTURE
Double coils of DNA combined with protein.
Exist in pairs: autosome and sex chromosomes.
Genes (segments of DNA chain) arranged along chromosome.

SEX CHROMOSOMES
In female: one X inactivated and appears attached to nuclear membrane.
In male: Y chromosome appears as bright fluorescent spot in intact cell.

Cell Division

MITOSIS
No reduction in chromosomes; daughter cells identical with parent cell.
Characteristic of somatic cells.
Sequence:
> *Prophase: chromosomes shorten, nuclear membrane breaks down, and spindle forms.*
> *Metaphase: chromosomes line up in middle of cell.*
> *Anaphase: chromosomes pull apart.*
> *Telophase: two daughter cells reform.*

MEIOSIS
Chromosomes reduced by half and modified by crossover.
Characteristic of germ cells.
Sequence:
> *First meiotic division: homologous chromosomes synapse and exchange segments.*
> *Homologous chromosomes separate, and daughter cells reform, each containing one member of homologous pair.*
> *Chromosomes reduce by half.*
> *Second meiotic division: like mitosis, but each cell has only 23 chromosomes.*

Gametogenesis

SPERMATOGENESIS
Spermatogonia (46 chromosomes) form primary spermatocytes (forty-six chromosomes).
Each primary spermatocyte forms two secondary spermatocytes (23 chromosomes).

Each secondary spermatocyte forms two spermatids (23 chromosomes).
Spermatids mature into sperm.

OOGENESIS
Oogonia (46 chromosomes) form primary oocytes (46 chromosomes) in fetal ovaries.
Primary oocyte forms primary follicle and begins prophase of meiosis but does not carry it through.
> *Many follicles degenerate during infancy and childhood. About one-half million persist.*
Follicle matures under influence of FSH-LH, and one is ovulated each cycle.
> *Primary oocyte completes first meiotic division to form secondary oocyte (23 chromosomes) and polar body (23 chromosomes).*
> *Secondary oocyte completes second meiotic division if fertilized to form mature ovum (23 chromosomes) and polar body (23 chromosomes).*

COMPARISON OF SPERMATOGENESIS AND OOGENESIS
Spermatogenesis:
Four sperm from each precursor cell.
Continual: always fresh sperm.
Oogenesis: One ovum from each precursor.
All precursors form before birth and remain in prophase until ovulated.
Ova ovulated late in reproductive life more prone to abnormal chromosome separation.

Chromosome Analysis

METHOD OF ANALYSIS
Blood cells cultured and lymphocytes induced to divide.
Cells arrested in metaphase and caused to swell.
Stained smears prepared.
Chromosomes arranged to form karyotype.

Genes and Inheritance

GENES
Exist in pairs (alleles), one on each chromosome.
Homozygous: alleles the same.
Heterozygous: alleles different.
Expression of genes varies.

Recessive: gene expressed in homozygous state.
Dominant: gene expressed in heterozygous state.
Codominant: both alleles expressed.
Sex-linked genes.
   Carried on X chromosome.
   Female has two X. Either can carry abnormal gene.
      Not clinically affected if acquires abnormal X
      because effect offset by gene on normal X.
   Male has only one X (hemizygous). Acquires heredi-
      tary disease if receives X chromosome contain-
      ing defective gene.

GENE IMPRINTING
Identical genes contributed by male and female parent
   to offspring may have different effects.
Genes modified during gametogenesis.
Manifestations of some hereditary diseases depends on
   which parent contributed the abnormal gene.

MITOCHONDRIAL GENES AND INHERITANCE
Some of the genes that code for ATP-generating enzymes
   are located in mitochondrial DNA. Ova contain many
   mitochondria, and sperm contain very few.
Mutations of mitochondrial DNA may affect ATP
   generation.
Some diseases are caused by mitochondrial DNA mutations and are transmitted by the mitochondria in the
   ova of the female parent.

Genes of the Histocompatibility (HLA) Complex

STRUCTURE AND FUNCTION
Important in organ transplantation.
Four linked gene loci on chromosome 6 designated
   HLA-A, *HLA-B*, *HLA-C*, and *HLA-D*.

Multiple alleles at each gene locus.
Genes control antigens on cells.
Genes on each chromosome 6 are transmitted as set
   called a haplotype.

INHERITANCE
Each child receives one haplotype from each parent.
Four different combinations of haplotype possible in children.
Probability is one in four that two children of same parents
   will possess same HLA haplotype.

HLA AND SUSCEPTIBILITY TO DISEASE
Genes controlling immune response associated with HLA
   complex.
Certain HLA types less capable of regulating immune
   response are prone to develop specific types of autoimmune diseases.

Genes and Recombinant DNA Technology (Genetic Engineering)
Technique inserts foreign gene into bacterial plasmid or
   yeast cell.
Microorganism produces desired protein.
Complex technology.
Principles applicable to understanding molecular basis
   of genetic disease.
Principles applicable to prenatal diagnosis of genetic
   disease.

Gene Therapy
Gene introduced into cell with genetic defect to compen-
   sate for missing or dysfunctional gene.
Procedure has great potential but also many limitations.
Limited applications at present time.

CHAPTER 4

Inflammation and Repair

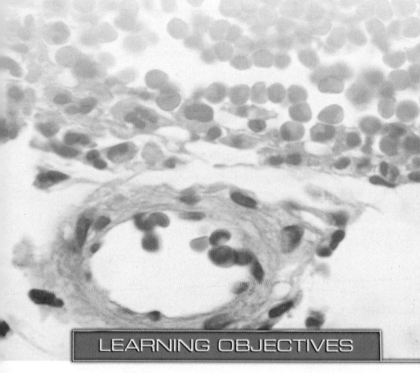

1 List the characteristics and clinical manifestations of an acute inflammation. Differentiate inflammations on the basis of their component of fluid and inflammatory cells (serous, purulent, fibrinous, and hemorrhagic inflammations).

2 Describe the possible outcomes of an inflammatory reaction.

3 Name the chemical mediators of inflammation. Explain how they interact to intensify the inflammatory process.

4 Describe the harmful effects of inflammation. Explain why it is sometimes necessary to suppress the inflammatory process.

5 Compare inflammation and infection. Name some of the terms used to describe infections.

The Inflammatory Reaction

The inflammatory reaction is a nonspecific response to any agent that causes cell injury. The agent may be physical (such as heat or cold), chemical (such as a concentrated acid or alkali or another caustic chemical), or microbiologic (such as a bacterium or virus). The inflammatory reaction is characterized by both local and systemic effects, as indicated diagrammatically in FIGURE 4-1.

Local effects consist of dilatation (expansion) of blood vessels and increased vascular permeability. Leukocytes (white blood cells) are attracted to the site of injury. They adhere to the endothelium of the small blood vessels, force their way

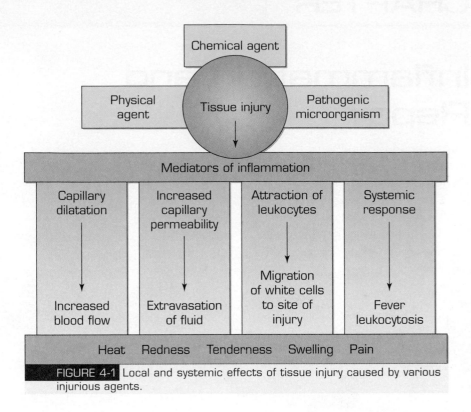

FIGURE 4-1 Local and systemic effects of tissue injury caused by various injurious agents.

through the walls, and migrate to the area of tissue damage (FIGURE 4-2). The characteristic signs of inflammation are heat, redness, tenderness, swelling, and pain. The increased warmth and redness of the inflamed tissues are caused by dilatation of capillaries and slowing of blood flow through the vessels. Swelling occurs because the extravasation (leakage) of plasma from the dilated and more permeable vessels causes the volume of fluid in the inflamed tissue to increase (FIGURE 4-3). The tenderness and pain are secondary to irritation of sensory nerve endings at the site of the inflammatory process.

The polymorphonuclear leukocyte is the most important cell in the acute inflammatory response. It is an actively phagocytic cell that is attracted to the area by the cell injury. Mononuclear cells (monocytes, macrophages) appear later in the inflammation reaction. One of their major functions is to clean up the debris produced by the inflammatory process. These cells are also active in chronic inflammatory reactions.

The fluid mixture of protein, leukocytes, and debris that forms during the inflammatory process is called **exudate**. Its proportions of protein and inflammatory cells vary in different exudates, and the appearance of the exudate will also vary. It is convenient to describe an exudate as serous, purulent, fibrinous, or hemorrhagic based on its appearance. If the exudate consists primarily of fluid containing very little protein, the term serous exudate is used. If a large amount of serous fluid accumulates in injured tissues—as, for example, after a severe burn of the skin—blisters may form (FIGURE 4-4). An exudate consisting largely of inflammatory cells

Exudate
(ex′yū-dāt)
The fluid, leukocytes, and debris that accumulate as a result of an inflammation.

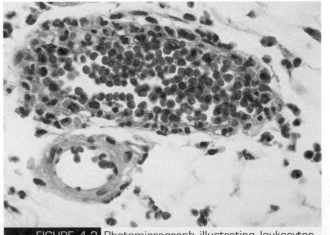

FIGURE 4-2 Photomicrograph illustrating leukocytes adherent to capillary endothelium and migrating through wall to site of tissue injury (original magnification × 160).

is called a purulent exudate, and the creamy yellow exudate is called pus. The term fibrinous exudate is used if the fluid in the exudate is rich in a blood protein called fibrinogen, which coagulates and forms fibrin, producing a sticky film on the surface of the inflamed tissue (FIGURE 4-5). (The proteins concerned in the coagulation of the blood are considered in the discussion on abnormalities of blood coagulation.) A hemorrhagic exudate occurs when the inflammatory process had ruptured many small capillaries, allowing red blood cells to escape into the tissues so that the exudate appears bloody.

If a fibrinous exudate involves two surfaces in close proximity, such as adjacent loops of small intestine, the surfaces may stick together. This type of inflammation often heals by ingrowth of fibrous tissue, which binds the adjacent surfaces together by means of fibrous bands called **adhesions** (FIGURE 4-6).

If the inflammatory process is severe, systemic effects become evident. The individual feels ill, and the temperature is elevated. The bone marrow accelerates its production of leukocytes so that the number of leukocytes circulating in the bloodstream increases. The liver produces several proteins called acute phase proteins that are released into the bloodstream in response to tissue injury or inflammation,

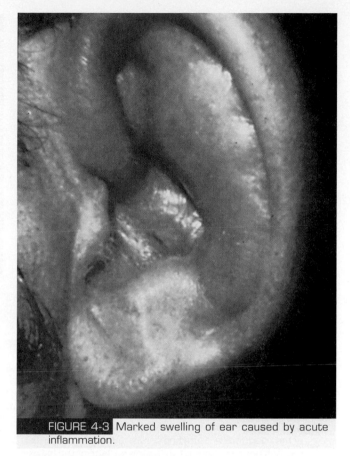

FIGURE 4-3 Marked swelling of ear caused by acute inflammation.

which help protect the body from the tissue injury caused by the inflammation. The best known of these proteins is called C reactive protein, which is often measured to monitor the activity of diseases characterized by tissue inflammation.

Adhesions
(ad-hē′shuns)
Bands of fibrous tissue that form subsequent to an inflammation and bind adjacent tissues together.

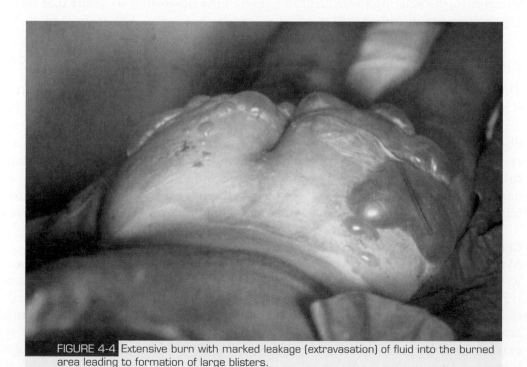

FIGURE 4-4 Extensive burn with marked leakage (extravasation) of fluid into the burned area leading to formation of large blisters.

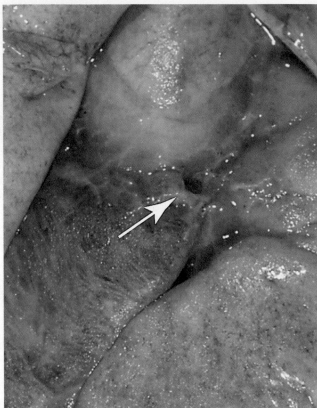

FIGURE 4-5 Fibrinous inflammation involving the surface of the heart (epicardium) and pericardium. The pericardial sac has been opened to expose the surface of the heart, which appears rough because fibrin has accumulated on the epicardium. The *arrow* indicates a large aggregate of fibrin adjacent to the right atrial appendage.

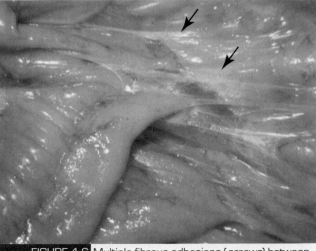

FIGURE 4-6 Multiple fibrous adhesions (*arrows*) between loops of small intestine resulting from previous abdominal inflammation.

The outcome of an inflammation depends on how much tissue damage has resulted from the inflammation. If the inflammation is mild, it soon subsides, and the tissues return to normal. This process is called **resolution**. If the inflammatory process is more severe, tissue is destroyed to some extent and must be repaired (FIGURE 4-7). During healing, damaged cells are replaced, and the framework of the injured tissue is repaired as an ingrowth of cells produces connective tissue fibers and new blood vessels. Scar tissue replaces large areas of tissue destruction (FIGURE 4-8). Sometimes, the scarring subsequent to a severe inflammation is so severe that function is seriously disturbed (FIGURE 4-9).

CHEMICAL MEDIATORS OF INFLAMMATION

The inflammatory reaction is a nonspecific, stereotyped response to tissue injury and is much the same no matter what caused the injury. For example, an injury caused by dropping a book on your foot produces the same type of inflammatory response as does a severe sunburn in the same region. The reason is because the inflammatory response is not directly caused by the tissue injury. It is caused by chemical agents called mediators of inflammation that are formed and released when the tissue is damaged. Some mediators are derived from cells, and others are formed from proteins in the blood plasma that accumulate in the injured area.

Cell-Derived Mediators

Mast cells, a major source of cell-derived mediators, are specialized cells that are widely distributed throughout the connective tissues of the body. Their cytoplasm is filled with granules containing histamine and other chemicals. If tissue is injured, the mast cells discharge their granules, liberating the chemicals to initiate the inflammatory process. Histamine is a potent **vasodilator** (*vas* = blood vessel + *dilate* = expand) and also greatly increases vascular permeability. Blood platelets also contain histamine and another mediator called **serotonin,** which are released when platelets

Resolution
A regression of an inflammatory process without significant tissue destruction and with return of the tissues to normal.

Mast cell
A specialized connective tissue cell containing granules filled with histamine and other chemical mediators.

Vasodilator
A substance that dilates blood vessels.

Serotonin
(sĕr-o-tō′-nin)
A vasoconstrictor mediator of inflammation released from platelets.

adhere to collagen fragments at the site of tissue injury. Other important cell-derived mediators are a group called **prostaglandins** (so named because compounds of this type were first isolated from the prostate gland) and a group of similar compounds called **leukotrienes**. These biologically active compounds are synthesized by cells from arachidonic acid present in cell membranes in response to stimuli that induce inflammation, and they function as mediators that intensify the inflammatory process.

Mediators from Blood Plasma

Blood plasma contains various protein substances that circulate as inactive compounds and leak from the permeable capillaries into the area of tissue damage where they become transformed (activated) by a complex process into chemical mediators. One important group of mediators formed in this way is called **bradykinins** (or simply kinins). The series of reactions that leads to the formation of bradykinins is triggered by one of the proteins concerned with blood coagulation, which is activated by the tissue injury.

Mediators of inflammation are also formed from another group of blood proteins called complement. Complement consists of several separate protein components, designated C_1 through C_9, that interact in a regular sequence to yield a series of by-products, some of which function as mediators of inflammation. Complement is activated when an antigen combines with an antibody but may also be activated in other ways that do not require an antigen–antibody interaction. The various functions of the complement system are considered in connection with immunity, hypersensitivity, allergy, and autoimmune diseases.

FIGURE 4-10 illustrates how the various mediators interact. The release of mediators from any source not only initiates the inflammatory process but also induces release of more mediators from other sources, setting off a "chain reaction" that intensifies the inflammatory process.

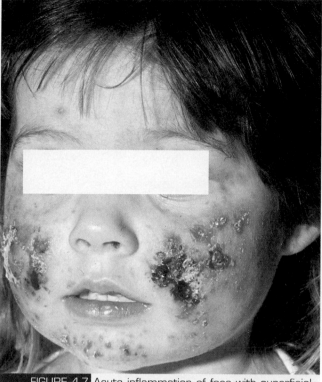

FIGURE 4-7 Acute inflammation of face with superficial necrosis of skin. Crusts of dried exudate (scabs) have formed on skin surface.

Prostaglandin
(pros-ta-glan'din)
A complex derivative of a fatty acid (prostanoic acid) that has widespread physiologic effects.

Leukotriene
(lōō-kō-try'-ēn)
A prostaglandin-like mediator of inflammation.

Bradykinin
(brā-dē-kī'nin)
A chemical mediator of inflammation derived from components in the blood plasma.

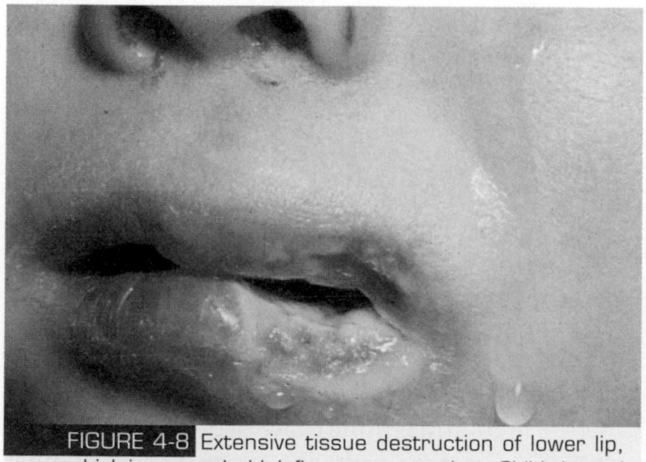

THE ROLE OF LYSOSOMAL ENZYMES IN THE INFLAMMATORY PROCESS

The cytoplasm of phagocytic neutrophils and monocytes that are attracted to the site of inflammation by chemical mediators contains granules called lysosomes (*lysis* = dissolving + *soma* = body). Lysosomes contain potent enzymes that

FIGURE 4-8 Extensive tissue destruction of lower lip, which is covered with inflammatory exudate. Child chewed an electric light cord, exposing bare wire, and sustained a severe electrical burn of lip.

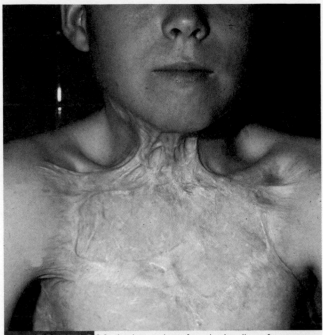

FIGURE 4-9 Marked scarring after the healing of a severe burn, which has restricted motion of neck and arms. Skin grafting was required to improve function.

are capable of digesting the material brought into the cytoplasm of the cells by phagocytosis. During phagocytosis, bacteria or other foreign materials become enclosed within vacuoles in the cell cytoplasm, and the lysosomes dissolve the material by discharging their enzymes into the vacuoles, as described in the discussion on cells and tissues (FIGURE 2-2).

In the course of any inflammatory reaction, many neutrophils and monocytes are damaged or destroyed, and their lysosomal enzymes are released. Some lysosomal enzymes also escape from intact leukocytes during phagocytosis. Much of the tissue injury in an area of inflammation is a result of the destructive effect of the lysosomal enzymes released from leukocytes. The tissue injury in turn generates more mediators, and this induces further inflammatory changes.

INFLAMMATION CAUSED BY ANTIGEN–ANTIBODY INTERACTION

Antibodies are one of the body's defense mechanisms. This is discussed in immunity, hypersensitivity, allergy, and autoimmune diseases. When antigen and antibody interact, an intense inflammatory reaction with marked tissue necrosis often follows. The interaction of antigen and antibody activates complement, and the mediators generated from complement activation induce the inflammatory reaction. Large numbers of leukocytes are attracted to the site, and the release of potent lysosomal enzymes from the leukocytes is the chief cause of the tissue damage.

HARMFUL EFFECTS OF INFLAMMATION

The tissue injury that results from an inflammation is due in part to the injurious agent and in part to the inflammatory reaction itself. In most cases, the inflammatory process is self-limited and subsides when the harmful agent has been eliminated. At times, however, an inflammatory process may persist and cause extensive, progressive tissue injury. If this occurs, it is sometimes necessary to suppress the inflammatory process by administering adrenal corticosteroid hormones to reduce the tissue damage that would result if the inflammatory process were not restrained. (Suppression of the immune response is considered in the discussion on immunity, hypersensitivity, allergy, and autoimmune diseases.)

Infection
Inflammation caused by a disease-producing organism.

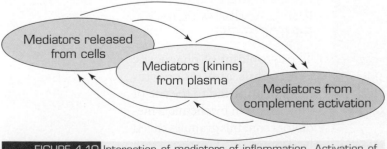

FIGURE 4-10 Interaction of mediators of inflammation. Activation of mediators from any source also leads to the formation of mediators from other sources, which intensifies the inflammatory reaction.

Infection

TERMINOLOGY OF INFECTION

The term **infection** is used to denote an inflammatory process caused by disease-producing organisms. A number of different terms are used to refer to infections in various sites. Generally, the

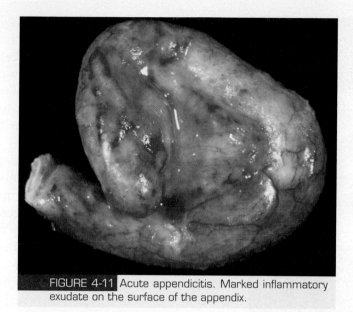

FIGURE 4-11 Acute appendicitis. Marked inflammatory exudate on the surface of the appendix.

ending *-itis* is appended to the name of the tissue or organ in order to indicate an infection or inflammatory process. For example, the terms appendicitis (FIGURE 4-11), hepatitis, colitis, and pneumonitis refer to inflammation of the appendix, liver, colon, and lung, respectively. An acute spreading infection at any site is called **cellulitis** (FIGURE 4-12). Usually, this term is used to refer to an acute infection of the skin and deeper tissues. The term **abscess** is used when an infection is associated with breakdown of the tissues and the formation of a localized mass of pus (FIGURE 4-13). If a localized infection spreads into the lymphatic channels draining the site of inflammation, the term **lymphangitis** is used. **Lymphadenitis** refers to infection in the regional lymph nodes draining the primary site of infection. The term **septicemia** is used to refer to an overwhelming infection in which pathogenic bacteria gain access to the bloodstream.

FACTORS INFLUENCING THE OUTCOME OF AN INFECTION

In any infection, the invading organism is pitted against the defenses of the body. Bacteria and other microbiologic agents vary in their ability to cause disease. Many are not harmful to humans. Others, capable of causing human disease, are called **pathogenic** (*pathos* = disease + *genic* = producing) organisms. The term **virulence**

Cellulitis (sell-ū-lī′tis)
An acute spreading inflammation affecting the skin or deeper tissues.

Abscess (ab′sess)
A localized accumulation of pus in tissues.

Lymphangitis (limf′an-jī′tis)
An inflammation of lymph vessels draining a site of infection.

Lymphadenitis (limf-a-den-ī′tis)
An inflammation of lymph nodes draining a site of infection.

Septicemia (sep-ti-sē′mē-yuh)
An infection in which large numbers of pathogenic bacteria are present in the bloodstream.

Pathogenic (path-ō-jen′ik)
Capable of producing disease.

Virulence (vir′u-lenz)
The ability of an organism to cause disease.

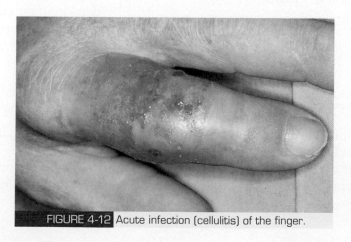

FIGURE 4-12 Acute infection (cellulitis) of the finger.

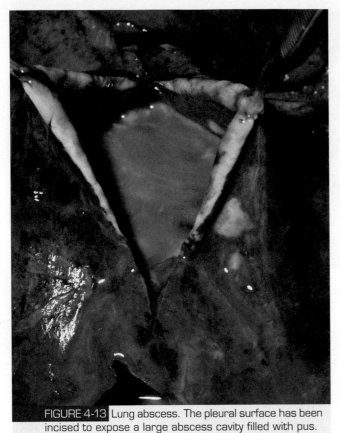

FIGURE 4-13 Lung abscess. The pleural surface has been incised to expose a large abscess cavity filled with pus.

refers to the ease with which a pathogenic organism can overcome the defenses of the body. A highly virulent organism is one that is likely to produce progressive disease in the majority of susceptible individuals. In contrast, an organism of low virulence is capable only of producing disease in a highly susceptible individual under favorable circumstances.

The outcome of any infection depends on two factors: the virulence of the organism combined with the numbers ("dosage") of the invading organisms and the resistance of the infected individual (often called the **host**). These may be considered balanced against one another, as indicated diagrammatically in FIGURE 4-14. When large numbers of organisms of high virulence are introduced into the body, especially when host resistance is lowered, the balance is tipped in favor of the invader, and progressive or fatal disease develops. When the virulence or dosage of the organism is low or the body's resistance is high, the balance is tipped in favor of the host. The infection is then overcome and healing occurs.

Chronic Infection

Sometimes, the organism and host are evenly matched. Neither can gain the advantage; the result is a stalemate. Clinically, this results in a chronic infection, characterized by a relatively quiet, smoldering inflammation that is usually associated with vigorous attempts at healing on the part of the host.

Host
Individual infected with a disease-producing organism.

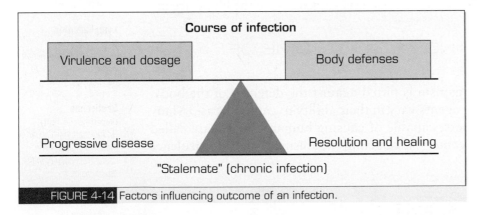

Course of infection

| Virulence and dosage | | Body defenses |

Progressive disease | | Resolution and healing

"Stalemate" (chronic infection)

FIGURE 4-14 Factors influencing outcome of an infection.

The balance between the host and the invader is precarious. The infection may flare up at times when the pathogen obtains a temporary advantage, or it may become quiescent at other times when the defenses of the host gain the upper hand. Lymphocytes, plasma cells, and monocytes are the predominant cells in chronic inflammatory processes.

QUESTIONS FOR REVIEW

1. What is the inflammatory reaction? What are its clinical manifestations?
2. What factors influence the outcome of an infection?
3. What are mediators of inflammation? How do they function?
4. What is meant by the following terms: *chronic infection, pathogenic, complement*?

SUPPLEMENTARY READINGS

Charo, I. F., and Ransohoff, R. M. 2006. The many roles of chemokines and chemokine receptors in inflammation. *New England Journal of Medicine* 354:610–21.

▶ Chemokines are small protein molecules (cytokines) that attract neutrophils and monocytes to sites of inflammation. Several research projects are underway to explore ways to minimize leukocyte-mediated tissue damage in persons with long-standing chronic diseases by drugs that block the cytokines that attract leukocytes.

Hotchkiss, R. S., and Karl, I. E. 2003. The pathophysiology and treatment of sepsis. *New England Journal of Medicine* 348:138–50.

▶ Sepsis is the inflammatory response to an infection. Many factors contribute to mortality, and ways to improve survival are considered.

Johnston, R. B., Jr. 1988. Current concepts: Immunology. Monocytes and macrophages. *New England Journal of Medicine* 318:747–52.

▶ Describes the structure and function of the mononuclear phagocyte system. Monocytes form in the marrow, have a half-life of about 3 days in the blood, and then migrate to the tissues where they live for several months. They are activated by lymphokines from T lymphocytes.

Kumar, V., Abbas, A. K., Fausto, N., et al. 2010. *Robbins and Cotran pathologic basis of disease*, 8th ed. Philadelphia: Elsevier Saunders.

▶ A standard textbook with detailed treatment of the inflammatory reaction in all of its aspects

OUTLINE SUMMARY

The Inflammatory Reaction

CHARACTERISTICS OF THE INFLAMMATORY REACTION
Dilatation of blood vessels.
Migration of leukocytes through vessel walls to the site of inflammation.
Increased capillary permeability.
Extravasation of fluids.

CLINICAL MANIFESTATIONS OF INFLAMMATION
Heat and redness: dilated blood vessels.
Swelling: accumulation of fluid and exudate.
Tenderness and pain: irritation of nerve endings.

TYPES OF INFLAMMATION REACTIONS
Serous inflammation: chiefly fluid exudate.
Purulent inflammation: chiefly inflammatory cells.
Fibrinous inflammation: exudate rich in protein, which coagulates.
Hemorrhagic inflammation: many capillaries ruptured, allowing escape of red cells.

SYSTEMIC EFFECTS OF INFLAMMATION
Patient feels ill.
Elevated temperature.
Leukocytosis.

OUTCOME OF INFLAMMATION
Resolution: inflammation subsides and tissues return to normal.
Repair: replacement of damaged cells and tissues.
Large areas of destruction replaced by scar tissue.
Mediators intensify inflammatory process and generate more mediators.

CHEMICAL MEDIATORS OF INFLAMMATION
Mast cells: discharge granules containing mediators.
Kinins form from blood proteins leaking into inflamed area.
Activation of complement generates mediators.

THE ROLE OF LYSOSOMAL ENZYMES IN THE INFLAMMATORY PROCESS
Lysosomal enzymes released from leukocytes cause tissue injury.
Injury generates more mediators, which promotes further inflammation and tissue injury.

INFLAMMATION CAUSED BY ANTIGEN–ANTIBODY INTERACTION
Interaction activates complement, leading to formation of mediators. This attracts leukocytes.
Lysosomal enzymes from leukocytes cause tissue injury.

HARMFUL EFFECTS OF INFLAMMATION

Inflammation usually subsides.

Persisting inflammation may cause severe tissue injury.

It may be necessary to suppress inflammatory reaction by corticosteroids to reduce tissue damage.

Infection

AN INFLAMMATION CAUSED BY A PATHOGENIC ORGANISM

Terms used to name infections:

  Named by adding -itis to name of affected organ.

  Cellulitis: acute spreading infection.

  Abscess: tissue breakdown forming pus pockets.

  Lymphadenitis: inflammation of draining lymph nodes.

  Septicemia: bloodstream infection.

Factors influencing outcome:

  Virulence of organism.

  Dosage.

  Resistance of host's body.

CHRONIC INFECTION

Organisms and host evenly balanced.

Lymphocytes and plasma cells predominate.

http://health.jbpub.com/humandisease/9e

Human Disease Online is a great source for supplementary human disease information for both students and instructors. Visit this website to find a variety of useful tools for learning, thinking, and teaching.

Immunity, Hypersensitivity, Allergy, and Autoimmune Diseases

1 List the basic features of cell-mediated and humoral immunity. Explain the role of lymphocytes in the immune response.

2 Compare immunity and hypersensitivity. Explain why it is sometimes necessary to suppress the immune response and describe how this is accomplished.

3 List the five classes of antibodies and explain how they differ from one another.

4 Describe the pathogenesis of allergic manifestations and the role of IgA in allergy. Compare the methods of treatment.

5 Summarize the theories concerning the pathogenesis of autoimmune disease, the clinical manifestations, and the methods of treatment.

The Body's Defense Mechanisms

The body has two separate defense mechanisms for dealing with pathogenic microorganisms and other potentially harmful substances. One mechanism consists of the inflammatory reaction, which is a nonspecific response to any harmful agent and includes phagocytosis of the material by neutrophils and macrophages. The second, which depends on the immune system, consists of the development of an acquired immunity. The two mechanisms complement one another and function together to protect an individual from disease.

Acquired immunity, which develops after contact with a pathogenic microorganism, is only one manifestation of a person's capacity to react to a large number

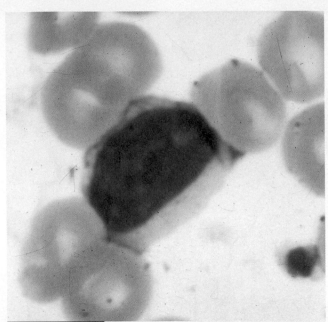

FIGURE 5-1 Structure of mature lymphocyte in the peripheral blood (original magnification × 1,000).

Humoral immunity
Immunity associated with formation of antibodies produced by plasma cells.

Cell-mediated immunity
Immunity associated with population of sensitized lymphocytes.

Hypersensitivity
A state of abnormal reactivity to a foreign material.

Autoantibody
(aw′tō-an′ti-bod-ē)
An antibody formed against one's own cells or tissue components.

Autoimmune disease
A disease associated with formation of cell-mediated or humoral immunity against the subject's own cells or tissue components.

Lymphokine
(limf′ō-kīn)
A soluble substance liberated by lymphocytes.

Cytokine
A general term for any protein secreted by cells that functions as an intercellular messenger and influences cells of the immune system. Cytokines are secreted by macrophages and monocytes (monokines), lymphocytes (lymphokines), and other cells.

of foreign antigens. There are two different types of acquired immunity: humoral immunity and cell-mediated immunity.

Humoral immunity is associated with the production of antibodies that can combine with and eliminate the foreign material. Humoral immunity is the body's major defense against many bacteria and bacterial toxins. **Cell-mediated immunity** is characterized by the formation of a population of lymphocytes that can attack and destroy the foreign material. It is the main defense against viruses, fungi, parasites, and some bacteria. Cell-mediated immunity is the mechanism by which the body rejects transplanted organs and eliminates the abnormal cells that sometimes arise spontaneously in cell division.

Acquired immunity is often associated with a stage of altered reactivity to bacterial products or foreign material, leading to an intense inflammatory reaction at the site of contact with the foreign antigen. This increased responsiveness is called **hypersensitivity**. For example, contact with the tubercle bacillus leads to cell-mediated immunity and is also associated with the development of tissue hypersensitivity to antigens of the tubercle bacillus. An individual who displays hypersensitivity to an organism or its products usually possesses some degree of immunity as well. However, many diseases are associated with the development of an acquired immunity without demonstrable hypersensitivity.

Normally, a person develops an immune response not against cell proteins in his or her own cells and tissues (called self-antigens) but only against foreign antigens (called non–self-antigens) because the body has developed a tolerance to the self-antigens present within it. Any lymphocytes that are inadvertently programmed in the course of prenatal development to react against self-antigens are destroyed or inactivated or their functions are suppressed.

However, there are some diseases that result when our own immune system attacks us, producing groups of destructive lymphocytes and injurious antibodies directed against our own cells and tissues, which may cause considerable organ damage. Antibodies directed against us are called **autoantibodies** (*auto* = self), and the diseases resulting from tissue damage caused by our own immune system are called **autoimmune diseases**.

Immunity

THE ROLE OF LYMPHOCYTES IN ACQUIRED IMMUNITY

The important cells of the immune system are the lymphocytes (FIGURE 5-1), which respond to foreign antigens, and the macrophages and related cells that process the antigen and "present" it to the lymphocytes.

The various cells of the immune system communicate with one another and produce many of their effects by secreting soluble protein (peptide) chemical messengers. Those secreted by lymphocytes are called **lymphokines**. The general term **cytokines** is used to designate any chemical messengers that take part in any function of the immune system, and some cytokines have specific names. Those that act by interfering with the multiplication of viruses within cells are called **interferons**. Those that send regulatory signals between cells of the immune system are called **interleukins**. Cytokines that can destroy foreign or abnormal cells are called **tumor necrosis factors**, so named because they can destroy tumor cells, although their destructive functions are not restricted to tumor cells.

DEVELOPMENT OF THE LYMPHATIC SYSTEM

Development of Immune Competence
The precursor cells of the lymphocytes are formed initially from stem cells in the bone marrow, and they eventually develop into either of two groups of lymphocytes, depending on where they undergo further development and "learn" their functions—a process called developing immune competence. In the fetus, some of these precursor cells migrate from the marrow into the thymus, where they undergo further maturation and develop into cells that are destined to form a specific type of lymphocyte called **T** (thymus-dependent) **lymphocytes**. Other lymphoid cells remain within the bone marrow, where they differentiate and develop into cells destined to form a second specific type of lymphocyte called **B** (bone marrow) **lymphocytes**.

The programming process by which lymphocytes acquire immune competence involves a rearrangement of genes within the developing B and T lymphocytes. Each programmed lymphocyte develops antigen receptors on its cell membrane that enable the lymphocyte to "recognize" and respond to a specific antigen. The antigen receptors of B lymphocytes are immunoglobulin (antibody) molecules, each a copy of the antibody that the B lymphocyte will eventually produce when stimulated by the appropriate antigen. T lymphocytes develop somewhat different types of receptors, but they serve the same functions as those on B cells. When the programming process has been completed, many millions of different T and B cells have formed, each programmed to recognize and respond to a different antigen. Although a single lymphocyte can respond to only a single antigen, there is such an enormous population of lymphocytes that some member of the "immunologic response team" can respond to any antigen the individual may ever encounter.

Migration and Circulation of Lymphocytes
Before birth, the precursor cells of both T and B lymphocytes migrate into the spleen, lymph nodes, and other sites. Here they proliferate to form the masses of mature lymphocytes that populate the various lymphoid organs.

T lymphocytes are usually classified into two major groups based on the type of protein molecules, called CD (cluster of differentiation) antigens, on their cell membranes. Lymphocytes containing CD4 antigens are usually called T4 lymphocytes, and those with CD8 antigens are called T8 lymphocytes. As described later, each group of T lymphocytes has different functions and responds somewhat differently when stimulated by an antigen.

Lymphocytes vary in their life span. Some have only a short survival time, but others live for many years. Lymphocytes do not remain localized within lymphoid organs. They continually recirculate between the bloodstream and the various lymphoid tissues. T and B lymphocytes are both present in the circulation and can be distinguished by special techniques.

About two-thirds of the circulating lymphocytes are T lymphocytes, and most of the rest are B lymphocytes. From about 10 to 15% of the circulating lymphocytes, however, have neither T nor B cell receptors. These cells are called **natural killer cells** or simply **NK cells**. Their major targets are virus-infected cells and cancer cells, which they can attack and destroy by secreting destructive lymphokines, even though they

Interferon
(in-tur-fēr′on)
A broad-spectrum antiviral agent manufactured by various cells in the body.

Interleukin-2
(inter-lōō′kin)
A lymphokine that stimulates growth of lymphocytes.

Tumor necrosis factor
A cytokine that can destroy foreign or abnormal cells.

T lymphocyte
A type of lymphocyte associated with cell-mediated immunity.

B lymphocyte
A lymphocyte that differentiates into plasma cells and is associated with humoral immunity.

Natural killer cells
Lymphocytes capable of destroying foreign or abnormal cells, although they have not had any prior antigenic contact with the cells.

NK cells
An abbreviation for natural killer cells.

have not been previously exposed to the foreign antigens that they are attacking. Furthermore, NK cells can destroy the target cells as soon as they are encountered, in contrast to T and B cells, which need time to become activated and function effectively. Although NK cells are not actually part of either the cell-mediated or the humoral immune defense systems, their functions are to some extent regulated by the immune system. NK cells are related to cell-mediated immunity because they are activated and function much more effectively when stimulated by lymphokines secreted by T lymphocytes. They are also related to humoral immunity because some types of NK cells possess cell membrane receptors for antibody molecules, which makes it easier for the NK lymphocytes to attach to and destroy target cells coated with antibodies.

RESPONSE OF LYMPHOCYTES TO FOREIGN ANTIGENS

Entry of a foreign antigen into the body triggers a chain of events that involves interactions between T and B lymphocytes and macrophages or similar antigen-processing cells. Macrophages are monocytes that have left the bloodstream and taken up permanent residence in the tissues throughout the body where they phagocytose and process antigens. Another important group of widely distributed antigen-processing cells is called dendritic cells, named from their long cytoplasmic processes that resemble the dendrites of a nerve cell. T and B lymphocytes respond differently to foreign antigens. T lymphocytes can only respond to processed antigens, but B lymphocytes can process intact antigens and display antigen fragments on their cell membranes. The interactions between antigen and antigen-processing cells involve three phases:

1. Recognition of the foreign antigen
2. Proliferation of the lymphocytes programmed to respond to the antigen, forming a large group (clone) of cells
3. Destruction of the foreign antigen by the lymphocytes that have responded to the antigen

FIGURE 5-2 summarizes the role of lymphocytes in acquired immunity. The first step in the immune defense reaction is the interaction of lymphocytes with the antigen that they have been programmed to recognize. The antigen must first be "processed" and displayed on the cell membrane of the antigen-processing cell before the immune response can be set in motion. Antigens are very large molecules. Only small fragments of the processed antigen called antigenic determinants or epitopes are displayed, not the entire molecule. When appropriately stimulated, B lymphocytes proliferate and mature into antibody-forming plasma cells, and T lymphocytes proliferate to form a diverse population of cells that both regulate the immune response and generate a cell-mediated immune reaction to eliminate the antigenic material.

Initial contact with a foreign antigen is followed by a lag phase of a week or more before an immune response is demonstrated. This lag corresponds to the time required for processing the antigen and for the lymphocytes to respond. After the body's immune mechanisms have reacted to a foreign antigen, however, some of the lymphoid cells retain a "memory" of the antigen that induced sensitization. They pass this information to succeeding generations of lymphocytes. Consequently, any later contact with the same antigen provokes a renewed proliferation of sensitized lymphocytes or antibody-forming plasma cells.

Role of Major Histocompatibility Proteins in Displaying Processed Antigen

The major histocompatibility (MHC) proteins play an essential role in "presenting" processed antigen to the responding cells of the immune system in order to generate

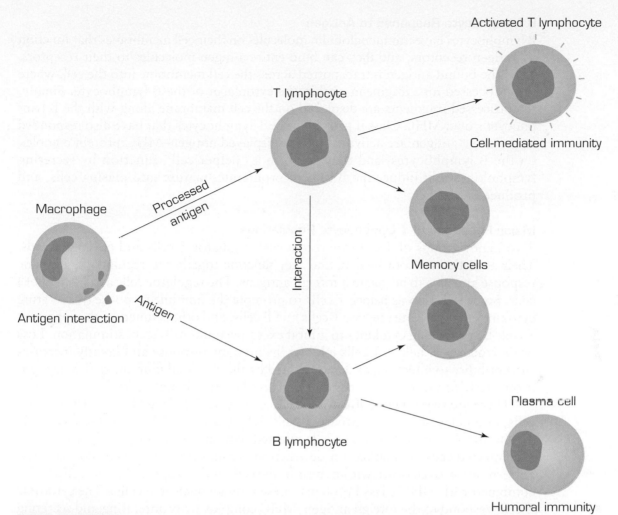

FIGURE 5-2 Interaction of cell-mediated and humoral immunity. Macrophage processes and presents processed antigen fragments to T lymphocyte; B lymphocyte processes intact antigen and displays fragments of the same antigen on its cell membrane. T lymphocyte, which has responded to the same antigen, stimulates the B lymphocyte to proliferate, mature into plasma cells, and make antibodies.

an immune response. The MHC proteins are carbohydrate–protein (glycoprotein) molecules on the surface of cells that distinguish the cells of one person from those of another. As described in the discussion on chromosomes, genes, and cell division, there are two major classes of MHC proteins: MHC Class I proteins are present on all nucleated cells; MHC Class II proteins are restricted to B lymphocytes, macrophages and related antigen-processing cells, and some activated T lymphocytes. The main function of the MHC proteins is to serve as a carrier for the processed foreign antigen fragments on the surface of cells to which the immune system can respond.

T Lymphocyte Response to Antigen

T lymphocytes are unable to respond to a foreign antigen until a macrophage or similar macrophagelike antigen-processing cell has phagocytosed the antigen, digested it, and displayed on its cell membrane the antigen fragments combined with its own MHC Class II proteins. In response to the displayed antigen-MHC Class II proteins, the T lymphocyte having the corresponding antigen receptors responds by proliferating and forms a group (clone) of identical T cells. The macrophages are also activated when they process and present antigen to T cells, and they secrete a cytokine that stimulates the T cells to proliferate.

B Lymphocyte Response to Antigen

B lymphocytes have immunoglobulin molecules on their cell membranes that function as antigen receptors, and they can bind entire antigen molecules to their receptors. Then the bound antigen is transported across the cell membrane into the cell, where it is processed into fragments within the cytoplasm of the B lymphocyte. Finally, the processed fragments are displayed on the cell membrane along with the B lymphocyte's own MHC Class II proteins. The T lymphocytes that have also responded to the same antigen are activated by the displayed antigen–MHC protein complex on the B lymphocytes, and they perform a "helper cell" function by secreting lymphokines that induce the B cells to proliferate, mature into plasma cells, and produce antibodies.

Major Functions of T Lymphocyte Populations

Two major groups of T cells are recognized: regulator T cells and effector T cells. Their activities are coordinated, and they function together to regulate the immune response and also to act against foreign antigens. The regulator cells are T4 (CD4+) cells. Some function as helper T cells to promote the immune response by secreting cytokines that activate effector T cells and B cells, and others function as suppressor T cells by producing cytokines to inhibit excessive immune system stimulation. Loss or destruction of helper T cells inhibits the immune response and greatly increases susceptibility to infection, as demonstrated by the acquired immune deficiency syndrome (AIDS) caused by a virus that destroys helper T lymphocytes.

Effector T cells
Cytotoxic and delayed hypersensitivity T cells that protect the body by attacking and destroying body cells infected with bacteria or viruses.

There are two types of **effector T cells**: cytotoxic T cells, which are T8 (CD8+) cells, and delayed hypersensitivity T cells, which are T4 (CD4+) cells. Cytotoxic T cells attack and destroy body cells infected with viruses or intracellular bacteria. The infected cells are marked for destruction because some of the viral or bacterial antigens are broken down within the infected cells and transported to the cell surface combined with MHC Class I proteins (present on all nucleated cells). The cytotoxic T cells respond to the foreign antigen–MHC complex by proliferating and secreting cytokines that destroy the infected cells. Cytotoxic T cells can also attack cancer cells, which display antigens different from normal cell antigens combined with MHC Class I proteins, and they are also responsible for the rejection of transplanted organs, which also contain foreign antigens.

Delayed hypersensitivity cells, also called sensitized T cells, are produced by a subgroup of helper T cells. The delayed hypersensitivity T cells respond to foreign antigens processed by macrophages or similar cells by accumulating at the site of the antigenic material, where they secrete a variety of lymphokines that attract macrophages, activate them, and stimulate them to secrete additional cytokines, including interferon and tumor necrosis factor. Some of the lymphokines also stimulate cytotoxic T cells and NK cells, both of which also secrete destructive cytokines. In this way, the delayed hypersensitivity reaction generates an intense inflammatory response directed against the antigens that stimulated the response.

In addition to regulator and effector T cells, a population of long-lived memory cells is also generated that can initiate a rapid cell-mediated immune response on later contact with the same antigen. TABLE 5-1 summarizes the classification and functions of the immune system cells.

Relation of MHC Proteins to Effector T Cell Responses

The two types of effector T cells are restricted in their ability to respond to processed antigens complexed and presented with MHC proteins. Cytotoxic T cells, which are T8 (CD8+) cells, can respond only to antigens complexed with MHC Class I proteins displayed on infected host cells, indicating to the immune system that some of the body's

TABLE 5-1

Classification and functions of immune system cells

Cell function	Cell type	Action of cell
Antigen processing	Macrophages, B lymphocytes, dendritic cells	Process antigen and present to lymphocytes
Regulate immune response	Regulator T cells (CD4+)	Cytokines regulate immune system activity
Promote cytotoxic immune response	Cytotoxic T cells (CD8+)	Produce cytokines that destroy foreign or abnormal cells displaying antigen fragments combined with MHC Class I antigens
Promote delayed hypersensitivity response	Delayed hypersensitivity T cells (CD4+)	Respond to antigen-processing cells presenting foreign antigen fragments combined with MHC Class II antigens; produce cytokines that activate and stimulate macrophages, cytotoxic T cells, and NK cells
Destroy virus-infected cells and cancer cells	NK cells	Cytokine-mediated cell destruction; no previous contact with antigen required
Produce antibodies	Plasma cells	Antigen processed by B lymphocytes and presented to responding T cells stimulates B lymphocytes to mature into plasma cells and make antibodies

own cells have been infected and should be destroyed. In contrast, delayed hypersensitivity cells, which are T4 (CD4+) cells, can respond only to processed antigen displayed on macrophages or related cells along with MHC Class II proteins, signaling the immune system cells to become activated in order to deal with the threat. Consequently, the manner in which the processed antigen is displayed determines which type of effector T cell will respond to the complexed antigen. Cytotoxic T cells are "designed" to attack and destroy infected host cells or other antigenically foreign or abnormal cells. Delayed hypersensitivity T cells function by orchestrating an intense inflammatory reaction to any type of foreign antigen, including micro-organisms such as the tubercle bacillus that are phagocytosed by macrophages. Activated macrophages, assisted by lymphoid cells, are the cells that play a major role in eliminating the antigenic material.

Immune-Response Genes

The ability to generate an immune response is under genetic control. Genes called **immune-response genes**, which are closely associated with the HLA complex on chromosome 6 in the discussion on chromosomes, genes, and cell division, control the

Immune-response genes
Genes on chromosome 6 that control the immune response to specific antigens.

immune response by regulating T cell and B cell proliferation. In this way, the genes regulate the intensity of the cell-mediated immune reaction and control the synthesis of antibody molecules. As a result, they influence resistance to infection and resistance to tumors. They also influence the likelihood of acquiring an autoimmune disease.

THE ROLE OF COMPLEMENT IN IMMUNE RESPONSES

Complement functions along with the immune system to destroy or inactivate all types of foreign antigens, including invading micro-organisms. As described in the discussion on inflammation and repair, complement can be activated in two ways: the classical pathway, which is triggered by antigen–antibody interactions, and the alternative pathway, in which complement is activated by bacterial cell wall material or products generated during the inflammatory reaction. When complement is activated, the complement components interact to accomplish several important functions. Some components function as mediators of inflammation. Other components coat the surface of invading bacteria, which makes them easier for macrophages and neutrophils to phagocytose. Finally, the interaction of the complement components generates a large molecule called an attack complex, which destroys the target micro-organism or abnormal cell by "punching holes" in its cell membrane (FIGURE 5-3).

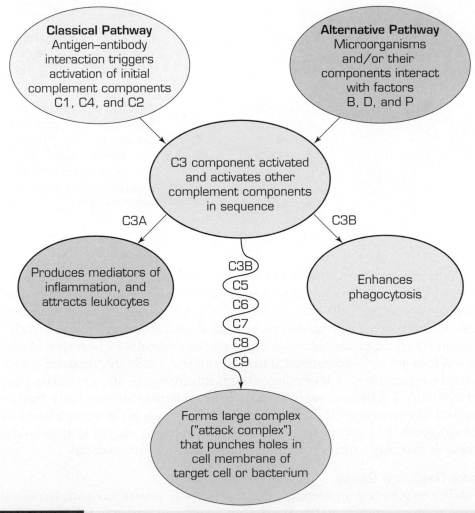

FIGURE 5-3 Components and pathways of complement activation that "complement" the body's immune defenses. Individual components named C1 through C9 and factors B, D, and P.

Antibodies (Immunoglobulins)

Antibodies are globulins produced by plasma cells and are usually called **immu-noglobulins** to emphasize their role in immunity. There are five different classes of immunoglobulins:

1. Immunoglobulin M (IgM)
2. Immunoglobulin G (IgG)
3. Immunoglobulin A (IgA)
4. Immunoglobulin D (IgD)
5. Immunoglobulin E (IgE)

Although the immunoglobulins differ somewhat from one another in their chemical composition, molecular weight, and size, they all have the same basic structure: two matched pairs of polypeptide (protein) chains joined by chemical bonds (FIGURE 5-4). One pair is called heavy chains. The second pair is only half as long as the heavy chains and is called light chains.

The arrangement of the Ig chains somewhat resembles the appearance of a fork. The ends of the Ig chains that combine with the antigen can be compared with its prongs. The "prong" end of the immunoglobulin molecule, which is different in each antibody, is called the variable part of the molecule. It is this part that imparts specificity to the molecule. Because of its structure, the antibody can react only with the specific antigen that induced its formation. The constant part of the chain, which can be compared with the handle of the fork, is the same for each major class of antibody. The "handle" end does not combine with antigen but determines other properties of the antibody, such as the ability to activate complement or fix to the surface of cell membranes.

All Ig molecules have the same basic four-chain unit structure, but some immunoglobulins characteristically aggregate to form clusters of two, three, or five individual units. For example, IgM is usually a cluster of five individual units, and IgA is usually a pair of units.

An antibody molecule is not a rigid structure. The junction of its constant and variable parts is quite flexible and is called the hinge region. This feature allows the variable end of the Y-shaped molecule to adapt to the configuration of the antigen that it is binding. Treatment with enzymes breaks an immunoglobulin molecule into three fragments. The variable region yields two fragments called the F_{ab} fragments (antibody-combining fragments), each consisting of a light chain and the associated part of the heavy chain. The other fragment is the constant region of the molecule and is called the F_c fragment (constant fragment).

Immunoglobulin
(im'mū-nō-glob'u-lin)
An antibody protein.

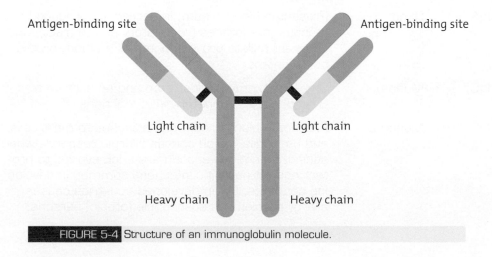

Antigen-binding site   Antigen-binding site

Light chain   Light chain

Heavy chain   Heavy chain

FIGURE 5-4 Structure of an immunoglobulin molecule.

IgM is present in the blood as a cluster of five individual molecules (a pentamer) joined together in a star-shaped configuration with the antigen-binding ends projecting outward and the opposite ends of the molecules directed toward the center of the cluster. As a pentamer, IgM forms a very large antibody cluster that is very efficient in combining with large particulate antigens such as fungi; it is often called a macroglobulin because of its large size and high molecular weight. IgM molecules are also found as single (monomeric) molecules attached, with their antigen-binding sites protruding, to the cell membranes of B lymphocytes, where they function as the antigen receptors on the surface of B lymphocytes. IgG is a much smaller antibody molecule and is the principal type of antibody molecule formed in response to the majority of infectious agents. IgA is produced by antibody-forming cells located in the respiratory and gastrointestinal mucosa. It is present in secretions of the respiratory and gastrointestinal tracts. IgA apparently functions by combining with potentially harmful ingested or inhaled antigens, forming antigen–antibody complexes that cannot be absorbed. In this way, IgA prevents the antigens from inducing sensitization. IgD is found on the cell membranes of B lymphocytes, along with the monomeric form of IgM and is present in only minute quantities in the blood. IgE is normally present in only small quantities in the blood of most persons, but its concentration is greatly increased in allergic individuals.

TABLE 5-2 summarizes the types and functions of the various immunoglobulins.

TABLE 5-2

Types and functions of immunoglobulins

Immuno-globulin	Usual type of secretion	Properties and functions
IgM	Pentamer	First Ig formed in response to foreign antigen (primary immune response). Present in bloodstream but not in tissues. Large pentamer antibody cluster very effective for combining with foreign antigen.
IgG	Monomer	Most prevalent Ig produced rapidly in large amounts (secondary immune response) to replace IgM. Found in blood and tissues. Crosses placenta to protect fetus until infant immune system can produce antibodies.
IgA	Dimer	Present in bloodstream, in secretions produced by mucous membranes (respiratory and GI tract), and in breast milk to provide maternal antibody protection to infant.
IgD	Monomer	Small amount in bloodstream and on surface of B lymphocytes. Undetermined functions.
IgE	Monomer	Present in bloodstream and attaches to mast cells and basophils, which causes allergic response when sensitizing antigen encountered. IgE evolved to protect against parasitic infections common in developing countries, but in developed countries causes allergy problems in susceptible (atopic) persons.

Hypersensitivity Reactions: Immune System–Related Tissue Injury

The immune system, while protecting us from foreign antigens that could harm us, may also damage the tissues where the immune response occurs. The desirable effect, which eliminates the foreign antigen, is called **immunity**. The undesirable effect, which is the associated tissue damage, is called **hypersensitivity**. Both are manifestations of the same process. The situation could be compared with the successful efforts of firefighters in putting out a potentially destructive house fire but at the same time breaking some windows and causing some water damage to the house and furniture.

It is conventional to classify the various types of hypersensitivity reactions based on how the immune system caused the injury (TABLE 5-3). Four different types of hypersensitivity reactions, usually designated by roman numerals, are recognized. The first three types are related to antibodies formed in response to antigenic material, and the fourth type is a cell-mediated hypersensitivity reaction. This section deals with the various mechanisms of immunologic injury. Specific examples of immune-mediated organ damage will be considered in connection with the disease of the various organ systems.

Immunity
Resistance to disease.

Hypersensitivity
A state of abnormal reactivity to a foreign material.

TABLE 5-3

Mechanisms of immunologic injury

Type	Mechanism	Examples
I: Immediate hypersensitivity	IgE antibodies fix to mast cells and basophils. Later contact with sensitizing antigen triggers mediator release and clinical manifestations.	Localized response: hay fever, food allergy, etc. Systemic response: bee sting or penicillin anaphylaxis, etc.
II: Cytotoxic hypersensitivity reactions	Antibody binds to cell or tissue antigen, and complement is activated, which damages cell, causes inflammation, and promotes destruction of antibody-coated cell by phagocytosis.	Autoimmune hemolytic anemia Blood transfusion reactions Rh hemolytic disease Some types of glomerulonephritis
III: Immune complex disease	Circulating antigen–antibody complexes form, which activate complement and cause inflammatory reaction.	Some types of glomerulonephritis Lupus erythematosus Rheumatoid arthritis
IV: Delayed (cell-mediated) hypersensitivity	Sensitized (delayed hypersensitivity) T cells release lymphokines that attract macrophages and other inflammatory cells.	Tuberculosis Fungus and parasitic infections Contact dermatitis

TYPE I. IMMEDIATE HYPERSENSITIVITY REACTIONS: ALLERGY AND ANAPHYLAXIS

Type I hypersensitivity reactions follow contact with foreign antigens that induce formation of specific IgE antibodies in the sensitized person. IgE has the unusual property of attaching to the surface of mast cells and similar cells circulating in the blood called basophils. The IgE attaches itself to the cell membrane by means of the F_c end of the molecule (the "handle of the fork"). If the sensitized person is later exposed to the sensitizing antigen, the antigen attaches to the free antibody-combining sites (the "prongs of the fork") on the IgE molecules. The union of antigen and antibody causes the cells to release their cytoplasmic granules filled with histamine, prostaglandins, and other potent chemical mediators. Immediate hypersensitivity reactions either may be localized, called allergic reactions, or may evoke a widespread systemic reaction, called **anaphylaxis**.

Allergy

Individuals who develop localized IgE-mediated reactions are predisposed to form specific IgE antibodies (become allergic) to ragweed, other plant pollens, and various other antigens that do not affect most persons. The allergy-prone individual is called an **atopic person**. The sensitizing antigen is called an **allergen**, and the allergic manifestations are localized to the tissues that are exposed to the allergens—for example, swollen itchy eyes, stuffy nose, and sneezing in a ragweed-sensitive person (FIGURE 5-5).

Because histamine is one of the mediators released from the IgE-coated cells, antihistamine drugs (which block the effects of histamine) often relieve many of the allergic symptoms. A more specific method of treating an allergic individual consists of immunizing the person to the offending allergen by repeated subcutaneous injections of the antigen that induced the allergy, such as an extract of ragweed pollen in a ragweed-sensitive person. This method of treatment, which is called **desensitization**, induces the formation of specific IgA and IgG antibodies against the offending allergen. The IgA and IgG act by combining with the allergen before it can affix to the cell-bound IgE and trigger the release of mediators. In a ragweed-sensitive person, for example, the ragweed-specific IgA present in the secretions of the respiratory tract combines with some of the inhaled ragweed antigen and helps prevent absorption of the allergen. At the same time, the ragweed-specific IgG circulating in the bloodstream combines with much of the absorbed ragweed antigen before it can interact with the IgE on the surface of the mast cells and basophils. Because less antigen is available to combine with cell-bound IgE and thereby trigger release of mediators, the allergic manifestations are minimized.

Anaphylaxis and Anaphylactoid Reactions

A severe generalized IgE-mediated hypersensitivity reaction may be life threatening and is called anaphylaxis. The condition results from an initial exposure to a substance (allergen) that induces the sensitization in a susceptible person. Commonly implicated allergens include penicillin, bee stings, peanuts, latex products, as well as various other sensitizing agents. Once sensitization has occurred, a later exposure to the sensitizing antigen triggers widespread mediator release from IgE-coated mast cells and basophils. This release may lead to a fall in blood pressure with circulatory collapse and is often accompanied by severe respiratory distress caused by mediator-induced spasm of smooth muscle in the walls of the bronchioles, which restricts air flow into and out of the lungs. Prompt treatment of this immunologic catastrophe with epinephrine and other appropriate agents is essential. A similar condition called an **anaphylactoid reaction** resembles an anaphylactic reaction but is not caused by IgE and occurs after the first contact with a foreign substance, possibly by stimulating mast cells directly or by activating complement. Aspirin, other nonsteroidal

Anaphylaxis
(a-nä-fil-aks'is)
A severe generalized IgE-mediated hypersensitivity reaction characterized by marked respiratory distress and fall in blood pressure.

Atopic
(ā-top'ik)
Having a genetic predisposition to certain allergic conditions such as hay fever and asthma.

Allergen
(al'ler-jen)
A substance capable of inducing an allergic reaction in a predisposed individual.

Desensitization
A method of inducing a diminished response to allergens by inducing the formation of specific IgG and IgA antibodies.

Anaphylactoid reaction
(a-na-fil-ack-toyd)
A hypersensitivity reaction resembling anaphylaxis but not caused by IgE antibodies.

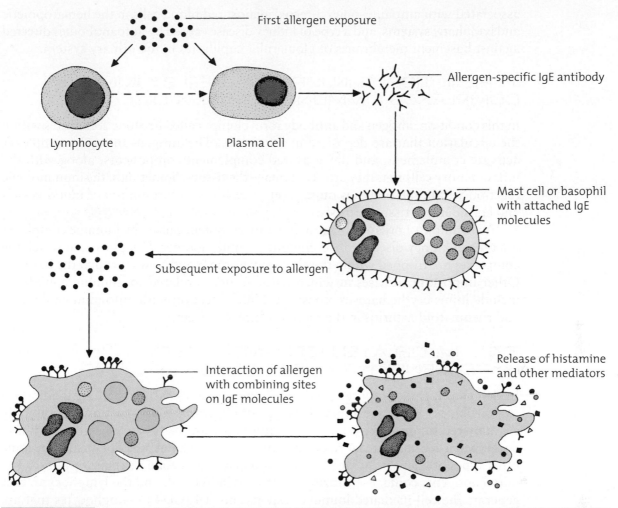

First allergen exposure

Lymphocyte

Plasma cell

Allergen-specific IgE antibody

Mast cell or basophil with attached IgE molecules

Subsequent exposure to allergen

Interaction of allergen with combining sites on IgE molecules

Release of histamine and other mediators

FIGURE 5-5 Pathogenesis of allergy. First exposure to allergen induces formation of specific IgE antibody in susceptible individual, which binds to mast cells and basophils by nonantigen receptor end of molecule. Subsequent exposure to allergen leads to an antigen–antibody interaction, liberating histamine and other mediators from mast cells and basophils. These mediators induce allergic manifestations.

anti-inflammatory drugs, some antibiotics, and radiopaque iodine-containing contrast material used for x-ray examinations may trigger an anaphylactoid reaction. The treatment is the same as for an anaphylactic reaction.

TYPE II. CYTOTOXIC HYPERSENSITIVITY REACTIONS

In this type of hypersensitivity reaction, antibody formed against a cell or tissue antigen binds to the surface of the target cell or tissue. The antigen–antibody reaction activates complement, and products of complement activation directly or indirectly damage the target. The complement components interact to form a large molecule called an attack complex that directly damages the target cell membrane. Inflammatory cells also are attracted and contribute to the tissue injury by releasing destructive enzymes; they may also destroy the antibody-coated target cells by phagocytosis.

Examples of Type II reactions include transfusion reactions caused by administration of incompatible blood, hemolytic disease of newborn infants caused by Rh incompatibility in prenatal development, some types of chronic hemolytic anemia associated with autoantibodies directed against red blood cells in the hematopoietic and lymphatic systems, and a type of kidney disease caused by autoantibodies directed against basement membranes of glomerular capillaries in the urinary system.

TYPE III. TISSUE INJURY CAUSED BY IMMUNE COMPLEXES ("IMMUNE COMPLEX DISEASE")

In this condition, antigen and antibody form clumps called immune complexes within the circulation that are deposited in the tissues. The antigen–antibody complexes activate complement, and the activated complement components, along with the inflammatory cells that they attract, damage the tissues. Sometimes, the immunologic reaction within the tissues is quite severe and leads to thrombosis of blood vessels and considerable tissue necrosis.

An example of organ damage in the urinary system caused by immune complexes is a type of kidney disease called immune-complex glomerulonephritis, in which the complexes are trapped within the glomeruli as the blood flows through the kidneys. Other important diseases in which tissue injury is related to immune complexes include lupus erythematosus, considered in connection with autoimmune disease, and rheumatoid arthritis in the musculoskeletal system.

TYPE IV. DELAYED (CELL-MEDIATED) HYPERSENSITIVITY REACTIONS

In delayed hypersensitivity reactions, T lymphocytes rather than antibodies are responsible for the tissue injury. This type of hypersensitivity reaction is commonly encountered in persons who have been infected with the tubercle bacillus and have developed a cell-mediated immune reaction directed against the organism, but some other types of bacteria, as well as fungi and parasites, evoke a similar response. The initial antigenic contact sensitizes the affected individual, and the lymphocytes that generate the cell-mediated immune response are T4 (CD4+) lymphocytes that are called delayed hypersensitivity T cells or, simply, sensitized T cells. After sensitization has occurred, any subsequent contact with the sensitizing antigen induces proliferation of T4 cells that accumulate at the site of antigen contact. The sensitized T cells secrete cytokines that attract and activate macrophages and other lymphocytes and incite an inflammatory reaction.

Delayed hypersensitivity reactions may also follow skin exposure to poison ivy, as well as various drugs, cosmetics, and chemicals. These agents combine with normal skin proteins to form a complex that induces sensitization. Any later skin contact with the offending agent that induced the initial sensitization provokes an intense cell-mediated inflammatory reaction in the skin, a condition called contact dermatitis.

Unlike immediate hypersensitivity reactions, which are mediated by antibodies, a cell-mediated inflammatory reaction requires from 24 to 48 hours to develop, the delay being the time necessary for sensitized T cells to accumulate at the site and generate an inflammatory reaction. Because this type of reaction takes place in persons who have been infected with the tubercle bacillus, a delayed hypersensitivity reaction is sometimes called tuberculin type hypersensitivity. The commonly used Mantoux skin test to detect infection with the tubercle bacillus is based on the presence or absence of a delayed hypersensitivity reaction to proteins of the tubercle bacillus. If an individual has had a previous contact with the tubercle bacillus, injection of a small test dose of proteins from the tubercle bacillus leads to an inflammatory reaction at the injection site. A positive test, however, only indicates a previous infection with the organism and development of cell-mediated immunity, along with associated hypersensitivity to the tubercle bacillus, but does not necessarily indicate that the person has active tuberculosis.

Suppression of the Immune Response

REASONS FOR SUPPRESSION

Cell-mediated and humoral immune responses protect against potentially harmful micro-organisms and other foreign substances. These same immunologic mechanisms may at times have undesirable effects:

1. They may be directed against the individual's own cells or tissue components, leading to autoimmune diseases.
2. They are responsible for the rejection of transplanted organs.
3. They lead to Rh hemolytic disease in newborn infants.

METHODS OF SUPPRESSION

It is sometimes necessary to suppress the immune response to treat certain autoimmune diseases, to perform organ transplants, and to prevent Rh hemolytic disease. There are many types of immunosuppressive agents that have found wide application in clinical medicine. The main types of immunosuppressive agents that are commonly used by physicians are as follows:

1. Radiation
2. Immunosuppressive drugs that impede cell division or cell function
3. Adrenal corticosteroid hormones
4. Immunoglobulin preparations

Radiation and Immunosuppressive Drugs

Radiation destroys normal cells. It exerts its immunosuppressive effect by destroying lymphoid tissue, which plays a key role in both cell-mediated and humoral immunity. There are several types of drugs that can suppress the immune response. **Cytotoxic drugs** (*cyto* = cell + *toxic* = poisonous) act by suppressing growth and division of lymphocytes. Lymphoid tissue is especially susceptible to the inhibitory effect of these drugs. **Antimetabolites,** as the name implies, inhibit important cellular metabolic functions, thereby inhibiting cell proliferation and suppressing the inflammatory reaction. Another important immunosuppressive drug called cyclosporine is often used to suppress the immune response in patients who have received organ transplants. The drug selectively inhibits T lymphocytes by interfering with the formation of a lymphokine called interleukin-2, which stimulates T lymphocyte proliferation. As a result, cell-mediated immune responses are suppressed with little effect on humoral immune responses or on the inflammatory reaction. (Cytotoxic drugs and antimetabolites are also used to treat some types of leukemia and malignant tumors, as described in the discussion on neoplastic disease.)

Cytotoxic drugs
(sī-tō-tok′sik)
Producing cell necrosis or destruction.

Antimetabolite
(an-ti-met-ab′o-līte)
A substance that competes with or replaces another substance (metabolite) required for cell growth or multiplication.

Corticosteroids

Adrenal corticosteroids act in several ways. They suppress the inflammatory response and impair phagocytosis. They also inhibit protein synthesis, thereby suppressing the growth and division of lymphocytes and inhibiting antibody formation by plasma cells.

Antibodies as Immunosuppressive Agents

Antibodies themselves may suppress or inhibit an immune response under certain circumstances. For example, injections of immunoglobulins appear to be a safe, effective treatment for many autoimmune neuromuscular diseases, although the optimal dose and frequency of administration are still being investigated. The immunoglobulins act by interfering with the generation of cytotoxic T cells, cytokines, and autoantibodies.

Eliminating a foreign antigen before the immune system can respond to the antigen is another effective way to suppress an immune response and is used routinely to prevent hemolytic disease of newborn infants caused by Rh incompatibility. Post-delivery administration of Rh immune globulin containing potent Rh antibodies to an Rh-negative mother who has given birth to an Rh-positive infant eliminates any antigenic Rh-positive fetal cells that may have entered the mother's bloodstream during delivery. Because the antigenic fetal cells are rapidly removed from the mother's circulation, the mother does not form Rh antibody, and Rh hemolytic disease is prevented in subsequent pregnancies. This application is described in connection with prenatal development and diseases associated with pregnancy.

TISSUE GRAFTS AND IMMUNITY

Rejection
An immunologic process characterized by destruction of a transplanted organ.

An individual will accept a graft of his or her own tissue or that of an identical twin, but not that of another person, because a graft from another person contains HLA antigens foreign to the recipient. The body "recognizes" the foreign antigens in the transplant, which becomes infiltrated by lymphocytes and macrophages and is eventually destroyed. This process is called **rejection** of the transplanted organ, and it is a manifestation of a cell-mediated immune reaction. Physicians who are treating kidney failure by transplantation can keep a foreign kidney from being rejected by inhibiting the recipient's immunologic defenses, using drugs that suppress the immune response. Transplantation of kidneys and other organs has been successful because it is usually possible to suppress the body's immune responses sufficiently to allow the transplanted organ to survive.

Autoimmune Diseases

The reasons why an individual forms an autoantibody to his or her own cells or tissue components are not well understood. Unfortunately, after an individual develops an autoimmune disease, it usually "doesn't go away." Although the affected person experiences periods when the disease is in remission or the manifestations are controlled by treatment, the disease persists and often progresses. Three major mechanisms have been postulated to explain the pathogenesis of autoimmune diseases:

1. Alteration of the patient's own (self) antigens that causes them to become antigenic and provoke an immune reaction
2. The formation of cross-reacting antibodies against foreign antigens that also attack the patient's own antigens
3. Defective regulation of the immune response by regulator T lymphocytes

The subject's own antigens may be altered by a viral infection or an infection with some other microbiologic agent in such a manner that the immune system no longer recognizes the antigen as a self-antigen, and an immune reaction is generated against the altered antigen (FIGURE 5-6A). Alternatively, some drug or medication ingested by the patient may change the structure of a self-antigen so that it is perceived as foreign and generates an immune response. Cross-reacting antibodies may induce organ damage when an antibody is formed against a foreign antigen, such as an invading bacterium, that shares antigenic determinants with some of the subject's

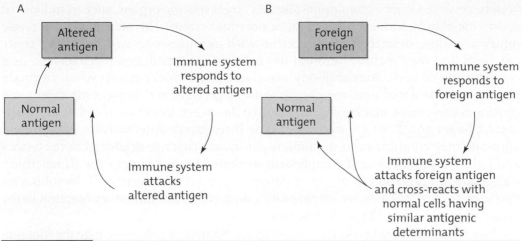

A

Altered antigen

Normal antigen

Immune system responds to altered antigen

Immune system attacks altered antigen

B

Foreign antigen

Normal antigen

Immune system responds to foreign antigen

Immune system attacks foreign antigen and cross-reacts with normal cells having similar antigenic determinants

FIGURE 5-6 Two mechanisms postulated to induce autoimmunity. **A**, Normal self-antigens altered, generating an immune response. **B**, Immune response directed against foreign antigen cross-reacts with similar antigenic determinants in normal self-antigens.

own cell or tissue antigens. As a result, the antibody that formed against the antigenic determinants in the foreign antigen cross-reacts with similar antigenic determinants in the subjects own tissues, leading to tissue injury (FIGURE 5-6B). The harmful effects of a cross-reacting antibody are demonstrated clearly by a newly described nervous system disease called **progressive inflammatory neuropathy** that occurred in workers at some Midwestern pork-processing plants. The affected persons worked in an area of the plant where pig brains were removed from the animal cranial cavities by using a high-pressure, compressed-air system that sprayed aerosolized pig brain tissue and blood into the air. Some of the employees inhaled small bits of pig tissue. Their immune systems responded by forming antibodies against the pig tissues, which contain antigens similar to those in human tissues. As a result, the anti-pig antibodies also attacked the nerve tissue of the affected employees, leading to the pain, numbness, and weakness associated with the disease.

Three factors appear to predispose to autoimmune diseases:

Progressive inflammatory neuropathy
An autoimmune neurologic disease caused by inhalation of pig brain tissue.

1. A genetic component, which in part is related to the genes on chromosome 6, which code for our own unique self-antigens. These are the same antigens that are involved in presenting processed antigen to lymphocytes by macrophages or other antigen-processing cells. Certain HLA types appear to be associated with an increased susceptibility to specific autoimmune diseases.
2. A gender component, as many autoimmune diseases occur much more frequently in women than in men.
3. An infection component in a genetically predisposed individual, as the onset of many autoimmune diseases appears to be associated with a recent infection, often a viral infection. An infection in a person with a chronic autoimmune disease may also cause a flare-up of disease.

AUTOIMMUNE DISEASE MANIFESTATIONS AND MECHANISMS OF TISSUE INJURY

The manifestations of autoimmune disease depend on which cells or tissue components are targeted for attack by the immune system. Some autoimmune diseases attack specific tissues throughout the body, such as bone, cartilage, connective tissue, blood vessels, or skin. Other autoimmune diseases target specific organs, such as individual endocrine glands, kidney, liver, lung, or nervous system. The mechanisms of tissue injury are those described in connection with immune-mediated hypersensitivity reactions and may include humoral mechanisms, cell-mediated mechanisms, or a combination of both. Autoantibody-associated tissue injury results when antibody becomes attached to the cell membrane of the target cells, activating complement and causing complement-mediated destruction of the target, usually assisted by activated macrophages and killer lymphocytes (Type II reaction). Alternatively, antigen and antibody may combine to form immune complexes that are deposited in the tissues and induce a similar type of complement-mediated tissue injury (Type III reaction). Cell-mediated destruction of target tissues is caused by sensitized T lymphocytes that secrete lymphokines, which generate a destructive inflammatory reaction in the target tissue or organ (Type IV reaction).

Not all autoantibodies destroy target tissue. Sometimes, they derange the function of the target but do not destroy it. The thyroid gland, for example, may be attacked by two different types of autoantibodies. One type destroys thyroid cells and impairs thyroid function, causing hypothyroidism. Another type stimulates the thyroid cells and makes them hyperfunction, causing hyperthyroidism.

In general, treatment of autoimmune disease is not very satisfactory. Various methods of treatment have been used to minimize inflammation and tissue damage, to suppress the function of the immune system, and to block the destructive effects of cytokines produced by T lymphocytes and macrophages.

TABLE 5-4 summarizes the features of some of the more important diseases in which autoantibody formation appears to play a role. These diseases are considered in greater detail in subsequent chapters.

CONNECTIVE TISSUE (COLLAGEN) DISEASES

The fibrous connective tissue that forms the framework of all tissues in the body is called collagen. The term connective tissue disease, or collagen disease, is used to describe a group of diseases characterized by necrosis and degeneration of collagen fibers throughout the body. In many instances, autoantibodies directed against antigens present in various cells and tissues can be detected in the serum of affected individuals, and aggregates of antigen combined with antibody (termed antigen–antibody complexes) can be identified at the sites of tissue damage. Often, large numbers of lymphocytes and plasma cells accumulate in the affected tissues. These cells are presumed to be responsible for the tissue injury by means of cell-mediated immune reactions and formation of autoantibodies. Therefore, the connective tissue diseases are usually classified as autoimmune diseases.

The clinical features of a connective tissue disease depend on the organ system affected and the extent of the injury to the tissues. Involvement of the connective tissue of the joints and periarticular tissues is manifested by swelling, pain, and tenderness in the joints. FIGURE 5-7 compares the cellular structure of a normal joint lining with a diseased one. Connective tissue diseases that affect the cardiovascular system cause collagen fibers of the heart valves to swell and degenerate (leading to valve injury). The heart muscle becomes inflamed. The connective tissue in the myocardium becomes necrotic, and destructive lesions occur in the small- and medium-sized blood vessels. Renal manifestations include inflammation and scarring of the glomeruli, damage to the glomerular basement membrane, and consequent leakage of protein and red blood cells into the urine. Severe glomerular damage impairs renal function and may eventually lead to renal insufficiency. Injury to the connective tissue of the lungs, pleura, and pericardium leads to pleural and pericardial pain, sometimes with

TABLE 5-4

Etiology and clinical manifestations of common autoimmune diseases

	Probable pathogenesis	Major clinical manifestations
Rheumatic fever	Antistreptococcal antibodies cross-react with antigens in heart muscle, heart valves, and other tissues.	Inflammation of heart and joints
Glomerulonephritis	Some cases caused by antibodies formed against glomerular basement membrane; other cases caused by antigen–antibody complexes trapped in glomeruli.	Inflammation of renal glomeruli
Rheumatoid arthritis	Antibodies formed against serum gamma globulin.	Systemic disease with inflammation and degeneration of joints
Autoimmune blood diseases	Autoantibodies formed against platelets, white cells, or red cells; in some cases, antibody apparently is formed against altered cell antigens, and antibody reacts with both altered and normal cells.	Anemia, leukopenia, or thrombocytopenia, depending on nature of antibody
Lupus erythematosus, scleroderma, and related collagen diseases	Various autoantibodies cause widespread injury to tissues and organs.	Systemic disease with manifestations in several organs
Thyroiditis (Hashimoto thyroiditis)	Antithyroid antibody causes injury and inflammatory cell infiltration of thyroid gland.	Hypothyroidism
Diffuse toxic goiter (Graves disease)	Autoantibody mimicking thyroid-stimulating hormone (TSH) causes increased output of thyroid hormone.	Hyperthyroidism
Diabetes (Type 1)	Autoantibodies and activated T lymphocytes destroy pancreatic islet beta cells	Diabetes mellitus caused by insulin deficiency
Pernicious anemia	Autoantibodies destroy gastric mucosa cells	Macrocytic anemia and nervous system damage resulting from adequate absorption of vitamin B_{12}
Vasculitis (various types of blood vessel inflammation)	Autoantibody-mediated damage to small, medium, and large blood vessels	Blood vessel damage interferes with blood vessel function and blood supply to tissues
Various skin conditions and diseases causing loss of skin pigment or skin blisters	Some autoantibodies damage pigment-producing cells in skin; others attack intercellular connections between skin cells	Pigment cell loss causes areas of skin depigmentation (vitiligo); blisters result from loss of skin intercellular connections
Myasthenia gravis	Autoantibodies destroy acetylcholine receptors at muscle–nerve junctions	Muscle weakness resulting from inadequate transmission of impulses from nerves to muscles

A

B

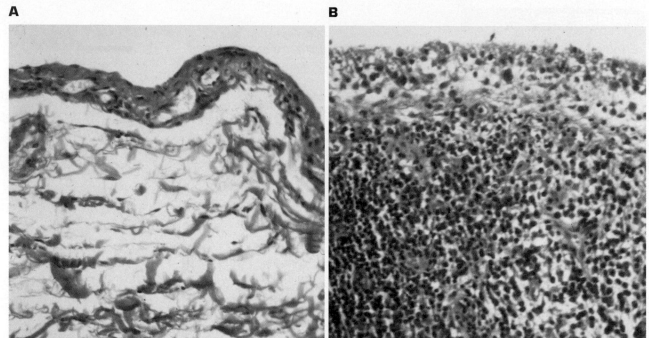

FIGURE 5-7 Comparison of normal joint lining **A**, with joint lining in one type of connective tissue disease **B**, The lining of the affected joint is heavily infiltrated with lymphocytes and plasma cells, and the joint injury is secondary to the inflammatory reaction (original magnification × 400).

Hemolytic anemia
An anemia caused by increased blood destruction.

Leukopenia
(lōō-kō-pē′ni-uh)
An abnormally small number of leukocytes in the peripheral blood.

accumulation of fluid in the serous cavities. Autoantibodies directed against one or more of the formed elements in the blood may cause anemia caused by destruction of red blood cells (**hemolytic anemia**), reduction in platelets (thrombocytopenia), or a decrease in the number of white blood cells (**leukopenia**).

LUPUS ERYTHEMATOSUS

One of the more common connective tissue diseases is called lupus erythematosus. This disease is seen most frequently in young women and is characterized by widespread damage to fibrous connective tissue in the skin, articular tissues, heart, serous membranes (pleura and pericardium), and kidneys. The skin rash often has a characteristic appearance and is called a *malar rash* because it affects both cheeks (*mala* = cheek) joined by an extension across the bridge of the nose. The rash is also sometimes called a *butterfly rash* from its fancied resemblance to a butterfly with spread wings (FIGURE 5-8). Hemolytic anemia, leukopenia, and thrombocytopenia are frequent hematologic manifestations of lupus; these are caused by autoantibodies. Many patients die of renal failure resulting from the severe renal glomerular injury.

Patients with lupus develop a variety of autoantibodies directed against cells and tissues, including antinucleoprotein antibodies and antibodies directed against red cells, white cells, platelets, and plasma proteins. Circulating antigen–autoantibody complexes (immune complexes) form and are deposited in kidney glomeruli, blood vessels, and other tissues. Complement is

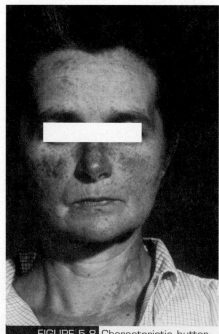

FIGURE 5-8 Characteristic butterfly rash in woman with lupus erythematosus.

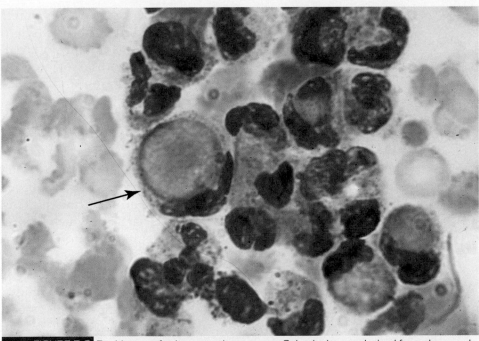

FIGURE 5-9 Positive test for lupus erythematosus. Spherical mass derived from damaged nucleus (*arrow*) engulfed by neutrophil (original magnification × 1,000).

activated, which generates an inflammatory reaction where the immune complexes are deposited. A characteristic feature of lupus erythematosus is the presence of antinucleoprotein antibodies in the patient's blood, which can be demonstrated by various methods. The original technique consisted of incubating the patient's blood serum with intact white blood cells. The antinucleoprotein antibodies damage many of the leukocytes, causing swelling and loss of structural detail in the cell nuclei. The damaged nuclei are converted into large, homogeneous, spherical "blobs" of blue-staining nuclear debris that becomes surrounded and phagocytized by polymorphonuclear leukocytes. The phagocytized spherical mass fills the cytoplasm of the cell and displaces the nucleus to the edge of the cell, resulting in the characteristic appearance called an LE cell. This classic method of demonstrating antinucleoprotein antibodies was described in 1948 by Hargraves and two associates from the Mayo Clinic in Minnesota and now is primarily of historical interest. The test has been superseded by newer, more sensitive techniques, but the method does clearly illustrate the damaging effect of nucleoprotein antibodies on intact cell nuclei (FIGURE 5-9).

The pathogenesis of lupus is not well understood but appears to be initiated by some event, possibly a viral infection or other antigenic stimulation in a genetically predisposed individual that damages normal MHC antigens so that they are no longer recognized as self-antigens by the immune system. Helper T lymphocytes and B lymphocytes directed against the abnormal self-antigens are activated. The helper T lymphocytes stimulate the B lymphocytes to proliferate. Then the B lymphocytes form the various autoantibodies and generate the antigen–autoantibody complexes that are responsible for the organ damage characteristic of this disease.

SCLERODERMA (SYSTEMIC SCLEROSIS)

Another connective tissue disease with widespread systemic manifestations has some lupuslike features and other manifestations that resemble rheumatoid arthritis.

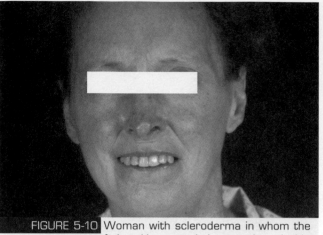

FIGURE 5-10 Woman with scleroderma in whom the appearance of the skin around the mouth and chin reflects loss of normal skin flexibility.

The disease is characterized by diffuse fibrosis (sclerosis) in the skin and internal organs with associated organ dysfunction and formation of characteristic autoantibodies. Usually, the disease is called scleroderma instead of systemic sclerosis to emphasize its effect on the skin and deeper tissues. The fibrous tissue proliferation thickens the facial skin, which reduces its flexibility, and also extends into the subcutaneous fat and skin appendages (sweat glands, sebaceous glands, and hair follicles). As the thickened skin becomes less mobile, facial movements associated with normal speech and expression become more difficult (FIGURE 5-10). Although the skin changes may be a source of concern, usually they are not life threatening. Unfortunately, the organ damage caused by the fibrosis can be devastating. The kidneys, esophagus, heart, and lungs are the most frequently and severely affected. Pulmonary fibrosis leads to serious respiratory complications and is the most frequent cause of death in severely affected persons.

QUESTIONS FOR REVIEW

1. What is meant by the following terms: *acquired immunity*, *cell-mediated immunity*, *humoral immunity*, and *hypersensitivity*?
2. What is the role of the lymphocyte in acquired immunity? What is the role of the macrophage?
3. How does the physician manipulate the body's immune reaction to allow kidney transplantation?
4. What is meant by the following terms: *B lymphocyte*, *T lymphocyte*, and *lymphokine*?
5. What are immunoglobulins? What is their basic structure? How do they function?
6. What is meant by the following terms: *light chains*, *macroglobulin*, and *allergy*?
7. What is an autoantibody? What are some of the postulated mechanisms that result in autoantibody formation? What is the effect of autoantibody directed against the patient's own blood cells?
8. What is a connective tissue disease? What are its manifestations? What is an LE cell?
9. What are antigen–antibody complexes? How do they cause tissue injury?
10. How can the immune response be suppressed? Why is this sometimes necessary?

SUPPLEMENTARY READINGS

Dalakas, M. C. 2004. Intravenous immunoglobulin in autoimmune neuromuscular diseases. *Journal of the American Medical Association* 19:2367–75.

► Injections of immunoglobulins are a safe, effective treatment for many autoimmune neuromuscular diseases, although the optimal doses and frequency of administration are still being investigated. The immunoglobulins act by interfering with virtually all of the processes that generate the cytotoxic cells, cytokines, and autoantibodies responsible for autoimmune damage to the target organ or tissue, such as interference with T cell functions, suppression of cytokines, suppression of autoantibody production by B cells, and interference with its ability to bind to its target.

Delves, P. J., and Roitt, I. M. 2000. The immune system. *New England Journal of Medicine* 343:37–49, and 343:108–17.

► A review of current knowledge on this complex system.

Gabrielli, A., Avvedimento, E. V., and Krieg, T. 2009. Scleroderma. *New England Journal of Medicine* 360:1989–2003.

► Scleroderma is a serious autoimmune disease characterized by skin and organ fibrosis preceded by vasculitis, pulmonary hypertension, sometimes associated with lupuslike and rheumatoid arthritislike manifestations, usually associated with autoantibodies directed against various tissue components. The kidneys, esophagus, heart, and lungs are the most frequently and severely affected. Pulmonary involvement is the most frequent cause of death.

Klein, J., and Sato, A. 2000. The HLA system. *New England Journal of Medicine* 343:702–9, and 343:782–6.

► A review of current knowledge about our system of self-antigens, how they function, and the abnormalities of genes linked to the HLA complex. The roles of the HLA system in cancer and transplantation are considered.

OUTLINE SUMMARY

The Body's Defense Mechanisms

Immunity

CHARACTERISTICS OF IMMUNE RESPONSE
Depends on lymphocytes and antigen-processing cells.
Specific populations of lymphocytes perform specific functions.
Cells of immune system communicate and produce their effects by secreting cytokines.

TYPES OF IMMUNITY

AUTOIMMUNITY

DEVELOPMENT OF THE LYMPHATIC SYSTEM
Immature lymphocytes develop immune competence in thymus (T lymphocytes) or bone marrow (B lymphocytes).
Lymphocytes are programmed to develop receptors for the antigens that they will eventually recognize.

T lymphocytes are classified into major groups based on CD antigens on cell membranes.
NK cells lack T or B receptors and can destroy infected or abnormal cells without prior antigenic contact.

RESPONSE OF LYMPHOCYTES TO FOREIGN ANTIGENS
B lymphocytes can respond to intact antigen and proliferate with T cell help.
T lymphocytes require macrophage-processed antigen in order to respond.
Antigens are presented to responding cells complexed with MHC proteins.

TYPES OF RESPONDING T CELLS
Helper T cells: promote immune response.
Cytotoxic T cells: attack and destroy infected cells, cancer cells, transplants.
Delayed hypersensitivity cells: attract and activate macrophages, cytotoxic T cells, NK cells.
Memory cells: set aside to respond rapidly if the same antigen is encountered again.
Response of effector T cell is determined by type of MHC protein displayed with processed antigen.

GENETIC CONTROL OF ABILITY TO GENERATE IMMUNE RESPONSE
THE FUNCTION OF COMPLEMENT

Antibodies (Immunoglobulins)

STRUCTURE

Composed of two light and two heavy chains.
Constant part of molecule determines class of antibody.
Variable part of molecule determines specificity.
Five types of immunoglobulins.

IgM: forms large complex pentamer.
IgG: principal antibody formed against majority of infectious agents.
IgA: produced by cells in respiratory and gastrointestinal tracts. Combines with antigens to prevent absorption.
IgD: on surface of lymphocytes.
IgE: increased in allergic persons. Attaches to mast cells and basophils.

Hypersensitivity Reactions: Immune System–Related Tissue Injury

Cell-tissue injury resulting from immune response.
Classified on pathogenesis of injury.

TYPE I. IMMEDIATE HYPERSENSITIVITY

Localized response: allergy.

Tendency to form IgE antibodies to antigens that do not sensitize most individuals.
IgE attaches to mast cells and basophils.
Subsequent contact with allergen leads to antigen–antibody interaction with release of mediators and allergic manifestations.
Antihistamines block some effects.
Desensitization induces formation of IgA and IgG, which combine with allergen before it can interact with IgE.

Systemic response: anaphylaxis.
Generalized mediator release from mast cells and basophils may be life threatening.
Prompt treatment essential.

TYPE II. CYTOTOXIC HYPERSENSITIVITY

Antibody attaches to cell or tissue antigen.
Complement activated and cell-tissue damage follows.

TYPE III. IMMUNE COMPLEX DISEASE

Circulating antigen–antibody complexes deposited in tissues.
Complement activated and cell-tissue injury follows.

TYPE IV. DELAYED HYPERSENSITIVITY

Sensitized T lymphocytes secrete cytokines that attract lymphocytes, macrophages, and other inflammatory cells, which produce tissue injury.

Mantoux test based on delayed hypersensitivity response to proteins from tubercle bacillus as indication of previous infection.

Suppression of the Immune Response

UNWANTED EFFECTS OF IMMUNE RESPONSE

Autoimmune disease.
Rejection of transplanted organs.
Rh hemolytic disease in newborn infants (discussed in prenatal development and diseases associated with pregnancy).

METHODS FOR SUPPRESSING THE IMMUNE RESPONSE

Radiation: destroys lymphocytes.
Cytotoxic drugs: suppress growth of lymphocytes.
Adrenal corticosteroids: suppress inflammatory reaction, impair phagocytosis, and inhibit protein synthesis.
Antibodies: prevent body from reacting to corresponding antigen.

TISSUE GRAFTS AND IMMUNITY

Graft contains foreign antigens.
Lymphocytes recognize foreign antigen and attempt to eliminate (rejection).
Immune response must be suppressed to prevent rejection of transplant.

Autoimmune Diseases

PATHOGENESIS

Antibodies formed to altered antigens and react with normal antigens.
Antibodies formed to foreign antigens and cross-react with normal tissue antigens.
T lymphocytes fail to control immune response.

TREATMENT

Corticosteroids.
Cytotoxic drugs.

CONNECTIVE TISSUE (COLLAGEN) DISEASES

Clinical features:

Autoimmune disease characterized by necrosis and degeneration of fibrous connective tissue.
Clinical features depend on organs affected.

LUPUS ERYTHEMATOSUS

A connective tissue disease of young women.
Associated with formation of autoantibodies and immune complexes.

SCLERODERMA (SYSTEMIC SCLEROSIS)

Autoimmune disease characterized by progressive fibrosis of skin and internal organs with associated organ damage.

http://health.jbpub.com/humandisease/9e

Human Disease Online is a great source for supplementary human disease information for both students and instructors. Visit this website to find a variety of useful tools for learning, thinking, and teaching.

CHAPTER 6

Pathogenic Microorganisms

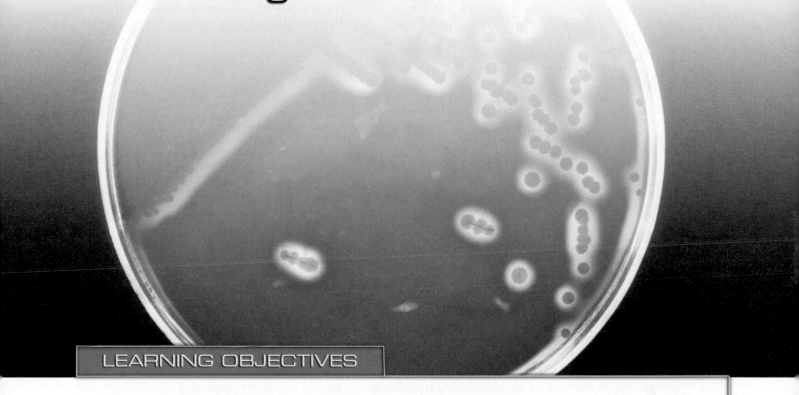

1 Explain the characteristics by which bacteria are classified. List and describe the major groups of pathogenic bacteria.

2 Describe the mechanism by which antibiotics inhibit the growth and metabolism of bacteria. Explain the adverse effects of antibiotics.

3 Describe the procedures used in antibiotic sensitivity testing and explain the principles by which the results are interpreted.

4 Explain the mode of action of virus infections and describe how the body's response to viral infection leads to recovery.

5 List the common infections caused by chlamydiae, mycoplasmas, and rickettsiae.

6 Discuss the spectrum of infections caused by fungi. Explain the factors that predispose to systemic infections. Describe the methods used to treat fungus infections.

Types of Harmful Microorganisms

The human species coexists with a large number of microorganisms. In most instances, we and our microbiologic associates live in harmony. Of the wide spectrum of organisms found in nature, only a relatively small proportion cause disease in humans. These pathogenic microorganisms are classified into several large groups:

1. Bacteria
2. Viruses
3. Chlamydiae
4. Rickettsiae and Ehrlichiae

    5. Mycoplasmas
    6. Fungi

In addition, humans serve as host to a number of animal parasites capable of causing illness or disability. The various organisms that are injurious to humans vary in their ability to cause disease. A small number of microbiologic agents are extremely virulent. Others are of very low virulence and are capable of causing disease only when the body's normal defenses have already been weakened by a debilitating illness.

Bacteria

CLASSIFICATION OF BACTERIA

Bacteria are classified on the basis of four major characteristics:

    1. Shape
    2. Gram-stain reaction
    3. Biochemical and cultural characteristics
    4. Antigenic structure

Shape

A bacterium may be spherical (coccus) or rod shaped (bacillus), or it may have a spiral or corkscrew shape. Cocci may grow in clusters (staphylococci), in pairs (diplococci), or in chains (streptococci).

Gram-Stain Reaction

In the Gram-stain method, a dried, fixed suspension of bacteria, prepared on a microscope slide, is stained first with a purple dye and then with an iodine solution. Next, the slide is decolorized with alcohol or another solvent; it is then stained with a red dye. Bacteria that resist decolorization and retain the purple stain are called gram-positive, whereas those that have been decolorized and accept the red counterstain are termed gram-negative. By means of the Gram-stain method, organisms may be characterized as either gram-positive or gram-negative (FIGURE 6-1A).

B

A

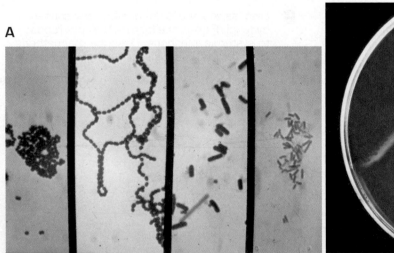
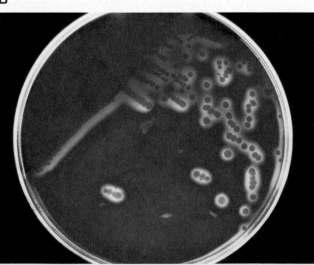

FIGURE 6-1 **A**, Appearance of bacteria as seen in Gram stains. From left to right: gram-positive cocci in clusters (staphylococci), gram-positive cocci in chains (streptococci), gram-positive bacilli, gram-negative bacilli (original magnification × 1,000). **B**, Bacteriologic culture plate (blood agar) containing colonies of hemolytic staphylococci. Enzymes produced by the bacteria break down (hemolyze) the blood cells in the culture medium, which causes the clear zones surrounding the colonies.

Biochemical and Cultural Characteristics

Some bacteria are quite fastidious and can be grown only on enriched media under carefully controlled conditions of temperature and acidity (pH). Other bacteria are hardy and capable of growing on relatively simple culture media under a wide variety of conditions.

Many bacteria grow best in the presence of oxygen (aerobic organisms). Some bacteria are able to grow only in the absence of oxygen or under extremely low oxygen tension. These are called anaerobic (without oxygen) bacteria. Others grow equally well under either aerobic or anaerobic conditions.

Many bacteria have special structural characteristics. Some bacteria have **flagella**: hairlike processes covering their surface. Flagella give a bacterium its motility; organisms that lack flagella are nonmotile. Some bacteria form **spores**: spherical structures formed within the bacterial cell. Spores can survive under conditions that would kill an actively growing bacterium. They may be considered a dormant, extremely resistant bacterial modification that forms under adverse conditions. Spores can germinate and give rise to actively growing bacteria under favorable conditions.

Most bacteria have distinct biochemical characteristics. Some types of bacteria are capable of fermenting carbohydrates and can bring about many different biochemical reactions under suitable cultural conditions. Each type of bacterium has its own "biochemical profile," which aids in its identification.

Flagellum
(fla-jel′um)
A whiplike process that propels an organism or sperm.

Spores
A highly resistant spherical structure produced by some bacteria to assure survival under adverse conditions.

Antigenic Structure

Each type of bacterium contains a large number of antigens associated with the cell body, the capsule of the bacterium, and the flagella (in the case of motile organisms). The antigenic structure can be determined by special methods, defining a system of antigens unique for each group of bacteria.

IDENTIFICATION OF BACTERIA

The methods of classifying bacteria can be applied to the identification of a specific bacterium. Let us assume, for example, that an organism has been isolated from the blood of a patient with a febrile illness. By means of the Gram-stain reaction, the organism is identified as a gram-negative bacillus. The cultural characteristics indicate that it is not a fastidious organism and is capable of growing on a wide variety of culture media at various temperatures; moreover, it grows well both in the presence of oxygen and under anaerobic conditions. The organism is motile and does not form spores.

At this point, the number of possible organisms consistent with these characteristics has been reduced to relatively few gram-negative bacteria. The number of possibilities is narrowed still further by various biochemical tests indicating that the bacterium does not ferment lactose but is able to ferment glucose and certain other sugars. These and other biochemical tests support the conclusion that the organism is a type of pathogenic bacterium, called Salmonella, found in the gastrointestinal tract and capable of causing a typhoidlike febrile illness. The bacterial antigens within the cell body and flagella of the bacteria can be identified to determine the exact type of Salmonella responsible for the patient's illness.

Once the organism has been identified, the clinician can begin proper treatment and can institute proper isolation and control procedures based on the means by which the disease is transmitted.

MAJOR CLASSES OF PATHOGENIC BACTERIA

This section summarizes important bacteria that infect humans and the principal diseases that they cause. These major groups of pathogenic bacteria and their

Gram-stain reactions are given in TABLE 6-1. The diseases caused by these organisms are described in the following section and summarized in TABLE 6-2.

Staphylococci

Staphylococci are normal inhabitants of the skin and nasal cavity and normally are not pathogenic. Some staphylococci, however, are pathogens, and some strains may be extremely virulent. Pathogens usually can be distinguished from nonpathogenic staphylococci by the appearance of their colonies on media containing blood (blood agar plates). Pathogenic staphylococci produce zones of complete hemolysis around the growing colonies (FIGURE 6-1B), in contrast to nonpathogenic staphylococci which do not hemolyze red cells.

Pathogenic staphylococci are a common cause of boils, other skin infections, and postoperative wound infections.

Occasionally, staphylococci cause serious pulmonary infections and other types of systemic infections. Staphylococcal infections often pose a serious problem in hospitals because the organisms are widely distributed and many hospitalized patients are unusually susceptible to infection. Many patients have had recent surgical operations; others have various chronic diseases associated with impairment of the body's normal defenses against bacterial infection. Some strains of staphylococci are highly resistant to antibiotics, and infections caused by antibiotic-resistant staphylococci are extremely difficult to treat.

Streptococci

There are many kinds of streptococci, and their pathogenicity varies. These organisms are classified on the basis of their serologic group designated by a capital letter,

TABLE 6-1

Important pathogenic bacteria

Type	Gram-stain reaction	
	Gram-positive	**Gram-negative**
Cocci	Staphylococci Streptococci Pneumococci	Gonococci Meningococci
Bacilli	*Corynebacteria* *Listeria* *Bacilli* *Clostridia*	*Haemophilus* *Gardnerella* *Francisella* *Yersinia* *Brucella* *Legionella* *Salmonella* *Shigella* *Campylobacter* Cholera bacillus Colon bacillus (*Escherichia coli*) and related organisms
Spiral organisms	*Treponema pallidum* *Borrelia burgdorferi*	
Acid-fast organisms	Tubercle bacillus Leprosy bacillus	

TABLE 6-2

Summary of major bacterial pathogens and the diseases they cause

Cocci	Disease
Staphylococcus aureus	Various localized and systemic infections
Beta hemolytic streptococcus, Group A	Pharyngitis, systemic infections, skin and muscle necrosis. Hypersensitivity response to organism causes rheumatic fever, nephritis.
Beta hemolytic streptococcus, Group B	Urinary tract and wound infections, systemic infection. Newborn infection acquired from vaginal organisms in mother.
Streptococci, other groups	Wound and urinary tract infections.
Streptococcus pneumoniae (Pneumococcus)	Middle ear and sinus infections. Systemic infection. Lobar pneumonia. Meningitis.
Neisseria gonorrhoeae (Gonococcus)	Genital tract infections. Bacteremia causing endocarditis, osteomyelitis, septic arthritis.
Neisseria meningiditis (Meningococcus)	Meningococcal meningitis.

Aerobic gram-positive rods	
Corynebacterium diphtheriae	Diphtheria. Clinical manifestations caused by toxin production.
Listeria monocytogenes	Systemic infection. Pregnant women may infect fetus. Persons with impaired immune system are very susceptible.

Aerobic spore-forming rods	
Bacillus anthracis	Primarily a disease of animals. People infected from contact with wool or animal products. Localized and systemic infection. Potential germ warfare agent.

Anaerobic spore-forming rods	
Clostridium perfringens	Gas gangrene. Muscle necrosis and hemolytic anemia caused by toxin. Gas formation in infected tissues.
Clostridium tetani	Tetanus (lockjaw) caused by toxin-induced spasm of voluntary muscles.
Clostridium botulinum	Botulism. Neuroparalytic toxin produced in improperly processed or canned foods.
Clostridium difficile	Antibiotic-associated colitis. Loss of normal intestinal flora caused by antibiotics allows overgrowth of Clostridia. Toxin produced by Clostridia damage bowel mucosa.

Gram-negative rods	
Haemophilus influenzae	Pulmonary infections. Meningitis in susceptible children.

continues

TABLE 6-2

Summary of major bacterial pathogens and the diseases they cause (cont.)

Gram-negative rods	Disease
Yersinia pestis	Plague. Disease of wild rodents transmitted to humans by fleas. Causes systemic infection. Can spread person-to-person if infection spreads to lungs (pneumonic plague).
Brucella species	Brucellosis. Febrile illness from contact with infected animals or consumption of raw milk from infected animals.
Francisella species	Tularemia. Febrile illness acquired from flesh of infected animals, usually wild rabbits, or transmitted to humans by bite of infected ticks or deer flies.
Legionella pneumophila	Legionnaires' disease. Organisms live in water and cause pulmonary infection in persons who inhale aerosolized droplets from showers, air conditioners, or other water sources. No person-to-person spread.
Salmonella species	Gastroenteritis and systemic infections. Infection acquired from contaminated food or water sources.
Shigella species	Dysentery with frequent watery stools. Spread by person-to-person contact, or by contaminated food and water.
Campylobacter species	Gastroenteritis. May cause systemic infection. Infects many animals. Humans infected from contaminated water, undercooked meat or poultry, or contact with infected animals.
Escherichia coli	Gastroenteritis, urinary tract and systemic infections. Some strains (O157:H7) produce toxins that cause hemolytic anemia and kidney damage.
Spiral organisms	
Treponema pallidum	Syphilis. Considered in the discussion on communicable diseases.
Borrelia burgdorferi	Lyme disease, transmitted from rodents to humans by ticks. Causes febrile illness and arthritis with lesion at site of tick bite.
Acid-fast bacteria	
Mycobacterium tuberculosis	Pulmonary tuberculosis. Considered in the discussion on the respiratory system.
Mycobacterium avium complex	A normally nonpathogenic organism that may cause an opportunistic infection in AIDS patients. See Case 8-3 in the discussion on communicable diseases.

and on the type of hemolysis the organism produces when grown on a solid medium containing blood. Generally, both the letter group and the type of hemolysis are specified when describing a streptococcus.

The serologic classification, called the Lancefield system, places the streptococci into twenty major groups based on differences in the carbohydrate antigens present in their cell walls. These groups are designated A through H and K through V, with most of the streptococci of medical importance in groups A, B, and D. The classification based on hemolysis describes the organisms as producing either alpha hemolysis, beta hemolysis, or no hemolysis on blood agar plates. Usually, both the Lancefield group and the type of hemolysis are specified when describing a streptococcus.

Alpha hemolytic streptococci (or simply alpha streptococci) produce green discoloration of the blood immediately around the colony and are often called *Streptococcus viridans* because of this growth characteristic (*viridans* = green). These organisms are normal inhabitants of the mouth and throat and usually are not pathogenic. They cannot be classified in the Lancefield system because they lack the carbohydrate antigen possessed by other streptococci.

Beta hemolytic streptococci (or simply beta streptococci) produce a narrow zone of complete hemolysis around the growing colony. One of the most important beta streptococci is in Lancefield group A and is called a group A beta streptococcus. Many group A beta streptococci are extremely pathogenic, causing streptococcal sore throat, scarlet fever, serious skin infections, and infections of the uterus after childbirth. Some produce a toxin that causes a toxic shock syndrome similar to that caused by toxin-producing staphylococci. One particularly virulent toxin-producing group A beta streptococcal strain causes a rapidly progressive, destructive infection of the subcutaneous tissues and the fibrous tissue (fascia) covering the adjacent muscles. This condition, called necrotizing fasciitis, may be complicated by necrosis (gangrene) of the overlying skin and by necrosis of the muscles in the infected area (streptococcal myositis).

In addition to causing infections in various tissues, some strains of group A beta streptococci are capable of inducing a state of hypersensitivity in susceptible individuals, leading to development of rheumatic fever or a type of kidney disease called glomerulonephritis. These diseases are considered in greater detail in the sections on the circulatory system (discussion on the cardiovascular system) and kidneys (discussion on the urinary system). Fortunately, group A beta streptococci still remain quite sensitive to penicillin and other antibiotics.

Beta streptococci in other Lancefield groups are also of medical importance. Group B beta streptococci may cause urinary tract and wound infections, but they are of greatest importance as a cause of serious infections in newborn infants. They often inhabit (colonize) the rectum and vagina of pregnant women, and the infant may become infected during labor and delivery. Because of the potential hazard of a life-threatening infection in an infant born to a mother colonized by group B beta streptococci, routine rectal and vaginal cultures to detect the organism are recommended for all pregnant women late in pregnancy. Those women who are colonized are treated with intravenous antibiotics during labor to reduce the risk of a serious group B beta streptococcal infection in the infant.

Group D streptococci and streptococci of other Lancefield groups may also cause various types of infections, but it is the group A beta streptococcus that is responsible for almost all of the late immunologic complications: rheumatic fever and glomerulonephritis.

Closely related to group D streptococci but classified separately are organisms that inhabit the intestinal tract called enterococci (*enteron* = bowel). These organisms are often very resistant to multiple antibiotics. Consequently, a wound or urinary tract infection caused by an enterococcus may be very difficult to treat.

Pneumococci

Pneumococci (*Streptococcus pneumoniae*) are gram-positive cocci and are classified with the streptococci. They grow in pairs and short chains and have certain biochemical characteristics setting them apart from other streptococci. Pneumococci are a common cause of bacterial pneumonia.

Gram-Negative Cocci

Most gram-negative cocci are nonpathogenic members of the genus *Neisseria* and are normal inhabitants of the upper respiratory passages. This group has two pathogenic members. The meningococcus (*Neisseria meningitidis*) causes a type of meningitis (inflammation of the membranes surrounding the brain and spinal cord) that frequently occurs in epidemics. The gonococcus (*Neisseria gonorrhoeae*) causes gonorrhea. This disease is transmitted by sexual contact and is discussed in greater detail in the discussion on communicable diseases.

Gram-Positive Bacilli

There are several important groups of gram-positive rod-shaped bacteria that can be subdivided on the basis of their oxygen requirements and on their ability to form spores. The two important groups of non–spore-forming aerobic bacteria are *Corynebacteria* and *Listeria*. The two important groups of spore-forming organisms are *Bacilli*, which are aerobic microorganisms, and *Clostridia*, which are anaerobic organisms.

Aerobic Non–Spore-Forming Gram-Positive Organisms. *Corynebacteria* are a large group of microorganisms. Most are nonpathogenic inhabitants of the skin and other squamous epithelium-lined body surfaces (mucous membranes). However, one member of this group (*Corynebacterium diphtheriae*) causes diphtheria. The organism causes an acute ulcerative inflammation of the throat and produces a potent toxin that can injure heart muscle and nerve tissue.

One important member of the *Listeria* group of microorganisms, called *Listeria monocytogenes*, can cause a very serious infection. The organism is widely distributed in nature: in the soil, on plants, and in the intestinal tract of people and animals. The organism may contaminate dairy products, raw vegetables, and other food products such as soft cheeses, hot dogs, and delicatessen foods. People become infected by eating *Listeria*-contaminated foods, and the persons at greatest risk for serious infections are infants and older people, pregnant women, and persons whose immune system is impaired. *Listeria* infection is a very serious systemic illness that may be complicated by spread of the organism to the brain and meninges, causing a meningitis or brain abscess. In pregnant women, the organism may also spread through the placenta to infect the unborn infant, leading to intrauterine fetal death or life-threatening infection of the infant.

Aerobic Spore-Forming Gram-Positive Organisms. Spore-forming aerobes are called *Bacilli*. Only one member of this group is highly pathogenic. This organism is *Bacillus anthracis*, which causes anthrax.

Anthrax is primarily a disease of animals that is rare in the United States, but is a more common animal infection in some other countries. Anthrax spores are highly resistant, can survive for many years in the soil, and can contaminate the hair, wool, or other tissues of animals from countries where anthrax is prevalent. If anthrax spores enter the body of a susceptible animal or person, the spores can germinate to form very large numbers of rapidly growing bacteria, which causes the disease anthrax.

Inhalation of anthrax spores from spore-contaminated wool, yarn, or other animal products causes a severe life-threatening pulmonary and systemic infection with an extremely high mortality. The spores germinate within the pulmonary alveoli, actively proliferate, and produce lethal toxins that cause extensive tissue destruction. Other spores are ingested by macrophages and transported to regional lymph nodes, where they continue to germinate and produce toxins. A vaccine to immunize against anthrax has been available for many years, and it is recommended for people at high risk of exposure to anthrax, such as veterinarians and employees of textile mills that process imported wool or similar animal products. The US military establishment has been quite concerned that anthrax spores may be used as a germ warfare agent because inhalation of spores is potentially lethal.

Concerns about the use of anthrax spores as a bioterrorism germ warfare agent became a reality in 2001 when a letter containing anthrax spores was mailed to a US senator, processed at a postal facility in Washington, DC, and opened in a senate office building. The spores contaminated the postal facility and senate office building, caused acute inhalation anthrax in five postal workers who worked in the facility where the letter was processed, and also exposed a number of persons who worked in the office building.

Persons who may have been exposed to anthrax spores require a prolonged course of antibiotics to prevent development of pulmonary anthrax because antibiotics effective against the germinated form of the anthrax bacillus are not effective against the spore form of the organism, and many spores do not germinate as soon as they are inhaled. Some are ingested by macrophages and transported to the regional lymph nodes, where they may continue to germinate for as long as 2 months after the initial exposure. The long course of antibiotics is required in order to destroy the antibiotic-sensitive vegetative bacteria as they germinate at various times from antibiotic-resistant spores.

Anaerobic Spore-Forming Gram-Positive Organisms. Anaerobic spore-forming bacilli are called *Clostridia*. These are normal inhabitants of the intestinal tract of animals and humans and are also found in the soil. Members of this group produce potent toxins and cause several important diseases. Some *Clostridia* cause gas gangrene. Some cause tetanus (lockjaw). Some cause botulism, and others cause an intestinal infection.

Gas gangrene, caused by *Clostridium perfringens* and related organisms, develops in dirty, spore-contaminated wounds. These anaerobic organisms germinate and proliferate in dead or devitalized tissues, especially in wounds where considerable necrosis of tissue has taken place. The *Clostridia* produce large amounts of gas by fermenting the necrotic tissues, and they also release powerful toxins that destroy tissues and cause widespread systemic effects.

Another clostridial species, *Clostridium tetani*, produces a potent toxin that causes spasm of voluntary muscles. The common term "lockjaw" comes from the marked rigidity of the jaw muscles that is a common feature of the disease. Tetanus may be fatal because of respiratory failure resulting from spasm of the muscles concerned with respiration.

Clostridium botulinum produces a potent neuroparalytic toxin. **Botulism** can generally be traced to eating improperly processed or canned foods in which the organism has grown and produced toxin. Botulism is actually a poisoning caused by the ingestion of toxin in food rather than a bacterial infection. Although botulism was more common when home canning was prevalent, outbreaks of botulism have been traced to contamination of canned tuna fish and canned soup prepared in commercial canneries.

Clostridium difficile is the organism responsible for the intestinal infection called *antibiotic-associated colitis* that sometimes follows use of broad-spectrum antibiotics and is considered in the discussion on the gastrointestinal tract.

Botulism
(bo'-chôô-lizm)
Food poisoning caused by ingestion of a neurotoxin produced by an anaerobic spore forming bacillus Clostridium botulinum *growing in improperly canned or preserved food.*

Gram-Negative Bacteria

There are many gram-negative organisms of clinical importance. Several different groups cause important diseases in humans. These are named *Haemophilus, Francisella, Yersinia, Brucella,* and *Legionella.* Members of the genus *Haemophilus* are normal inhabitants of the respiratory tract. One member of this group, *Haemophilus influenzae,* sometimes causes meningitis in infants and young children. Occasionally, it produces respiratory infections in patients with chronic lung disease. Another closely related organism was previously classified as *Haemophilus* but has been renamed *Gardnerella.* In conjunction with other bacteria, this organism causes a common vaginal infection called *nonspecific vaginitis* (discussion on the female reproductive system). One member of the genus *Yersinia* is responsible for bubonic plague. A member of the genus *Francisella* produces a somewhat similar illness called *tularemia.* Members of the genus *Brucella* cause disease in cattle, goats, and hogs that can be transmitted to people from contact with meat or other tissues from infected animals, or from drinking unpasteurized milk from infected cows or goats. In humans, the disease is a febrile illness without any specific features and responds to appropriate antibiotics. *Legionella* causes a serious respiratory illness called *Legionnaires disease.*

Other gram-negative organisms of medical importance include a number of closely related organisms that live in the gastrointestinal tract of people and animals. Other members of this group are free-living organisms, widely distributed in nature. Important pathogenic members of the group include Salmonella, Shigella, Campylobacter, and the cholera bacillus (*Vibrio cholerae*). These organisms cause various types of febrile illness and gastroenteritis. The organisms are excreted from the gastrointestinal tract in the feces of infected patients and are transmitted by contaminated food or water.

An organism closely related to *Campylobacter* but recently designated *Helicobacter* is of medical importance because it appears to cause chronic inflammation of the stomach lining (chronic gastritis) and stomach ulcers. This organism is considered in connection with the gastrointestinal tract (discussion on the gastrointestinal tract).

Other members of this large group are of only limited pathogenicity but sometimes produce disease when they are outside of their normal habitat in the gastrointestinal tract. These organisms may cause wound infections, urinary tract infections, and pulmonary infections in susceptible individuals. The best-known enteric bacterium is the colon bacillus (*Escherichia coli*), which is the predominant organism found within the intestinal tract of humans and animals. Some strains of the colon bacillus can produce various toxins that can cause intestinal symptoms ranging from a choleralike diarrhea to a dysentery-like acute inflammation of the intestinal tract. One well-known pathogenic strain is designated *E. coli 0157:H7*, the numbers referring to the antigens contained in the bacterial cell and its flagellae. This organism's toxin causes an acute inflammation of the colon characterized by bloody diarrhea and abdominal pain. Sometimes there is also an associated destruction of the patient's red blood cells, with marked anemia and impaired renal function with renal failure, called the hemolytic uremic syndrome. This pathogenic organism is present in the intestinal tract of infected cattle, and people usually become infected by consuming contaminated, incompletely cooked beef or by drinking raw milk. A recent outbreak of more than 500 cases, traced to a fast food restaurant chain, was caused by consumption of improperly cooked hamburgers prepared from beef contaminated with the organism.

Spiral Organisms

The spiral organisms can cause a wide variety of illnesses. The best-known member of this group is *Treponema pallidum,* which causes syphilis—one of the sexually transmitted diseases. These diseases are considered in the discussion on communicable diseases. Another spiral organism in this group is *Borrelia burgdorferi*, which causes **Lyme disease**. Named after a town in Connecticut where the disease was first recognized, it is now widespread in North America, Europe, and Australia. Transmission to humans is by the bite of an infected tick (*Ixodes dammini* and other *Ixodes* species). Most infections occur in the summer when exposure to ticks is frequent. Untreated Lyme disease typically progresses through three stages. In the first stage, a roughly circular, localized skin rash appears at the site of the tick bite and is frequently associated with flulike symptoms of fever, chills, and headaches, along with muscular and joint aches and pain. The rash and other manifestations eventually subside, but weeks or months later, many patients develop various neurologic, cardiac, and joint manifestations, which characterize the second stage of the disease. The third stage, which eventually develops in some untreated patients, is characterized by chronic arthritis and various neurologic problems. Diagnosis is usually made by means of various serologic tests, and the disease is usually treated with a tetracycline antibiotic.

Lyme disease
(lī′m)
A tick-borne systemic infection caused by a spiral organism, Borrelia burgdorferi, *characterized by neurologic, joint, and cardiac manifestations.*

Acid-Fast Bacteria

Acid-fast bacteria have a waxy capsule that is stained with difficulty by means of certain red dyes. After the organism has been stained, the stain-impregnated capsule resists decolorization with various acid solvents. This property, attributable to the capsule, is the reason for the term acid-fast, used to refer to this type of organism. Acid-fast bacteria cause a special type of chronic inflammatory reaction, called a chronic granulomatous inflammation, rather than the polymorphonuclear inflammatory reaction usually seen with bacterial infections.

The best-known acid-fast bacterium is the tubercle bacillus (*Mycobacterium tuberculosis*) responsible for tuberculosis. Mycobacteria, other than the tubercle bacillus, may at times cause a tuberculosis-like disease affecting lungs, lymph nodes, or skin, and some may cause severe systemic infections in immunocompromised persons. (Disseminated infection caused by *Mycobacterium avium* complex in persons with the acquired immune deficiency syndrome is described in the discussion on communicable diseases.) Another acid-fast bacterium (*Mycobacterium leprae*) causes leprosy.

ANTIBIOTIC TREATMENT OF BACTERIAL INFECTIONS

The discovery of antibiotic compounds and their widespread use to treat various types of infections has been one of the great advances in medicine. Antibiotics are substances that destroy bacteria or inhibit their growth. They are useful clinically because of their ability to injure bacterial cells without producing significant injury to the patient.

The bacterial cell is a complex structure containing genetic material, a protein-synthesizing mechanism, numerous enzyme systems concerned with intracellular metabolic functions, a semipermeable cell membrane, and a rigid cell wall. The bacterial genetic material is arranged as a circular DNA molecule that is attached to the cell membrane. Some bacteria also contain smaller circular DNA molecules, called plasmids, that contain genes coding for various properties useful to bacteria but often harmful to the persons infected by the bacteria. Such properties include resistance to antibiotics, toxin production, and formation of soluble factors that inhibit growth of normal bacterial flora, so the plasmid-bearing bacterium has a growth advantage over the bacterial flora with which it must compete. Antimicrobial substances act by

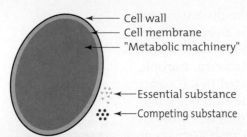

- Cell wall
- Cell membrane
- "Metabolic machinery"

- Essential substance
- Competing substance

FIGURE 6-2 Various sites of action of antibiotics. Antibiotics may act by disrupting the bacterial cell wall, by disturbing the functions of the cell membrane, or by interfering with the intracellular "metabolic machinery." Some antimicrobial drugs are not directly injurious to the bacterial cell, but compete with essential substances required for bacterial growth and multiplication.

interfering with the structure or function of the bacterial cell in one or more of the following ways (FIGURE 6-2):

1. Inhibition of cell-wall synthesis
2. Inhibition of cell-membrane function
3. Inhibition of metabolic functions
4. Competitive inhibition

Inhibition of Cell-Wall Synthesis

The bacterial cell has a high internal osmotic pressure, and the rigid outer cell wall maintains the shape of the bacterium. In some respects, the function of the cell wall can be compared with a corset or girdle supporting the enclosed cell. Penicillin and several other antibiotics act by inhibiting the synthesis of the bacterial cell wall so that the cell body is exposed. Because of the high osmotic pressure inside the bacterium, the relatively unsupported cell swells and eventually ruptures.

Inhibition of Cell-Membrane Function

The cell membrane is a semipermeable membrane surrounding the bacterial protoplasm. It controls the internal composition of the cell by regulating the diffusion of materials into and out of the cell. Some antibiotics act by inhibiting various functions of the cell membrane. Loss of the selective permeability of the cell membrane leads to cell injury and death.

Inhibition of Metabolic Functions

Some antibiotics interfere with nucleic acid or protein synthesis by bacteria so that the organisms are unable to carry out essential metabolic functions.

Competitive Inhibition

Some antibiotics resemble important compounds required by bacteria for growth and multiplication. The bacteria are unable to distinguish between the essential compound and the antibiotic that resembles it, but the antibiotic cannot be substituted for the required compound in the metabolic process. When the bacteria use the "wrong" compound rather than the "correct" substance, bacterial metabolism is disrupted, leading to inhibition of bacterial growth.

ANTIBIOTIC SENSITIVITY TESTS

In selecting antibiotics to treat a bacterial infection, the practitioner is aided by laboratory tests called antibiotic sensitivity tests. These tests measure, under standardized conditions, the ability of the antibiotic to inhibit the growth of the organism isolated from the patient. One method, called a tube dilution sensitivity test, consists of preparing various dilutions of antibiotics in test tubes and inoculating the tubes with the organism to be tested. The tubes are then incubated for a period of time in order to permit growth of the organism. Finally, determination of the highest dilution of antibiotic that inhibits the growth of the organism indicates the sensitivity of the organism to the drug.

Another method of sensitivity testing consists of inoculating the organism on a bacteriologic plate containing a culture medium. One then places several filter paper disks on the plate, each containing a standardized concentration of a different antibiotic. Next, the plate is incubated to allow the organism to grow. During incubation, the antibiotics in the disks diffuse into the surrounding culture. If the

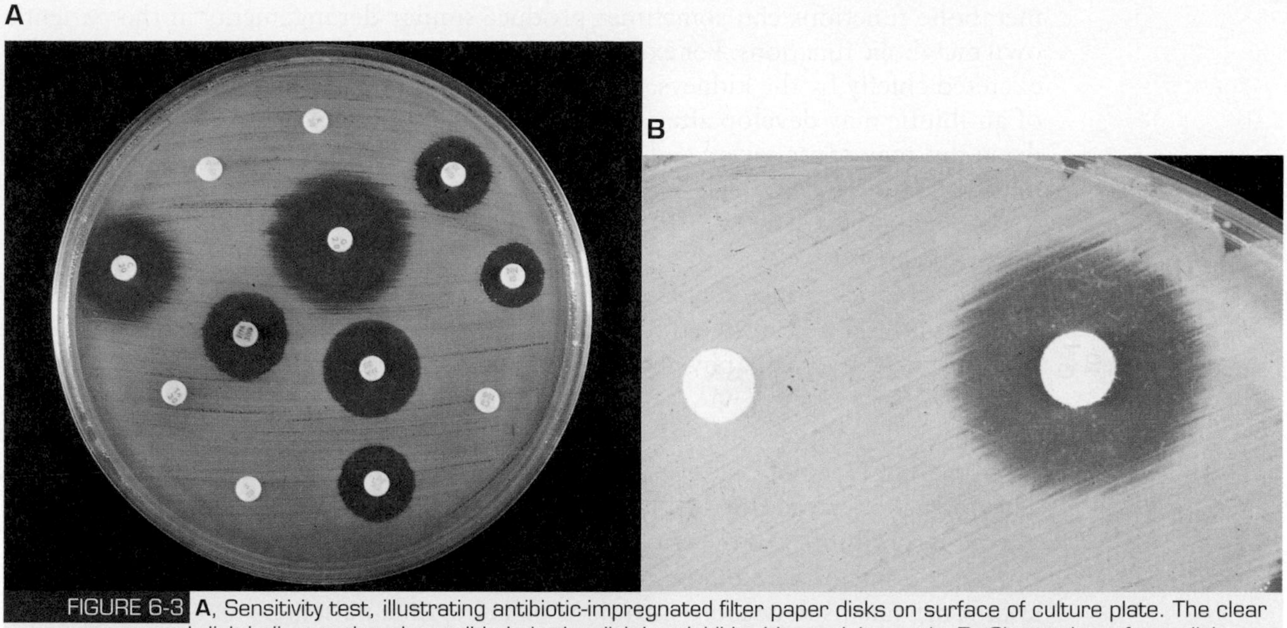

A

B

FIGURE 6-3 **A**, Sensitivity test, illustrating antibiotic-impregnated filter paper disks on surface of culture plate. The clear zone around disk indicates that the antibiotic in the disk has inhibited bacterial growth. **B**, Closer view of two disks on plate. The antibiotic contained in the disk on the *left* fails to inhibit growth of organism, which is *resistant* to antibiotic. The clear zone around antibiotic on the *right* indicates that the antibiotic in the disk inhibits the growth of the organism, which is *sensitive* to the antibiotic.

antibiotic is capable of inhibiting the organism, the organism is unable to grow in the area around the disk, and a circular clear zone free of bacterial growth appears (FIGURE 6-3). The organism is said to be sensitive to the antibiotic. On the other hand, if the growth of the organism is not influenced by the antibiotic, growth will not be inhibited around the disk, and the organism is said to be resistant to the antibiotic. The diameter of the zones of inhibition around the disks further indicates the sensitivity of the organism. The tube dilution and disk diffusion sensitivity test methods yield comparable results. The two methods are standardized so that the diameter of the zone of inhibition obtained by the disk diffusion method correlates with the antibiotic concentration required to inhibit the organism, as measured by the tube dilution method.

A bacteriology laboratory report that the organism is sensitive to a given antibiotic means that the organism probably can be inhibited by giving the patient the usual therapeutic dose of that drug. A report that the organism is resistant to an antibiotic indicates that a therapeutic dose of antibiotic is unlikely to inhibit the growth of the organism.

It should be emphasized, however, that the sensitivity of an organism to an antibiotic is only one factor influencing a patient's response to an infection. Other factors include the patient's own resistance and the antibiotic's ability to diffuse in sufficient quantities into the site of the infection.

ADVERSE EFFECTS OF ANTIBIOTICS

Toxicity

Antibiotics are useful because they are much more toxic to bacteria than they are to the patient. Antibiotics vary in their effects on people, but all are toxic to some degree. Some injure the kidneys; others injure nerve tissue or the blood-forming tissues. Penicillin and other antibiotics that act by interfering with bacterial cell-wall synthesis are relatively nontoxic, probably because the body cells have no structure comparable to the bacterial cell wall. Some antibiotics that interfere with bacterial metabolic functions can sometimes produce similar derangements in the patient's own metabolic functions. For example, tetracycline is a relatively nontoxic antibiotic, excreted chiefly by the kidneys. If renal function is impaired, very high blood levels of antibiotic may develop after administration of the usual therapeutic doses of the drug; this may cause severe and often fatal impairment of the patient's own cellular metabolic functions.

Hypersensitivity

Some antibiotics induce a marked hypersensitivity that can lead to a fatal reaction if the drug is later administered to a sensitized patient. Penicillin is capable of inducing extremely severe anaphylactic reactions, although the antibiotic itself has a very low toxicity.

Alteration of Normal Bacterial Flora

The normal bacterial flora in the oral cavity, the colon, and other locations may be altered by antibiotics. If the normal bacteria are destroyed, there may be overgrowth of resistant bacteria and fungi previously controlled by the normal flora. These resistant organisms may cause infections in susceptible patients.

Development of Resistant Strains of Bacteria

Some bacteria that are initially sensitive to antibiotics eventually become resistant. There are two ways in which an organism becomes resistant. It may undergo a spontaneous mutation that conveys resistance, or it may acquire a plasmid that contains resistance genes from another bacterium.

Spontaneous mutations do not occur frequently in cell division, but many bacteria divide so rapidly that spontaneous mutations can present a problem if the rapidly dividing bacteria are not quickly eliminated by the antibiotic. After a mutation that conveys antibiotic resistance occurs, the mutant organism has an advantage over its antibiotic-sensitive counterpart because it can flourish in the presence of the antibiotic while the antibiotic-sensitive organisms are eliminated.

Plasmid-acquired resistance can be a major problem because the transferred plasmid may convey resistance to multiple antibiotics, and plasmid transfers can take place between bacteria of different types. In this process, a bacterium with antibiotic-resistant genes carried on one of its plasmids (the donor) extends a thin cytoplasmic tube to contact another bacterium (the recipient), "reels in" the bacterium that it has contacted, and passes a copy of its plasmid to the recipient bacterium. Now both bacteria possess antibiotic-resistance plasmids, which they in turn can pass to other bacteria.

There are a number of mechanisms by which resistant bacteria can circumvent an antibiotic's effect. Such mechanisms include (1) developing enzymes to destroy the antibiotic, (2) either changing their cell-wall structure so that the antibiotic is unable to get into the cell or developing mechanisms to expel the antibiotic as soon as it enters the cell and before it can disturb bacterial functions, (3) changing their intracellular "metabolic machinery" so that the antibiotic is no longer able to disturb bacterial functions.

A few examples serve to illustrate the ingenuous adaptations of bacteria that thwart our efforts to eliminate them. A bacterium that is penicillin sensitive may develop an enzyme, penicillinase, that inactivates the antibiotic and allows the bacterium to survive in the presence of the drug. An antibiotic that acts against an enzyme required for a bacterial function, such as constructing a cell wall, may be rendered ineffective if the bacterium slightly alters the structure of its enzyme so that the antibiotic can no longer bind to the enzyme and inactivate it. An antibiotic that attaches to bacterial ribosomes, preventing protein synthesis, may be rendered ineffective if the bacterium slightly changes the structure of the ribosome so that the antibiotic can no longer act against it.

Widespread use of an antibiotic predisposes to the development of resistant strains. This may complicate the treatment of patients who become infected with antibiotic-resistant organisms. Staphylococci, in particular, have raised this problem because many strains isolated from hospital patients have been found to be highly resistant to a large number of antibiotics. Treatment of gonorrhea also has been complicated by the development of a high degree of penicillin resistance in many strains of gonococci; consequently, prolonged courses of therapy and much larger doses of antibiotic are required to eradicate the infections. Even the pneumococcus is no longer uniformly sensitive to penicillin, as it was in the past. Some strains are resistant to penicillin and other drugs normally used against them. Resistant strains of tubercle bacilli also have developed, hindering treatment of tuberculosis with antituberculosis drugs. On the other hand, some bacteria still remain quite sensitive to antibiotics. For example, group A beta streptococci remain sensitive to penicillin, despite widespread use of penicillin to treat streptococcal infections. *Treponema pallidum*, the organism responsible for syphilis, also has remained quite sensitive to penicillin, even though the drug has been used to treat syphilis for many years.

Chlamydiae

The chlamydiae are very small, gram-negative, nonmotile bacteria that were once thought to be large viruses. They are deficient in certain enzymes, and can live only as parasites inside of the cells of the individual that they infect. They are taken into the cells of the host by phagocytosis, where they divide to form large intracytoplasmic clusters of organisms called **inclusion bodies**. These resemble inclusion bodies formed in some viral diseases. Their growth can be inhibited by various antibiotics that inhibit protein synthesis, such as tetracycline and erythromycin. Some strains of chlamydiae are also inhibited by sulfonamide drugs.

Inclusion bodies
Spherical structures in the nucleus or cytoplasm of virus-infected cells.

Chlamydiae cause several different types of diseases. The most common chlamydial disease affects the genital tract and is transmitted by sexual contact. In the male, it causes an inflammation of the urethra called *nongonococcal urethritis*. In the female, it causes an inflammation of the uterine cervix that may spread to the fallopian tubes and ovaries as well. If a mother has a chlamydial infection of the cervix, infected secretions may get into her infant's eyes during childbirth and cause an inflammation called *inclusion conjunctivitis*. The name is based on the fact that characteristic inclusions can be demonstrated in the infected cells of the infant's conjunctiva. Other chlamydiae cause pulmonary infections. One species causes a disease of birds called psitticosis that is transmissible to humans and is manifested clinically as a type of pneumonia. Another species of chlamydiae causes an uncommon sexually transmissible disease called lymphogranuloma venereum. This disease is characterized by marked enlargement and inflammation of the lymph nodes in the groin and around the rectum.

Rickettsiae and Ehrlichiae

Rickettsiae are very small intracellular bacteria that can only multiply within the cells of an infected person. Many small animals and dogs are infected. The rickettsiae are transmitted to humans by insect bites, and they multiply in the endothelial cells of small blood vessels, which become swollen and necrotic, leading to thrombosis, rupture, and necrosis. Clinically, a rickettsial infection usually causes a febrile illness, often associated with a skin rash. Typhus and Rocky Mountain spotted fever are the most common rickettsial diseases. These organisms are sensitive to some antibiotics (tetracyclines and chloramphenicol). Similar organisms transmitted by ticks infect white blood cells rather than endothelial cells and are called Ehrlichiae (named after a famous immunologist, Paul Ehrlich). There are several species. Some infect neutrophils and others infect monocytes. The infected white cells contain small, compact clusters of organisms called morulae (singular, morula), which can be identified in blood smears. The disease called ehrlichiosis is a febrile illness similar to infections caused by rickettsiae and may be associated with a skin rash. Ehrlichiosis can be treated successfully with a tetracycline antibiotic but differs from rickettsial diseases in that ehrlichiosis does not respond to chloramphenicol.

Mycoplasmas

The mycoplasmas are very small bacteria that are very fragile because they lack a cell wall. One member of this group causes a type of pneumonia called primary atypical pneumonia. Mycoplasmas respond to the antibiotics tetracycline and erythromycin.

Viruses

Capsid
(kap′sid)
The protein covering the central nucleic acid core of a virus.

....

Capsomere
(kap′sō-mēr)
One of the subunits that make up the protein shell (capsid) of a virus.

Viruses are the smallest infectious agents. A typical virus consists of a molecule of nucleic acid (either DNA or RNA), its genome, enclosed within a protein shell called a **capsid**. The capsid is made of subunits called **capsomeres**, which are arranged in a precise geometric fashion around the genome. Many viruses are also covered by an outer lipid envelope acquired from the cytoplasm of the host cell when the virus buds from the cell that it has infected. Projections from the surface of the virus allow the virus to attach to the cell that it will infect. Viruses vary greatly in size. The smallest are only slightly larger than protein molecules, whereas the largest viruses approach the size of a bacterium.

The nucleic acid of the virus genome may be arranged in either a single or a double strand and the complexity of the viral genome varies. Some viruses have as many as 400 genes within their nucleic acid structure, whereas others have as few as eight. Viruses have few metabolic enzymes and therefore must rely on the cells of the infected person to carry out their activities. When a virus invades the cell, the viral genome directs the metabolic processes of the cell to synthesize more virus particles. In many respects, the virus may be likened to a criminal who takes over a business, forcing it to function for the criminal's benefit rather than for the benefit of the owner (FIGURE 6-4).

CLASSIFICATION OF VIRUSES

An older classification of viruses was based on the major clinical features of the viral infection, and viruses were classified on the basis of the portion of the body or organ system in which the viral infection produced the most prominent clinical manifestations. A more modern classification categorizes viruses on the basis of their nucleic acid structure, size, structural configuration, and biologic characteristics. In this classification, several large groups of viruses are recognized, and a large number of viruses are identified in each group. TABLE 6-3 presents a simplified classification of viruses and the diseases they cause.

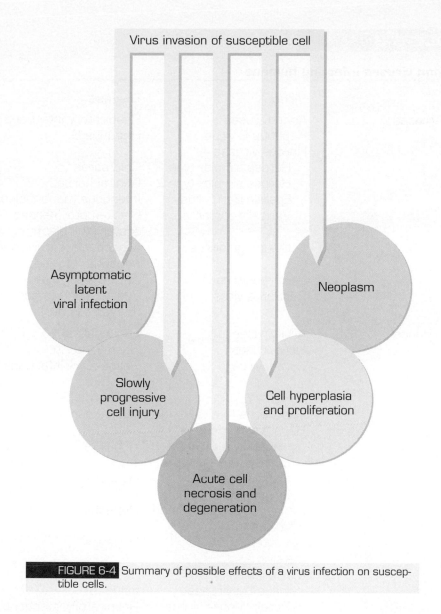

FIGURE 6-4 Summary of possible effects of a virus infection on susceptible cells.

MODE OF ACTION

A distinction is sometimes made between a viral infection and a viral disease. A condition in which a virus infects a cell without causing any evidence of cell injury is considered a latent viral infection. Many viruses are capable of coexisting with normal cells in lymphoid tissue and the gastrointestinal tract, and probably in other sites, without causing cellular injury. Such viruses are able to live for long periods within the cells of the infected host while they continually discharge virus particles. Other viruses are more virulent and regularly produce cell injury, manifested by necrosis and degeneration of the infected cell. This is called a cytopathogenic effect. Some cytopathogenic effects are shown in FIGURES 6-5 and 6-6. Some viruses induce cell hyperplasia and proliferation rather than cell necrosis. These effects are shown in FIGURES 6-7 and 6-8. Many viruses induce various combinations of cell damage and cell hyperplasia.

Under certain circumstances, a latent asymptomatic viral infection may become activated, leading to actual disease. The herpes virus, which infects both the oral cavity and the genital tract, may persist in the tissues of the host for many years.

TABLE 6-3

Common viruses infecting humans

	Virus	Disease
DNA viruses	Adenoviruses	Respiratory infections
	Hepatitis B virus	Hepatitis B
	Herpes viruses	
	Herpes simplex type 1	Cold sores
	Herpes simplex type 2	Genital herpes
	Epstein-Barr virus	Infectious mononucleosis
	Varicella-zoster virus	Chicken pox, herpes zoster (shingles)
	Cytomegalovirus	Mononucleosis-like illness, hepatitis
	Herpesvirus 8	Kaposi's sarcoma
	Papilloma virus	Warts, condylomas (benign tumors)
RNA viruses	Arboviruses	Encephalitis
	Noroviruses	Gastroenteritis
	Coronavirus	Respiratory infections
		Severe acute respiratory syndrome (SARS)
	Hantavirus (bunyavirus)	Acute respiratory illness
	Hepatitis viruses	
	Hepatitis A virus (picornavirus)	Hepatitis
	Hepatitis C virus (flavivirus)	Hepatitis
	Hepatitis D virus (coated with HbsAg)	Hepatitis
	Hepatitis E virus (calicivirus)	Hepatitis
	Myxoviruses	
	Influenza viruses	Influenza
	Parainfluenza viruses	Respiratory infections, croup
	Respiratory syncytial viruses	Respiratory infections
	Measles virus	Measles
	Mumps virus	Mumps
	Picornaviruses	
	Coxsackie viruses	Pharyngitis, myocarditis, pericarditis
	Echoviruses	Respiratory infections, gastroenteritis
	Hepatitis A virus	Hepatitis A
	Polioviruses	Poliomyelitis
	Rhinoviruses	Respiratory infections
	Rabies virus (rhabdovirus)	Rabies
	Retroviruses	
	HIV	AIDS
	HTLV 1	Adult T-cell leukemia
	Rubella virus (togavirus)	German measles

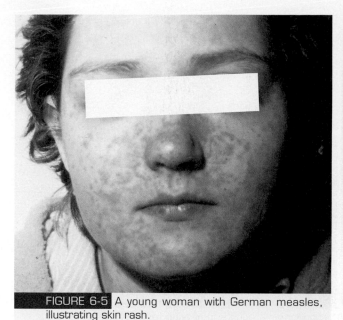

FIGURE 6-5 A young woman with German measles, illustrating skin rash.

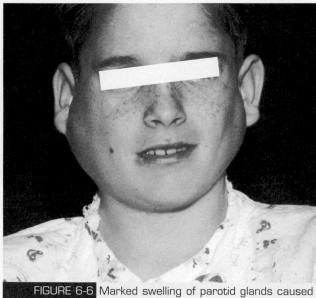

FIGURE 6-6 Marked swelling of parotid glands caused by the mumps virus.

The virus periodically becomes activated and causes crops of painful vesicles that may recur during an intercurrent febrile illness, when the patient's immunologic defenses have been disrupted by a neoplasm or by various other diseases, or sometimes for no apparent reason (FIGURE 6 9).

Another member of the herpes group of viruses is the varicella-zoster virus, named from its two different manifestations. The initial contact with the virus causes chicken pox (varicella), which is an extremely contagious disease characterized by an itchy

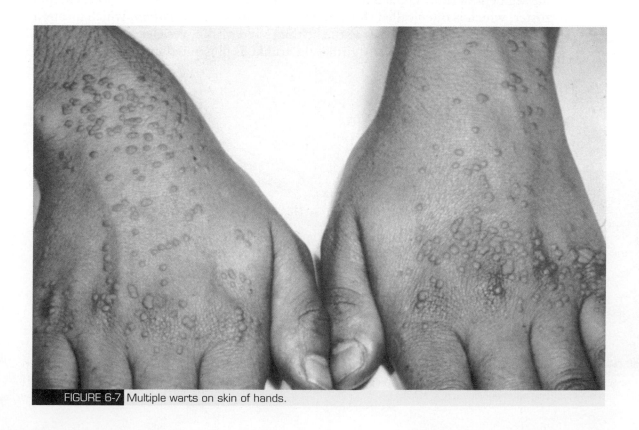

FIGURE 6-7 Multiple warts on skin of hands.

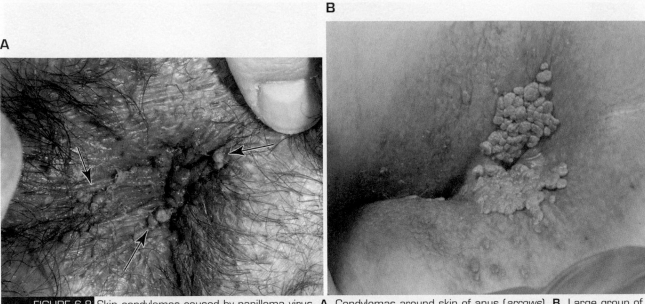

FIGURE 6-8 Skin condylomas caused by papilloma virus. **A**, Condylomas around skin of anus (*arrows*). **B**, Large group of condylomas involving skin of buttocks around gluteal cleft.

Herpes zoster
A skin rash caused by re-activation of the varicella-zoster virus that caused chicken pox.

Shingles
Another name for herpes zoster.

skin rash that usually soon subsides without any serious complications. A person who has had chicken pox develops an immunity and cannot contract chicken pox again. However, the virus is not eradicated by the immune system and remains dormant within sensory nerve ganglia. Sometimes the virus becomes active again within a sensory ganglion many years later and then travels in the nerve associated with the ganglion to the skin, where it causes a characteristic bandlike vesicular skin rash in the segment of skin supplied by the sensory nerve. The recurrent infection is **herpes zoster**, which is often called **shingles**, from a Latin word, *cingulum*, which means a belt or girdle. The term refers to the beltlike band of skin vesicles along the course of a spinal nerve that partially girdles the trunk, as illustrated in FIGURE 6-10.

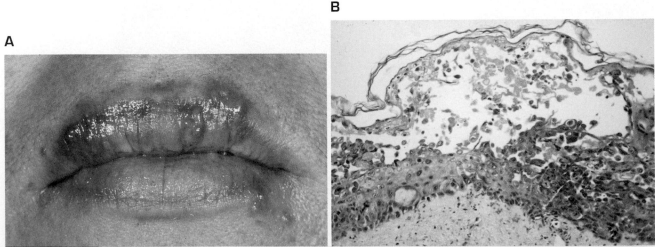

FIGURE 6-9 Herpes virus infection. **A**, Recurrent oral herpes caused by herpes virus type 1. **B**, Section of small herpes blister (vesicle). The superficial skin layer is almost completely destroyed, and a superficial ulcer will form when the surface epithelium sloughs (original magnification × 100).

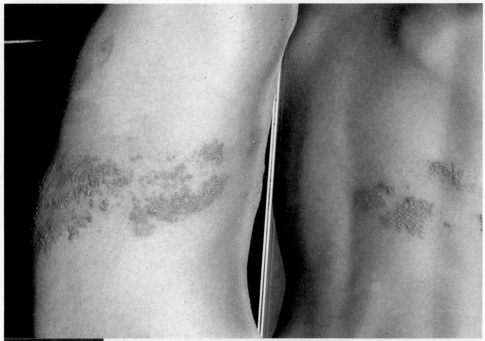

FIGURE 6-10 One type of herpes virus infection (called *shingles* or *herpes zoster*) characterized by clusters of vesicles that occur in a segment of skin (dermatome) supplied by a sensory nerve. The subject was photographed beside a mirror in order to illustrate the bandlike distribution of the rash in the segment of skin supplied by a spinal nerve.

Herpes zoster is a late complication of the varicella-zoster virus (VZV) infection and can be complicated by chronic pain in the distribution of the previously affected nerve, which is called post–herpes-zoster neuralgia. Chicken pox had been a very common disease before the introduction of a live virus varicella-zoster vaccine in 1996. Over 95% of persons living in the United States had developed chicken pox by the time they were 20 years old, and they were at risk for later reactivation of the virus followed by development of herpes zoster. However, they had also developed a cell-mediated immune response resulting from chicken pox, which tended to suppress reactivation of the latent virus. When chicken pox was prevalent, previously infected adults who later were exposed to chicken pox–infected children, received additional exposures to the virus, which functioned as booster doses to maintain their cell-mediated immunity. In the postvaccination era, childhood chicken pox did not occur very often, and the cell-mediated immunity of previously infected adults declined as they age, which increased the risk that the latent virus might become activated to cause herpes zoster and its associated complications.

A live virus vaccine called Zostavax was developed to help prevent herpes zoster and is recommended for older adults to help boost their immunity against VZV. The vaccine provided an immunologic response similar to one achieved when previously infected adults were exposed to children with chicken pox. A clinical investigation compared the frequency of herpes zoster in a large group of older adults who received the herpes zoster vaccine with a comparable unvaccinated group, which indicated a 55% reduction of herpes zoster in the vaccine-treated group. Although the vaccine helps prevent herpes zoster, it does not prevent all cases and it is not effective once herpes zoster has developed. To treat patients with herpes zoster, a number of medications similar to acyclovir (used to treat oral and genital herpes) are helpful to shorten the duration and severity of herpes zoster and may also reduce the pain often associated with the skin rash.

Inclusion bodies
Spherical structures in the nucleus or cytoplasm of virus-infected cells.

Interferon
(in-tur-fēr'on)
A broad-spectrum antiviral agent manufactured by various cells in the body.

Humoral immunity
Immunity associated with formation of antibodies produced by plasma cells.

Cell-mediated defense mechanism
The defense against foreign antigens provided by a population of T lymphocytes that can attach and destroy the foreign antigens.

Inclusion Bodies in Viral Disease

Tissues that are infected with virus frequently contain spherical, densely staining structures called **inclusion bodies** (FIGURE 6-11). These are present within the nucleus or the cytoplasm or both locations. Inclusion bodies consist of masses of virus or products of virus multiplication. The presence of inclusion bodies may be of considerable diagnostic aid in recognizing viral infection and determining the type of viral disease present.

BODILY DEFENSES AGAINST VIRAL INFECTIONS

The body responds to a viral infection by forming a protein substance called **interferon** and by activating **humoral immunity** and **cell-mediated defense mechanisms**.

Formation of Interferon

Interferon is a general term for a group of carbohydrate-containing proteins produced by cells in response to viral infection and was named from its ability to "interfere" with viral multiplication. Interferon functions as a nonspecific, "broad-spectrum" antiviral agent. It inhibits not only the virus that induced its formation, but other viruses as well. This is in contrast with the behavior of a specific antiviral antibody, which reacts only to the virus that induced its formation. Many cells are capable of producing interferon, but monocytes and lymphocytes are the primary sources. Several different interferons are produced, each designated by a Greek letter. Interferons provide a rapid "first-line" defense against a viral infection. By slowing viral growth during the early phase of the infection, the infected person is allowed time to mobilize humoral and cell-mediated responses directed against the invading virus.

In addition to their antiviral activity, interferons have other actions concerned with regulation of the immune system and cell growth. These functions are considered in the discussion on neoplastic disease.

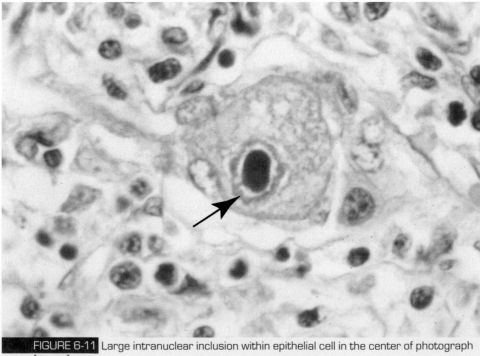

FIGURE 6-11 Large intranuclear inclusion within epithelial cell in the center of photograph (*arrow*).

Humoral and Cell-Mediated Immunity in Viral Infections

The body also forms specific antiviral antibodies that are capable of inactivating viruses and may actually destroy virus particles in the presence of complement. Antiviral antibodies cannot combine with the virus, however, unless the virus particles are discharged into the extracellular fluid where they are exposed to the action of the antibody. Consequently, antiviral antibodies are relatively inefficient in combating viruses that spread directly from cell to cell because the virus particles remain within the infected cells and are protected from the antibody. For example, persons who have recurrent fever blisters caused by the herpes virus possess antibodies to the virus, but the antibody is often unable to eradicate the intracellular virus particles.

In addition to producing specific antiviral antibodies, the immune defenses of the host are directed against the virus-infected cells. This occurs because viruses that invade cells often induce the formation of new antigens on the surface of the infected cells. These antigens are recognized as foreign by the host's immune defenses and induce both humoral and cell-mediated immune reactions directed against the virus-infected cells. Antibodies are formed that affix to the infected cells and destroy them in the presence of complement. Sensitized lymphocytes release lymphokines, which damage the cells, and they also produce interferon, which inhibits the multiplication of viruses. Chemical mediators that induce an acute inflammatory reaction also are liberated (discussion on inflammation and repair). In many viral infections, much of the tissue injury is caused, not by proliferation of the virus within the cells of the host, but by the inflammation and tissue destruction caused by the body's attempts to rid itself of the virus-infected cells.

TREATMENT WITH ANTIVIRAL AGENTS

Because viruses are simple structures lacking a cell wall, a cell membrane, and the complex "metabolic machinery" of bacteria, they are not susceptible to the disruptive actions of antibiotics. Some chemotherapeutic agents that are active against viruses have been developed, however. In many cases, their mechanisms of action are similar to those of compounds used to treat cancer (discussion on neoplastic disease). Some antiviral agents active against DNA viruses either block synthesis of DNA or induce the formation of an abnormal, nonfunctional DNA, thereby preventing virus multiplication. Another agent active against RNA viruses causes the formation of an abnormal messenger RNA that disrupts viral multiplication. Unfortunately, many compounds that block viral multiplication by such mechanisms also have a similar adverse effect on the host cells and may be as toxic to the host as to the virus. For this reason, antiviral agents have had limited application in clinical medicine.

Newer antiviral agents are being developed, however, that are less toxic and promise to be more useful. One such drug is effective against some infections caused by the herpes group of viruses. The drug is activated within the virus-infected cells by a viral enzyme to yield the active antiviral compound that selectively inhibits synthesis of viral DNA within the cells in which the virus is replicating.

Fungi

Fungi are plantlike organisms without chlorophyll and are subdivided into two large groups: yeasts and molds. Yeasts are small ovoid or spherical cells that reproduce by budding. Molds, when grown on suitable media at room temperature, form large colonies composed of multiple branching filamentous structures called **hyphae** (singular, hypha) (FIGURE 6-12). The matted mass of hyphae, which is called a **mycelium**, is responsible for the characteristic appearance of the colony

Hyphae
(hī′fāy)
Filamentous branching structures formed by fungi.

Mycelium
(mī-sē′lē-yum)
Matted mass of hyphae forming a fluffy colony characteristic of fungi.

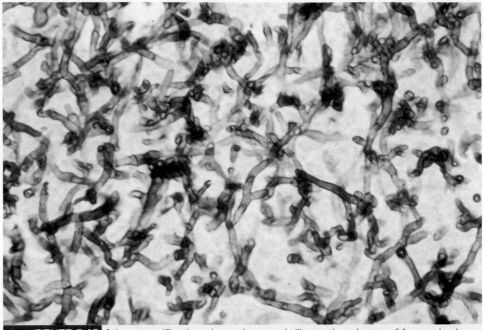

FIGURE 6-12 A low-magnification photomicrograph illustrating cluster of fungus hyphae (original magnification × 160).

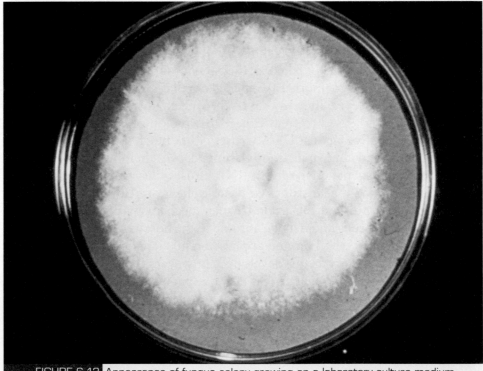

FIGURE 6-13 Appearance of fungus colony growing on a laboratory culture medium.

(FIGURE 6-13). Some pathogenic fungi exhibit two different growth phases, forming typical mycelial colonies on laboratory culture media but forming small yeastlike structures in the tissues of the infected individual.

Some fungi live on the skin and only occasionally cause minor discomfort. Others are found in small numbers in the oral cavity, gastrointestinal tract, and vagina, where they live in harmony with the normal bacterial flora. Most fungi have a limited ability to cause disease. Under special circumstances, however, fungi may produce serious localized or systemic infections in susceptible individuals. Two major factors predispose to systemic fungal infections: disturbance in the normal bacterial flora and impaired immunologic defenses.

After intensive therapy with broad-spectrum antibiotics, the normal bacterial flora of the oral cavity, colon, vagina, and other areas may be altered or completely eradicated, disturbing the normal balance between the bacterial flora and fungi. Normally, the predominance of the bacterial flora holds the fungi in check. When the bacteria are eliminated, the fungi may proliferate and cause disease.

Patients with various types of chronic debilitating diseases may be susceptible to fungal infections. Infections of this type are also encountered in patients whose immunologic defense mechanisms have been depressed by various drugs and chemicals or by radiation therapy. Patients with certain types of cancer, particularly those treated with cytotoxic drugs, may also develop systemic fungal infections.

SUPERFICIAL FUNGAL INFECTIONS

The common superficial fungal infections of the skin are caused by a group of fungi called **dermatophytes,** which grow on the skin. They cause itchy, scaling skin lesions on the scalp and on other parts of the body. Some have been given such picturesque, popular names as "athlete's foot" and "jock itch." A common superficial fungal infection of the mucous membranes is caused by a yeastlike fungus called *Candida albicans.* This organism is a common cause of vaginal infections, producing symptoms of itching and vaginal discharge (FIGURE 6-14). Pregnant women and women taking oral contraceptive pills seem more susceptible to *Candida* infection, as are persons treated with broad-spectrum antibiotics such as tetracycline. A number of antifungal drugs are available that can be applied locally to treat infections caused by dermatophytes and *Candida.*

Dermatophyte
(der-mat′o-fīt)
A fungus that causes a superficial infection of the skin.

Histoplasmosis
(his′tō-plas-mō′sis)
An infection caused by the fungus Histoplasma capsulatum.

HIGHLY PATHOGENIC FUNGI

Although most fungi are at best only potential pathogens of low virulence, two are highly infectious and frequently produce disease in humans. They can be identified by biopsy or by culture of infected tissues. The fungus *Histoplasma capsulatum,* which is found in many parts of the United States, causes the disease **histoplasmosis.** This organism is found in the soil. People become infected by inhaling dust containing spores of the fungus. In most cases, the fungus produces an acute, self-limited respiratory infection. Less commonly, the organism causes a more chronic pulmonary infection similar to tuberculosis. In some cases, a progressive, disseminated, sometimes fatal disease develops. Another fungus, *Coccidioides immitis,* which is found in parts of California and elsewhere in the southwestern part

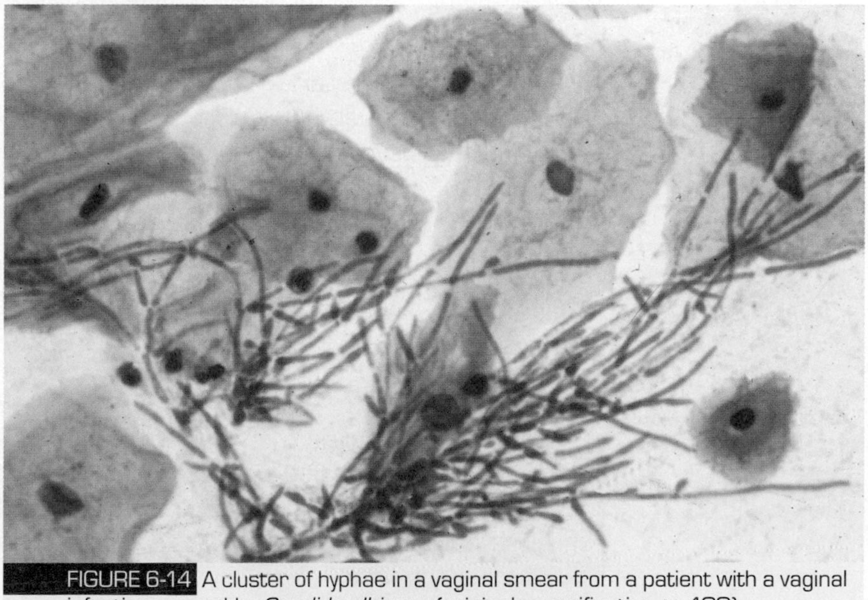

FIGURE 6-14 A cluster of hyphae in a vaginal smear from a patient with a vaginal infection caused by *Candida albicans* (original magnification × 400).

Coccidioidomycosis
(kok-sid-ē-oy′dō-
mī-kō′sis)
*A disease caused by
the pathogenic fungus*
Coccidioides immitis.

of the United States, causes the disease **coccidioidomycosis.** As in the case of histoplasmosis, humans become infected by inhaling dust that contains fungus spores. The symptoms are similar to those of histoplasmosis. Coccidioidomycosis is usually manifested as an acute pulmonary infection, but sometimes the fungus causes chronic or severe progressive systemic disease.

OTHER FUNGI OF MEDICAL IMPORTANCE

Blastomycosis
(blast-ō-mīkō′sis)
*A systemic fungus infec-
tion caused by the fungus*
Blastomyces dermatiditis.

Two other pathogenic fungi of medical importance are *Blastomyces dermatitidis,* which causes the disease **blastomycosis,** and *Cryptococcus neoformans,* which causes *cryptococcosis.* Infections caused by these organisms are less common than either histoplasmosis or coccidioidomycosis. Both organisms are found in the soil, and infection is caused by inhalation of dust containing the organisms.

Clinically, blastomycosis is similar to histoplasmosis and coccidioidomycosis. Most infections are acute and self-limited. Occasionally, the fungus causes a more chronic pulmonary infection or a widespread systemic disease.

Cryptococcus neoformans is a yeastlike organism that has a large mucoid capsule. The organism initially causes a pulmonary infection but then may be transported in the bloodstream to the meninges of the brain, where it causes a chronic meningitis. The organisms can be identified in smears and cultures of spinal fluid.

TREATMENT OF SYSTEMIC FUNGAL INFECTIONS

Acute pulmonary infections caused by fungi frequently subside spontaneously and do not require treatment. Chronic or progressive systemic fungal infections are treated with various antifungal antibiotics, as illustrated by the following cases.

CASE 6-1

A young man who had resided for a short time in the southwestern United States consulted his physician and was found to have a dense infiltrate in the upper lobe of the lung with the formation of a cavity, suggesting tuberculosis. However, cultures of sputum for tubercle bacilli were negative. A specimen from the affected area was obtained by means of a flexible bronchoscope, and material for culture also was obtained. *Coccidioides immitis* was cultured from the involved area. Biopsy revealed only nonspecific chronic inflammation. No organisms were identified in the biopsy specimen. The patient was treated with an antifungal antibiotic and made an uneventful recovery.

CASE 6-2

A 39-year-old diabetic man was admitted to the hospital with cough and fever, and chest x-ray revealed a large area of consolidation in the left lung (FIGURE 6-15). Bronchial biopsy revealed nonspecific chronic inflammation, but cultures revealed growth of *Blastomyces dermatitidis.* The patient responded to treatment with antifungal antibiotics.

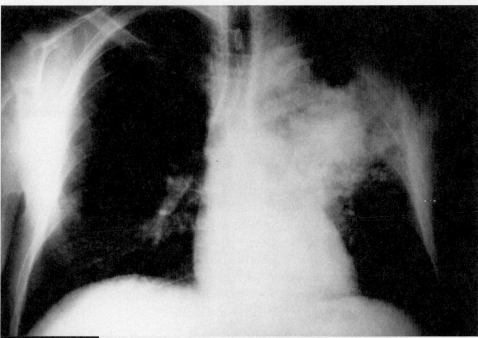

FIGURE 6-15 Chest x-ray illustrating a blastomycosis of the left lung (*right side* of photograph), which appears as a dense (white) area occupying the upper part of the lung. The right lung (*left side* of photograph) appears normal (case 6-2).

QUESTIONS FOR REVIEW

1. By what standards are bacteria classified? Name the classifications.
2. What is the Gram-stain test procedure? What important diseases are caused by the following bacteria: staphylococci, beta streptococci, pneumococci, gonococci, and acid-fast bacteria?
3. What is meant by the following terms: *granulomatous inflammation*, *gram-positive organism*, and *Legionella*?
4. How do antibiotics inhibit the growth of bacteria? How does penicillin kill bacteria?
5. How do bacteria become resistant to an antibiotic?
6. What are some of the potential harmful effects of antibiotics?
7. What is meant by the following terms: *competitive inhibition*, *sensitivity test*, *resistant organism*, and *cell membrane*?
8. How does a viral infection affect a susceptible cell?
9. What is a latent (asymptomatic) viral infection? Give an example.
10. What is meant by the following terms: *inclusion body*, *chlamydiae*, and *mycoplasma*?
11. What factors render a patient susceptible to an infection by a fungus of low pathogenicity?
12. What are the names of the two highly pathogenic fungi? What type of disease do they produce?
13. A young woman receives a course of antibiotics and soon afterward develops a vaginal infection caused by a fungus. Why?

SUPPLEMENTARY READINGS

Centers for Disease Control and Prevention. 2001. Update: Outbreak of acute febrile respiratory illness among college students—Acapulco, Mexico, March 2001. *Morbidity and Mortality Weekly Report* 50:359–60.

▶ 229 students from 44 colleges in 22 states who went to Acapulco during spring developed acute histoplasmosis characterized by cough, shortness of breath, chest pain, or headache. They stayed at several different hotels during spring break, but one hotel was associated with the largest number of cases.

Centers for Disease Control and Prevention. 2000. Coccidioidomycosis in travelers returning from Mexico—Pennsylvania. *Morbidity and Mortality Weekly Report* 49:1004–6.

▶ 35 church members from two cities in Pennsylvania spent a week in Mexico to construct a church, and 27 developed acute coccidioidomycosis (CM) within 2 weeks after returning home. Travel to endemic areas is becoming more frequent and presents a special risk to elderly and persons with impaired immunity, who may develop severe pulmonary disease or widely disseminated disease.

Centers for Disease Control and Prevention. 2001. Coccidioidomycosis in workers at an archeologic site—Dinosaur National Monument, Utah, June–July 2001. *Morbidity and Mortality Weekly Reports* 50:1005–8.

▶ Under the direction of National Park Service (NPS) archaeologists, six student volunteers and two leaders worked at an archaeological site. All eight team members and two NPS archaeologists developed acute coccidioidomycosis with pulmonary symptoms and abnormal chest x-rays, and eight were hospitalized.

Colditz, G. A., Brewer, T. F., Berkey, C. S., et al. 1994. Efficacy of BCG vaccine in the prevention of tuberculosis. Meta-analysis of the published literature. *Journal of the American Medical Association* 271:698–702.

▶ BCG vaccination produces cell-mediated immunity against the tubercle bacillus and reduces the risk of infection.

Inglesby, T. V., O'Toole, T., Henderson, D. A., et al. 2002. Anthrax as a biological weapon, 2002: Updated recommendations for management. *Journal of the American Medical Association* 287:2236–52.

▶ Inhalation anthrax follows germination of spores in the alveoli. Macrophages ingest the spores, and some are destroyed. Surviving spores are transmitted to mediastinal lymph nodes. A long course of antibiotics is required because antibiotics are not effective against spores, and spores may continue to germinate for some time after the spores enter the body. Penicillin, doxycycline, and ciprofloxacin are appropriate antibiotics.

Klevens, R. M., Morrison, M. A., Nadle, J., et al. 2007. Invasive methicillin-resistant *Staphylococcus aureus* infections in the United States. *Journal of the American Medical Association* 298:1763–71.

▶ Invasive methicillin-resistant staphylococcal infections (MRSA) were classified as either healthcare associated (in hospital facilities or in community-based healthcare facilities) or community associated (patients without healthcare risk factors for MRSA). Invasive MRSA is a major public-health problem related to healthcare but has spread into the community and is no longer confined to healthcare institutions.

Omer, S. B., Salmon, D. A., Orenstein, W. A., et al. 2009. Vaccine refusal, mandatory immunization, and the risks of vaccine-preventable diseases. *New England Journal of Medicine* 360:1981–88.

▶ The success of an immunization program depends on high rates of acceptance and coverage. Rates of refusal of immunization are increasing, and clustering of refusals leads to outbreaks of vaccine-preventable diseases. Children with exemptions from school immunization requirements, which is a measure of vaccine refusal, are at increased risk for measles and pertussis. In turn, they can infect others who are too young to be vaccinated, cannot be vaccinated for medical reasons, or were vaccinated but did not achieve a sufficient immunologic response. Clinicians can play a crucial role in promoting vaccination by respectfully listening to parents' concerns and discussing the risks and benefits of immunization.

Phares, C. R., Lynfield, R., Farley, M. M., et al. 2008. Epidemiology of invasive group B streptococcal disease in the United States, 1999–2005. *Journal of the American Medical Association* 299:2056–65.

▶ Revised disease-prevention guidelines have led to a lower incidence of group B streptococcal disease in infants, but has been associated with a greater number of invasive streptococcal disease cases in older children and adults. The increased frequency affects black populations of all age groups, as well as pregnant women.

Whitley, R. J. 2009. A 70-year-old woman with shingles: Review of herpes zoster. *Journal of the American Medical Association* 302:73–80.

▶ Herpes zoster is a common late complication of the varicella-zoster virus (VZV) exposure and can be complicated by chronic pain in the distribution of the previously affected nerve (post–herpes-zoster neuralgia). As the cell-mediated immunity of previously infected adults directed against VZV declines as they age, the risk increases that a latent virus may become activated to cause herpes zoster and its associated complications. The currently available vaccine to prevent herpes zoster in adults acts by boosting the subject's cell-mediated immune response to VZV. Although the vaccine helps prevent herpes zoster, it is not effective once herpes zoster has developed. A number of medications similar to acyclovir (used to treat oral and genital herpes) are helpful to shorten the duration and severity of herpes zoster and may also reduce the pain often associated with the skin rash.

OUTLINE SUMMARY

Types of Harmful Microorganisms

Bacteria

CLASSIFICATION

Shape: coccus, bacillus, spiral.
Gram stain: gram-positive and gram-negative.
Biochemical and cultural characteristics:
aerobic and anaerobic.
Spore formation.
"Biochemical profile" aids identification.
Antigenic structure: antigens in cell body, capsule, flagella.

DISEASES CAUSED BY PATHOGENIC BACTERIA

Staphylococci: inhabit skin and nasal cavity; cause boils, pulmonary infection.

Streptococci:
Alpha streptococci: normal inhabitants of respiratory tract.
Beta streptococci: cause strep sore throat, scarlet fever, skin infections, uterine infections.
Gamma streptococci: limited pathogenicity.
Pneumococci: pneumonia.
Gram-negative cocci:
Meningococci cause meningitis.
Gonococci cause gonorrhea.
Gram-positive bacilli:
Aerobic: diphtheria bacillus, Listeria.
Anaerobic: clostridia cause gas gangrene, tetanus, botulism.
Gram-negative bacteria: a large diverse group that causes various systemic and intestinal infections.
Spiral organisms: syphilis, Lyme disease.
Acid-fast organisms: tuberculosis.

Antibiotic Treatment of Bacterial Infection

Inhibits cell wall synthesis.
Inhibits cell membrane function.
Inhibits metabolic functions of bacterium.
Competitive inhibition.

ANTIBIOTIC SENSITIVITY TESTS

Tube dilution: measures highest dilution inhibiting growth in test tube.
Disk method: inhibition of growth around disk indicates sensitivity to antibiotic.

BACTERIAL RESISTANCE TO ANTIBIOTICS

Bacteria develop enzymes that inactivate antibiotic—for example, penicillinase.
Bacteria develop other mechanisms that circumvent effects of antibiotics.

ADVERSE EFFECTS OF ANTIBIOTICS

Toxicity: almost all have some toxicity, which varies with the antibiotic.
Hypersensitivity: may cause fatal reaction if given to sensitized patient.
Alteration of normal bacterial flora: disturbs normal bacterial flora and allows overgrowth of pathogens.
Development of resistant strains: may complicate treatment.

INDICATIONS FOR ANTIBIOTICS

Infection caused by susceptible organisms.
Should not be administered if not indicated because of potential adverse effects.

Chlamydiae

CHARACTERISTICS

Gram-negative nonmotile bacteria.
Deficient in enzymes and can only live in host tissue.
Form inclusion bodies in infected cells.

CHLAMYDIAL DISEASES

Nongonococcal urethritis.
Inclusion conjunctivitis.
Pulmonary infections.
Lymphogranuloma venereum.

Rickettsiae and Ehrlichiae

CHARACTERISTICS

Intracellular parasites transmitted to humans by insect bites.
Multiply in endothelial cells of blood vessels or in white cells.
Cause febrile illness with skin rash.
Respond to some antibiotics.

Mycoplasmas

CHARACTERISTICS

Fragile bacteria lacking cell wall.
Cause primary atypical pneumonia.
Respond to some antibiotics.

Viruses

STRUCTURE

Either DNA or RNA.
Genome enclosed in capsule.
Size and complexity of genome varies with virus.
Virus lacks metabolic enzymes and relies on metabolic processes of host for survival.

MODE OF ACTION

Invades host cell and produces various effects.
 Asymptomatic.
 Acute cell necrosis.
 Cell hyperplasia and proliferation.
 Slowly progressive cell injury.
 Neoplasia.
Inclusion bodies formed are caused by masses of viral particles.

BODILY DEFENSES AGAINST VIRAL INFECTIONS

Formation of interferon: "broad-spectrum" antiviral agents.
Cell-mediated immunity and humoral defenses.

CLASSIFICATION OF VIRUSES

Nucleic acid structure: either DNA or RNA.
Size, structural configuration, and biologic characteristics.

ANTIVIRAL AGENTS

Block viral multiplication or prevent virus from invading cell.
Limited use because of toxicity and limited effectiveness.

Fungi

TYPES OF FUNGAL INFECTIONS

Superficial fungal infections.
 Dermatophytes: athlete's foot, jock itch.
Mucous membranes: *Candida* causes vaginitis.
Highly pathogenic fungi: *Histoplasma* and *Coccidioides* cause acute or chronic pulmonary infection, occasionally progressive systemic infection.
Other systemic fungal diseases of medical importance.
 Blastomycosis: similar to histoplasmosis.
 Cryptococcus: occasionally causes chronic meningitis.

TREATMENT OF FUNGAL INFECTIONS

Superficial fungal infections respond to various medications.
Acute systemic fungal infections treated with antifungal antibiotics.

http://health.jbpub.com/humandisease/9e

Human Disease Online is a great source for supplementary human disease information for both students and instructors. Visit this website to find a variety of useful tools for learning, thinking, and teaching.

Animal Parasites

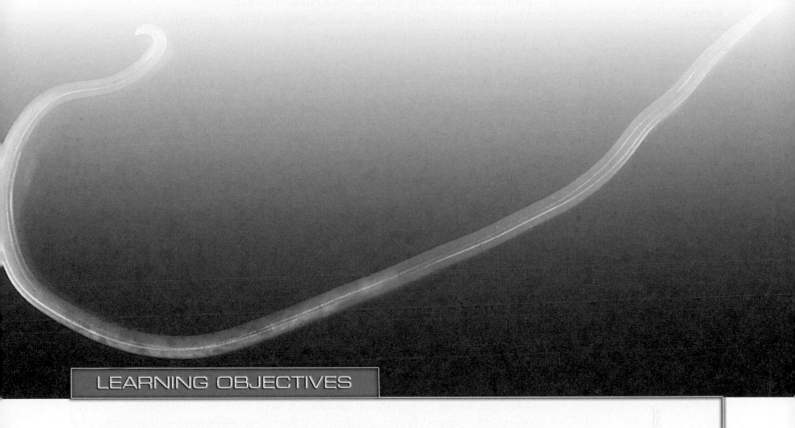

1 List the common parasitic infections that affect humans.

2 Explain how these infections are acquired.

3 Describe their clinical manifestations, and explain their clinical significance.

The Parasite and Its Host

Animal parasites are organisms that have become adapted to living within or on the body of another animal, called the **host**. These organisms are no longer capable of free-living existence. Many animal parasites have a complex life cycle. An immature form of a parasite may spend a part of its cycle within the body of an animal or fish (the intermediate host) before the mature parasite eventually takes up residence within the body of the final host (the definitive host). In general, many animal parasites live within the intestinal tract and discharge eggs in the feces. Transmission is favored by conditions of poor sanitation and by relatively high temperature and humidity, which enhance survival of the parasite in its infective stage. Therefore, many

Host
Individual infected with a disease-producing organism.

Protozoa
(prō-tō-zō′uh)
Simple one-celled animal parasites, such as the plasmodium causing malaria.

Metazoa
(me′tuh-zō-uh)
Complex multicelled animal parasites, such as worms and flukes.

Arthropod
(är′thrō-pod)
Invertebrate animal with jointed limbs and segmented body, such as insect and spider. Important arthropods that parasitize humans include the crab louse and the organism causing scabies.

parasitic infections are common in tropical climates but are much less frequent in cold or temperate climates. Specific drugs are available to treat almost all parasitic infections effectively.

Animal parasites may be classified into three large groups:

1. **Protozoa**, which are simple, one-celled organisms
2. **Metazoa**, which are more complex, multicellular structures
3. **Arthropods**, which are small insects

Infections Caused by Protozoa and Related Organisms

Some of the more important protozoal infections in humans include:

1. Malaria, caused by various species of *Plasmodium*.
2. Babesiosis, usually caused by *Babesia microti*, a malaria-like parasite.
3. Amebic dysentery, caused by a pathogenic ameba, *Entamoeba histolytica*.
4. Genital tract trichomonad infections, caused by the parasite *Trichomonas vaginalis*.
5. Giardiasis, caused by *Giardia lamblia*, which infects the small intestine.
6. Toxoplasmosis, caused by *Toxoplasma gondii*, which may infect the fetus and cause congenital malformations.
7. Cryptosporidiosis, caused by a parasite called *Cryptosporidium parvum*, which parasitizes the intestinal tract and can cause severe diarrhea.
8. Pneumocystis pneumonia, caused by *Pneumocystis Jiroveci*, a parasite that does not cause disease in immunocompetent persons but causes a severe, sometimes fatal pulmonary infection in persons with acquired immune deficiency syndrome (AIDS). Recently, the organism was reclassified as a fungus based primarily on its nucleic acid structure, but it does not resemble the other disease-causing fungi described elsewhere in this book. The disease caused by this reclassified organism is considered in the discussion on respiratory system.

MALARIA

Malaria is caused by several species of the protozoan parasite *Plasmodium*, which has a complicated life cycle. The parasite is transmitted to humans by the bite of the Anopheles mosquito, which breeds in swampy lowland areas. The name malaria dates to the time when the disease was thought to be caused by breathing night air near lowland marshes and swampy areas (*malo* = bad + *aria* = air). After the parasite and its mosquito vector were recognized, it became apparent that the marshy areas were mosquito breeding grounds, and the evening hours were the times when the mosquitoes were most active.

The parasites first begin their development within the liver and then invade the red blood cells of the host. There they multiply, feeding on the hemoglobin, which becomes degraded to a product called malarial pigment. Soon, the rapidly multiplying parasites destroy the red cells that they have invaded, releasing masses of new parasites along with red-cell debris and malarial pigment into the circulation. This event is associated with an elevated temperature and a shaking chill ("chills and fever"). The newly liberated parasites in turn attack other red cells, and the cycles of invasion–multiplication–red-cell destruction continue. The time taken for each species of parasite to complete its cycle is quite constant. Consequently, the episodes of chills and fever tend to occur at regular intervals every 48 or 72 hours, depending on the species. Besides suffering repeated, periodic chills and fever, infected individuals frequently become anemic because of the excessive red-cell destruction. Often their spleens also enlarge because phagocytic cells in the spleen proliferate and become filled with debris and malarial pigment. In one type of malaria, clumps of parasitized red cells may plug small blood vessels in the brain, heart, or other vital organs. This serious complication impedes blood flow to the affected organs and may be fatal. Diagnosis of malaria is established by demonstrating the parasite in properly prepared and stained slides made from the blood of the infected patient.

Malaria is a major health problem in many parts of the world. It is widespread in many Third World countries, including parts of Africa, Asia, Central America, and South America. More than 100 million people are afflicted at any given time, and about one million people die of the disease each year. Few infectious diseases have had such a profound effect on the social and economic development of countries. Malaria is no longer a problem in the United States, Canada, and Europe. Most cases of malaria in the United States are contracted by persons who have traveled to areas where malaria occurs frequently and become ill after returning home. Malaria is also sometimes transmitted by blood transfusion if the donor carries the parasite. Malarial infections have also been contracted by drug abusers who share contaminated syringes and needles. Various antimalarial drugs are available to prevent infection when traveling in an endemic area and to treat an established infection. Unfortunately, parasites are becoming resistant to some antimalarial drugs, which makes treatment more difficult.

CASE 7-1

An American family had been vacationing in a resort outside the United States. After returning to their own country, several members became ill with chills and fever. Examination of the blood smears revealed malarial parasites. The affected family members received a course of antimalarial therapy and made an uneventful recovery.

BABESIOSIS

Babesiae are tick-borne protozoal parasites that infect a wide variety of wild and domestic animals and birds, and they sometimes also infect people. Human infections have been documented in North America, Europe, and many other countries. The first documented infections in the United States occurred in Nantucket Island in Massachusetts, but now babesia infections are more widely distributed throughout the United States. In North America, the organism that infects people is *Babesia microti*, which is usually transmitted from small rodents to people by the same ticks that transmit Lyme disease (discussion on pathogenic microorganisms). The organism parasitizes red cells where the babesiae multiply and eventually rupture the parasitized red cells, releasing the parasites to invade and proliferate in other red cells. The *Babesia microti* infection causes a malaria-like illness characterized by chills, fever, and anemia resulting from destruction of red cells by the parasites. The diagnosis of the infection is established by identifying the parasites within the infected red cells, which must be distinguished from malaria parasites that they resemble. The severity of the babesial infection varies in different individuals, and the blood filtration function of the spleen plays an important role in controlling the infection by eliminating many of the parasites as blood flows through the spleen. Most infected individuals have a mild illness and recover without complications. However, if the infected person has had a splenectomy, the proliferation of the parasites is unchecked by the spleen, and these unfortunate persons develop a severe and sometimes fatal infection. Several drugs are available to treat the infection.

AMEBIASIS

Amebiasis is an infection of the intestinal tract by a pathogenic ameba, *Entamoeba histolytica*. The life cycle of the parasite includes an active, motile, vegetative phase (called a trophozoite) and a relatively resistant cystic phase. Humans become infected by ingesting cysts of the parasite in contaminated food and water. The motile phase of the parasite develops from the cyst and invades the mucosa of the colon, producing mucosal ulcers and causing symptoms of inflammation of the colon. Occasionally, the amebas are carried to the liver in the portal circulation and may cause amebic hepatitis or amebic liver abscess.

GENITAL TRACT INFECTIONS CAUSED BY TRICHOMONADS

The trichomonads are small motile parasites. One species, *Trichomonas vaginalis*, sometimes causes an acute inflammation of the vagina characterized by itching, burning, and a profuse, frothy vaginal discharge. The infection can be transmitted to the male by sexual intercourse and causes an inflammation of the urethra.

CASE 7-2

A young woman complained of vaginal itching and profuse vaginal discharge. Examination revealed redness of the vaginal mucosa and abundant yellow vaginal secretions. Microscopic examination revealed large numbers of trichomonads and leukocytes in the secretions (FIGURE 7-1). The patient was treated with an antiparasitic drug (metronidazole). Because the disease is transmitted by sexual intercourse, the patient's sexual partner also was treated.

GIARDIASIS

Giardia lamblia is a small, pear-shaped parasite that inhabits the duodenum and upper jejunum. The parasite attaches to the mucosa, causing an intestinal inflammation manifested by crampy abdominal pain, distention, and watery diarrhea. Parasites are present in the stools of infected individuals, and the disease is usually transmitted by means of contaminated food and water. The infection is relatively common in certain parts of Russia, and many American tourists traveling there have

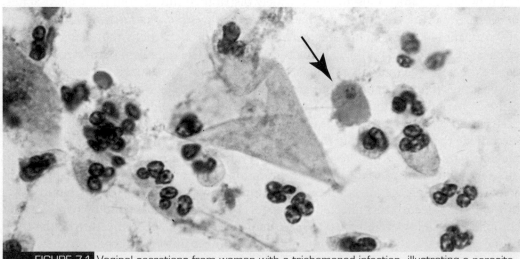

FIGURE 7-1 Vaginal secretions from woman with a trichomonad infection, illustrating a parasite (*arrow*) and many neutrophils (original magnification × 400).

been infected. Several epidemics of giardia infection caused by contaminated water supplies have occurred in the United States.

TOXOPLASMOSIS

Toxoplasma gondii is a small intracellular parasite that infects a large number of birds and animals as well as humans. Many cats are infected with the parasite and excrete an infectious form of the organism in their stools. The parasite is frequently present in the flesh of cattle and many other animals. People acquire Toxoplasma infections by ingesting raw or partially cooked meat that is infected with the parasite or by contact with infected cats who excrete in their feces an infectious form of the parasite called an oocyst. Usually the infection does not cause symptoms in healthy adults. About 50% of the adult population has had a previous inapparent infection and is immune. The importance of toxoplasmosis is related to its effect on the fetus. If a susceptible (nonimmune) woman acquires a Toxoplasma infection during pregnancy, the parasite may be transmitted to the fetus. Infection of the fetus causes severe injury to fetal tissues and often leads to congenital malformations that are described in the discussion on congenital and hereditary disease.

Toxoplasmosis is also a risk to immunocompromised persons, as are other parasitic infections. The disease may result either from a first exposure to the parasite or from reactivation of an infection acquired many years previously, as illustrated by the following case.

Toxoplasma gondii
(tähk′sō-plas′muh gän′dē-ī)
A small intracellular parasite of birds, animals, and humans. Causes the disease toxoplasmosis.

CASE 7-3

A 55-year-old HIV-antibody-positive man consulted his physician because of recent onset of confusion, dizziness, and seizures. Neurologic examination was normal, but CT scans of the head revealed multiple spherical nodules throughout both cerebral hemispheres. Examination of the spinal fluid was normal. Biopsy of one of the nodules revealed the characteristic appearance of toxoplasmosis, which was associated with some surrounding cerebral edema and reactive proliferation of astrocytes (FIGURE 7-2). The toxoplasmosis was considered to be a reactivation of a prior infection, and appropriate treatment was started to control the infection.

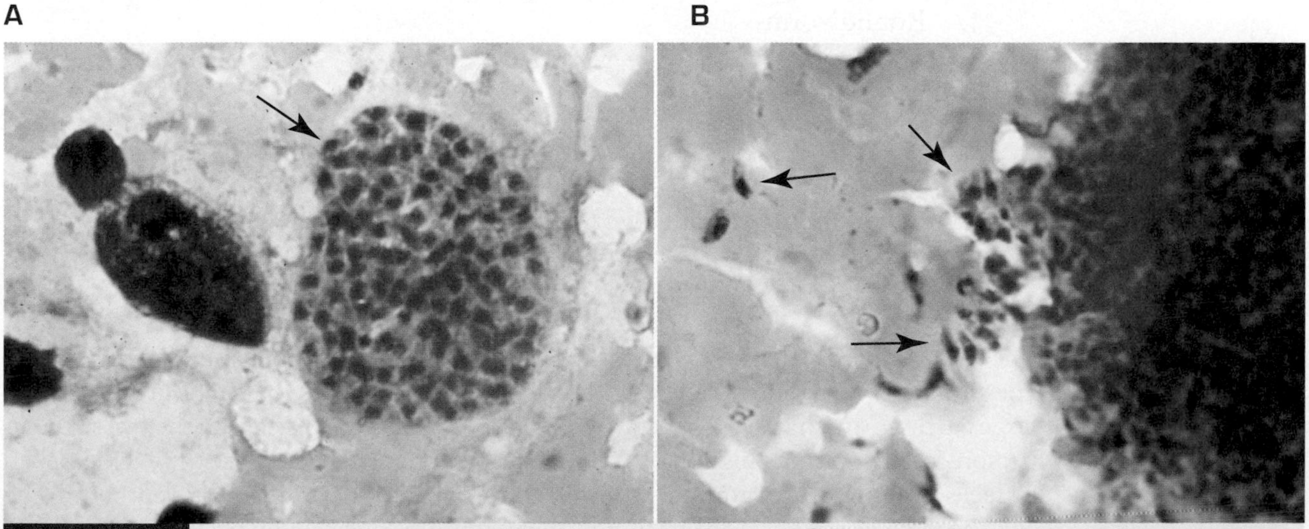

A B

FIGURE 7-2 A cerebral toxoplasmosis demonstrated by brain biopsy. **A**, Cyst composed of a large cluster of organisms (*arrow*) (original magnification × 400). **B**, Higher magnification view illustrating disruption of the cyst wall with extruded sickle-shaped parasites (*arrow*) (original magnification × 1,000).

CRYPTOSPORIDIOSIS

Cryptosporidium parvum, an organism closely related to Toxoplasma, has been recognized recently as a very important cause of severe diarrhea in both immuno-competent and immunocompromised persons. The organism infects cattle, other farm animals, and people who excrete in their fecal material large numbers of the infectious forms of the parasites called oocysts. Fecal material from farm animals can contaminate surface water flowing into rivers and lakes, and oocysts have been identified in from 65 to 85% of surface water samples tested throughout the United States. The infectious oocyst has a thick wall and is quite small, only about half the size of a red blood cell. It is highly resistant to chlorination of water supplies and can be removed from municipal water supplies only by filtration. People can become infected by ingesting oocysts in unfiltered municipal water supplies, from oocyst-contaminated water in swimming pools, or by person-to-person fecal–oral transmission in the same way that other intestinal infections are transmitted. The infection is easily transmitted person to person in households and in child day care facilities.

When oocysts are ingested, the cyst wall disintegrates in the intestinal tract, releasing the infectious parasite, which multiplies and infects the intestinal epithelial cells. The parasite is very infectious. Only a few oocysts are enough to cause an infection, and persons with diarrhea excrete large numbers of oocysts in their stool. Persons with normal immune defenses experience an acute self-limited diarrhea when infected with the parasite, but persons with AIDS and other immunocompromised persons develop a severe chronic life-threatening diarrhea. Unfortunately, there is no specific treatment for the infection.

Several large epidemics of cryptosporidiosis have been traced to municipal water supplies where filtration of water to eliminate oocysts either was not performed or was inadequate. The largest recent epidemic occurred in Milwaukee in 1993 in which 400,000 people became ill from a municipal water supply. Small, swimming-pool–related epidemics also have been reported. In these cases, the oocyst contamination of the pool water was caused by persons with cryptosporidial diarrhea using the pool; oocysts contaminating the perianal skin of these people were released into the pool water and infected other swimmers. The major features of these protozoal infections are summarized in TABLE 7-1.

Metazoal Infections

The three large groups of metazoal parasites are:

1. Roundworms
2. Tapeworms
3. Flukes

ROUNDWORMS

The three most important roundworms that parasitize human beings are the *Ascaris*, the pinworm, and the *Trichinella* worm.

Ascaris

The *Ascaris lumbricoides* is the most commonly encountered parasitic worm, infecting an estimated one billion people worldwide. It is a large roundworm, about the size of a large earthworm, that lives in the intestinal tract and discharges eggs in the feces. Direct person-to-person transmission of *Ascaris* eggs does not occur because the eggs expelled in feces are immature, and a 2- to 3-week maturation period is required before the eggs become infectious. Maturation of the immature eggs usually occurs in the soil, as when fecal material is defecated on the ground if toilet facilities are not available or if a child is not toilet trained, or when fecal material is used to fertilize the soil for growing

TABLE 7-1

Common protozoal infections

Disease	Source of infection	Manifestations	Diagnosis	Treatment
Malaria	Mosquito bite	Chills and fever Anemia	Identify parasite in red cells	Antimalarial drugs
Babesiosis	Deer tick bite	Chills and fever Anemia	Identify parasite in red cells	Various drugs available
Amebiasis	Ingestion of parasite in contaminated food or water	Cramps and diarrhea. Sometimes hepatitis.	Identify parasite or cysts in stool	Various drugs available
Giardiasis	Ingestion of parasite in contaminated food or water	Cramps and diarrhea	Identify parasite in stool. Other tests also available	Antiparasite drug (Metronidazole)
Cryptosporidiosis	Food or water contaminated with parasite cysts. Recreational water (swimming pools).	Cramps and diarrhea	Identify parasite cysts in stool	No anti-parasite drugs available. Treat symptoms.
Trichomoniasis	Vaginal secretions containing parasite	Profuse vaginal discharge	Identify parasite in vaginal secretions	Anti-parasite drug (Metronidazole).
Toxoplasmosis	Eating meat containing parasites. Contact with feces of infected cats.	Causes disease in AIDS patients. Pregnant woman may transmit infection to fetus.	Identify parasite (usually biopsy required)	Drugs available to prevent disease in AIDS patients. Otherwise no treatment required

vegetables or other farm products, as is done in some countries. The mature eggs can survive in the soil for many years, and later contact with egg-contaminated soil may transfer eggs to hands, then to food or beverages, and finally into the intestinal tract.

When mature *Ascaris* eggs are ingested, the larval worms are released from the eggs within the intestinal tract, and the small larval worms burrow through the intestine, enter the circulatory system, and are carried in the circulation throughout the body. They are then filtered out in various organs and tissues. The larvae that lodge in the lung burrow through the alveolar walls and migrate into the bronchi, are coughed up, and eventually are swallowed, finding their way again into the small intestine where they grow to maturity. The stage characterized by the passage of *Ascaris* larvae through the lungs and other tissues is called the phase of larval migration and may be associated with fever, cough, and inflammation of the lungs. Adult worms living in the small intestine may at times wander from their usual location. They may migrate upward and be coughed up or vomited, or they may pass out through the nose. At times, they may enter and block the bile ducts or plug the appendix. Rarely, a large mass of worms may completely block the lumen of the small intestine. An *Ascaris* infection is identified by detecting worm eggs in the fecal material of an infected person or by identifying an adult worm as illustrated in Cases 7-4 and 7-5, which illustrate the migratory behavior of the *Ascaris* worm.

Dogs and cats may be infected with a similar type of roundworm; the animal worm occasionally causes disease in humans. Infection by the animal worm is most common in children who are in close contact with an infected animal. The children

CASE 7-4

A young woman complained of a "funny feeling" in the back of her throat and coughed up a large *Ascaris* worm. The organism, which normally inhabits the small intestine, had migrated through the stomach and esophagus into the pharynx and was subsequently expelled (FIGURE 7-3).

CASE 7-5

A child was admitted to the hospital with symptoms suggesting acute appendicitis, and an appendectomy was performed. When the base of the appendix was cut away from the colon during the removal, an *Ascaris* was found stuck in the appendix and was transected during the removal of the appendix (FIGURE 7-4). The symptoms of appendicitis apparently had been caused by the worm lodged in the lumen of the appendix.

transfer the eggs to their mouths by means of contaminated hands, toys, or other objects. The eggs hatch within the intestinal tract, and the larvae invade the tissues of the host, undergoing a phase of larval migration, which may be associated with systemic symptoms. However, the larvae that have been ingested by a foreign host are eventually destroyed within the tissues of the host and never reach maturity within the intestinal tract. Unfortunately, the larvae can survive for several months and produce symptoms related to their migration before they are eventually destroyed.

Pinworms

Pinworm
A small parasitic worm infecting humans. Lives in lower bowel and causes perianal pruritus.

The small roundworm *Enterobius vermicularis* is usually called simply the **pinworm** because of its small size, which generally measures less than 1 cm in length. Pinworm infections are very common, second only to *Ascaris* infections in frequency, and often infect children, who may harbor a large number of worms in their intestinal tract. Often the infection spreads from the child to the rest of the family members. The infection is acquired from ingesting worm eggs that are transferred to the hands from contaminated bedclothes or other objects. The worms hatch in the duodenum and then travel to

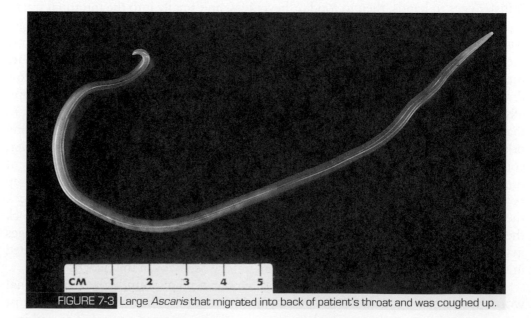

FIGURE 7-3 Large *Ascaris* that migrated into back of patient's throat and was coughed up.

the colon, where they take up residence. Female egg-laden worms migrate out of the colon through the anus, often at night while the child is asleep, and deposit their eggs on the perianal skin. Sometimes recently deposited eggs may hatch near the anus, and worms on the perineal skin may travel back through the anus into the colon. Occasionally, a worm may migrate into the vagina instead of the anus and may travel through the genital tract until it is eventually destroyed by the body's defenses, but this is uncommon. The main symptoms of pinworm infection are intense anal and perianal itching caused by irritation resulting from the migration of the worm. Pinworm eggs are usually not found in fecal material. The diagnosis of a pinworm infection is made by identifying the eggs deposited by migrating worms on the perianal skin. Usually, a piece of Scotch tape is applied to the skin, and any pinworm eggs present stick to the tape. Then the sticky side of the tape is attached to a glass slide, and the slide is examined microscopically for pinworm eggs. Sometimes a worm that has left the colon to deposit eggs can be identified by examining the perianal skin, as illustrated in Case 7-6. The disease is more a nuisance than a threat to life, as illustrated by the following case.

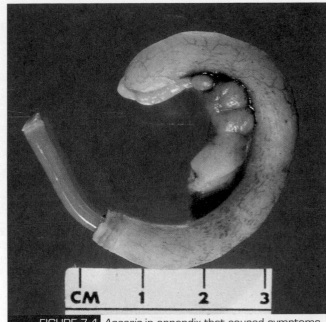

FIGURE 7-4 *Ascaris* in appendix that caused symptoms suggesting appendicitis. The head of a worm had entered the appendix, and the worm was transected when the appendix was removed.

CASE 7-6

An 8-year-old girl who had recently attended a slumber party at a neighbor's house began to experience perianal and vulvar itching which at times awakened her at night. On such occasion, her mother examined the perineum after she had been awakened by the itching and found a small 1 cm long worm moving around the perianal area. The mother collected the worm on a piece of Scotch tape and brought it to her physician for evaluation.

It was a pinworm, and the eggs within the worm had the typical appearance of pinworm eggs. She was treated with an appropriate medication to eradicate the worms, and the other family members also were treated.

Trichinella

Another small roundworm, *Trichinella spiralis*, causes a severe parasitic infection called *trichinosis*. The organism parasitizes not only humans, but also a wide variety of animals. Larval forms of the *Trichinella* are encapsulated as small cystic structures within the muscles of the infected human or animal host. People usually become infected by eating improperly cooked pork or meat from another *Trichinella*-infected animal. After the infected meat has been ingested, the larvae are released from their cysts and develop into mature parasitic worms in the small intestine. The worms then burrow into the intestinal mucosa and produce larvae, which gain access to the circulation and are carried throughout the body. They are filtered out in various tissues, where they incite an intense inflammatory reaction. The parasites that lodge in the muscles of the infected individual become encapsulated, forming small cysts within the muscle (FIGURE 7-5). These cysts are the infectious form of the parasite. The phase of larval migration is associated with severe systemic symptoms, and there may also be symptoms referable to disturbed function of organs that have been heavily infiltrated by the parasites. Extremely heavy parasitic infestations may be fatal.

A   **B**

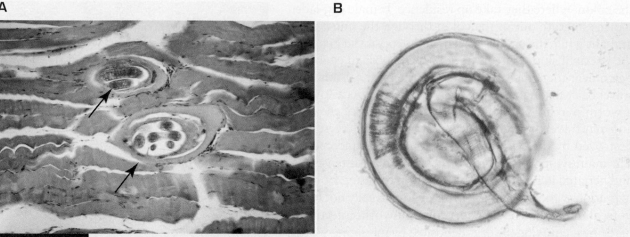

FIGURE 7-5 Trichinosis. **A**, Biopsy of skeletal muscle showing encysted larvae surrounded by fibrous capsules. Each cyst measures about 1 mm in diameter (original magnification × 100). **B**, Higher magnification view of unstained coiled larva with the capsule removed (original magnification × 400).

TAPEWORMS

Tapeworms are long, ribbonlike worms that sometimes grow to a length of several feet. They inhabit the intestinal tract. In general, tapeworms cause no great inconvenience to the individual carrying them except for depriving the host of the food that nourishes the worm. Three species of tapeworms are recognized: the pork tapeworm, the beef tapeworm, and the fish tapeworm. Humans become infected by eating the flesh of an infected animal that contains the larval form of the parasite.

FLUKES

Flukes are thick, fleshy, short worms that are provided with suckers for the attachment to the host. They have a complex life cycle involving one or more intermediate hosts. Flukes are classified according to the area of the body in which the development of the adult flukes is completed and the eggs are deposited. Some species of flukes live within the intestinal tract; others live within the liver; and one species lives within the lung. Some flukes called Schistosomes, or blood flukes, live within the portal venous system and its tributaries or within the veins draining the bladder, where they cause serious damage to the surrounding tissues. Fluke infections are an important cause of illness and disability in some Asiatic countries, but human fluke infections are not seen in the United States or Canada.

Although human fluke infections do not occur in North America, some animal schistosomes can infect humans but are more a nuisance than a cause of serious illness. Birds and mammals, infected with their own specific species of schistosomes, excrete them in their droppings into lakes and other bodies of water, where they develop into the infectious form of the parasite. People who swim in bird or animal schistosome-contaminated lakes may be "attacked" by the parasites, which can penetrate the skin of the swimmers. The parasites cause discrete areas of acute pruritic inflammation at the site where they entered the skin. They cannot cause a systemic infection, however, because humans are not the normal host for the parasite, and the parasites are destroyed in the skin by the body's immune defenses. The condition is called *schistosome dermatitis* but is more commonly referred to as "swimmers itch." Many lakes in North America and some saltwater beaches are contaminated by bird or animal schistosomes, and the problems they cause are illustrated in Case 7-7. The major features of these metazoal infections are summarized in (TABLE 7-2).

CASE 7-7

A middle-aged man, who had a summer cabin in Wisconsin, spent the morning swimming and working on his dock. Soon afterward he developed multiple very itchy nodules on the skin of his legs (FIGURE 7-6). He consulted a physician who diagnosed "swimmers itch" and prescribed some medication to relieve the itching.

TABLE 7-2

Characteristics of common metazoal parasites

Parasite	Source of infection	Parasite characteristics	Result of infection
Large round-worm *Ascaris lumbricoides*	Eggs expelled in stool require 2–3 weeks before eggs are infectious. Infection acquired from eggs in soil by hands directly to mouth or by egg contaminated food or beverages.	Larvae hatch in bowel, enter bloodstream, lodge in tissues, travel from lung to trachea and into throat, are swallowed and mature in bowel.	Mature worms move around in bowel, may block appendix or bile duct, or several worms may form a ball that blocks the intestine.
Pinworm *Enterobius vermicularis*	Worms live in colon and migrate out anus at night to lay eggs, which contaminate peri-anal tissues.	Eggs contaminate hands, bed clothes, and other surfaces. Eggs on hands spread infection through families and to others.	Heavy infection may cause itching and disturb sleep. Occasionally, worm may migrate into vagina instead of anus.
Small roundworm *Trichinella spiralis*	Cyst of parasite in flesh of animals. Eating improperly cooked meat releases larvae to mature in small intestine.	Worms produce larvae that enter bloodstream and lodge in tissues. Larvae in muscle form cysts.	Larval migration causes severe inflammation in affected organs. Heavy infection may be very hazardous.
Tapeworm *Taenia species*	Long ribbonlike worms acquired from eating meat of infected beef, pork, or fish.	Larvae mature in intestine can become several feet long and live for a long time.	Worms consume our food but usually do not cause any major problems.
Fluke Bird or animal *Schistosomes*	Complex life cycle that forms the infectious form of the parasite. Hazardous schistosomes do not occur in the United States.	Schistosome can invade skin of person swimming in contaminated water.	Schistosome lesions called "swimmers itch" but systemic infection does not occur.

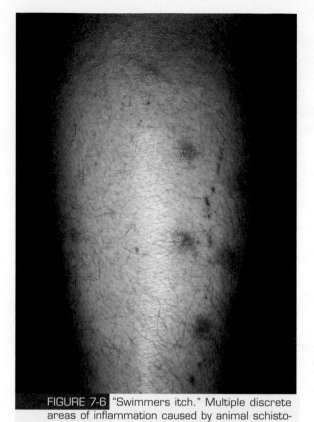

FIGURE 7-6 "Swimmers itch." Multiple discrete areas of inflammation caused by animal schistosomes penetrating skin of calf.

Crab louse
A parasite of the pubic area; causes intense itching.

Arthropods

There are two common parasitic skin infestations: scabies and lice. Both are transmitted by close physical contact and are often spread by sexual contact. Both infestations respond promptly to treatment with antiparasitic medications applied to the skin.

SCABIES

Scabies is caused by a small parasite called *Sarcoptes scabiei*, which burrows in the superficial layers of the skin, where it lays eggs that hatch in a few days. The infestation causes intense itching. The tracks made by the parasites as they burrow in the skin appear as fine, wavy, dark lines in the skin measuring from 1 mm to 1 cm in length. Common sites of involvement are the base of the fingers, the wrists, the armpits, the skin around the nipples, and the skin around the belt line.

CRAB LOUSE INFESTATION

Of the various types of lice that may infest the body, the most common and best known is the **crab louse** (*Phthirus pubis*), which lives in the anal and genital hairs (FIGURE 7-7). The organism also causes intense itching. The louse lays eggs that become attached to the hair shafts. Diagnosis is established by identifying either the parasite or the eggs.

CASE 7-8

A young man complained of intense itching in the pubic area. Examination revealed small crab lice in the pubic hair (FIGURE 7-7) and numerous eggs attached to the hair shafts. Both the patient and his sexual partner were treated with an antiparasitic drug (Kwell).

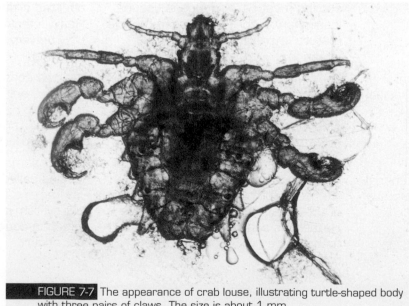

FIGURE 7-7 The appearance of crab louse, illustrating turtle-shaped body with three pairs of claws. The size is about 1 mm.

QUESTIONS FOR REVIEW

1. What are some of the more important protozoal infections?
2. How is malaria transmitted?
3. What is trichinosis? How is it transmitted?
4. What are the more important worm infestations? What are their manifestations?
5. What are "crabs"? What symptoms do they cause? How are they acquired?
6. How do people become infected with pinworms? How do they acquire an *Ascaris* infection?
7. How does malaria differ from babesiosis?

SUPPLEMENTARY READINGS

Blumenthal, D. S. 1977. Intestinal nematodes in the United States. *New England Journal of Medicine* 297:1437–9.
► Worm infections are common in rural communities in the southeastern United States and among immigrants from tropical countries. Manifestations, diagnosis, and treatment are described.

Centers for Disease Control and Prevention. 1994. *Cryptosporidium* infections associated with swimming pools—Dane County, Wisconsin, 1993. *Morbidity and Mortality Weekly Report* 43:561–3.
► Members of a swim team became infected from a swimming pool. Measures to prevent such infections are discussed.

Chen, X. M., Keithly, J. S., Paya, C. V., et al. 2002. Cryptosporidiosis. *New England Journal of Medicine* 346:1723–31.
► An update on the organism's life cycle, clinical features, diagnosis, and management.

Hayes, E. B., Matte, T. D., O'Brien, T. R., et al. 1989. Large community outbreak of cryptosporidiosis as a result of contamination of filtered water supply. *New England Journal of Medicine* 320:1372–6.
► Parasites in municipal supply caused large community outbreak.

Keiser, J., and Utzinger., J. 2008. Efficacy of current drugs against soil-transmitted helminth infections: Systematic review and meta-analysis. *Journal of the American Medical Association* 299:1937–48.
► *Ascaris* is the most important worm transmitted from contact with egg-contaminated soil. Current approaches to treatment of soil-associated worm infections are considered and recommendations for treatment are provided.

Krick, J. A., and Remington, J. S. 1978. Toxoplasmosis in the adult—an overview. *New England Journal of Medicine* 298:550–3.
► Asymptomatic toxoplasmosis occurs in a large percentage of the population. It may cause an illness resembling infectious mononucleosis, and it can cause a fatal infection in an individual whose immune defenses have been suppressed. An important cause of congenital abnormalities caused by intrauterine infection.

Mac Kenzie, W. R., Hoxie, N. J., Proctor N. E., et al. 1994. A massive outbreak in Milwaukee of *Cryptosporidium* infection transmitted through the public water supply. *New England Journal of Medicine* 331:161–7.
► Documents a huge outbreak with some deaths related to this parasite in unfiltered water.

Olliaro, P., Cattani, J., and Wirth, D. 1996. Malaria, the submerged disease. *Journal of the American Medical Association* 275:230–3.
► Malaria is an increasing worldwide problem and is becoming harder to control because the organisms are becoming resistant to antimalarial drugs. About 1,000 new cases are reported annually in the United States, usually acquired outside the country by travelers, military personnel, and immigrants from malaria-endemic countries, but a small number of cases are acquired in the United States.

OUTLINE SUMMARY

Animal Parasites

CLASSIFICATION

Protozoa: simple one-celled organisms.
Metazoa: complex, multicelled.
Arthropods: small insects that infest skin.

Protozoal Infections

MALARIA

Transmission by mosquito, occasionally by blood transfusion or hypodermic syringes of illicit drug users.
Parasites invade red blood cells and cause febrile illness with red-cell destruction.

BABESIOSIS

Tick-borne protozoal parasite.
Causes malaria-like symptoms.
Persons without spleen have severe infection.

AMEBIASIS

Transmission by contaminated food or water.
Invades colon with mucosal ulcers.
Occasionally causes liver abscesses.

TRICHOMONAD INFECTIONS

Cause vaginal infection.
Transmission by sexual intercourse.

GIARDIASIS

Transmission by contaminated food and water.
Causes inflammation of small intestine with crampy pain and diarrhea.

TOXOPLASMOSIS

Parasite in flesh of animals.
Infection acquired by eating incompletely cooked meat or from contact with cats who excrete infectious form of parasite.
Toxoplasma infection of pregnant women may be transmitted to fetus and cause intrauterine injury.

CRYPTOSPORIDIOSIS

Animal parasite excreted in stool and contaminates surface water.
Infectious oocysts resistant to chlorination. Can be eliminated only by water filtration.

People infected from ingestion of unfiltered water from municipal water supplies, swimming pool water, or direct person-to-person spread. Organisms infect small intestine and cause diarrhea, which can be chronic and severe in AIDS patients.
No specific treatment available.

Metazoal Infections

ROUNDWORMS

Ascaris
   Not transmitted person-to-person.
   Ingested eggs hatch in intestine.
   Larvae migrate into circulation and migrate through tissues.
   Worms lodging in lung are coughed up, swallowed, and mature in intestine.
Pinworms
   Worms live in colon.
   Migrate out of anus and lay eggs.
   Cause itching as a result of worm migration.
   Transmitted by ingestion of eggs on hands and in bedclothes.
Trichinella
   Parasite in flesh of pigs and other animals.
   Human beings usually infected by eating improperly cooked pork.
   Worms hatch in intestine; larvae enter circulation and are filtered out in tissues.
   Worm migration causes systemic symptoms, eosinophilia, and evidence of disturbed organ function.

TAPEWORMS

Live in intestinal tract and consume nutrients ingested by host.

FLUKES

Short, fleshy worms that live in liver, intestine, or lung.
Human fluke infections not seen in the United States and Canada.
Bird or animal flukes (schistosomes) may cause skin inflammation (dermatitis) in people who swim in schistosome-infested water.

Arthropods

SCABIES

Small parasite burrows in skin, lays eggs, and causes severe itching.

Spread by close physical or sexual contact.

Responds to antiparasitic medications.

CRAB LOUSE

Lives in pubic hair and lays eggs that are attached to hair shafts.

Causes intense itching.

Spread by close physical and sexual contact.

Responds to antiparasitic medications.

http://health.jbpub.com/humandisease/9e

Human Disease Online is a great source for supplementary human disease information for both students and instructors. Visit this website to find a variety of useful tools for learning, thinking, and teaching.

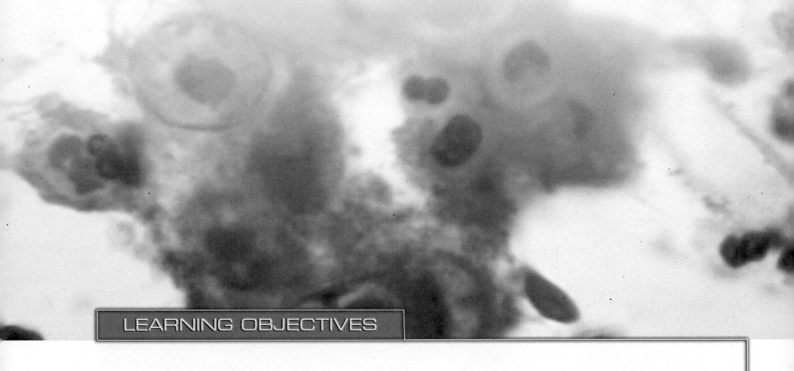

Communicable Diseases

1 Explain how communicable diseases are transmitted and controlled.

2 List the common sexually transmitted diseases. Describe their major clinical manifestations, complications, and methods of treatment.

3 Describe the symptoms of herpes infection in men and women. Explain the effects on sexual partners. Describe how herpes may affect a fetus or newborn infant of an infected mother.

4 Understand the pathogenesis of human immunodeficiency virus infections, the groups affected, and the effects of the virus on the immune system. List the major clinical manifestations of the infection, the significance of a positive test for antibody to the virus, and methods of preventing spread of the infection.

Communicable disease
A disease transmitted from person to person.

Endemic disease
(en-dem′ik)
A communicable disease in which small numbers of cases are continually present in a population.

Epidemic disease
(ep-i-dem′ik)
A communicable disease affecting concurrently large numbers of persons in a population.

Methods of Transmission and Control

An infectious disease that is readily transmitted from person to person is considered a **communicable disease**. Such a disease is said to be **endemic** (*en* = within + *demos* = population) if small numbers of cases are continually present in the population. It reaches **epidemic** proportions (*epi* = upon + *demos* = population) when relatively large numbers of people are affected. Sometimes an endemic disease may flare up and assume epidemic proportions.

METHODS OF TRANSMISSION

A communicable disease may be transmitted from person to person by either direct or indirect methods. Direct transmission is either by direct physical contact or by means of droplet spread, such as by coughing or sneezing. Indirect transmission of an infectious agent is accomplished by some intermediary mechanism, such as transmission in contaminated water or by means of insects. A few communicable diseases are primarily diseases of animals and are transmitted to humans only incidentally.

For a communicable disease to perpetuate itself, there must be a continuous transmission of the infectious agent from person to person by either direct or indirect methods. Therefore, in order to eradicate or control the disease, the chain of transmission must be broken at some point (FIGURE 8-1).

METHODS OF CONTROL

This section deals with some of the methods that can be applied to control communicable diseases. In practice, multiple methods of control are applied whenever possible.

Immunization

If a large proportion of the population can be immunized against a communicable disease, the disease will eventually die out because there will be very few susceptible persons in the population. Smallpox is an example of a disease that has been eliminated worldwide because of widespread immunization. Poliomyelitis is another disease that has been virtually eradicated in the United States as a result of widespread immunization of persons at risk.

Immunization can also be used to protect susceptible persons entering a foreign country where a communicable disease is endemic. The immunized person will no longer be susceptible to the disease, even though the disease is widespread in the native population.

Identification, Isolation, and Treatment of Infected Persons

Sick persons are identified and treated promptly in order to shorten the time during which they can infect others. Isolation of infected persons prevents contact with susceptible persons and stops the spread of the disease. Identification, isolation, and treatment are the primary methods used to control diseases when effective methods of immunization are not available. In some cases, these measures are difficult to accomplish because some diseases produce relatively few symptoms in the infected individual. For example, the person infected with tuberculosis or a sexually transmitted disease may spread the disease to others, but his or her own disease may not be recognized and treated because the person does not feel ill and does not seek medical treatment.

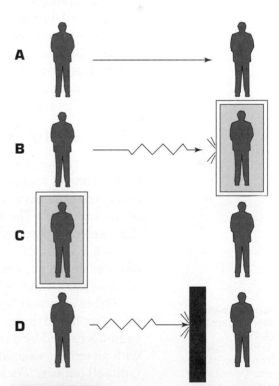

FIGURE 8-1 Methods of eradicating or controlling a communicable disease. **A,** Unimpeded direct or indirect transmission of a communicable disease from person to person. **B,** Immunization protects a susceptible person by conferring resistance to infection. **C,** Isolation and prompt treatment of the infected person prevent the spread of disease to susceptible persons. **D,** Control of means of indirect transmission blocks spread of infectious agent.

Control of Means of Indirect Transmission

Various control measures can be instituted, depending on the manner by which the infectious agent is transmitted. Where the transmission is by means of contaminated food or water, methods of control include chlorination of water supplies and establishment of effective sewage treatment facilities, control of food handlers, and standards for monitoring the manufacture and distribution of commercially prepared foods. When a disease is transmitted by insects, either between people or between infected animals and people, it is necessary to eradicate or control the insects that transmit the disease. When a disease is spread from animals to people, control of the animal source of infection also is required.

Requirements for Effective Control

Application of effective control measures requires knowing the cause of the disease and its method of transmission. If this information is not available, control measures are often ineffective. For example, bubonic plague, the "black death" of the Middle Ages, decimated entire populations because the people understood neither the cause of the disease nor how it was transmitted and therefore were unable to protect themselves from its ravages. We now know that plague is primarily a disease of rats and other rodents, that it is caused by a bacterium, and that it is transmitted to people by insects. In some cases, the plague bacillus causes a pulmonary infection in people. When this occurs, direct transmission from person to person can be through droplet spread, causing an extremely contagious and highly fatal pulmonary infection called *pneumonic plague*. In some parts of the United States, plague infection still persists in some rodent populations, but plague is no longer a serious problem because the disease can be largely prevented in people by controlling the infected animal population and by instituting measures that prevent close contact between potentially infected rodents and people. Transmission from person to person is prevented by prompt isolation and treatment of infected persons.

Sexually Transmitted Diseases

Sexually transmitted diseases are communicable diseases that spread primarily by sexual contact and have reached epidemic proportions. They can be transmitted by sexual relations between heterosexual partners and by sexual acts between individuals of the same sex. The four major sexually transmitted diseases are syphilis, gonorrhea, genital herpes infection, and genital chlamydial infections (TABLE 8-1). In a class by itself because of its devastating consequences and high mortality is the **acquired immune deficiency syndrome** (AIDS), which is transmitted by both homosexual and heterosexual contacts and by blood and secretions from infected persons.

Other common but less serious sexually transmitted diseases are anal and genital warts (condylomas) caused by the papilloma virus (see FIGURE 6-8), nonspecific vaginitis caused by pathogenic micro-organisms such as *Gardnerella* in conjunction with anaerobic vaginal bacteria, and trichomonal vaginitis caused by the protozoan (animal) parasite *Trichomonas vaginalis*. Other diseases including scabies and crabs in animal parasites, hepatitis in the liver, and some gastrointestinal tract infections are also sometimes transmitted sexually.

SYPHILIS

Syphilis, caused by the spirochete **Treponema pallidum**, is a very serious sexually transmitted disease because it may cause severe damage in almost any organ of the body. If the disease is not treated, it progresses through three stages called primary, secondary, and tertiary syphilis. Each stage has its own characteristic clinical manifestations.

Acquired immune deficiency syndrome (AIDS)
An infection caused by the human immunodeficiency virus. The virus attacks and destroys helper T lymphocytes, which compromises cell-mediated immunity, leading to increased susceptibility to infection and some tumors.

Treponema pallidum
(trep-pō-nē'muh pal'lid-dum)
The spiral organism causing syphilis.

TABLE 8-1

Comparison of four major sexually transmitted diseases

	Syphilis	Gonorrhea	Herpes	Chlamydia
Organism	*Treponema pallidum*	Gonococcus (*Neisseria gonorrhoeae*)	Herpes virus	*Chlamydia trachomatis*
Major clinical manifestations	Primary: chancre Secondary: systemic infection with skin rash and enlarged lymph nodes Tertiary: late destructive lesions in internal organs	Urethritis Cervicitis Pharyngitis Infection of rectal mucosa (proctitis)	Superficial vesicles and ulcers on external genitalia and in genital tract Regional lymph nodes often enlarged and tender	Cervicitis Urethritis
Tests used to establish diagnosis	Demonstration of treponemas in chancre Serologic tests	Culture of organisms from sites of infection Nonculture tests also available	Demonstration of intranuclear inclusions in infected cells Virus cultures Serologic tests in some cases	Detection of chlamydial antigens in cervical/urethral secretions Fluorescence microscopy Cultures Nonculture tests also available
Major complications	Damage to cardiovascular system and nervous system in tertiary syphilis may be fatal	Disseminated bloodstream infection Tubal infection with impaired fertility Spread of infection to prostate and epididymides	Spread from infected mother to infant	Tubal infection with impaired fertility Epididymitis
Treatment	Antibiotics	Antibiotics	Antiviral drug shortens infection but not curative	Antibiotics

Primary Syphilis

Contact with an infected partner enables the treponemas to penetrate the mucous membranes of the genital tract, oral cavity, or rectal mucosa, or to be introduced through a break in the skin. The organisms multiply rapidly and spread throughout the body. After an incubation period of several weeks, a small ulcer called a chancre develops at the site of inoculation. It is easily seen if it is on the penis or vulva, but it may be undetected if it is within the vagina, oral cavity, or rectum.

The chancre, which is swarming with treponemas and is highly infectious, persists for about 4–6 weeks and eventually heals even if the disease is untreated. Even though the chancre has healed, however, the treponemas are widely disseminated through the body and continue to multiply.

Secondary Syphilis

The secondary stage of syphilis begins several months after the chancre has healed. The infected individual develops manifestations of a systemic infection characterized by elevated temperature, enlargement of lymph nodes, a skin rash, and shallow ulcers on the mucous membranes of the oral cavity and genital tract. This stage of the disease also is extremely infectious because the skin and mucous membrane lesions contain large numbers of treponemas. The secondary stage persists for several weeks and, like the chancre, eventually subsides even if no treatment is administered. Some subjects experience one or more recurrences of secondary syphilis, but each recurrence subsides spontaneously.

Tertiary Syphilis

After the second stage subsides, the infected individual appears well for a variable period of time, but the organisms are still active and may cause irreparable damage to the cardiovascular and nervous systems and to other organs as well. Chronic inflammation and scarring of the aortic valve lead to valve malfunction and heart failure. Often, the aortic wall just above the aortic valve also is damaged by the treponemas. This weakens the aortic wall, causing it to balloon out and eventually rupture. Degeneration of fiber tracts in the spinal cord caused by syphilis impairs sensation and disturbs walking. Damage to the brain by the treponemas causes mental deterioration and eventual paralysis. The late manifestations of the disease, which can appear as long as 20 years after the initial infection, are called tertiary syphilis. This stage is not generally communicable because the organisms are relatively few and are confined to the internal organs.

Diagnosis and Treatment

Two different types of laboratory tests are used to diagnose syphilis:

1. Demonstration of treponemas, by means of microscopic examination, in fluid squeezed from the ulcerated surface of the chancre. Specialized techniques and equipment are required.
2. Blood tests, called serologic tests for syphilis, that detect the various antibodies produced in response to a treponemal infection. The serologic tests become positive soon after the chancre appears and remain positive for many years.

Both types of tests are widely used; each has specific applications and limitations. Microscopic examination of material from a suspected chancre establishes the diagnosis of syphilis several weeks before a blood test will show positive results. On the other hand, if the chancre is in an inaccessible location and escapes detection, a positive blood test may be the only indication of syphilis in an individual who does not exhibit symptoms of active infection.

Syphilis can be treated successfully by penicillin and some other antibiotics. Treatment stops the progression of the disease and prevents serious late complications.

Congenital Syphilis

A syphilitic mother may transmit the disease to her unborn infant. The intrauterine infection may cause death of the fetus, or the infant may be born with congenital syphilis. The treponemas seem to be less able to pass through the placenta to infect the fetus during the first few months of pregnancy. Early in pregnancy, the placental villi are covered by a double layer of epithelium and contain more connective tissue compared with their appearance later in pregnancy, which may account for their reduced permeability. An infected mother should be treated as soon as the maternal infection is identified without regard to the stage of her pregnancy, but it is unlikely that the fetus will be infected if treatment is started during the early months of the pregnancy.

GONORRHEA

Gonorrhea, caused by the gonococcus *Neisseria gonorrhoeae*, is one of the most common communicable diseases (FIGURE 8-2). The organism primarily infects mucosal surfaces: the linings of the urethra, genital tract, pharynx, and rectum. Symptoms of infection appear about a week after exposure, and the clinical manifestations differ in the two sexes.

Gonorrhea in the Female
In the female, the gonococci infect chiefly the mucosa of the uterine cervix and the urethral mucosa. The gonococcal infection may also spread into Bartholin glands, which are located adjacent to the vaginal orifice. The cervical infection usually causes profuse vaginal discharge; the urethral involvement is manifested by pain and burning on urination. Some women, however, have few or no symptoms of infection but are nevertheless capable of transmitting the disease to their sexual partners.

The gonococcal infection may also spread upward from the cervix through the uterus into the fallopian tubes, where it causes an acute salpingitis (*salpinx* = tube). Sometimes, the tubal infection is followed by the formation of an abscess within the fallopian tube or an abscess involving both the tube and the adjacent ovary.

Gonococcal salpingitis is manifested by abdominal pain and tenderness together with elevated temperature and leukocytosis. Scarring following the tubal infection may delay transport of the fertilized ovum through the fallopian tube, causing the pregnancy to develop in the tube instead of the uterus, a condition called an ectopic pregnancy (described in the discussion on prenatal development and diseases associated with pregnancy). Complete obstruction of both tubes by scar tissue completely blocks the transport of a fertilized ovum through the tubes and leads to sterility.

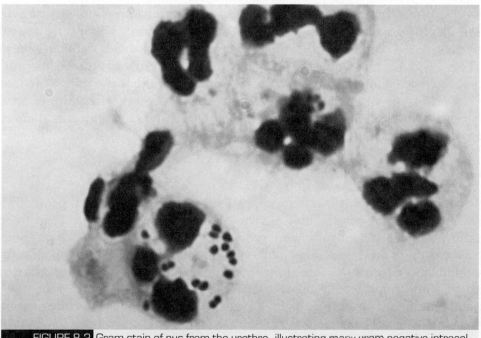

FIGURE 8-2 Gram stain of pus from the urethra, illustrating many gram-negative intracellular diplococci characteristic of gonorrhea (original magnification × 1,000).

Gonorrhea in the Male

In the male, gonococci cause an acute inflammation of the mucosa of the anterior part of the urethra. The infection is usually manifested by a purulent urethral discharge and considerable pain on urination, but occasionally the infected male may have relatively few symptoms, although he is still capable of infecting others. However, gonorrhea is less likely to be asymptomatic in men than in women.

From the anterior urethra, the infection often spreads by direct extension into the posterior urethra, prostate, seminal vesicles, vasa deferentia, and epididymides. An infection in both epididymides and vasa deferentia may lead to sterility because the scarring after the infection may obstruct the duct system and thus block transport of sperm into the seminal fluid.

Extragenital Gonorrhea

Recently, the incidence of gonococcal infection in extragenital sites has increased. Gonoccocal infection of the rectal mucosa causes anorectal pain and tenderness associated with purulent bloody mucoid discharge from the rectum. Rectal infection results from contamination of the rectal mucosa either by infected vaginal secretions or from anal intercourse. Gonococcal infection of the pharynx and tonsils results from oral–genital sex acts. The infection may be asymptomatic but often causes a sore throat.

Disseminated Gonococcal Infection

In a small proportion of infected patients, the organism gains access to the bloodstream and spreads throughout the body. This serious complication is characterized by elevated temperature, joint pain, multiple small abscesses in the skin, and sometimes infections of the joints, tendons, heart valves, and covering of the brain (meninges).

Diagnosis and Treatment

Diagnosis of gonorrhea is established by culturing gonococci from suspected sites of infection: urethra, cervix, rectum, and pharynx. Gonococci may also be cultured from the bloodstream in disseminated gonococcal infection. A non–culture-based test to identify gonococci (called a nucleic acid amplification test) is also available. The test is based on the identification of groups of nucleic acids in the organism.

Formerly, most infections responded to penicillin. Now, many strains produce an enzyme (penicillinase) that inactivates penicillin so that the antibiotic is ineffective, and some strains have also become resistant to other antibiotics as well. Consequently, selection of an appropriate antibiotic to treat a gonococcal infection is more difficult than in the past.

HERPES

The herpes simplex virus is one of several herpes viruses that infect people. There are two forms of the herpes simplex virus, designated type 1 and 2. Type 1 herpes usually infects the oral mucous membrane, where it causes the familiar fever blisters. Most individuals are infected in childhood, and most adults have antibodies to the virus, indicating a previous infection. Type 2 herpes virus usually infects the genital tract, and infections usually occur after puberty. However, the two types are not restricted in their distribution. Type 1 virus may cause genital infections, and type 2 virus may infect the oropharyngeal mucous membrane.

Genital herpes virus infection has increased significantly in recent years. Most genital infections (80%) are caused by type 2 virus. Genital tract infections caused by type 1 virus also have become more common (20%), probably because more people are engaging in oral–genital sexual practices.

The lesions caused by the viral infection usually appear within a week after sexual exposure. They consist of clusters of very small, painful blisters (vesicles) that soon rupture, forming painful shallow ulcers that often coalesce. The lesions contain large quantities of virus and are infectious to sexual contacts. Usually the lymph nodes draining the infected areas are swollen and tender. In men, the vesicles usually appear on the glans or shaft of the penis (FIGURE 8-3). In women, the lesions may be quite extensive (FIGURE 8-4). They may be on the vulva, in the vagina, or on the cervix. Vulvar lesions are quite painful, but those deep in the vagina or on the cervix may cause little discomfort because these regions are relatively insensitive. The ulcers heal slowly in a few weeks. However, the virus persists in the tissues of the infected person and may flare up periodically, causing recurrent infections. Some patients have repeated flare-ups for several years after the initial infection.

Active herpetic ulcers shed large amounts of virus, and sexual partners of patients with active lesions are readily infected. Unfortunately, patients without active lesions also may excrete small amounts of virus periodically and infect their sexual partners even though they have no lesions or symptoms of infection.

Diagnosis and Treatment

Herpes can usually be suspected from the clinical appearance of the lesions and can be confirmed by smears obtained from the lesions, which reveal the characteristic intranuclear inclusions in infected cells (FIGURE 8-5). The most reliable diagnostic test is culture of the virus from the ulcers and vesicles, and facilities for virus culture are now widely available.

Cold compresses applied to the affected areas and pain-relieving medications reduced discomfort. Now, antiviral drugs are available that shorten the course and reduce the severity of an acute infection, but antiviral drugs do not eradicate the virus. Depending on the severity of the infection, they can be administered intravenously or orally or applied as an ointment to the lesions. Patients with frequent and disabling

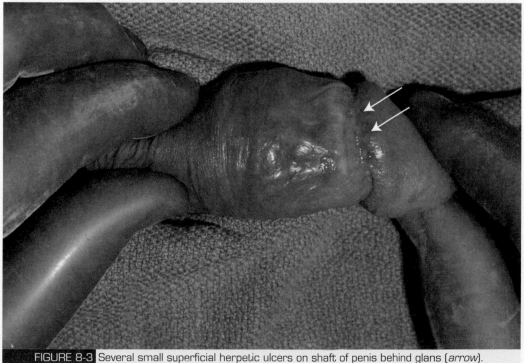

FIGURE 8-3 Several small superficial herpetic ulcers on shaft of penis behind glans (*arrow*).

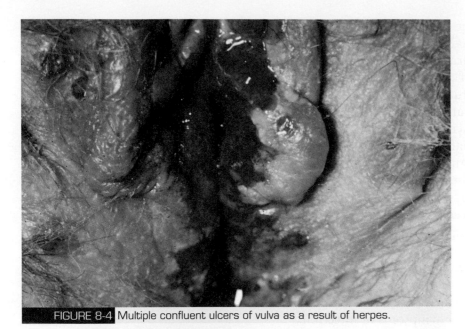

FIGURE 8-4 Multiple confluent ulcers of vulva as a result of herpes.

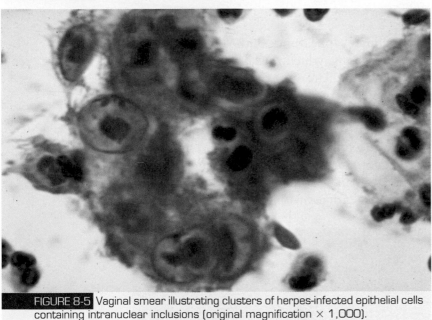

FIGURE 8-5 Vaginal smear illustrating clusters of herpes-infected epithelial cells containing intranuclear inclusions (original magnification × 1,000).

recurrent infections sometimes benefit from long-term oral treatment, which seems to reduce the frequency and severity of recurrences.

Herpes Infection and Pregnancy
A pregnant woman with a genital herpes infection may infect her infant. If the mother has active herpetic lesions in her genital tract, the infant may acquire the virus when passing through the genital tract during delivery. Consequently, a mother with an active infection is usually delivered by cesarean section in order to prevent infection of the newborn infant, which is likely if the infant is delivered vaginally.

GENITAL CHLAMYDIAL INFECTIONS

Genital tract infections caused by pathogenic micro-organisms such as *Chlamydia trachomatis* are now the most common sexually transmitted disease, and it has been estimated that there are between 3 and 4 million new cases each year. Part of this increase reflects the availability of new diagnostic tests that enable the physician to recognize chlamydial infections in patients who have few symptoms and whose cases probably would previously have gone undetected.

Chlamydia causes much the same type of inflammation and clinical symptoms as gonorrhea. In women, the initial infection is usually in the uterine cervix and is associated with moderate vaginal discharge. Men often develop acute inflammation of the urethra associated with frequency and burning on urination, which is called *nongonococcal urethritis*. Like gonorrhea, the chlamydial infection may spread to the fallopian tubes in women, followed by scarring and impaired fertility, and may cause acute epididymitis in men. As in gonorrhea, many infected persons may have no symptoms of infection but are still able to infect their sexual partners and may develop complications related to the spread of the infection to other parts of the genital tract.

Diagnosis and Treatment
Highly sensitive specific tests are available that can detect chlamydial antigens in cervical secretions and secretions from the male urethra, and the tests can also be

performed on urine. Chlamydia can also be identified in smears prepared from cervical or urethral material, stained by special techniques, and examined microscopically. Nucleic acid amplification tests, similar to the tests used to identify gonococci, can also be used to diagnose a chlamydial infection by identifying characteristic groups of chlamydial nucleic acids. Positive tests for chlamydia have been found from 10 to 20% of young sexually active women attending family planning clinics and from 17 to as high as 46% of clients attending sexually transmitted disease clinics. The infection responds to tetracycline antibiotics. Both the client and her partner should be treated.

Human Immunodeficiency Virus Infections and AIDS

AIDS is a devastating disease that cripples the body's immune system by attacking and destroying helper T lymphocytes, making the affected persons susceptible to a number of unusual infections and malignant tumors. AIDS is the end-stage and most serious manifestation of an infection caused by a virus called the human immunodeficiency virus or simply HIV. There are actually two viruses that cause AIDS, designated HIV-1 and HIV-2. HIV-1 is the virus that causes AIDS in most parts of the world, but HIV-2 infections are more prevalent in West Africa. Although HIV infection often is regarded as a sexually transmitted disease, many HIV infections are transmitted in other ways. Consequently, this disease is considered separately here not only because of the various ways that it can be transmitted but also because of the devastating effects of the virus on the people who are infected.

The first cases of the disease that we now call AIDS were identified in 1981 in a small group of homosexual men with an unusual opportunistic lung infection. HIV was identified in 1983, and a blood test to detect HIV infection became available in 1985. Today, we know a lot about the virus and how it damages the immune system, and we know how to avoid becoming infected. Unfortunately, the disease continues to spread because we do not know how to eradicate the virus even though we can slow the multiplication of the virus and arrest the progression of the disease that it causes. Worldwide, millions of people are infected, and the numbers continue to increase.

HIV AND ITS TARGET

HIV is an RNA virus that belongs to a class of viruses called retroviruses. The viral RNA and an important enzyme called reverse transcriptase are enclosed within a protein coat (capsid), forming the core of the virus. The core is surrounded by an envelope, composed of a double layer of lipid molecules, that was acquired from the cell membrane of the infected cell when the virus budded from the cell. The target of the HIV virus is the CD4 protein present on the cell membranes of helper T lymphocytes, as well as on monocytes, macrophages, and similar macrophagelike cells in the skin, lymph nodes, and within the central nervous system. The CD4 protein functions as a receptor for the virus to which the virus attaches. When the virus binds to the cell, the virus envelope fuses with the cell membrane, and the virus enters the cell. Once inside the cell, the virus makes a DNA copy of its own RNA genetic material by means of its reverse transcriptase enzyme, and the DNA copy is inserted into the genetic material of the infected cell, a process assisted by another viral enzyme called HIV integrase, and the viral genes direct the synthesis and assembly of more virus. The final stages of virus production requires a viral enzyme called HIV protease, which cuts and assembles the virus protein into small segments that surround the viral RNA, forming the infectious virus particles that bud from the infected cells. As the virus particles bud from the cells, they become coated by part of the cell membranes of the infected cells. The newly formed virus particles attack other susceptible cells within the lymphoid tissue throughout the body, where the virus replicates (proliferates) and releases more virus particles to infect still more susceptible cells. Helper T lymphocytes, which are the primary targets for the virus, are damaged and many are killed. Monocytes, however, which are also attacked, are quite resistant and survive, but the virus continues to replicate within the monocytes, releasing virus particles that infect other cells. In addition, the monocytes function as vehicles to transport the virus throughout the body and into the nervous system to infect the brain.

MANIFESTATIONS OF HIV INFECTION

During the early stages of the infection, large amounts of virus can be detected in the blood and body fluids of the infected person, and large numbers of virus-infected lymphocytes are present in lymph nodes and other lymphoid tissue throughout the body. During this phase, many infected persons develop a mild febrile illness. The body responds to the infection by forming anti-HIV antibodies and by generating cytotoxic T lymphocytes. The amount of virus in the blood and body fluids declines as the acute phase of the infection subsides, but unfortunately, the body's defenses are not able to eliminate the virus, and the infection enters a more chronic phase. However, there is no latent or dormant phase where the virus remains inactive. Very large numbers of virus particles are produced continuously, which infect and destroy CD4+ cells (helper T cells). Large numbers of virus particles also circulate in the bloodstream, and the amount of virus in the blood correlates with the magnitude of the infection in the body's lymphoid tissue.

The body responds to the destruction of CD4+ cells by stepping up production of more CD4+ cells to replace those killed by the virus. Cytotoxic (CD8+) T cells directed against the virus proliferate in an attempt to restrain the viral multiplication and the helper T cell destruction. Eventually, the rate at which CD4+ cells are replaced cannot keep up with rate of destruction, and the functions of the immune system begin to decline.

Generally, anti-HIV antibodies appear from 1 to as long as 6 months after the initial infection. Unfortunately, the antibodies cannot eradicate the virus or reduce its infectivity. Nevertheless, a confirmed positive test for virus antibodies is a useful test to indicate that a person has been infected with HIV, is infectious to others, and is at risk of damage to the immune system from the infection.

There are many different strains of HIV. Some appear to be quite aggressive, given that the disease in some infected persons appears to progress relatively rapidly. In contrast, a few strains appear to be relatively benign because some fortunate individuals who have been infected with HIV for many years do not show any evidence that their immune systems have been damaged.

Current antiviral treatment has greatly improved the outcome of an HIV infection, which now can be controlled for many years by appropriate treatment. Unfortunately, although the proliferation of the virus and associated damage to the immune system can often be suppressed, current antiviral drugs cannot completely eliminate the virus, which persists indefinitely in the tissues of the infected host. Current drug therapy has changed HIV infection from a relatively rapidly progressing fatal disease to a more slowly progressive chronic disease that can be controlled but cannot be cured. TABLE 8-2 summarizes the sequence of events in HIV infection and their significance.

TABLE 8-2

Sequence of events in HIV infections and their significance

Event	Significance
HIV invades CD4+ cells and becomes part of cell DNA	Individual is infected for life
Virus proliferates in infected cells and sheds virus particles	Virus present in blood and body fluids
Body forms anti-HIV antibody	Antibody is a marker of infection but is not protective
Progressive destruction of helper T cells	Compromised cell-mediated immunity
Immune defenses collapse	Opportunistic infections Neoplasms

MEASUREMENT OF VIRAL RNA AND CD4 LYMPHOCYTES AS AN INDEX OF DISEASE PROGRESSION

Although HIV replicates in lymph nodes and not in the blood, the amount of viral RNA in the blood reflects the extent of viral replication in the lymphoid tissue throughout the body and can vary from over a million virus particles per milliliter of blood plasma in a patient with an acute infection to extremely low levels in a patient being treated successfully with agents effective against the virus.

A determination of the number of helper T lymphocytes in the blood allows one to estimate the extent of damage to the immune system. Normally, there are from about 800 to 1,200 helper T (CD4+) lymphocytes per microliter of blood, but this number declines progressively as the disease advances. When this number falls to about 500 cells per microliter of blood, the patient becomes at risk of opportunistic infections, and by the time the helper T lymphocyte count falls below 200 per microliter, the infected person is at very high risk of major complications from the disease.

COMPLICATIONS OF AIDS

The impaired cell-mediated immunity leads to two very serious problems: a greatly increased susceptibility to infection and a predisposition to various malignant tumors.

Infections

Many of the viruses, fungi, parasites, and other pathogens that attack AIDS patients do not usually cause disease in healthy persons. (Infections of this type are often called **opportunistic infections** because the pathogens normally do not have an opportunity to cause serious disease in persons whose immune systems are intact.) One of the most common AIDS-related opportunistic infections is pneumonia in the respiratory system caused by the fungus parasite *Pneumocystis jiroveci*. Another relatively common and serious systemic infection is caused by a normally nonpathogenic acid-fast bacterium called *Mycobacterium avium* complex. Other serious infections are the parasitic infections toxoplasmosis and cryptosporidiosis, described in the discussion on animal parasites.

Opportunistic infection (op-por-too-nis'tik) *An infection in an immunocompromised person caused by an organism that is normally nonpathogenic or of limited pathogenicity.*

AIDS patients are also at risk for acquiring widespread, rapidly progressive tuberculosis or histoplasmosis—infections that normally are held in check by persons with normal immune systems. Many of the symptoms exhibited by patients with AIDS such as fever, cough, shortness of breath, weight loss, and enlarged lymph nodes are the result of the severe infections that afflict these unfortunate individuals. TABLE 8-3 lists some of the more common, severe, and often life-threatening infections in AIDS patients.

Malignant Tumors

The malignant tumors common in AIDS patients also are related to failure of the immune system, which helps to protect persons from neoplastic disease such as tumors as well as infections. The most common malignant tumor in AIDS patients, which is rare in other persons, is Kaposi sarcoma, which is caused by a herpes virus designated human herpesvirus 8. This tumor, which is composed of immature connective tissue cells (fibroblasts) and blood capillaries intermixed with inflammatory and phagocytic cells, forms hemorrhagic nodules in the skin, mouth, lymph nodes, and internal organs (FIGURE 8-6). Malignant tumors of B lymphocytes also are common, as are cancers of the mouth, rectum, and uterine cervix.

PREVALENCE OF HIV INFECTION IN HIGH-RISK GROUPS

The Centers for Disease Control and Prevention (CDC) estimates that more than 1 million people are infected with HIV in the United States and about 15,000 new infections occur each year. The largest group of infected persons is homosexual and bisexual men who engage in sexual activity with other group members who are designated by the CDC as men who have sex with men (MSM). Although MSM accounts for only about 4% of the male population aged 13 years and older, new HIV infections occur 44 times more frequently in MSM than in heterosexual men. This group accounts for over half of the million HIV-infected people. This is the only group in the United States in whom HIV infections are increasing. In contrast, new infections have declined among heterosexual men and injection drug users.

The distribution of HIV cases among the various high-risk groups is indicated in TABLE 8-4. Most HIV cases are found in homosexual or bisexual males and intravenous drug abusers, and these two groups make up about 53% of all HIV cases.

TABLE 8-3

Common infections in HIV patients	
Viruses	Herpes, cytomegalovirus, Epstein-Barr virus (infectious mononucleosis)
Fungi	Histoplasmosis, coccidioidomycosis, aspergillosis, *Candida* infections, *Pneumocystis jiroveci* pneumonia
Protozoa	Amebiasis, cryptosporidiosis, toxoplasmosis
Mycobacteria	Tuberculosis, *Mycobacterium avium-intracellulare* infections

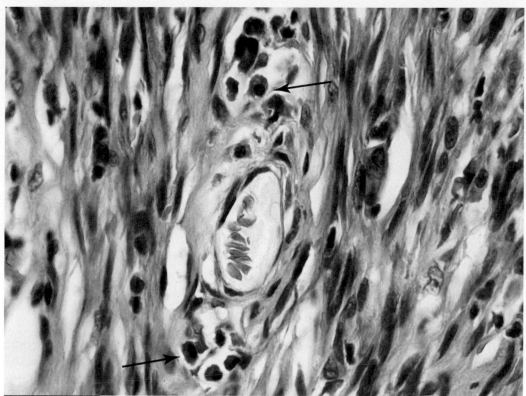

FIGURE 8-6 Kaposi sarcoma, illustrating proliferating spindle-shaped connective tissue cells (fibroblasts) surrounding a small blood vessel in the center of the field. Plasma cells (*arrow*) are intermixed with connective tissue cells (original magnification × 400).

Heterosexual HIV-infected persons make up another 31% of the total, and women account for about 25% of new HIV infections each year.

There are also some striking ethnic differences in the prevalence of HIV infections and AIDS. There is a disproportionately large number of AIDS cases in minority groups. African Americans and Hispanics comprise about 25% of the US population, but they account for about 69% of all AIDS cases.

HIV Transmission by Blood and Body Fluids

Transmission of the virus requires contact with body fluids containing virus infected cells or free virus particles. Much of the virus is contained within lymphocytes and

TABLE 8·4

Distribution of HIV cases by risk group	
Risk group	Percentage of total AIDS cases
Homosexual and bisexual men	53
Homosexual and bisexual men who are also intravenous drug users	4
Heterosexual drug abusers	12
Heterosexual HIV-infected persons	31

Data from Hall H. J., Song, R., Rhodes, P., et al. 2008. Estimation of HIV incidence in the United States. *Journal of the American Medical Association* 300, 520–9.

monocytes, with smaller amounts within the extracellular fluid. The amount of virus in body fluids varies with the stage of the disease and the source of the body fluids. Blood, seminal fluid, cervical and vaginal secretions, and breast milk generally contain large amounts of virus and are considered quite infectious, whereas urine, stool, saliva, tears, and perspiration usually contain little virus and are much less infectious. Transmission of the virus is usually either by sexual contact or by means of infected blood or blood products, but the virus may also be passed from an infected mother to her newborn infant.

Sexual Transmission.   Among male homosexuals and bisexuals, transmission of the virus is chiefly by anal intercourse, which injures anal tissues and permits intermixing of infected blood and seminal fluid. Heterosexual partners of infected persons become infected by sexual intercourse because semen of infected males and vaginal secretions of infected women contain the virus. Many prostitutes of both sexes are infected, either from drug abuse or sexual contacts, and sexual contacts with prostitutes are very risky. Many Haitians of both sexes, as well as persons from central Africa, are infected. In these countries, the infection is transmitted chiefly by heterosexual intercourse, and both sexes are equally affected.

Transmission by Blood and Blood Products.   Intravenous drug abusers become infected by sharing needles and syringes contaminated with blood from an infected person. Persons with hemophilia acquired the infection from blood products administered to treat their coagulation defect. Transfusion recipients were infected from contaminated blood received before laboratory tests were available to screen donors for evidence of infection.

Mother-to-Infant Transmission.   Infected maternal blood or cervical–vaginal secretions are the source of infection of newborn infants born to infected mothers, and the likelihood of fetal infection depends to some extent on how much virus is present in the mother's blood and body fluids. Consequently, all infected pregnant women should receive highly active antiviral therapy to suppress HIV multiplication. With effective antiviral therapy, the amount of virus in the maternal blood can be reduced to an extremely low level, which greatly reduces the risk of fetal HIV infection.

PREVENTION AND CONTROL OF HIV INFECTION

Individuals infected with the virus are at risk of late complications, which eventually occur in a significant number of persons. Infections and tumors in AIDS patients can be treated, but treatment of the underlying viral infection has been hampered by lack of a drug that can eliminate the virus. Several drugs are available that can impede viral replication and slow the progression of the disease. Much effort is being directed toward finding ways to control or eradicate the virus and toward developing a vaccine to immunize against the virus, but at present, there are no major breakthroughs on the horizon. The only really effective way to control the disease is to prevent further spread of the infection. This means that each individual must assume responsibility for his or her own behavior if the relentless spread of the disease is to be contained.

1. Uninfected persons should avoid sexual contacts with persons in high-risk groups or known to be infected with the virus (TABLE 8-5).
2. Members of high-risk groups should limit their number of sexual partners, practice "safe sex," which requires the use of condoms to reduce the risk of transmitting the infection, and avoid sexual practices such as unprotected anal intercourse and oral–genital contact, which can spread the virus.

TABLE 8-5

Groups at high risk of immunodeficiency virus infection

1. Homosexual or bisexual men

2. Present or past intravenous drug abusers

3. Persons with clinical or laboratory evidence of HIV infection

4. Persons born in countries where heterosexual transmission plays the major role in spreading the infection

5. Male or female prostitutes and their sexual partners

6. Sexual partners of infected persons

3. Persons at high risk of infection should not donate blood in order to prevent transmission of the virus by blood transfusion. Blood banks now screen donor blood for antibodies to the AIDS virus (as well as the hepatitis virus) and reject the blood for transfusion if antibodies are detected. The screening tests, however, will not reliably exclude all infected donors because some persons who have been recently infected may not have yet formed anti-bodies.

4. Infected women planning to become pregnant should consider the risks of pregnancy based on the stage of the HIV disease and the risks of mother-to-infant transmission of HIV, which can be greatly reduced but not completely eliminated by antiviral drugs.

TREATMENT OF HIV INFECTION

When to Treat

When to start treatment requires one to balance the advantages of suppressing viral multiplication against the cost, side effects, and inconvenience of treatment. Intensive treatment of HIV infection is called highly active antiretroviral therapy (HAART), which involves multiple drugs that must be taken on a precise schedule for life in order to arrest the progression of the disease. Side effects related to the drugs are relatively frequent and may be severe, and drug resistance may occur, especially if the multiple drugs are not taken as prescribed. However, effective antiviral therapy inhibits viral multiplication, reduces the amount of virus in the circulation, and helps the immune system to recover.

The current goal of treatment is to suppress virus replication completely for as long as possible by using a potent combination of antiviral drugs, with periodic determination of the number of virus particles in the blood to measure response to therapy.

In general, most physicians believe that persons with high concentrations of virus in their blood should be treated even though the number of CD4+ cells in the blood is still normal and they have no symptoms of infection. Persons with a large amount of virus in their blood have a large amount of replicating virus in their lymphoid tissue, which is destroying their CD4+ cells. Suppressing virus multiplication helps preserve the function of the immune system and reduces the likelihood of spreading the infection to an uninfected partner, which also slows the spread of HIV to other people in the community.

Drugs to Treat HIV Infections

Many drugs are now available to treat HIV infections, and more are being developed. Treatment schedules are being revised continually as new drugs are developed and as physicians gain experience with the advantages and side effects of various drug combinations. The anti-HIV drugs are classified into six groups based on the phase of the viral life cycle inhibited by the drugs:

1. Non-nucleoside reverse transcriptase inhibitors
2. Nucleoside reverse transcriptase inhibitors (nucleoside analogs)
3. Protease inhibitors
4. HIV entry inhibitors
5. HIV integrase inhibitors
6. Fixed dose combination tablets containing two or more anti-HIV drugs that can be from different drug classes (TABLE 8-6).

Each class of drug attacks a different phase in the HIV life cycle. Generally, a combination of drugs is given. Such combinations usually are very effective for inhibiting viral replication and maintaining the function of the immune system and can help restore an immune system that has already been damaged by the virus. Although combination drug therapy can reduce the level of virus in the circulation to extremely low or undetectable levels, such therapy has not been shown to eradicate the virus in the lymphoid tissues of the body. Infected persons must be willing to continue lifelong treatment with various combinations of potent antiviral drugs to inhibit virus proliferation, even though the virus cannot be destroyed. Other drugs are also available that interfere with specific phases of virus proliferation.

How the Drugs Act

Nonnucleoside reverse transcriptase inhibitors bind directly to reverse transcriptase and block DNA polymerase, which is required to convert viral RNA to DNA so that it can be incorporated into the nucleus of the infected cell.

Nucleoside reverse transcriptase inhibitors (**nucleoside analogs**) interrupt the formation of viral DNA from RNA by substituting a nucleoside analog (a "look-alike" compound) that resembles one of the normal nucleosides used by the virus to construct DNA. The virus cannot distinguish the analog from the "normal" nucleoside that it

Nonnucleoside reverse transcriptase inhibitors
Drugs used to treat HIV infections that bind to reverse transcriptase, blocking DNA polymerase that converts RNA to DNA.

Nucleoside reverse transcriptase inhibitors
Nucleoside analogs ("look alike compounds") that resemble the normal nucleosides that a virus uses to construct DNA. Synthesis is disrupted when the analog substitutes for the required nucleoside.

TABLE 8-6

Method of action on anti-HIV drugs

Class of anti-HIV drug	Method of action
1. Non-nucleoside reverse transcriptase inhibitor	Blocks DNA polymerase that converts viral RNA to DNA
2. Nucleoside reverse transcriptase inhibitor	Substitutes a faulty nucleoside for normal nucleoside, which interrupts viral DNA synthesis
3. Protease inhibitor	Inhibits the viral enzyme that cuts and assembles the protein surrounding viral RNA
4. HIV entry inhibitor	Inhibits HIV entry into cell to cause infection
5. HIV integrase inhibitor	Inhibits the protein that inserts (integrates) HIV into the DNA of infected cell
6. Fixed dose combination anti-HIV drugs	Two or more drugs of different classes work together to impede HIV infection

resembles. When the virus tries to incorporate the "look-alike" compound into the viral DNA, the viral DNA synthesis is interrupted and unable to continue.

Protease inhibitors block the enzyme that cuts the viral protein into short segments and assembles the protein segments around viral RNA to form the infectious virus particle. Inhibition of the protease enzyme leads to release of disorganized and noninfectious virus particles. HIV entry inhibitors block entry of HIV into the cell, and integrase inhibitors inhibit the viral enzyme *integrase* that is needed to insert HIV genetic material into the DNA of the infected cell.

Protease inhibitors
Drugs used to treat HIV infection that block the enzyme that cuts the viral protein into segments and assembles them around the viral RNA to form the infectious virus particle. As a result, the virus particle is improperly constructed and is not infectious.

Case Studies

The following cases illustrate some of the clinical features and medical problems encountered in AIDS patients.

CASE 8-1

A 62-year-old woman, whose husband has hemophilia and had been treated with antihemophilic globulin, was hospitalized because of low-grade fever, cough, sweating, and a 35-lb weight loss over the previous 6 weeks. Chest x-ray revealed a bilateral pneumonia. A blood test for antibodies to the HIV was positive, and lung biopsy obtained by bronchoscopy revealed *Pneumocystis jiroveci* pneumonia. The patient was treated with appropriate antibiotics.

This patient had been infected with the HIV through sexual intercourse with her husband, who had become infected previously from blood products used to treat his hemophilia.

CASE 8-2

A 30-year-old HIV-positive homosexual male had been treated previously for various AIDS-related complications. Recently, he had experienced fever, fatigue, and weight loss. Physical examination revealed many large lymph nodes in the neck, armpits, and groin. A chest x-ray revealed no evidence of pneumonia. Lymph node biopsy revealed large numbers of mononuclear phagocytic cells filling the lymph node, and special stains revealed that the phagocytes were packed with acid-fast organisms (FIGURE 8-7). Biopsy of the bone marrow revealed similar focal clusters of mononuclear cells within the marrow, and marrow culture yielded *Mycobacterium avium* complex. Treatment with appropriate antibiotics was begun.

CASE 8-3

A 39-year-old HIV-positive homosexual male with multiple sexual partners had been treated on several occasions for *Candida* infections of the mouth and intermittent chronic diarrhea. Recently, he developed a red vascular nodule in his oral cavity that was biopsied and interpreted as Kaposi sarcoma. The implications of this diagnosis were explained to the patient, and he was advised of the precautions necessary to prevent the spread of the HIV infection to others. He was referred to another physician for further treatment.

A

B

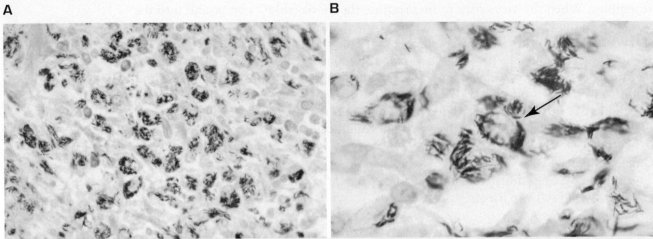

FIGURE 8-7 Disseminated *Mycobacterium avium* complex infection (Case 8-2). **A**, Acid-fast organisms that fill the cytoplasm of large mononuclear phagocytes (macrophages) throughout the node, as demonstrated by special stains. **B**, High-magnification view of the mycobacteria. The nucleus of a mononuclear phagocyte (*arrow*) surrounded by masses of organisms in the cytoplasm appears in the center of the field. Large clumps of organisms fill the cytoplasm of other phagocytes in the field, obscuring the nuclei of the phagocytes (original magnification × 1,000).

QUESTIONS FOR REVIEW

1. How are communicable diseases transmitted? How are they controlled?
2. What is meant by the following terms: *epidemic disease, endemic disease, immunization,* and *sexually transmitted disease?*
3. How is syphilis transmitted? What are its clinical manifestations?
4. How is gonorrhea transmitted? What are its clinical manifestations? What is nongonococcal urethritis?
5. What are the manifestations of herpes infection of the genital tract?
6. What are the manifestations of chlamydial infection of the genital tract? How are chlamydial infections diagnosed and treated?
7. What is AIDS? What is its cause? What are its clinical manifestations? What groups are at high risk of infection, and how do they become infected? How can the spread of the infection be prevented or minimized?
8. What is the significance of a positive test for HIV antibody?

SUPPLEMENTARY READINGS

Bhaskaran, K., Hamouda, O., Sannes, M., et al. 2008. Changes in the risk of death after HIV seroconversion compared with mortality in the general population. *Journal of the American Medical Association* 300:51–9.

▶ Mortality rates for HIV-infected persons have become much closer to mortality rates in the general population for the first 5 years after becoming infected, apparently related to the introduction of highly active antiretroviral therapy. This is not sustained after 5 years, probably related to problems in drug toxicity, HIV drug resistance, and less adherence to therapy.

Centers for Disease Control and Prevention. 2007. Symptomatic early neurosyphilis among HIV-positive men who have sex with men—four cities, United States, January 2002–June 2004. *Morbidity and Mortality Weekly Report* 56:625–8.

▶ Symptomatic early neurosyphilis is a rare manifestation of syphilis, which usually occurs within the first 12 months after infection and is characterized by manifestations of meningitis, disturbed cranial nerve functions, and inflammation of cerebral blood vessels leading to strokelike symptoms caused by interruption of blood flow to the brain. Symptomatic neurosyphilis almost completely disappeared in the late 1940s, coincident with widespread use of penicillin to treat syphilis, but reappeared in the late 1980s among HIV-positive men who had sex with other men (MSM). Syphilis-infected subjects are at increased risk of symptomatic neurosyphilis, which is likely to be more severe, progress more rapidly, and is more difficult to treat. Clinical manifestations and response to treatment are described.

Cooper, D. A., Maclean P., and Finlayson, R. 1985. Acute AIDS retrovirus infection: Definition of a clinical illness associated with seroconversion. *Lancet* 1:537–40.

▶ Describes clinical features of acute infectious mononucleosislike illness caused by the AIDS virus.

Goulder, P. J. R., and Walker, B. D. 2002. HIV-1 superinfection: A word of caution. *New England Journal of Medicine* 347:756–8.

▶ An HIV-1 infection with one strain of virus does not protect against a new infection with a different strain of virus, and the infection with a new virus strain may precipitate a rapid progression of HIV disease. To prevent a second infection with a different virus strain, an HIV–positive person should use the same "safe-sex" precautions that an uninfected person should use.

Greene, J. B., Sidhu, G. S., Lavin, S., et al. 1982. *Mycobacterium avium-intracellulare.* A cause of disseminated life-threatening infection in homosexuals and drug abusers. *Annals of Internal Medicine* 97:539–46.

▶ Systemic infections caused by normally nonpathogenic mycobacteria may occur in persons with AIDS and often are resistant to most commonly used antimycobacterial drugs.

Kovacs, J. A., and Masur, H. 2000. Prophylaxis against opportunistic infections in patients with human immunodeficiency infections. *New England Journal of Medicine* 342:1416–29.

▶ Persons with counts above 200 CD4 cells are at low risk of opportunistic infections. No prophylactic therapy is 100% effective; prophylaxis is available against many infections, and maintenance therapy is usually required. However, additional maintenance anti-tuberculosis treatment is not required if a patient has been treated successfully for tuberculosis. Relapses are rare among treated patients with drug-sensitive tuberculosis, but such patients may acquire a new infection with a drug-resistant tubercle bacillus.

McArthur, J. C. 1987. Neurologic manifestations of AIDS. *Medicine* 66:407–37.

▶ Reviews the neurologic complications in 186 patients with HIV infection and biologic properties of the human immunodeficiency virus.

Thompson, M. A., Aberg, J. A., Cahn, P., et al. 2010. Antiretroviral treatment of adult HIV infection: 2010 recommendations of the International AIDS Society—USA panel. *Journal of the American Medical Association* 304:321–33.

▶ Increasing evidence indicates immune system damage begins in the early asymptomatic phase of HIV infection. The risks associated with antiretroviral therapy (ART) have decreased. Many AIDS patients have very high HIV-1 RNA and rapid CD4 cell count decline are reasons to start ART regardless of CD4 cell count. HIV also increases mortality from coexisting HBV or HCV infection and is also associated with an increased risk of cardiovascular disease. Widespread use of ART has nearly eliminated mother-to-child transmission, and ART has reduced the risk of transmission of HIV to an uninfected partner. Plasma HIV-1 RNA should be monitored frequently and treatment should be changed if levels rise, indicating failure to suppress the virus, and new therapy should be instituted. The goal is to achieve plasma HIV-1 RNA below the detection level of the most sensitive HIV test available. Increasing evidence indicates immune system damage begins in the early asymptomatic phase of HIV infection. If levels rise, indicating failure to suppress the virus, new therapy should be instituted.

OUTLINE SUMMARY

Methods of Transmission

Direct: Physical contact or droplet spread.
Indirect: Contaminated food or water; insects.

Methods of Control

IMMUNIZATION
Renders population nonsusceptible.
Disease incidence declines or disease dies out because no susceptible host.

IDENTIFICATION, ISOLATION, AND TREATMENT OF INFECTED PERSONS
Identification shortens time of infectivity.
Isolation often not effective because infected persons not recognized.

CONTROL OF MEANS OF INDIRECT TRANSMISSION
Control of food and water supplies.
Control of food handlers.
Control of insect population.
Control of animal sources.

REQUIREMENTS FOR EFFECTIVE CONTROL
Know cause.
Know method of transmission.

Sexually Transmitted Diseases

SYPHILIS
Primary stage: chancre at site of infection will eventually heal without treatment.
Secondary stage:
  Follows primary after several months.
  Characterized by fever, rash, and large lymph nodes.
  Subsides without treatment.
Tertiary stage: late destructive lesions in nervous system and heart.
Congenital:
  Acquired by newborn infant of infected mother.
  May cause fetal death or live-born infected infant.
  Treatment of mother early in pregnancy prevents fetal infection.

GONORRHEA
A surface infection of mucous membranes: genital tract, rectum, pharynx.
May spread to upper genital tract in both sexes.
Extragenital gonorrhea occurs frequently.
Occasional systemic infection affects joints, skin, heart valves, brain.

HERPES
Clinical features:
  May be caused by either type 1 or type 2 herpes virus.
  Causes vesicles that form ulcers.
  Recurrences occur frequently.
  No curative treatment.
Diagnosis of herpes:
  By clinical features.
  Smears reveal inclusions.
  Virus cultured from lesions.
  Serologic tests reveal antibodies.
  Herpes in pregnancy: may infect infant during delivery. Rarely causes intrauterine infection leading to congenital abnormalities.
  Frequency of herpes infection: significant increase recently, mostly HSV-2 infections.

CHLAMYDIAL INFECTIONS
Clinical features:
  Most common sexually transmitted disease.
  Many patients are asymptomatic.
  Infects uterine cervix. May spread to fallopian tubes followed by scarring and impaired fertility.
  Causes nongonococcal urethritis in men; may spread to cause epididymitis.
Diagnosis and treatment:
  Rapid tests detect chlamydial antigens in infected secretions.
  Chlamydia can be demonstrated in specially stained smears of secretions by microscopy.
  Infection responds to antibiotics.

HUMAN IMMUNODEFICIENCY VIRUS INFECTIONS AND AIDS
Nature of the disease:
  Virus cripples immune system.
  AIDS is most devastating manifestation of infection.
  Asymptomatic or milder infections in many persons.
Effect of the virus on T cells:
  RNA virus invades helper T lymphocytes and monocytes.

Virus makes DNA copy of its own RNA genetic material.

Viral DNA copy inserted into DNA of infected cell and directs production of virus particles in cell.

Virus buds from cell and infects other helper T lymphocytes.

Virus particles appear in blood and body fluids, which are infectious to others.

Antibody response to virus:

Antibodies formed within 1–6 months.

Antibodies are evidence of infection but do not eradicate virus.

Early manifestations of infection:

Most have no symptoms initially.

Some have brief illness resembling infectious mononucleosis.

Generalized lymph node enlargement.

Nonspecific symptoms: fever, weakness, fatigue, weight loss.

AIDS:

Pathogenesis:

Destruction of helper T cells.

Impaired cell-mediated immune defenses.

Humoral immunity less affected.

Complications of AIDS:

Infections:

Opportunistic infections—Pneumocystis jiroveci, Mycobacterium avium complex, and others.

Widespread infections caused by organisms usually controlled by normal persons.

Malignant tumors:

Kaposi sarcoma.

Malignant tumors of B lymphocytes.

Cancers of oral cavity and rectum.

AIDS in high-risk groups:

Homosexual/bisexual males.

Intravenous drug abusers.

Hemophiliacs.

Heterosexual partners of infected persons.

Children born to infected mothers.

Small percentage of infected persons do not fit into high-risk groups.

Manner of virus transmission in high-risk groups:

Sexual contact:

Primarily anal intercourse and oral–genital contact in homosexuals or bisexuals.

Heterosexual partners of infected persons infected by sexual intercourse.

Prostitutes frequently infected.

Spread primarily by heterosexual contacts in Haiti and central Africa. Both sexes equally infected.

Blood and blood products:

Intravenous drug abusers infected by contaminated needles and syringes.

Those with hemophilia infected from blood products.

Transfusion recipients infected from blood prior to routine screening of blood for AIDS virus.

Mother-to-infant transmission:

Infected maternal blood and/or cervicovaginal secretions infect newborn.

Risk of transmission reduced by: administration of antiretroviral drugs during pregnancy and delivery and to infant after birth avoiding nursing; administration of antiretroviral drugs to mother during pregnancy; elective cesarian delivery.

PREVENTION AND CONTROL OF HIV INFECTION

Avoid sexual contact with high-risk persons.

Practice "safe sex" and limit number of sexual partners.

High-risk groups should not donate blood because screening tests to exclude infected blood cannot detect infected persons who have not yet formed antibody to virus.

TREATMENT OF HIV INFECTION

Goal is to suppress viral multiplication by potent antiretroviral drug therapy.

Many drugs available given in combination, each targeting different phase of virus life cycle.

Intensive treatment inhibits virus, retards progression of disease, and may restore damaged immune system but does not eradicate virus.

Intensive early therapy has drawbacks: toxicity and possible drug resistance that may preclude later use of drugs when they may be required later in course of disease.

http://health.jbpub.com/humandisease/9e

Human Disease Online is a great source for supplementary human disease information for both students and instructors. Visit this website to find a variety of useful tools for learning, thinking, and teaching.

Congenital and Hereditary Diseases

1. List the common causes of congenital malformations and their approximate incidence.

2. List four abnormalities of sex chromosomes, and describe their clinical manifestations.

3. Describe some of the common genetic abnormalities, and explain four methods of transmission.

4. Compare the methods of transmission and clinical manifestations of phenylketonuria and hemophilia.

5. Describe some of the more important malformations resulting from intrauterine injury.

6. Explain the process of amniocentesis.

7. Explain multifactorial inheritance. Give an example of a multifactorial defect, and describe the relevant factors.

8. List the causes of Down syndrome, and describe its clinical manifestations. Give reasons why it is important to identify a carrier of a 14/21 chromosome translocation.

9. Understand the various methods available to make a diagnosis of a congenital abnormality in the fetus.

Causes of Congenital Malformations

Congenital
Present at birth.

There are many congenital and hereditary diseases. Their clinical manifestations range from minor, inconsequential defects to severe malformations that are incompatible with extrauterine life. A *hereditary* or *genetic* disease may be defined as one resulting from a chromosome abnormality or a defective gene. The term **congenital** disease or malformation refers to any abnormality that is present at birth (*congenitus* = with birth), even though it may not be detected until some time after birth; this broad category encompasses all abnormalities caused by disturbed prenatal development, regardless of their nature. Congenital defects are recognized in about 2–3% of all newborn infants. In an additional 2–3%, developmental defects are not recognized at birth but become apparent as the infants grow older. Major malformations are also found in from 25 to 50% of spontaneously aborted embryos and fetuses and in stillborn infants.

Four major factors are known to induce congenital malformations:

1. Chromosomal abnormalities
2. Abnormalities of individual genes
3. Intrauterine injury to the embryo or fetus by drugs, radiation, maternal infection, or other harmful environmental factors
4. Environmental factors acting on a genetically predisposed embryo

Chromosomal Abnormalities

Chromosomal abnormalities leading to congenital malformations may result from failure of homologous chromosomes in the germ cells to separate normally, from abnormal breaks and rearrangements of chromosomes in the germ cells as they are maturing (gametogenesis), and occasionally from failure of chromosomes to separate normally in the fertilized ovum (zygote) as the cells divide by mitosis during early prenatal development.

Occasionally, homologous chromosomes in germ cells fail to separate from one another in either the first or the second meiotic division. This is called *nondisjunction*. It causes abnormalities in the distribution of chromosomes between germ cells (FIGURE 9-1). One of the two germ cells derived from the abnormal chromosome division has an extra chromosome, and the other cell lacks a chromosome. Nondisjunction may involve either the sex chromosomes or the autosomes. If it occurs during gametogenesis, one daughter cell will have 24 chromosomes, and the other will have 22. If a gamete having an abnormal number of chromosomes fuses with a normal gamete during fertilization, the resulting zygote will either have an extra chromosome or be lacking one of the homologous

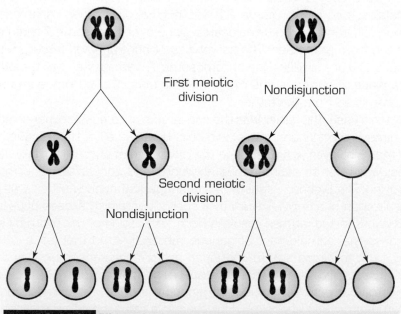

FIGURE 9-1 Effects of nondisjunction in meiosis, leading to formation of gametes with an extra or missing chromosome. Only the chromosome pair involved in nondisjunction is illustrated. *Left,* Nondisjunction at second meiotic division. *Right,* Nondisjunction at first meiotic division.

Trisomy
The presence of an extra chromosome within a cell; having three of a given chromosome instead of the usual pair.

....

Monosomy
A condition of a cell in which one chromosome of a homologous pair is missing.

....

Translocation
A transfer of a piece of one chromosome to a nonhomologous chromosome.

pair of chromosomes. The presence of an extra chromosome in a cell is called a **trisomy** (*tri* = three + *soma* = body) of the chromosome present in triplicate. Absence of a chromosome is called a **monosomy** (*mono* = one) of the missing chromosome.

CHROMOSOME DELETIONS AND TRANSLOCATIONS DURING GAMETOGENESIS

Sometimes a chromosome breaks in the course of meiosis, and the broken piece is lost from the cell. This is called a chromosome deletion. In some cases, the broken piece is not lost but becomes attached to another nonhomologous chromosome with which it is carried along during meiosis. A misplaced chromosome or part of a chromosome attached to another chromosome is called a **translocation** (*trans* = across + *locus* = place). In a reciprocal translocation, pieces of chromosomes (containing different sets of genes) are reciprocally exchanged between two nonhomologous chromosomes. Such an accident does not disturb the function of the cell because there is no loss or gain of genetic material. However, if the translocation occurs in a germ cell, an egg or sperm containing either a deficiency or an excess of chromosomal material may form during meiosis. If such a chromosomally abnormal gamete unites with a normal gamete during fertilization, the fertilized ovum (zygote) contains an abnormal amount of chromosomal material. Many abnormal zygotes are spontaneously aborted, but some survive and give rise to defective fetuses, as illustrated by the following case from the medical literature.

CASE 9-1

A mother gave birth to an infant with multiple congenital abnormalities and had two subsequent pregnancies. Both terminated in spontaneous abortions about 8 weeks after conception. Chromosome studies were performed on both parents, the liveborn infant, and the two aborted fetuses. The mother's karyotype was normal. The father's karyotype revealed that a piece of one chromosome 7 had been translocated to chromosome 21. In the offspring with the congenital abnormalities, one chromosome 21 was normal. The other chromosome 21 was abnormal, containing a translocated piece of chromosome 7 that had been transmitted from the father. The karyotypes of both aborted fetuses also were abnormal and were similar. One chromosome 7 was normal, but the other was lacking a piece of chromosome material. This abnormal chromosome also had been transmitted from the father.

In this case, the father was the carrier of a chromosomal abnormality that did not disturb the function of his own cells because all of the genetic material was normal. However, it did result in the formation of chromosomally abnormal gametes, which led to spontaneous abortions and congenital abnormalities in the offspring. The liveborn infant with the congenital abnormalities was derived from fertilization of a normal ovum by a sperm containing excess genetic material. The two aborted fetuses resulted from fertilization of the ovum by a sperm lacking a normal complement of genetic material. A normal fetus could have resulted if the fertilizing sperm contained normal chromosomes 7 and 21 and would also result from fertilization by a sperm containing the 7-21 translocation chromosome because the amount of genetic material was normal even though the chromosome was abnormal. However, the fetus would be a carrier of the translocation chromosome, as was the father. FIGURE 9-2 illustrates how the chromosomes can be distributed to the fetus based on the possible chromosomes provided by the fertilizing sperm.

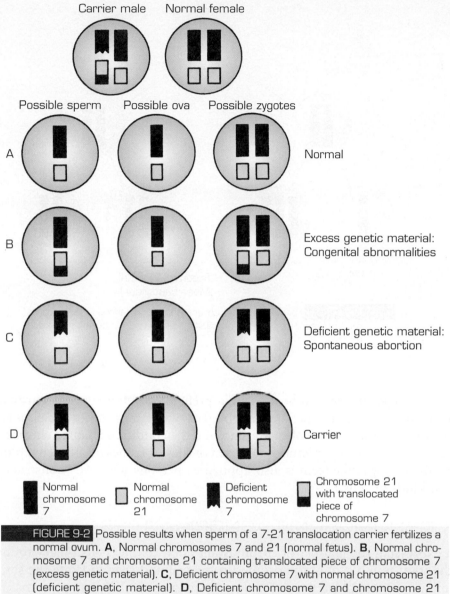

Carrier male   Normal female

Possible sperm   Possible ova   Possible zygotes

A   Normal

B   Excess genetic material:
Congenital abnormalities

C   Deficient genetic material:
Spontaneous abortion

D   Carrier

Normal chromosome 7 | Normal chromosome 21 | Deficient chromosome 7 | Chromosome 21 with translocated piece of chromosome 7

FIGURE 9-2 Possible results when sperm of a 7-21 translocation carrier fertilizes a normal ovum. **A**, Normal chromosomes 7 and 21 (normal fetus). **B**, Normal chromosome 7 and chromosome 21 containing translocated piece of chromosome 7 (excess genetic material). **C**, Deficient chromosome 7 with normal chromosome 21 (deficient genetic material). **D**, Deficient chromosome 7 and chromosome 21 containing the translocated piece of chromosome 7 (abnormal chromosomes but normal genetic material).

The literature contains many descriptions of clinical abnormalities that are associated with extra chromosomes, chromosome translocation, or loss of entire chromosomes or portions of chromosomes. Identification of chromosomal abnormalities is possible when the chromosomes are abnormal in size or configuration or when an abnormality is identified in the band pattern on the arms of the chromosomes.

CHROMOSOME NONDISJUNCTION IN THE ZYGOTE

Failures of chromosome separation are not restricted to germ cells. Sometimes, the chromosomes fail to separate during mitosis in one of the cells of the zygote during prenatal development. When this occurs during mitosis, the cell lacking the chromosome is unable to survive, but the cell with the extra chromosome continues to divide along with the other chromosomally normal cells. As a result, the embryo eventually becomes composed of a population of normal cells and another population of cells having a chromosome trisomy (FIGURE 9-3). The relative proportions of

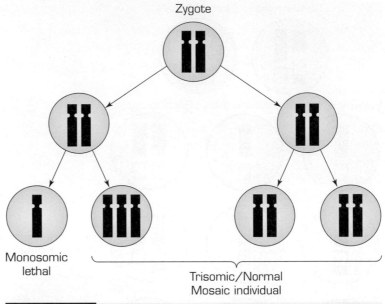

Zygote

Monosomic
lethal

Trisomic/Normal
Mosaic individual

FIGURE 9-3 Formation of two chromosome populations (chromosome mosaic) resulting from chromosome nondisjunction during mitosis in the zygote.

the two cell types depend on how early in prenatal development the chromosome nondisjunction occurred. A person composed of two or more types of cells is called a chromosomal mosaic or, simply, a mosaic, and the condition is called chromosomal mosaicism. (A mosaic is a picture composed of tiles or stones of different colors and shapes. By analogy, the term is also applied to persons who are "constructed" of different kinds of cells.)

SEX CHROMOSOME ABNORMALITIES

When expressing the number of chromosomes in a cell, it is customary to indicate first the total number of chromosomes in the cell and then indicate the sex chromosomes. For example, a normal male is designated 46,XY, and a normal female is 46,XX. Variations from the normal number of sex chromosomes are often associated with some reduction of intelligence. The Y chromosome directs masculine sexual differentiation, and its presence is almost invariably associated with a male body configuration regardless of the number of X chromosomes present. An extra Y chromosome does not cause any significant changes in the appearance of the affected individual, because the Y chromosome carries little genetic material other than genes concerned with male sexual differentiation. If the Y chromosome is absent, the body configuration is female.

The effect of extra X chromosomes depends on the sex of the individual. The presence of one or more extra X chromosomes adversely affects masculine development but has very little effect on the female, because the additional X chromosomes are inactivated and appear as extra sex chromatin bodies attached to the nuclear membrane of the cell.

Several syndromes result from abnormalities in the number or structure of the sex chromosomes. The two most common that occur in the female are (1) **Turner syndrome**, which usually results from an absence of one X chromosome (genotype 45,X), and (2) triple X syndrome, which results from an extra X chromosome (genotype 47,XXX).

Turner syndrome
A congenital syndrome usually caused by absence of one X chromosome in the female.

The two most common syndromes in the male are (1) **Klinefelter syndrome**, which results from an extra X chromosome (genotype 47,XXY), and (2) the XYY syndrome, which results from an extra Y chromosome (genotype 47,XYY).

The principal characteristics of these syndromes are summarized in TABLE 9-1.

Turner Syndrome

Turner syndrome, which results from an X chromosome abnormality, occurs less often than other sex chromosome abnormalities because most embryos lacking an X chromosome are aborted spontaneously. The reported frequency of about 1 in 2,500 female births represents only the very small proportion of the embryos surviving to be born alive. Most persons with Turner syndrome have only 45 chromosomes since they lack one X chromosome (designated 45,X) and are sex-chromatin negative since their cells lack a sex chromatin (Barr) body. Sometimes both X chromosomes are present, but one X chromosome is abnormal. The karyotype of many persons with Turner syndrome reveals that they have another population of cells in addition to their 45,X cells, which is called chromosome mosaicism.

FIGURE 9-4 illustrates the appearance of a girl with Turner syndrome. The body configuration is female but abnormal, and secondary sex characteristics have not developed. Characteristic features include short stature, broad neck with prominent lateral skin folds, broad chest lacking breast development, and widely spaced nipples. The uterus is small, and the ovaries consist only of bands of fibrous tissue. Sometimes, congenital abnormalities of the cardiovascular system are also present.

Triple X Syndrome

The presence of an extra X chromosome in the cells of the female is a relatively common abnormality. It has an incidence of about 1 in 850 female births. Usually there are no specific abnormalities of body form because the extra X chromosome is inactivated and appears on the nuclear membrane of the cell as an extra sex chromatin (Barr) body. Sexual development is generally normal. Fertility and intelligence may be either normal or somewhat decreased.

Klinefelter Syndrome

Having an incidence of about 1 in 750 male births, Klinefelter syndrome results from the presence of extra X chromosomes in the male (usual genotype 47,XXY).

Klinefelter syndrome
(klīn'felt-er)
A congenital syndrome caused by an extra X chromosome in the male. Characterized by testicular atrophy, sterility, feminine body configuration, and subnormal intelligence.

TABLE 9-1

Syndromes resulting from an abnormal complement of sex chromosomes

	Usual genotype	Approximate incidence	Unusual number of Barr bodies	Unusual number of Y fluorescent bodies	Fertility
Turner syndrome	45,X	1:2,500 females	0	0	Sterile
Triple X syndrome	47,XXX	1:850 females	2	0	Usually not impaired
Klinefelter syndrome	47,XXY	1:750 males	1	1	Usually sterile
XYY syndrome	47,XYY	1:850 males	0	2	Usually not impaired

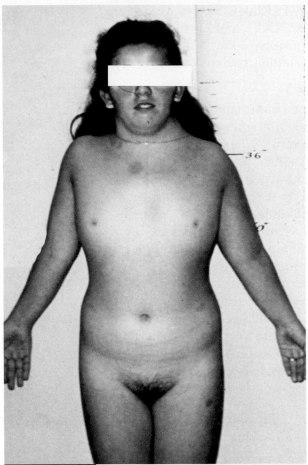

FIGURE 9-4 Child with Turner syndrome, illustrating a broad neck resulting from prominent lateral skin folds, a broad chest with widely spaced nipples, and a short stature.

FIGURE 9-5 illustrates the characteristic appearance of a subject with this chromosomal abnormality. The external genital organs are male, but the testicles are atrophic. Usually, no spermatozoa are produced, and the individual is sterile. The body configuration is somewhat feminine, and there may be moderate breast hypertrophy. Intelligence tends to be subnormal; however, many men with Klinefelter syndrome function reasonably well in society, and some are able to hold responsible positions. Because of the extra X chromosome, the cells contain a sex chromatin body (Barr body) as well as a Y fluorescent body.

XYY Syndrome

The sex chromosomal abnormality known as XYY syndrome has an incidence of about 1 in 850 male births. It may be associated with some reduction of fertility and intelligence. The individuals are usually taller than normal, but there are no specific abnormalities of body configuration. Some persons of this genotype may exhibit aggressive and antisocial behavior.

The Fragile X Syndrome (X-Linked Mental Deficiency)

This condition, although not related to an excess or deficiency of a sex chromosome, is associated with a characteristic abnormality of the X chromosome. The condition is called the fragile X syndrome or X-linked mental deficiency and is second only to Down syndrome as a major cause of mental deficiency. The X chromosome abnormality is a constricted area on the long arm of the chromosome near its tip, causing the tip of the long arm to look like a small round knob connected to the rest of the chromosome by a narrow stalklike constriction. The constricted area is quite fragile compared with the rest of the chromosome and is often broken in the course of preparing a chromosome karyotype, which is how the designation "fragile X chromosome" originated.

The gene responsible for the fragile X syndrome has been identified and named FMR1 (for **F**ragile X **M**ental **R**etardation-1) or simply fragile X gene, and the gene product is called fragile X mental retardation protein (FMRP). In normal persons, the first part of the fragile X gene contains groups (sequences) of the three nucleotides cytosine–guanine–guanine arranged in that order from 6 to as many as 50 times (CGG repeating sequences, often just called repeats). A greater number of repeats is abnormal, and the larger the number, the more marked is the mental deficiency. Individuals in whom the gene contains from 50 to 530 CGG repeats are considered to have a premutation of the gene, which means that the gene is abnormal but that the number of repeats is not markedly increased. A gene containing from 530 to 4,000 or more CGG repeats is very abnormal, which is called a full mutation of the gene. The great excess of CGG repeats causes mental retardation because the large number of repeats blocks the function of the gene. As a result, no gene product is produced, which interferes with the formation and function of synapses within the nervous system and is apparently the cause of the mental retardation. Moreover, the number of CGG repeats in the fragile X gene tends to increase progressively, and the mental deficiency becomes progressively more pronounced as the gene is passed from parent to offspring in successive generations. Expansion of the gene from a premutation to a full mutation is more likely to occur when the gene is transmitted to the child from the mother rather than from the father because the increase in the number of CGG repeats (gene amplification) occurs in the mother's ova during oogenesis but not in the father's sperm during spermatogenesis.

When a woman transmits the gene, the number of CGG repeats in the transmitted X chromosome becomes greatly increased (amplified) during oogenesis so that her gametes contain more repeats than she has in her own somatic (body) cells. Consequently, the degree of mental deficiency in the offspring who received the chromosome may be more marked than that of the mother who transmitted the fragile X gene. In contrast, when a man carrying the fragile X passes it to his daughter, the number of CGG repeating sequences in the fragile X gene that the daughter receives does not increase significantly, and the severity of the mental deficiency in the daughter may be no greater than that of the father because the number of repeats does not increase during spermatogenesis as it does in oogenesis.

A diagnosis of fragile X syndrome should be considered in any mentally retarded person. The preferred diagnostic test is DNA analysis, which can identify greatly increased number of CGG repeats in the gene characteristic of a full mutation. Cytogenetic studies to identify the constriction on the X chromosome is a relatively insensitive method for diagnosing the fragile X syndrome because the test will not detect all affected individuals. Nevertheless, cytogenetic studies are also helpful because they may detect other clinically important chromosomal abnormalities.

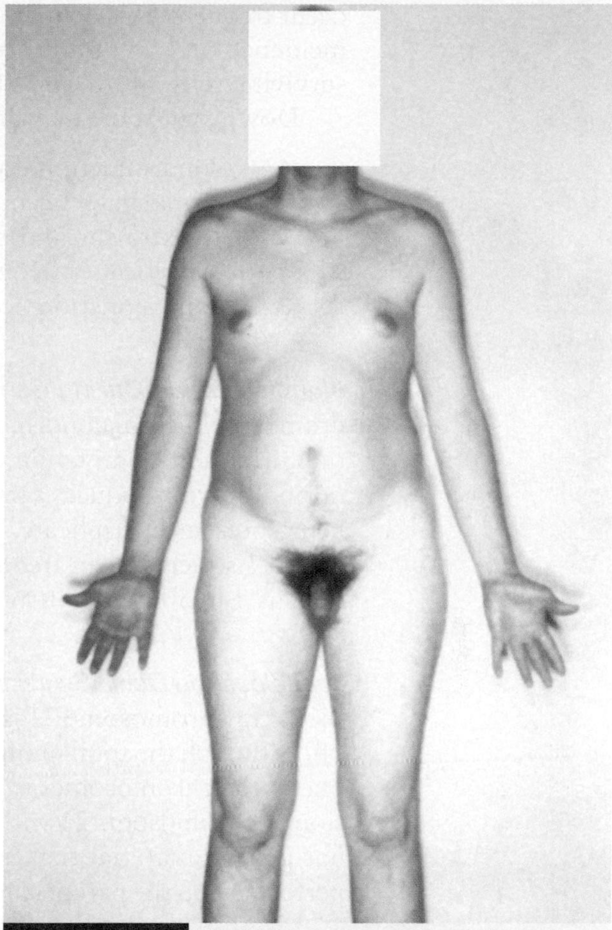

FIGURE 9-5 Klinefelter syndrome. The patient's body configuration is male, although there is slight breast hypertrophy (Courtesy of the estate of Dr. Robert Gorlin).

AUTOSOMAL ABNORMALITIES

Absence of an autosome results in the loss of so many genes that development is generally not possible and the embryo is aborted. Deletion of a small part of an autosome may be compatible with development, but it usually results in multiple severe congenital abnormalities in the infant. The most common autosomal trisomy seen in newborn infants is that of the small chromosome 21, which causes **Down syndrome**. Trisomy of a larger chromosome, such as chromosome 13 or chromosome 18, is less frequent and is associated with multiple severe congenital malformations. Trisomy of other large autosomes is almost invariably lethal.

Down syndrome
A congenital syndrome caused by an extra chromosome 21.

Down Syndrome
Down syndrome is the most common chromosomal abnormality, having an incidence of about 1 in 600 births. It is characterized by mental deficiency and a characteristic facial expression caused by the upward-slanting eyes and the prominent skin folds extending from the base of the nose to the inner aspects of the eyebrows (FIGURE 9-6). Other abnormalities of body form also are seen. Congenital cardiac malformations

occur frequently, as do major congenital defects in other organ systems. The reported incidence of 1 in 600 births represents only the proportion of abnormal fetuses surviving to term. About 70% of trisomy 21 fetuses do not survive to be liveborn.

Down syndrome may arise as a result of three possible conditions:

1. Nondisjunction during gametogenesis, leading to the formation of an abnormal gamete containing an extra chromosome 21
2. An extra chromosome 21 acquired as part of a translocation chromosome (translocation Down syndrome)
3. Nondisjunction occurring in the zygote

Nondisjunction During Gametogenesis. In about 95 percent of cases, Down syndrome results from nondisjunction of chromosome 21 during oogenesis, which causes the formation of an ovum containing an extra chromosome 21. Fertilization by a normal sperm produces a zygote containing 47 chromosomes, with chromosome 21 being present in triplicate. Down syndrome resulting from nondisjunction during oogenesis increases in frequency with advancing maternal age. The incidence is as high as 1 in 50 in the offspring of women over 40 years.

Translocation Down Syndrome. In a small number of persons with Down syndrome, the extra chromosome 21 is attached to another chromosome, usually chromosome 14. Although the total number of chromosomes is not increased in these individuals, one of the chromosomes is actually a composite chromosome resulting from the fusion of chromosome 21 with another chromosome; consequently, the affected person has genetic material that is equivalent to 47 chromosomes. Chromosome studies performed on the parents of children with translocation Down syndrome often reveal normal chromosomes in the cells of both parents. In these instances, the translocation apparently occurred as an accident in the germ cells of one parent during gametogenesis and is not present in other germ cells or in somatic cells. In other instances, the translocation chromosome can be identified in the karyotype of one of the parents, who is a carrier of the abnormal chromosome. The carrier parent has only 45 chromosomes because one chromosome is represented by a fusion of chromosome 21 with another chromosome.

The recognition of a translocation carrier is important because the carrier is capable of transmitting the abnormal chromosome to his or her children, resulting in translocation Down syndrome. However, the translocation chromosome is not always transmitted, as shown in FIGURE 9-7, which demonstrates the possible outcome of a pregnancy involving a female carrier of a 14/21 translocation chromosome. As indicated, the ova of the carrier parent can possess any one of four chromosome types, depending on how chromosomes 14 and 21 are distributed in the reduction divisions of the oocyte. Because there is only one chromosome 14 that can be distributed to the ovum independent of chromosome 21, an ovum can receive either the normal chromosome 14 (ova A

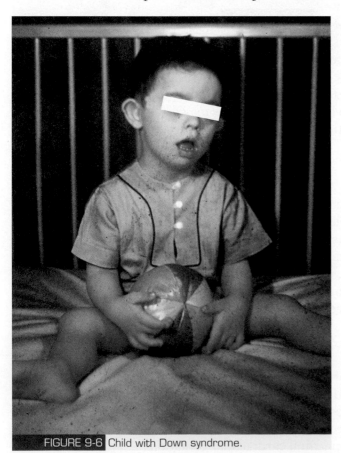

FIGURE 9-6 Child with Down syndrome.

and C) or the translocation chromosome (ova B and D). Because only one chromosome 21 can be distributed to the ovum (the other being carried with chromosome 14 as the translocation chromosome), some ova will receive the single chromosome 21 (ova A and D), but others will fail to receive this chromosome (ova B and C). The consequences of fertilization of these various possible ova by normal spermatozoa are indicated. In the first example (A), union of a normal ovum with a normal sperm produces a normal zygote containing 46 chromosomes. In the second example (B), a zygote containing 45 chromosomes results from fertilization, one chromosome being represented by the translocation chromosome. The individual derived from this zygote will be normal but will be a carrier of the translocation chromosome. In example C, the zygote lacks one chromosome 21 and is unable to survive. Fertilization of the ovum containing the translocation chromosome (example D) produces a zygote containing an excess of chromosome 21 material, resulting in a translocation Down syndrome.

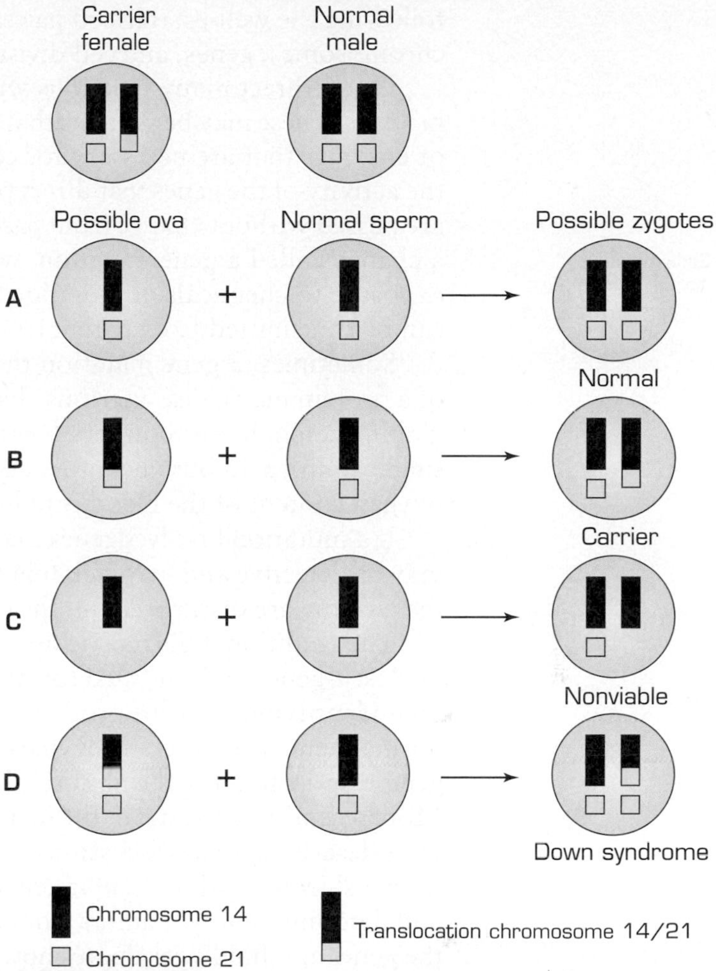

Nondisjunction in the Zygote. In a few individuals with Down syndrome, only some of the cells exhibit the characteristic trisomy 21. Other cells have a normal component of chromosomes, which is called a mosaic Down syndrome, resulting from nondisjunction during mitosis of a normal cell to form a trisomy 21

FIGURE 9-7 Possible ova produced by a female carrier of a 14/21 translocation chromosome and possible zygotes that could result from fertilization by normal sperm.

cell and another cell lacking chromosome 21, which does not survive. Both the normal cells and the trisomy 21 cells continue to proliferate, and both cell populations are present in the developing embryo, as described previously and illustrated in FIGURE 9-3. Individuals with mosaic Down syndrome suffer less disability than those in whom all of the cells contain an extra chromosome 21.

Trisomy of Other Autosomes

Trisomy of chromosome 13 is associated with multiple severe developmental abnormalities, the most conspicuous being cleft lip and palate, abnormal development of the skull and brain, abnormal eye development, congenital heart defects, and polydactyly (extra fingers and toes). Trisomy of chromosome 18 also is associated with multiple severe congenital malformations. Both chromosomal trisomies are usually fatal in the neonatal period or in early infancy.

Genetically Transmitted Diseases

Genetically determined diseases are the result of abnormalities of individual genes on the chromosome. The chromosomes themselves appear normal, and the chromosome karyotype is normal. Transmission of the abnormal gene is from parent to offspring, following the well-established patterns of inheritance described in the discussion on chromosomes, genes, and cell division.

Genes direct many functions within the cell. Some genes direct the synthesis of proteins. These may be proteins that form the structure of the cell (structural proteins) or enzymes that are necessary for cell function. Other genes function by regulating the activity of the genes that direct protein synthesis. Normally, genes are stable and are passed without change from parent to offspring. Occasionally, a gene undergoes a change called a **gene mutation**, which may occur spontaneously or as a result of exposure to chemicals or radiation. After a mutation has occurred in a germ cell, it can be transmitted from parent to offspring.

Gene mutation
A change in the structure of a gene, which may alter its functions.

Sometimes, a gene mutation that induces only a minor change in the structure of a protein may cause a serious change in its properties. For example, sickle hemoglobin (hemoglobin S) differs from normal hemoglobin (hemoglobin A) only in a single amino acid but undergoes crystallization within the red blood cells when the oxygen content of the blood is reduced.

If a mutation involves genes that control the synthesis of an enzyme, the enzyme may be defective and may lack functional activity. Metabolic processes regulated by the enzyme are disturbed, and the cell is unable to function normally.

The traditional diagnostic approach to genetic disease, based on the principles of classic genetics, is directed toward first identifying the abnormality in the patient, then identifying the gene product that is responsible for the disease, such as an abnormal hemoglobin or an enzyme deficiency, and finally, attempting to identify the gene responsible for the abnormal gene product that caused the cell dysfunction. More recently, as a result of the many advances in recombinant DNA technology that were described in the discussion on chromosomes, genes, and cell division, there has been a shift toward molecular genetics in which one first identifies the mutant gene and determines how it differs from the normal gene, then determines the product of the gene, and finally, evaluates how the abnormal gene and its gene product disrupt the functions of the cell. This approach has led to great advances in the prenatal diagnosis of many genetic diseases, as described later in the chapter.

Most hereditary diseases are transmitted on autosomes. A few are carried on sex chromosomes (TABLE 9-2).

AUTOSOMAL DOMINANT INHERITANCE

A dominant gene expresses itself in the heterozygous state. If either parent carries an abnormal dominant gene, either the abnormal gene or the corresponding normal allele may be passed to the offspring. Consequently, there is one chance in two that the offspring will receive the abnormal gene and will be affected with the hereditary disease. A common example of a genetic disease transmitted in this manner is achondroplasia, a type of dwarfism in which the limbs are disproportionately short (discussion on the musculoskeletal system). A second example is one type of congenital polycystic kidney disease, which is characterized by the formation of multiple cysts throughout both kidneys that progressively enlarge and eventually destroy renal function (discussion on the urinary system). A third genetic disease of this type is multiple neurofibromatosis, a condition characterized by the formation of multiple tumors that arise from peripheral nerves (discussion on the nervous system).

AUTOSOMAL RECESSIVE INHERITANCE

A trait transmitted as an autosomal recessive is expressed only in the homozygous individual. Many diseases characterized by an enzyme deficiency within the cell are

TABLE 9-2

Mode of inheritance, pathogenesis, and major manifestations of some common genetic diseases

Abnormality	Mode of inheritance	Defect	Manifestations
Phenylketonuria	Recessive	Phenylalanine hydroxylase deficiency	Mental retardation
Tay-Sachs disease	Recessive	Hexosaminidase A deficiency	Mental retardation, motor weakness, blindness
Cystic fibrosis of pancreas	Recessive	Dysfunction of mucous and sweat glands, thick mucus obstructs bronchioles, pancreatic ducts, and bile ducts	Chronic broncho-pulmonary infections as a result of bronchial obstruction by mucus; pancreatic and liver dysfunction as a result of thick mucous obstruction of excretory ducts
Achondroplasia	Dominant	Disordered bone growth at ends of long bones (epiphyses)	Dwarfism with disproportionately short limbs
Congenital polycystic kidney disease	Dominant	Maldevelopment of nephrons and collecting tubules causes formation of multiple cysts in kidneys	Renal failure
Multiple neurofibromatosis	Dominant	Multiple tumors arise from peripheral nerves	Disfigurement and deformities caused by tumors; predisposition to malignant change in tumors
Sickle cell trait	Codominant	Red cells contain mixture of normal (A) and sickle (S) hemoglobin	None
Sickle cell anemia	Codominant	Red cells contain no normal hemoglobin	Severe anemia and obstruction of blood flow to organs by masses of sickled red cells
Hemophilia	X-linked recessive	Deficiency of protein required for normal coagulation of blood	Uncontrolled bleeding into joints and internal organs after minor injuries

transmitted in this manner. The hereditary disease results only if both alleles are abnormal and no enzyme is produced. Therefore, in order for the offspring to be affected, both parents must carry the abnormal gene, and both must transmit the gene to the offspring. Consequently, when both parents carry an abnormal recessive gene, there is one chance in four that the mother will give birth to an abnormal infant who is homozygous for the defective gene. If only one parent transmits the recessive gene, the infant will be a carrier of the abnormal gene but will be normal because the normal allele will direct the synthesis of enough enzymes to keep the cell functioning normally. The many recognized types of genetically determined enzyme defects are sometimes called inborn errors of metabolism. Two of the more important ones are phenylketonuria and Tay-Sachs disease.

Phenylketonuria

Phenylalanine is an essential amino acid present in dietary protein. Much of it is converted in the body to tyrosine, which the body uses to make thyroid hormone, melanin, and other important compounds. A deficiency of the enzyme phenylalanine hydroxylase, which is required for normal metabolism of the amino acid phenylalanine, causes a disease called phenylketonuria. The enzyme deficiency causes no difficulty while the infant is still within the uterus being nourished by the mother. Soon after birth, however, the infant begins to drink milk. Because milk protein contains abundant phenylalanine, which the infant is unable to metabolize, this amino acid accumulates in the infant's blood and is excreted in the urine. The affected infant is able to convert some phenylalanine into phenylpyruvic acid (and other metabolites) by means of other metabolic pathways that do not require phenylalanine hydroxylase (FIGURE 9-8). Phenylpyruvic acid accumulates in the blood and is excreted in the urine along with phenylalanine. Permanent mental deficiency results from the disturbed phenylalanine metabolism, but it can be prevented by restricting the dietary intake of phenylalanine. Phenylketonuria can be detected in the newborn infant by means

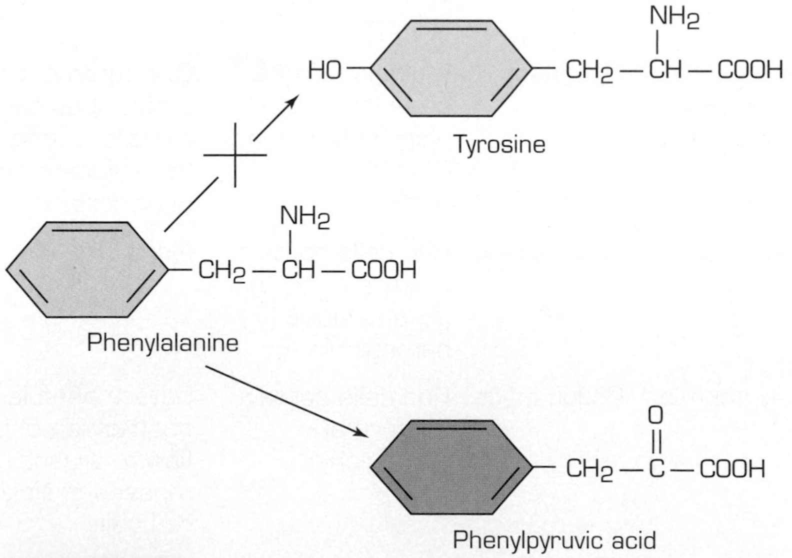

FIGURE 9-8 Metabolic defects in phenylketonuria. Infants with this disorder lack the enzyme phenylalanine hydroxylase, and their bodies are unable to hydroxylate phenylalanine to form tyrosine. Some phenylalanine is converted into phenylpyruvic acid (substitution of a keto group for the amino group in the molecule) by other metabolic pathways. Permanent mental deficiency results from disturbed phenylalanine metabolism and can be prevented by restricting dietary intake of phenylalanine.

of a screening laboratory test capable of detecting the elevated level of phenylalanine in the blood. It can be confirmed by more detailed testing to detect the presence of phenylpyruvic acid and other metabolites that also are derived from the disturbed metabolism of phenylalanine. This disease is a cause of preventable mental deficiency; thus, a routine screening test to detect phenylketonuria is an important requirement for all newborn infants.

Many children with phenylketonuria maintained on a restricted diet have matured normally and have reached childbearing age. Many no longer adhere to a phenylalanine-restricted diet and have very high levels of phenylalanine and its metabolites in their blood. If a woman with phenylketonuria is considering a pregnancy, it is essential that she resume a phenylalanine-restricted diet because a high blood phenylalanine and its metabolites can cross the placenta and damage the developing fetal brain, leading to mental deficiency in her infant, and also injure other developing organ systems.

Tay-Sachs Disease

Tay-Sachs disease occurs primarily in the offspring of Jewish parents who carry the defective gene. The clinical manifestations result from absence of a lysosomal enzyme called hexosaminidase A. The enzyme deficiency causes a lipid called a ganglioside to accumulate within the lysosomes of nerve cells in the brain, spinal cord, autonomic nervous system, and retina of the eye, causing cell dysfunction and, eventually, degeneration of the affected nerve cells. Clinically, the disease is characterized by progressive mental deterioration, neurologic dysfunction, and blindness. Onset of symptoms begins by about 6 months of age, and the disease is invariably fatal by the time the child is 3 or 4 years old.

Carriers of the abnormal gene can be detected by means of the low levels of hexosaminidase A in their serum and in their leukocytes. Tests for this enzyme can be used for screening. Surveys have indicated that the carrier rate is relatively high in some Jewish populations (those of Eastern European origin). In these groups, about 1 in 30 individuals carry the abnormal gene.

Tay-Sachs disease can be diagnosed prenatally by examining fetal cells obtained by amniocentesis. The applications and limitations of this diagnostic procedure are described later in this chapter.

Other Genetic Diseases

Two other relatively common and important diseases that are transmitted by autosomal recessive inheritance are cystic fibrosis of the pancreas and hemochromatosis. Cystic fibrosis, manifested by dysfunction of mucous and sweat glands, is considered in the pancreas and diabetes mellitus discussion in conjunction with diseases of the pancreas. Hemochromatosis is characterized by excessive absorption of iron, which accumulates within the body and disrupts organ functions and is considered in the hematopoietic and lymphatic systems discussion.

CODOMINANT INHERITANCE

If both alleles of a pair are fully expressed in the heterozygous state, the genes are said to be codominant. This type of transmission is illustrated by the genes responsible for the synthesis of **sickle (S) hemoglobin** and other abnormal hemoglobins. These genes are alleles of the gene that directs the synthesis of normal (A) hemoglobin. An individual heterozygous for the sickle hemoglobin gene will have approximately equal quantities of sickle hemoglobin and normal hemoglobin in the red cells. This condition is called sickle cell trait and usually causes no difficulties. Significant clinical manifestations are apparent, however, if the individual is homozygous for the sickle cell gene, and

Sickle hemoglobin
An abnormal hemoglobin that crystallizes under reduced oxygen tension.

no normal hemoglobin is formed. This leads to a serious hereditary anemia called sickle cell anemia. This subject is considered in the hematopoietic and lymphatic systems discussion.

X-LINKED INHERITANCE

A few hereditary diseases are transmitted on the X chromosome. The best-known example is the disease hemophilia, which is caused by a deficiency of protein called antihemophilic globulin, which is required for normal blood coagulation. This disease is described in the discussion on abnormalities of blood coagulation. The female parent carries the defective gene on one of her X chromosomes and can transmit either the normal X chromosome or the one containing the defective gene to her offspring. The child will be born normal if the normal X chromosome is received. If the mother transmits the abnormal X chromosome, its effect depends on the sex of the offspring. A female child will appear normal because the defective gene on the X chromosome is paired with a normal allele on the other X chromosome. However, she will be a carrier of the abnormal gene and can transmit it to her own children. In contrast, a male child will have hemophilia. Because a male has only one X chromosome, he lacks the normal allele possessed by a female carrier. Consequently, the abnormal X-linked gene functions like a dominant gene when paired with the Y chromosome.

Although female carriers of the mutant gene appear normal and generally produce adequate antihemophilic globulin, they produce less than normal amounts of this protein. The subnormal production is related to the random inactivation of one of the X chromosomes, as described in the discussion on chromosomes, genes, and cell division. Consequently, a carrier female has two populations of cells concerned with synthesis of antihemophilic globulin. Synthesis is normal in the cells in which the X chromosome containing the mutant gene is inactivated but deficient in the cells in which the X chromosome containing the normal gene is inactivated. The amount of antihemophilic globulin produced by a carrier female depends on the relative proportions of the two cell types: functioning cells that produce antihemophilic globulin and nonfunctional cells in which the functional gene is carried on the X chromosome that has been inactivated.

Intrauterine Injury

The embryo or fetus may be injured by drugs, radiation, or an infection that disrupts prenatal development and leads to congenital malformations. The effects of the injury inflicted on the developing embryo vary depending on the nature of the harmful agent and the stage of gestation. The embryonic period from the third to the eighth week after conception, when the organ systems are forming, is the time when the embryo is most vulnerable to the injurious effects of environmental agents.

HARMFUL DRUGS AND CHEMICALS

Many drugs are known to harm the developing embryo. The classic example is thalidomide, which was widely used in Europe in the 1960s to treat nausea and vomiting associated with pregnancy (morning sickness) but was never marketed in the United States. The drug produced a highly characteristic malformation in which the bones of the extremities were much reduced or absent, the hands or feet arising from the trunk (FIGURE 9-9). Either upper or lower limbs or all four extremities were affected, depending on the time when the drug was taken during pregnancy. In addition to causing limb defects, the drug also caused malformations of the heart, gastrointestinal

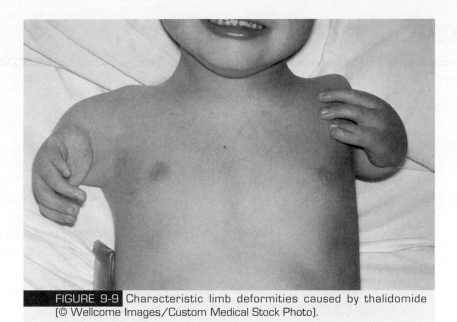

FIGURE 9-9 Characteristic limb deformities caused by thalidomide (© Wellcome Images/Custom Medical Stock Photo).

tract, eyes, and ears. The correlation between thalidomide and congenital malformations was eventually determined because of the unusual type of limb malformations produced by the drug but, unfortunately, not until thousands of infants had been damaged by this drug. The thalidomide tragedy clearly demonstrated to the medical profession the disastrous effects of a supposedly innocuous drug taken by a mother during a critical phase of embryonic development.

Despite the extreme hazard of thalidomide to the fetus, the drug has some properties that make it potentially useful for treating some diseases. The drug blocks the formation of blood vessels and impedes the formation of a cytokine called tumor necrosis factor, which damages cells and tissues (discussion on immunity, hypersensitivity, allergy, and autoimmune diseases). Recently, the U.S. Food and Drug Administration (FDA) has approved the use of thalidomide for very limited clinical indications. Because of the extreme hazard of the drug on fetal development, physicians prescribing the drug are required to take great precautions to be certain that the patient is not pregnant and will not become pregnant while taking the drug.

Many other drugs, although less hazardous than thalidomide, may also cause congenital malformations. Currently, all drugs used in the United States are rated in five categories by the U.S. FDA according to the degree of possible risk to the fetus balanced against the drug's potential benefit to the patient (TABLE 9-3). Ratings range from "A" for drugs that are generally considered safe for use in pregnancy through "D" for drugs that may injure the fetus but are of enough benefit to the patient that the benefit of the drug to the patient outweighs the risk to the fetus. "X"-rated drugs are contraindicated in pregnancy because the severe risk to the fetus outweighs any possible benefit to the patient.

Even cigarettes and alcoholic beverages are not without risk. Cigarette smoking leads to retarded intrauterine growth with birth of smaller than normal infants and premature births. Heavy alcohol consumption during pregnancy can result in a characteristic pattern of developmental abnormalities called the fetal alcohol syndrome. Affected infants are both physically and mentally retarded, exhibit abnormal cranial and facial development, and may have other congenital malformations affecting the genital tract and cardiovascular system. Consequently, women with severe drinking

TABLE 9-3

Five categories of all drugs used in the United States rated by the FDA according to degree of possible risk to the fetus

Category	Interpretation
A	No risk to fetus demonstrated in well-controlled studies in humans.
B	No evidence of risk to fetus. Either animal studies show risk but human studies do not or there are no adequate human studies but animal studies do not indicate risk.
C	Risk to fetus cannot be ruled out. No human studies available to assess risk. Animal studies either are not available or indicate possible risk.
D	Positive evidence of risk to fetus; however, drug is needed to treat patients, and no safer alternative drug is available. Potential benefit to patients outweighs risk to fetus.
X	Absolutely contraindicated in pregnancy. Severe risk to fetus greatly outweighs any possible benefit to patients.

problems should be cautioned not to become pregnant until their alcoholism is controlled. Even small amounts of alcohol may put the fetus at risk, and it is generally considered unsafe for a pregnant woman to consume any alcohol during pregnancy.

Drugs such as heroin, methadone, and cocaine used by a pregnant woman impair fetal growth and development and may lead to congenital malformation, as well as to addiction in both the fetus and the mother. The infant born to an addicted mother may experience narcotic withdrawal symptoms within a few days after delivery. Maternal cocaine use may also disturb blood flow through the placenta, leading to intrauterine fetal death, as described in the discussion on prenatal development and diseases associated with pregnancy.

Some drugs that are well tolerated by the mother may cause manifestations of drug toxicity in the fetus because the fetus lacks an efficient means of detoxifying and excreting these drugs. Some drugs may slow the growth rate of the fetus (intrauterine growth retardation), resulting in the birth of a smaller than normal infant. Other drugs retard fetal growth and cause congenital malformations as well.

Some drugs may leave their mark on the developing fetus even though the harmful effects are not immediately apparent. The antibiotic tetracycline, when taken by a pregnant woman, is deposited in the developing teeth of the fetus, causing yellow-brown discoloration of the enamel and sometimes also disturbing the development of the enamel. The abnormality is not apparent until the teeth erupt (discussion on the gastrointestinal tract).

Because of the established relation between drugs and congenital defects, most physicians recommend that pregnant women refrain from indiscriminate use of drugs or other medications, especially during the early part of pregnancy when the embryo is especially vulnerable. Many new drugs and antibiotics are not recommended for use in pregnancy because the possible effects of the drugs on the developing embryo are not known.

RADIATION

Exposure of a pregnant woman to radiation may harm the fetus. Consequently, x-ray examinations or diagnostic tests using radioactive materials are avoided during pregnancy.

MATERNAL INFECTIONS

Some infections acquired by a pregnant woman may injure the developing fetus. Three infectious agents are known to be important causes of congenital malformations and may also cause a chronic systemic infection of the fetus:

1. The virus of German measles (*rubella*)
2. The virus of cytomegalic inclusion disease (*cytomegalovirus*)
3. The protozoan parasite *Toxoplasma gondii*

Rubella

Rubella is a mild illness that is usually acquired in childhood; 90% of women of childbearing age have already had the disease or have been immunized and are immune. If a susceptible woman acquires rubella during pregnancy, the virus may infect the embryo, leading to either spontaneous abortion of severely affected embryos or congenital malformations in many of the embryos that survive. Common malformations resulting from prenatal rubella infection include congenital cataracts, cardiac malformations, deafness, and neurologic disturbances. The earlier in the pregnancy, the greater the hazard to the developing embryo. In cases in which the mothers contract rubella in the first month of pregnancy, as many as 50% of their infants develop congenital malformations. The incidence declines to about 25% when infection occurs in the second month and to about 10% when the infection occurs later in pregnancy. The virus may also cause a chronic progressive infection in the fetus. When this occurs, the affected infant is born with evidence of an active systemic disease characterized by enlargement of the liver and spleen, anemia, and reduced numbers of platelets in the blood (thrombocytopenia). The low platelet levels usually lead to multiple small hemorrhages in the skin (called *thrombocytopenic purpura*). Rubella virus can be isolated from the tissues and secretions of the infected infants. It may persist in the infant's tissues for 6 months or longer after delivery.

Cytomegalic Inclusion Disease

The name of the cytomegalovirus (*cyto* = cell + *megalos* = large) derives from its characteristic property of producing marked enlargement of the cells it infects. The infected cells also contain characteristic large, basophilic, intranuclear inclusions, causing the virus-infected cell to have a distinctly characteristic histologic appearance (FIGURE 9-10). Cytomegalovirus infection is very common and is usually asymptomatic. More than

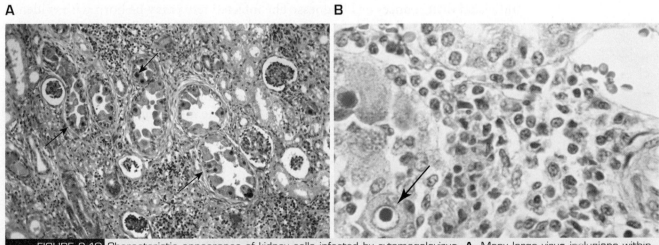

A **B**

FIGURE 9-10 Characteristic appearance of kidney cells infected by cytomegalovirus. **A**, Many large virus inclusions within enlarged kidney tubule cells (*arrows*) (original magnification × 100). **B**, High-magnification view illustrating virus infected cells (*arrow*) in kidney tubules with many chronic inflammatory cells in adjacent tissue (original magnification × 400).

50% of women of childbearing age have had a previous cytomegalovirus infection and have formed antibodies against the virus, but latent cytomegalovirus persists within the tissues of the infected woman and may become reactivated during pregnancy, leading to intermittent excretion of virus in cervical and vaginal secretions throughout the pregnancy. The fetus may become infected either from a new maternal infection acquired during pregnancy or from reactivation of a prior maternal infection. A newly acquired maternal infection poses the greatest risk to the fetus. The virus may cause severe fetal damage characterized by injury to the brain and eyes, leading to failure of the brain to develop normally (microcephaly), mental retardation, and blindness. The cytomegalovirus may also cause a chronic systemic infection of the fetus similar to that caused by the rubella virus, and the virus can be identified in the tissues of the infected infant.

A reactivation of a previous maternal infection is less hazardous to the fetus and may produce only relatively mild symptoms. The fetus may be infected within the uterus before delivery, at the time of delivery from virus in cervical and vaginal secretions, or during nursing from virus excreted in breast milk.

Other Virus Diseases in Pregnancy

The herpes simplex virus, the same virus that causes fever blisters, may at times cause congenital infections similar to those produced by cytomegalovirus, leading to malformations of the nervous system. Some other viruses may occasionally be transmitted to the fetus and cause disease in the fetus, but they are not usually associated with congenital malformations.

Toxoplasmosis

Toxoplasma gondii is a small, ovoid, intracellular parasite described in the discussion on animal parasites. Adults acquired the infection by eating raw or partially cooked meat that is infected with the parasite or by contact with infected cats, which excrete an infectious form of the organism (oocysts) in their feces. As with cytomegalovirus infection, more than 50% of women of childbearing age have had a previous inapparent infection and have formed antibodies to the parasite. These women are immune, and the prior infection does not put the fetus at risk.

A hazard to the fetus exists if a susceptible mother acquires the infection during pregnancy. In the fetus, the parasite causes severe injury to the brain and eyes, leading to abnormal development of the brain (microcephaly); obstruction of the ventricles of the brain, causing hydrocephalus (discussion on the nervous system); and visual disturbances or blindness. The infected fetus may be born with evidence of a systemic toxoplasma infection that is clinically quite similar to that caused by rubella and the cytomegalovirus.

It is possible to determine by laboratory tests whether a pregnant woman is susceptible to toxoplasma. A susceptible pregnant woman should avoid eating incompletely cooked meat and should exercise caution in contact with cats. Pregnant women with cats are generally advised to adopt the following precautions.

1. Wash hands after handling cats, especially before eating.
2. Have the cat-litter box emptied daily by someone else (to avoid contact with oocysts).
3. Do not permit indoor cats to go outside because cats allowed to roam outdoors have a higher risk of acquiring a toxoplasma infection.
4. Do not allow outdoor cats or stray cats to enter the house because they are very likely to be infected with toxoplasma.
5. Do not feed cats raw meat products because they may become infected in this way.

The following case illustrates the clinical features of a systemic infection of the fetus that resulted from an inapparent infection of the mother during pregnancy (FIGURE 9-11).

Rubella virus, cytomegalovirus, toxoplasma, and occasionally the herpes virus all produce a similar type of infection in the fetus, and it may not be possible to determine clinically which agent caused the disease unless the infectious agent can be identified by histologic examination, culture, or serologic methods.

Multifactorial Inheritance

Many congenital defects do not result from single gene abnormalities and are not entirely caused by environmental factors. Rather, they result from the combined effects of multiple genes interacting with environmental agents. This type of inheritance is called **multifactorial inheritance**.

Many of the phases of embryologic development, such as the formation of the heart or palate, are regulated by multiple genes. Because embryos differ in their genetic makeup, they also vary somewhat in the rates at which the various organs and other embryonic structures are formed. These genetic variations will influence the susceptibility of an embryo to drugs or other environmental factors that disturb the normal process of development. Susceptible embryos are likely to develop congenital malformations if they are exposed to harmful environmental agents, whereas genetically resistant embryos remain unaffected under similar circumstances.

Some of the common defects in which inheritance is multifactorial include cleft lip and palate, some congenital cardiac malformations, clubfoot, congenital dislocation of the hip,

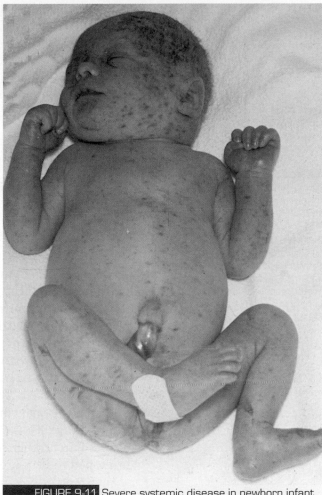

FIGURE 9-11 Severe systemic disease in newborn infant caused by an inapparent infection of the mother during pregnancy, as described in Case 9-2.

Multifactorial inheritance
Inheritance of a trait or condition related to the combined effect of multiple genes rather than a single gene, as in mendelian inheritance.

CASE 9-2

The patient was an infant girl at 36-weeks' gestation. The skin was covered with numerous small hemorrhages, and the abdomen was markedly distended because of extreme enlargement of both the liver and the spleen. The infant was moderately anemic, and the platelet count was significantly reduced, which accounted for the widespread hemorrhages in the skin. The infant was considered to be seriously ill as a result of a prenatal infection acquired from the mother. Diagnostic possibilities considered were congenital rubella, cytomegalic inclusion disease, systemic herpes virus infection, or toxoplasmosis. The infant died from widespread infection about 5 hours after examination before further diagnostic studies could be undertaken. The autopsy revealed the infection was caused by the cytomegalovirus.

Anencephaly
(an-en-seff'uh-lē)
A congenital malformation: absence of brain, cranial vault, and scalp as a result of defective closure of the neural tube.

....

Spina bifida
(spī'-nuh bif'fid-duh)
Incomplete closure of vertebral arches over the spinal cord, sometimes associated with protrusion of meninges and neural tissue through the defect (cystic spina bifida).

....

Alpha fetoprotein
(al'fuh fē'tō-prō'tēn)
Protein produced by fetal liver early in gestation. Sometimes produced by tumor cells. Level is elevated in amnionic fluid when fetus has neural tube defect.

and certain congenital abnormalities of the nervous system called **anencephaly** and **spina bifida**. These multifactorial malformations have an incidence among newborn infants of from 1 in 500 to 1 in 2,000, depending on the malformation. The incidence is much higher, approximately 1 in 25, if one parent has the same type of congenital malformation or if other children born to the same parents have the malformation. This is because the genes that the parents are transmitting render their offspring more susceptible to disturbances in embryologic development, leading to specific types of congenital abnormalities.

Prenatal Diagnosis of Congenital Abnormalities

A wide variety of approaches are available to identify congenital abnormalities in the fetus. They fall into several groups:

1. Tests on maternal blood to screen for possible fetal abnormalities.

    These tests measure the concentration of three substances that are normally present in the blood of pregnant women. Abnormal results may indicate a fetal abnormality. One of the first maternal blood screening tests measured a protein called **alpha fetoprotein** (AFP). The protein, produced by the fetus, diffuses into the amnionic fluid and then into the mother's blood. AFP is elevated when the fetus has a major central nervous system abnormality called an open neural tube defect, as described in the discussion on the nervous system. Later, it was observed that maternal blood AFP is often lower than normal when the mother is carrying a fetus with Down syndrome or a trisomy of some other autosome, although we do not know why this occurs. Later, other screening tests were added, and a battery of tests was developed to help predict the possibility of a congenital fetal abnormality.

    Currently, screening tests are offered to all pregnant women, not just to older women who are at higher risk for chromosomal abnormalities. Most Down syndrome infants are born to younger women because they conceive a much greater proportion of infants than do older women. Restricting prenatal screening to older women will fail to detect many Down syndrome infants. Screening tests, however, may at times yield false-positive results, and positive screening test results should always be confirmed by amniocentesis and fetal chromosome studies.

2. Examination of amnionic fluid.

    Products secreted into the fluid by the fetus, such as AFP, may indicate a congenital fetal abnormality. An abnormal volume of amnionic fluid, either an excess (polyhydramnios) or a deficiency (oligohydramnios) as described in the discussion on prenatal development and diseases associated with pregnancy, may also suggest a fetal abnormality.

3. Examination of fetal cells.

    Fetal cells can be obtained by amniocentesis or by a procedure called chorionic villus sampling. Cytogenetic studies of fetal cells can detect chromosomal abnormalities. Genetic abnormalities also can be identified by biochemical tests performed on fetal cells or by analysis of DNA obtained from fetal cells.

4. Ultrasound examination of the fetus.

    By about 16-weeks' gestation, ultrasound examination, described in the discussion on general concepts of disease: principles of diagnosis, can visualize the limbs and all of the major organs, including the brain and spinal cord, kidneys, bladder, and heart. The examination can detect major structural abnormalities of the nervous system called neural tube defects (anencephaly and spina bifida) and congenital hydrocephalus (discussion on the nervous system). Other structural abnormalities can also be identified, including such defects as congenital obstruction of the urinary tract, failure of the kidneys to develop, or failure of the limbs to form normally.

The procedure is usually also performed before amniocentesis or chorionic villus sampling in order to check for any fetal abnormalities, to locate the position of the placenta, and to guide placement of the needle for aspirating amnionic fluid during amniocentesis.

AMNIOCENTESIS

Fetal cells can be obtained easily from amnionic fluid because the cells in the fluid are of fetal origin. The cells can be grown in the laboratory by tissue culture techniques, and the karyotype of the cells can be determined. In this way, abnormalities in the number or structure of the fetal chromosomes can be determined, and analysis of fetal DNA makes it possible to identify a large number of genetic diseases, including those listed in TABLE 9-2. The list of genetic disease that can be identified prenatally continues to grow along with the rapid advances in the field of molecular genetics. One also can determine the concentration in amnionic fluid of a protein called AFP, which is high when the fetus has a neural tube defect. This subject is considered in the nervous system discussion.

Amniocentesis is usually performed between the 14th and 18th week of pregnancy, although amniocentesis as early as the 12th to 13th week of pregnancy is available in some medical centers (FIGURE 9-12). A needle is inserted through the mother's abdominal wall directly into the amnionic sac, and a small amount of amnionic fluid is withdrawn.

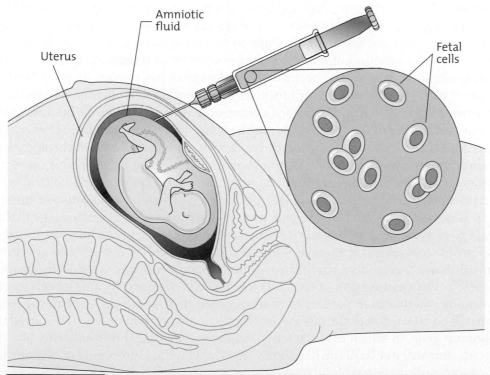

FIGURE 9-12 Amniocentesis. Amnionic fluid containing some free cells derived from the fetus is withdrawn. The fetal cells can be grown in tissue culture so that their karyotype and many of their metabolic functions can be determined. Studies of fetal DNA can also be performed in selected cases (from: Alters, S. 2000. *Biology, Understanding Life, 3rd ed.* Boston: Jones & Bartlett Learning).

TABLE 9-4

Main indications for amniocentesis or chorionic villus sampling

1. Maternal blood tests (triple screen) indicating increased risk of fetal chromosome abnormality
2. Maternal age older than 35 years
3. Previous infant born with Down syndrome or other chromosomal abnormality
4. Known translocation chromosome carrier, or other chromosome abnormality in either parent
5. Risk of fetal genetic disease that can be detected by fetal cell biochemical or DNA analysis

TABLE 9-4 summarizes the main indications for the procedure. At present, the main indication for amniocentesis is to confirm a chromosomal abnormality suggested by abnormal prenatal screening tests or to determine the karyotype of the fetus carried by a woman age 35 years or older who has declined prenatal screening tests. Some older women decline screening tests because even the most comprehensive battery of screening tests cannot detect all affected fetuses. However, many older women want to be absolutely certain that their fetus does not have Down syndrome or some other chromosomal abnormality, which can only be guaranteed by examination of fetal chromosomes by amniocentesis or chorionic villus sampling. Consequently, even if the woman were to have screening tests and the results were positive, she would still want to have an examination of fetal chromosomes obtained by amniocentesis or chorionic villus sampling. On the other hand, if the screening test were negative, she would still want the negative test confirmed by a fetal chromosome study. Therefore, an older woman often may not see any advantage to screening tests because she already has decided to have chromosome studies no matter what result the screening tests provide. Amniocentesis should also be performed if the woman has previously given birth to an infant with Down syndrome or other chromosomal abnormality. It also should be performed if the woman is a carrier of a translocated chromosome 21 because of the very high incidence of Down syndrome in the offspring of a translocation carrier. The procedure is also indicated if one of the parents has some other type of chromosomal abnormality, such as in Case 9-1. Amniocentesis should be performed if there is a history of an inherited disease that can be identified by examination of fetal cells. For example, examination of fetal DNA is indicated when both parents are carriers of an abnormal gene, such as the gene responsible for Tay-Sachs disease, the thalassemia gene associated with defective hemoglobin synthesis, or the hemoglobin gene responsible for sickle cell anemia. (Diseases characterized by defective or abnormal hemoglobins are considered in the hematopoietic and lymphatic systems discussion.) In these cases, examination of fetal DNA from cells obtained by amniocentesis can determine whether both parents have transmitted their abnormal gene to the fetus, who will be affected with the disease, or whether only one parent has transmitted the abnormal gene, in which case the fetus will carry only one abnormal gene, like the parents, but will not have the hereditary disease. Finally, amniocentesis is indicated when screening maternal blood tests indicate an increased risk of a fetal abnormality.

If an abnormal fetus is identified by means of a prenatal amnionic fluid study, the parents are advised of the nature of the abnormality and its possible effects on the offspring. They must then reach a decision as to whether to terminate the pregnancy or allow it to continue to term.

CHORIONIC VILLUS SAMPLING

Chorionic villus sampling also can be used to obtain fetal cells for evaluation and in general provides the same type of information as does amniocentesis, although no amnionic fluid is obtained for chemical examination. (Chorionic villi are frondlike structures that form part of the placenta and attach to the lining of the uterus, described in the discussion on prenatal development and diseases associated with pregnancy.) The usual procedure involves passing a small catheter through the cervix to the site where the villi are attached to the uterus and suctioning out a small quantity of villi with a syringe.

Chorionic villus sampling has some advantages over amniocentesis because it can be performed at 8- to 10-weeks' gestation, which is earlier than amniocentesis can be performed, and results can be obtained earlier. If a congenital abnormality is detected and the patient wants to terminate the pregnancy, the abortion can be performed earlier in pregnancy, which carries less risk than one performed midway through the pregnancy. There are disadvantages, however. Chorionic villus sampling is technically more difficult than amniocentesis, and complications from the procedure leading to spontaneous abortion are more frequent than with amniocentesis. Moreover, in some instances, chorionic villus sampling may injure the embryo. There appears to be a slight increase of limb deformities in fetuses that have undergone chorionic villus sampling early in pregnancy.

QUESTIONS FOR REVIEW

1. What are the consequences of chromosome nondisjunction? What is Down syndrome?
2. What is the karyotype of an individual with Down syndrome? Klinefelter syndrome? Turner syndrome? What is the fragile X syndrome?
3. What is the approximate incidence of congenital abnormalities? What are the major causes of congenital abnormalities? What types of maternal infections may cause congenital abnormalities in the infant?
4. What is amniocentesis? How is it used in prenatal diagnosis of congenital malformations? What type of congenital malformations may be detected by this method? In which group of patients is amniocentesis most widely used?

SUPPLEMENTARY READINGS

Bass, H. N., Crandall, B. F., and Marcy, S. M. 1973. Two different chromosome abnormalities resulting from a translocation carrier father. *Journal of Pediatrics* 83:1034–40.
► Describes the transmission of abnormal sets of genes to offspring from a father who is a carrier of a balanced translocation.

Benn, P. A., and Chapman, A. R. 2009. Practical and ethical considerations of noninvasive prenatal diagnosis. *Journal of the American Medical Association* 301:2154–6.

► Newer tests under development are based on fetal DNA in maternal blood derived from trophoblast cells, which can be used as a noninvasive test for a fetal chromosome abnormality, which may be able to substitute for amniocentesis or chorionic villus sampling. However, the procedure would need to be validated by comparing the results of the new procedure with amniocentesis.

Centers for Disease Control and Prevention. 1995. Chorionic villus sampling and amniocentesis: Recommendations for prenatal counseling. *Morbidity and Mortality Weekly Report* 44 (No. RR-9):1–11.

▶ Chorionic villus sampling carries a small risk of limb deformities probably caused by disruption of the blood supply to the limbs related to the procedure. Risk is from 0.03 to 0.10%, with greater risk if the procedure is performed prior to 10-weeks' gestation. The procedure also carries a greater risk of spontaneous abortion than does amniocentesis.

Clarren, S. K. 1981. Recognition of fetal alcohol syndrome. *Journal of the American Medical Association* 245:2436–9.

▶ Heavy maternal alcohol consumption causes characteristic congenital malformations in the offspring, which are described in the article.

Copel, J. A., and Bahado-Singh, R. O. 1999. Prenatal screening for Down's syndrome—a search for the family's values. *New England Journal of Medicine* 341:521–2.

▶ First trimester screening, second trimester screening, or more sensitive sequential integrated screening tests combining both first and second trimester results are available. The decision as to the type of screening depends on the woman's personal values.

▶ If a woman plans to terminate a Down syndrome pregnancy, she will opt for confirmation of an abnormal screening test results by chorionic villus sampling, followed by pregnancy termination during the first trimester, which is a much safer procedure for the mother. A woman who plans not to terminate a Down pregnancy may follow up with a second trimester screening test, and an abnormal test result can be followed by an amniocentesis, which will determine the fetal karyotype. If the karyotype is normal, Down syndrome is excluded. If the karyotype reveals a chromosome abnormality, the mother has time to come to terms with her baby's condition. On the other hand, if she later decides to terminate the pregnancy, this is still possible but at greater risk to the mother than a first-trimester termination.

Haddow, J. E., Palomaki, G. E., Knight, G. J., et al. 1998. Screening of maternal serum for fetal Down's syndrome in the first trimester. *New England Journal of Medicine* 338:955–61.

▶ Two blood tests and an ultrasound test performed at 9–12 weeks' gestation can be used to detect Down syndrome in the first trimester. The concentration chorionic gonadotropin (hCG) in maternal blood is higher than normal; the concentration of another maternal blood component called pregnancy-associated protein A (PAP-A) is lower than normal; and the fetal neck skinfold thickness measured by ultrasound (nuchal translucency measurement) is thicker in a fetus with Down syndrome than in unaffected fetuses. The PAP-A change rapidly during the first trimester, so the exact gestational age of the fetus needs to be determined precisely by ultrasound measurement to determine the proper gestation-related concentration of PAP-A with which to compare the woman's test result. If the woman plans to terminate a suspected Down syndrome pregnancy, the screening test results can be confirmed by chorionic villus sampling, and the termination can be accomplished more safely in the first trimester. Alternatively, she may choose to wait for additional blood testing early in the second trimester. The combined first and second trimester screening test results have a low rate of false-positive tests, and the woman may elect not to have an amniocentesis if the screening tests are normal. However, if she wants to be absolutely certain that the fetus is normal, only an amniocentesis can provide the answer.

Kaback, M., Lim Steele, J., Dabholkar, D., et al. 1993. Tay-Sachs disease—carrier screening, prenatal diagnosis, and the molecular area. An international perspective, 1970 to 1993. The International TSD Data Collection Network. *Journal of the American Medical Association* 270:2307–15.

▶ The international experience with carrier screening and prenatal diagnosis.

Little, B. B., Snell, L. M., Klein, V. R., et al. 1989. Cocaine abuse during pregnancy: Maternal and fetal implications. *Obstetrics and Gynecology* 73:157–60.

▶ A review article outlining major problems and complications from cocaine abuse.

O'Donnell, W. T., and Warren, S. T. 2002. A decade of molecular studies of fragile X syndrome. *Annual Review of Neuroscience* 25:315–38.

▶ A review of current knowledge, including how the fully mutated *FMR1* gene may affect formation and function of synapses in the nervous system. The greatly increased number of CGG repeats characteristic of a full mutation blocks the function of the *FMR1* gene so that no gene product (FMRP) is produced. Expansion of the gene from a premutation to a full mutation is likely to occur when the gene is transmitted to the child from the mother rather than from the father.

Ouellette, E. M., Rosett, H. L., Rosman, N. P., et al. 1977. Adverse effects on offspring of maternal alcohol abuse during pregnancy. *New England Journal of Medicine* 297:528–30.

▶ Describes fetal alcohol syndrome.

Rosengren, J. 1990. Alcohol. A bigger drug problem. *Minnesota Medicine* 73:33–4.

▶ Describes the harmful effects of alcohol on the fetus.

Simpson, J. L. 2005. Choosing the best prenatal screening protocol. *New England Journal of Medicine* 353:2068–70.

▶ Most pregnant women prefer the option of prenatal screening for Down syndrome and avoiding the possible risk of amniocentesis. First semester screening, including an ultrasound measurement of the skinfold thickness at the back of the fetal neck is more effective than second trimester screening, and combining both screening tests increases the detection rate of Down syndrome to 97%, with a 5% false-positive rate. However, if the woman's goal of screening is 100% detection of a fetal trisomy, even the most comprehensive screening cannot guarantee this result, and amniocentesis or chorionic villus sampling may be preferable.

Stagno, S., Pass, R. F., Cloud, G., et al. 1986. Primary cytomegalovirus infection in pregnancy. Incidence, transmission to fetus, and clinical outcome. *Journal of the American Medical Association* 256:1904–8.

▶ Primary CMV infection during pregnancy poses a significant risk of intrauterine transmission, and an adverse outcome is more likely when the infection occurs within the first half of gestation.

Waisbren, S., Hanley, W., Levy, H. L., et al. 2000. Outcome at age 4 years in offspring of women with maternal phenylketonuria: The maternal PKU collaborative study. *Journal of the American Medical Association* 283:756–62.

▶ Maternal phenylketonuria puts the infant at risk for impaired development, congenital malformations, and mental retardation. The risk can be minimized by a phenylalanine restricted diet and close control of maternal phenylalanine blood levels.

OUTLINE SUMMARY

Causes of Congenital Malformations

Pathogenesis of Congenital Malformation

CHROMOSOMAL ABNORMALITIES

Nondisjunction leading to trisomy, deletions, and translocations during gametogenesis and in the zygote.

Sex chromosome abnormalities:

Klinefelter syndrome: genotype 47,XXY with sex chromatin body. Infertility, testicular atrophy, breast hypertrophy.

47,XYY syndrome: reduced intelligence and aggressive behavior.

Fragile X syndrome: important cause of mental deficiency.

Turner syndrome: genotype 45,X lacking sex chromatin body. Abnormal body configuration.

Triple X syndrome: genotype 47,XXX with extra sex chromatin body. No specific somatic abnormalities.

Abnormalities of autosomes:

Down syndrome:

Mental deficiency, characteristic facial expression, often congenital cardiac malformation.

Caused by nondisjunction during gametogenesis, chromosome translocation, or nondisjunction in zygote.

GENETICALLY TRANSMITTED DISEASES

Gene mutation involving structural protein or enzyme: phenylketonuria and sickle hemoglobin disorders.

Transmission:

Autosomal: dominant, recessive, or codominant.

Sex-linked: male affected if carrying X chromosome containing defective gene. Female may be carrier but is unaffected.

INTRAUTERINE INJURY

Harmful drugs (e.g., thalidomide).

Radiation.

Maternal infections: German measles (rubella), cytomegalovirus, other viral diseases, toxoplasmosis.

INTERACTION OF GENETIC AND ENVIRONMENTAL FACTORS

Susceptible embryo develops malformation if exposed to environmental agents. Resistant embryo unaffected. Parents are transmitting sets of genes that increase susceptibility to embryologic disturbances.

Prenatal Diagnosis

APPLICATION

Maternal blood tests to screen for congenital abnormalities.

Detect chromosomal abnormalities and some genetic abnormalities.

Analysis of fetal DNA—an important diagnostic test when indicated.

Detect nervous system defects (alpha fetoprotein analysis).

TECHNIQUE

Perform amniocentesis as early as 12 weeks.

Culture amnionic cells (of fetal origin) and determine karyotype.

Biochemical analysis where indicated.

Alpha fetoprotein analysis where indicated.

Analysis of fetal DNA when indicated.

Chorionic villus sampling: provides same information as amniocentesis. Has some advantages and some disadvantages compared with amniocentesis.

CHAPTER 10

Neoplastic Disease

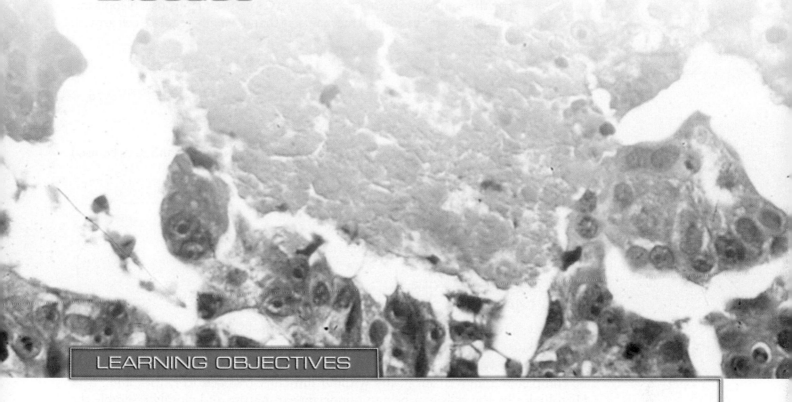

LEARNING OBJECTIVES

1 Compare the general characteristics of benign and malignant tumors. Explain how tumors are named. List the common exceptions to standard terminology.

2 Summarize the features of the principal types of lymphoma.

3 Differentiate between infiltrating and in situ carcinoma. Explain the role of the Pap smear in early diagnosis of neoplasm.

4 Explain how leukemias are classified. Describe the clinical manifestations of each type and its response to treatment.

5 Differentiate myeloma from leukemia. Describe its clinical manifestations, and explain how it is diagnosed.

6 Explain the mechanisms of the body's immunologic defenses against tumor.

7 Summarize the principal modalities of tumor treatment, including advantages, disadvantages, and common side effects of each technique.

8 Describe the applications and limitations of tumor-associated antigens in the diagnosis and treatment of patients with tumors.

9 Compare the incidence and survival rates for various types of malignant tumors. Explain the mechanisms of late recurrence. Define the role of adjuvant therapy in preventing late recurrence.

10 Understand the role of activated oncogenes and disturbance in suppressor gene function on the pathogenesis of tumors.

Tumors: Disturbed Cell Growth

Normal life processes are characterized by continuous growth and maturation of cells, and all cells are subject to control mechanisms that regulate their growth rate. This ongoing growth process serves the purpose of replacing cells that have been injured or have undergone degenerative changes. In contrast, a neoplasm (*neo* = new + *plasm* = growth) is an overgrowth of cells that serves no useful purpose. Neoplasms appear not to be subject to the control mechanisms that normally regulate cell growth and differentiation.

Tumors

CLASSIFICATION AND NOMENCLATURE

Tumor
A benign or malignant overgrowth of tissues that serves no normal function.

The terms neoplasm and **tumor** have essentially the same meaning and may be used interchangeably. There are two large classes of neoplasms:

1. Benign tumors
2. Malignant tumors

TABLE 10-1 compares the major characteristics of the two classes.

COMPARISON OF BENIGN AND MALIGNANT TUMORS

Generally, a benign tumor grows slowly and remains localized. Although it pushes surrounding normal tissue aside, it does not infiltrate surrounding tissues or spread by blood and lymphatic channels to distant sites. Usually, a benign tumor can be completely removed surgically without difficulty (FIGURES 10-1, 10-2, and 10-3). Histologically, the cells in a benign tumor appear mature and closely resemble the normal cells from which the tumor was derived.

In contrast to a benign tumor, a malignant neoplasm is composed of less well-differentiated cells (FIGURE 10-4), grows more rapidly, and infiltrates the surrounding tissues rather than growing by expansion (FIGURE 10-5). Frequently, the infiltrating strands of tumor find their way into the vascular and lymphatic channels. Bits of tumor may be carried in the lymphatics to reach the lymph nodes, where they establish secondary sites of tumor growth not connected with the original tumor (FIGURE 10-6). Eventually, the tumor may spread widely throughout the lymphatic channels. Tumor cells may also gain access to the bloodstream and be carried to distant sites, leading to secondary tumor deposits throughout the body. The process by which a tumor spreads some

TABLE 10-1

Comparison of benign and malignant tumors		
	Benign tumor	**Malignant tumor**
Growth rate	Slow	Rapid
Character of growth	Expansion	Infiltration
Tumor spread	Remains localized	Metastasis by bloodstream and lymphatics
Cell differentiation	Well differentiated	Poorly differentiated

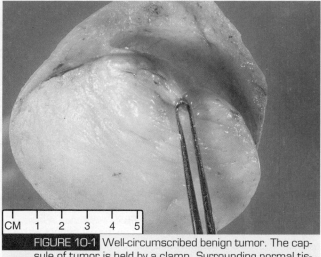

FIGURE 10-1 Well-circumscribed benign tumor. The capsule of tumor is held by a clamp. Surrounding normal tissues have retracted, indicating an absence of infiltration.

A

B

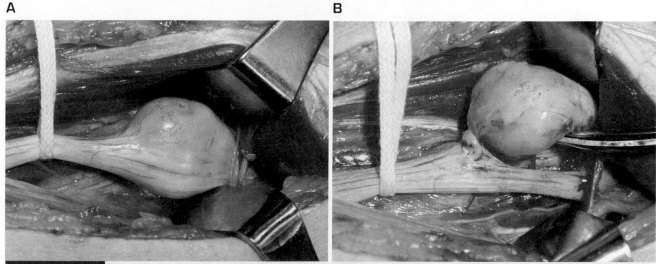

FIGURE 10-2 **A**, Benign tumor (neuroma) arising from the sciatic nerve. **B**, Tumor dissected from surrounding nerve. The cleavage plane is easily established, indicating that the tumor is sharply circumscribed and does not infiltrate the adjacent nerve.

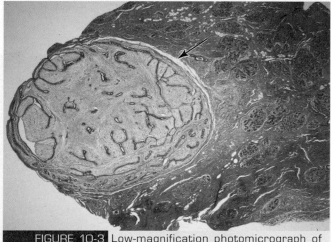

FIGURE 10-3 Low-magnification photomicrograph of benign breast tumor (fibroadenoma). Note the sharp demarcation between the tumor and surrounding breast tissue (*arrow*).

A

B

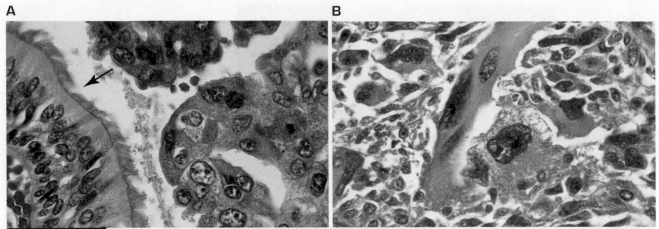

FIGURE 10-4 Cellular abnormalities in malignant tumors. **A**, Biopsy of a bronchus from a patient with lung carcinoma, comparing normal respiratory epithelium (*arrow*) with clusters of neoplastic cells from a lung carcinoma. Cancer cells grow in a haphazard pattern and exhibit great variation in size and structure. **B**, Malignant tumor of smooth muscle (leiomyosarcoma), illustrating large, bizarre, elongated tumor cells showing little resemblance to normal smooth muscle cells from which the tumor arose.

A

B

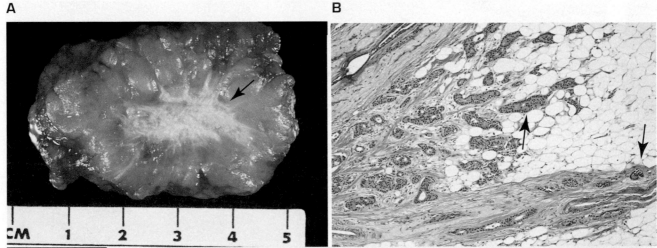

FIGURE 10-5 Breast carcinoma. **A**, Breast biopsy illustrating breast carcinoma (*arrow*) infiltrating adjacent fatty tissue of breast. There is no distinct demarcation between tumor and normal tissue. **B**, Low-magnification photograph illustrating the margin of infiltrating breast carcinoma. Small clusters of tumor cells (*arrows*) infiltrate adipose tissues of breast (original magnification × 2O).

A

B

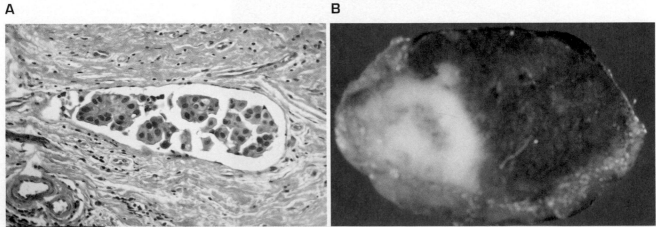

FIGURE 10-6 Lymphatic spread of carcinoma. **A**, Cluster of tumor cells in lymphatic vessel (original magnification × 4OO). **B**, Deposit of metastatic carcinoma (white mass within node) that has spread via lymphatic channels into a small regional lymph node.

distance from the primary site is called **metastasis** (*meta* = beyond + *stasis* = standing), and the secondary deposits are called metastatic tumors (FIGURE 10-7). If a malignant tumor is not eradicated promptly, it may eventually become widely disseminated throughout the body and may kill the patient. Benign tumors do not metastasize.

Tumors are named and classified according to the cells and tissues from which they originate. Therefore, understanding the primary tissue classifications explained in the discussion on cells and tissues: their structure and function in health and disease is helpful in understanding the names of tumors. Tumor nomenclature is not completely uniform, but certain generalizations are possible.

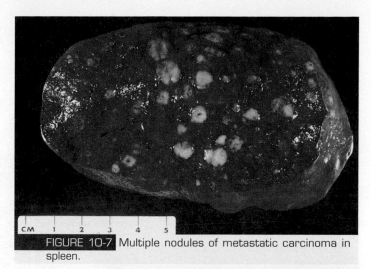

FIGURE 10-7 Multiple nodules of metastatic carcinoma in spleen.

BENIGN TUMORS

A benign tumor that projects from an epithelial surface is usually called a **polyp** or **papilloma** (FIGURE 10-8). Most other benign tumors are named by adding the suffix *-oma* to the prefix that designates the cell of origin, as shown in TABLE 10-2. For example, a benign tumor arising from glandular epithelium is called an adenoma. A benign tumor of blood vessels is an angioma (FIGURE 10-9), and one arising from cartilage is designated a chondroma.

MALIGNANT TUMORS

There are many types of malignant tumors, but all can be classified into three groups: (1) carcinomas, (2) sarcomas, or (3) leukemias. The term cancer is a word used to indicate any type of malignant tumor.

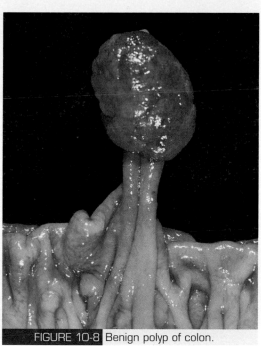

FIGURE 10-8 Benign polyp of colon.

TABLE 10-2

Common prefixes used to name tumors

Prefix	Meaning
Adeno-	Gland
Angio-	Vessels (type not specified)
Chondro-	Cartilage
Fibro-	Fibrous tissue
Hemangio-	Blood vessels
Lymphangio-	Lymph vessels
Lipo-	Fat
Myo-	Muscle
Neuro-	Nerve
Osteo-	Bone

Metastasis
The spread of cancer cells from the primary site of origin to a distant site within the body.

Polyp
A descriptive term for a benign tumor projecting from an epithelial surface.

Papilloma
(pap-pil-ō'muh)
A descriptive term for a benign tumor projecting from an epithelial surface.

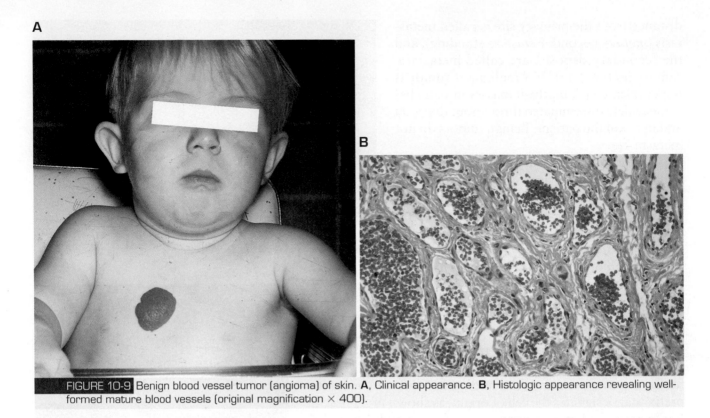

FIGURE 10-9 Benign blood vessel tumor (angioma) of skin. **A**, Clinical appearance. **B**, Histologic appearance revealing well-formed mature blood vessels (original magnification × 400).

It is generally agreed that a malignant tumor starts from a single cell that has sustained some type of damage to its genome that causes it to proliferate abnormally, forming first a clone of identical cells and, if unchecked, eventually developing into a distinct tumor. Cells of malignant tumors exhibit behavior that is quite different from that of normal cells. They do not respond to normal growth regulatory signals from other cells, and they continue to proliferate when there is no need to do so. Indeed, some cancer cells actually secrete growth factors to stimulate their own growth. As they grow, they acquire properties that allow them to flourish at the expense of the surrounding normal cells. They secrete enzymes that break down normal cell and tissue barriers, which allows them to infiltrate into adjacent tissues, invade lymphatic channels and blood vessels, and eventually spread throughout the body. Moreover, the proliferating tumor cells do not "wear out" and die after a specific number of cell divisions, as normal cells do. They become "immortal" and can proliferate indefinitely.

A **carcinoma** is any malignant tumor arising from surface, glandular, or parenchymal (organ) epithelium. (The term is not applied, however, to malignant tumors of endothelium or mesothelium, which behave more like malignant connective tissue tumors.) A carcinoma is classified further by designating the type of epithelium from which it arose. For example, a malignant tumor arising from the transitional epithelium of the urinary bladder is called a transitional cell carcinoma of the bladder. A carcinoma arising from the glandular epithelium of the pancreas is termed an adeno-carcinoma of the pancreas (*aden* = gland), and a tumor arising from the squamous epithelium of the esophagus is called a squamous cell carcinoma of the esophagus.

Sarcoma is a general term referring to a malignant tumor arising from primary tissues other than surface, glandular, or parenchymal epithelium. The exact type of sarcoma is specified by prefixing the term designating the cell of origin. For example, a malignant tumor of cartilage is designated as a chondrosarcoma. Fibrosarcoma, liposarcoma, myosarcoma, osteosarcoma, and angiosarcoma indicate, respectively, malignant tumors of fibroblasts, fat cells, muscle cells, bone-forming cells, and blood vessels.

Carcinoma
(kär-sin-ō′-mah)
A malignant tumor derived from epithelial cells.

Sarcoma
(sar-kō′muh)
A malignant tumor arising from connective and supporting tissues.

The term **leukemia** is applied to any neoplasm of blood-forming tissues. Neoplasms arising from the precursors of white blood cells usually do not form solid tumors. Instead, the abnormal cells proliferate diffusely within the bone marrow, where they overgrow and crowd out the normal blood-forming cells. The neoplastic cells also "spill over" into the bloodstream, and large numbers of abnormal cells circulate in the peripheral blood.

TABLE 10-3 summarizes the general principles used to name both benign and malignant tumors.

VARIATIONS IN TERMINOLOGY

There are some inconsistencies and exceptions to the general principles of nomenclature. Exceptions are encountered in the naming of lymphoid tumors, skin tumors arising from pigment-producing cells within the epidermis, certain tumors of mixed cellular components, and certain types of tumors composed of primitive cells seen in children. In other cases, names of tumors seem to follow no rules or general principles. The student should not be unduly concerned about the exceptions or unusual situations but should attempt to grasp the general principles of naming tumors.

Lymphoid Tumors

All neoplasms of lymphoid tissue are called **lymphomas**. With extremely rare exceptions, these tumors are malignant (FIGURE 10-10). Therefore, the term lymphoma without qualification refers to a malignant, not a benign, tumor. Often, to avoid confusion, the term malignant lymphoma, rather than simply lymphoma, is used.

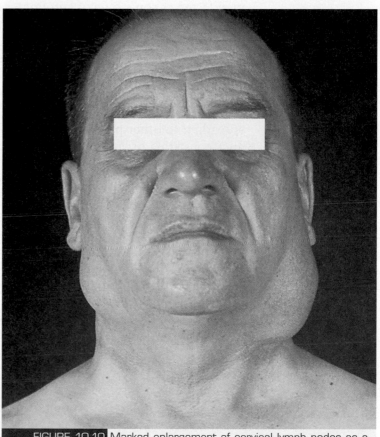

FIGURE 10-10 Marked enlargement of cervical lymph nodes as a result of malignant lymphoma.

Leukemia
(lōō-kē′mē-yuh)
A neoplastic proliferation of leukocytes.

Lymphoma
(limf-ō′muh)
A neoplasm of lymphoid cells.

TABLE 10-3

General principles of naming tumors

General term	Meaning
Polyp, papilloma	Any benign tumor projecting from surface epithelium.
____ + oma (suffix)	A benign tumor. The prefix designates primary tissue of origin.
Carcinoma	Malignant tumor arising from surface, glandular, or parenchymal epithelium (but not endothelium or mesothelium).
Sarcoma	Malignant tumor of any primary tissue other than surface, glandular, and parenchymal epithelium.
Leukemia	Neoplasm of blood cells.

Over 80% of lymphomas arise from B cells. Most of the rest come from T cells, and a few originate from NK cells (natural killer cells) or histiocytes. The neoplastic cells of most lymphomas arise from early precursor stages in the development of mature B and T cells, and the tumors sometimes resemble masses of neoplastic precursor B or T cells that have failed to mature normally. The abnormal proliferation of lymphoid cells may also disrupt the normal functions of the immune system, which may be manifested either as an impairment of the body's immune defenses resulting in increased susceptibility to infection or as an abnormal immune response manifested as some type of autoimmune disease.

Lymphomas are subdivided into two major groups: Hodgkin's lymphoma, more often called **Hodgkin's disease**, and non-Hodgkin's lymphoma. Hodgkin's lymphoma has several features that are quite different from other lymphomas. The disease frequently occurs in young adults, in contrast to non-Hodgkin's lymphoma, which usually affects much older persons. The disease usually starts in a single lymph node or small group of nodes and then spreads to adjacent nodes before eventually spreading to other parts of the body. The tumor has a variable histologic appearance consisting of large atypical B cells called **Reed-Sternberg cells** intermixed with lymphocytes, plasma cells, eosinophils, and fibrous tissue. The Reed-Sternberg cells make up only a small proportion of the total cells in the tumor, but they secrete cytokines that attract the other cells, which become intermixed with the Reed-Sternberg cells. The typical Reed-Sternberg cell is a large cell that characteristically contains either a single nucleus or two nuclei that appear as mirror images of each other. Each nucleus contains a large nucleolus surrounded by a clear halo (FIGURE 10-11). Several different histologic types of Hodgkin's disease are recognized that differ somewhat in their clinical behavior and prognosis. A person with Hodgkin's lymphoma usually first becomes aware of a painless enlargement of a single lymph node or group of nodes. In more advanced cases, several groups of nodes may be involved. Previously, patients with early stage Hodgkin's disease were treated with radiation therapy to the enlarged lymph nodes which was quite successful in most patients, but unfortunately the disease recurred in some radiotherapy-treated patients. Now most patients are treated with courses of chemotherapy consisting of four drugs (doxorubicin, bleomyxin, vinblastine, and dacarbazine) as well as radiotherapy to the involved areas and the combined therapy approach has been very successful.

All other lymphomas are grouped together under the general term of non-Hodgkin's lymphomas. Most are B-cell lymphomas that are quite variable in their

Hodgkin's disease
One type of lymphoma.

Reed-Sternberg cell
The characteristic cell of Hodgkin's disease, containing two "mirror image" nuclei with prominent nucleoli.

A   B

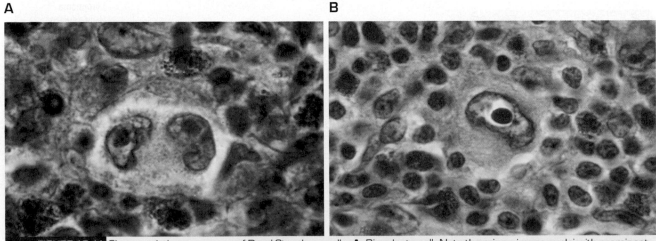

FIGURE 10-11 Characteristic appearance of Reed-Sternberg cells. **A,** Binucleate cell. Note the mirror image nuclei with prominent nucleoli. **B,** Cell with single nucleus illustrating prominent nucleolus and perinuclear halo (original magnification × 400).

appearance, behavior, and prognosis. Most patients have widespread disease by the time the lymphoma is diagnosed, and it is difficult to cure the lymphoma because the tumor cells have already spread throughout the body. Some tumors are very aggressive and grow rapidly, whereas other tumors that appear somewhat similar grow more slowly. Some lymphomas respond reasonably well to specific anticancer drugs, whereas others do not. Moreover, some lymphomas, which initially were composed of mature, slowly growing cells, may transform abruptly into aggressive rapidly growing tumors composed of very immature cells.

The variable appearance and sometimes poor correlation between histologic appearance and biologic behavior have created difficulties when attempting to classify lymphomas. Various classifications have been proposed to provide a better guide to prognosis and treatment. One classification is based on the size, shape, and growth pattern of the neoplastic cells. Lymphomas can also be classified into prognostic groups based on their histologic appearance. The most recent classification divides lymphomas into four large groups based on the type of cells giving rise to the tumor (T cells, B cells, NK cells, or histiocytes) and the maturity of the cells, with many subgroups within each of the four major groups. This classification system helps the physician determine the specific type of non-Hodgkin's lymphoma affecting the patient, which also helps determine the prognosis and the appropriate type of treatment.

Skin Tumors

Most skin tumors arise either from the keratin-forming cells or from the pigment-producing cells of the epidermis. The keratin-forming cells are called **keratinocytes**. The deepest layer of keratinocytes adjacent to the dermis consists of cuboidal cells called basal cells that proliferate and give rise to the upper layers of cells, which are called squamous cells. Interspersed among the keratinocytes are the skin cells that normally produce pigment and are responsible for normal skin color. These are called **melanocytes**, and the black pigment that they produce is called **melanin**. The common benign pigmented skin lesion that is derived from melanin-producing cells is called a **nevus**, a Latin word that means "birthmark" (FIGURE 10-12). The malignant counterpart is called a **melanoma** (or malignant melanoma), the name being derived from the pigment elaborated by the cells.

Keratinocytes can give rise to benign proliferations, called keratoses, and two types of skin carcinomas. One type, called a basal cell carcinoma, is composed of clusters of infiltrating cells that resemble the normal basal cells of the epidermis. It is a rather indolent, slowly growing tumor that can be locally destructive but rarely metastasizes. The other type, composed of abnormal infiltrating squamous cells, is called a squamous cell carcinoma and is a more aggressive tumor that sometimes metastasizes. Both types generally can be cured by complete surgical excision and carry a very good prognosis. Excessive sunlight exposure predisposes to the development of all types of skin cancer, including the potentially lethal melanoma, and also predisposes to the development of some types of keratoses, as well as causing skin damage and premature aging of the skin (FIGURE 10-13).

Keratinocyte
(ker-u-tin′ō-cyte)
A keratin-forming cell in the epidermis.

Melanocyte
(me-lan′o-cyte)
Melanin-producing cell in the epidermis.

Melanin
Dark pigment found in the skin, in the middle coat of the eye, and in some other regions.

Nevus (nē′vus)
A benign tumor of pigment-producing cells.

Melanoma
(mel-uh-nō′muh)
A malignant tumor of pigment-producing cells.

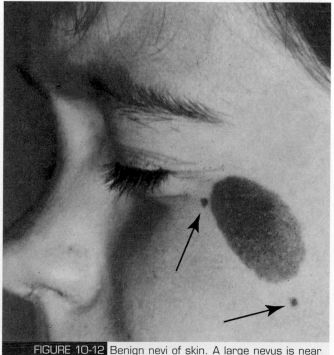
FIGURE 10-12 Benign nevi of skin. A large nevus is near the eye, and two smaller adjacent nevi are shown (*arrows*).

A

B

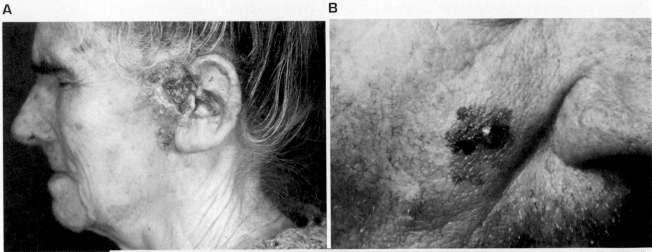

FIGURE 10-13 Common skin cancers caused by excessive sun exposure. **A**, Cancer arising from keratinocytes (basal cell carcinoma). **B**, Cancer arising from melanocytes (malignant melanoma).

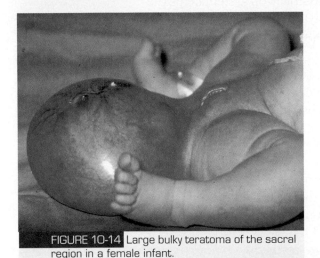

FIGURE 10-14 Large bulky teratoma of the sacral region in a female infant.

Tumors of Mixed Components (Teratomas)

A **teratoma** is a tumor derived from cells that have the potential of differentiating into many different types of tissue (bone, muscle, glands, epithelium, brain tissue, and hair). Frequently, such tumors consist of poorly organized mixtures of many tissues. Teratomas often arise in the reproductive tract but may also develop in some other locations. Because a teratoma may be either benign or malignant, one must specify the type, calling the tumor either a benign teratoma or a malignant teratoma (FIGURE 10-14). A common type of cystic benign teratoma arising in the ovary is usually called a **dermoid cyst** (FIGURE 10-15).

Teratoma
(tăr-uh-tō′muh)
A tumor of mixed cell components.

....

Dermoid cyst
(derm′oyd)
A common type of benign cystic teratoma that commonly arises in the ovary.

A

B

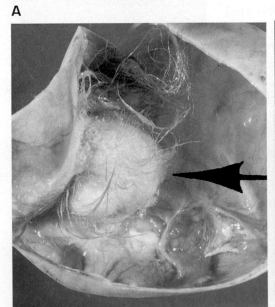
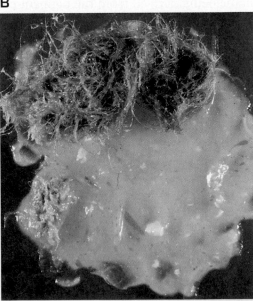

FIGURE 10-15 **A**, Cystic teratoma (dermoid cyst) of ovary. The cyst is lined by skin containing sweat and sebaceous (oil secreting) glands, and the skin surface is covered by hair. The *arrow* indicates a nodule in the cyst wall containing fat, muscle, and bone. **B**, Contents of cyst, consisting of matted hair and oil derived from skin lining the cyst.

Childhood Primitive Cell Tumors

Certain unusual and relatively rare tumors encountered in children may arise in the brain, retina of the eye, adrenal gland, kidney, liver, or genital tract. Primitive cell tumors of this type are named from the site of origin, with the suffix *-blastoma* added (*blast* = a primitive cell + *oma* = tumor). Thus, a primitive cell tumor arising from the retina of the eye is a retinoblastoma (FIGURE 10-16) and one of hepatic origin is called a hepatoblastoma. A primitive cell tumor of the kidney, however, is usually called a **Wilms tumor** rather than a nephroblastoma.

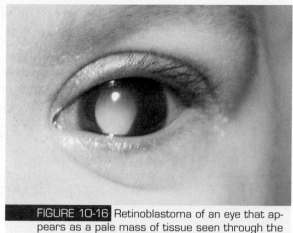

FIGURE 10-16 Retinoblastoma of an eye that appears as a pale mass of tissue seen through the dilated pupil.

NECROSIS IN TUMORS

Tumors derive their blood supply from the tissues they invade. Malignant tumors frequently induce new blood vessels to proliferate in the adjacent normal tissues to supply the demands of the growing tumor. However, a malignant tumor may outgrow its blood supply. When this occurs, the parts of the tumor with the poorest blood supply undergo necrosis (FIGURE 10-17). If the tumor is growing within an organ such as the lung or kidney and is surrounded by normal tissue, the blood supply is best at the junction of tumor and adjacent normal tissue and poorest in the center of the tumor, which often degenerates. In contrast, if the malignant tumor is growing outward from an epithelial surface, such as the colon, the best blood supply is at the base of the tumor. The poorest blood supply is at the surface, which frequently becomes necrotic and sloughs, leaving a shallow crater covered with degenerated tissue and inflammatory exudate (FIGURE 10-18). Often, small blood vessels are exposed in the ulcerated base of the tumor. Blood may ooze continuously from these vessels, eventually leading to anemia from chronic blood loss. Sometimes the ulcerated tumor may be the source of a severe hemorrhage.

Wilms tumor
A malignant renal tumor of infants and children.

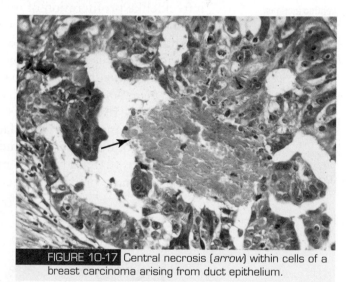

FIGURE 10-17 Central necrosis (*arrow*) within cells of a breast carcinoma arising from duct epithelium.

A   B

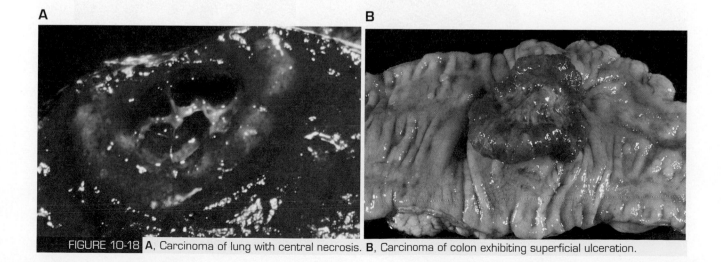

FIGURE 10-18 **A**, Carcinoma of lung with central necrosis. **B**, Carcinoma of colon exhibiting superficial ulceration.

NONINFILTRATING (IN SITU) CARCINOMA

Infiltration and metastasis are two characteristic features of malignant tumors. However, we now know that many carcinomas arising from surface epithelium remain localized within the epithelium for many years before evidence of infiltration into the deeper tissues or spread to distant sites becomes apparent. This has been well documented for squamous cell carcinoma of the cervix (FIGURE 10-19). Noninfiltrating tumors have also been recognized in many other locations, including the breast (discussion on the breast), urinary tract, colon, and skin. The term carcinoma in situ (in-site carcinoma) is used for this type of neoplasm. In situ carcinoma can be completely cured by surgical excision or other treatment that eradicates the abnormal epithelium, and this is the stage most favorable to successful treatment.

PRECANCEROUS CONDITIONS

Actinic keratosis

(ak-ti′-nik ke-rä-tō′sis)
A precancerous warty proliferation of squamous epithelial cells in sun-damaged skin of older persons.

Lentigo maligna

A precancerous, pigmented skin lesion arising from proliferation of atypical melanin-producing epithelial cells (melanocytes).

Leukoplakia

A white patch of hyperplastic and usually atypical squamous epithelium on the oral mucosa or genital tract mucosa.

Sometimes the term precancerous is used when referring to conditions that have a high likelihood of eventually developing into cancer. Prolonged exposure to sunlight, for example, not only causes premature aging of the skin, but also causes small, crusted, scaly patches to develop on sun-exposed skin called **actinic keratoses** ("actinic" refers to sun rays). Untreated, many keratoses eventually develop into skin cancers. Another precancerous condition resulting from prolonged sun exposure is a frecklelike proliferation of melanin-producing cells in the skin called **lentigo maligna** (a Latin term meaning "malignant freckle"). They are so named because many eventually become transformed into melanomas. Precancerous, thick white patches descriptively called **leukoplakia** (*leuko* = white + *plakia* = patch) may develop in the mucous membranes of the mouth as a result of exposure to tobacco tars from pipe or cigar smoking or from use of smokeless tobacco (snuff and chewing tobacco) and may give rise to squamous cell cancers of the oral cavity. Somewhat similar precancerous changes may take place in the epithelium of the vulva (discussion on the female reproductive system) and may eventuate into vulvar cancer. Some types of colon polyps that are prone to malignant change also are considered precancerous. There are many precancerous conditions, of which these are only a few examples.

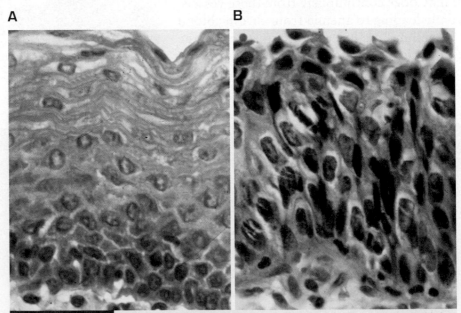

A   **B**

FIGURE 10-19 Normal cervical stratified squamous epithelium **A**, compared with in situ carcinoma of cervix **B**. Note the nuclear abnormalities characteristic of carcinoma. The tumor has not yet infiltrated the underlying tissues (original magnification × 400).

Precancerous conditions should always be treated appropriately in order to prevent malignant change, which occurs in many, but not all, cases.

Etiologic Factors in Neoplastic Disease

VIRUSES

Many types of tumors in animals are caused by viruses and can be readily transmitted by appropriate methods to animals of the same or a different species. In some instances, a single type of virus is capable of producing many different types of tumors in various species of animals. At least some of the cancers in humans also appear to be caused by viruses. Some unusual types of leukemia and lymphoma are caused by a virus called the human T cell leukemia–lymphoma virus (HTLV-1), which is related to the virus that causes the acquired immune deficiency syndrome (AIDS). Kaposi's sarcoma in AIDS patients is caused by a herpes virus, designated human herpesvirus 8 (HHV-8). Some strains of the papilloma virus that cause genital condylomas (discussion on the female reproductive system) appear to predispose to cervical carcinoma and are also responsible for some squamous cell carcinomas of the mouth, throat, and larynx (oropharyngeal carcinomas). Chronic viral hepatitis (discussion on the liver and the biliary system) predisposes to primary carcinoma of the liver. Some types of nasophyngeal carcinoma and some types of lymphoma appear to be related to Epstein-Barr virus infections, the virus that causes infectious mononucleosis.

GENE AND CHROMOSOMAL ABNORMALITIES

The basic process common to all neoplasms is an alteration of the genes on the chromosomes of a cell so that the cell no longer responds to normal control mechanisms and proceeds to proliferate without regard for the needs of the body. In the body, many billions of cells are dividing all the time. They are also continually subjected to radiation, various chemical carcinogens (cancer-producing substances), or other agents that can alter the structure of genes. A change in the gene's structure is called a **mutation** (*muto* = change), and the mutated gene may function differently from a normal gene.

Three large groups of genes play important roles in regulating cell functions, and derangements of these genes are associated with formation of tumors. The first group comprises **proto-oncogenes**. The second group consists of **tumor suppressor genes**, and the third group is the **DNA repair genes** (TABLE 10-4).

Mutation
(mū-tā′shun)
An alteration in a base sequence in DNA; may alter cell function. Transmitted from parents to offspring only if mutation is in gametes.

Proto-oncogene
(pro-to-on′-koh-jēn)
A normal gene that regulates some aspect of cell growth, maturation, or division.

Tumor suppressor gene
A gene that suppresses cell proliferation.

DNA repair genes
Genes that monitor and correct errors in DNA replication during cell division.

TABLE 10-4

Gene mutations that disrupt cell function

Gene	Normal function	Malfunction
Proto-oncogene	Promotes normal cell growth	Point mutation, amplification, or translocation forms an oncogene, resulting in unrestrained cell growth
Paired tumor suppressor genes	Inhibit cell proliferation	Both genes inactivated in same cell promotes cell proliferation
Paired DNA repair genes	Correct errors in DNA duplication	Gene inactivation increases mutation rate

Proto-Oncogenes

Human chromosomes contain a number of normal "growth genes" that promote some aspect of cell growth, differentiation, or mitotic activity. They are called proto-oncogenes; they are closely related to genes carried by viruses that cause tumors in experimental animals, and they are named from the tumor viruses that they resemble. A proto-oncogene is a normal gene that regulates some normal growth function in a cell, but a proto-oncogene can undergo a mutation or become translocated to another chromosome where its functions are deranged. Either event can convert a normally functioning proto-oncogene into an **oncogene** (*onkos* = tumor), an abnormally functioning gene that stimulates cell growth excessively and leads to unrestrained cell proliferation. An oncogene is a "gene that causes cancer."

Conversion of a proto-oncogene into an oncogene (activation of an oncogene) may consist of a change in only a single nucleotide in the DNA of the gene, which is called a point mutation, or the mutation may generate multiple copies of the same gene, called gene amplification, which greatly increases the activity of the gene. Translocation to another chromosome activates an oncogene because of the way in which genes are related on individual chromosomes. A specific gene, such as one that regulates some aspect of cell growth or mitotic activity, is influenced by other nearby genes that either suppress or stimulate its activities. Cell growth and differentiation are normal when the proto-oncogene ("growth gene") and its neighbors function together in an orderly manner, but may be deranged if this relation is disturbed. For example, the translocation may bring the proto-oncogene to a new location on another chromosome where it is freed from the inhibitory genes that formerly controlled its activities. Alternatively, the translocation may bring the proto-oncogene to a new location on another chromosome adjacent to another gene that stimulates its functions.

Tumor Suppressor Genes

These are groups of different genes that function to suppress cell proliferation. Loss of suppressor gene function by mutation or another event disrupts cell functions and can lead to unrestrained cell growth. Suppressor genes exist in pairs at corresponding gene loci on homologous chromosomes, and both suppressor genes must cease to function before the cell malfunctions.

Tumor suppressor genes may also play a role in determining how many times a cell can divide before it involutes and dies. In some cases, loss of a tumor suppressor gene function may allow the cell to proliferate indefinitely rather than dying after a predetermined number of cell divisions, as normal cells do.

Loss of function of specific tumor suppressor genes has been correlated with specific tumors, and the suppressor genes are often named from the tumors with which they have been associated.

DNA Repair Genes

DNA repair genes are part of the cell's "quality control" and repair system. These genes regulate the processes that monitor and repair any errors in DNA duplication that may occur when the cell's chromosomes are duplicated in the course of cell division; they are also concerned with the repair of DNA that has been damaged by radiation, chemicals, or other environmental agents. Any change in the normal arrangement of DNA nucleotides on the DNA chain constitutes a DNA mutation. Consequently, failure of DNA repair gene function increases the likelihood of DNA mutations within the affected cell. A high mutation rate within cells predisposes to tumors because some mutations may affect cell functions that promote unrestrained cell growth.

Oncogene
(on′-koh-jēn)
An abnormally functioning gene that causes unrestrained cell growth leading to formation of a tumor. Results from mutation or translocation of a proto-oncogene.

Like tumor suppressor genes, DNA repair genes also exist in pairs in homologous chromosomes, and both must become nonfunctional before the repair functions regulated by the genes are compromised. Persons with an inherited mutation of a DNA repair gene are at increased risk of some tumors because if a spontaneous mutation of the other gene occurs, the affected cell is no longer able to regulate cell growth properly. Uncontrolled cell proliferation results and gives rise to a tumor.

Genes Regulating Apoptosis

Another group of genes plays a more limited role in regulating cell functions by influencing the survival time of cells. Normal cells live for a variable period of time, depending on the cell type. Then the cell dies and is replaced by a new cell. The predetermined death of a cell is regulated by genes within the cell and is called programmed cell death or **apoptosis**. If the genes regulating programmed cell death fail to function properly, the cells don't die as they should and continue to accumulate, eventually forming a tumor. Some lymphoid tumors, for example, appear to result primarily from an accumulation of long-surviving lymphocytes within lymph nodes rather than excessively rapid proliferation of lymphocytes.

Apoptosis
(ah-pop-toe'-sis, or ah-po-toe'-sis)
Programmed cell death that occurs after a cell has lived its normal life span.

Multistep Progression of Genetic Changes Leading to Cancer In most cases, cancers do not result from mutation of a single gene, but rather are the result of multiple genetic "insults" to the genome characterized by activation of oncogenes along with loss of function of one or more tumor suppressor genes. The transition, for example, from a benign polyp of the colon to an invasive colon cancer requires activation of an oncogene (called ras) and inactivation of three distinct tumor suppressor genes (designated *APC, DCC,* and *p53*).

After a cell has been deregulated and has formed a tumor, additional random genetic changes may take place in the tumor cells, which is indicative of the instability of the tumor cell genome. Often, individual genes may undergo additional mutations or they may reduplicate themselves by gene amplification, forming multiple copies of a single gene. Chromosomes may fragment; pieces of chromosomes may be lost from the cells or be translocated to other chromosomes. Some of these mutations in the unstable tumor cell genome may produce new mutant cells that exhibit more aggressive growth than the original tumor cells, and the new mutant may eventually outgrow the other cells in the tumor. Clinically, this event may be manifested by more rapid growth and aggressive behavior of the tumor, and often the tumor may become less responsive to the anticancer drugs that formerly could control it.

Chromosomal Abnormalities Not all gene alterations that activate oncogenes or inactivate tumor suppressor genes can be identified from examination of the tumor cell chromosomes. Point mutations do not change chromosome structure, but translocations relocate large pieces of chromosomes and change their structure, as do deletions of chromosome material and amplification of individual genes. Some chromosomal abnormalities occur quite frequently in specific tumors and may be of diagnostic value. Others may give some indication of how aggressively a tumor may behave. The best-known neoplasm-associated chromosomal abnormality, which is called Philadelphia or Ph1 chromosome (named after the city where it was discovered), can be demonstrated in the white cells of patients with chronic granulocytic leukemia (described in the section on leukemia). The abnormality is a reciprocal translocation of broken end pieces between chromosomes 9 and 22. In this translocation, a proto-oncogene (designed *abl*) on chromosome 9 is moved to a position on chromosome 22. There it becomes fused with another gene (called *bcr*) to form

Tyrosine kinase
*Enzyme that produces
multiple effects concerned
with cell growth and cell
division.*

a composite gene (*bcr/abl*) that directs the synthesis of an uncontrolled extremely active **tyrosine kinase** enzyme that produces multiple effects concerned with cell growth and cell division. It is the excessive unregulated activity of this enzyme that stimulates the unrestrained proliferation of white blood cells characteristic of chronic granulocytic leukemia (FIGURE 10-20). The same type of translocation also occurs in some patients with acute lymphocytic leukemia, but the composite gene *bcr/abl* resulting from the translocation is slightly different, which leads to a different and more aggressive type of lymphoma.

FAILURE OF IMMUNOLOGIC DEFENSES

The basic processes common to all neoplasms are gene mutations within a cell that deregulate the cell, causing it to proliferate abnormally. Many environmental factors can induce mutations. A mutant cell often produces different cell proteins not present in a normal cell. These mutant-gene–encoded proteins are recognized as abnormal by the immune system, which attempts to destroy the abnormal cell by means of various cell-mediated and humoral mechanisms. Apparently, mutations leading to neoplastic transformation of cells are relatively common, but the body recognizes the altered cells as abnormal and destroys them as soon as they are formed. Only a tiny percentage of abnormal cells ever develop into clinically apparent tumors. Therefore, one may consider a tumor to manifest in part a failure of the body's immune defenses. This concept is supported by evidence that individuals with congenital deficiencies of immunologic defense mechanisms have a higher than expected incidence of tumors. Tumors also occur frequently in persons whose immune responses have been deliberately suppressed by drugs or other substances.

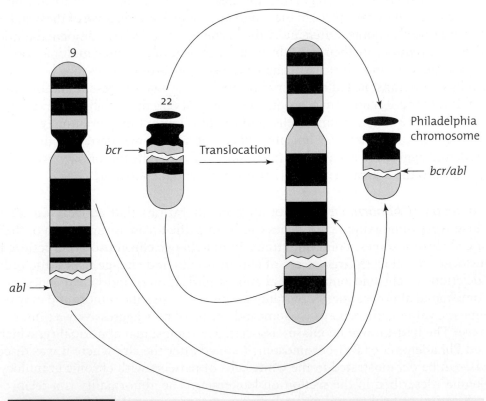

FIGURE 10-20 Reciprocal translocation between broken pieces of chromosomes 9 and 22, forming the Philadelphia chromosome containing the composite gene that disrupts normal cell functions.

FIGURE 10-21 illustrates the interrelation of the factors concerned with the defense against tumors. On one hand, abnormal cells arise and tend to proliferate, leading to tumors. On the other hand, the immune–defense mechanisms destroy these abnormal cells before they can prove hazardous to the body. Tumors result when the defense mechanisms fail. Fortunately, in most instances, the immune surveillance system eliminates the "bad" cells as soon as they appear. Although the immune-defense mechanisms are quite efficient in eliminating abnormal cells before they develop into a tumor, they are much less effective in eliminating an established tumor.

HEREDITY AND TUMORS

Although there is no strong hereditary predisposition to most common malignant tumors, hereditary factors do play a small role in some common tumors. A person whose parent or sibling has been afflicted with a breast, colon, or lung carcinoma has about a three times greater risk of developing a similar tumor than do other people. The predisposition is apparently the result of a multifactorial inheritance pattern in which the individual at risk has inherited sets of genes that influence some hormonal- or enzyme-regulated biochemical process within the body that slightly increases the susceptibility to a specific cancer. The increased risk may be caused by genetic

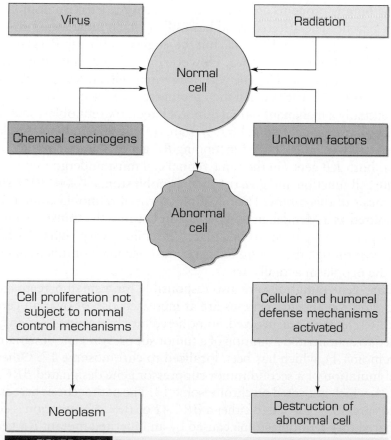

FIGURE 10-21 Factors leading to neoplastic transformation of cells counterbalanced by immunologic defense against neoplasm. Conversion of a normal cell into an abnormal one requires activation of oncogenes and inactivation of tumor suppressor genes, which renders the cell unresponsive to normal control mechanisms that regulate cell growth. Generally, multiple step-by-step mutations are required to transform a normal cell into a cancer cell.

differences in various biochemical or physiologic activities that influence cell functions, such as

1. Differences in circulating hormone levels that could influence cell growth rates
2. Variations in the rate at which the cell can metabolize and inactivate cancer-causing chemicals to which the cells are exposed
3. Variations in the ability to repair DNA that has been damaged by injurious agents
4. Variations in the efficiency of the immune system in eliminating abnormal cells as they arise

Heredity does play an important role in some tumors. The classic example is retinoblastoma, an uncommon childhood tumor illustrated in Figure 10-16. This tumor is also a typical example of how tumor suppressor genes control cell function and how loss of control can cause a tumor. Retinoblastoma is a malignant tumor of primitive retinal cells occurring in infants and children that is caused by loss of function of tumor suppressor genes called *RB* genes. Normal *RB* genes exist in pairs, one on each of the homologous pair of chromosome 13, and both *RB* genes must be nonfunctional in a retinal cell before a tumor arises. About half the retinoblastomas are hereditary; the rest occur sporadically, without any hereditary predisposition. The hereditary form of retinoblastoma is prone to occur if a child inherits a defective nonfunctional *RB* gene from a parent. The affected child has only a single functioning *RB* gene in all body cells, including those in the retina, but the single functioning *RB* gene is sufficient to maintain control of cell functions. However, if a chance mutation occurs in the remaining single functional *RB* gene within a retinal cell, all *RB* gene function in the affected cell is lost. The affected cell then proliferates to form a clone of unregulated cells and eventually a malignant retinal tumor. Hereditary retinoblastomas may occur in both eyes because retinal cells in both eyes are equally vulnerable to similar random *RB* gene mutations in other single functioning *RB* genes. In the sporadic form of retinoblastoma, both *RB* genes in the same retinal cell must undergo mutation in order to deregulate cell function and give rise to a retinoblastoma. FIGURE 10-22 summarizes the pathogenesis of this tumor. The hereditary form of retinoblastoma is considered to be transmitted as a Mendelian dominant trait because the transmission of a single defective *RB* gene from parent to child places the child at very high risk of developing this tumor, even though the second *RB* gene must become nonfunctional in a retinal cell before the neoplasm actually arises.

Hereditary gene mutations are also responsible for a small percentage of breast carcinomas, and the affected persons are at increased risk of ovarian carcinoma as well. Two different genes are involved. Some hereditary breast and ovarian carcinomas can be traced to an inherited mutation of a tumor suppressor gene designated *BRCA1* (breast carcinoma 1), which has been localized to chromosome 17. Other cases are related to a mutation of a second tumor suppressor gene designated *BRCA2* (breast carcinoma 2), which is located on chromosome 13. The pathogenesis hereditary breast and ovarian carcinoma related to either a *BRCA1* or *BRCA2* mutation is comparable to that of hereditary retinoblastoma caused by an inherited mutant *RB* gene as illustrated in FIGURE 10-22. *BRCA* mutations are considered to be inherited as dominant traits because the inheritance of a single *BRCA* mutant gene from either parent is responsible for the increased susceptibility to both breast and ovarian carcinomas.

A condition called multiple polyposis of the colon, also a dominant trait, is characterized by the formation of multiple polyps throughout the colon, and usually one or more of them eventually becomes malignant. Another condition transmitted as

Hereditary **Sporadic**

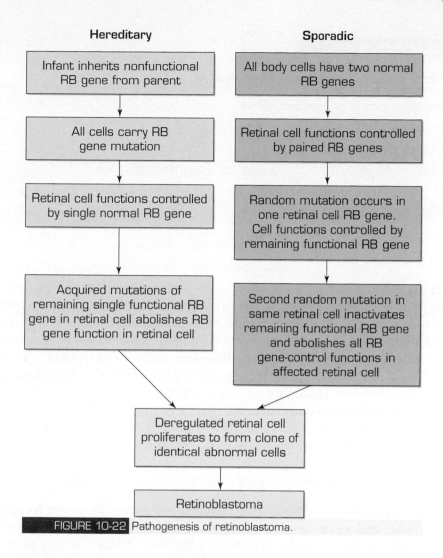

Hereditary	Sporadic
Infant inherits nonfunctional RB gene from parent	All body cells have two normal RB genes
All cells carry RB gene mutation	Retinal cell functions controlled by paired RB genes
Retinal cell functions controlled by single normal RB gene	Random mutation occurs in one retinal cell RB gene. Cell functions controlled by remaining functional RB gene
Acquired mutations of remaining single functional RB gene in retinal cell abolishes RB gene function in retinal cell	Second random mutation in same retinal cell inactivates remaining functional RB gene and abolishes all RB gene-control functions in affected retinal cell

Deregulated retinal cell proliferates to form clone of identical abnormal cells

Retinoblastoma

FIGURE 10-22 Pathogenesis of retinoblastoma.

an autosomal dominant trait is called multiple neurofibromatosis (discussion on the nervous system). Many of the nerves throughout the body give rise to benign tumors called neurofibromas, and often one of these tumors eventually undergoes malignant change. Still, another hereditary tumor syndrome, also an autosomal dominant transmission, is called multiple endocrine adenomatosis and is characterized by the formation of adenomas arising in several different endocrine glands, as the name indicates.

There are many other examples of tumors related to hereditary gene mutations, but it is important to remember that they make up only a small fraction of the benign and malignant tumors afflicting humans.

Diagnosis of Tumors

EARLY RECOGNITION OF NEOPLASMS

The American Cancer Society publicizes a number of signs and symptoms that should arouse suspicion of cancer (TABLE 10-5). In general, any abnormality of form or function may be an early symptom of a neoplasm and should be investigated by a physician. For example, a lump in the breast, an ulcer on the lip, or a change in the character of a wart or mole may be considered an abnormality of form. Menstrual bleeding in a postmenopausal woman or a change in bowel habits manifested by constipation or diarrhea is an abnormality of function.

TABLE 10-5

American Cancer Society warning signals

1. Change in bowel or bladder habits
2. A sore that does not heal
3. Unusual bleeding or discharge
4. A thickening or lump in the breast or elsewhere
5. Indigestion or difficulty in swallowing
6. An obvious change in wart or mole
7. A nagging cough or hoarseness

A complete medical history and physical examination by the physician are the next steps in evaluating suspected abnormalities. The physical examination may include special studies such as an examination of the rectum and colon by means of a special instrument, a vaginal examination and Pap smear in women, examination of the esophagus and stomach with special devices, and various types of x-ray studies.

If a tumor is discovered, exact diagnosis requires biopsy or complete excision of the suspected tumor. Histologic examination of the tissue by the pathologist will provide an exact diagnosis and serve as a guide to further treatment. If the tumor is benign, simple excision is curative. If the tumor is malignant, a more extensive operation or another kind of treatment may be required.

CYTOLOGIC DIAGNOSIS OF NEOPLASMS

Tumors shed abnormal cells from their surfaces, and these cells can be recognized in the body fluids and secretions that come into contact with the tumor (FIGURE 10-23). Often the abnormal cells can be recognized when the neoplasm is only microscopic in size and is still confined to the surface epithelium. These observations have been applied to the cytologic diagnosis of tumors. The method is named after the physician who played a large part in developing and applying cytologic methods, Dr. George Papanicolaou. The microscopic slides of the material prepared for cytologic examination are called Papanicolaou smears or, simply, **Pap smears**.

In carcinoma of the uterine cervix, abnormal cells can often be found in the vaginal secretions. They are more readily identified, however, in smears prepared from material that has been gently scraped from the epithelium of the cervix surrounding the cervical opening (external os) by means of a small, disposable wooden spatula. Usually, secretions for study are also obtained from the cervical canal at the same time. Widespread application of cytologic methods has led to much earlier detection of cervical carcinoma than had previously been possible and has played a significant role in reducing mortality from carcinoma of the uterine cervix. Cytologic methods can also be applied to the diagnosis of neoplasms in other locations by examining

Pap smear
A study of cells from various sources, commonly used as a screening test for cancer.

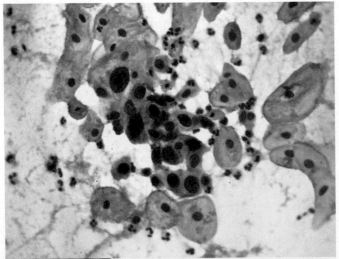

FIGURE 10-23 Photomicrograph of Pap smear, illustrating cluster of abnormal cells from in situ carcinoma of cervix. Cells appear much different from adjacent normal squamous epithelial cells (original magnification × 160).

sputum, urine, breast secretions, and fluids obtained from the pleural or peritoneal cavities. However, cytology has been most valuable in the early diagnosis of cervical cancer. It should be emphasized, however, that an abnormal cervical Pap smear indicates only that the cervical epithelium is shedding atypical or abnormal cells. It does not necessarily indicate a diagnosis of cancer because some benign diseases are occasionally associated with desquamation of atypical cells. A Pap smear should be considered as a screening procedure, and an atypical or abnormal smear should be followed by further studies, which may include a biopsy and histologic examination of the tissue to establish an exact diagnosis. This subject is considered further in the discussion on the female reproductive system.

Cytologic Diagnosis by Fine-Needle Aspiration

Cells for cytologic study can also be obtained by aspirating material from organs or tissues by means of a fine needle attached to a syringe and preparing slides from the aspirated material. This technique is often used to evaluate nodules in the thyroid or breast, and often one can determine whether the nodule is benign or malignant from the appearance of the aspirated cells, avoiding the need for a biopsy. Suspected tumors in the lung, liver, pancreas, kidney, and other internal organs also can be examined by fine-needle aspiration. When attempting aspiration from internal organs, one must precisely determine the location of the suspected tumor by means of a CT scan or other x-ray examination or by ultrasound and insert the needle into the suspected tumor under x-ray guidance. In general, the diagnostic accuracy of fine-needle aspiration is not as good as an actual biopsy but often is adequate for diagnosis and avoids a major surgical operation, which would be required to obtain tissue for biopsy.

FROZEN-SECTION DIAGNOSIS OF NEOPLASMS

Many times, it is important that a surgeon learn immediately whether a tumor discovered in the course of an operation is benign or malignant because the extent of resection performed may depend on the nature of the neoplasm. Often, the surgeon must also find out during the operation whether a tumor has been excised completely or whether it has spread to lymph nodes or distant sites. A pathologist can provide the surgeon with a rapid histologic diagnosis and other information by means of a special technique called a **frozen section**. In this method, a portion of the tumor or other tissue to be examined histologically is frozen solid at a subzero temperature. A thin section of the frozen tissue is cut by means of a special instrument called a microtome, and slides are prepared and stained. The slides can then be examined by the pathologist, and a rapid histologic diagnosis can be made. The entire procedure takes only a few minutes.

TUMOR-ASSOCIATED ANTIGEN TESTS

Some cancers secrete substances called **tumor-associated antigens**. These are either absent from normal mature tissues or present only in trace amounts. Most tumor-associated antigens are carbohydrate–protein complexes (glycoproteins) that are secreted as a coating on the surface of the cancer cells. Some of the glycoprotein gains access to the circulation, where it can be detected by means of specialized laboratory tests performed on the blood of patients with cancer.

A well-known tumor-associated antigen is a substance called **carcinoembryonic antigen (CEA)**, so named because it resembles a glycoprotein antigen secreted by the cells lining the fetal intestinal tract. It has been postulated that cancer cells elaborate CEA because they are immature and have acquired some properties of fetal cells that adult cells do not have (FIGURE 10-24).

Frozen section
A method of rapid diagnosis of tumors used by the pathologist; tissue is frozen solid, cut into thin sections, stained, and examined microscopically.

Tumor-associated antigen
An antigen associated with growing tumor cells, which serves as an indicator of tumor growth in the body.

Carcinoembryonic antigen (CEA)
(kär'sin-ō-em-bry-on'ik)
A tumor-associated antigen that resembles the antigen secreted by the cells of the fetal gastrointestinal tract.

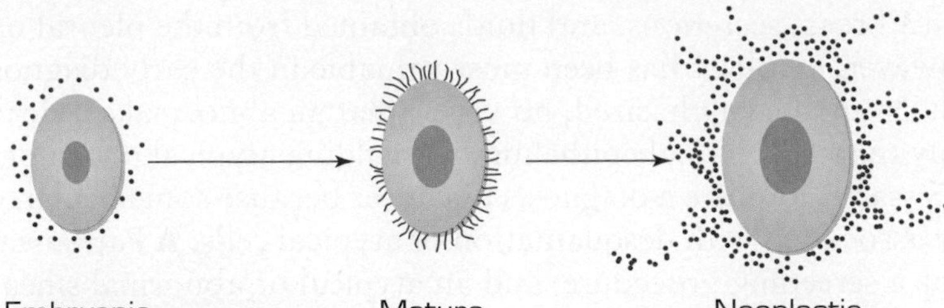

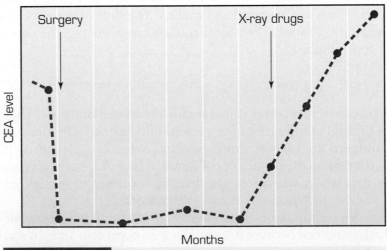

Embryonic   Mature   Neoplastic

FIGURE 10-24 Relation of carcinoembryonic antigen (CEA) to embryonic cells. Embryonic cell (*left*) produces a specific type of carbohydrate–protein coating in its surface. Coating is replaced by a different type in a mature cell (*center*). Neoplastic cell (*right*) reverts to a more primitive state and resumes production of embryonic coating material, which enters circulation and often can be detected in blood of patient with invasive carcinoma.

Not all malignant tumors secrete CEA. Moreover, elevation of CEA levels is not specific for any one type of cancer. CEA is produced by most malignant tumors of the gastrointestinal tract and pancreas, but it is also secreted by many cancers of the breast and lung and by other cancers as well. The amount of CEA secreted is related to the size of the tumor. CEA is usually not elevated in the blood of persons with small, early cancers, but the levels are often quite high in persons with large tumors or tumors that have metastasized. When CEA is elevated in a patient with cancer, the level falls after the tumor has been removed and often rises again if the tumor recurs or metastasizes (FIGURE 10-25). One can perform serial determinations of CEA to monitor the course of patients with CEA-secreting tumors. If CEA falls after removal of the tumor and later becomes elevated, this usually means that the tumor has recurred and indicates that additional treatment is needed. Slight elevations of CEA are sometimes detected in patients with diseases other than cancer. This does not detract from the usefulness of the CEA test, however, because the CEA levels are usually much lower than in patients with malignant tumors.

Other products secreted by tumor cells that can be used to monitor tumor growth are discussed in the discussion on the male reproductive system. They include **alpha fetoprotein,** a protein produced by fetal tissues but not normally produced by adult cells, and **human chorionic gonadotropin,** the hormone normally produced by the

Alpha fetoprotein
(al′fuh fē′tō-prō′tēn)
Protein produced by fetal liver early in gestation. Sometimes produced by tumor cells. Level is elevated in amnionic fluid when fetus has neural tube defect.

Human chorionic gonadotropin (HGC)
(kōr-ō-on′ik gō-na-dō-trō′pin)
A hormone made by the placenta in pregnancy having actions similar to pituitary gonadotropins. Same hormone is made by neoplastic cells in some types of malignant testicular tumors.

FIGURE 10-25 The use of CEA to monitor response to therapy. An elevated CEA level falls after resection of colon cancer and then rises when tumor recurs, indicating the need for additional treatment.

placenta in pregnancy, which are often elevated in patients with testicular carcinoma. Alpha fetoprotein is also frequently elevated in patients with primary carcinoma of the liver. Prostatic-specific antigen (PSA), produced by prostatic epithelial cells, often is elevated in the bloodstream of men with prostatic carcinoma. The PSA test often is used as a screening test to detect early prostate carcinoma before symptoms develop and also to monitor the response to treatment. Many other tumor-associated substances have been described (sometimes called tumor markers), which are used to monitor patients with various types of lung, breast, and ovarian carcinoma.

Treatment of Tumors

Benign tumors are completely cured by surgical excision. Malignant tumors are much more difficult to treat. Four major forms of treatment are directed against malignant tumors:

1. Surgery
2. Radiotherapy
3. Hormones
4. Anticancer drugs (chemotherapy)

The method of treatment depends on the type of tumor and its extent, and sometimes several methods are combined. In many cases, treatment eradicates the cancer, and the patient is cured. In less favorable cases, cure is no longer possible, but the growth of the cancer is arrested and life is prolonged. Before a course of treatment is selected, usually further information is needed, which is obtained by grading and staging the tumor, as described in the following section.

GRADING AND STAGING MALIGNANT TUMORS

After a biopsy has established the diagnosis of a malignant tumor, the selection of the appropriate treatment is based on the characteristics of the tumor cells and the extent of the tumor. Grading the tumor is attempting to predict the behavior of the tumor from the biopsy material based on the differentiation of the tumor cells, their growth rate based on the number of mitoses, and any characteristics of the tumor cells that would influence the type of treatment selected, such as the response of the tumor cells to estrogen in the case of a breast carcinoma (as described in the discussion on the breast). Staging the tumor is determining whether the tumor is still localized or has spread to regional lymph nodes or distant sites, which is very useful additional information to guide selection of the best treatment. For example, a small well-differentiated breast carcinoma that responds to estrogen and has not spread to the regional lymph nodes would be treated differently from a large, poorly differentiated carcinoma that does not respond to estrogen and has already spread to distant sites. Often, the various characteristics of a tumor identified by grading and staging are expressed in a classification called the TNM system. The *T* refers to the characteristics of the tumor, which is graded in terms of tumor size and differentiation as T1 through T4, with T0 used to indicate a noninvasive (in situ) carcinoma. *N* refers to the spread of tumor to regional lymph nodes, with N0 indicating no spread, and N1 through N3 indicating progressively greater lymph node spread. *M* refers to distant metastasis, with M0 indicating no distant spread and M1 and M2 indicating progressively more extensive distant metastases.

Grading and staging are useful not only for selecting treatment, but also as an indication of prognosis as well as being useful in clinical research studies. For example, if a study were evaluating the effectiveness of a new anticancer chemotherapy treatment in one group of patients compared with the response to the current treatment method in another group, both groups of patients should have the same TNM classification to ensure that any difference in response to treatment was based on the treatment and not on differences in the stage of disease between the two patient groups.

SURGERY

Many malignant tumors are treated by wide surgical excision of the tumor and the surrounding tissues, usually with removal of the regional lymph nodes that drain the tumor site. This treatment is successful if the tumor has not already spread to distant sites. Unfortunately, many cancers have already metastasized when first detected and may no longer be curable by surgery alone. Other methods of treatment must be used—frequently in combination with surgery.

RADIOTHERAPY

Malignant lymphomas and some epithelial tumors are quite radiosensitive and can be destroyed by radiotherapy rather than by surgical excision. In some cases, antibodies can be used to deliver radiotherapy to the tumor cells. Antibodies can be prepared in animals then can attach to specific cells, such as B lymphocytes, and can be labeled with radioactive iodine and administered to patients with B cell lymphomas that have spread throughout the body. The isotope-labeled antibody can seek out the B cells, attach to them, and destroy them wherever they are located. In other cases, radiation and surgery are combined. For example, radiation may be administered preoperatively to reduce the size of a tumor, thereby facilitating its surgical resection; in other instances, radiotherapy is given after a malignant tumor has been resected (cut out) in order to destroy any cancer cells that may have been left behind. Radiotherapy is also used to control the growth of widespread tumors and to treat deposits of metastatic tumor that cause pain and disability. The treatment relieves symptoms and makes the patient more comfortable, even though the cancer is not curable.

HORMONE THERAPY

Some malignant tumors require hormones for their growth and are called hormone responsive. They regress temporarily if deprived of the required hormone. For example, many prostate tumors require testosterone and are inhibited by removal of the testes (eliminating the source of testosterone) or by administration of estrogens (which suppresses testosterone secretion). Many breast carcinomas in postmenopausal women are estrogen responsive and can be controlled by drugs that block estrogen so that the tumor cells are no longer stimulated by estrogen.

Adrenal cortical hormones (corticosteroids) also inhibit the growth of many malignant tumors. Corticosteroids inhibit protein synthesis, thereby suppressing the growth and division of the tumor cells. Tumors of the lymphatic tissues are especially susceptible to the effects of corticosteroids.

ANTICANCER DRUGS

Cancer cells, like normal cells, synthesize deoxyribonucleic acid (DNA) from various precursors. The DNA directs the production of the various forms of ribonucleic acid (messenger RNA, transfer RNA, and ribosomal RNA), and the RNA in turn takes part in the synthesis of enzymes and other proteins that are necessary for cell function. Anticancer drugs impede the growth and division of cells by disrupting some phase of this complex process.

The various drugs differ in their mechanisms of action. Some inhibit the synthesis of either DNA or RNA. Others alter the structure of DNA or disturb its function. Still, others inhibit protein synthesis or prevent the mitotic spindle from forming, and thus, the cell cannot divide. Frequently, several different anticancer drugs are administered simultaneously, each drug blocking a different phase in the cell's metabolic processes. Another group of anticancer drugs act by suppressing the proliferation of the blood vessels that nourish the tumor, thereby inhibiting tumor growth by interfering with its blood supply.

Most anticancer drugs work best against fast-growing tumors that contain large numbers of actively growing and dividing cells. They are usually less effective against slowly growing tumors because only relatively small numbers of the tumor cells are in the stages of cell growth or division that are susceptible to the injurious effects of the drugs.

One important group of anticancer drugs is called **alkylating agents**. These drugs interact with both strands of the paired DNA chains in the nucleus and bind them together so that they cannot separate. This reaction is called cross-linking of the DNA chains. It disrupts the function of DNA because the chains must separate for duplication of the DNA chains and for synthesis of RNA. Alkylating agents also disturb cell function by altering the structure of the DNA chains. In contrast to most anticancer drugs, these agents are effective against nondividing ("resting") cells as well as actively growing cells.

Another large group of anticancer drugs is called **antimetabolites**. They resemble essential compounds required for cell growth and multiplication, but they cannot be used by the cell. Therefore, they disrupt the cell's metabolic processes. (Some antimicrobial agents inhibit bacterial growth in this way, as described in the section on competitive inhibition in the discussion on pathogenic microorganisms.)

Most anticancer drugs are quite toxic. They injure normal cells as well as cancer cells and must be administered very carefully in order to assure maximum damage to tumor cells without irreparable injury to normal cells. Lymphoid tissue is quite susceptible to the destructive effects of these potent drugs, and consequently, one unavoidable side effect of anticancer drugs is impairment of cell-mediated and humoral immunity.

Recently, several less toxic and more cell-specific anticancer drugs have been developed that function by blocking the action of specific cell components that stimulate the tumor cells. Some of these drugs suppress tumor growth by blocking growth factor receptors on the surface of the tumor cells so that growth factors produced by normal cells cannot attach to the receptors and stimulate the tumor cells. Other drugs inhibit the functions of important intracellular proteins, such as the enzyme tyrosine kinase, that in various ways stimulate cell proliferation.

ADJUVANT CHEMOTHERAPY

Sometimes surgical resection of a cancer appears to be successful, but metastases appear several years later and eventually prove fatal. The operation fails to eradicate the tumor because small, unrecognized metastases have already spread throughout the body. Even though the main tumor has been removed, the minute metastases continue to grow until eventually they form many large, bulky deposits of metastatic tumor that kill the patient.

In order to forestall the development of late metastases, a current trend is to administer a course of anticancer drugs after surgical resection of some tumors. This is called **adjuvant chemotherapy** (*adjuvare* = to assist). The drugs destroy any small, undetected foci of metastatic tumor before they become large enough to produce clinical manifestations. In some cases, adjuvant chemotherapy combined with surgery appears to achieve better results than surgery alone. Many anticancer drugs are quite toxic, however, and the potential benefits of adjuvant chemotherapy must be weighed against the harmful effects of the drugs on normal tissues.

Alkylating agent
(al'kil-ā-ting)
An anticancer drug that disrupts cell function by binding DNA chains together so that they cannot separate.

Antimetabolite
(an-ti-met-ab'o-līte)
A substance that competes with or replaces another substance (metabolite) required for cell growth or multiplication.

Adjuvant chemotherapy
(ad'joo-vent)
Anticancer chemotherapy administered after surgical resection of a tumor in an attempt to destroy any small undetected foci of metastatic tumor before they become clinically detectable.

IMMUNOTHERAPY

The immune system has evolved a number of ways to deal with abnormal cells that can proliferate and form tumors and to deal with established tumors.

1. Cytotoxic T cells recognize antigens on tumor cells that are displayed along with the cells' own MHC Class I proteins and can damage the tumor cells by secreting destructive lymphokines.
2. Natural-killer lymphocytes can attack and destroy tumor cells without prior antigenic stimulation, and some killer lymphocytes specialize in attacking antibody-coated tumor cells.
3. Activated macrophages can destroy tumor cells by phagocytosis and by secreting tumor necrosis factor along with other cytokines that stimulate lymphocytes to attack tumor cells.
4. Antibodies formed against tumor cell antigens can affix to tumor cells and activate complement; products of complement activation attract lymphocytes and macrophages and form destructive attack complexes that damage the cell membranes of the tumor cells.

Despite the array of immunologic defenses, many tumors circumvent or overwhelm the body's immune defenses, and thus, they become ineffective and no longer retard the growth of the tumor. Some tumor cells produce little or no MHC Class I protein. Because cytotoxic T cells can recognize tumor cell antigens only if they are displayed along with MHC Class I proteins, the lymphocytes cannot attack the tumor cells because they cannot recognize the tumor antigens without the associated MHC Class I proteins. Some tumor cells thwart the immune system because the tumor cells release large amounts of soluble tumor-specific antigens that saturate the body to such an extent that the lymphocytes are no longer capable of responding to the tumor-specific antigens on the surface of the tumor cells. In addition, the chemotherapy and irradiation used to treat tumors also suppress the body's immune responses. When the patient's immune capacity is impaired for any reason, attempts have been made to stimulate the body's immune system so that it can deal more effectively with the tumor in order to improve the patient's prognosis. Treatment of tumors by stimulating the body's immune defenses is called **immunotherapy**. Nonspecific immunotherapy is directed toward bolstering the patient's own immune defenses so that the patient can deal more effectively with the tumor. Specific immunotherapy directs the immune system against the specific antigens present in the patient's own tumor.

Immunotherapy
(im'mū-nō-ther'uh-pē)
Treatment given to retard growth of a disseminated malignant tumor by stimulating to body's own immune defenses.

Nonspecific Immunotherapy

Initially, attempts were made to stimulate the immune system nonspecifically by immunizing the patient with vaccines prepared from various types of bacteria or bacterial products, but this approach had very limited success and was associated with serious complications.

More recent approaches have consisted of the administration of various cytokines that either stimulate cells of the immune system or act against the tumor cells. The two cytokines that have been used with greatest success against tumors are **interferon** and **interleukin-2**.

Interferon
(in-tur-fēr'on)
A broad-spectrum antiviral agent manufactured by various cells in the body.

Interleukin-2
(inter-lōō'kin)
A lymphokine that stimulates growth of lymphocytes.

Interferon   Interferon is the name given to a group of carbohydrate-containing, "broad-spectrum" antiviral protein substances produced by cells in response to viral infection (discussion on pathogenic microorganisms), but interferon has other functions. It regulates the functions of the immune system and regulates cell growth, inhibiting the growth of rapidly dividing cells. These latter properties have led to the use of interferon for treating tumors as well as viral infections. After methods for producing interferon commercially were developed, large quantities of interferon became available for clinical use, and studies were undertaken in patients with various tumors in order to evaluate the usefulness of this material. To date, the best results have been obtained in patients with a relatively rare type of leukemia called "hairy cell" leukemia (so named because of the hairlike processes projecting from the cytoplasm of the tumor cell). Interferon has also produced responses in some patients with other types of leukemia, multiple myeloma (described later in this chapter), some lymphomas, and some widely disseminated carcinomas that had not responded to other methods of treatment. Interferon has the advantage of being much less toxic than many anticancer drugs, and treatment by intramuscular injection several times per week is usually well tolerated.

Interleukin-2   Interleukin-2 is a lymphokine produced by T cells. It stimulates natural-killer cells and cytotoxic T cells that can destroy tumor cells, but it has no direct effects against the tumor cells. Interleukin-2 is administered in multiple courses and has produced beneficial effects in the treatment of metastatic melanoma and renal cell carcinoma. High doses of interleukin-2 produce a variety of toxic effects that limit its use to some extent.

Interleukin-2 has also been administered along with lymphocytes obtained from the patient, an approach called cell transfer immunotherapy. One method is to collect blood from the patient and incubate the blood with interleukin-2 in the laboratory, which stimulates the lymphocytes to proliferate and generates a large population of natural-killer lymphocytes. Then the lymphocytes (which are called lymphokine-activated killer cells) are infused into the patient to seek out and destroy the tumor.

Other Cytokines   Various other cytokines have been produced by genetic engineering and are undergoing clinical evaluation. They include tumor necrosis factor and a cytokine produced by macrophages called interleukin-1, which has antitumor activity.

Specific Immunotherapy

Specific immunotherapy targets the patient's own tumor cells for attack. Three different approaches appear promising: (1) administration of cytotoxic T lymphocytes directed against the tumor, which are called tumor-infiltrating lymphocytes; (2) administration of tumor vaccines; and (3) administration of antitumor antibodies.

Tumor-Infiltrating Lymphocyte Therapy   This is a specific type of cell transfer immunotherapy in which the lymphocytes infused back into the patient are obtained from the patient's own tumor. These lymphocytes are actually infiltrating the tumor and are trying to destroy it, and they are obtained when the tumor is biopsied or excised. The tumor-infiltrating lymphocytes contain a large concentration of cytotoxic T lymphocytes specifically targeted against the antigens in the patient's own tumor, as well as numbers of natural-killer lymphocytes that also can destroy tumor cells. The lymphocytes from the tumor are grown in the laboratory with interleukin-2 to stimulate growth of the lymphocytes and then infused back into the patient to attack and destroy the tumor. This approach has been used with some success to treat metastatic malignant melanoma.

Tumor Vaccines   Tumor vaccines prepared from the patient's own tumor also have been used to immunize the patient against the tumor in an effort to reduce the likelihood that the tumor will recur or metastasize after it has been resected. Tumor cells are obtained from the resected tumor, grown in the laboratory, and then killed so that they cannot proliferate in the patient but can still generate an immune response. They are then used to prepare a vaccine that will stimulate an immune response to the resected tumor. Tumor vaccines have been used as an additional treatment after resection of a malignant melanoma or a colon carcinoma when the patient is considered at high risk of recurrence.

Tumor Antibody Therapy   In this approach, antibodies are prepared against tumor cell antigens, and then the antibodies are linked to some antitumor drug or toxin that can kill tumor cells. The antibodies with attached drug or toxin are then infused back into the patient to seek out and destroy the tumor cells without damaging normal cells.

Results of Immunotherapy

Results of immunotherapy have been mixed. There have been some notable successes, as in the use of interferon therapy for one type of leukemia called hairy cell leukemia. Some types of immunotherapy have produced gratifying results in persons with specific types of widespread tumors when no other methods of treatment were available to control the tumor. No single method works against all types of tumors, and ongoing clinical trials continue to assess the applications and limitations of these various methods. Unfortunately, most patients treated with immunotherapy have advanced diseases, and often the body's immune defenses are incapable of dealing with such large amounts of tumor even when stimulated by immunotherapy.

Leukemia

Leukemia
(lōō-kē′mē-yuh)
*A neoplastic proliferation
of leukocytes.*

The term **leukemia** refers to a neoplasm of hematopoietic tissue. In contrast to solid tumors, which form nodular deposits, leukemic cells diffusely infiltrate the bone marrow and lymphoid tissues, spill over into the bloodstream, and infiltrate throughout the various organs of the body. The leukemic cells may be mostly mature, or they may be extremely primitive. The overproduction of white cells in leukemia may be revealed in the peripheral blood by a very high white blood count. In some cases of leukemia, however, the proliferation of the white cells is largely confined to the bone marrow, and there is no significant increase in the number of white cells in the bloodstream.

CLASSIFICATION OF LEUKEMIA

Leukemia is classified on the basis of both the cell type and the maturity of the proliferating cells. Any type of hematopoietic cells can give rise to leukemia, but the most common types are granulocytic, monocytic, and lymphocytic. Leukemia developing from stem cells that would normally give rise to the leukocytes containing specific granules (neutrophils, eosinophils, and basophils) is called granulocytic leukemia. Monocytic leukemia develops from precursor cells that give rise to monocytes. Lymphocytic leukemia is derived from lymphoid precursor cells. Various subclassifications have been established within these major groups on the basis of the characteristics of the cell membranes and the enzymes present within the leukemic cells, as determined by highly specialized techniques.

If the leukemia cells are mostly primitive forms, the leukemia is classified as acute leukemia (FIGURE 10-26), and if the cells are mostly mature, the leukemia is classified as chronic leukemia. In chronic granulolcytic leukemia, most of the circulating cells are maturing granulocytes and neutrophils, and there are few primitive cells (FIGURE 10-27). In chronic lymphocytic leukemia, the circulating cells are mostly mature lymphocytes (FIGURE 10-28). Another type of leukemia also arises from lymphoid cells and has some unusual features. Cytoplasmic processes projecting from the cells give the cells a distinctive appearance, which is responsible for the descriptive term hairy cell leukemia, which is applied to this condition (FIGURE 10-29).

In most instances, the total number of white blood cells in the peripheral blood is significantly above normal. Occasionally, however, the marrow may be crowded

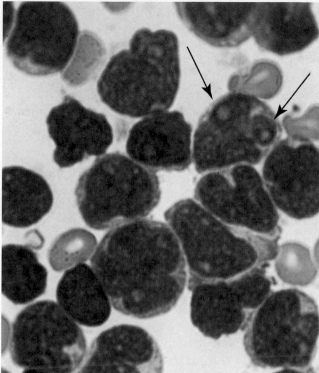

FIGURE 10-26 A photomicrograph of a blood smear from a patient with acute leukemia. The nuclei of the white cells have fine chromatin structure and prominent nucleoli indicating immaturity (*arrows*). Nuclei are irregular in size and configuration (original magnification × 1,000).

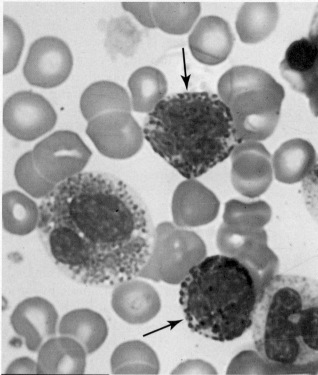

FIGURE 10-27 Chronic granulocytic leukemia. Most of the cells in the photomicrograph are mature. Note the basophils (*arrows*), the eosinophil (left of *arrows*), and the two neutrophils (right of *arrows*) (original magnification × 1,000).

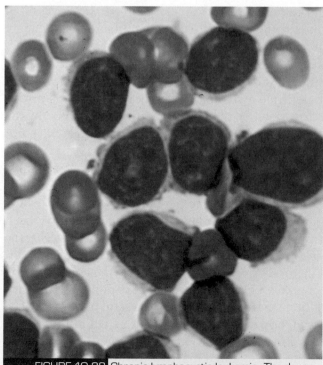

FIGURE 10-28 Chronic lymphocyctic leukemia. The dense nuclear chromatin structure indicates that the lymphocytes are mature (compare with Figure 10-26). The total white count is elevated (original magnification × 1,000).

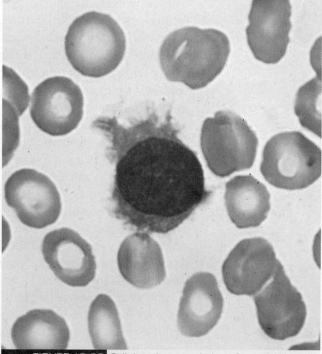

FIGURE 10-29 Cellular characteristics of neoplastic cell in "hairy cell" leukemia. Uniform nuclear chromatin and scanty cytoplasm with multiple cytoplasmic process (original magnification × 1,000).

with abnormal cells, but the number of white blood cells in the blood is normal or decreased. This variety of leukemia is sometimes called aleukemic leukemia. The term is merely descriptive and does not denote a type of leukemia with any special clinical features or any difference in prognosis.

Generally, the classifications by cell type and maturity are used together. Thus, one may speak of chronic granulocytic leukemia, acute lymphocytic leukemia, or acute monocytic leukemia. The term aleukemic is sometimes added if the number of white cells in the circulating blood is reduced.

CLINICAL FEATURES AND PRINCIPLES OF TREATMENT

The clinical features of leukemia are of two kinds: those caused by impairment of bone marrow function and those caused by infiltration of the viscera by leukemic cells. The overgrowth of leukemic cells in the bone marrow often crowds out normal bone marrow cells. This leads to anemia as a result of inadequate red cell production, bleeding caused by thrombocytopenia, and infection resulting from inadequate numbers of normal white blood cells, which are an important part of the body's defenses against pathogenic organisms.

The leukemic cells not only infiltrate the bone marrow, but also spread into the spleen, liver, lymph nodes, and other tissues. In chronic leukemia, the evolution of the disease proceeds at a relatively slow pace and often can be well controlled by treatment for long periods of time. Therefore, the patient with chronic leukemia may survive for many years in relatively good health. In contrast, acute leukemia is often a rapidly progressive disease. Symptoms of bone marrow infiltration and visceral infiltration make their appearance early and are quite conspicuous. In some patients with acute leukemia, the abnormal proliferation of the leukemic cells can be stopped for a variable period of time by various anticancer drugs, and the patient appears to have completely recovered. An arrest of the disease induced by therapy is called a remission. In many cases, however, the patient undergoes a relapse, and the disease ultimately proves fatal. Acute leukemia in children responds better to anticancer chemotherapy than acute leukemia in adults, and some children have been completely cured by intensive therapy.

Some patients with acute leukemia can be treated successfully by a bone marrow transplant from a compatible donor. Marrow transplantation has also been used successfully to treat patients with multiple myeloma, widespread lymphoma affecting the bone marrow, Hodgkin's disease when the bone marrow is infiltrated by the neoplasm, and other neoplastic diseases affecting the bone marrow that have not responded to treatment.

Before performing a marrow transplant, the patient's own bone marrow cells must be destroyed by anticancer (cytotoxic) drugs and radiation treatment. Then the bone marrow cells to be transplanted are injected into the patient's bloodstream where they become established in the patient's bone marrow whose own cells have been destroyed in order to receive the transplanted bone marrow. Within a few weeks, the donor's blood cells (stem cells) in their new location begin to produce mature red cells, white cells, and platelets. Several methods can be used to increase the concentration of stem cells in the donor's bone marrow before the transplant is performed, which assures that there will be sufficient bone marrow cells for a successful transplant. The marrow transplant is a foreign tissue, however, and the patient's own immunologic defenses must be suppressed (discussion on immunity, hypersensitivity, allergy, and autoimmune diseases) in order for the transplanted marrow to survive.

The transplant patient also faces another problem related to immunologic differences between the cells of the donor and those of the patient, which is called a graft-versus-host reaction. The donor lymphocytes in the transplanted marrow recognize the patient's cells as antigenically different and attempt to destroy them, leading to various clinical manifestations, including skin rash, liver injury, and gastrointestinal symptoms. This is the reverse of the usual situation in which the patient tries to reject the transplant. Here, the transplant tries to reject the patient! A less intense cytotoxic drug and irradiation treatment used successfully to perform bone marrow transplants on persons with sickle cell anemia can also be used to treat selected patients with myeloma and other hematopoietic diseases. The treatment modification has reduced the frequency of graft-versus-host disease and also increased the long-term survival of treated patients.

Although marrow transplantation is an important advance, it is not always successful. Patients may develop life-threatening infections related to the immunosuppression required to maintain the transplant, and in some patients, the leukemia recurs, arising from the patient's surviving leukemic cells that were not destroyed by the prior chemotherapy and radiation.

Newer transplantation methods are being developed in which the patient's own marrow is used for transplantation, which is called an autologous bone marrow transplant (*auto* = self). One approach comprises collecting the patient's own marrow while the patient is in remission, treating the marrow to destroy any surviving leukemic cells, and storing the marrow in liquid nitrogen for later use should the patient develop recurrent leukemia. If this occurs, the patient's leukemic marrow is destroyed by anticancer drugs and radiation, and the stored leukemic-free marrow is reinfused into the patient as a transplant. Because the transplant is the patient's own marrow, immunosuppression is not required, and complications related to immunosuppression are avoided. Autologous bone marrow transplants have also been used to treat patients with acute leukemia when no compatible marrow transplant donor is available. In this situation, the leukemic patient's marrow is collected in the same way as marrow is from a donor. Then the patient is treated with chemotherapy and radiation to destroy the diseased marrow. Meanwhile, the patient's previously collected marrow is treated with specific antibodies that destroy the leukemic cells without affecting the normal marrow cells. Then the treated marrow is returned to the patient, and if all goes well, the leukemia-free marrow becomes reestablished and functions normally.

Not all leukemic patients are suitable candidates for bone marrow transplantations, and many patients require some type of chemotherapy. The types of chemotherapy drugs used and the treatment schedules are being evaluated and adjusted continually. As new drugs become available, their effectiveness and side effects are compared with drugs currently used, and treatment schedules may be readjusted as required in order to provide the maximum benefit to the patient. Patients with Philadelphia chromosome-positive chronic granulocytic leukemia and those with Philadelphia chromosome-positive lymphocytic leukemia can often be treated successfully with a drug that inhibits the hyperactive tyrosine kinase enzyme produced by the composite *bcr/abl* gene. Blocking the activity of this dysfunctional enzyme suppresses the proliferation of the leukemic cells.

PRECURSORS OF LEUKEMIA: THE MYELODYSPLASTIC SYNDROMES

For many years, it has been recognized that acute leukemia in older patients may not have an abrupt onset but is preceded by a period lasting from several months to several years in which the affected patients have only a moderate anemia, sometimes associated with reduced white cells (leukopenia) and low blood platelets (thrombocytopenia). Examination of the bone marrow of these patients reveals variable degrees of disturbed growth and maturation of red cells, white cell precursors, and megakaryocytes but not leukemia. This condition has been called preleukemia, although it was realized that not all patients with bone marrow maturation disturbances of this type develop leukemia, and one could not reliably predict which patients would eventually become leukemic. Recently, these conditions have been grouped together under the general term **myelodysplastic syndromes** (*myelo* = marrow + *dysplasia* = disturbed growth). Several different types have been described that differ somewhat in their clinical and hematologic manifestations. In general, the more severe the maturation disturbance in the bone marrow, the greater the likelihood that leukemia would eventually occur. Unfortunately, there is no specific treatment available for most patients with these conditions, although some patients with severe "preleukemic" changes in their bone marrow have been treated successfully by bone marrow transplantation.

Multiple Myeloma

Multiple myeloma is a neoplasm arising from plasma cells within the bone marrow (FIGURE 10-30). In many ways, it resembles leukemia, but the neoplastic plasma cell proliferation is generally confined to the bone marrow. Infiltration of the viscera by the abnormal plasma cells is unusual; outpouring of large numbers of plasma cells into the peripheral blood also is uncommon. The abnormal plasma cells either may infiltrate the bone marrow diffusely or may form discrete tumors that weaken the bone, leading to spontaneous fractures, pain, and disability (FIGURE 10-31).

Normal plasma cells produce antibody proteins (**immunoglobulins**), as described in the discussion on immunity, hypersensitivity, allergy, and autoimmune diseases. In myeloma, the neoplastic cells also often produce large amounts of protein. This greatly increases blood proteins and, correspondingly, blood viscosity. The protein produced by the myeloma cells is generally a single type of immunoglobulin, usually IgG. In some patients, the production of immunoglobulins also is abnormal, and an excess of light chains is produced. Any light chains that are not incorporated into

Myelodysplastic syndrome
(my′elo-dis-plas′tik)
A disturbance of bone marrow function that is characterized by anemia, leukopenia, and thrombocytopenia and that may be a precursor to leukemia in some patients.

Multiple myeloma
(my-el-ō′muh)
A malignant neoplasm of plasma cells.

Immunoglobulin
(im′mū-nō-glob′u-lin)
An antibody protein.

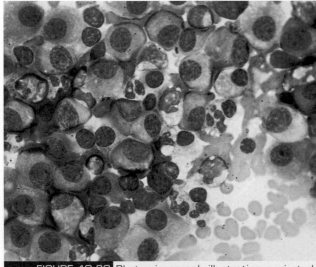

FIGURE 10-30 Photomicrograph illustrating aspirated bone marrow from a patient with multiple myeloma. Almost all cells are immature plasma cells containing large eccentric nuclei and abundant cytoplasm (original magnification × 400).

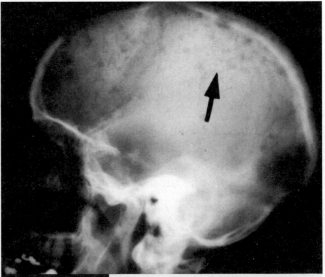

FIGURE 10-31 A skull x-ray from a patient with multiple myeloma. Multiple punched-out areas in skull bones (*arrow*) result from bone destruction caused by nodular masses of neoplastic plasma cells growing in bone marrow.

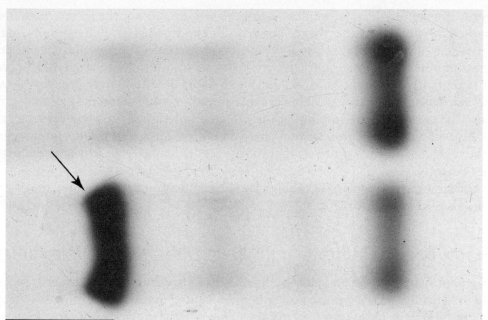

FIGURE 10-32 An examination of serum proteins by a special technique (*electrophoresis*) that separates serum proteins into various fractions. The upper pattern is from normal serum, with the dense albumin band at the *far right* in the photograph and the less intensely stained globulin bands to the left of the albumin band. The lower pattern is from a patient with multiple myeloma. The *arrow* indicates densely stained homogeneous globulin band representing large amounts of a single type of globulin protein produced by the abnormal plasma cells.

the immunoglobulin molecules are excreted in the urine. The myeloma protein can be identified in the blood (FIGURE 10-32), and the free light chains can be identified in the urine by special laboratory tests.

Masses of coagulated myeloma protein may accumulate within the patient's own tissues, and thus the function of the affected tissues is severely impaired. Some patients with myeloma die of kidney failure because masses of protein produced by the plasma cells infiltrate the kidneys and block the renal tubules.

A number of different drugs and treatment schedules are used to treat myeloma. Thalidomide and similar drugs derived from thalidomide have been quite effective, primarily by suppressing the proliferation of the blood vessels that support the growth of the myeloma cells. Radiotherapy may also be useful for treating localized areas of bone destruction caused by myeloma. In highly selected patients, a bone marrow transplant may improve the patient's survival but usually does not cure the patient.

PRECURSORS OF MULTIPLE MYELOMA

Increased Monoclonal Protein of Uncertain Significance

In many patients who eventually develop multiple myeloma, blood protein abnormalities can be demonstrated long before the characteristic features of the disease appear. The condition is an asymptomatic **premyeloma** phase of several years duration characterized by a relatively small number of plasma cells in the bone marrow and a single small but uniform (homogeneous) protein band identified by serum protein electrophoresis. There are no clinical manifestations of multiple myeloma. The condition may not be recognized unless routine blood chemistry tests reveal the protein abnormality, which is caused by a group (clone) of plasma cells derived from a single precursor plasma cell in which all the plasma cells in the group produce an

Premyeloma
An early stage of multiple myeloma in which plasma cell proliferation in the bone marrow is only slightly increased and only minor blood protein abnormalities are present.

identical protein, which is usually a gamma globulin. Often, the term *monoclonal gammopathy* is used to describe the abnormal homogeneous band. Eventually, many of these cases slowly evolve into more pronounced bone marrow plasma cell proliferation and finally into characteristic features of multiple myeloma. However, this precursor condition occurs in adults ages 65 or older and may progress slowly over many years. In many patients, the plasma cell proliferation may not progress to myelomas during the lifetime of the affected individual. In some respects, the monoclonal plasma cell proliferation phase preceding multiple myeloma is analogous to the myelodysplastic syndrome that may precede the development of leukemia in older persons.

Once the plasma cell proliferation has evolved into multiple myeloma, the disease responds poorly to treatment.

Survival Rates in Neoplastic Disease

Malignant neoplasms are a leading cause of disability and death. Cancer is second only to heart disease as a cause of death in the United States, accounting for almost 23% of all deaths in this country. Of the cancers affecting major organs, lung carcinoma is a common malignant tumor in men, and breast carcinoma is the most frequent in women. Carcinoma of the intestine is quite common in both sexes. The survival rate for patients with malignant tumors depends on whether the disease has been diagnosed and treated early, before it has spread. The chances for survival are significantly reduced if the tumor has metastasized to regional lymph nodes or to distant sites.

The curability of the various types of cancer can be assessed in terms of 5-year survival rates, which range from more than 95% for patients with thyroid cancer to a discouraging 5% for those with pancreatic carcinoma (TABLE 10-6). Attempts are being made continually to improve survival rates by means of earlier diagnosis and more effective therapy. Unfortunately, 5-year survival does not necessarily indicate

TABLE 10-6

Malignant neoplasms: 5-year survival rates

Type of neoplasm	5-Year survival (%) White	5-Year survival (%) Black	Type of neoplasm	5-Year survival (%) White	5-Year survival (%) Black
Thyroid	97	94	Kidney	65	66
Melanoma	93	75	Non-Hodgkin's lymphoma	64	54
Uterus, cervix	73	63	Ovary	45	39
Uterus, body	85	60	Multiple myeloma	33	32
Breast	90	77	Leukemia	49	47
Bladder	83	65	Stomach	22	23
Larynx	67	52	Lung	15	12
Prostate	100	98	Esophagus	16	11
Hodgkin's disease	87	81	Pancreas	5	5
Colon-rectum	65	55			

Cases diagnosed 1996–2002. Survival for all ages with survival for whites and blacks listed separately. Average survival for both sexes used when neoplasm occurs in both sexes.
Data from *CA: A Cancer Journal for Clinicians*. 2007. 57:43–66.

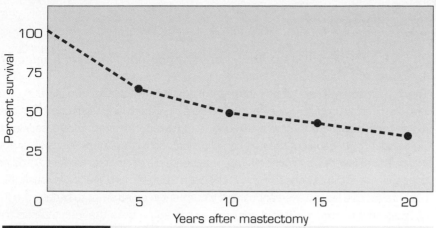

FIGURE 10-33 Continuing mortality from breast carcinoma after mastectomy as a result of late recurrences of carcinoma, as described in text (data from J. Berg and G. Robbins. *Surg Gynecol Obstet* June 1966).

that the patient is cured because some types of malignant tumors may recur and prove fatal many years after initial treatment. Breast carcinoma and malignant melanomas are two such tumors that are prone to late recurrence. For breast carcinoma, for example, the overall 5-year survival rate in one large group of patients followed for many years is approximately 65% (although more recent 5-year survival data indicated in Table 10-6 reveal higher survival rates). The 10-year rate in this group is only 50% because of late recurrences and metastases. Even after 10 years, a small proportion of patients eventually die of their original tumor (FIGURE 10-33). In such cases, the tumor had already spread by the time it was first recognized and treated, but the metastatic deposits were held in check by the body's immune defense mechanisms. The recurrence was caused by an eventual failure of the body's defenses, which allowed the tumor to become reactivated.

QUESTIONS FOR REVIEW

1. What are the major differences between a benign and a malignant tumor (see Table 10-1)?
2. How are tumors named? What are the common prefixes used in naming tumors? How would you name the following tumors: a benign tumor of fat, a malignant tumor of muscle, a malignant tumor of squamous epithelium, a benign tumor of glandular epithelium arising from the surface of the colon and projecting into the lumen, a malignant tumor of cartilage?
3. How does the body defend itself against abnormal cells that arise spontaneously in the course of cell division? What is the consequence of failure of these defense mechanisms (see Figure 10-21)?
4. What is a lymphoma? What is the difference between a nevus and a melanoma? What is a teratoma?
5. What is a Pap smear? How is it used in the early diagnosis of tumors? What is the significance of a Pap smear containing atypical cells?
6. What is a frozen section? How is it used in the diagnosis of tumors? How are neoplasms treated?
7. What is leukemia? What are its major clinical manifestations? How is leukemia classified? What is the difference between multiple myeloma and leukemia?

Armitage, J. O. 2010. Early-stage Hodgkin's lymphoma. *The New England Journal of Medicine* 363:653–62.

▶ The 5-year survival rate of patients with Hodgkin's lymphoma is over 90%. However, long-term follow-up of surviving patients reveals significant long-term complications, including second malignant tumors, leukemia, and radiation-related cardiovascular disease. Consequently, because of the late complications occurring many years after successful treatment of Hodgkin's lymphoma, more patients die of late treatment-related complications than from the disease for which they were treated many years previously. Now many patients receive less intense anticancer treatment in an attempt to reduce the frequency of treatment-related complications, but at the same time the less intense treatment must not reduce the successful results of chemotherapy and radiation treatment.

Artandi, S. E. 2006. Telomeres, telomerase, and human disease. *The New England Journal of Medicine* 355:1195–97.

▶ Telomeres (*telos* = end + *meros* = part) are repeating DNA segments on the ends of chromosomes. Telomeres shorten progressively with each cell division as the terminal repeating DNA segments are lost until eventually the telomeres become so short that they lose their ability to protect the ends of the chromosomes, and the telomere-depleted cell is recognized by the cell DNA repair system and is eliminated. Progressive telomere shortening limits the number of cell divisions that a normal cell can perform, which limits its longevity and, in turn, affects the survival of the various cell populations that make up an individual.

▶ Recently, an enzyme called telomerase has been identified that can restore telomeres, which greatly extends the life span of the cell by allowing the cell to divide repeatedly without "wearing out." Most human tumors contain telomerase enzyme, which allows them to proliferate indefinitely.

Black, W. C., and Baron, J. A. 2007. CT screening for lung cancer: Spiraling into confusion? *Journal of the American Medical Association* 297:995–97.

▶ A discussion of the different conclusions reached on the value of CT scans to detect early lung carcinoma. One study revealed a threefold increase in the number of lung cancer cases and a tenfold increase in lung cancer resections related to CT scans but no decrease in advanced lung cancer cases, which indicated that CT scanning has no effect on mortality. Another study revealed an 88% 10-year survival in early lung carcinoma detected by CT, which decreased mortality by 80%. The author indicates that early detection of disease does not necessarily reduce mortality; it only detects the tumor earlier, which leads to a longer interval between initial diagnosis and death from the tumor.

Connors, J. M. 2005. Radioimmunotherapy—Hot new treatment for lymphoma. *The New England Journal of Medicine* 352:496–98.

▶ Most patients with B-cell lymphomas have widespread disease by the time the lymphoma is diagnosed, and it is difficult to cure the lymphoma because the tumor cells have already spread throughout the body. Recently, antibodies directed against B cells and labeled with a radioisotope have been used to seek out and destroy the B-lymphoma cells wherever they are located in the body. Studies on a selected group of patients have yielded encouraging results.

Dantal, J., and Soulillou, J. P. 2005. Immunosuppressive drugs and the risk of cancer after organ transplantation. *The New England Journal of Medicine* 352:1371–73.

▶ Immunosuppressive therapy, which is essential for survival of organ transplants, has some important limitations: cardiovascular disease, infections, and cancer. Many of the cancers result from activation of oncogenic viruses: lymphomas related to EB virus, Kaposi's sarcoma caused by human herpesvirus 8, and skin cancer caused by human papilloma virus. Most immunosuppressive agents favor cancer development, but a few actually reduce cancer risk by suppressing cell proliferation. Hopefully, effective combinations of immunosuppressive drugs can prevent organ rejection and also reduce cancer risk.

D'Souza, G., Kreimer, A. R., Viscidi, R., et al. 2007. Case-control study of human papillomavirus and oropharyngeal cancer. *The New England Journal of Medicine* 356:1944–56.

▶ The association between some types of oropharyngeal cancer and HPV infections appears to be firmly established. HPV type 16 (one of the same types responsible for cervical HPV infections and cervical carcinoma) also occurs frequently associated with oropharyngeal carcinoma.

Geenen, M. M., Cardous-Ubbink, M. C., Kremer, L. C., et al. 2007. Medical assessment of adverse health outcomes in long-term survivors of childhood cancer. *Journal of the American Medical Association* 297:2705–15.

▶ Improved survival of children with cancer has been associated with multiple treatment-related complications. Long-term follow-up revealed a large number of late complications. Seventy-five percent had one or more late complications. Twenty-four point six percent had five or more complications. The highest complication rates occurred in radiotherapy-treated children.

Gooley, T. A., Chien, J. W., Pergam, S. A., et al. 2010. Reduced mortality after allogeneic hematopoietic-cell transplantation. *The New England Journal of Medicine* 363:2091–101.

▶ Over the past decade, advances have been made in the care of patients undergoing transplantation. We found that less intense cytotoxic chemotherapy and radiation treatment resulted in better results because of less organ damage, infection, and severe graft-versus-host disease.

Harousseau, J. L., and Moreau, P. 2009. Autologous hematopoietic stem-cell transplantation for multiple myeloma. *The New England Journal of Medicine* 360:2645–54.

▶ A description of the evolution of plasma cell proliferation into myeloma and various methods of treatment, including details of bone marrow transplantation and its effects on patient survival.

Hoagland, H. C. 1995. Myelodysplastic (preleukemia) syndromes: The bone marrow factory failure problem. *Mayo Clinic Proceedings* 70:673–77.

▶ A review of classification, clinical features, cytogenetic abnormalities, diagnosis, and management.

Jacobs, A. D., Champlin, R. E., and Golde, D. W. 1985. Recombinant alpha-2-interferon for hairy cell leukemia. *Blood* 65:1017–20.

▶ Interferon is a highly effective therapy for hairy cell leukemia.

Jemal, A., Siegel, R., Ward, E., et al. 2007. Cancer statistics, 2007. *CA: A Cancer Journal for Clinicians* 57:43–66.

▶ Extensive cancer data from the American Cancer Society, including most recent 5-year survival rates of cancers diagnosed 1996–2002.

Krause, D. S., and Van Etten, R. A. 2005. Tyrosine kinases as targets for cancer therapy. *The New England Journal of Medicine* 353:172–87.

▶ Tyrosine kinase (TK) enzymes perform many functions concerned with cell growth and differentiation, and unrestrained cell proliferation follows if TK malfunctions, as occurs in chronic myelogenous leukemia. Several other tumors result from disturbed

TK function. TK can also be inhibited by blocking its receptor using a monoclonal antibody. Some toxic effects related to TK-directed therapy may be related to inhibition of TK activity in normal tissues.

Landgren, O., and Waxman, A. J. 2010. Multiple myeloma precursor disease. *Journal of the American Medical Association* 304:2397–404.

► Myeloma is often preceded by blood protein abnormalities which may slowly evolve into the characteristic features of multiple myeloma.

OUTLINE SUMMARY

Tumors: Disturbed Cell Growth

Classification and Nomenclature

BENIGN TUMORS
Descriptive: polyp, papilloma.
Tissue of origin + *oma*.

MALIGNANT TUMORS
Cancer: general term.
Carcinoma: arising from surface, glandular, or parenchymal epithelium.
Sarcoma: solid tumor arising from other primary tissues.
Leukemia: neoplasm of blood-forming tissues.

Comparison of Benign and Malignant Tumors

BENIGN TUMORS
Grow slowly.
Grow by expansion.
Remain localized.
Cells well differentiated.

MALIGNANT TUMORS
Grow more rapidly.
Grow by infiltration.
Metastasize.
Cells not well differentiated.

Variations in Terminology

LYMPHOID TUMORS
Lymphoma: a malignant lymphoid tumor.
Classification:
   Hodgkin's disease: characteristic Reed-Sternberg cells.
   Non-Hodgkin's lymphoma: well-differentiated and poorly differentiated.

SKIN TUMORS
From melanocytes:
   Benign: nevus.
   Malignant: melanoma.

From keratinocytes:
   Benign: keratoses.
   Malignant: basal cell carcinoma, squamous cell carcinoma.
Sun exposure damages skin and predisposes to development of tumors.

TUMORS OF MIXED COMPONENTS (TERATOMAS)
Frequently occur in reproductive tract.
Must specify as either benign or malignant.

PRIMITIVE CELL TUMORS
Arise from persisting groups of primitive cells.
Named from tissue of origin + *blastoma*.

Necrosis in Tumors

PATHOGENESIS
Tumor outgrows blood supply.
Necrosis occurs in center of deeply placed tumor.
Necrosis occurs on the surface of tumors growing from epithelial surface.

Noninfiltrating (In Situ) Carcinoma

CHARACTERISTICS
Remains localized for many years.
Frequently occurs in cervix, but encountered in other locations as well.
Most favorable stage for cure.

PRECANCEROUS CONDITIONS
Characteristics:
   Nonmalignant conditions with tendency to eventually become malignant.
   Treatment prevents progression.
Common precancerous conditions:
   Actinic keratosis: arises in sun-damaged skin and may form skin cancers.
   Lentigo maligna: arises in sun-damaged skin and may lead to melanoma.
   Leukoplakia: affects oral mucosa, usually caused by exposure to tobacco tars. May affect vulva (Chapter 17).
   Some colon polyps.

Etiologic Factors in Neoplastic Disease

VIRUSES
Some animal tumors are caused by viruses.
Some human tumors also may be virus induced.

GENE AND CHROMOSOME ABNORMALITIES
Activation of oncogenes and inactivation of tumor suppressor genes deregulates cell, which proliferates to form tumor.
Translocation or deletion may change the relation of genes on the chromosome, disturbing cell regulation and growth functions.
Philadelphia chromosome is the best-known abnormality.
>   *Reciprocal translocation of ends of chromosomes 9 and 22.*
>   *Oncogene on translocated piece of chromosome 9 exhibits increased activity.*

FAILURE OF IMMUNOLOGIC DEFENSES
Body produces abnormal cells periodically.
Immune defenses eliminate abnormal cells.
Failure of elimination may allow overgrowth, forming malignant tumors.

HEREDITY AND TUMORS
No strong hereditary predisposition to most tumors.
Slightly increased susceptibility in relatives of cancer patients may be caused by multifactorial inheritance pattern.
Some breast carcinomas have strong hereditary background, owing to inheritance of mutant gene.
Rare tumors:
>   *Autosomal dominant inheritance:*
>   *Some retinoblastomas.*
>   *Multiple polyposis of colon.*
>   *Neurofibromatosis.*
>   *Multiple endocrine adenomas.*

Only small fraction of all tumors affecting humans.

Diagnosis of Tumors

EARLY RECOGNITION
An abnormality of form or function requires evaluation by physician.
If abnormality discovered, perform biopsy or excise.
Excision of benign tumor is curative; malignant tumor may require further treatment.

CYTOLOGIC DIAGNOSIS
Tumor cells shed from the surface or can be scraped from the epithelial surface.
Abnormal smear indicates need for further studies but not diagnostic of neoplasm.

FROZEN-SECTION DIAGNOSIS
Means of rapid evaluation of abnormal tissue obtained at surgery.
Permits immediate decision about proper course of treatment.

TUMOR-ASSOCIATED ANTIGEN TESTS
Carbohydrate–protein complexes secreted by tumor cells.
Can be detected in the blood.
Used to monitor response to treatment.

Treatment of Tumors
Pretreatment tumor grading and staging helps determine prognosis, helps select the most appropriate treatment, and provides useful information for future clinical research studies.

SURGERY
Extensive resection of tumor with draining lymph nodes.
Not curative if tumor has already metastasized to distant sites.

RADIOTHERAPY
Lymphomas and some epithelial tumors treated primarily by radiotherapy.
May be used in conjunction with surgery.
Useful for pain relief.

HORMONES
Hormone-dependent tumors undergo temporary regression when deprived of required hormones.
Some tumors inhibited by hormones, corticosteroids, estrogens.

ANTICANCER DRUGS
Impede processes concerned with cell growth and cell division.
Most effective against rapidly growing tumors.
>   *Alkylating agents.*
>   *Antimetabolites.*

Some drugs act by blocking cell growth factor receptors or inhibit intracellular enzymes that promote cell growth.

ADJUVANT CHEMOTHERAPY
Used after surgical resection of tumor.
Attempts to eradicate small metastases before they become apparent clinically.

IMMUNOTHERAPY
Nonspecific immunotherapy:
>   *Interferon:*
>>   *Interferon regulates cell growth and functions of immune system in addition to antiviral activity.*
>>   *Large quantities available from commercial production.*
>>   *Best results in hairy cell leukemia, but useful for causing regression of some other neoplasms.*
>>   *Low toxicity.*
>   *Interleukin-2:*
>>   *Stimulates production of natural killer cells that attack tumor.*
>>   *Best results in metastatic melanoma and renal cell carcinoma.*
>   *Other cytokines under investigation.*

Specific immunotherapy:
>   *Tumor-infiltrating lymphocytes:*
>>   *Cytotoxic T cells attack patient's own tumor.*
>>   *Some success in treating metastatic melanoma.*
>   *Tumor vaccines:*
>>   *Vaccine prepared from patient's own tumor induces immune response.*
>>   *Used as additional treatment after melanoma or colon cancer if patient at high risk of recurrence.*

Tumor antibody therapy:
Antibodies prepared against tumor antigens and coupled with antitumor drug or toxin.
Antibody infused into patient and damages tumor cells without injuring normal cells.

Leukemia

CLASSIFICATION

By cell type: granulocytic, lymphocytic, or monocytic.
By maturity of cells: acute (primitive cells) or chronic (mature cells).
By number of circulating white cells: descriptive term *aleukemic* indicates low white count in peripheral blood.

CLINICAL FEATURES/PRINCIPLES OF TREATMENT

As a result of impaired bone marrow function: anemia, thrombocytopenia, and infections caused by reduced numbers of mature functional leukocytes.
As a result of infiltration of organs: splenomegaly, hepatomegaly, lymphadenopathy.
Chronic leukemia well controlled by treatment; relatively long survival.
Acute leukemia difficult to treat and has poor prognosis in many cases; childhood leukemia has better prognosis and may be cured by treatment.
Bone marrow transplant available in selected patients.
Philadelphia chromosome positive subjects respond to drug that inhibits the hyperactive intracellular tyrosine kinase enzyme that promotes cell growth.

Preleukemia/Myelodysplasia

MANIFESTATIONS

Disturbed growth and maturation of marrow cells.
Anemia, leukopenia, thrombocytopenia.
May be precursor of leukemia in some patients.

Multiple Myeloma

CHARACTERISTICS

A neoplasm of plasma cells.
Differs somewhat from leukemia.
Nodular deposits of plasma cells in bone.
Plasma cells produce protein.
Usually no visceral infiltration.
May be preceded by "premyeloma"

Premyeloma

CHARACTERISTICS

An early stage of multiple myeloma characterized by only slightly increased plasma cell proliferation in bone marrow along with slightly increased but abnormal blood protein.

Survival Rates in Neoplastic Disease

NATURE OF PROBLEM

Cancer is leading cause of disability and mortality.
Survival rates vary from 4% to 95%, depending on tumor.
Early diagnosis and treatment may enhance survival.
Some tumors may recur many years after treatment.

CHAPTER 11

Abnormalities of Blood Coagulation

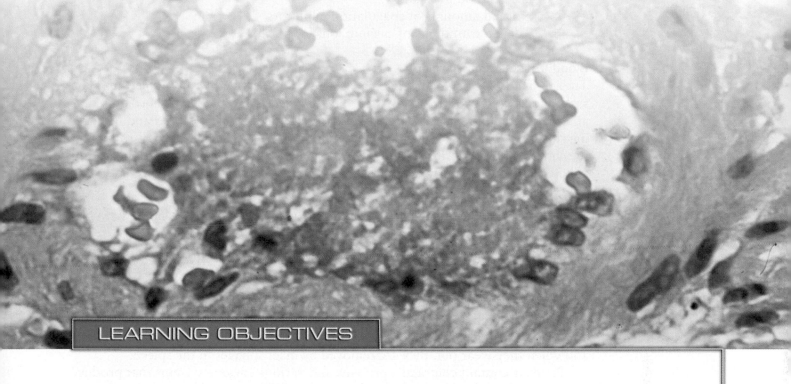

LEARNING OBJECTIVES

1 Describe the functions of blood vessels and platelets in controlling bleeding.

2 Explain the three phases of coagulation, and list the coagulation factors involved.

3 Describe the laboratory tests used to evaluate hemostasis.

4 List the most common clinically significant disturbances of hemostasis and describe their clinical manifestations.

Hemostasis

If a person cuts his or her finger with a knife, the cut bleeds, but the bleeding soon stops and healing ensues. The body has a complex mechanism for causing blood to clot when and where it is necessary, while keeping the blood fluid within the capillaries and larger blood vessels.

FACTORS CONCERNED WITH HEMOSTASIS

The proper functioning of the hemostatic mechanism depends on the proper integrated functioning of the five major factors that affect hemostasis:

1. Integrity of the small blood vessels
2. Adequate numbers of structurally and functionally normal platelets
3. Normal amounts of coagulation factors (proteins present in small quantities in the blood plasma)
4. Normal amounts of coagulation inhibitors
5. Adequate amounts of calcium ions in the blood

Blood Vessels and Platelets

The small blood vessels and blood platelets function together to prevent bleeding. The small blood vessels are the body's first line of defense. If a blood vessel is injured, it automatically contracts (reflex vasoconstriction), narrowing its caliber and facilitating closure of the vessel by a blood clot. Injury to the vessel also leads to disruption of the endothelium, exposing the underlying connective tissue. Platelets accumulate and adhere to the site of injury, where they perform three important functions:

1. They plug the defect in the vessel wall.
2. They liberate chemical compounds (vasoconstrictors) that cause the vessel to contract and compounds that cause platelets to aggregate.
3. They release substances (phospholipids) that initiate the process of blood coagulation.

Platelets, which play an essential role in blood coagulation, are very small fragments of the cytoplasm from large precursor cells in the bone marrow called megakaryocytes. Platelets have an average survival in the circulation of about 10 days, and when they wear out, they are removed by macrophages in the spleen.

Platelets contain contractile proteins and various enzyme systems that produce products essential for normal platelet functions. When platelets come in contract with a roughened or damaged endothelial surface, they undergo a dramatic change. They swell and become sticky. Long processes (pseudopods) extend from their cytoplasm, and they release various products that cause further platelet swelling and platelet aggregation to form a platelet plug. Activation of platelets also starts the blood coagulation process, as illustrated in FIGURE 11-1.

Platelets play a very important part in preventing bleeding from capillaries. Small breaks in the walls of capillaries occur frequently, but the defects are promptly sealed by platelets, and bleeding does not occur. However, if the quantity of platelets in the blood is seriously reduced, as occurs in some diseases, the "platelet sealing mechanism" is impaired. As a result, the affected individual develops multiple small pinpoint areas of bleeding (called **petechiae** or petechial hemorrhages) in the skin and deeper tissues resulting from leakage of blood through minute defects in the capillary endothelium.

Petechia (pe-tē′kēy-uh)
A small pinpoint hemorrhage caused by decreased platelets, abnormal platelet function, or capillary defect.

Plasma Coagulation Factors

The blood plasma contains several different proteins called coagulation factors, which are designated by both name and roman numerals. When these factors are activated, they interact to produce a blood clot. The process of blood coagulation is a chain reaction in which each component of the chain is formed from an inactive precursor in the blood, and each activated component in turn activates the next member of the chain. The process has been compared with what happens when the first in a long chain of dominoes is knocked over. Tipping the first domino represents the initiation of the clotting mechanism, and the fall of the last domino represents the formation of a firm blood clot.

The process of blood coagulation is a highly complex and bewildering sequence of interactions involving plasma and tissue components, platelets, and calcium. At the risk of oversimplifying its complexities, however, it is convenient to divide it into three phases for descriptive purposes (Figure 11-1).

Phase 1 leads to the formation of **thromboplastin**, which may be produced by either of two different mechanisms. One mechanism depends on the interaction of platelets and plasma coagulation factors. If the wall of a blood vessel is injured, platelets accumulate at the site and release a phospholipid that interacts with plasma components to form thromboplastin. This is called the intrinsic system because the thromboplastin is produced from substances present in the bloodstream. Tissues also have thromboplastic activity, and thromboplastin is also liberated from injured tissues. This is called the extrinsic system because the thromboplastin is not derived from the blood but primarily from tissue outside of the vascular compartment.

Actually, the intrinsic and extrinsic pathways are not completely independent. Usually both pathways are activated at the same time when tissues are injured, and both pathways interact to initiate the blood clotting process.

The conversion of prothrombin into thrombin takes place in phase 2. The thromboplastin formed in either the intrinsic or the extrinsic system interacts with additional plasma factors and platelet phospholipid to form a complex (called prothrombin

Thromboplastin
(throm-bō-plas'tin)
A component formed during blood coagulation from interaction of platelets and plasma components (intrinsic system) *or liberated from injured tissues* (extrinsic system).

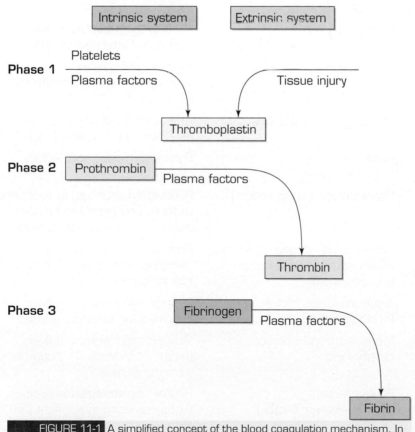

FIGURE 11-1 A simplified concept of the blood coagulation mechanism. In the intrinsic system, plasma factors (XII, XI, and IX) are activated, and they interact with factor VIII and platelets to yield intrinsic thromboplastin. In the extrinsic system, tissue injury yields extrinsic thromboplastin that reacts with a plasma factor (VII). Then the thromboplastin formed by either the intrinsic or extrinsic system interacts with additional components (factors V, X, and platelet phospholipid) to form the complex (prothrombin activator) that converts prothrombin into thrombin in the second phase. Thrombin converts fibrinogen into fibrin in the third phase.

Thrombin
A coagulation factor formed by activation of prothrombin in the process of blood coagulation.

Fibrinogen
(fī-brin′ō-jen)
A precursor in plasma converted into fibrin by thrombin during blood coagulation.

Fibrin
The meshwork of protein threads that form during the clotting of the blood.

Fibrin monomer
(mä′nō-mer)
A derivative of fibrinogen that polymerizes to form the fibrin clot during blood coagulation.

activator) that converts the prothrombin into thrombin. Prothrombin is a protein manufactured in the liver. It is split into several fragments by thromboplastin. One of these is the active component **thrombin**, an enzyme capable of digesting protein. The formation of thrombin from prothrombin requires other plasma coagulation factors (called accessory factors) that function by speeding the rate of the conversion.

Phase 3 leads to the conversion of **fibrinogen** into **fibrin** by thrombin. Fibrinogen is a high molecular weight protein produced by the liver. Thrombin splits off a part of the fibrinogen molecule, forming a smaller molecule called **fibrin monomer**. The fibrin monomer molecules then become joined end to end (polymerized) to form long strands of fibrin, and the fibrin strands also become linked together side to side. Another plasma factor (fibrin stabilizing factor) acts by strengthening the bonds between the fibrin molecules and increasing the strength of the fibrin clot. The blood clot is the end stage in the clotting process. It consists of an interlacing meshwork of fibrin threads containing entrapped plasma, red cells, white cells, and platelets.

TABLE 11-1 summarizes the coagulation factors and their role in the clotting process.

TABLE 11-1

Coagulation factors

Factor number	Name	Functions
I	Fibrinogen	Protein synthesized in liver; converted into fibrin in phase 3
II	Prothrombin	Protein synthesized in liver (requires vitamin K); converted into thrombin in phase 2
III	Tissue thromboplastin	Released from damaged tissue; required in extrinsic phase 1
IV	Calcium ions	Required throughout entire clotting sequence
V	Proaccelerin (labile factor)	Protein synthesized in liver; required to form prothrombin activator in both intrinsic and extrinsic phase 1
VII	Serum prothrombin conversion accelerator (stable factor, proconvertin)	Protein synthesized in liver (requires vitamin K); functions in extrinsic phase 1
VIII	Antihemophilic factor (antihemophilic globulin)	Protein synthesized in liver; required for intrinsic phase 1
IX	Plasma thromboplastin component	Protein synthesized in liver (requires vitamin K); required for intrinsic phase 1
X	Stuart factor (Stuart-Prower factor)	Protein synthesized in liver (requires vitamin K); required to form prothrombin activator in both intrinsic and extrinsic phase 1
XI	Plasma thromboplastin antecedent	Protein synthesized in liver; required for intrinsic phase 1
XII	Hageman factor	Protein required for intrinsic phase 1
XIII	Fibrin-stabilizing factor	Protein required to stabilize the fibrin strands in phase 3

Coagulation Inhibitors and Fibrinolysins

Coagulation factors are counterbalanced by various coagulation inhibitors that restrict the clotting process to a limited area. One coagulation inhibitor called protein C and another called protein S function together to inactivate two coagulation factors (V and VIII). Another important member of this group is antithrombin, which inhibits not only thrombin but also several other activated coagulation factors generated in the clotting process.

An equally important control system is one that dissolves fibrin after it has formed. A precursor compound in blood plasma called plasminogen (profibrinolysin) is activated to form plasmin (fibrinolysin), which dissolves fibrin in blood clots. The fibrinolytic system is activated at the same time that the coagulation process is initiated, and thrombin produced in the coagulation process also activates this system. Another important plasminogen activator is a substance called tissue plasminogen activator, which is released from endothelial cells in the region where the clot is forming. As described in the discussion on cardiovascular system, tissue plasminogen activator or another plasminogen activator called streptokinase, produced by streptococci, is administered intravenously to dissolve blood clots in the coronary arteries of patients who have had a recent heart attack. Prompt administration of one of these plasminogen activators within a few hours after onset of symptoms dissolves the clot and restores flow through the artery, which minimizes heart muscle damage resulting from the blockage.

Calcium and Blood Coagulation

Adequate amounts of calcium ions (Ca^{2+}) are required in all phases of blood coagulation, and blood will not clot in the absence of calcium. However, there are no diseases in which a disturbance of blood coagulation results from an abnormally low level of blood calcium because calcium levels sufficiently low to affect blood coagulation would be incompatible with life.

Clinical Disturbances of Blood Coagulation

Disturbances of blood coagulation may be classified as one of four major categories:

1. Abnormalities of small blood vessels
2. Abnormalities of platelet function
3. Deficiency of one or more of the plasma coagulation factors
4. Liberation of thromboplastic material into the circulation

ABNORMALITIES OF SMALL BLOOD VESSELS

Some rare diseases characterized by abnormal bleeding have been found to result from abnormal function of the small blood vessels. Normally, small blood vessels contract after injury, helping to seal the defect by a blood clot. Sometimes this function is defective, leading to excessive bleeding. In a few other rare diseases, the small blood vessels are abnormally formed and cannot function properly.

ABNORMALITIES OF PLATELET NUMBERS OR FUNCTION

A decrease in platelets is called **thrombocytopenia** (*thrombus* = clot + *cyte* = cell + *penia* = deficiency). This decrease may be a result of injury or disease of the bone

Thrombocytopenia
(throm′bō-sī-tō-pē′ny-yuh)
A deficiency of platelets.

marrow, which damages the megakaryocytes in the marrow, the precursor cells of the platelets. In other cases, thrombocytopenia occurs because the bone marrow has been infiltrated by leukemic cells or by cancer cells that have spread to the skeletal system and the megakaryocytes have been crowded out by the abnormal cells. Thrombocytopenia may also occur if antiplatelet autoantibodies destroy the platelets in the peripheral blood (as seen in some autoimmune diseases). Sometimes platelets are normal in quantity but abnormal in function, and so they are ineffective in initiating the clotting process.

Bleeding associated with defective or inadequate platelets is generally manifested by small petechial hemorrhages rather than by large areas of hemorrhage (FIGURE 11-2A).

DEFICIENCY OF PLASMA COAGULATION FACTORS

Hematoma
A large circumscribed collection of blood in body tissues.

Deficiencies of plasma coagulation factors often lead to large areas of hemorrhage called **hematomas** (*heme* = blood + *oma* = swelling) (FIGURE 11-2B). Deficiencies of factors concerned with the first phase of coagulation are usually hereditary and are relatively rare. Only three hereditary bleeding diseases occur with any frequency. Hemophilia, an X-linked hereditary disease affecting males, is the most common and best known. Clinically, the disease is characterized by episodes of hemorrhage in joints and internal organs after minor injury. There are two forms of hemophilia. Both have the same clinical manifestations and X-linked method of transmission. The most common type, which is called hemophilia A or classic hemophilia, is characterized by a decrease in coagulation factor VIII, which is also called antihemophilic factor. Its method of inheritance was considered in the discussion on congenital and hereditary diseases. The less common form of hemophilia is called hemophilia B or Christmas disease. It is caused by a deficiency of coagulation factor IX, which is also called Christmas factor (named after an affected patient, not the holiday). Both factors VIII and IX, which are produced in the liver, are required in the first phase of coagulation.

A | B

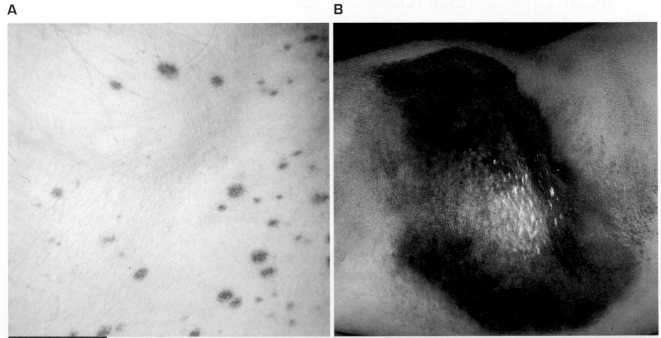

FIGURE 11-2 Characteristics of bleeding in patients with disturbed hemostatic function. **A**, Petechial hemorrhages indicative of thrombocytopenia or defective platelet function. **B**, A large hemorrhage (hematoma) associated with a deficiency of plasma coagulation factors.

A third hereditary bleeding disease is called von Willebrand disease and is usually transmitted as a Mendelian dominant trait. This disease also is characterized by excessive bleeding after a minor injury, but usually the bleeding is not in the joints, as is so characteristic of hemophilia. The manifestations of von Willebrand disease result from a deficiency of a large protein molecule that is produced primarily by the endothelial cells lining blood vessels. This factor is required in order for platelets to adhere to the vessel wall at the site of injury. The protein is also released into the bloodstream, where it forms a complex in the circulation with factor VIII, and it is needed in order to maintain a normal level of factor VIII in the blood.

Von Willebrand's factor functions by adhering to the vessel wall where the endothelium is disrupted, forming a latticelike framework that allows platelets and coagulation factors to adhere, interact, and form a blood clot.

The level of factor VIII is low in patients with von Willebrand disease, as it is in hemophilia A, but for a different reason. Patients with von Willebrand disease can synthesize factor VIII, but an adequate level of von Willebrand's factor is required to form a complex with factor VIII and maintain a normal amount of factor VIII in the circulation. The factor VIII deficiency in von Willebrand disease occurs because the affected persons lack adequate amounts of circulating von Willebrand's factor with which the factor VIII can combine.

Because von Willebrand's factor is also required in order for platelets to adhere at the site of vascular injury, some platelet functions also are disturbed in persons with this disease, which can be identified by special laboratory tests.

Patients with hemophilia A, hemophilia B, and von Willebrand disease who have bleeding episodes can be treated by administration of factor concentrates prepared from human blood plasma. A factor VIII concentrate prepared by recombinant DNA technology also has become available and can be used to treat patients with classic hemophilia.

Disturbances affecting the second phase of blood coagulation result from a deficiency of prothrombin or various accessory coagulation factors that are required for the conversion of prothrombin into thrombin. These factors are produced in the liver, and vitamin K is required for the synthesis of most of these factors (called vitamin K–dependent factors). Vitamin K is synthesized by intestinal bacteria and also can be obtained from foods, especially green leafy vegetables. It is a fat-soluble vitamin, and bile is required for its absorption.

A disturbance of blood coagulation caused by a deficiency of prothrombin or related factors suggests four possibilities:

1. Administration of anticoagulant drugs
2. Inadequate synthesis of vitamin K
3. Inadequate absorption of vitamin K
4. Severe liver disease

Anticoagulant drugs such as warfarin and similar compounds are sometimes used to treat patients who have shown an increased tendency to develop blood clots in their leg veins, such as patients having a total hip or total knee replacement procedure or other surgical procedures that increase their risk of forming leg vein clots. The drug is also given to patients with some types of heart disease in which blood clots tend to form within the cardiac chambers and to patients with some types of artificial heart valves to prevent clot formation within the artificial valve, which would disrupt the function of the valve. The amount of warfarin or related anticoagulant given to the patient must be monitored closely to reduce blood coagulability sufficiently to prevent unwanted blood clots forming in the heart chambers, leg veins, or other locations without reducing the coagulation factors to such an extent that spontaneous bleeding occurs. Anticoagulant drugs act by inhibiting the synthesis of biochemically active vitamin K–dependent factors. Inadequate synthesis of vitamin K also occurs if the intestinal bacteria have been eradicated by prolonged antibiotic therapy, as sometimes occurs in seriously ill, hospitalized patients. Another cause of inadequate uptake of vitamin K is blockage of the common bile duct by a gallstone or tumor, preventing bile from entering the intestine to promote absorption of the vitamin. Patients with severe liver diseases have deficiencies of prothrombin and accessory factors because the liver is so badly damaged that it can no longer synthesize adequate amounts of coagulation factors.

Intramuscular administration of vitamin K corrects coagulation disturbances resulting from Coumadin anticoagulants, inadequate synthesis of vitamin K, or insufficient absorption of the vitamin. The coagulation disturbance associated with severe liver disease does not respond because the diseased liver is no longer capable of synthesizing sufficient coagulation factors to provide efficient hemostasis.

Another vitamin K–deficient group is newborn infants who lack the intestinal bacteria to make the vitamin and are not yet eating foods that contain the vitamin. They are at risk for serious bleeding called *hemorrhagic disease of the newborn*. In order to prevent this condition, all newborn infants routinely receive a vitamin K injection to prevent spontaneous bleeding caused by lack of the vitamin.

A number of other anticoagulant drugs are available that interfere with some other phase of the coagulation mechanism, which may have advantages over warfarin in specific clinical situations, such as an antithrombin drug that impedes the second phase of blood coagulation. Some newer anticoagulant drugs act by interfering with factor X in the first phase of blood coagulation. The anticoagulant can be given as a standard daily dose without requiring laboratory tests, which simplifies the patient's treatment.

LIBERATION OF THROMBOPLASTIC MATERIAL INTO THE CIRCULATION

In a number of diseases associated with shock, overwhelming bacterial infection, or extensive necrosis of tissue, products of tissue necrosis and other substances with thromboplastic activity are liberated into the circulation, leading to widespread intravascular coagulation of the blood (FIGURE 11-3). In the process of clotting, platelets and the various plasma coagulation factors are utilized, and the levels of these components in the blood drop precipitously.

In order to defend itself against widespread intravascular clotting, the body activates the fibrinolysin system; this dissolves clots and prevents potentially lethal obstruction of the circulatory system by massive intravascular coagulation. The breakdown products produced during degradation of the fibrin act as additional inhibitors of the clotting process.

The net effect of these various events is a bleeding disturbance, sometimes in a patient already seriously ill because of an underlying disease that caused the blood-clotting mechanism to be activated. This abnormal bleeding state is called **disseminated intravascular coagulation syndrome** or **consumption coagulopathy**. The latter term alludes to consumption of the clotting factors as a result of the pathogenic coagulation process. FIGURE 11-4 summarizes the pathogenesis of this bleeding syndrome.

RELATIVE FREQUENCY OF THE VARIOUS COAGULATION DISTURBANCES

In one group of 350 hospitalized patients with bleeding problems that I studied, most of the disorders were caused by inadequate numbers of platelets or abnormal platelet function. Next in frequency were coagulation disturbances caused by

Disseminated intravascular coagulation syndrome
A disturbance of blood coagulation as a result of activation of the coagulation mechanism and simultaneous clot lysis.

Consumption coagulopathy
See disseminated intravascular coagulation syndrome.

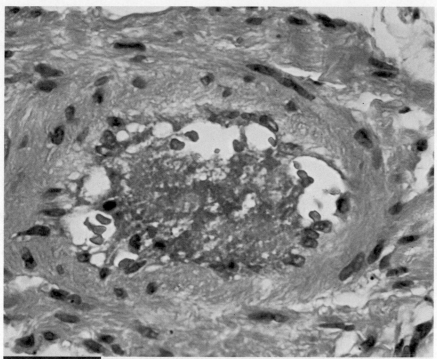

FIGURE 11-3 Fibrin thrombus in small blood vessel of patient with disseminated intravascular coagulation syndrome (original magnification × 400).

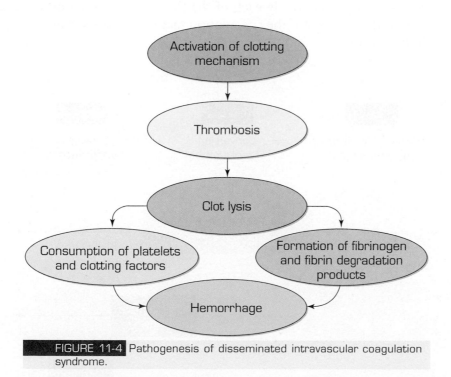

FIGURE 11-4 Pathogenesis of disseminated intravascular coagulation syndrome.

deficient formation of coagulation factors in patients with liver disease. In acutely ill patients, the majority of acquired coagulation disturbances are the result of disseminated intravascular coagulation, with depletion of both platelets and plasma coagulation factors.

Laboratory Tests to Evaluate Hemostasis

Several laboratory tests can evaluate the overall efficiency of the coagulation process, detect the presence of inhibitors of coagulation, and estimate the number and function of the platelets (FIGURE 11-5).

The number of platelets in the blood can be estimated by examining the blood smear, and more precise data can be obtained by a numerical platelet count. Special tests also are available to evaluate platelet function. The function of the capillaries in the hemostatic process is evaluated by the bleeding time, which reflects the time it takes for a small, standardized skin incision to stop bleeding.

A few relatively simple tests can be used to evaluate the various proteins concerned with blood coagulation (coagulation factors). The time it takes for blood to clot in a test tube under standard conditions is a crude and relatively insensitive test that measures the overall efficiency of the clotting process. Three other tests are more often used to evaluate the coagulation system. The tests, which are performed on plasma obtained from blood collected in tubes containing an anticoagulant, are the partial thromboplastin time, the prothrombin time, and the thrombin time. Each test measures a different phase of the coagulation process. When the tests are used together, one can assess separately each of the three phases of blood coagulation and can identify the location of the coagulation factor deficiency if any of the tests yield an abnormal result.

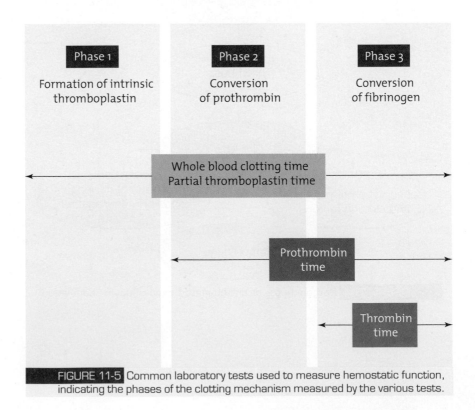

FIGURE 11-5 Common laboratory tests used to measure hemostatic function, indicating the phases of the clotting mechanism measured by the various tests.

The **partial thromboplastin time (PTT) test** measures the time it takes for blood plasma to clot after a lipid substance is added to the plasma along with calcium to start the clotting process. The lipid added is similar to the lipid material released from platelets to initiate the first phase of blood coagulation, which in turn is followed by activation of the second and third phases of the coagulation process. If a plasma factor in any of the three coagulation phases is deficient, the coagulation process is slowed, and the partial thromboplastin time is prolonged.

The **prothrombin time test** measures the time it takes for blood plasma to clot after adding a commercially available preparation of thromboplastin made from rabbit brain along with calcium to start the coagulation. The thromboplastin added to start the reaction is essentially the same material as the thromboplastin produced by the interaction of platelets and plasma coagulation factors in the first phase of blood coagulation. A normal prothrombin time test indicates that the second and third phases of blood coagulation are normal. If the prothrombin time is prolonged, an abnormality in either the second or third stages of coagulation is indicated. The abnormality cannot be in the first phase of blood coagulation because the first phase is concerned with the formation of intrinsic thromboplastin, and thromboplastin has already been supplied as the test reagent. The first phase has been bypassed, and the test is only measuring the coagulation factors involved in the second and third phases. The prothrombin time test is commonly used to monitor the effect of Coumadin anticoagulants administered to patients in order to reduce the coagulability of the blood. When using the test to monitor the amount of Coumadin to give to a patient who is taking Coumadin to reduce the coagulability of the blood, it is essential that any clinical laboratory performing the test obtains the same result. If the results of a test varied depending on the laboratory performing the test, the physician prescribing the Coumadin would have great difficulty determining how much to give. The physician might give too much, which could cause bleeding, or not enough, which would be undesirable by increasing the coagulability of the patient's blood. The problem was solved by standardizing the thromboplastin against an international standard to achieve uniformity, and the prothrombin time result is reported by comparing the patient's result with normal controls obtained using a standardized thromboplastin.

The **thrombin time test** bypasses the first two phases of blood coagulation. One determines the clotting time of plasma after the addition of thrombin, which is normally generated in the second phase of the clotting process. Therefore, the test primarily measures the level of fibrinogen, which may be deficient in some conditions. The level of fibrinogen can also be measured directly by other tests, and one can also test for fibrinogen and fibrin degradation products, which are increased if fibrinolysis is excessive.

In the event that abnormalities are detected in any phase of coagulation, it is necessary to determine whether they have occurred because a coagulation factor is deficient or because an inhibitor is impairing the action of the factor. If necessary, one can also determine the concentrations of the various factors.

Case Studies

The following cases illustrate the spectrum of coagulation abnormalities encountered in clinical medicine. The cases also illustrate how laboratory tests can help to determine the nature of the abnormality and suggest a proper course of treatment.

Partial thromboplastin time (PTT) test
(throm-bō-plas'tin)
A test that measures the overall efficiency of the blood coagulation process.

Prothrombin time test
A test that measures the phase of the coagulation mechanism after the formation of thromboplastin.

Thrombin time test
A laboratory test measurement that determines the concentration of fibrinogen in the blood by determining the clotting time of the blood plasma after addition of thrombin.

CASE 11-1

FACTOR VIII DEFICIENCY A 10-month-old child was admitted to the hospital through the emergency room because he was bleeding profusely from a cut under the lip that he received when falling. The history revealed easy bruising since birth but no episodes of bleeding into the joints, and the child was considered by the parents to be in good health.

Physical examination revealed ecchymoses over the left chest and a small bruise on the abdomen. Small bruises were noted on both lower extremities. Laboratory studies revealed moderate anemia and normal platelets. Coagulation studies revealed a normal plasma prothrombin time, but the partial thromboplastin time was significantly prolonged.

The bleeding was controlled by applying pressure for about 10 minutes. The next day, the child had a tarry stool, apparently caused by swallowed blood. After this, the stools became normal in color, and no further bleeding was noted.

In this case, the abnormal partial thromboplastin time indicated an abnormality of blood coagulation, but the normal prothrombin time indicated that the abnormality was not in the second or third stages of coagulation. Therefore, the defect must have been in the first phase, which suggests either hemophilia or von Willebrand disease as diagnostic possibilities. Further tests showed a very low level of factor VIII (antihemophilic factor), and additional diagnostic tests established the diagnosis of von Willebrand disease.

CASE 11-2

VITAMIN K DEFICIENCY A 55-year-old woman was admitted to the hospital with a severe staphylococcal pneumonia that was complicated by an accumulation of pus in the left pleural cavity. She received intensive antibiotic therapy. She was unable to take food or fluid orally because of severe nausea and vomiting and was maintained almost entirely on intravenous fluids. It was difficult to maintain a satisfactory fluid balance and nutrition. After several weeks in the hospital, she developed bleeding from her urinary tract and rectal bleeding.

Coagulation studies revealed a prolonged partial thromboplastin time, and prolonged plasma prothrombin time (27 seconds, control 13 seconds). The patient was given a vitamin K preparation. Both the partial thromboplastin time and the prothrombin time returned to normal, and she had no further bleeding.

In this case, the coagulation data indicate an acquired depression of vitamin K–dependent coagulation factors primarily caused by deficient synthesis of vitamin K by intestinal bacteria, which were eliminated by the intensive antibiotic treatment. The excellent response to vitamin K confirmed the diagnosis.

CASE 11-3

CHRONIC LIVER DISEASE A 57-year-old man was admitted to the hospital because of bleeding from his urinary tract. Blood coagulation studies revealed a prolonged partial thromboplastin time and prothrombin time. The plasma prothrombin time was 18 seconds (control 13 seconds). Other studies revealed that his liver function was very abnormal. The prothrombin time did not return to normal after administration of a vitamin K preparation. A needle biopsy of the liver revealed a type of chronic liver and biliary system disease called *cirrhosis*.

Here the abnormality was localized to the second stage of blood coagulation. Failure to respond to vitamin K suggested chronic liver disease rather than vitamin K deficiency or a decrease in coagulation factors caused by anticoagulant therapy. The needle biopsy confirmed the presence of chronic liver disease.

CASE 11-4

DISSEMINATED INTRAVASCULAR COAGULATION SYNDROME AS A RESULT OF RETAINED DEAD FETUS A 36-year-old pregnant woman was admitted to the hospital at 38 weeks' gestation. She had not felt fetal movement for the previous month, and no fetal heart tones were detected by her physician. Coagulation studies revealed prolonged partial thromboplastin time and prothrombin time. Fibrinogen was markedly reduced. The patient's blood contained high levels of fibrinogen and fibrin degradation products. Labor was induced, and delivery was accomplished with very little loss of blood. The next day, the fibrinogen returned to normal, and all coagulation studies were within normal limits.

In this case, all of the coagulation factors were decreased because they had been used up in the coagulation process induced by release of thromboplastic material into the maternal circulation from the retained dead fetus. The high levels of fibrinogen and fibrin degradation products were the result of activation of the fibrinolytic system—the body's defense against a potentially lethal intravascular coagulation process.

QUESTIONS FOR REVIEW

1. How does blood clot?
2. What are some of the common disturbances of blood coagulation?
3. What is thrombocytopenia? What type of bleeding is produced when platelets are markedly reduced? What types of diseases are associated with thrombocytopenia?
4. What types of diseases produce abnormalities in the first phase of blood coagulation?
5. What is the consequence of liberation of thromboplastic material into the circulation?
6. What laboratory tests are used to evaluate the coagulation of blood?
7. A patient with a bleeding tendency has a prolonged partial thromboplastin time with a normal prothrombin time. In what phase of the clotting process is the disturbance located? Name one possible disease that could produce these findings.
8. What are the effects of Coumadin anticoagulants on the clotting mechanism? How do they work? What laboratory test can be used to monitor the effect of the anticoagulant?

SUPPLEMENTARY READINGS

Ansell, J. E., Kurnar, R., and Deykin, D. 1977. The spectrum of vitamin K deficiency. *Journal of the American Medical Association* 238:40–2.
  ► A common problem, especially in postoperative patients and those with cancer or renal failure. Treatment with parenteral vitamin K confirms the diagnosis and stops bleeding.

Crowley, L. V. 1968. Diagnosis of blood clotting disorders in a community hospital. *The Journal—Lancet* 88:295–302.
  ► Thrombocytopenia, chronic liver disease, and disseminated intravascular coagulation were the common problems when this article was written in 1968, and more recent data reveal comparable distribution of coagulation problems in community hospital patients.

Hylek, E. M. 2010. Therapeutic potential of oral factor Xa inhibitors. *New England Journal of Medicine* 363:2559–61.
  ► Two factor Xa inhibitors, which do not require laboratory test monitoring, have proven very useful as prophylaxis against venous thromboembolism in patients undergoing total hip replacement and is much safer than warfarin; Xa inhibitors may also be useful to prevent atrial thrombi in patients with atrial fibrillation.

Kumar, V., Abbas, A. K., Fausto, N., et al. 2010. *Robbins and Contran pathologic basis of disease.* 8th ed. Philadelphia: Elsevier Saunders.
  ► Good section on coagulation.

Lassen, M. R., Gallus, A., Raskob, G. E., et al. 2010. Apixaban versus enoxaparin for thromboprophylaxis after hip replacement. *New England Journal of Medicine* 363:2487–98.
  ► Among patients undergoing hip replacement, treatment with apixaban (a factor X antagonist) compared with enoxaparin (a low molecular weight heparin) was associated with lower rates of venous thrombosis without increased bleeding.

Hemostasis

FACTORS CONCERNED WITH HEMOSTASIS

Blood vessels and platelets
Reflex contraction of blood vessels after injury.
Platelets adhere to site of injury: plug vessel, liberate vaso-constrictors, release phospholipids to initiate clotting.
Small breaks in capillaries are sealed by platelets as they occur.
Plasma Coagulation Factors
Phase 1: generation of prothrombin activator:
   Intrinsic system: components derived from blood.
   Extrinsic system: tissue injury yields tissue thrombo-plastin.
Phase 2: formation of thrombin.
Phase 3: formation of fibrin.
Coagulation Inhibitors
Calcium
Required for all phases of coagulation.
No clinical disturbances of coagulation caused by low calcium.

Clinical Disturbances of Blood Coagulation

ABNORMALITIES OF SMALL BLOOD VESSELS

Abnormal function of small blood vessels.
Abnormal structure of small blood vessels.

ABNORMALITIES OF PLATELET NUMBERS OR FUNCTION

Thrombocytopenia:
   As a result of bone marrow infiltration.
   As a result of autoantibodies.
Defective platelet function.

DEFICIENCY OF PLASMA COAGULATION FACTORS

First phase:
   Usually congenital.
   Hemophilia is best-known defect.

Second phase:
   Administration of anticoagulant drugs.
   Inadequate synthesis of vitamin K.
   Inadequate absorption of vitamin K.
   Severe liver disease.
Liberation of thromboplastic material into circulation:
   Activation of coagulation mechanism by products of tissue injury.
   Intravascular coagulation.
   Activation of fibrinolysin.
   Consumption of coagulation factors and platelets.
   Products of fibrin breakdown have anticoagulant activity.

FREQUENCY OF COAGULATION DISTURBANCES

Frequently a result of inadequate platelets or defective platelet function.
Chronic liver disease.
Disseminated intravascular coagulation syndrome.

Laboratory Tests to Evaluate Hemostasis

PLATELETS

Platelet count.
Examination of blood smear for platelet numbers.

OVERALL EVALUATION OF COAGULATION MECHANISM

Clotting time of whole blood.
Partial thromboplastin time.

SECOND AND THIRD STAGES

Evaluation by prothrombin time.
Test bypasses first stage of blood coagulation.

THIRD STAGE

Thrombin time.
Determine fibrinogen and fibrin degradation products.

---

http://health.jbpub.com/humandisease/9e

Human Disease Online is a great source for supplementary human disease information for both students and instructors. Visit this website to find a variety of useful tools for learning, thinking, and teaching.

CHAPTER 12

Circulatory Disturbances

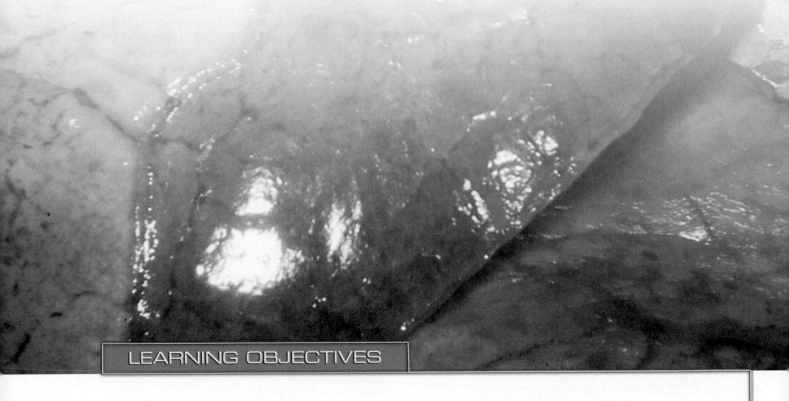

LEARNING OBJECTIVES

1 Describe the causes and effects of venous thrombosis.

2 Explain the pathogenesis of pulmonary embolism. Describe the clinical manifestations and compare the techniques of diagnosis.

3 Describe the causes and effects of arterial thrombosis.

4 List the four factors regulating the circulation of fluid between capillaries and interstitial tissue. Explain the major clinical disturbances leading to edema.

5 Describe the pathogenesis of the hypercoagulable state sometimes seen in patients with carcinoma.

Intravascular Blood Clots

Normally, blood does not clot within the vascular system. Under unusual circumstances, however, intravascular clotting may occur because of one or more of the following factors:

1. Slowing or stasis of the blood flow
2. Damage to the walls of the blood vessel
3. An increase in the coagulability of the blood

An intravascular clot is called a thrombus; the condition is termed **thrombosis**. Intravascular thrombi may form within veins or arteries and occasionally within the heart itself. A clot in the vascular system may become detached and may be carried in the circulation. Such a clot is termed an embolus (*embolus* = plug or stopper); the condition is termed **embolism**. Depending on where the blood clot was formed initially, the embolus may be carried into either the pulmonary circulation or the systemic arterial circulation. Eventually, it is arrested in an artery of smaller caliber than the diameter of the clot. When the embolus plugs the vessel, it blocks the blood flow to the tissue beyond (distal to) the obstruction, and the damaged tissue may undergo necrosis if the collateral blood supply is inadequate. The area of tissue breakdown is called an **infarct** or infarction.

Thrombosis
A blood clot formed within the vascular system.

Embolism
(em′bō-lizm)
A condition in which a plug composed of a detached clot, mass of bacteria, or other foreign material (embolus) occludes a blood vessel.

Infarct (in′färkt)
Necrosis of tissue caused by interruption of its blood supply.

Venous Thrombosis and Pulmonary Embolism

Formation of blood clots within leg veins is primarily a result of slowing or stasis of the blood in the veins. This is likely to occur during periods of prolonged bed rest or after a cramped position has been maintained for a long period of time. Under these circumstances, the "milking action" of the leg musculature, which normally promotes venous return, is impaired, leading to stasis of the blood. Varicose veins or any condition preventing normal emptying of veins predisposes an individual to thrombosis by causing venous stasis.

Postoperative thrombosis in leg veins is a common problem. The surgical patient is susceptible to venous thrombosis because of the combined effects of venous stasis resulting from inactivity and increased blood coagulability resulting from an increased concentration of coagulation factors. (Blood coagulation factors usually increase as a result of tissue injury or necrosis from any cause.)

A venous thrombosis may partially block venous return in the leg, making the leg swell. However, the major complication of venous thrombosis is related to detachment of the clot from the wall of the vein. The thrombus often is not firmly attached to the vein wall. It may break loose, forming an embolus that is carried rapidly up the inferior vena cava into the right side of the heart. From there, it is ejected into the pulmonary artery, where it may become lodged in either the main pulmonary artery or one of its branches. The clinical manifestations of a pulmonary embolism depend on the size of the embolus and where it lodges in the pulmonary artery.

LARGE PULMONARY EMBOLI

A large embolus that completely blocks the main pulmonary artery or its two major branches obstructs the flow of blood through the lungs (FIGURE 12-1). The right side of the heart becomes overdistended with blood because blood cannot be expelled into the lungs. The pulmonary artery leading to (proximal to) the obstructing embolus also becomes overdistended with blood, and the pressure in the pulmonary artery rises. Because less blood flows through the lungs into the left side of the heart, the left ventricle is unable to pump an adequate volume of blood to the brain and other vital organs. The systemic blood pressure falls, and the patient may go into shock. Blood still flows into the lungs from the bronchial arteries, which arise from the descending aorta and interconnect with the pulmonary arteries by means of collateral channels. This flow normally prevents infarction of the lung (FIGURE 12-2).

Clinically, the patient becomes very short of breath, and the skin and mucous membranes assume a bluish coloration (cyanosis) because of inadequate oxygenation

A　**B**

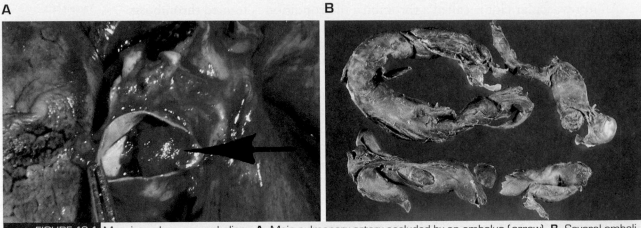

FIGURE 12-1 Massive pulmonary embolism. **A**, Main pulmonary artery occluded by an embolus (*arrow*). **B**, Several emboli filled both pulmonary arteries and obstructed blood flow to lungs.

of the blood. If the massive embolism is not immediately fatal, some blood may be able to flow around the embolus and circulate through the lungs, because the caliber of the pulmonary artery is increased by overdistention, and the high arterial pressure forces blood around the site of obstruction. In favorable circumstances, the embolus is eventually dissolved by the body's normal clot-dissolving mechanisms, and blood flow through the pulmonary artery is restored. In unfavorable cases, however, thrombus material builds up on the surface of the obstructing embolus and enlarges it. The sluggishly flowing blood in the branches of the pulmonary artery distal to the obstructing embolus may also become thrombosed. These events further impair pulmonary blood flow and may ultimately cause death several days after the initial embolization.

SMALL PULMONARY EMBOLI

If emboli are small, they may pass through the main pulmonary arteries and become impacted in the peripheral branches, usually in the arteries supplying the lower lobes of the lungs. Smaller emboli impede the flow of blood through the lungs and raise pulmonary artery pressure, but they have a less devastating effect than large emboli.

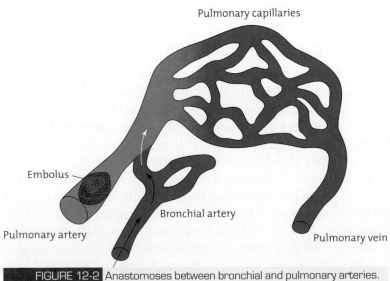

Pulmonary capillaries

Embolus

Bronchial artery

Pulmonary artery

Pulmonary vein

FIGURE 12-2 Anastomoses between bronchial and pulmonary arteries. The presence of an alternative pathway for blood flow often prevents infarction of the lung when the pulmonary artery is blocked by an embolus.

Frequently, the segment of lung supplied by the obstructed pulmonary artery undergoes necrosis, resulting in a pulmonary infarct. The alveolar septa break down, and blood flows from the ruptured capillaries into the pulmonary alveoli, which become distended with blood. The typical infarct is a wedge-shaped hemorrhagic area that extends to the pleural surface (FIGURE 12-3). Infarction does not always follow a pulmonary embolism because anastomoses between the bronchial artery and pulmonary artery distal to the obstruction provide an alternative pathway for blood flow. If the pulmonary venous pressure is elevated, however, as occurs in heart failure or when the lungs are poorly expanded, an adequate collateral circulation often does not develop and the lung becomes infarcted.

The clinical manifestations of smaller pulmonary emboli are quite variable and are frequently minimal if the lung does not become infarcted. Common symptoms of pulmonary infarction are difficulty in breathing (dyspnea), pleuritic chest pain, cough, and expectoration of bloody sputum. The chest pain occurs because the pleura overlying the infarct become inflamed and rubs against the overlying parietal pleura as the

A

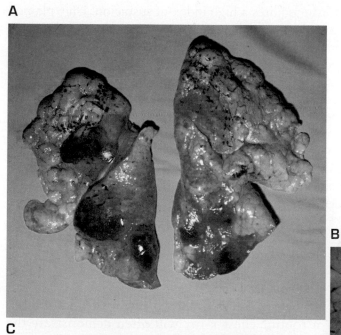

C

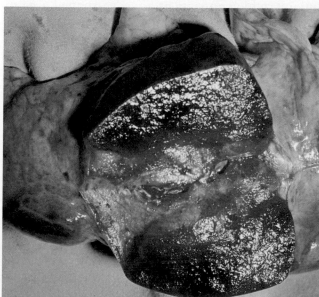

B

FIGURE 12-3 **A**, Multiple hemorrhagic pulmonary infarcts in both lungs. **B**, Closer view of infarct illustrating typical wedge-shaped hemorrhagic area that extends to pleural surface. **C**, Cut surface of pulmonary infarct, illustrating the hemorrhage in the infarcted lung segment and the sharp demarcation between infarct and adjacent normal lung tissue.

lung expands and contracts during respiration. The cough is caused by irritation of the bronchi in the injured area. The bloody sputum appears because blood escapes from the infarcted segment of lung into the bronchi and is subsequently coughed up.

SEPTIC PULMONARY EMBOLI

Sometimes, thrombi form in pelvic veins as a result of a bacterial infection in adjacent pelvic organs, as may occur after a uterine infection, and the bacteria may spread to infect the venous thrombi as well. If an infected thrombus breaks loose and causes a pulmonary infarct, the bacteria transported to the lung in the embolus invade the infarcted tissue, which breaks down to form a lung abscess. An infected embolus is called a septic embolus. If a patient sustains a pulmonary infarct owing to a septic embolus, the usual manifestations of pulmonary infarction are overshadowed by those of the systemic infection and the pulmonary abscess.

DIAGNOSIS OF PULMONARY EMBOLISM

A diagnosis of pulmonary embolism requires a high index of suspicion. Unexplained dyspnea, cough, or pleuritic chest pain in a predisposed patient may be the only manifestations of a pulmonary embolism. These symptoms should alert the physician to undertake further diagnostic studies. Sometimes, a blood test is helpful to confirm the physician's clinical impression of a possible pulmonary embolism. The test (called the *d-dimer test*) measures a by-product formed when fibrin within a blood clot is being broken down (fibrinolysis) by the body's normal clot-dissolving process, which would be activated in response to an intravascular thrombus or embolus. If the d-dimer concentration is not elevated, the possibility of a pulmonary embolism is less likely. On the other hand, an elevated d-dimer concentration would support the physician's clinical evaluation, and further studies are required. Some of the more useful tests are required. Some of the more useful studies are chest x-ray, radioisotope lung scans, and pulmonary angiography using either a standard radiologic method or a computed tomography (CT) procedure.

Chest X-Ray

If the embolus has caused pulmonary infarction, a routine chest x-ray will often demonstrate the infarct, which appears as a wedge-shaped area of increased density in the lung (FIGURE 12-4). Because emboli cannot be visualized on x-ray films, the lung will appear normal if it is not infarcted.

Radioisotope Lung Scan

To perform a radioisotope lung scan, one first injects a peripheral vein with a solution of specially prepared albumin labeled with a radioisotope. The injected material flows through the lung and is filtered out in the pulmonary capillaries. The radioactivity in the lungs, which is related to pulmonary blood flow, is then recorded by special instruments. If pulmonary blood flow is normal, the isotope is uniformly distributed throughout both lungs, and a uniform pattern of radioactivity appears on the lung scan. When blood flow to a part of the lung is blocked by an embolism, however, the

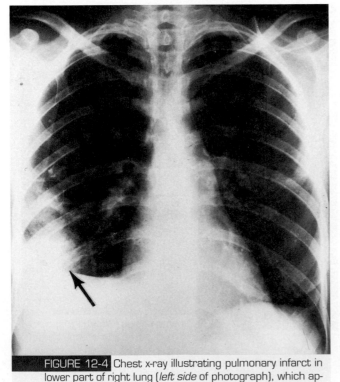

FIGURE 12-4 Chest x-ray illustrating pulmonary infarct in lower part of right lung (*left side* of photograph), which appears as an area of increased density (*arrow*). The opposite lung appears normal.

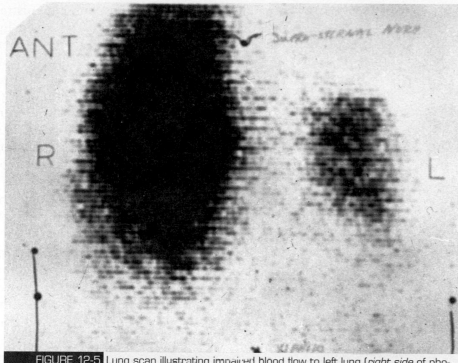

FIGURE 12-5 Lung scan illustrating impaired blood flow to left lung (*right side* of photograph), representing decreased radioactivity. Radioactivity of the opposite lung is normal (*uniform dark appearance*), indicating normal pulmonary blood flow.

isotope does not flow into the portion of lung supplied by the blocked artery, and no radioactivity is detected in the affected part of the lung. The isotope study does not actually demonstrate the embolus; it indicates only that a part of the lung has a reduced blood supply. Nevertheless, the isotope study does detect the abnormal pulmonary blood flow caused by the embolus (FIGURE 12-5). Consequently, the lung scan will be abnormal even when the lung is not infarcted, and the routine chest x-ray appears normal.

Pulmonary Angiography

The definitive diagnostic method to identify a pulmonary embolism is a pulmonary angiogram, which directly visualizes the pulmonary artery and its branches. A catheter is inserted into a vein in the arm and advanced up the vein through the superior vena cava, into the right side of the heart, and out the pulmonary artery. A radiopaque material is then injected into the artery through the catheter, and the flow of the material through the pulmonary arteries is visualized by means of serial x-ray films. If the pulmonary artery or one of its branches is completely obstructed by an embolus, no contrast material flows into the blocked vessel (FIGURE 12-6). If the embolus does not completely obstruct the artery, some contrast medium flows around the embolus, which appears as a filling defect in the column of contrast material within the partially occluded vessel. New advanced CT equipment can provide similar information and does not require insertion of a catheter into the pulmonary artery, although an intravenous injection of radiopaque contrast material is required. The equipment can monitor the flow of contrast material through the pulmonary artery and its branches and can detect an obstruction of blood flow within the pulmonary circulation, indicating a pulmonary embolus.

TREATMENT OF PULMONARY EMBOLISM

Treatment of patients with pulmonary embolism includes general supportive care and administration of anticoagulants. Heparin, which has an immediate effect, is

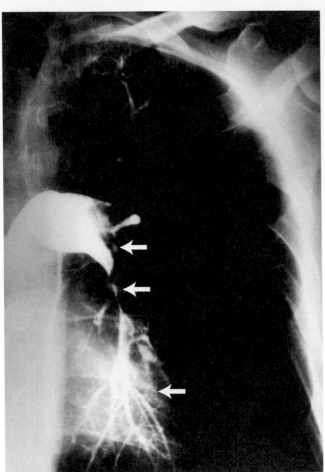

FIGURE 12-6 An angiogram used to identify pulmonary embolism illustrated by view of the left lung and pulmonary artery. A catheter has been inserted into the pulmonary artery and radiopaque contrast material injected. Flow of contrast material is almost completely blocked (*upper arrow*) by a large pulmonary embolus obstructing the left main pulmonary artery. Only a thin trickle of contrast material flows around the embolus (*middle arrow*) to fill the pulmonary artery branches supplying part of the lower lobe (*lower arrow*).

generally used initially, followed by administration of coumadin-type anticoagulants, which act by depressing hepatic synthesis of coagulation factors. The purpose of anticoagulant therapy is twofold: (1) to prevent recurrent pulmonary emboli by preventing the formation of more thrombi in leg and pelvic veins and (2) to prevent thrombus formation in branches of the pulmonary artery distal to the embolism. If adequate therapy is given, further thromboembolism is prevented, and the embolus will slowly dissolve. Rarely, if the patient has sustained a massive embolus and is in critical condition because blood flow through a main pulmonary artery is blocked, it is necessary to remove the embolus surgically or dissolve the embolus rapidly by administering clot-dissolving (thrombolytic) drugs. These are the same drugs that are given to a heart attack patient in order to dissolve a thrombus blocking a coronary artery (discussion on the cardiovascular system).

If the patient continues to have pulmonary emboli despite adequate anticoagulant therapy, it may be necessary to perform surgery on the inferior vena cava to interrupt the passage of clots from the peripheral veins to the lungs. Generally, the operative procedure consists of either complete or partial interruption of the vena cava below the level of the renal veins. Complete interruption is accomplished by surgical ligation of the vein. Partial interruption has been performed by various methods in such a way as to allow normal blood flow and yet trap emboli.

The following case illustrates the clinical features of a large pulmonary embolism treated successfully by anticoagulant therapy.

CASE 12-1

A 26-year-old woman consulted her physician because of cough and marked shortness of breath. Physical examination revealed that she was in severe respiratory distress with a dry, hacking cough. Her lips and fingernails were slightly cyanotic, indicating poor oxygenation of the blood. Chest x-ray revealed prominent pulmonary arteries but no evidence of pulmonary consolidation suggesting an infarct. The oxygen saturation of the arterial blood was reduced, which was compatible with a pulmonary embolus. An angiographic study revealed that the left main pulmonary artery was occluded by a pulmonary embolus. The patient received anticoagulant therapy and supplementary oxygen. Her condition gradually improved. Past medical history was significant in that the patient was taking a relatively high-estrogen contraceptive pill for control of a menstrual irregularity. The pill apparently predisposed her to thrombosis of a leg vein, which was followed by a pulmonary embolus.

Arterial Thrombosis

Blood flow in arteries is rapid, and intravascular pressure is high; so stasis of blood is not a factor in arterial thrombosis. The main cause of arterial thrombosis is injury to the wall of the vessel, usually secondary to arteriosclerosis. The arteriosclerotic deposits cause ulceration and roughening of the lining of the artery, and thrombi form on the roughened area. The effects of arterial thrombus formation depend on the location and size of the artery that has become obstructed. Blockage of a coronary artery frequently causes infarction of the heart muscle and consequent "heart attack." If a major artery supplying the leg is occluded, the extremity undergoes necrosis, usually called **gangrene** (FIGURE 12-7). (This differs from gas gangrene, which is caused by a species of *Clostridium*.) Occlusion of an artery to the brain leads to infarction of a portion of the brain, commonly called a "stroke."

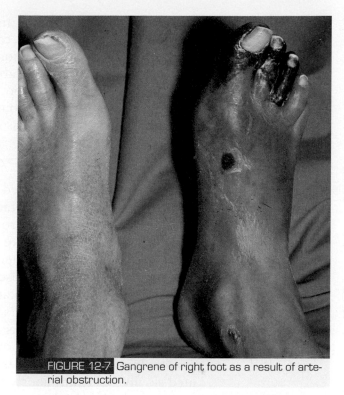

FIGURE 12-7 Gangrene of right foot as a result of arterial obstruction.

Intracardiac Thrombosis

Occasionally, blood clots may form within the heart itself. Thrombi may form within the atrial appendages when heart function is abnormal, as in heart failure, or when the atria are not contracting normally. Thrombi may also form on the surfaces of heart valves that have been damaged as a result of disease. Occasionally, thrombi may form on the internal lining of the ventricle adjacent to an area where the heart muscle is infarcted. Intracardiac thrombi may become dislodged and may be carried into the systemic circulation, resulting in infarction of the spleen, kidneys, brain, or other organs. The symptoms produced depend on the size and location of the infarction.

Gangrene
(gang-grēn′)
Term has two different meanings. Refers to (1) infection caused by gas-forming anaerobic bacteria (gas gangrene) or (2) necrosis of an extremity caused by interruption of its blood supply (ischemic gangrene).

Clostridium
(klä-strid′ē-yum)
Anaerobic gram-positive spore-forming rod-shaped bacterium.

Thrombosis Caused by Increased Blood Coagulability

In some conditions, the concentration of various blood coagulation factors is elevated, increasing the coagulability of the blood and predisposing the individual to intravascular clotting. After injury or operation, products of tissue necrosis with thromboplastic activity stimulate the synthesis of many clotting factors. This increases the likelihood of postoperative thrombosis in leg veins.

The estrogen in contraceptive pills has been found to stimulate synthesis of coagulation factors, raising their concentration and predisposing the women who use the pills to both venous and arterial thrombosis. This observation has led to concern about the safety of "the pill" when used for long periods of time.

Hereditary gene mutations affecting the synthesis of coagulation factors may also increase blood coagulability and the risk of venous thrombosis. One is a relatively common mutation, present in about 5% of the population, that codes for synthesis of coagulation factor V. This is one of the factors involved in the conversion of prothrombin to thrombin in the second phase of blood coagulation. Normal factor

V is inactivated by a coagulation inhibitor called protein C, which terminates its activity. The abnormal factor, called factor V Leiden (after a city in the Netherlands), is more resistant to inactivation, which prolongs the activity of the mutant factor, thereby increasing the coagulability of the blood and the risk of venous thrombosis. The other significant mutation, found in 2% of the population, affects a gene regulating synthesis of prothrombin. The mutation leads to a higher than normal level of prothrombin and is also associated with an increased risk of venous thrombosis.

THROMBOSIS IN PATIENTS WITH CANCER

Many patients with advanced cancer have elevated platelets and increased concentrations of coagulation factors in their blood, and they are predisposed to both venous and arterial thromboses. This tendency results from the release of thromboplastic materials into the circulation from deposits of tumor. The same basic mechanism induces hemorrhage in patients with a disseminated intravascular coagulation syndrome (discussed on abnormalities of blood coagulation). The variations in clinical manifestations result from differences in the rate at which the thromboplastic material enters the circulation. In the acute process, a large quantity of thromboplastic material is rapidly released into the circulation. Platelets and coagulation factors are consumed faster than they can be replenished, and bleeding results. In patients with widespread cancer, the thromboplastic material is liberated slowly but continuously from the tumor. The blood coagulation mechanism is activated, and clot lysis occurs. Production of coagulation factors and platelets increases in response to an increased demand, but the body overcompensates. Production exceeds destruction, which leads to a hypercoagulable state. FIGURE 12-8 compares these two processes.

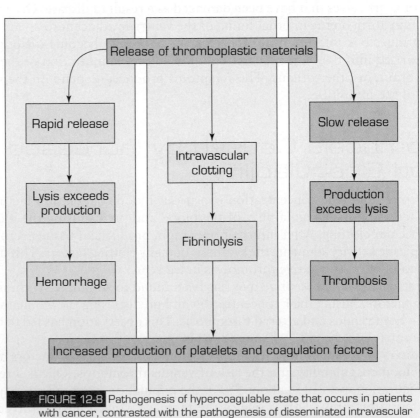

FIGURE 12-8 Pathogenesis of hypercoagulable state that occurs in patients with cancer, contrasted with the pathogenesis of disseminated intravascular coagulation syndrome. Different clinical manifestations reflect differing rates of fibrinolysis and compensatory regeneration of hemostatic components.

Embolism as a Result of Foreign Material

Most emboli are caused by blood clots, but other materials occasionally gain access to the circulation. Fat, air, and foreign particles within the vascular system may sometimes cause serious difficulties.

FAT EMBOLISM

After a severe bone fracture, fatty bone marrow and surrounding adipose tissue may be disrupted. The emulsified fat globules may be sucked into the veins and carried into the lungs, leading to widespread obstruction of the pulmonary capillaries. Some of the fat may be carried through the pulmonary capillaries and may reach the systemic circulation, eventually blocking small blood vessels in the brain and other organs.

AMNIONIC FLUID EMBOLISM

This condition is an uncommon but devastating complication of pregnancy that usually occurs during labor when the pressure of uterine contractions forces a large volume of amnionic fluid through a tear in fetal membranes into a torn uterine vein at the site of a cervical or uterine laceration. The amnionic fluid, which contains desquamated fetal epithelial cells and hair, fatty material (vernix), debris from the fetal respiratory and gastrointestinal tract, and thromboplastic material, is carried in the maternal venous circulation to the lungs, where it plugs the pulmonary capillaries. Manifestations are severe dyspnea, shock, and often an acute disseminated intravascular coagulation syndrome induced by the thromboplastic material in the amnionic fluid (Figure 12-8).

AIR EMBOLISM

Sometimes, a large amount of air is sucked into the venous circulation after a chest wound with injury to the lung. Air may also be accidentally injected into the circulation in attempts at abortion by persons without medical training. The air is carried to the heart and accumulates in the right heart chambers, preventing filling of the heart by returning venous blood. As a result, the heart is unable to pump blood, and the individual dies rapidly of circulatory failure.

EMBOLISM OF PARTICULATE FOREIGN MATERIAL

Various types of particulate material may be injected into veins by drug abusers, who crush and dissolve tablets intended for oral use and inject the material intravenously. The material is usually trapped within the small pulmonary blood vessels, producing symptoms of severe respiratory distress caused by obstruction of the pulmonary capillaries by the foreign material.

Edema

The term **edema** refers to accumulation of fluid in the interstitial tissues. Edema is most conspicuous in the skin and subcutaneous tissues of the dependent parts of the body and is usually noted first in the legs and ankles. When the edematous tissue is compressed by indenting the tissue with the fingertips, the fluid is pushed aside, leaving a pit or indentation that gradually refills with fluid. This characteristic is responsible for the common term pitting edema. Fluid may also accumulate in the pleural cavity (**hydrothorax**) or in the peritoneal cavity (**ascites**).

Edema may result from any condition in which the circulation of extracellular fluid between the capillaries and the interstitial tissues becomes disturbed.

Edema
(e-dē′muh)
Accumulation of an excess of fluid in the interstitial tissues.

Hydrothorax
(hī-drō-thor′ax)
Accumulation of fluid in the pleural cavity.

Ascites
(a-si′tēz)
Accumulation of fluid in the abdominal cavity.

FACTORS REGULATING FLUID FLOW BETWEEN CAPILLARIES AND INTERSTITIAL TISSUE

The flow of fluid through the interstitial space depends on four factors:

1. The capillary hydrostatic pressure, which tends to filter fluid from the blood through the capillary endothelium.

2. The permeability of the capillaries, which determines the ease with which the fluid can pass through the capillary endothelium.

3. The osmotic pressure exerted by the proteins in the blood plasma (called colloid osmotic pressure), which tends to attract fluid from the interstitial space back into the vascular compartment. Osmotic pressure, which was considered in cells and tissues: their structure and function in health and disease discussion, may be defined as the property causing fluid to migrate in the direction of a higher concentration of molecules. The osmotic pressure of the plasma depends primarily on the concentration of the plasma proteins. Because the capillaries are impermeable to protein, the protein tends to draw water from the interstitial fluid into the capillaries and to hold it there.

4. The presence of open lymphatic channels, which collect some of the fluid forced out of the capillaries by the hydrostatic pressure of the blood and return the fluid to the circulation.

FIGURE 12-9 illustrates the mechanism by which fluid flow is regulated through interstitial tissues.

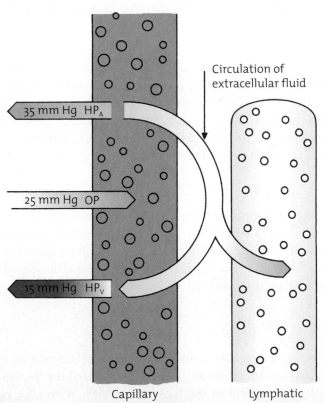

FIGURE 12-9 Factors regulating the flow of fluid through the interstitial tissues, as described in the text. HP$_A$, hydrostatic pressure at the arterial end of the capillary. HP$_V$, hydrostatic pressure at the venous end of the capillary. OP, osmotic pressure. Pressures are indicated in millimeters of mercury (mm Hg). Fluid is forced from the arterial end of the capillary because the hydrostatic pressure exceeds the osmotic pressure. At the venous end of the capillary, the hydrostatic pressure is lower than the osmotic pressure and fluid returns. Lymphatic channels also collect some of the fluid forced from the capillaries by the hydrostatic pressure.

Flow of Fluid Into and Out of Capillaries

The pressure of the blood at the arterial end of the capillary is higher than the colloid osmotic pressure, which causes fluid to be filtered through the endothelium of the capillaries into the interstitial space. The capillary endothelium acts as a semipermeable membrane and limits the rate at which fluid is filtered from the blood. At the venous end of the capillary, the hydrostatic pressure is lower than the colloid osmotic pressure, and fluid tends to diffuse back into the capillaries. In this way, the fluid containing dissolved nutrients is carried from the blood into the interstitial tissues to nourish the cells, and waste products are returned to the circulation for excretion.

PATHOGENESIS AND CLASSIFICATION OF EDEMA

Increased Capillary Permeability

Normally, the endothelium of the capillaries limits the amount of fluid filtered from the blood. If the capillaries are excessively permeable, filtration of fluid into the interstitial space is greater than normal. Increased capillary permeability is responsible for the swelling of the tissues associated with an acute inflammation such as a boil or a severe sunburn. Some systemic diseases also cause a generalized increase in capillary permeability, which leads to widespread edema of the subcutaneous tissues (FIGURE 12-10).

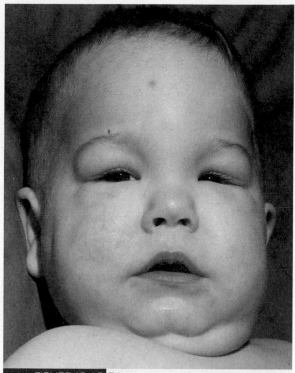

FIGURE 12-10 Edema as a result of increased capillary permeability. Note the swelling of the eyelids and face.

Low Plasma Proteins

If the concentration of plasma proteins is decreased, the colloid osmotic pressure is reduced correspondingly. Consequently, less fluid is attracted back into the capillaries, and the fluid accumulates in the tissues. A low concentration of plasma proteins may result from excessive loss of plasma proteins in the urine, as occurs in patients with some types of kidney disease or from inadequate synthesis of plasma proteins as a result of malnutrition or starvation (FIGURE 12-11). Hypoproteinemia caused by inadequate protein intake may be encountered in patients with chronic debilitating diseases who are unable to eat an adequate amount of food and in patients with intestinal diseases in whom assimilation of food is impaired.

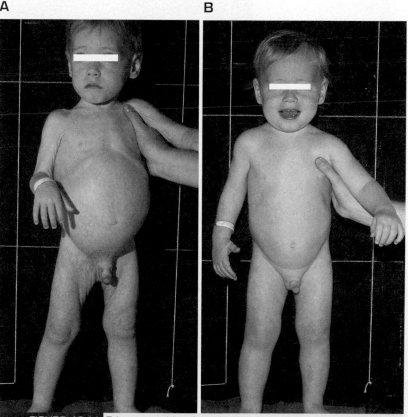

FIGURE 12-11 Edema resulting from low plasma proteins as a result of malnutrition. **A**, Child prior to treatment, illustrating emaciation, abdominal distention caused by accumulation of fluid in the peritoneal cavity, and edema of legs. **B**, Same child after treatment by a nutritious high-protein diet.

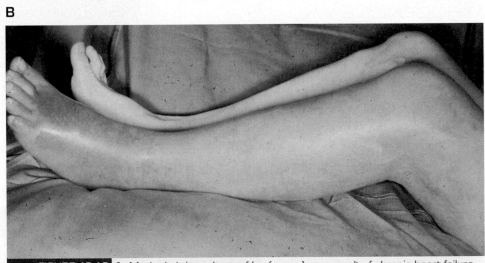

FIGURE 12-12 **A**, Marked pitting edema of leg (*arrow*) as a result of chronic heart failure. **B**, Localized edema of left leg caused by venous obstruction. Right leg appears normal.

Increased Hydrostatic Pressure

Increased pressure in the veins draining the capillaries is reflected as a higher than normal pressure at the venous end of the capillaries. As a result, more fluid is filtered from the capillaries, causing it to accumulate in the tissues. A localized increase in venous pressure may be encountered if the veins draining a part of the body become compressed, twisted, or obstructed by a blood clot that fills the lumen. More commonly, the increased venous pressure is a manifestation of heart failure, and the pressure is elevated in all the systemic veins (FIGURE 12-12).

Lymphatic Obstruction

Sometimes, lymphatic channels draining a part of the body become obstructed because of disease. The obstruction blocks a pathway by which fluid is returned from the interstitial space into the circulation and leads to edema in the region that is normally drained by the obstructed lymphatic vessels (FIGURE 12-13).

Shock

Shock is a general term to describe any condition in which the blood pressure is too low to provide adequate blood flow to the body cells and organs, and is a serious,

Shock
A general term for any condition leading to such a marked fall of blood pressure that body tissues do not receive an adequate amount of oxygen, most often caused by acute blood loss or severe infection (sepsis).

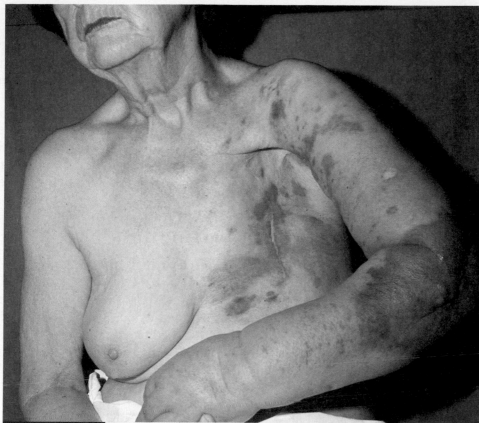

FIGURE 12-13 Severe edema of arm resulting from long-standing lymphatic obstruction. The patient had a radical operation for breast carcinoma many years previously. Scarring in the axilla blocked lymphatic drainage from the arm, leading to chronic edema. The dark discolored areas in the skin of the chest wall and upper limb are caused by a malignant tumor of lymphatic vessels (lymphangiosarcoma), which sometimes complicates chronic lymphedema.

potentially life-threatening condition. Shock results from a disproportion between the volume of blood in the circulatory system and the capacity of the vascular system that carries the blood. Blood pressure falls if the volume of blood filling the circulatory system falls or if marked dilation of blood vessels expands the capacity of the vascular system to such an extent that the existing blood volume is insufficient to fill the vessels adequately.

CLASSIFICATION

Often shock is classified in four categories based on its cause (pathogenesis).

1. Hypovolemic shock is caused by low blood volume, leading to a corresponding drop in blood pressure. Most cases result from a large hemorrhage that significantly reduces the circulating blood volume, but any excessive depletion of body fluids such as fluid losses from a severe burn, from severe diarrhea, or from excessive fluid loss in urine resulting from diuretics can also reduce blood volume as fluid shifts from the vascular compartment into the depleted extravascular body fluids.

2. Cardiogenic shock is caused by inadequate or impaired cardiac pumping function, which reduces cardiac output. Cardiogenic shock usually is a complication of a myocardial infarction, but the pumping function of the heart can also be impaired if the heart is compressed by accumulation of

blood or fluid within the pericardial sac, which prevents filling of the heart in diastole, or by other conditions that cause acute heart failure.

3. Septic shock results from excessive dilation of the body's blood vessels, in which the volume of circulating blood is insufficient to fill adequately the greatly expanded capacity of the blood vessels. Marked vasodilation results from the severe infection in which microbial toxins and mediators of inflammation that are released at the site of infection dilate the vessels.

4. Anaphylactic shock (described in the discussion on immunity, hypersensitivity, allergy, and autoimmune diseases) also results from excessive vasodilation caused by the widespread release of mediators of inflammation from mast cells and basophils, which is often followed by circulatory collapse.

PROGNOSIS AND TREATMENT

The outcome of shock depends on its cause and how quickly it is recognized and treated. Treatment consists of administering drugs that raise blood pressure by constricting blood vessels, restoring blood volume by intravenous fluids or blood if the shock is caused by a severe hemorrhage, and treating the underlying condition that leads to the shock. Unfortunately, septic shock or cardiogenic shock in an elderly patient with other medical problems has a very poor prognosis.

QUESTIONS FOR REVIEW

1. What is the difference between a thrombus and an embolus? What is an infarct?
2. What factors predispose to venous thrombosis? What is the major complication of a thrombus in a leg vein?
3. What factors predispose to arterial thrombosis?
4. What are the causes and effects of intracardiac thrombi?
5. What conditions predispose to thrombosis by increasing the coagulability of the blood?
6. What factors regulate the flow of fluid between capillaries and interstitial tissue? What are the major causes of edema?
7. What coagulation disturbances may be encountered in patients with tumors?
8. What is the difference between a pulmonary embolus and a pulmonary infarct? What are the clinical manifestations of a pulmonary infarct?

SUPPLEMENTARY READINGS

Alperin, J. B. 1987. Coagulopathy caused by vitamin K deficiency in critically ill, hospitalized patients. *Journal of the American Medical Association* 258:1916–9.
   ▶ Vitamin K deficiency in hospitalized patients is common and can be misdiagnosed as disseminated intravascular coagulation syndrome. It can be prevented by prophylactic vitamin K in seriously ill patients receiving antibiotics.

Blom, J. W., Doggen, C. J., Osanto, S., et al. 2005. Malignancies, prothrombotic mutations, and the risk of venous thrombosis. *Journal of the American Medical Association* 293:715–22.
   ▶ Patients with cancer have a sevenfold greater risk of venous thrombosis than a comparable control group of patients, especially in the first few months after diagnosis and in the presence of distant metastases. Two hereditary gene mutations increase the

risk even more by greatly increasing the coagulability of the blood. One is a relatively common mutation of a gene coding for the synthesis of coagulation factor V called *factor V Leiden*. Normal factor V is inactivated by a coagulation inhibitor called *protein C* during coagulation of the blood, but factor V Leiden is less efficiently inhibited. Mutation of another gene that regulates prothrombin synthesis leads to a higher than normal concentration of prothrombin in the blood.

Goldhaber, S. Z. 2005. Multislice computed tomography for pulmonary embolism—a technological marvel. *New England Journal of Medicine* 352:1812–4.

▶ CT scanning of the chest has revolutionized the diagnostic approach to pulmonary embolism and has largely replaced radioisotope lung scans to evaluate suspected pulmonary emboli.

Hull, R. D. 2006. Diagnosing pulmonary embolism with improved certainty and simplicity. *Journal of the American Medical Association* 295:213–5.

▶ Ultrasound has supplanted venography for diagnosing a deep vein thrombosis. Spiral CT provides information about a possible pulmonary embolus. D-dimer is a degradation product of fibrin, which is elevated if there is a leg vein thrombus, and rapid tests are available. Judicious application of these methods improves diagnostic accuracy and allows the clinician to detect a pulmonary embolus or exclude the possibility with more assurance than was available previously.

Litin, S. C., and Gastineau, D. A. 1995. Current concepts in anticoagulant therapy. *Mayo Clinic Proceedings* 70:266–72.

▶ Discusses various anticoagulation strategies for treating venous thromboembolic disease and methods for monitoring anticoagulant therapy.

Miller, G. H., and Feied, C. F. 1995. Suspected pulmonary embolism. The difficulties of diagnostic evaluation. *Postgraduate Medicine* 97:51–8.

▶ Discusses the use of various diagnostic procedures in the diagnosis of pulmonary embolism.

OUTLINE SUMMARY

Intravascular Blood Clots

Thrombosis and Embolism

PATHOGENESIS
Slowing or stasis of blood flow.
Damage to wall of blood vessel.
Increased coagulability of blood.

TERMINOLOGY
Thrombosis: intravascular clot.
Embolus: detached clot carried in circulation.
Infarct: tissue necrosis caused by interruption of blood supply.

Venous Thrombosis

PREDISPOSING FACTORS
Stasis of blood in veins.
Varicose veins.
Increased blood coagulability.

Pulmonary Embolism

LARGE PULMONARY EMBOLI
Obstructs main pulmonary artery or major branches.
Obstructs blood flow to lungs.
Causes severe dyspnea and cyanosis.
May cause shock and sudden death.
Usually lung is not infarcted because adequate collateral blood flow is provided by bronchial arteries.

SMALL PULMONARY EMBOLI
Become impacted in peripheral branches of pulmonary artery.
Collateral circulation may be inadequate, and lung infarct develops.
Causes chest pain, cough, and bloody sputum secondary to infarct.

DIAGNOSIS
Chest x-ray: detects infarct, not embolus.
Lung scan: detects impaired lung perfusion secondary to embolus.
Pulmonary angiography: detects blocked pulmonary artery.

TREATMENT
Anticoagulants.
Operation on inferior vena cava to prevent passage of clots if anticoagulants ineffective.

SEPTIC PULMONARY EMBOLI
Thrombi form in pelvic veins after pelvic infection.
Bacteria invade thrombi.
Infected thrombus is transported to lungs and causes pulmonary infarct.
Bacteria in clot invade infarct, which becomes infected and forms lung abscess.

Arterial Thrombosis
PATHOGENESIS
Roughening of arterial wall caused by arteriosclerosis.
Thrombus forms on roughened surface.

CLINICAL MANIFESTATIONS DEPEND ON VESSEL AFFECTED
Heart attack.
Stroke.
Gangrene of extremity.

Intracardiac Thrombosis
LOCATION
Atrial appendage: in heart failure.
Heart valves: secondary to valve injury.
Left ventricle: secondary to infarct of heart muscle.

Thrombosis Caused by Increased Blood Coagulability
PREDISPOSING FACTORS
Postoperative increase in coagulation factors.
Estrogens in contraceptive pills.
Malignant tumors: induce hypercoagulable state.

Embolism as a Result of Foreign Material
SOURCES
Fat embolism: after fracture.
Amnionic fluid embolism during labor.
Air embolism: after chest injury.
Particulate material: associated with illicit drug use.

Edema
FACTORS REGULATING FLOW OF FLUID BETWEEN CAPILLARIES AND INTERSTITIAL TISSUE
Hydrostatic pressure.
Capillary permeability.
Osmotic pressure.
Open lymphatic channel.
PATHOGENESIS AND CLASSIFICATION
Increased capillary permeability.
Low plasma proteins:
  Excess protein loss: kidney disease.
  Inadequate synthesis: malnutrition.
Increased hydrostatic pressure:
  Heart failure.
  Localized venous obstruction.
Lymphatic obstruction.

Shock
BLOOD PRESSURE TOO LOW TO SUPPLY BODY
Classified by pathogenesis.
Hypovolemic shock: low blood volume.
Cardiogenic shock: impaired cardiac pumping function.
Septic shock: excessive vasodilation.
Anaphylactic shock: excessive vasodilation.

PROGNOSIS DEPENDS ON EARLY RECOGNITION AND RAPID APPROPRIATE TREATMENT

CHAPTER 13

The Cardiovascular System

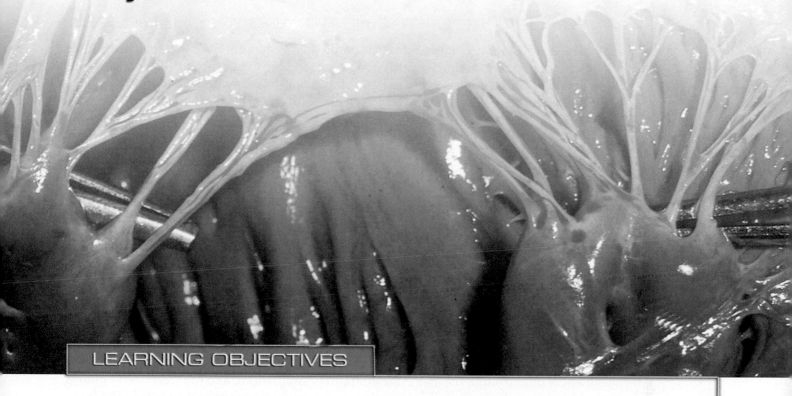

LEARNING OBJECTIVES

1 Explain the basic anatomy and physiology of the heart as they relate to the common types of heart disease.

2 Describe the common causes of congenital heart disease and valvular heart disease. Explain the effects of these diseases. Describe the methods of treating congenital and acquired valvular heart disease.

3 Describe the pathogenesis of coronary heart disease. List the four most important risk factors. Describe the clinical manifestations of coronary heart disease. Explain the methods of treatment and their rationales.

4 List the major complications of myocardial infarction and describe their clinical manifestations.

5 Explain the general principles applied to the diagnosis and treatment of coronary heart disease and myocardial infarction.

6 Explain the current concepts regarding the effect of diet on coronary heart disease. Describe how cholesterol is transported by lipoproteins. Distinguish between "good" and "bad" cholesterol.

7 Describe the adverse effects of hypertension on the cardiovascular system and the kidneys.

8 Differentiate between pathogenesis of acute and chronic heart failure. Describe the pathogenesis of each, and list the principles of treatment.

9 Differentiate between the pathogenesis and clinical manifestations of arteriosclerotic and dissecting aneurysms of the aorta. Explain the principles of treatment.

10 List the common diseases affecting veins, their clinical manifestations, and methods of treatment.

Cardiac Structure and Function

The heart is a muscular pump that propels blood through the lungs and to the peripheral tissues. Heart disease is caused by a disturbance in the function of the cardiac pump. A working knowledge of the normal structure and function of the heart is essential to an understanding of the various types of heart disease.

STRUCTURE OF THE HEART AND ITS CHAMBERS

The heart is a cone-shaped muscular pump that weighs about 350 g, enclosed within a fibrous sac called the pericardial sac located in the mediastinum. The pericardium is lined by a layer of mesothelial cells that is continuous with a similar layer of mesothelial cells covering the external surface of the heart.

The heart is composed of three layers: (1) the epicardium consisting of a layer of mesothelial cells overlying a small amount of loose fibrous and adipose tissue; (2) the myocardium, a thick layer of muscle that forms the bulk of the heart; and (3) the endocardium, a thin layer of endothelial cells that lines the chambers and covers the surfaces of the heart valves. The heart is divided into four chambers by partitions. The two upper chambers are separated by the interatrial septum into the right and left atria, which receive venous blood returning to the heart. The two lower chambers are separated by the interventricular septum into the right and left ventricles. The right ventricle pumps blood through the pulmonary artery to the lungs, where it is oxygenated and returned to the left atrium, and the left ventricle pumps oxygen-rich blood throughout the body, which is then collected into veins and returned to the right atrium. Although the right and left cardiac chambers work together, no direct communications normally exist between the chambers on the right and left sides of the heart, and it is convenient clinically to consider each half as an independent structure. The "right heart" circulates blood into the pulmonary artery and through the lungs (the pulmonary circulation), and the "left heart" pumps blood into the aorta for distribution to the various organs and tissues in the body (the systemic circulation) (FIGURE 13-1).

The atrial and ventricular muscle is arranged in bundles that encircle the heart and attach to a layer of dense fibrous tissue called the fibrous framework of the heart located between the atria and ventricles, which also extends into the upper part of the interventricular septum and surrounds the openings of the cardiac valves. The fibrous framework separates the atrial muscle fibers from those in the ventricles so that the atrial and ventricular muscles can function independently. Contraction of cardiac muscle reduces the size of the atria or ventricles, raising the pressure of the blood within the compressed chambers, which squeezes blood out of the chambers. The fibrous framework also provides a firm support to which the heart valves can attach, and contains a small opening to allow the atrioventricular bundle (bundle of His), which is part of the impulse conducting system, to carry impulses to the ventricles.

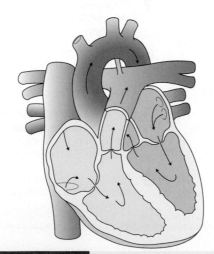

FIGURE 13-1 Normal blood flow through the right and left cardiac chambers: the pulmonary and systemic circulations.

CARDIAC VALVES

The flow of blood into and out of the cardiac chambers is controlled by a system of valves that normally permits flow in only one direction. The **atrioventricular (AV) valves** are flaplike valves surrounding the orifices between atria and ventricles. The free margins of the valves are connected to the papillary muscles of the ventricular walls by narrow, stringlike bands of fibrous tissue called the *chordae tendineae* (FIGURE 13-2A). These bands prevent the valves from prolapsing into the atria during ventricular systole. The **semilunar valves** surrounding the orifices of the aorta and pulmonary artery are positioned so that the free margins of the valves face upward. This structural arrangement defines cuplike pockets between the free margins of the valves and the roots of the blood vessels to which the valves are attached (FIGURE 13-2B).

Atrioventricular (AV) valve
(a′trē-o-ven-trik′ū-lar)
The flaplike heart valve located between the atrium and ventricle.

Semilunar valve
The cup-shaped valve located between the ventricles and the aorta or pulmonary artery.

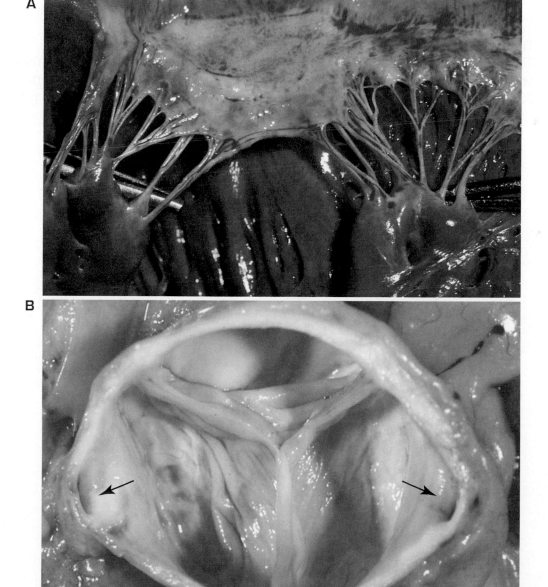

FIGURE 13-2 **A,** Normal mitral valve, illustrating thin chordae extending from valve leaflets to papillary muscles. **B,** Aortic valve viewed from above, illustrating a cup-shaped configuration of valve leaflets. Note the openings of coronary arteries (*arrows*) arising from base of aorta adjacent to aortic valve leaflets.

When the heart relaxes in diastole, the chordae produce tension on the valves and pull the atrioventricular valves apart. When the ventricles contract, the chordae are no longer under tension, and the force of the blood flow pushes the valves together so that no blood flows from the ventricles into the atria. During ventricular contraction, the semilunar valves are forced apart by the jets of blood leaving the ventricles. When ventricular contraction ceases, the weight of the column of ejected blood forces the valves back into position, preventing reflux of blood into the ventricles during diastole. The atrioventricular and semilunar valves function reciprocally. Ventricular contraction relaxes tension on the chordae, causing the atrioventricular valves to close at the same time that the jets of blood open the semilunar valves. Closure of the semilunar valves in diastole is also associated with opening of the atrioventricular valves. FIGURE 13-3 illustrates the reciprocal action of the two sets of valves, which is responsible for the unidirectional flow required for normal cardiac function.

BLOOD SUPPLY TO THE HEART

The Left and Right Coronary Arteries

The heart is supplied by two large coronary arteries that arise from the aortic sinuses at the root of the aorta (FIGURE 13-4). The left coronary artery is a short vessel that soon divides into two major branches. The left anterior descending artery descends

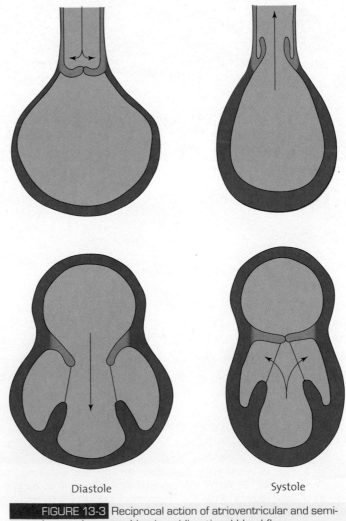

Diastole

Systole

FIGURE 13-3 Reciprocal action of atrioventricular and semilunar valves, resulting in unidirectional blood flow.

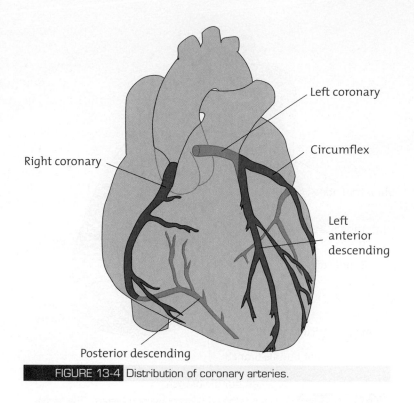

Left coronary

Circumflex

Right coronary

Left anterior descending

Posterior descending

FIGURE 13-4 Distribution of coronary arteries.

to supply the front of the heart and the anterior part of the interventricular septum. The circumflex artery swings to the left (*circum* = around + *flex* = bend) to supply the left side of the heart. The right coronary artery swings to the right, supplying the right side of the heart, and then descends to supply the back of the heart and the posterior part of the interventricular septum. Each coronary artery gives off many branches that supply the heart muscle. The terminal branches of the coronary arteries frequently communicate with each other by means of connections called **anastomoses**. Because of these connections, obstruction of one of the arteries does not necessarily completely interrupt the blood flow to the tissues supplied by the blocked vessel. There may be enough blood flow through anastomoses with other arteries to supply the heart muscle. This is called a **collateral circulation**.

CONDUCTION SYSTEM OF THE HEART

The impulses that cause the heart to beat are initiated and propagated by groups of specialized muscle cells that depolarize spontaneously, which is called the conduction system of the heart (FIGURE 13-5). Impulses normally are generated in the sinoatrial (SA) node, which is located in the right atrium near the opening of the superior vena cava. Small bundles of fibers called internodal tracts connect the SA node to the atrioventricular (AV) node, which is located posteriorly in the lower part of the atrial septum. The atrioventricular bundle (bundle of His) is the continuation of the AV node, which transmits the impulse to the ventricles by passing through a small opening in the fibrous framework of the heart, the fibrous tissue that separates the atrial muscle from the ventricular muscle. After entering the ventricles, the AV bundle divides into right and left bundle branches in the upper part of the interventricular septum, then descends in the septum and extends into the ventricles, where they terminate as Purkinje fibers that activate the heart muscle. The depolarization rate is also influenced by the autonomic nervous system. Sympathetic nervous system impulses increase the rate, and parasympathetic impulses slow it. The normal rhythm established by the cardiac conduction system is often called a normal sinus rhythm

Anastomosis
(ä-nas-ta-mō′sis)
A communication between two blood vessels or other tubular structures. Also refers to a surgical connection of two hollow tubular structures, such as the divided ends of the intestine or a blood vessel (surgical anastomosis).

Collateral circulation
An accessory circulation capable of delivering blood to a tissue when the main circulation is blocked, as by a thrombus or embolus.

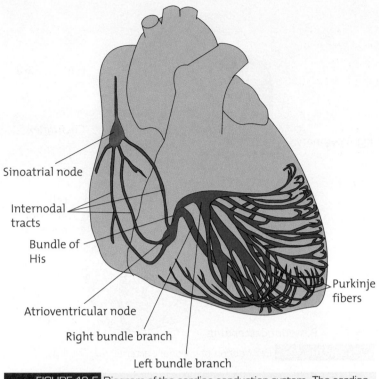

Sinoatrial node

Internodal tracts

Bundle of His

Atrioventricular node

Right bundle branch

Left bundle branch

FIGURE 13-5 Diagram of the cardiac conduction system. The cardiac impulse originates in the SA node and is conducted to the ventricles via the inter-nodal tracts, the AV node, the bundle of His, and the right and left bundle branches, which terminate in the network of Purkinje fibers.

Purkinje fibers

to emphasize that the normal cardiac rhythm is controlled by the sinoatrial node (which is often called simply the sinus node).

Although any part of the conduction system can depolarize spontaneously and generate an impulse, the SA node normally functions as the cardiac pacemaker because it depolarizes about 60 to 70 times per minute, which in turn depolarizes the other parts of the conduction system that depolarize at a slower rate. However, if impulse transmission from the SA node is interrupted by damage to the conduction system, the AV node, which discharges at about 50 times per minute, can take over, and if this system fails, then the bundle or bundle branches can initiate impulses but at a still slower rate of about 30 to 40 times per minute.

THE CARDIAC CYCLE

The sequence of events that occurs during a single contraction and relaxation of the cardiac chambers is called a cardiac cycle. During diastole, both the atria and ventricles are relaxed, the chambers are dilated, and the pressure of the blood within the chambers is very low. In a normal person at rest, each ventricle in diastole contains about 120 ml of blood, and much of the blood that fills the ventricles flows passively into the ventricles through the open atrioventricular valves. Atrial systole expels an additional 30 ml of blood into the ventricles. If the heart rate is normal, the additional blood pumped into the ventricles by atrial contractions is not essential for reasonably normal cardiac function because most of the blood flows into the ventricles during diastole. Atrial systole delivers a relatively small additional amount. However, the additional blood pumped into the ventricles during atrial systole becomes progressively more important as the heart rate increases, which shortens the length of diastole and reduces the volume of blood flowing passively into the ventricles. Atrial systole makes a much greater contribution to ventricular filling when the heart beats rapidly.

The ventricles contract following completion of atrial systole, ejecting blood into the aorta at high pressure and into the pulmonary artery at much lower pressure. Both ventricles contract at the same time, and each ventricle ejects the same volume of blood. Only about 70 ml is ejected from each ventricle during a systolic contraction, which is called the stroke volume, and is about 60% of the blood contained within the ventricles. The percentage of the ventricular volume ejected during systole is called the ejection fraction, and this measurement is often used when evaluating patients with heart failure.

Cardiac output is the output of blood from a single ventricle in 1 minute, and is the product of the stroke volume (about 70 ml) multiplied by the heart rate (about 72 beats per minute), which equals about 5,000 ml per minute. This is approximately the total blood volume of the average adult. During vigorous activity, the normal heart of a healthy young person can double its stroke volume and greatly increase its heart rate, which can increase cardiac output from 4 to 7 times over resting cardiac output.

BLOOD VESSELS

The heart pumps blood into a system of conduction, distribution, and collection tubes that differ in both their structure and function. It is convenient to consider them as four separate groups:

1. Large elastic arteries conduct the blood to various locations throughout the body. They distend as blood is ejected from the heart during systole and recoil during diastole to maintain flow between contractions.
2. Arterioles are smaller vessels with muscular walls that function like a nozzle on a garden hose to regulate flow from the large arteries into the capillaries. They lower the pressure and dampen the amplitude of the pulsations.
3. Capillaries are thin endothelium-lined channels that deliver nutrients to cells and remove waste products.
4. Veins return blood to the heart under low pressure and usually travel with the arteries.

A separate system of channels carrying fluid called lymph is part of the lymphatic system. Its functions and relation to the circulatory system are considered in the discussion on circulatory disturbances.

BLOOD PRESSURE

The flow of blood in the arteries is a result of the force of ventricular contraction. The pressure within the arteries varies rhythmically with the beating of the heart. The highest pressure is reached during ventricular contraction as blood is ejected into the aorta and its branches (systolic pressure). The pressure is lowest when the ventricles are relaxed (diastolic pressure), and the recoil of the stretched arteries provides the force to propel the blood between contractions. The peripheral arterioles regulate the rate of blood flow into the capillaries by varying the degree of arteriolar constriction. In many respects, the effect is analogous to the resistance to outflow of water from a garden hose, which can be varied by tightening or loosening the nozzle on the hose. Because of the resistance offered by the arterioles, the blood pressure during cardiac diastole does not fall to zero but declines slowly as blood leaves the large arteries through the arterioles into the capillaries.

The elasticity of the large arteries also influences the systolic pressure. Some of the pressure rise caused by the blood ejected from the ventricle is absorbed by the stretch of the arteries so that the systolic pressure does not rise as high as would occur if the arteries were more rigid and unable to stretch normally. In summary, the systolic blood pressure is a measure of the force of ventricular contraction as blood is ejected into the large arteries. The diastolic pressure is a measure of the rate of "run off" of blood into the capillaries, which is governed by the peripheral resistance caused by the small arterioles throughout the body. The mean (average) pressure of blood in the large arteries is approximately midway between systolic and diastolic pressure.

The Electrocardiogram

The electrocardiogram (ECG) is a measure of the electrical activity of the heart as measured on the surface of the body by means of electrodes attached to the legs, arms, and chest. Voltage differences are recorded as a series of upward (positive) and downward (negative) deflections that form a characteristic pattern of deflections named in order: P, Q, R, S, and T (FIGURE 13-6). The P wave reflects the initial wave of depolarization associated with atrial systole. The Q, R, and S waves, called collectively as the QRS complex, reflect the depolarization of the ventricles, which is followed by ventricular systole. The T wave represents repolarization of the ventricles during diastole. The time interval from the beginning of the P wave to the beginning of the QRS complex, which is called the PR interval, reflects the time required for the depolarization wave to pass through the AV bundle from the atria to the ventricles.

Usually, the positive and negative deflections are recorded on calibrated graph paper, each horizontal line representing a standard voltage difference and each vertical line representing a standard time interval. However, the ECG tracing also can be displayed on a fluorescent screen, as when continuously monitoring a patient in a coronary care unit.

The ECG is a valuable diagnostic aid that can identify characteristic disturbances in the heart rate or rhythm and abnormalities in the conduction of impulses through the heart. The ECG can also identify heart muscle injury, as occurs following a heart attack, and can also determine the extent of the damage to the heart muscle.

CARDIAC ARRHYTHMIAS

The orderly depolarization and repolarization of the conduction system that directs the contraction and relaxation of the atria and ventricles do not always function perfectly, which leads to disturbances in the heart rate or rhythm, called cardiac arrhythmias.

Atrial Fibrillation

One of the more common abnormal cardiac rhythms is a condition called atrial fibrillation (AF), in which the atria fail to contract normally. The condition often occurs in older persons, especially those with cardiovascular disease or chronic pulmonary disease, but may also occur in persons whose thyroid glands produce an excess of thyroid hormone (hyperthyroidism) and in a few other conditions. Occasionally, AF occurs in apparently normal healthy persons for no apparent reason.

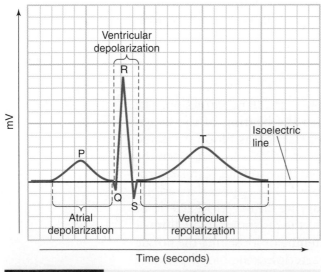

FIGURE 13-6 Characteristic features of a normal electrocardiogram.

AF starts as an abnormal focus of electrical activity in the atrium, which abruptly evolves into multiple areas of depolarization throughout the atria that stimulate atrial muscle fibers continuously in a haphazard disorganized manner at a very rapid rate of up to 400 impulses per minute. The intense disorderly stimulation of multiple groups of atrial muscle fibers causes the atrial muscle to quiver ineffectively instead of contracting normally. The abnormal electrical impulses are also relayed to the AV node, which is overwhelmed and unable to respond to such a large number of stimuli. Only a relatively small number of impulses are able to travel through the AV node and AV bundle (bundle of His) to reach the ventricles, which beat irregularly at about 140 to 160 times per minute (FIGURE 13-7A). At such a fast ventricular contraction rate, the duration of diastole is very short. The duration of diastole also varies from beat to beat because the rate at which impulses can be delivered to the ventricles from the quivering atria is not uniform. As a result, the time available for ventricular filling in diastole also varies from beat to beat, which causes the volume of blood filling the ventricles and ejected during each ventricular contraction (stroke volume) to vary. Some of the ventricular contractions occur before the ventricles are adequately filled with blood, and the volume of blood ejected may not always be enough to be detected as a pulse in the radial artery at the wrist. Consequently, the radial pulse detects fewer beats per minute than the number of ventricular contractions per minute heard with a stethoscope placed on the chest. This discrepancy is called a pulse deficit. The diagnosis of atrial fibrillation is made by examination of the ECG, which reveals a lack of P waves and indicates that the atria are not contracting normally, associated with some variability in the QRS complexes related to the variable ventricular stroke volumes, as manifested by the pulse deficit (Figure 13-7A).

A

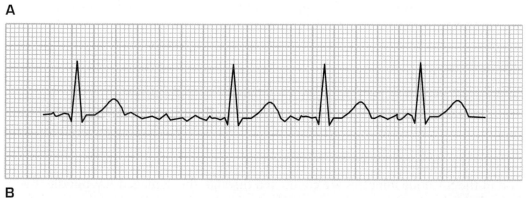

B

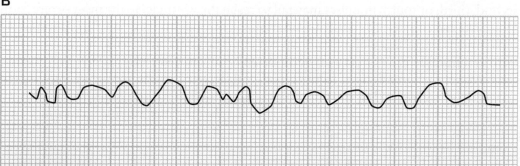

FIGURE 13-7 **A**, Atrial fibrillation illustrating absence of distinct P waves together with irregular ventricular rate, usually 140 to 160 beats per minute. **B**, Ventricular fibrillation illustrating extremely abnormal chaotic cardiac rhythm without any evidence of synchronized electrical impulses. (From Garcia, T. B., and Holtz, N. E. 2003. Introduction to 12-Lead ECG. Boston: Jones and Bartlett Publishers.)

Treatment of Atrial Fibrillation

The rapid irregular heart rate shortens the time available for ventricular filling in diastole, and the lack of normal atrial contractions further compromises ventricular filling. The cardiac output falls, which may not be well tolerated by a person with pre-existing cardiovascular disease.

The first treatment step is to improve the cardiac output by slowing the heart rate, which provides more time for passive ventricular filling during diastole. This can be accomplished by giving a medication that impedes the transmission of impulses through the AV node and bundle so that fewer impulses reach the ventricles. A digitalis preparation can be used (digoxin), but other pharmacologic agents are also effective.

When the heart rate has been slowed, the next step is to restore a normal heart rhythm by terminating the fibrillation. This can be accomplished either by an electrical cardioversion, which involves the application of an electrical shock by paddles applied to the patient's chest to terminate the arrhythmia, or by pharmacologic therapy, which uses drugs that terminate the arrhythmia by interfering with some phase in the abnormal impulse formation to "break up" the arrhythmia. Once the normal rhythm is restored, the patient may need to continue taking some medication to maintain the normal rhythm.

Further details on the management of atrial fibrillation and its complications along with two case studies illustrating both acute atrial fibrillation and chronic atrial fibrillation are available at the web site that accompanies this text at http://health.jbpub.com/humandisease/9e.

Ventricular Fibrillation

In contrast to atrial fibrillation, ventricular fibrillation is incompatible with life because the ventricles are unable to contract normally and the circulation ceases (FIGURE 13-7B). Ventricular fibrillation sometimes occurs following a heart attack. If recognized promptly, it is often possible to stop the fibrillation by delivering an electric shock to the heart by means of electrodes applied to the chest. The procedure usually causes the ventricles to resume normal contractions.

Heart Block

Heart block is a delay or complete interruption of impulse transmission from the atria to the ventricles. Usually, the condition results from arteriosclerosis of the coronary arteries in which parts of the conduction system fail to receive an adequate blood supply. In the mildest form, heart block is manifested only as a delay in the conduction of impulses from the atria to the ventricles, as indicated by a prolonged PR interval in the electrocardiogram. In a more marked degree of block (incomplete heart block), not all the SA node impulses are conducted through the damaged AV bundle. Every second, third, or fourth impulses may fail to reach the ventricle. In the most severe form (complete heart block), conduction of impulses through the AV bundle is completely interrupted. Impulses originating in the SA node cause the atria to contract normally, but the impulses are not transmitted normally to the ventricles. When this occurs, the conduction system distal to the block "takes over" as the source of impulses to activate the ventricles, but the impulses are generated at a much slower rate of 30 to 40 per minute. The extremely low ventricular rate may not provide sufficient blood flow to the brain, resulting in periodic episodes of dizziness or loss of consciousness. Complete heart block is treated by implanting an artificial pacemaker that consists of a small electrode inserted into the heart through a vein such as the subclavian vein and positioned in the ventricle. The electrode is connected to a small device containing a battery that is implanted beneath the skin of the chest. The device can be programmed to generate impulses that stimulate ventricular contractions at a predetermined rate. Many different types of pacemakers are available, each having specific applications.

Heart Disease as a Disturbance of Pump Function

For a pump to function properly, several conditions are required:

1. The pump must be properly constructed so that it is free of mechanical defects.
2. The pump must have a system of valves that is properly synchronized to allow unidirectional flow. If valves do not function properly, the force of the pump stroke is dissipated, and effective pumping is impaired.
3. The pump must have an adequate fuel supply. It will not run properly if the fuel line is dirty or plugged.
4. The pump must be used within its rated capacity. One must not use a pump rated at 3 horsepower to perform a job requiring a 10-horsepower pump. Either the pump will not function at all, or it will wear out very rapidly.
5. The pump motor must function smoothly and efficiently. If the motor functions erratically, the efficiency of the pump is reduced greatly.

The heart is a muscular pump that is subject to the same requirements as any mechanical pump. Each type of heart disease can be roughly compared with one of the derangements that would impair the function of a mechanical pump (TABLE 13-1).

Congenital heart disease corresponds to faulty pump construction. The term valvular heart disease indicates that heart valves have been damaged by rheumatic fever or other diseases, and so they fail to open and close properly. It is comparable to a malfunction in the unidirectional valve system of a mechanical pump. Coronary heart disease is a result of deposits of fatty material in the arterial walls that narrow their lumens and eventually may completely block the flow of blood through the arteries. This type of heart disease corresponds to failure of a mechanical pump caused by a dirty or plugged fuel line. Hypertensive heart disease results when the heart is forced to pump blood at high pressure against an excessively high resistance in the peripheral arterioles and corresponds to overloading a mechanical pump. Primary myocardial disease corresponds to malfunction of the pump motor.

THE ROLE OF ECHOCARDIOGRAPHY IN DIAGNOSIS OF CARDIOVASCULAR DISEASE

Ultrasound examinations described in the discussion on general concepts of disease: principles of diagnosis have many applications in medicine. An ultrasound examination of the cardiovascular system is usually called an **echocardiogram**. The procedure can identify valve and chamber abnormalities, and the dimensions of a narrowed valve orifice can be calculated from the rate of flow through the valve.

Echocardiogram
(eko'-kar-dē-o-gram')
A record obtained from an ultrasound examination of the heart and related blood vessels; used to assist in the diagnosis of cardiovascular disease.

TABLE 13-1

Heart disease compared with mechanical pump dysfunctions

Mechanical abnormality	Comparable heart disease
Faulty pump construction	Congenital heart disease
Faulty unidirectional valves	Valvular heart disease
Dirty or plugged fuel line	Coronary heart disease
Overloaded pump	Hypertensive heart disease
Malfunctioning pump	Primary myocardial disease

Abnormal blood flow patterns between chambers can be detected. On the other hand, if a cardiac valve abnormality is suspected because a faint heart murmur was heard during a routine physical examination and the echocardiogram is normal, the subject can be reassured that there are no cardiovascular problems. Some faint murmurs result from turbulent blood flow within a normal heart, which are called functional murmurs. The subject need not restrict his or her activities based on the information obtained from the echocardiogram. A normal echocardiogram can exclude a valve abnormality, an abnormal communication between adjacent atria or between adjacent ventricles, or an abnormal communication between the major blood vessels leaving the heart.

Congenital Heart Disease

CARDIAC DEVELOPMENT AND PRENATAL BLOOD FLOW

The heart undergoes a complex developmental sequence. It is formed from a tube that undergoes segmental dilatations and constrictions along with considerable growth and change in configuration. Eventually the individual chambers, valves, and large arteries develop, culminating in the final structural characteristics of a normal fully developed heart.

As the heart is developing, the blood flow through the fetal heart differs from its final postdelivery flow pattern. Much of the blood flow in the pulmonary artery is diverted away from the lungs, which are nonfunctional in the fetus, and used instead to supply other fetal tissues. One bypass called the **ductus arteriosus** is a large communication connecting the pulmonary artery with the aorta that shunts much of the blood pumped into the pulmonary artery directly into the aorta. As soon as the infant is born and begins to breathe air, the lungs expand and the ductus arteriosus constricts, which blocks blood flow through the ductus arteriosus. Consequently, pulmonary artery blood can flow only into the newly-expanded lungs, and the non-functional ductus eventually becomes converted into a fibrous cord called the ligamentum arteriosum. The other bypass is an opening in the atrial septum called the **foramen ovale**, which maintains blood flow between the two atria as the atrial septum is developing. Blood flow across the foramen ovale is controlled by a flap of atrial tissue on the left atrial side of the septum that covers (overlaps) the opening in the foramen ovale. In this position, the flap functions as a one-way valve that allows blood to flow from the right atrium into the left atrium but does not allow flow in the opposite direction (FIGURE 13-8). The right-to-left flow is determined by pressure differences between the two chambers. In the fetus, the blood pressure is higher in the right atrium than in the left atrium because only a relatively small volume of blood flows through the lungs and is returned to the left atrium. Most is directed into the aorta through the ductus arteriosus. After birth, the left atrial pressure rises when the lungs expand and a large volume of blood flows through the lungs and into the left atrium. The higher left atrial pressure presses the flap valve against the left atrial surface of the septum, closing the communication between the atria. Usually, the tissue flap fuses with the atrial septum to form a solid partition between the two atria. Often, the fusion is incomplete but no flow of blood from right to left atria is possible as long as the left atrial pressure exceeds the pressure in the right atrium, which holds the flap against the atrial septum.

A diagram and additional details on the prenatal fetal circulation and the postnatal circulatory adjustments are available at the web site that accompanies this text at http://health.jbpub.com/humandisease/9e.

Ductus arteriosus
A fetal artery connecting the pulmonary artery with the aorta that permits pressure determined blood flow from pulmonary artery into the aorta, bypassing blood flow to the nonfunctional fetal lungs.

Foramen ovale
An opening in the atrial septum covered by a one-way flap valve regulated by pressure differences between the atria, permitting blood flow from right to left atrium but not in the opposite direction, thereby bypassing blood flow from right cardiac chambers to the nonfunctional fetal lungs.

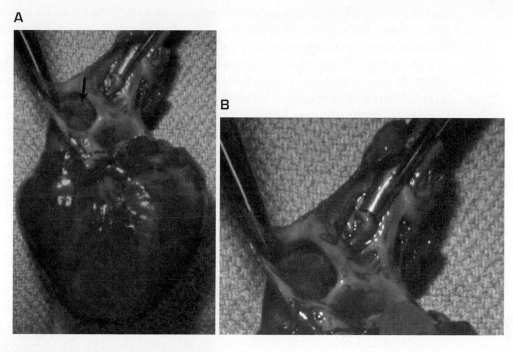

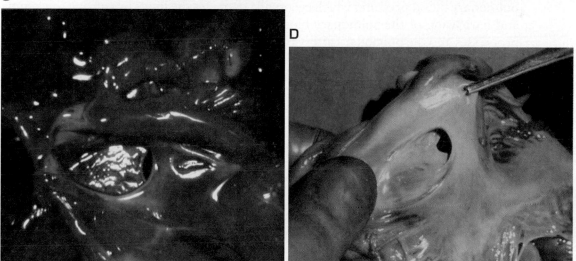

FIGURE 13-8 Structure and function of the foramen ovale. **A**, Overview of fetal heart with the right atrium opened to show the atrial septum. The foramen ovale appears as a depression in the right atrial surface of the septum (*arrow*). **B**, Closer view of foramen ovale, illustrating flap of atrial septum tissue forming the base of the foramen, which would be displaced toward the left atrium by the higher pressure of blood in the right atrium, allowing blood to flow into the left atrium. **C**, View of septal surface of the fetal right atrium stretched to reveal the free margin of the flap of septal tissue, which would be displaced by the higher right atrial pressure in the fetus, allowing blood to flow into the left atrium. **D**, Similar view of stretched right atrium from adult heart with patent foramen ovale to illustrate how a high right atrial pressure allows blood to flow from right to left atrium but normally would prevent left-to-right blood flow when the flap is in its normal position.

PATHOGENESIS AND MANIFESTATIONS
OF CONGENITAL HEART DISEASE

Sometimes the heart fails to develop normally. Partitions between cardiac chambers may be defective. The cardiac valves may be malformed, or the large vessels entering and leaving the heart may not communicate normally with the appropriate atrium or ventricle. Some viral infections, such as German measles or other maternal illnesses during the early phases of fetal development, may cause improper development of the heart as well as other organs. Some drugs or medications taken by the mother may disrupt normal fetal development. Some chromosomal abnormalities, such as Down syndrome, also are frequently associated with abnormal cardiac development. Genetic factors may also account for some cardiac abnormalities, but often the reason for a congenital abnormality cannot be determined.

The effect of a structural abnormality depends on the nature of the defect and its effect on the circulation of blood. Most persons with congenital heart abnormalities have a heart murmur caused by turbulent flow of blood within the heart, related to the cardiac malformation. Many congenital heart abnormalities result from abnormal communications between the systemic and pulmonary circulations that permit blood to be shunted between the adjacent chambers. The amount of blood shunted and the direction of the shunt depend on the size of the opening between the chambers, and the blood pressure difference between the chambers determines the direction of flow.

Most shunts are left-to-right shunts from left cardiac chambers (systemic circulation) into right cardiac chambers (pulmonary circulation). A left-to-right shunt mixes oxygenated blood from the left cardiac chambers with deoxygenated blood in the right chambers, but the admixture does not affect the oxygen content of the blood delivered to the tissues by the left ventricle. The amount of blood shunted depends on the size of the septal defect. A small defect shunts very little blood and has no significant effect on cardiovascular function. However, a large septal defect can shunt a large volume of blood, which puts an additional burden on the right ventricle, which is overfilled by the shunted blood. The larger volume of blood pumped into the lungs raises the pulmonary blood pressure, which eventually damages the lungs by causing thickening and narrowing of the pulmonary blood vessels. As the pulmonary vascular damage progresses and the pulmonary artery pressure continues to rises, the right ventricle has to work even harder to overcome the increasing resistance to blood flow through the lungs. The higher right ventricular pressure also causes the right atrial pressure to rise, reducing the pressure differences between the left and right atria. Consequently, the amount of blood shunted from the left to the right atrium also falls. Little or no blood shunting occurs when left and right atrial pressures equalize, and if right atrial pressure exceeds left atrial pressure, blood shunts between the atria in the opposite direction.

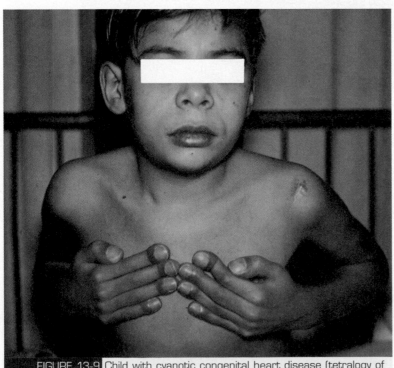

FIGURE 13-9 Child with cyanotic congenital heart disease (tetralogy of Fallot) illustrating cyanosis of skin and prominent clubbing of fingers caused by deoxygenated blood mixing with oxygenated blood (right-to-left shunt).

In contrast, right-to-left shunts mix poorly oxygenated blood from the right cardiac chambers with normally oxygenated blood contained in the left cardiac chambers, which reduces the oxygen content of the blood pumped by the left ventricle to supply the body. The affected person's activities usually are severely restricted because of the low oxygen content of the arterial blood. The skin and mucous membranes acquire a blue color called cyanosis, which is caused by the low oxygen saturation of arterial blood, and congenital cardiovascular abnormalities associated with cyanosis are grouped together under the general term cyanotic congenital heart disease. Usually the finger tips and toes become swollen (called clubbing). The condition results from overgrowth of connective tissue and blood vessels at the tips of the fingers and toes caused by the low oxygen content of the arterial blood (FIGURE 13-9). The poorly oxygenated blood also stimulates the bone marrow to increase red cell production (called polycythemia) in an attempt to increase oxygen delivery to the tissues, which unfortunately has some disadvantages. The heart has to work harder to pump the more viscous blood, and the increased blood viscosity also predisposes to formation of blood clots within the circulation.

COMMON CARDIOVASCULAR ABNORMALITIES

The more common and important cardiovascular abnormalities fall into four major groups:

1. Failure of the normal fetal bypass channels to close.
2. Atrial and ventricular septal defects.
3. Abnormalities that obstruct blood flow through the heart, pulmonary artery, or aorta.
4. Abnormal formation of the aorta and pulmonary artery, or abnormal connection of the arteries to the appropriate ventricles.

Patent Ductus Arteriosus

Normally the ductus closes spontaneously soon after birth in full-term infants. A large patent ductus shunts blood from the aorta into the pulmonary artery and causes the same clinical manifestations and complications as an intracardiac left-to-right shunt, and is treated by surgical closure of the ductus.

Patent Foramen Ovale

The foramen ovale normally becomes nonfunctional after birth, caused by the rapid postdelivery changes in atrial pressures. The left atrial pressure rises when pulmonary blood flow increases after the ductus arteriosus closes. The higher left atrial pressure pushes the flap valve of the foramen ovale against the atrial septum, where it usually fuses with the septum.

In newborn infants, the foramen ovale may remain patent and functional if the infant has a congenital cardiac abnormality that is associated with a high right atrial pressure, which forces right-to-left blood flow through the foramen ovale.

In about 25% of adults the flap valve does not fuse completely, but the foramen ovale remains nonfunctional as long as the left atrial pressure remains higher than the right atrial pressure. Some uncommon late neurologic problems have been identified that may be related to a patent foramen ovale, which will be considered in the discussion on the nervous system.

Atrial and Ventricular Septal Defects

Usually, an atrial septal defect results from defective development of the partitions that divide the atria, and the defect is located in the middle of the septum at the site usually occupied by the foramen ovale. Small defects in children often close spontaneously. Larger defects should be closed, which usually can be accomplished using a device inserted into the heart through a peripheral vein. Sometimes an open surgical procedure is required to place a patch over the defect. Ventricular septal defects are also very common (FIGURE 13-10).

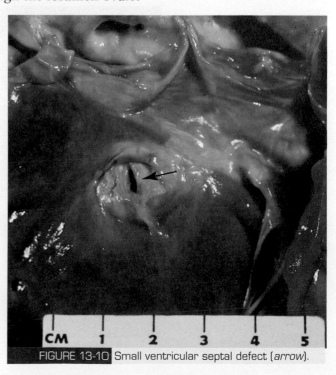

FIGURE 13-10 Small ventricular septal defect (arrow).

Many are less than 3 mm in diameter and often close spontaneously, but larger defects require surgical closure.

Generally, all large septal defects need to be closed because of the harmful effects of a large open left-to-right shunt on the heart and pulmonary blood vessels, as described previously.

Pulmonary or Aortic Valve Stenosis Caused by Semilunar Valve Maldevelopment

Abnormal development of the semilunar valve leaflets narrows the valve opening, which can vary from 2 to 10 ml diameter, and the degree of obstruction depends on the diameter of the orifice (FIGURE 13-11). Pulmonary stenosis obstructs outflow from the right ventricle, and aortic stenosis impedes outflow from the left ventricle. Treatment consists of dilating the valve opening by inserting a balloon-like device into the narrow valve opening.

Coarctation of the Aorta

Coarctation is a Latin word meaning narrowing, and the term describes a localized narrowing of the proximal aorta that restricts blood flow into the distal aorta. Usually, the constriction is located distal to the origin of the large arteries arising from the arch of the aorta. The blood pressure in the aorta and its branches proximal to the coarctation is much higher than normal because the heart has to pump blood at a much higher pressure in order to deliver blood through the narrowed segment of aorta, but the higher pressure is not adequate to deliver a normal volume of blood through the constriction. The pressure and volume of blood flowing into the aorta distal to the coarctation are both lower than normal, and a collateral circulation develops to bypass the obstruction. Branches of the subclavian arteries proximal to the coarctation communicate with chest arteries distal to the coarctation (intercostal arteries) to deliver blood into the aorta distal to the obstruction. A subject with a coarctation may appear normal except for high blood pressure identified when measuring pressure in the brachial arteries, but lower-than-normal blood pressure in the arteries of the lower extremities. Often, a coarctation is first identified during a

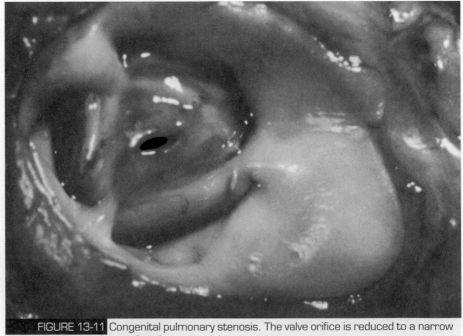

FIGURE 13-11 Congenital pulmonary stenosis. The valve orifice is reduced to a narrow slit, obstructing outflow from the right ventricle.

medical examination for an unrelated condition in which an unexpected hypertension is detected. Usually, the narrowed segment of aorta is relatively short and can be treated by resecting the constricting segment and reconnecting the aorta so that its caliber is normal throughout its entire length.

The Tetralogy of Fallot and Transposition of the Great Arteries

Both of these conditions result from abnormal division of a single channel called the truncus arteriosus, which extends from the developing ventricles and will be divided by a partition to form the aorta and the pulmonary artery. The partition, called the aorticopulmonary septum, takes a spiral course as it divides the truncus arteriosus, which is why the aorta and the pulmonary artery spiral around each other as they attach to their respective ventricles. The two abnormalities caused by abnormal division of the truncus arteriosus are relatively common, and both cause intermixing of deoxygenated blood with oxygenated blood, which leads to marked cyanosis and related problems, as described in the subject illustrated in Figure 13-9.

The tetralogy of Fallot results if the aorticopulmonary septum divides the truncus unequally. As a result, the pulmonary artery is smaller than it should be and the aorta is too large; the upper part of the ventricular septum, which is formed in part from the aorticopulmonary septum, does not connect properly to the aorta and the pulmonary artery that extend from the ventricles. The failed connection results in a large ventricular septal defect that is straddled by the enlarged aorta and receives blood ejected from both ventricles. The four abnormalities composing the tetralogy are (1) a ventricular septal defect, (2) pulmonary stenosis, (3) an enlarged aorta that overrides the septal defect, and (4) right ventricular hypertrophy that develops as a consequence of the pulmonary stenosis. In this condition, poorly oxygenated blood in the right ventricle flows through the septal defect to mix with blood from the left ventricle flowing into the aorta, which overrides the septal defect. Treatment consists of enlarging the opening of the narrowed pulmonary artery and closing the septal defect.

Transposition of the great arteries results if the aorticopulmonary septum divides the truncus arteriosus without following its normal spiral course when it divides the truncus into the aorta and pulmonary artery. Consequently, the aorta and pulmonary artery develop parallel to each other. The aorta becomes located to the right of the pulmonary artery instead of behind and to the left of the pulmonary artery, which changes the relationship of the arteries to their "correct" ventricles. The aorta becomes connected to the right ventricle and the pulmonary artery attaches to the left ventricle, which severely disrupts blood flow in both the pulmonary and systemic circulations. The right ventricle pumps blood into the aorta (instead of the pulmonary artery) to be distributed to the body, and the blood is returned by the superior and inferior vena cava to the right atrium. Consequently, the body is supplied by poorly oxygenated blood that is continuously circulated in the systemic circulation. In contrast, the left ventricle pumps oxygenated blood into the pulmonary artery (instead of the aorta), which returns in the pulmonary veins to the left atrium. The flow of oxygenated blood remains confined to the pulmonary circuit, where it serves no useful purpose. After birth, the condition is not compatible with life unless there is a communication that permits some intermixing of blood between the pulmonary and systemic circulations such as a patent foramen ovale, atrial septal defect, or ventricular septal defect (FIGURE 13-12). Generally, such communications do not provide enough oxygenated blood to supply the infant's needs.

The current treatment of this condition is called the arterial switch operation, which involves cutting across the bases of the aorta and pulmonary artery above their attachments to the ventricles. Then the aorta is connected to the left ventricle, and the pulmonary artery is attached to the right ventricle. It is also necessary to reposition the coronary

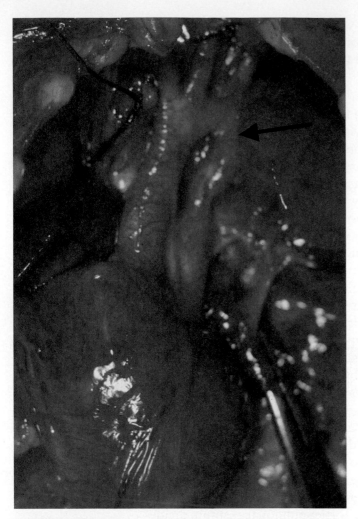

FIGURE 13-12 Transposition of the great arteries showing the parallel course of the aorta and pulmonary artery. Aorta is located to the right of the pulmonary artery (*left* of photograph) and is connected to the right ventricle, and the pulmonary artery is attached to the left ventricle. Some intermixing of blood between the aortic and pulmonary circulations is achieved by the large patent ductus arteriosus (*arrow*), and also by the foramen ovale, which is not demonstrated in the photograph.

Rheumatic fever
A disease caused by hypersensitivity to antigens of the beta streptococcus, characterized by fever, joint pains, and inflammation of heart valves and muscle.

arteries so that they are connected properly to the artery supplying blood to the left ventricle.

TABLE 13-2 summarizes the principal features of the congenital cardiovascular malformations described in this section, which are also illustrated in FIGURE 13-13.

PREVENTION OF CONGENITAL HEART DISEASE

The only way to prevent congenital heart disease is to attempt to protect the developing fetus from intrauterine injury during the early phases of pregnancy when it is extremely vulnerable. The factors that may cause intrauterine fetal injury are discussed in the discussion on congenital and hereditary diseases.

Valvular Heart Disease

Rheumatic fever is much less frequent now than formerly. As a result, rheumatic valvular heart disease has also declined, and other conditions that cause valve malfunction have assumed greater importance. These include various degenerative conditions of the aortic valve and an abnormality of the mitral valve that causes it to prolapse into the atrium during ventricular systole.

RHEUMATIC FEVER AND RHEUMATIC HEART DISEASE

Rheumatic fever is a complication of infection by the group A beta hemolytic streptococcus, the organism responsible for streptococcal sore throat and scarlet fever. This disease, encountered most commonly in children, is a febrile illness associated with inflammation of connective tissue throughout the body, especially in the heart and joints. Clinically, the affected individual has an acute arthritis affecting multiple joints (which is why the disease is called "rheumatic" fever) and evidence of inflammation of the heart.

Rheumatic fever is not a bacterial infection but a type of hypersensitivity reaction induced by various antigens present in the streptococcus. This reaction develops several weeks after the initial streptococcal infection. It is uncertain exactly how the streptococcus induces the development of rheumatic fever. Apparently, some persons form antibody against antigens present in the streptococcus, and the antistreptococcal antibody cross-reacts with similar antigens in the individual's own tissues. The antigen–antibody reaction injures connective tissue and is responsible for the febrile illness. Fortunately, rheumatic fever develops in only a small proportion of persons with group A beta streptococcal infections.

TABLE 13-2

Features of common congenital cardiovascular abnormalities

Abnormality	Physiologic disturbance	Complications	Treatment
Patent ductus arteriosus	Aorta to pulmonary artery shunt	Pulmonary hypertension	Ligate or excise ductus
Patent foramen ovale	Right-to-left atrial shunt	Usually nonfunctional as long as left atrial pressure exceeds right atrial pressure	Usually no treatment required
Atrial, ventricular, and combined septal defects	Left-to-right shunt	Pulmonary hypertension damages lungs. Right ventricular hypertrophy.	Close defect
Pulmonary stenosis	Obstructed outflow from right ventricle	Right ventricular hypertrophy	Dilate narrowed valve opening
Aortic stenosis	Obstructed outflow from left ventricle	Left ventricular hypertrophy	Dilate narrowed valve opening
Aortic coarctation	Obstructed flow into aorta distal to coarctation	Hypertension in arteries supplying head and upper limbs	Excise coarctation and reconnect aorta
Tetralogy of Fallot	Right-to-left shunt. Ventricular septal defect straddled by enlarged aorta. Pulmonary stenosis. Right ventricular hypertrophy.	Cyanosis. Polycythemia. Clubbing of fingers and toes.	Enlarge pulmonary artery opening. Close septal defect.
Transposition of great arteries	Aorta attached to right ventricle and pulmonary artery attached to left ventricle	Only communication between systemic and pulmonary circulations is through ductus arteriosus and foramen ovale	Reattach aorta and pulmonary artery to proper ventricles. Reposition coronary arteries.

Some patients with acute rheumatic fever die as a result of severe inflammation of the heart and consequent acute heart failure. In most instances, however, the fever and signs of inflammation eventually subside. Healing is often associated with some degree of scarring. In the joints and in many other tissues, scarring causes no difficulties, but scarring of heart valves may produce various deformities that impair function.

Unfortunately, rheumatic fever is likely to recur when the patient develops another streptococcal infection because any subsequent contact with the streptococcus reestablishes the sequence of hypersensitivity and connective tissue damage.

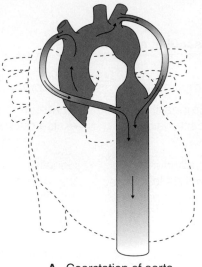

A. Coarctation of aorta

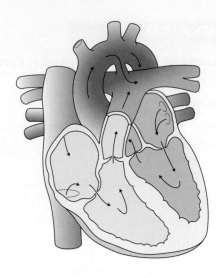

B. Patent ductus arteriosus

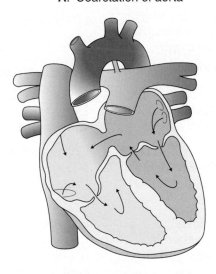

C. Atrial septal defect

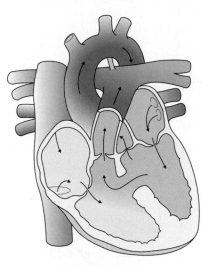

D. Ventricular septal defect

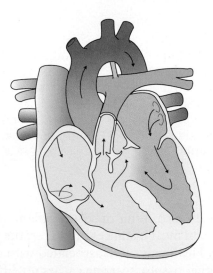

E. Tetralogy of Fallot

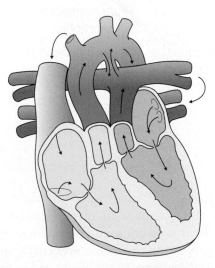

F. Transposition of great arteries

FIGURE 13-13 Blood flow patterns in six common congenital abnormalities described in this section. **A**, Aortic coarctation. **B**, Patent ductus arteriosus. **C**, Atrial septal defect. **D**, Ventricular septal defect. **E**, Tetralogy of Fallot. **F**, Transposition of the great arteries.

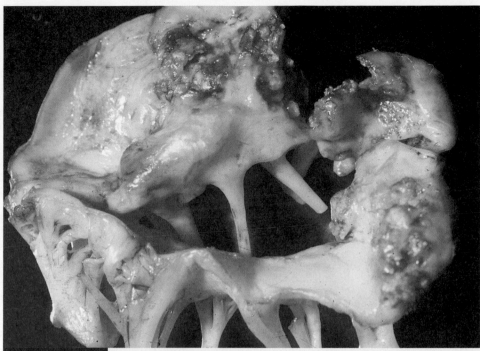

FIGURE 13-14 A poorly functioning scarred and calcified mitral valve resulting from valve damage caused by prior rheumatic fever. The valve was excised and replaced by an artificial heart valve.

Rheumatic heart disease, a complication of rheumatic fever, is caused by scarring of the heart valves subsequent to the healing of a rheumatic inflammation. This complication is relatively common and primarily affects the valves of the left side of the heart, the mitral and aortic valves (FIGURE 13-14). If the valve does not close properly, blood refluxes back through it (called regurgitation). Frequently, the damaged valve also does not open properly, and the valve orifice is narrowed. This is called a valve stenosis. Valve lesions impair cardiac function. When valvular stenosis is present, the heart must exert more effort than normal to force blood through the narrowed orifice. In regurgitation, a portion of the ventricular output is not expelled normally and leaks through the incompetent valve. This is a serious disadvantage because the heart must repump the volume of regurgitated blood to deliver the same amount of blood to the peripheral tissues.

An individual with a mild rheumatic valvular deformity that does not seriously interfere with cardiac function may experience little or no disability. However, a severe valve deformity may place a serious strain on the heart, eventually causing heart failure many years after the initial attack of rheumatic fever. When a person is seriously disabled by a rheumatic valvular deformity, it is possible to excise the abnormal, scarred heart valve surgically and replace it with an artificial valve.

Prevention of Rheumatic Heart Disease

Rheumatic heart disease can be largely prevented by treating beta streptococcal infection promptly, thereby forestalling the hypersensitivity state that causes rheumatic fever. Because a person who has once had rheumatic fever is susceptible to recurrent attacks after beta streptococcal infections, many physicians recommend that persons who have had rheumatic fever receive prophylactic penicillin therapy throughout childhood and young adulthood. Penicillin treatment prevents streptococcal infections and reduces the risk of recurrent rheumatic fever and further heart valve damage.

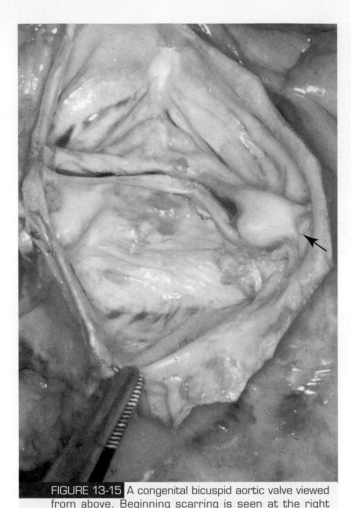

FIGURE 13-15 A congenital bicuspid aortic valve viewed from above. Beginning scarring is seen at the right margin of the valve (*arrow*).

NONRHEUMATIC AORTIC STENOSIS

In about 2% of all people, the aortic valve has two rather than the usual three cusps. This abnormality is called a congenital bicuspid aortic valve. The valve functions satisfactorily for a time but is subjected to unusual stress during opening and closing because of its bicuspid configuration. As a result, the valve gradually becomes thickened and may eventually become calcified after many years, leading to marked rigidity of the valve when a person reaches middle age (FIGURE 13-15). This condition is called aortic stenosis secondary to bicuspid aortic valve.

Fibrosis and calcification of the valve leaflets of a normal three cusp aortic valve may also occur in older persons, and sometimes the valve becomes so rigid that it is unable to open properly. This entity is called calcific aortic stenosis (FIGURE 13-16).

Mild degrees of aortic stenosis may not greatly compromise cardiac function, but severe aortic stenosis places a great strain on the left ventricle, which must expel blood through the greatly narrowed and rigid valve orifice. This leads to marked left ventricular hypertrophy and eventual heart failure. Treatment of severe aortic stenosis consists of surgically replacing the stenotic valve with an artificial heart valve.

Aortic stenosis usually is considered to be caused by degenerative changes in valve leaflet connective tissue, a consequence of the stresses placed on the

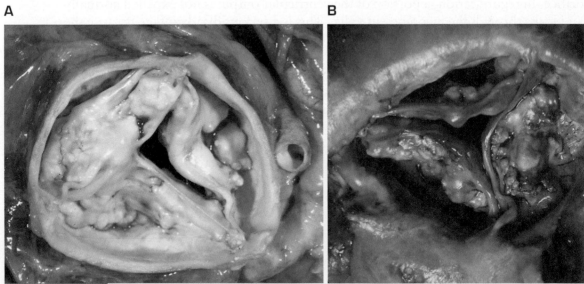

FIGURE 13-16 An aortic valve viewed from above, illustrating marked thickening and nodularity of valve leaflets. **A**, Partial fusion of valve cusps (*left side* of photograph). A normal coronary artery is seen in a cross section at right of aortic valve. **B**, Severe calcific aortic stenosis. Extensive calcium deposits within cusps severely limit valve mobility.

valve resulting from the repeated opening and closing of the valve leaflets over many years, followed by calcification that restricts valve mobility. More recent studies, however, have demonstrated deposits of lipids and accumulation of macrophages in the valve leaflets similar to the changes found in coronary atherosclerosis. On the basis of these studies, it now appears that the same risk factors that predispose to coronary artery disease, such as high cholesterol, diabetes, and hypertension, also may contribute to the valve changes leading to aortic stenosis. Control of these risk factors may retard or perhaps even prevent the fibrosis and calcification of the valve leaflets that impair valve function.

As our population ages, aortic stenosis is becoming one of the most common types of valvular heart disease. Case 13-1 describes a common clinical presentation of aortic stenosis and also illustrates the management of a patient with this condition.

MITRAL VALVE PROLAPSE

Mitral valve prolapse is a common condition, and only a very small percentage of persons ever develops any problems related to the prolapse. In this condition, one or both mitral leaflets are enlarged and redundant and prolapse into the left atrium during ventricular systole. Sometimes, the prolapsing free margins of the valve leaflets do

CASE 13-1

During a routine physical examination, a 73-year-old man was found to have a systolic murmur. He was in good health and had not had any serious illnesses in the past, and there was no history of previous rheumatic fever.

Physical examination was completely normal except for the heart murmur. Temperature, pulse, and blood pressure were all within normal limits. Routine laboratory tests and an electrocardiogram were all normal.

An echocardiogram was performed in order to determine the cause of the murmur and revealed that he had mild aortic stenosis. The aortic valve was calcified, and there was a mild to moderate restriction of the aortic valve opening. The aortic valve did not appear to be bicuspid, although this possibility could not be excluded completely. The aortic valve opening was calculated to be 1.2 sq. cm., in contrast to a normal valve opening which should be 3 to 4 sq. cm. when fully open. The mean pressure gradient across the aortic valve was 17 mm Hg, indicating that the pressure within the left ventricle during systole was higher than that in the aorta because outflow of blood from the left ventricle was impeded by the valve stenosis. Normally, there should be no pressure difference between the pressure in the aorta and the pressure within the ventricular chamber. However, there was as yet no significant hypertrophy of the left ventricle.

The patient was told that he had a mild degree of aortic stenosis that was likely to progress over time and that he probably would eventually require a valve replacement. He did not need to restrict his activities, but he was advised to take prophylactic antibiotics before any dental procedures or surgical procedures that could cause transient entry of bacteria into his circulation in order to reduce his risk of endocarditis. He was also advised to take one 81-mg aspirin tablet daily (a "baby aspirin" tablet) both to reduce his risk of coronary heart disease and also to prevent platelets from adhering to the roughened surface of the stenotic aortic valve. He was also advised to have the echocardiogram repeated in 2 years to evaluate possible progression of the stenosis.

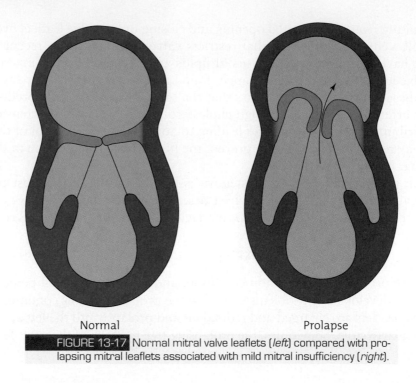

Normal   Prolapse

FIGURE 13-17 Normal mitral valve leaflets (*left*) compared with pro-lapsing mitral leaflets associated with mild mitral insufficiency (*right*).

not fit together tightly, which allows some blood to leak across the closed mitral valve into the atrium, which is called mitral regurgitation. The extent of the prolapse is quite variable, and the amount of blood that leaks into the left atrium through the prolaps-ing valve depends on how tightly the free margins of the prolapsing valve leaflets come together during ventricular systole (FIGURE 13-17).

The mitral valve leaflets, like other cardiac valve leaflets, are attached to a ring of dense connective tissue called the mitral annulus, which circumscribes the valve opening. The annulus is part of the fibrous framework of the heart to which the valves and cardiac muscle bundles are attached. Normally, the valve leaflets close at the level of the mitral annulus or just below the annulus. The closure position is determined by the length of the valve leaflets, the chordae to which the leaflets are attached, and the length of the papillary muscles.

When one listens to the heart sounds with a stethoscope, one first hears a click sound during systole when the leaflets come together, which is often followed by a faint systolic murmur caused by reflux of blood between the closed valve leaflets into the left atrium.

In some cases, the prolapse appears to be caused by degenerative changes in the con-nective tissue of the valve leaflets, which permits the affected valve leaflets to gradually stretch as a result of the degeneration of the valve connective tissue. Eventually, one or both leaflets may become enlarged and redundant. When this occurs, the stretched prolapsing mitral valve, held at its margin by the chordae, somewhat resembles an open parachute (FIGURE 13-18), and a significant amount of blood may reflux into the left atrium. The prolapsing valve may also produce excessive strain on the chordae and papillary muscles, which may provoke bouts of ventricular arrhythmia. Sometimes, the excessive stress causes one of the chordae to rupture.

SEROTONIN-RELATED HEART VALVE DAMAGE

Some uncommon types of heart valve damage seem to be related to high concen-trations of serotonin in the blood. Serotonin (5-hydroxytryptamine) is a biologic compound produced by many cells throughout the body and has many different

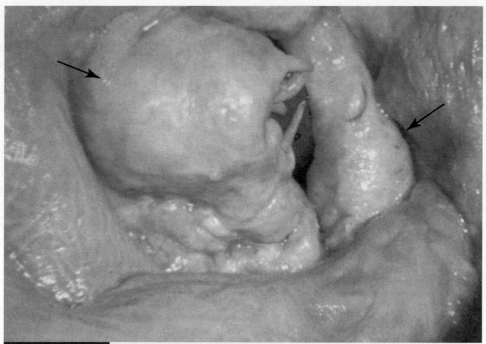

FIGURE 13-18 The interior of the left atrium viewed from above, illustrating prolapsing mitral valve leaflets ballooning into the left atrium (*arrows*). Prolapse was complicated by a rupture of mitral valve chorda tendinea.

functions. Serotonin produces different effects on body tissues and organs because there are several different types of serotonin receptors, and the biologic effects of serotonin in a specific tissue are governed by the characteristics of the receptor to which the serotonin attaches. (Usually, the receptor is designated by the chemical name of serotonin [5-hydroxytryptamine], abbreviated 5-HT, with the type of receptor indicated by a subscript, such as 5-HT_{2B}). Serotonin is produced by specialized cells (called neuroendocrine cells), which are scattered among the secretory and absorptive cells within the epithelium of the gastrointestinal tract, where the serotonin regulates some gastrointestinal functions. Similar neuroendocrine cells are also present in the epithelium of other organs. Platelets contain large amounts of serotonin, which constricts blood vessels to decrease bleeding when it is released along with histamine as platelets aggregate during blood coagulation. Serotonin is also released from nerve endings within the nervous system, where it is involved in the transmission of nerve impulses.

Sometimes, tumors arise from the neuroendocrine cells of the gastrointestinal tract or other organs and produce large amounts of serotonin. Patients with serotonin-producing tumors of this type often develop marked thickening of their heart valves caused by proliferation of connective tissue within the valves, which distorts the valves and impairs their functions. The heart valve damage occurs because the receptor to which the serotonin attaches (designated 5-HT_{2B}) stimulates the valve connective tissue cells (fibroblasts) to proliferate and form an excess of connective tissue fibers, which leads to fibrous thickening of the valves.

Some drugs and chemicals other than serotonin have a chemical structure that enables them to attach to heart valve serotonin receptors (5-HT_{2B}) and cause the same type of valve injury as serotonin. These drugs are called 5-HT_{2B} receptor agonists (*ago* = to act or do something) because they mimic the effects of serotonin. Some of these drugs are derived from ergot, which constricts blood vessels, and are used to treat persons with migraine headaches; other ergot-derived drugs are used to treat persons with a neurologic disease called Parkinson disease (described in the discussion on the nervous system). Two appetite suppressant drugs used together about 10 years ago to treat overweight and obese patients caused heart valve damage because one of the drugs stimulated proliferation of connective tissue in the heart valves by attaching to serotonin receptors (5-HT$_{2B}$) on the heart valves.

PROSTHETIC (ARTIFICIAL) HEART VALVES

A heart valve that has been so badly damaged by disease that it no longer can function adequately can be replaced by an artificial valve, which is usually called a prosthetic heart valve (*prosthesis* = replacement). There are two major types, mechanical valves and tissue valves. Each type has advantages and disadvantages, and no prosthetic valve can function as well as a normal heart valve. Mechanical valves, which are very durable, are composed of metal components. The valves are classified into three categories according to how they function: (1) a caged-ball valve, (2) tilting circular disk valve, or (3) a two leaflet (bi-leaflet) valve. The valves come in various sizes and the appropriate size is selected for the replacement. The periphery of all valves have a rim of synthetic flexible material for attachment of sutures to hold the valve in proper position when anchoring the valve within the heart after the patient's own dysfunctional valve has been removed. In all prosthetic valves, the opening and closing of the valve is governed by blood pressure differences on opposite sides of the valve, as in a normal heart valve.

In the **caged-ball valve** (FIGURE 13-19A), the ball is shown against the valve opening (orifice) at the base of the valve, which closes the valve. When used to replace an aortic valve, the column of blood ejected from the aorta during ventricular systole pushes the ball away from the valve opening at the base of the cage. When the blood pressure within the ventricle falls lower than the intra-aortic pressure during diastole, the ball returns to the base of the cage to close the valve opening, thereby preventing reflux of ejected blood from the aorta into the left ventricle. A lateral x-ray of a patient with a caged-ball prosthesis is illustrated in FIGURE 13-19B. The metal parts of the prosthesis are demonstrated but the ball is not radio-opaque.

In a **tilting disk valve** (FIGURE 13-19C), the circular disk is held within the valve by two struts that extend from the metal valve ring on opposite sides of the disk, which allows the disk to open or close the valve in response to blood pressure difference on opposite sides of the valve. When used to replace a mitral valve, the disk moves (tilts) away from the valve opening during diastole, allowing blood to flow from the left atrium into the left ventricle. During ventricular systole, the rising ventricular pressure pushes the disk against the valve opening to prevent reflux of blood into the left atrium.

In a **two leaflet valve**, the single circular disk of a tilting disk valve is replaced by two "half leaflets" that pivot on a hinge to open or close the valve, which perform essentially the same function as the tilting disk (FIGURE 13-19D). Despite the durability of mechanical valves, they have one disadvantage; blood clots can form on the metal parts of the prosthesis unless the patient takes an anticoagulant continuously to prevent formation of thrombi, which would disrupt the function of the prosthesis and could also lead to embolism of pieces of blood clot from the prosthesis, blocking major systemic arteries. Tissue valves, which more closely resemble normal valves, are composed of specially treated animal tissues, such as "pig valves." The patient does not have to take anticoagulants, since thrombi do not form on tissue valves, but they are not as durable as mechanical valves and tend to wear out in 10 to 15 years. Consequently, their use is usually limited to older individuals, such as elderly persons with severe calcific aortic stenosis.

Obviously, a prosthetic valve is not the same as a normal valve, and a person with a valve prosthesis has an increased risk of developing infective endocarditis, as

Caged-ball valve
An artificial heart valve consisting of a small ball in a metal cage in which the position of the ball in the cage determines the blood flow through the valve.

Tilting disk valve
An artificial heart valve in which the flow through the valve is determined by the position of a flat circular disk within the valve.

Two leaflet valve
An artificial heart valve in which the flow through the valve is determined by two flat "half moon" leaflets that pivot to open and close the valve.

A

B

C

D

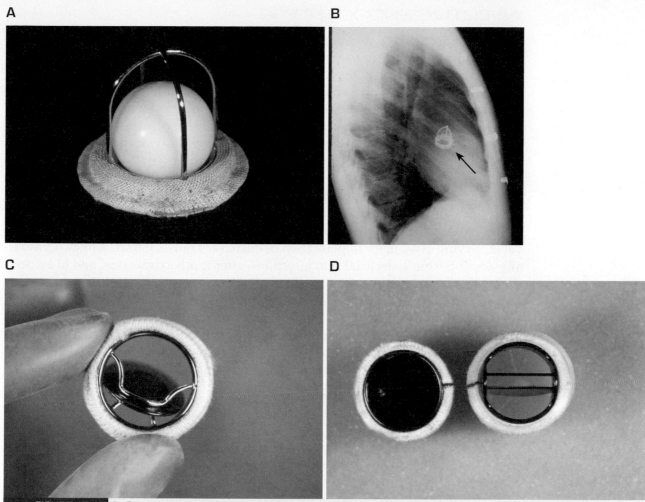

FIGURE 13-19 **A**, Caged ball valve. **B**, Lateral chest x-ray showing the caged ball valve positioned to replace the aortic valve. The base of the valve is positioned in the aortic valve opening with the cage extending into the base of the aorta (*arrow*). The ball is not radio-opaque and is not seen in the x-ray film. **C**, Tilting disk valve viewed from superior surface with the disc in open-valve position to allow flow from atrium to ventricle during diastole, as when replacing a mitral valve. **D**, Two views of two leaflet valves viewed from undersurface with leaflets closed (*left*) and opened (*right*).

described in the following section. Infection of a prosthetic heart valve is a very serious complication. If this unfortunate complication occurs, the infection is often at the site where the valve is attached to the myocardial tissues surrounding the valve opening.

Methods of Valve Replacement

The standard method for replacing a poorly functioning heart valve, such as a narrowed calcified aortic stenosis in an elderly patient, as illustrated by the valve in Figure 13-16, requires an extensive surgical procedure. The sternum must be divided and separated to reach the heart, followed by a cardiopulmonary bypass procedure assisted by a heart lung machine to divert blood from the heart while the calcified valve is removed and usually replaced by a tissue valve, such as a pig valve. Many elderly patients with other health problems in addition to aortic stenosis may be too ill for such an extensive procedure. Consequently, other less invasive procedures to replace heart valves are being developed, such as passing the replacement valve retrograde into the heart through the femoral artery, or directly into the left ventricle through a small chest incision. Advances in valve design and development of newer ways to place the valves in the heart should improve the safety of valve replacement.

INFECTIVE ENDOCARDITIS

Infective endocarditis is an infection of a heart valve, usually caused by bacteria but occasionally caused by other pathogens. In most cases, the infection is in the valves in the left side of the heart. It is customary to classify infective endocarditis into two groups: (1) subacute infective endocarditis, which is caused by organisms of low virulence, may be a complication of any type of valvular heart disease and is associated with relatively mild symptoms of infection; and (2) acute infective endocarditis, caused by highly virulent organisms that infect previously normal heart valves, is associated with symptoms of a severe systemic infection.

Subacute Infective Endocarditis

An abnormal or damaged valve is susceptible to infection because small deposits of agglutinated platelets and fibrin may accumulate on the roughened surface of the valve, serving as a site for implantation of bacteria. Transient bacteremias occasionally develop from superficial skin infections, after tooth extractions, and in association with various minor infections. In normal persons, transient bacteremia causes no problems because the organisms are normally destroyed by the body's defenses. However, an individual with a damaged valve runs the risk that bacteria may become implanted on the valve and incite an inflammation (FIGURE 13-20). Frequently, thrombi form at the site of the valve infection, and bits of thrombus may be dislodged and carried as emboli to other parts of the body, producing infarcts in various organs.

Antibiotic Prophylaxis to Prevent Endocarditis

Infective (bacterial) endocarditis is relatively uncommon, but it is a very serious disease. Persons with damaged heart valves or other cardiac abnormalities are at increased risk. Some surgical procedures and many dental procedures, such as cleaning and removal of dental plaque, tooth extractions, and root canal treatment, may

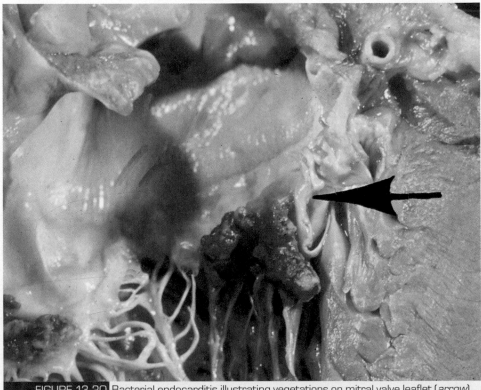

FIGURE 13-20 Bacterial endocarditis illustrating vegetations on mitral valve leaflet (*arrow*). Normal coronary artery is seen in cross section (*upper right*).

cause a shower of bacteria to be discharged into the bloodstream, which was considered a potential risk to patients with damaged or abnormal heart valves. Therefore, prophylactic antibiotics were given to susceptible persons about to undergo dental procedures because small deposits of agglutinated platelets and fibrin may have accumulated on the roughened surface of the valve, on which bacteria may implant. The American Heart Association provides guidelines regarding who should receive antibiotic prophylaxis, the types of surgical procedures requiring antibiotic prophylaxis, the recommended antibiotics to use, and the recommended dosage and duration of antibiotic treatment.

Recently, these guidelines were modified by a committee of physicians because the low risk of bacterial endocarditis in most persons with heart murmurs did not justify routine use of prophylactic antibiotics in all persons with heart murmurs. Now, prophylactic antibiotics are only recommended for dental patients who are at high risk of endocarditis. This latter group includes:

1. Persons with heart valve damage who have been treated previously for endocarditis
2. Persons in whom a diseased valve has been replaced by an artificial heart valve
3. Most persons who have had surgically treated congenital heart disease

Although the current recommendations are less restrictive, the committee concedes that possibly a very small number of cases of infective endocarditis could be prevented by a more liberal use of prophylactic antibiotics prior to dental procedures. Ultimately, the dental patient who has a heart murmur but is not at high risk of endocarditis must make the final decision about the use of prophylactic antibiotics, guided by the advice of the physician or dentist who is involved in the patient's care.

Acute Infective Endocarditis

Acute infective endocarditis results when highly pathogenic organisms spread into the bloodstream from an infection elsewhere in the body and infect a previously normal heart valve. Virulent staphylococci are a common cause of acute endocarditis and may cause considerable destruction of the affected valve (FIGURE 13-21).

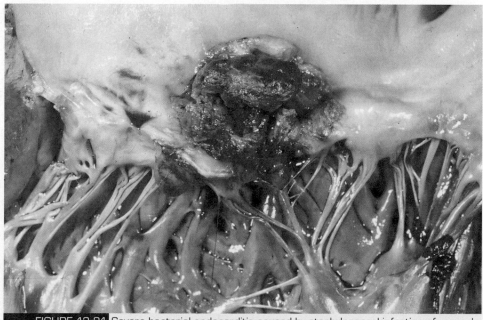

FIGURE 13-21 Severe bacterial endocarditis caused by staphylococcal infection of normal mitral valve. Infection has caused extensive destruction and perforation of valve leaflet.

CASE 13-2

A thirty-two-year-old hospital employee was admitted to the hospital because of chills and fever of about 2 weeks' duration. She was an intravenous cocaine user. Physical examination revealed numerous needle marks on the extremities and neck. Laboratory studies revealed increased numbers of polymorphonuclear leukocytes in the blood, suggesting an infection, and blood culture revealed *Staphylococcus aureus*. Special cardiac studies (echocardiograms) demonstrated a large vegetation on the tricuspid valve, and chest x-ray revealed multiple densities throughout both lungs, suggesting pulmonary infarcts secondary to emboli from the infected tricuspid valve. She eventually required surgical removal of the tricuspid valve and entered a drug treatment program.

Another group at high risk are intravenous drug abusers; in this group, the infection is usually in the tricuspid valve rather than the valves on the left side of the heart. Infection results from using unsterile materials to dissolve and inject the drug. In addition to bacterial contamination, undissolved particles and other debris contaminate the injected material. Intravenous injection carries the contaminated solution directly to the right side of the heart, where the particles and debris abrade the surface of the tricuspid valve. Platelets adhere to the site of injury and form thrombi, providing a favorable site for the injected microorganisms to implant and start an infection. Often, large bacteria-laden vegetations form on the valve. Pieces often break loose and are swept into the pulmonary arteries where they lodge in the lungs, causing multiple infected pulmonary infarcts and lung abscesses. Case 13-2 illustrates some of the clinical features of an acute endocarditis in a drug abuser.

Coronary Heart Disease

Coronary heart disease results from arteriosclerosis of the large coronary arteries. The arteries narrow owing to accumulation of fatty materials within the vessel walls. The lipid deposits, consisting of neutral fat and cholesterol, accumulate in the arteries by diffusion from the bloodstream. The initial event may be an injury to the endothelium of the vessel, which is followed by proliferation of cells within the inner layer of the arterial wall (called the intima) and accumulation of cholesterol and other lipids within their cytoplasm (FIGURE 13-22). Some of the cells accumulate so much cholesterol that it precipitates as crystals within the cytoplasm, disrupting the cells and causing cell necrosis. Cholesterol crystals, debris, and enzymes escape from the disrupted cells, inducing secondary fibrosis, calcification, and other degenerative changes in the arterial wall. The end result is an irregular mass of yellow, mushy debris that encroaches on the lumen of the artery and extends more deeply into the muscular and elastic tissue of the arterial wall. Often, the smooth internal lining of the vessel becomes ulcerated over the surface of the fatty deposits, leaving a roughened surface that predisposes to thrombus formation. The plaquelike deposit of material is called an atheromatous plaque or **atheroma** (*athere* = mush); the term for this type of arteriosclerosis is **atherosclerosis** (FIGURE 13-23).

The initial stage in the development of atherosclerosis is reversible, and the newly formed plaques are called unstable plaques. The later stages, characterized by crystallization of cholesterol and secondary degenerative changes, are irreversible. The plaques, which become surrounded by fibrous tissue, are called stable plaques, and the vessel becomes permanently narrowed (FIGURE 13-24).

Atheroma
(ah-ther-ō′muh)
A mass of lipids and debris that accumulates in the intima lining of an artery and narrows its lumen.

Atherosclerosis
A thickening of the lining (intima) of blood vessels caused by accumulation of lipids, with secondary scarring and calcification.

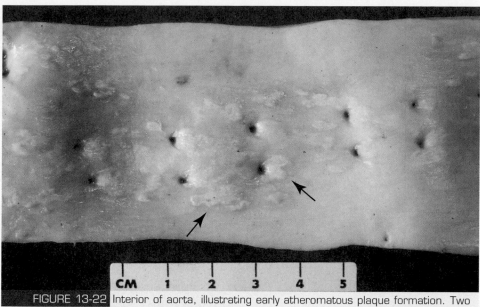

FIGURE 13-22 Interior of aorta, illustrating early atheromatous plaque formation. Two plaques are indicated by *arrows*. Circular openings are orifices of intercostal arteries.

RISK FACTORS

A number of factors are known to increase the risk of developing coronary heart disease and its associated complications. The four most important of these are (1) elevated blood lipids, (2) high blood pressure, (3) cigarette smoking, and (4) diabetes. If one risk factor is present, the likelihood of coronary heart disease and heart attacks is twice that in an individual lacking risk factors. If two risk factors are present, the risk increases fourfold, and if three factors are present, the risk of heart attack is seven times that for an individual with none.

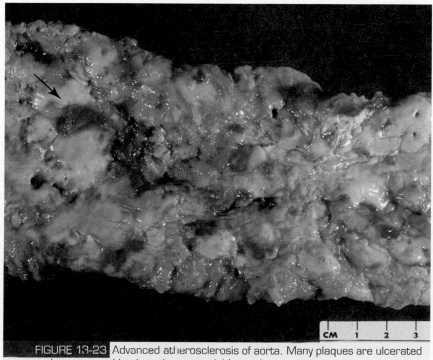

FIGURE 13-23 Advanced atherosclerosis of aorta. Many plaques are ulcerated and are covered by thrombus material (*arrow*).

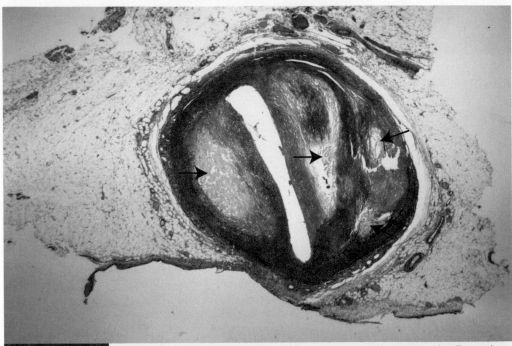

FIGURE 13-24 Low-magnification photomicrograph of coronary artery in cross section illustrating several stable atheromatous plaques (*arrows*) surrounded by dense fibrous tissue. Atheromatous deposits reduce lumen of artery to a narrow slit (original magnification × 40).

Other factors also may increase risk but play a less important role. Obesity increases the risk, but probably because an obese person usually has high blood lipids and elevated blood pressure. The personality of the individual may also play a role. One investigator has classified individuals on the basis of personality traits into two large groups. The type A person is aggressive, hard driving, and competitive and is thought to have a greater risk of coronary heart disease than the type B person, who is less aggressive and more easygoing.

MANIFESTATIONS

Ischemic heart disease
(iss-kē′mik)
Used synonymously with coronary heart disease. Designates heart disease as a result of inadequate blood flow through the coronary arteries.

If atherosclerotic plaques narrow the coronary arteries by 50% or more, the arteries may still be able to supply enough blood to the heart muscle if the individual is not very active and no excessive demands are placed on the heart (FIGURE 13-24). However, blood supply may become inadequate if the subject exerts himself or herself and the heart requires more blood to satisfy the increased demands. Myocardial ischemia is the term commonly used to describe a reduced blood supply to the heart muscle caused by narrowing or obstruction of the coronary arteries, and the term **ischemic heart disease** is frequently used interchangeably with coronary heart disease. Although the flow rate through a tube falls as the tube narrows, the decrease is related not directly to the tube diameter but to the fourth power of the diameter. Consequently, a moderate decrease in the caliber of a coronary artery causes a disproportionately large reduction in its flow rate (FIGURE 13-25).

The clinical manifestations of coronary heart disease are quite variable. Although many individuals are free of symptoms, some experience bouts of oppressive chest pain that may radiate into the neck or arms. The pain, which is caused by myocardial ischemia, is called angina pectoris, which means literally "pain of the chest." The usual type of angina is a midsternal pressure discomfort that occurs on exertion and subsides when the person rests or takes a nitroglycerine tablet, which dilates the coronary arteries and increases blood flow to the heart muscle. This kind of angina is often called stable angina to distinguish it from unstable angina, which is a manifestation of more severe and progressive narrowing of the coronary arteries. Unstable angina is characterized by episodes of pain that occur more frequently, last longer, and are less completely relieved by nitroglycerine.

A few patients exhibit another type of angina that characteristically occurs at rest rather than on exertion and is caused by a coronary artery spasm. This type of angina is usually called Prinzmetal's angina, named after the physician who first described it. Although angina is a common manifestation of coronary artery disease, it is not invariably present even though the coronary arteries are severely narrowed.

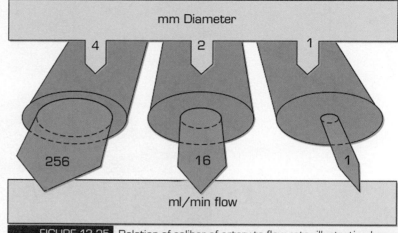

Flow rate varies with fourth power of lumen diameter

FIGURE 13-25 Relation of caliber of artery to flow rate, illustrating how a small reduction in diameter causes a disproportionately large drop in flow rate.

DIAGNOSIS OF CORONARY ARTERY DISEASE

Physicians can now evaluate the extent of coronary artery disease as well as the exact sites where the main coronary arteries are obstructed. This is accomplished by passing a catheter into the aorta and injecting a radiopaque dye directly into the orifices of the coronary arteries. The filling of the coronary arteries can be observed, along with the location and degree of arterial obstruction (FIGURE 13-26). This procedure is called a coronary angiogram (discussion on general concepts of disease: principles of diagnosis).

CORONARY DISEASE MANIFESTATIONS WITH APPARENTLY NORMAL CORONARY ARTERIES

Sometimes patients have symptoms of coronary artery disease, but coronary arteriograms reveal apparently normal coronary arteries or only evidence of small arteriosclerotic plaques that do not narrow the coronary arteries significantly. There are three possible reasons for the discrepancies between clinical manifestations and the apparently normal coronary angiograms.

1. There is arteriosclerosis of the coronary arteries, but the angiogram cannot detect it.

    For example, a coronary artery may be involved diffusely and uniformly by arteriosclerosis rather than forming discrete plaques that lead to localized narrowing of the artery, and the artery may appear to have a small lumen without evidence of disease. In other cases, isolated plaques may expand outward rather than extending into the lumen of the vessel and may escape detection.

2. The coronary arteries are normal, but marked sympathetic nervous system vasoconstrictor impulses may reduce myocardial blood flow by causing coronary artery spasm.

    This is the cause of the type of angina pectoris called Prinzmetal's angina, described previously. Other examples include stress-induced coronary artery

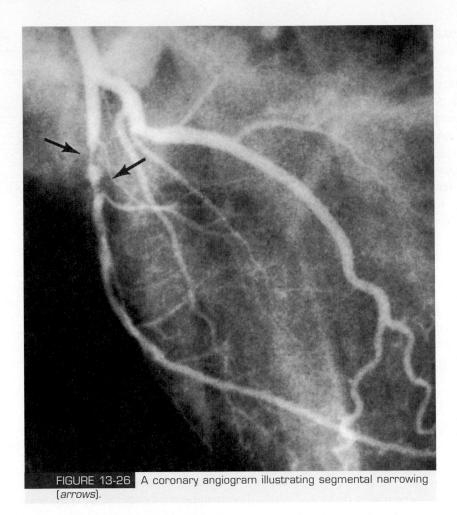

FIGURE 13-26 | A coronary angiogram illustrating segmental narrowing (*arrows*).

vasoconstriction, which may actually lead to myocardial damage, as documented in a recent study of 19 women without coronary artery disease. In these women, severe emotional stress caused coronary artery vasospasm and myocardial injury as demonstrated by abnormal electrocardiograms, elevated cardiac enzymes, and impaired left ventricular function.

3. The coronary arteries are normal, but the function of the coronary arterioles is not.

Normal coronary arterioles regulate blood flow to the heart muscle in response to myocardial oxygen requirements. When the arterioles are completely dilated, they can increase myocardial blood flow up to five times over basal levels when heart muscle needs more blood during exercise or exertion. In some persons, however, studies have demonstrated that the coronary arterioles are unable to dilate sufficiently to provide adequate blood to the heart muscle during exertion, which leads to symptoms of myocardial ischemia.

TREATMENT OF CORONARY ARTERY DISEASE

Medical Treatment

Medical treatment of coronary heart disease consists of administering drugs that reduce myocardial oxygen consumption and improve coronary circulation (antianginal drugs). If the patient exhibits cardiac irregularities, drugs that reduce myocardial irritability also are prescribed (antiar-rhythmial drugs). Factors that potentiate coronary artery disease also are controlled or eliminated as follows whenever possible (FIGURE 13-27):

1. Cessation of smoking, which has an adverse effect on the coronary circulation
2. Control of hypertension, which increases myocardial work and accelerates development of atherosclerosis
3. An "anti-coronary diet," which lowers levels of cholesterol and fat in the blood
4. Weight reduction
5. A program of graduated exercises, which seems to improve myocardial performance

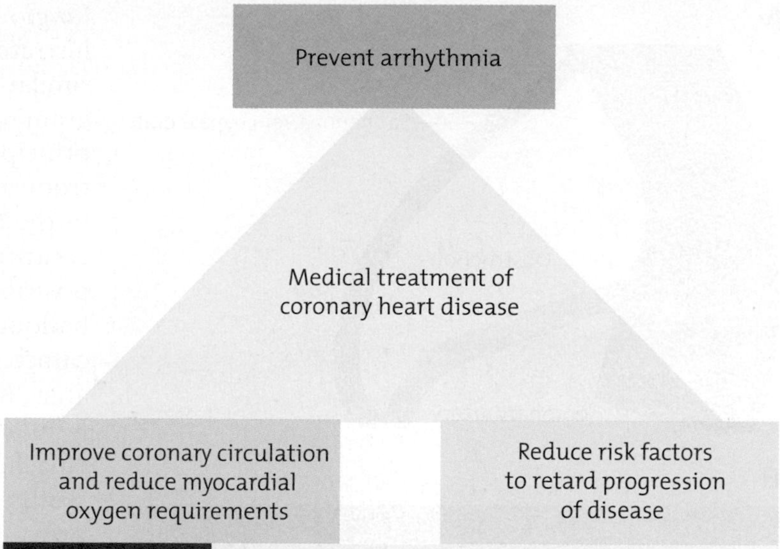

Prevent arrhythmia

Medical treatment of coronary heart disease

Improve coronary circulation and reduce myocardial oxygen requirements

Reduce risk factors to retard progression of disease

FIGURE 13-27 Principles of medical treatment of coronary heart disease.

Surgical Treatment

Several surgical approaches, called myocardial revascularization procedures, have been devised to improve blood supply to the heart muscle. Surgery is often recommended for patients who do not respond satisfactorily to medical treatment. The usual surgical method is to bypass the obstructions in the coronary arteries by means of segments of saphenous vein obtained from the patient's legs. The proximal ends of the grafts are sutured to small openings made in the aorta above the normal openings of the coronary arteries, and the distal ends are sutured into the coronary arteries beyond the areas of narrowing (FIGURE 13-28). Myocardial revascularization operations are generally reserved for patients with severe sclerosis of all three major coronary arteries, and usually grafts are used to bypass all three arteries. The operation alleviates or greatly improves symptoms of angina and may also improve survival in some groups of patients. Unfortunately, the high arterial pressure carried by the vein grafts sometimes causes the grafts to undergo progressive intimal thickening, which may lead to complete occlusion of the grafts. Many of the grafts eventually also develop the same type of atherosclerosis that occurred in the coronary arteries.

The internal thoracic arteries, which are more often called by their older name of internal mammary arteries, also can be used to bypass obstructed coronary arteries. The internal mammary arteries are paired arteries that arise from the aorta and descend along the undersurface of the thoracic cavity just lateral to the sternum. They can be dissected from their normal location and connected to the coronary arteries, thereby delivering blood directly from the aorta to the coronary arteries beyond the narrowed or blocked areas. Because the arteries are able to carry blood under much higher pressure than veins, artery grafts are less likely to become narrowed or obstructed. In some patients, both vein grafts and internal mammary arteries are used to restore adequate blood flow to the myocardium.

Coronary Angioplasty

Many patients with less extensive coronary artery disease can be treated successfully by dilating narrowed areas in the coronary arteries instead of bypassing them, thereby avoiding major surgery. The procedure is called coronary angioplasty

A

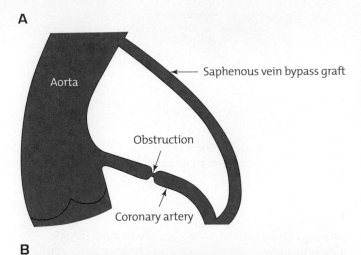

Aorta

Saphenous vein bypass graft

Obstruction

Coronary artery

B

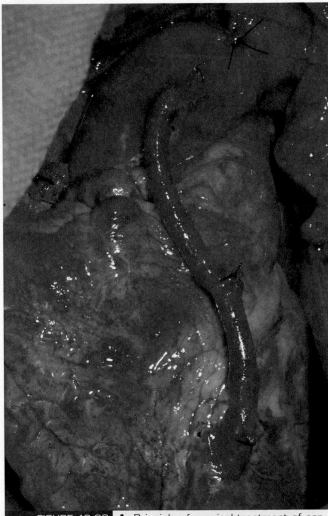

FIGURE 13-28 **A**, Principle of surgical treatment of coronary heart disease by means of saphenous vein grafts that bypass obstructions in coronary arteries. **B**, Vein graft extending from aorta above the origin of the coronary arteries to the anterior interventricular (descending) coronary artery distal to the site of arterial narrowing.

(*angio* = vessel + *plasty* = molding) and is illustrated in FIGURE 13-29. By means of a technique similar to that used to perform a coronary arteriogram (discussion on general concepts of disease: principles of diagnosis), a guiding catheter is introduced through the skin and into a large artery in the arm or leg, threaded under fluoroscopic control into the narrowed coronary artery, and positioned at the site of narrowing. Then the balloon catheter is threaded through the guide catheter until the balloon lies within the narrowed area. After the balloon is properly positioned, it is inflated briefly under very high pressure, which smashes the plaque and pushes it into the arterial wall, enlarging the lumen of the artery and improving blood flow to the myocardium. At first, the procedure was used to treat patients who had only a single narrowed artery, but it is now used to treat patients who have multiple obstructing plaques in their coronary arteries and can also be used to dilate saphenous vein grafts that have become narrowed or obstructed.

Successful dilatation of a narrowed coronary artery restores normal blood flow through the artery. Unfortunately, in about 35% of successfully treated patients, the stenosis recurs within 6 months after balloon angioplasty and may require redilatation. In an attempt to solve the problem of restenosis, most physicians now perform balloon angioplasty using a **stent**, which is a short, expandable metal mesh tube that is placed over the balloon catheter with the metal mesh collapsed. The stent expands as the balloon is inflated to enlarge the lumen of the artery and functions as a rigid support to help keep the vessel open (FIGURE 13-29). This procedure is usually supplemented by administration of drugs that prevent accumulation of platelets at the site where the stent was placed. The arterial wall responds to the metal stent by proliferation of connective tissue and smooth muscle cells that grow through the meshes in the stent and cover its inner surface, followed by gradual ingrowth of endothelial cells to provide a smooth interior lining for the stent. Consequently, platelets are less likely to adhere at the site of the stent placement and cause thrombosis of the stented vessel.

Although use of stents has been helpful, restenosis of the dilated artery still occurs in about 25% of patients, resulting from ingrowth of tissue extending from the inner layers of the stented artery into the lumen of the vessel between the meshes of the stent. In an attempt to avoid this problem, stents have been

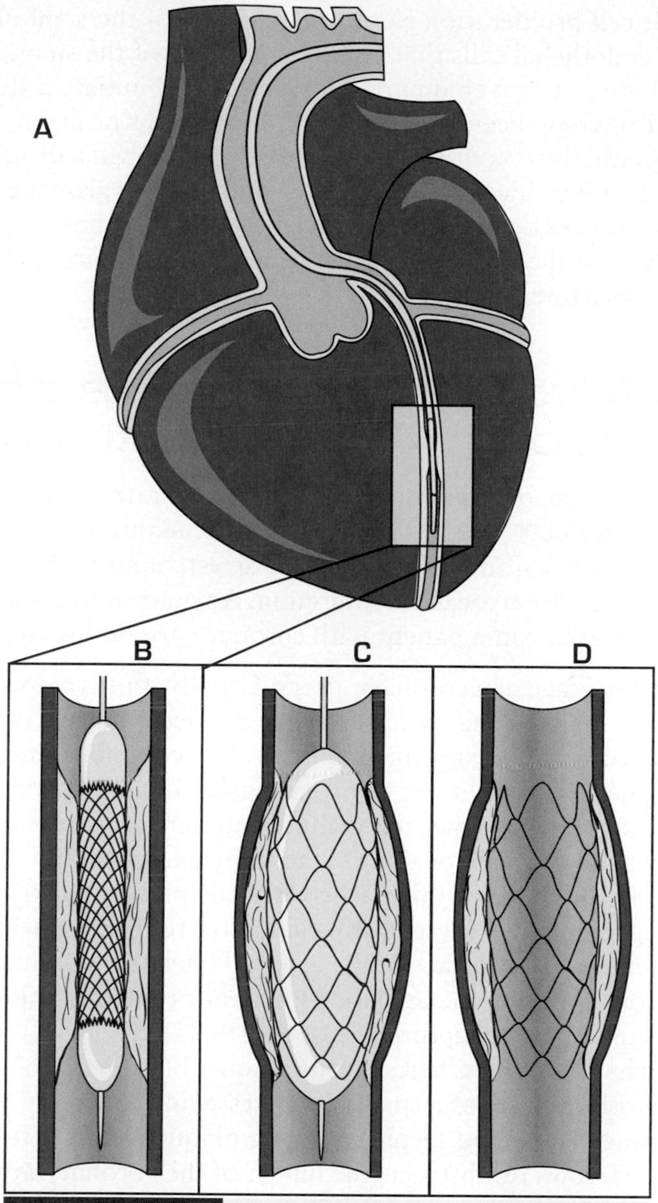

FIGURE 13-29 Principle of coronary angioplasty. **A,** An overview illustrating the positioning of the guide catheter at the site of narrowing in the coronary artery. **B,** A balloon catheter covered by unexpanded stent advanced through guide catheter and positioned within narrowed segment of artery. **C,** Balloon inflated, relieving arterial obstruction by smashing plaque and simultaneously expanding the stent. **D,** Balloon catheter withdrawn, leaving an expanded stent that forms a rigid support to maintain the caliber of the dilated artery.

Stent
An expandable metal hollow tubular device placed within the lumen of a structure such as a blood vessel, often used to expand the lumen of the vessel, where it functions as a support to prevent narrowing of the dilated vessel.

produced that are coated with drugs that suppress the cell proliferation responsible for narrowing the stented artery.

After a drug-releasing stent has been inserted in an artery, the patient is treated with antiplatelet drugs for several months to prevent formation of a thrombus within the lumen of the stented artery, as is also done when using bare metal stents. Drug-releasing stents are less prone to stenosis, but are slightly more likely to become thrombosed than are bare metal stents, which usually occurs after the antiplatelet drugs have been discontinued. Apparently, the chemicals in the drug-releasing stent that inhibit cell proliferation to prevent stenosis of the stent also impede the proliferation of endothelial cells that cover the interior of the stent. Consequently, platelets can adhere to uncovered parts of the stent and initiate a thrombosis after the antiplatelet drugs have been discontinued. To avoid this problem, treatment with antiplatelet drugs usually is continued for at least a year when a drug-releasing stent is used, in order to allow adequate time for the more slowly growing drug-inhibited endothelial cells to cover the interior of the stent. Currently, both types of stents are used successfully, and the type used depends on the preference of the cardiologist performing the procedure.

Severe Myocardial Ischemia and Its Complications: A "Heart Attack"

Severe and prolonged myocardial ischemia may precipitate an acute episode called a "heart attack" (see FIGURE 13-30). This event may be manifested as either cessation of normal cardiac contractions, called a **cardiac arrest**, or an actual necrosis of heart muscle, which is termed a **myocardial infarction**. Any one of four basic mechanisms may trigger a heart attack in a patient with coronary artery disease.

Cardiac arrest
Complete cessation of cardiac activity.

Myocardial infarction
(mī-o-kar′dī-ul in-färk′ shun)
Necrosis of heart muscle as a result of interruption of its blood supply. May affect full thickness of muscle wall (transmural infarct) or only part of the wall (subendocardial infarct).

1. Sudden blockage of a coronary artery. Usually, this is cause by a blood clot that forms on the roughened surface of an ulcerated atheromatous plaque. This is called a coronary thrombosis. A less common cause of blockage is an obstruction of the lumen by atheromatous debris. This sometimes occurs if a break develops in the endothelium and fibrous tissue covering a plaque, allowing the contents of the plaque to be extruded and block the lumen (FIGURE 13-31A). An unstable atheromatous plaque (lacking a fibrous cap covering the plaque) is especially vulnerable to rupture, which disrupts the endothelium-lined surface of the artery. Platelets accumulate, followed by activation of the blood coagulation mechanism and formation of a thrombus at the site of plaque rupture (FIGURE 13-31B).

2. Hemorrhage into an atheromatous plaque. Bleeding into a plaque usually results from rupture of a small blood vessel in the arterial wall adjacent to the plaque. The blood seeping into the plaque causes it to enlarge, which further narrows or obstructs the lumen of the coronary artery.

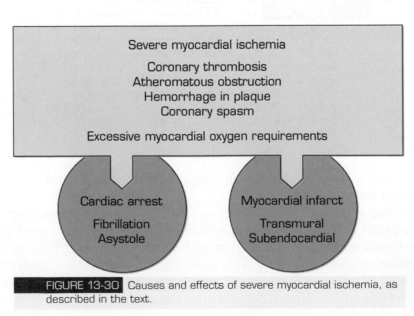

FIGURE 13-30 Causes and effects of severe myocardial ischemia, as described in the text.

A   B

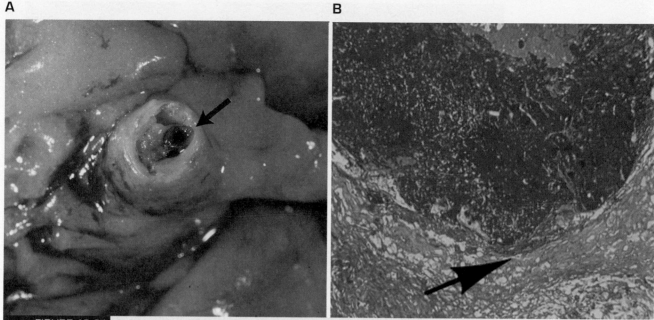

FIGURE 13-31 **A**, Marked atherosclerosis of coronary artery with thrombus blocking artery (*arrow*). **B**, Photomicrograph illustrating thrombosis of coronary artery at the site of a ruptured unstable atheromatous plaque. Note absence of fibrous tissue (*arrow*) covering the inner surface of the plaque.

3. Arterial spasm. A spasm of coronary arteries has been shown to occur adjacent to atheromatous plaques. This may be the mechanism that precipitates arterial obstruction in some patients with heart attacks.

4. *Sudden greatly increased myocardial oxygen requirements.* Vigorous activity such as running, snow shoveling, or tennis abruptly increases cardiac output, which in turn raises myocardial oxygen consumption. However, the sclerotic coronary arteries are incapable of delivering an adequate blood supply to the heart muscle, and severe myocardial ischemia develops.

Cardiac Arrest

Myocardial ischemia increases myocardial irritability, which may lead to disturbances of cardiac rhythm called cardiac **arrhythmias**. A cardiac arrest occurs when an arrhythmia induced by prolonged or severe myocardial ischemia disrupts the pumping of the ventricles. The most devastating arrhythmia is an uncoordinated quivering of the ventricles that is called ventricular fibrillation. It is the most common cause of cardiac arrest and sudden death in patients with coronary heart disease. Ventricular fibrillation is rapidly fatal because the normal pumping action of the ventricles ceases. If the condition is recognized promptly, it is often possible to stop the fibrillation by delivering an electric shock to the heart by means of electrodes applied to the chest. This procedure frequently causes the ventricles to resume normal contractions, but in many cases, ventricular fibrillation occurs without warning, and the patient dies before medical attention can be obtained. A less common cause of cardiac arrest is complete cessation of cardiac contractions, which is called asystole (*a* = without + *systole*).

Arrhythmia
(a-rith′mi-uh)
An irregularity of the heartbeat.

Myocardial Infarction

A myocardial infarct is a necrosis of heart muscle resulting from severe ischemia (FIGURE 13-32). It occurs when blood flow through one of the coronary arteries is insufficient to sustain the heart muscle and when collateral blood flow into the

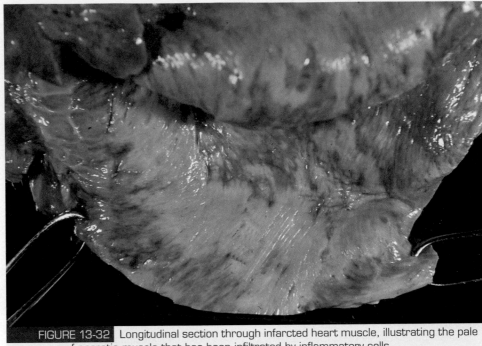

FIGURE 13-32 Longitudinal section through infarcted heart muscle, illustrating the pale zone of necrotic muscle that has been infiltrated by inflammatory cells.

ischemic muscle from other coronary arteries is inadequate. The infarction is usually associated with severe chest pain and often with shock and collapse.

The manifestations of a myocardial infarct results from partial to complete obstruction of a coronary artery, and prognosis is related to the amount of muscle damage, which often can be minimized by prompt treatment to restore blood flow to the damaged heart muscle.

An infarct may involve the full thickness of the muscular wall or only part of the wall. A full-thickness infarct extending from endocardium to epicardium is called a transmural infarct (*trans* = across + *muris* = wall) and is usually the result of thrombosis of a major coronary artery. If only a part of the wall undergoes necrosis, the term subendocardial infarct is used.

LOCATION OF MYOCARDIAL INFARCTS

Myocardial infarcts involve the muscle of the left ventricle and septum almost exclusively. Only rarely are the walls of the atria or right ventricle involved. This is because the left ventricle is much more vulnerable to interruption of its blood supply than are other parts of the heart. The left ventricular wall is much thicker than the walls of the other chambers, and it works much harder because it must pump blood at high pressure into the systemic circulation. Consequently, it requires a very rich blood supply. In contrast, the other chambers have much thinner walls, pump blood under much lower pressures, need a less abundant blood supply, and can usually "get by" by means of collateral blood flow if a major coronary artery is blocked.

The size and location of myocardial infarcts are determined by both the location of the obstructions in the coronary arteries and the amount of collateral blood flow. Generally, an obstruction of the left anterior descending artery leads to an infarct of the anterior wall and often of the adjacent anterior part of the interventricular septum as well. If the circumflex artery is blocked, it is usually the lateral wall that is damaged. Occlusion of the right coronary artery generally causes an infarction of the back wall of the left ventricle and adjacent posterior part of the interventricular septum. A block of the main left coronary artery, which fortunately is quite uncommon, causes an extensive infarction of both the anterior and the lateral walls of the left ventricle and is frequently fatal.

MAJOR COMPLICATIONS OF MYOCARDIAL INFARCTS

Patients who sustain a myocardial infarct are subject to a number of complications. The most important are

1. Disturbances of cardiac rhythm (arrhythmias)
2. Heart failure
3. Intracardiac thrombi
4. Cardiac rupture.

Complications are not inevitable, and prompt restoration of blood flow through the blocked artery can reduce the damage sustained by the heart muscle and improve the patient's prognosis.

Arrhythmias

Disturbances of cardiac rhythm are common subsequent to a myocardial infarct. The arrhythmias result from the extreme irritability of the ischemic heart muscle adjacent to the infarct and can frequently be controlled by drugs that reduce myocardial irritability. The most serious arrhythmia is ventricular fibrillation, which leads to cessation of the circulation. Another type of disturbance of cardiac rhythm occurs if the conduction system of the heart is damaged by the infarct. Conduction of impulses from the atria to the ventricles may be disturbed, which is called a **heart block**. The conduction disturbance may subside spontaneously as the infarct heals, but sometimes it is necessary to insert various types of electrodes directly into the heart in order to stimulate the ventricles to contract properly. A device of this type is called a cardiac pacemaker.

Heart block
Delay or complete interruption of impulse transmission from the atria to the ventricles.

Heart Failure

The ventricle may be so badly damaged that it is unable to maintain normal cardiac function, and the heart fails (Figure 13-32). Heart failure may develop abruptly (acute heart failure) or more slowly (chronic heart failure), as described in a subsequent section, and may be difficult to treat.

Intracardial Thrombi

If the infarct extends to involve the endocardium, thrombi may form on the interior of the ventricular wall and cover the damaged endocardial surface. This is called a mural thrombus (FIGURE 13-33). Bits of the thrombus may break loose and be carried as emboli into the systemic circulation, causing infarctions in the brain, kidneys, spleen, or other organs. Some physicians attempt to forestall this

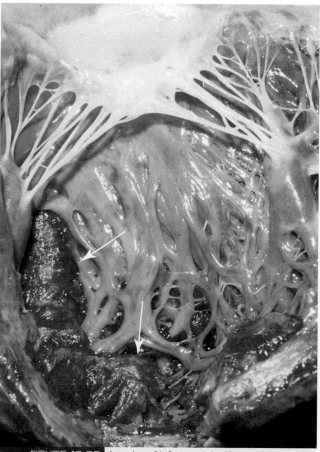

FIGURE 13-33 Interior of left ventricle, illustrating mural thrombus (*arrows*) adherent to endocardium adjacent to myocardial infarct. Normal mitral valve leaflets and chordae are seen on *top* of photograph.

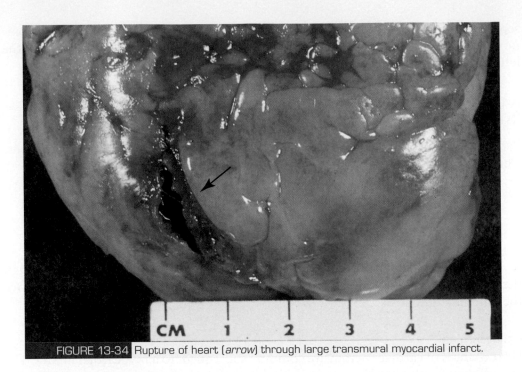

FIGURE 13-34 Rupture of heart (*arrow*) through large transmural myocardial infarct.

complication by administering anticoagulants when a patient has sustained a severe infarction.

Cardiac Rupture

If a patient sustains a transmural infarct, a perforation may occur through the necrotic muscle (FIGURE 13-34). This permits blood to leak through the rupture into the pericardial sac, and as the blood accumulates, it compresses the heart so the ventricles cannot fill in diastole. Eventually, the circulation ceases because the heart is no longer able to pump blood.

SURVIVAL AFTER MYOCARDIAL INFARCTION

The survival rate of patients who have had a myocardial infarct depends on many factors, the more important being (1) the size of the infarct, which is related to how rapidly the blood flow to the damaged muscle can be restored, (2) the patient's age, (3) the development of complications, and (4) the presence of other diseases that would adversely affect the patient's survival. Mortality rates vary from about 6% in patients who have had small infarcts and who do not develop heart failure to more than 50% in patients with large infarcts who develop severe heart failure. Major causes of death after myocardial infarction are fatal arrhythmia, heart failure, and cardiac rupture. Coronary care units staffed by specially trained personnel have reduced the mortality from cardiac arrhythmias, which are prone to occur in the first several days after myocardial infarction, but these facilities have not had any significant effect on the rates of death from heart failure or cardiac rupture.

If we consider all hospitalized patients as a group, about 95% survive and are able to leave the hospital. The data on survival, however, relate only to patients with myocardial infarction who are admitted to the hospital. They do not include patients with severe heart attacks who die suddenly or within a few hours. This is a significant number of patients because it is estimated that one-third of all deaths from heart attacks occur outside the hospital. On the other hand, the survival data also do not include patients with small infarcts that may not be detected clinically.

Many small myocardial infarcts cause relatively mild symptoms and heal without complications. The patients may ascribe the chest discomfort associated with the infarction to indigestion or other causes and never seek medical attention. Some studies indicate that as many as 25% of all patients with myocardial infarcts have very few symptoms and do not consult a physician.

DIAGNOSIS OF MYOCARDIAL INFARCTION

Diagnosis of myocardial infarction rests on evaluation and interpretation of the medical history, physical examination, and laboratory data. The clinical history may at times be inconclusive because severe angina may be quite similar to the pain of a myocardial infarction. Conversely, many patients who develop subendocardial myocardial infarcts may have minimal symptoms. Physical examination will usually not be abnormal unless the subject exhibits evidence of shock, heart failure, or a heart murmur as a result of papillary muscle dysfunction. Consequently, the physician must rely on specialized diagnostic studies to demonstrate infarction of heart muscle. The most helpful diagnostic aids are the electrocardiogram and determination of blood levels of various enzymes that leak from damaged heart muscle.

The Electrocardiogram

The **electrocardiogram** (ECG or EKG), which measures the transmission of electrical impulses associated with cardiac contraction, reveals rather characteristic abnormalities when heart muscle becomes infarcted. By means of the electrocardiogram, the physician can often determine the location and approximate size of the infarct. The process of healing can be followed by means of serial cardiograms. The electrocardiogram can also detect arrhythmias and various disturbances in the transmission of impulses through the cardiac conduction system.

Electrocardiogram
(ē lek-trō-kär′dē-ō-gram)
A technique for measuring the serial changes in the electrical activity of the heart during the various phases of the cardiac cycle. (Often called ECG or EKG.)

Blood Tests to Identify Cardiac Muscle Necrosis

Heart muscle is rich in proteins and enzymes that regulate the metabolic activities of cardiac muscle cells. When heart muscle is damaged, some of these components leak from the injured cells into the bloodstream, where they can be detected by laboratory tests on the blood of the affected patient. The most important proteins used as diagnostic tests of muscle necrosis are called troponin T and troponin I, which are not detectable in the blood of normal persons. Cardiac muscle damage causes the proteins to leak from the damaged cardiac muscle fibers.

Elevated troponin blood levels appear within 3 hours after muscle necrosis, with the highest levels attained within 24 hours, and the elevations persist as long as for 10 to 14 days. In general, the larger the infarct, the higher the troponin elevation and the longer it takes for the levels to return to normal. The pattern of rapid troponin rise and subsequent fall over the succeeding days is characteristic of myocardial necrosis. Troponin tests are so sensitive that even very small areas of muscle necrosis are sufficient to produce a positive test. Consequently, the troponin tests have become the preferred blood tests for evaluating patients with a suspected myocardial infarct because the tests can detect a very small area of heart muscle damage as well as a large myocardial infarct.

Another diagnostic test for heart muscle damage is measurement of the creatine phosphokinase (CK) enzyme present in heart muscle called CK-MB. The test is less sensitive than troponin tests but usually becomes positive when a large amount of heart muscle has been damaged. Consequently, the CK-MB has been used to assess the severity of the heart muscle damage. The original World Health Organization definition of a major myocardial infarction requires an elevated CK-MB test as well as an elevated troponin test result. Using both tests together was considered to help the clinician assess the extent of muscle damage because a small infarct which raises the sensitive troponin test may not elevate the less sensitive CK-MB test. Although the CK-MB is still used by some clinicians along with the troponin test, many cardiologists use only the troponin test as the preferred biochemical test of muscle necrosis. The test result is used in conjunction with the clinical features and the electrocardiogram to assess the patient's condition. Then this information is used to determine the most effective way to restore blood flow to the injured heart muscle.

THE ACUTE CORONARY SYNDROME CLASSIFICATION OF CORONARY ARTERY DISEASE: A GUIDE TO PROGNOSIS AND TREATMENT

This classification system assigns all patients with suspected inadequate blood flow to the heart muscle (myocardial ischemia) into three categories of progressively increasing severity based on the clinical manifestations, enzyme tests, and ECG findings under the general heading of *acute coronary syndromes*, often shortened to ACS. The term *myocardial infarction* is applied to any degree of heart muscle necrosis, which can vary from minor myocardial injury to extensive heart muscle damage resulting from complete obstruction of a large coronary artery. The categories, which also serves as a guide to prognosis and treatment, include (1) unstable angina without evidence of muscle necrosis, (2) non-ST segment elevation myocardial infarction, and (3) ST segment myocardial infarction.

The physician usually can assess the amount of heart muscle damage by correlating the changes in the ECG (FIGURE 13-35) and cardiac enzyme test results with the patient's clinical condition, which can be used to classify patients with chest pain into one of three groups called **acute coronary syndromes**. The information helps to guide proper treatment, and also provides an indication of the patient's prognosis (TABLE 13-3).

Acute coronary syndromes
A classification of patients with coronary artery disease complaining of chest pain into one of three separate groups (unstable angina, non-ST elevation myocardial infarction, and ST elevation myocardial infarction) based on ECG and cardiac enzyme tests, used to assess prognosis and guide treatment.

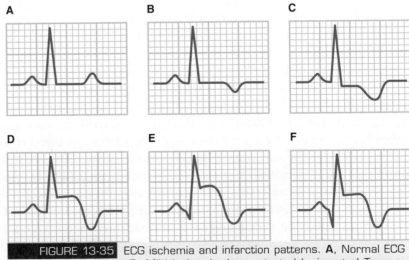

FIGURE 13-35 ECG ischemia and infarction patterns. **A**, Normal ECG for comparison. **B**, Mild ischemia demonstrated by inverted T wave. **C**, Moderate ischemia demonstrated by slight ST-segment depression and inverted T wave. **D** and **E**, ST-segment elevation myocardial infarction. **F**, ST-segment myocardial infarction with prominent Q wave indicating more severe myocardial damage. (Slightly modified from Garcia, T. B., and Holtz, N. E., 2003. *Introduction to 12-Lead ECG.* Boston: Jones and Bartlett Publishers.)

TABLE 13-3

Acute coronary syndrome (ACS) classification of coronary heart disease

Condition	ECG	Enzymes	Evaluation and treatment
Unstable angina	ST depression during angina returns to normal when angina subsides	Not elevated	Treat angina. May progress to minor myocardial damage. Consider adding anti-platelet and anticoagulant drugs. Minimize cardiovascular risk factors.
Non ST-segment elevation myocardial infarction	ST-segment depression	Troponin elevated. Creatine kinase not elevated, if test is performed.	Minor myocardial damage caused by atheromatous debris from ruptured coronary plaque blocking distal branches of artery, or artery partially blocked by thrombus. Treat with anticoagulant and antiplatelet drugs to keep artery open. Consider angioplasty (percutaneous coronary intervention) if anticoagulant-antiplatelet treatment is not successful.
ST-segment elevation myocardial infarction	ST-segment elevation	Troponin elevated. Creatine kinase also elevated if test is performed.	Artery completely blocked. Identify site of block by arteriogram and open blocked coronary artery preferably by angioplasty (percutaneous coronary intervention) as quickly as possible to salvage as much cardiac muscle as possible. If facilities not available for angioplasty, attempt to dissolve clot by thrombolytic drugs.

ST Segment Elevation Myocardial Infarction

Complete obstruction of a major coronary artery by a thrombus leads to a large transmural infarction. The extensive myocardial injury causes a characteristic elevation of the ST segment in the ECG, and is also associated with marked elevation of cardiac muscle enzymes that leak from the damaged muscle and can be detected in the bloodstream by laboratory tests. This type of myocardial infarct usually is named after its characteristic ECG pattern as a ST-segment elevation myocardial infarction, which sometimes is called by its acronym, STEMI.

A ST elevation myocardial infarction is a medical emergency and should be treated by an angioplasty or thrombolytic drugs to unblock the artery as soon as possible. The faster the blood flow can be restored through the blocked artery, the less severe the heart muscle damage and the better the prognosis.

Non-ST Segment Elevation Myocardial Infarction

Incomplete obstruction of a coronary artery causes less damage. The blood clot may not completely block the artery, or the atheromatous debris contained within a ruptured plaque may be extruded into the lumen and carried distally (downstream) to plug small arterioles and capillaries in the distribution of the ruptured plaque instead of completely occluding the artery. Some blood still flows to the damaged myocardium, which leads to a more favorable prognosis than a large transmural infarct. The ECG may show minor abnormalities but does not reveal the ST-segment elevation of a large infarct, and the rise of cardiac enzymes is less pronounced. The very sensitive troponin test result is elevated, but the less sensitive CK test result is normal.

Unstable Angina Without Evidence of Muscle Necrosis

Sometimes a patient with a history of stable angina begins to experience more severe chest pain, and it may be difficult clinically to determine whether the patient has unstable angina or is having a myocardial infarction. The ECG and enzyme tests will help make the distinction. The ECG may show minor abnormalities but does not show the ST-elevation pattern of a large infarct, and cardiac enzyme tests indicating muscle necrosis are not elevated. These features favor the diagnosis of unstable angina without evidence of muscle necrosis. The patient requires treatment with anti-angina drugs, but also anticoagulant and antiplatelet drugs, to prevent aggregation of platelets that may initiate a coronary thrombosis.

Restoring Blood Flow Through a Thrombosed Coronary Artery

Two different methods can be used to re-establish blood flow through a thrombosed coronary artery. Each has advantages and limitations. One method is thrombolytic (clot dissolving) treatment, which attempts to dissolve the clot, and the second is a procedure called percutaneous coronary intervention (often abbreviated PCI), which is another name for an angioplasty procedure that is used to open the artery and place a short expandable metal mesh tube called a stent at the site of the occlusion to hold the artery open. The angioplasty procedure is more effective than thrombolytic therapy, but requires a medical center staffed by personnel experienced with PCI procedures.

Thrombolytic Treatment

Thrombolytic therapy offers the advantage of ready availability. Any physician can perform the procedure in a hospital or emergency room setting, which is an advantage when there are no personnel available who are skilled in performing angioplasty procedures, and the additional time required to transfer the patient to a coronary care facility would delay attempting to open the artery and would lead to further myocardial necrosis. The disadvantages are that a significant number of patients are not suitable for thrombolytic therapy. The procedure is less effective than percutaneous coronary intervention, and in some patients may be complicated by a serious hemorrhage.

The thrombolytic method attempts to dissolve the clot by administering a thrombolytic (*thrombus* = clot + *lysis* = dissolving) drug intravenously. In many patients, good results are obtained and mortality is reduced if the drug can be given within 1 hour after the patient experiences the first symptoms of a heart attack.

The benefit of thrombolytic therapy decreases progressively as the time interval between coronary thrombosis and clot lysis lengthens. After about 6 hours, administration of a thrombolytic drug is of no benefit because by this time the heart muscle has progressed from ischemia to complete infarction, and it can no longer be salvaged by restoring blood flow through the occluded vessel.

Various thrombolytic drugs are available for intravenous administration. These include streptokinase and a more slowly acting streptokinase preparation and several preparations of tissue plasminogen activator. All act by converting plasminogen into plasmin, which is the fibrinolytic agent that dissolves the clot. (The coagulation and fibrinolytic mechanisms are described in the discussion on abnormalities of blood coagulation.) Each agent has advantages and disadvantages, and each is quite effective. Tissue plasminogen activator (TPA), which is produced commercially by recombinant DNA technology, is the same material that is normally produced by the endothelial cells of blood vessels to dissolve clots. It binds to the fibrin within the clot in the coronary artery, where it converts plasminogen into plasmin within the clot and dissolves the clot. Several types of TPA preparations are available.

Aspirin and heparin are often used along with thrombolytic agents. Aspirin reduces the tendency of platelets to aggregate and initiate the coagulation process at the site where the clot was dissolved. Heparin reduces the coagulability of the blood and decreases the likelihood that the clot will reform.

Although thrombolytic therapy improves survival and salvages myocardium, it also tampers with the body's coagulation mechanisms, and treatment may be complicated by serious bleeding episodes, including brain hemorrhage (hemorrhagic stroke) that can severely disable the patient or may even be fatal. Consequently, patients who are at greater than normal risk of hemorrhagic complications are not suitable candidates for thrombolytic therapy. In this group are (1) patients who have had a stroke or have any other disease affecting the cerebral blood vessels because they are at greater risk of a hemorrhagic stroke; (2) patients with severe hypertension, which increases the risk of a cerebral hemorrhage; (3) patients who have had a recent operation because the site of the operation may not be completely healed and may bleed if the clotting mechanism is disturbed; and (4) patients with any type of bleeding disorder or with any condition (such as a gastric or duodenal ulcer) in which thrombolytic therapy may precipitate bleeding.

Percutaneous Coronary Intervention (PCI)

The term percutaneous coronary intervention, often abbreviated as PCI, is used frequently to describe a coronary angioplasty (*angio* = vessel + *plasty* = molding), which is used to open a blocked coronary artery, and is the preferred method of treatment if the procedures can be performed by an experienced physician within 12 hours after onset of symptoms and within 90 minutes after the patient reaches the hospital or coronary care unit where PCI is to be performed. The procedure is quite similar to the angioplasty procedure used to dilate stenotic coronary arteries described previously and illustrated in FIGURE 13-29. The first step required to perform a PCI requires a coronary angiogram to identify the location of the blocked artery. A guiding catheter is introduced through the skin and into a large artery in the arm or leg, and threaded under fluoroscopic control to the openings of the coronary arteries at the base of the aorta. Next, a guidewire is inserted through the thrombus and atheromatous material that is obstructing blood flow through the artery. Then a balloon catheter covered by a collapsed expandable metal mesh tube called a stent is directed over the guide wire, passing through the clot and atheromatous debris obstructing blood flow through the artery. The balloon is inflated, which opens the artery and expands the stent to keep the artery open. Aspirin, heparin, and drugs that block platelet function are also given to prevent thrombus formation at the site of the reopened artery. Generally, blood flow through the artery can be restored in about 90% of the patients, as compared with dissolving the clot with thrombolytic drugs, which has only a 50 to 60% success rate. Unfortunately, although good flow is restored through the blocked artery, the PCI procedure may dislodge small bits of thrombus and atherosclerotic plaque debris from the arterial wall when the artery is opened, which is carried downstream to block small arterioles and capillaries. Consequently, blood flow to the heart muscle is reduced somewhat even though the flow through the artery has been restored. Coronary care units in many hospitals can evaluate a suspected myocardial infarction patient and proceed with a PCI if necessary in as little as 1 hour. Unfortunately, success of the PCI procedure depends on how long the artery has been obstructed before the patient reaches the coronary care unit, not on the elapsed time between the diagnosis and the treatment of a blocked coronary artery in the coronary care unit. Many patients delay seeking treatment for several hours after onset of symptoms, which reduces the chance of a successful outcome in patients with an ST elevation myocardial infarction caused by a completely blocked coronary artery.

The advantage of directly opening the blocked artery is the higher success rate when compared with thrombolytic therapy even though opening the artery does not always guarantee that the blood supply to the damaged heart muscle will be restored completely. The disadvantage is the need to reach a cardiac care facility staffed by highly trained personnel within a very short period of time. These facilities are readily available in large metropolitan communities but may not be easy to access in small communities or rural areas, and transferring the patient to a metropolitan coronary care unit consumes valuable time, which delays restoring blood flow through the blocked artery.

Nevertheless, transferring patients for PCI may still be advantageous, as demonstrated by a study involving 1,100 Canadian patients who were treated initially at a facility where PCI was not available. The patients were divided into two groups. The half underwent immediate transfer to a medical facility for angiography and PCI if needed. The other group received standard medical treatment for an acute myocardial infarction. The PCI patients did better than those receiving medical treatment. There were 11% deaths and infarct-related complications (coronary events) within the first 30 days after the infarction in the PCI group, which compared favorably with the 17% death and complication rate in the medical treatment group.

SUBSEQUENT TREATMENT AND PROGNOSIS OF MYOCARDIAL INFARCTION

After as much myocardium as possible has been salvaged by restoring flow through the occluded artery, further treatment of myocardial infarction consists of bed rest initially, gradually progressing to limited activity and then to full activity. Sometimes, the injured heart is quite irritable and prone to abnormal rhythms. Therefore, various drugs are often given to decrease the irritability of the heart muscle. Development of heart block may require insertion of a cardiac pacemaker. The patient who has sustained a myocardial infarction may develop intracardiac thrombi if the endocardium is injured or may develop thrombi in leg veins as a result of reduced activity. Therefore, some physicians also administer anticoagulant drugs to reduce the coagulability of the blood and thereby decrease the likelihood of thromboses and emboli. If the patient shows evidence of heart failure, various drugs are administered to sustain the failing heart.

Patients recovering from a myocardial infarct are at increased risk of sudden death from a fatal arrhythmia or another infarct, and the risk is greatest within the first 6 months after the infarct. The overall mortality rate within the first 30 days after a major myocardial infarction ranges from about 10% to as high as 25%, depending on the size of the infarct, the patient's condition, and any complications associated with the infarct. Many physicians treat postinfarct patients for at least 2 years with drugs that reduce myocardial irritability (called beta-blockers) because this seems to reduce the incidence of these postinfarct complications and improves survival. Ingesting a small amount of aspirin daily also is beneficial. As mentioned earlier, aspirin inhibits platelet function, making them less likely to adhere to roughened atheromatous plaques and initiate a thrombosis in the coronary artery. Some physicians also recommend insertion of a cardioverter-defibrillator in post-infarct patients considered at high risk of a cardiac arrest or fatal arrhythmia. The device continually monitors the patient's heart rhythm. If ventricular fibrillation or other life-threatening arrhythmia is detected, the device automatically administers an electric shock to terminate the arrhythmia.

Case Studies

The following three cases illustrate some of the clinical features and complications of myocardial infarctions.

CASE 13-3

A 74-year-old man was admitted to the emergency room because of severe oppressive chest pain of about 5 hours' duration. For the previous 2 weeks, he had also experienced episodes of less severe chest pain when he walked rapidly, but the pain soon subsided when he rested.

Physical examination revealed an older man in no acute distress. Heart sounds were normal. Lungs were clear. Blood pressure was 190/110 (normal about 120/80). Electrocardiogram showed the pattern of acute ST elevation myocardial infarction involving the anterior wall of the left ventricle.

Laboratory studies revealed elevated cardiac enzymes troponin and CK-MB.

Soon after admission, his blood pressure fell precipitously as a result of the severe myocardial damage, and the cardiac monitor recorded ventricular fibrillation. Resuscitative measures were unsuccessful.

An autopsy revealed severe arteriosclerosis of all coronary arteries. The left anterior descending coronary artery was occluded by a thrombus, and there was a large transmural anterolateral myocardial infarction. A myocardial perforation at the apex had permitted blood to fill the pericardial sac.

CASE 13-4

A 57-year-old man was admitted to the hospital from his place of employment. While at work he complained of a sweaty feeling and then lost consciousness. When he regained consciousness, he noted a constant, oppressive, substernal pain. In the preceding month, he had experienced similar episodes of substernal pain that would last for several minutes and disappear spontaneously. The pain was associated with a feeling of numbness in the arms. The patient had sustained a myocardial infarction 2 years earlier.

Physical examination and blood pressure were normal. An electrocardiogram showed changes of acute myocardial infarction involving the anterior wall and interventricular septum.

Soon after admission, his blood pressure dropped precipitously and the cardiac monitor recorded ventricular fibrillation. Resuscitation was unsuccessful.

The autopsy revealed old scarring in the posterior wall and the posterior portion of the interventricular septum in the distribution of the right coronary artery. There was a recent area of infarction in the anterior and lateral wall and in the anterior portion of the interventricular septum in the distribution of the anterior descending left coronary artery. The coronary arteries showed a variable degree of arteriosclerosis. The main left and circumflex arteries showed from 35 to 50% narrowing. The anterior descending left artery was 85 to 90% narrowed but was not occluded. The right coronary artery was occluded by old thrombus material that extended within the vessel for a distance of 7 to 8 cm. Lungs exhibited marked pulmonary edema.

CASE 13-5

A 52-year-old man experienced an episode of severe precordial pain associated with nausea and vomiting. He attributed this to indigestion and did not consult a physician. He remained at home on restricted activity but felt quite weak and experienced periodic episodes of sweating and chest pain. Eventually, he was able to be up and about around the house and felt somewhat better. While eating supper 2 weeks later, he experienced a sudden onset of weakness in the right arm and difficulty with speech. When he attempted to get up from the table, his right leg did not support him and he fell to the floor.

On admission to the hospital, he exhibited a paralysis of the right side of the body. His blood pressure was elevated (210/110). The remainder of the physical examination was normal.

The electrocardiogram showed the pattern of a recent anterior-wall myocardial infarction. Serum cardiac enzyme studies on admission, at 24 hours, and at 48 hours were all within normal limits because the myocardial infarct had occurred 2 weeks earlier. The elevated levels of enzyme activity had returned to normal by the time the patient entered the hospital.

The patient's disorder was treated as a recent myocardial infarction. A mural thrombus had apparently formed in the left ventricle at the site of the infarct. A piece of the clot had broken loose and had been carried as an embolus to the brain, where it had obstructed a cerebral artery and caused the paralysis. He made a satisfactory recovery but was left with some residual weakness and speech difficulty.

Additional Factors Influencing Cardiovascular Disease Risk

TAKING ASPIRIN TO REDUCE THE RISK OF CARDIOVASCULAR DISEASE

Aspirin is now widely used in clinical medicine to reduce the risk of heart attacks and strokes. Aspirin works by interfering with platelet function (discussion on abnormalities of blood coagulation). Aspirin permanently inactivates (acetylates) a platelet enzyme needed to produce a chemical compound called thromboxane A_2 that is released by platelets when they adhere to a roughened surface, which causes platelets to clump together and start the clotting process. Blocking platelet function by taking aspirin reduces the likelihood that platelets will adhere to the roughened surface of an atherosclerotic plaque in a coronary or cerebral artery and cause a blood clot to plug the artery.

Aspirin is rapidly absorbed from the stomach and small intestine. Peak levels are obtained in the blood within about 20 minutes after aspirin is ingested, and some inhibition of platelet function can be detected within an hour after the drug is taken. Although not all patients respond uniformly to the beneficial antiplatelet effects of aspirin, the platelets of most persons are extremely sensitive to aspirin. As little as 30 mg per day (less than one-half a baby aspirin) inactivates thromboxane A_2 production, which persists for the entire 10-day life span of the platelets. Because about 10% of the circulating platelets are replaced every 24 hours, after about 10 days almost no functionally normal platelets are present in the circulation.

Although taking aspirin to inactivate platelet function reduces the risk of cardiovascular disease as well as strokes caused by blood clots in cerebral blood vessels, aspirin use to reduce the risk of heart attacks slightly increases the risk of bleeding in the brain if the person does have a stroke.

COCAINE-INDUCED ARRHYTHMIAS AND MYOCARDIAL INFARCTS

Cocaine has very powerful effects on the cardiovascular system, and as the recreational use of cocaine has increased in recent years, so has the number of cocaine-related cardiac deaths.

The drug prolongs and intensifies the effects of sympathetic nerve impulses that regulate the heart and blood vessels. As a result, the heart beats faster and more forcefully, thereby increasing myocardial oxygen requirements. The heart muscle becomes more irritable, which predisposes to arrhythmias, and the peripheral arterioles constrict, which raises the blood pressure. Cocaine also constricts the coronary arteries and may induce coronary artery spasm, which leads to severe myocardial ischemia and may be followed by a myocardial infarction. Cocaine-related fatal arrhythmias and myocardial infarcts may occur in persons with normal coronary arteries, and cocaine users who already have some degree of coronary atherosclerosis are at even greater risk.

BLOOD LIPIDS AND CORONARY ARTERY DISEASE

The level of lipids in the blood has been shown to be an important factor in the pathogenesis of coronary atherosclerosis. The lipids of clinical importance are neutral fat (triglyceride) and cholesterol.

Neutral Fat

Chemically, a fat (triglyceride) is composed of three molecules of fatty acid combined with glycerol. A fatty acid consists of a long chain of carbon atoms joined together by shared (covalent) bonds. The end carbon in each fatty acid chain forms the carboxyl group (COOH), which is the acid group of organic molecules. Glycerol is a three-carbon alcohol containing a hydroxyl group (OH) attached to each carbon molecule. The carboxyl groups of the fatty acids are linked to the hydroxyl groups of glycerol, with loss of a molecule of water, in a linkage called an ester (FIGURE 13-36A).

A carbon atom has a valence of four, meaning that there are four sites on the carbon atom at which it can combine with other atoms. In the carbon chain of a fatty acid, each carbon atom in the chain is joined to the two adjacent carbon atoms by either a single or double covalent bond, and the remaining bonds are connected to hydrogen atoms.

A fat may be classified as saturated or unsaturated. In a saturated fat, each carbon atom in the chain is joined to the two adjacent carbon atoms, each by a single covalent bond, and the other two bonding sites are occupied by hydrogen atoms (FIGURE 13-36B). The three fatty acids attached to glycerol form long straight symmetrical molecules "packed" closely together and parallel to one another. This configuration gives rise to a compact, relatively dense fat molecule, which is why saturated fats have a high melting point and are solid at room temperature. Most animal fats such as butter, lard, and beef products are saturated fats.

Most vegetable oils and fats found in fish and poultry are unsaturated. In an unsaturated fat at least one of the three fatty acids in the molecule has a double bond between two adjacent carbon atoms in the carbon chain instead of a single bond, and the two carbon atoms flanking the double bond have only a single attached hydrogen atom instead of two, as in a saturated fat. If the fatty acid molecules contain more than one double bond, the term polyunsaturated fat is used. In almost all naturally occurring unsaturated fats, the hydrogen atoms attached to the carbons flanking the double bond are located on the same side of the carbon chain, which is called a cis configuration (FIGURE 13-36C). This arrangement "unbalances" the symmetry of the carbon chain and causes the chain to bend sharply at the double bond, which requires the bent chain to occupy more space in the triglyceride molecule (FIGURE 13-36E). Consequently, the fatty acids in the triglyceride molecule are less closely packed together and occupy more space than the molecules in a saturated fat, which is why unsaturated fats have a lower melting point and are liquid rather than solid at room temperature.

Trans Fats

A trans fat is unsaturated fat in which the hydrogen atoms attached to the carbons flanking the double bond in a fatty acid molecule are located on opposite sides of the carbon chain (FIGURE 13-36D), which is called a trans configuration (*trans* = across) and causes the carbon chain to maintain a more straight-line configuration, similar to that of a saturated fat instead of bending sharply at the double bond, which causes the fatty acid to adopt a straight-line configuration similar to that of a saturated fat (FIGURE 13-36F). Almost all trans fats are produced artificially by partial hydrogenation of vegetable oils at high temperature and pressure using a catalyst to facilitate the reaction. Partial hydrogenation adds hydrogen atoms to some of the double bonds that are converted to single bonds, but also changes many of the bonds from cis to trans configuration without hydrogenating the bonds, and may also change the location of some of the double bonds. The cis-to-trans change at the double bonds converts the bent fatty acid chains to straight chains, which causes the fatty acid molecules to resemble those in a saturated fat, and also changes a vegetable oil to a semisolid fat.

We know now that trans fats are "bad fats" because of their harmful effects on blood lipids. They are much more atherogenic (predisposing to atherosclerosis) than saturated fats and should be avoided as much as possible in our diets.

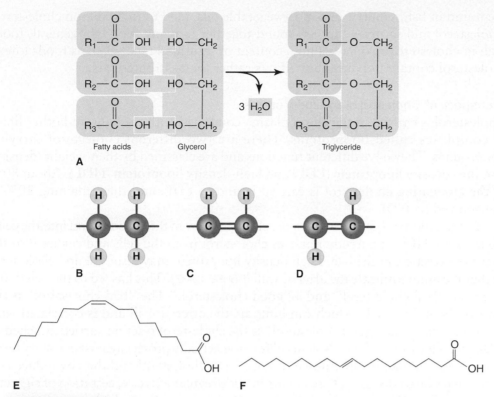

FIGURE 13-36 **A**, Structure of a triglyceride composed of 3 long fatty acid molecules (R1, R2, and R3) each containing 16 to 18 carbon atoms. The carboxyl groups of the fatty acids are joined to glycerol with loss of water molecules to form the triglyceride. **B**, Single bonds join carbon atoms in the triglyceride molecules of a saturated fat. **C**, Double bond in an unsaturated fat in which the hydrogen atoms are on the same side of the chain (cis configuration). **D**, Double bond in an unsaturated fat in which the hydrogen atoms are on opposite sides of the chain (trans configuration). **E**, Representation of the bent fatty acid chain at the site of a cis position double bond. **F**, Representation of the straight fatty acid chain structure caused by the trans position double bond, which is similar to the chains in a saturated fat.

High levels of neutral fat (along with cholesterol) in the blood promote atherosclerosis. Carbohydrate is converted readily into fat in the body, and much of the blood triglyceride is derived not from ingested fat but from ingested carbohydrate. In clinical medicine, most examples of high blood triglycerides can be traced to diets excessively high in carbohydrate. Sugar has been found to be more potent in elevating blood triglycerides than the more complex carbohydrates derived from cereals and other starches.

Cholesterol

Cholesterol is a complex carbon compound containing several ring structures and is classified as a sterol. Most cholesterol is present in the body in combination with fatty acids as cholesterol esters. Cholesterol is synthesized in the body and is also present in many foods. Normally, cholesterol is excreted in the bile into the gastrointestinal tract.

Much evidence indicates that a high dietary intake of cholesterol leads to high levels of blood cholesterol and premature atherosclerosis. Americans subsist on a diet relatively high in cholesterol; they also have one of the highest rates of death from coronary heart disease. In contrast, other populations whose diet is much lower in cholesterol have much lower rates of death from coronary heart disease.

The level of blood cholesterol is influenced not only by the amount of cholesterol in the diet, but also by the type of dietary fat. Saturated fats, the type found in meats and dairy products, tend to raise blood cholesterol, whereas unsaturated fats, which are found in fish, poultry, and most vegetable oils, tend to lower blood cholesterol. Cholesterol and saturated fat are found together in many foods. In general, foods high in cholesterol also have a high content of saturated fats, whereas foods low in cholesterol contain polyunsaturated fats rather than saturated fats.

Transport of Cholesterol by Lipoproteins

Lipoproteins
A lipid-protein complex that transports cholesterol and triglycerides in the blood stream to various locations throughout the body.

Low-density lipoprotein (LDL) cholesterol
(li-pō-prō'tēn kō-les'ter-all)
The fraction of cholesterol carried by low-density lipoproteins, which is correlated with atherosclerosis.

High-density lipoprotein (HDL) cholesterol
(li-pō-prō'tēn kō-les'ter-ol)
The fraction of cholesterol carried by high-density lipoprotein, which is correlated with protection against atherosclerosis.

Cholesterol is carried in the blood plasma combined with proteins and other lipids as complexes called **lipoproteins**. There are two different cholesterol-carrying lipoproteins. They have different functions and are classified by their weight (density) into **low-density lipoprotein (LDL)** and **high-density lipoprotein (HDL)**. About 80% of the circulating cholesterol is carried bound to LDL, and the remaining 20% is transported by HDL.

The function of LDL is to transport cholesterol from the bloodstream into the cells, whereas the HDL apparently removes cholesterol from the cells and carries it to the liver for excretion in the bile. High-density lipoprotein may also "tie up" cholesterol so that it cannot infiltrate the arterial wall (FIGURE 13-37). This has led to the belief that there is a "bad cholesterol" and a "good cholesterol." The "bad cholesterol" is the fraction bound to LDL, which can infiltrate the arterial wall and is correlated with atherosclerosis. The "good cholesterol" is the cholesterol fraction carried attached to HDL, and elevations of this cholesterol fraction actually protect against coronary heart disease. Several factors are known to raise HDL cholesterol and thereby reduce risk of coronary heart disease. These factors include regular exercise, cessation of cigarette smoking, and (surprisingly) a modest regular intake of alcoholic beverages.

Alteration of Blood Lipids by Change in Diet

Various studies have demonstrated that the levels of both cholesterol and triglycerides in the blood can be lowered by dietary change. These studies have also demonstrated that individuals maintained on a modified diet have a lower incidence of coronary artery disease than a comparable group subsisting on an average American diet.

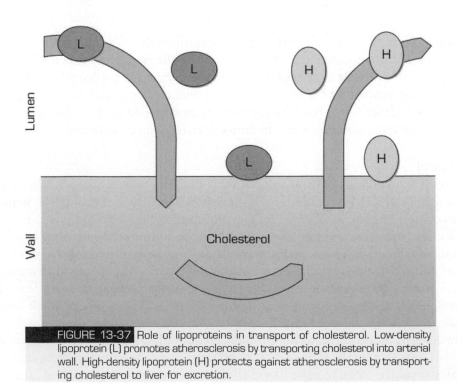

FIGURE 13-37 Role of lipoproteins in transport of cholesterol. Low-density lipoprotein (L) promotes atherosclerosis by transporting cholesterol into arterial wall. High-density lipoprotein (H) protects against atherosclerosis by transporting cholesterol to liver for excretion.

The diet (often called an "anti-coronary" diet) is modified by decreasing the amount of cholesterol and saturated fat and substituting foods containing polyunsaturated fats. This involves restricting the intake of animal fat and substituting fish and poultry. Carbohydrates are derived primarily from starches and cereals. The consumption of sugar and foods rich in sugar (pies, cakes, candies) is reduced. Alcohol consumption is restricted but not forbidden because of its favorable effect on HDL levels, which seems to protect against coronary heart disease. In addition to raising HDL, modest alcohol intake also helps protect against heart attacks by raising the level of circulating tissue plasminogen activator. This substance, which is one of the body's physiologic clot-dissolving components, is produced by the endothelial cells of blood vessels and diffuses into the circulation. Blood containing a higher concentration of tissue plasminogen activator has increased fibrinolytic activity. Consequently, any small clots that begin to form over atheromatous plaques in coronary arteries would be dissolved by the body's own tissue plasminogen activator before the clots become large enough to occlude the vessel.

Modifying the typical American diet is difficult because it requires breaking old dietary habits. However, some change in diet is desirable because it will significantly reduce the incidence of coronary artery disease. An "anti-coronary" diet is essential for individuals who have high levels of blood lipids because they run a greatly increased risk of death or disability from coronary artery disease.

It should be emphasized that the factors influencing the development of atherosclerosis are complex; an elevated level of blood lipids is only one of many factors concerned with atherogenesis. A number of other conditions, among them obesity, hypertension, cigarette smoking, and genetic factors, also predispose individuals to atherosclerosis.

C-REACTIVE PROTEIN AS A RISK FACTOR FOR CARDIOVASCULAR DISEASE

C-reactive protein (CRP) is one of several proteins produced by the liver and released into the bloodstream in response to tissue injury or inflammation. The protein is one of the body's nonspecific defenses against infection and also provides some protection against the harmful effects of inflammation by neutralizing various products produced by the cells that accumulate at the site of the inflammation. Measurement of CRP has been used for many years to monitor the activity of diseases associated with inflammation such as rheumatic fever and rheumatoid arthritis.

Recently, very sensitive tests have been developed that can detect slight CRP elevations in persons who do not appear to have evidence of an inflammatory or infectious disease. Several studies have demonstrated that an elevated CRP level in an otherwise normal person predicts an increased long-term risk of cardiovascular disease, probably because the elevated CRP is detecting the accumulation of macrophages, lymphocytes, lipids, and products of tissue injury within unstable plaques in coronary arteries. The CRP test has been proposed as an additional screening test to detect persons at risk of coronary artery disease, who then can be offered treatment to reduce their risk factors.

THE METABOLIC SYNDROME AND CARDIOVASCULAR DISEASE

The **metabolic syndrome**, which is also called the syndrome of insulin resistance, is a group of conditions and laboratory abnormalities that leads to development of cardiovascular disease and type 2 diabetes (described in the discussion on the pancreas and diabetes mellitus). The condition is characterized by obesity with concentration of fat around the abdomen (a waist circumference of over 40 in. in men and over

Metabolic syndrome
A group of conditions consisting of obesity, hypertension, elevated blood glucose and blood lipids, which predisposes to cardiovascular disease and diabetes.

35 in. in women, called an "apple shape" body configuration), hypertension, impaired carbohydrate tolerance that may progress to type 2 diabetes, and lipid abnormalities that predispose to coronary artery disease. The condition is estimated to affect about 23% of the adult population in the United States, and about half of those affected also have type 2 diabetes mellitus. Treatment consists of weight loss, a low-calorie and low-cholesterol diet, regular exercise, and appropriate drugs to treat lipid abnormalities and hypertension. Hopefully, treatment will prevent or slow the progression of cardiovascular disease and diabetes in persons with the metabolic syndrome.

HOMOCYSTEINE AND CARDIOVASCULAR DISEASE

Homocysteine is a sulfur-containing amino acid formed enzymatically from methionine, an essential amino acid that is abundant in animal protein. Homocysteine is then metabolized by other biochemical pathways in which vitamin B_6, vitamin B_{12}, and folic acid are required. Blood concentrations of homocysteine are higher in men than in premenopausal women but increase in women after the menopause. Renal function also influences homocysteine blood levels, which are elevated in persons with kidney disease.

Abnormal homocysteine metabolism is characteristic of a rare hereditary disease called *homocystinuria*. The disease results from a gene mutation leading to an enzyme defect that impairs the normal metabolism of homocysteine. Affected persons have an extremely high concentration of homocysteine in their blood and excrete the amino acid in their urine. The affected persons show evidence of marked vascular disease, which has its onset at a very young age. These manifestations include arteriosclerosis of coronary arteries and other major arteries, strokes, and blood clots in arteries and veins.

Because of the relationship of elevated homocysteine and premature vascular disease in persons with homocystinuria, investigators studied the relationship of homocysteine blood levels to cardiovascular disease in large groups of people. Numerous clinical studies have demonstrated that many persons with cardiovascular disease, strokes, and peripheral vascular disease have elevated homocysteine blood levels, and a high homocysteine blood level is a risk factor for arteriosclerosis, comparable to the increased risk associated with hypercholesterolemia, smoking, and hypertension.

In most persons in whom renal function is normal, the elevated homocysteine level seems to be related to a deficiency of vitamin B_6, vitamin B_{12}, or folic acid and can be corrected by vitamin supplements. A significant proportion of the population consumes insufficient amounts of both vitamin B_6 and folic acid.

Since vitamin B and folic acid supplements lower homocysteine blood levels, additional studies were undertaken to determine whether therapy with vitamin B_6, B_{12}, and folic acid would benefit patients with coronary artery disease who had already had a myocardial infarct. A large group of patients with severe cardiovascular disease received homocysteine-lowering vitamin therapy, and their outcomes were compared with a similar group of patients who did not receive vitamins. The homocysteine levels of the vitamin-treated group declined, but vitamin therapy did not reduce their risk of recurrent myocardial infarction or death from cardiovascular disease when compared with the untreated group. Moreover, the risk of a recurrent myocardial infarction was slightly higher in the vitamin-treated group, possibly because folic acid promotes cell proliferation and may have increased the size of some plaques by stimulating proliferation of cells within the plaques. Consequently, supplementary folic acid is no longer recommended for patients who have had a recent myocardial infarct. Supplementary folic acid is probably also inadvisable for patients who have had a stent inserted in one or more of their coronary arteries because cell proliferation in the arterial wall adjacent to the stent may encroach on the lumen of the stented artery and possibly lead to stenosis of the stented artery.

Hypertension and Hypertensive Cardiovascular Disease

PRIMARY HYPERTENSION

The ideal normal blood pressure should be below 120/80. A pressure consistently higher than 140/90 is called hypertension, and the higher the pressure, the greater are its harmful effects. Most cases of hypertension result from excessive vasoconstriction of the small arterioles throughout the body, which raises the diastolic pressure. Because of the high peripheral resistance, the heart needs to pump more forcefully in order to overcome the resistance created by the constricted arterioles and supply adequate blood to the tissues, which leads to a compensatory rise in systolic blood pressure. Therefore, both systolic and diastolic pressure rise when the primary problem is excessive arteriolar vasoconstriction. We do not really understand all of the factors responsible for this condition, which is called primary hypertension or essential hypertension, but we know that severe hypertension exerts injurious effects not only on the heart, but also on the blood vessels and kidneys.

Cardiac Effects

The heart responds to the increased workload resulting from the high peripheral resistance by becoming enlarged. Although the enlarged heart may be able to function effectively for many years, the cardiac pump is being forced to work beyond its "rated capacity." Eventually, the heart can no longer maintain adequate blood flow, and the patient develops symptoms of cardiac failure.

Vascular Effects

Because the blood vessels are not designed to carry blood at such a high pressure, the vessels wear out prematurely. Hypertension accelerates the development of atherosclerosis in the larger arteries. The arterioles also are injured; they thicken and undergo degenerative changes, and their lumens become narrowed. This process is termed **arteriolosclerosis**. Sometimes the walls of the small arterioles become completely necrotic owing to the effects of the sustained high blood pressure. Weakened arterioles may rupture, leading to hemorrhage. The brain is particularly vulnerable, cerebral hemorrhage being a relatively common complication of severe hypertension.

Arteriolosclerosis
(är-tēr-ē-ólo-skler-ō'-sis)
One type of arteriosclerosis characterized by thickening and degeneration of small arterioles.

Renal Effects

The narrowing of the renal arterioles decreases the blood supply to the kidneys, which, in turn, leads to injury and degenerative changes in the glomeruli and renal tubules. Severe hypertension may cause severe derangement of renal function and eventually leads to renal failure.

SECONDARY HYPERTENSION

In a small proportion of patients, the hypertension results from a known disease or condition such as chronic kidney disease (discussion on the urinary system), endocrine gland dysfunction such as a pituitary or an adrenal tumor, or a hyperactive thyroid gland (discussion on the endocrine glands). The high blood pressure associated with these conditions is called secondary hypertension because the cause of the hypertension is known. In many cases, successful treatment of the underlying condition cures the hypertension.

ISOLATED SYSTOLIC HYPERTENSION

As the name implies, isolated systolic hypertension is characterized by a mild to moderately elevated systolic pressure with a normal or even lower than normal diastolic pressure. This condition occurs primarily in older adults because the aorta and major arteries become less flexible with age. Consequently, when blood is ejected into the aorta during ventricular systole, the more rigid arteries are less able to stretch and absorb some of the force of the ejected blood. As a result, the systolic pressure is higher than it would be if the vessels were more flexible. The diastolic pressure remains normal because there is no excessive arteriolar vasoconstriction. Previously, this condition was considered to be less serious than hypertension in which both pressures were higher than normal, but unfortunately, more recent studies have demonstrated that isolated systolic hypertension causes the same harmful effects on the heart and blood vessels as primary and secondary hypertension.

TREATMENT OF HYPERTENSION

Although the reason for the hypertension cannot be determined in most instances, the blood pressure can be reduced to more normal levels, thereby lowering risk of complications of high blood pressure. This is accomplished by administering various drugs that lower the blood pressure by lessening the vasoconstriction of the peripheral blood vessels. This same approach is used to treat isolated systolic hypertension. Even though the cause of this condition is related to aging and increased rigidity of larger arteries, the same types of drugs used to treat primary and secondary hypertension are also effective.

Primary Myocardial Disease

In a small number of patients, heart disease results not from valvular or coronary disease or hypertension but from primary disease of the heart muscle itself. There are two major types of primary myocardial disease. One type results from inflammation of heart muscle and is called myocarditis. The other type, in which there is no evidence of inflammation, is designated by the noncommittal term cardiomyopathy (*cardio* = heart + *myo* = muscle + *pathy* = disease).

MYOCARDITIS

Myocarditis is characterized by an active inflammation in the heart muscle associated with injury and necrosis of individual muscle fibers. In the United States, most cases are caused by viruses. A few are caused by parasites, such as *Trichinella* (discussion on animal parasites) that lodge in the myocardium and cause an inflammation. Occasionally, other pathogens such as *Histoplasma* are responsible, especially in immunocompromised patients. Some cases are the result of a hypersensitivity reaction such as the myocarditis occurring in acute rheumatic fever.

The onset of myocarditis is usually abrupt and may lead to acute heart failure. Fortunately, in most cases, the inflammation subsides completely and the patient recovers without any permanent heart damage. There is no specific treatment other than treating the underlying condition that caused the myocarditis and decreasing cardiac work by bed rest and limited activity while the inflammation subsides.

CARDIOMYOPATHY

The general term cardiomyopathy encompasses two different conditions: dilated cardiomyopathy and hypertrophic cardiomyopathy. Both conditions are hereditary and transmitted as dominant traits. Often, the responsible gene mutations can be identified by genetic tests. Dilated cardiomyopathy is characterized by enlargement of the heart and dilatation of its chambers. The pumping action of the ventricles is greatly impaired which leads to chronic heart failure.

A   B

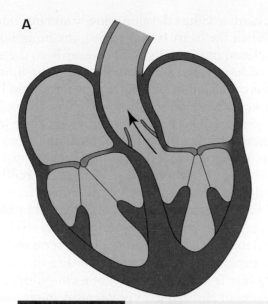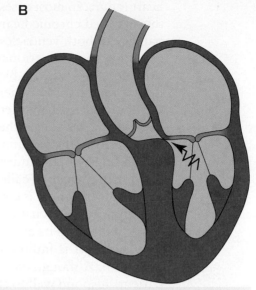

FIGURE 13-38 A comparison of normal cardiac function with malfunction characteristic of hypertrophic cardiomyopathy. **A**, Normal heart, illustrating unobstructed flow of blood from left ventricle into aorta during ventricular systole. **B**, Hypertrophic cardiomyopathy, illustrating obstruction to outflow of blood from left ventricle by hypertrophied septum, which impinges on anterior leaflet of mitral valve.

Hypertrophic cardiomyopathy is characterized by disarray of muscle fibers that intersect at odd angles with no apparent organized pattern and marked hypertrophy of heart muscle to such an extent that the thick-walled chambers become greatly reduced in size and do not dilate readily in diastole. Frequently, the muscle of the septum is hypertrophied to a greater extent than the rest of the myocardium and hinders outflow of the blood from the ventricle into the aorta. At times, the thick septum may actually impinge on the anterior mitral valve leaflet, intermittently completely blocking the outflow of blood from the left ventricle (FIGURE 13-38). This type of cardiomyopathy is often called idiopathic hypertrophic subaortic stenosis, usually abbreviated IHSS. The term indicates that the obstruction (stenosis) is located below the aortic valve (subaortic), resulting from myocardial hypertrophy (hypertrophic) of unknown cause (idiopathic).

Patients with IHSS frequently exhibit manifestations related to inadequate cardiac output, such as episodes of excessive fatigue and lightheadedness related to exertion. The characteristic myocardial hypertrophy with greatly thickened septum can be identified by echocardiography (discussion on general concepts of disease: principles of diagnosis). Treatment consists of administering drugs that slow the heart (allowing more time for ventricular filling) and reduce the force of ventricular contraction (which tends to reduce the degree of obstruction caused by the hypertrophied septum). Commonly used drugs are those that block the sympathetic nerve impulses that normally increase heart rate and the force of contraction (beta blockers) and those that decrease myocardial contractility by impeding the flow of calcium into myocardial cells (called calcium channel blocking agents). Persons who do not respond to medical treatment may require surgical resection of part of the thickened septum.

Heart Failure

Heart failure exists whenever the heart is no longer able to pump adequate amounts of blood to the tissues. It may result from any type of heart disease. Rapid failing of the heart, as when a large portion of muscle undergoes infarction, is called acute heart failure. In most cases, however, cardiac failure develops slowly and insidiously; this is called chronic heart failure. When the heart begins to fail, the pumping capability of both ventricles slowly declines, but initially not necessarily to the same extent. A disproportionate decline of left ventricular output causes the lungs to become engorged with blood, which is called left heart failure. The term right heart failure may be used when the right ventricle cannot "keep up" with the volume of venous blood being returned to the heart. The increased venous pressure in the distended veins causes the body tissues to accumulate fluid that usually is detected most easily in the feet and legs. When one compresses the swollen (edematous) skin with a fingertip, the indentation persists for a few minutes until the fluid refills the depression, which is called pitting edema. Because the most prominent feature in chronic heart failure is congestion of the tissues as a result of engorgement by blood, the physician often uses the term congestive heart failure when referring to chronic heart failure and its attendant clinical manifestations. Although the term indicates that the heart is failing, it does not necessarily indicate a severe life-threatening condition. Although chronic heart failure is a slowly progressing condition, many patients respond well to effective treatment and can live comfortably in reasonably good health for many years.

PATHOPHYSIOLOGY AND TREATMENT

Sometimes the terms "forward failure" and "backward failure" are used to describe the mechanisms leading to the development of heart failure. In forward failure, the initial effect of inadequate cardiac output is considered to be insufficient blood flow to the tissues. The inadequate renal blood flow results in retention of salt and water by the kidneys. (This effect is mediated indirectly through the adrenal glands.) Fluid retention, in turn, leads to an increased blood volume, and this is soon followed by a rise in venous pressure. The high venous pressure and high capillary pressure cause excessive transudation of fluid from the capillaries, leading to edema of the tissues. In backward failure, the inadequate output of blood is considered to cause "back up" of blood within the veins draining back to the heart, leading to increased venous pressure, congestion of the viscera, and edema. FIGURE 13-39 illustrates the interrelation of the various factors concerned in the development of cardiac failure. Probably, both forward failure and backward failure are present to some degree in every patient with heart failure. Treatment consists of diuretic drugs, which promote excretion of excess salt and water by the kidneys, thereby lowering blood volume. In addition, digitalis preparations are sometimes administered. They act to increase the efficiency of ventricular contractions. Other medications called ACE inhibitors are also frequently used. These drugs block an enzyme called angiotensin converting enzyme (abbreviated ACE), which is part of a renal regulatory mechanism called the renin–angiotensin-aldosterone system (discussion on the urinary system) that promotes retention of salt and water by the kidneys and raises blood pressure. Both of these effects are undesirable in heart failure patients, and blocking this mechanism by an ACE inhibitor has been shown to improve survival of patients in congestive heart failure.

COMPARISON OF SYSTOLIC AND DIASTOLIC DYSFUNCTION IN HEART FAILURE

The efficiency of ventricular function in heart failure patients can be measured, which allows the physician to determine whether the heart failure results primarily from inadequate ejection of blood from the ventricles in systole or from inadequate filling

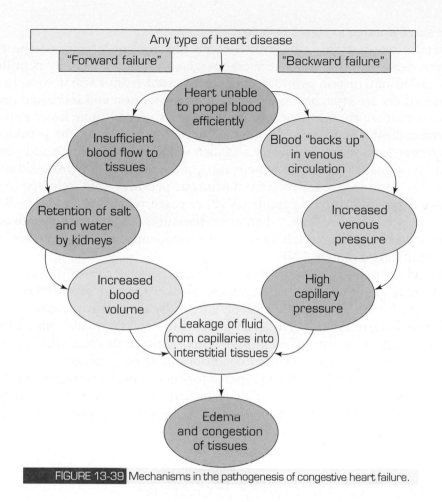

FIGURE 13-39 Mechanisms in the pathogenesis of congestive heart failure.

of the ventricles in diastole. In most patients with heart failure, the failing ventricles are distended with blood but are unable to expel a normal volume of blood during systole. Consequently, the left ventricular ejection fraction is significantly reduced and may fall from a normal value of about 60% to as low as 20%. This condition is called **systolic heart failure**.

In contrast, the main problem in some heart failure patients is not with the impaired ejection of blood in systole but with inadequate filling of the ventricles during diastole. In this condition, called **diastolic heart failure**, the volume of blood contained in the ventricles during diastole is lower than it should be, and the pressure of the blood within the chambers is elevated. This condition may occur in persons with marked hypertension in whom the thick hypertrophied left ventricular wall cannot relax enough in diastole to allow the left ventricular chamber to expand normally. Consequently, less blood can flow into the ventricle and the pressure of the blood within the ventricle is elevated. Some other less common conditions in which the ventricles are unable to relax normally in diastole may also reduce ventricular filling and raise intraventricular pressure. In all of these conditions, the left ventricle is underfilled in diastole (low end-diastolic volume), and the stroke volume is also low because there is a smaller volume of blood available in the chamber to be ejected. However, the ejection fraction is normal because both end-diastolic volume and stroke volume are reduced proportionately. Nevertheless, the cardiac output is inadequate to supply the body's needs. The clinical manifestations and methods of treatment of both systolic and diastolic heart failure are similar, although diuretics are the preferred treatment for patients with diastolic heart failure.

Systolic heart failure
Heart failure caused by inadequate ejection of blood from the ventricles during systole, in contrast to diastolic heart failure in which filling of the ventricles in diastole is inadequate.

Diastolic heart failure
Heart failure caused by inadequate filling of the ventricles during diastole, in contrast to systolic heart failure in which ejection of blood from the ventricles during systole is inadequate.

Natriuretic Peptides in Heart Failure

In heart failure patients, the unfavorable physiologic effects of the renin–angiotensin–aldosterone system are counteracted to some extent by peptide hormones called natriuretic peptides that are released from cardiac muscle fibers when the fibers are stretched as a result of overdistention and increased pressure within the cardiac chambers, as occurs in patients with chronic heart failure. As the name indicates (*natrium* = sodium + *uresis* = urination), the peptides promote urinary loss of salt and water and also reduce blood volume and pressure, effects that oppose those caused by activation of the renin–angiotensin–aldosterone system. The peptides are called atrial natriuretic peptide (ANP) released from the atria and B-type natriuretic peptide (BNP) released from the ventricles. Because ventricular pressures are higher than atrial pressures, the ventricular muscle cells are subjected to greater stretching forces. Consequently, BNP is of greater physiologic significance than is ANP.

A blood test to measure the level of BNP in a seriously ill patient who is very short of breath may help the physician determine whether the patient's marked dyspnea (shortness of breath) is caused by heart failure or by some other condition, such as lung disease. In heart failure, BNP is very high because the ventricular muscle fibers of the failing heart are overstretched. If BNP is not significantly elevated, the diagnosis of heart failure is unlikely, and other conditions must be considered to explain the patient's symptoms. BNP has been prepared for clinical use by recombinant technology and is sometimes used to treat patients in acute heart failure who are very short of breath. The intravenously administered BNP preparation promotes fluid loss and improves the patient's dyspnea.

Acute Pulmonary Edema

Acute pulmonary edema is a manifestation of acute heart failure and is a very serious life-threatening condition that requires immediate treatment. It is caused by a temporary disproportion in the output of blood from the ventricles. If the output of blood from the left ventricle is temporarily reduced more than the output from the right ventricle, the "right heart" will pump blood into the lungs faster than the "left heart" can deliver the blood to the peripheral tissues. This rapidly engorges the lungs with blood, raises the pulmonary capillary pressure, and produces transudation of fluid into the pulmonary alveoli. The patient becomes extremely short of breath because fluid accumulates within the alveoli, and oxygenation of the blood circulating through the lungs is impaired. The edema fluid becomes mixed with inspired air, forming a frothy mixture that "overflows" into the bronchi and trachea, filling the patient's upper respiratory passages. Treatment consists of supplementary oxygen to get more oxygen to the edematous pulmonary alveoli, intravenous diuretics and other medications to improve cardiac function by reducing the circulating blood volume, morphine to relieve anxiety, and measures directed toward correcting the underlying condition that precipitated the acute heart failure.

Aneurysms

An aneurysm is a dilatation of the wall of an artery or an outpouching of a portion of the wall. Most aneurysms are acquired as a result of arteriosclerosis, which causes weakening of the vessel wall. One type of aneurysm involving the cerebral arteries is the result of a congenital abnormality of the vessel wall and is considered in conjunction with the nervous system (discussion on the nervous system).

ARTERIOSCLEROTIC ANEURYSM

A small artery that undergoes arteriosclerotic change becomes narrowed and may eventually become thrombosed. A large artery such as the aorta has a diameter so large that complete obstruction is uncommon. However, atheromatous deposits tend to damage the wall of the aorta, reducing its elasticity and weakening the wall (FIGURE 13-40). The aortic wall tends to balloon out under the stress of the high pressure within the vessel. Aortic aneurysms usually develop in the distal part of the abdominal aorta, where the pressure is highest and the atheromatous change is most severe (FIGURES 13-41 AND 13-42). Usually, the interior of the aneurysm becomes covered with a layer of thrombus material, and the wall often becomes partially calcified.

As the name implies, arteriosclerosis is the major cause of arteriosclerotic aneurysms, but there appears to be some genetic predisposition as well, as 15 to 20% of patients with an aneurysm also have another affected family member. An aortic aneurysm usually enlarges slowly and does not produce symptoms initially. Because a small aneurysm is difficult to detect by physical examination, current guidelines recommend a routine ultrasound screening examination to identify an asymptomatic aneurysm in any adult older than age 65 who has risk factors that predispose to arteriosclerosis or who has a family history of an aortic aneurysm.

Aortic aneurysms are dangerous because they may rupture, leading to massive and often fatal hemorrhage. The normal cross-section diameter of the abdominal aorta is about 2 cm. An aneurysm exceeding about 5 cm in diameter may rupture

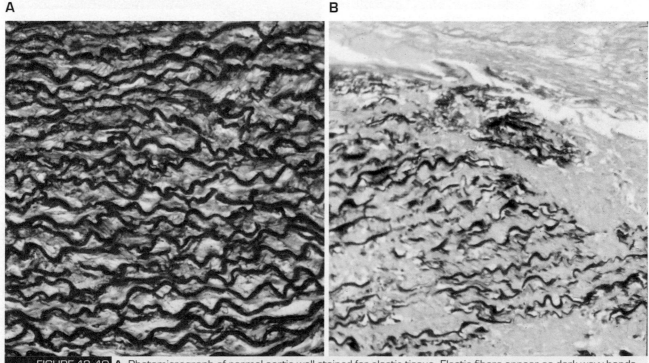

A

B

FIGURE 13-40 **A**, Photomicrograph of normal aortic wall stained for elastic tissue. Elastic fibers appear as dark wavy bands. **B**, Aortic wall from a patient with severe aortic atherosclerosis, illustrating marked fragmentation and destruction of elastic fibers, which weakens wall and predisposes to aneurysm (original magnification × 400).

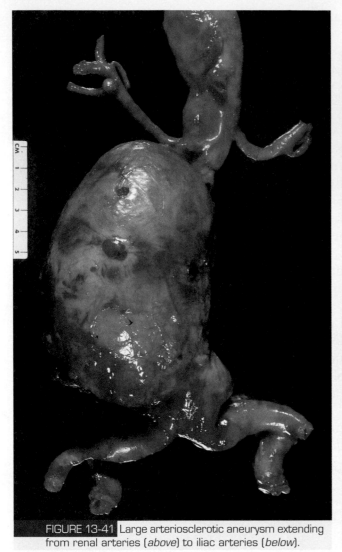

FIGURE 13-41 Large arteriosclerotic aneurysm extending from renal arteries (*above*) to iliac arteries (*below*).

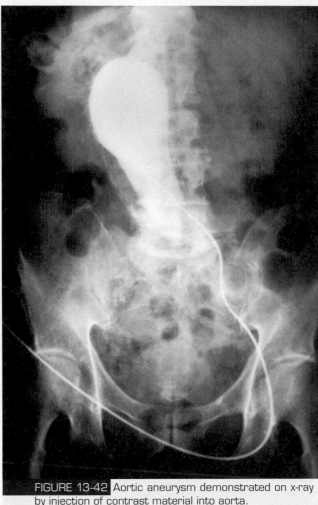

FIGURE 13-42 Aortic aneurysm demonstrated on x-ray by injection of contrast material into aorta.

Open surgical aneurysm repair
A surgical procedure in which an aortic aneurysm is opened; a graft is placed within the aneurysm sac and sutured to the aorta above and below the aneurysm so that the blood flows through the graft rather than through the aneurysm.

Endovascular aneurysm repair
A nonsurgical treatment of an abdominal aortic aneurysm in which the aneurysm graft is inserted through the femoral arteries, positioned within the aneurysm, and anchored within the aorta above and below the aneurysm.

and should be repaired. In general, the larger the aneurysm, the greater the likelihood of rupture (FIGURE 13-43).

The standard **open surgical aneurysm repair** procedure consists of opening the aneurysm and sewing a nylon or Dacron graft into the aorta above and below the aneurysmal segment so that the blood flowing through the aorta flows through the graft rather than through the aneurysm (FIGURE 13-44). It is not necessary to excise the aneurysm that has been bypassed by the graft, and usually the walls of the aneurysm are wrapped around the graft. This procedure is a well-established, reliable, and highly successful method of treatment, but it is a major surgical procedure and poses some risks to older patients who may have coronary artery disease and other medical problems.

In selected patients, an alternative method of treatment is available called **endovascular aneurysm repair** (*endo* = within + *vascular* = blood vessel). Two small incisions are made in the groins to expose the femoral arteries. A specially designed stent graft is inserted through the femoral arteries using a specially designed equipment to place the graft within the aneurysm under x-ray guidance. Then a balloon expands the stent graft, which has hooks or similar attachment devices to fix the graft to the aorta proximally, and to the aorta or iliac arteries distally (FIGURE 13-45). When properly fixed in position, blood flows through the graft instead of through the aneurysm. Two recently completed large studies comparing endovascular graft repair with standard surgical procedures appear to favor the endovascular graft, which had a lower mortality associated with the graft insertion than the surgical procedure, a shorter hospitalization, and fewer complications. However, the function of the graft after 3 years may not be as good as the open surgical procedure and may require additional treatment.

DISSECTING ANEURYSM OF THE AORTA

The thick middle layer of the aorta is called the media. It is composed of multiple layers of elastic tissue and muscle bonded together by fibrous connective tissue. Degenerative changes sometimes occur in the media, causing the layers to lose their cohesiveness and separate (FIGURE 13-46). Then the pulsatile force of the blood flowing through the aorta may cause the inner half of the aortic wall to pull away from the outer half in the region where the media has degenerated, and sometimes the inner lining (intima) tears as the media separates. This complication is especially likely to occur in persons with high blood pressure.

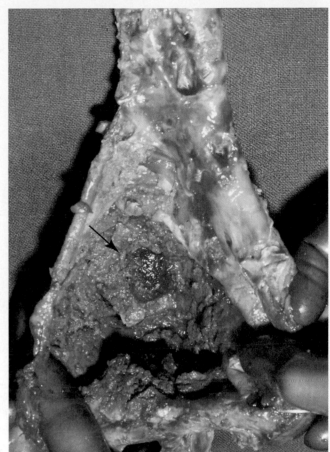

FIGURE 13-43 Interior of arteriosclerotic aneurysm, illustrating marked degenerative change in wall. Extremely thin area in wall (*arrow*) predisposes to rupture.

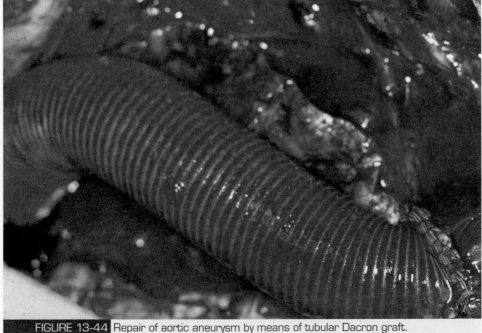

FIGURE 13-44 Repair of aortic aneurysm by means of tubular Dacron graft.

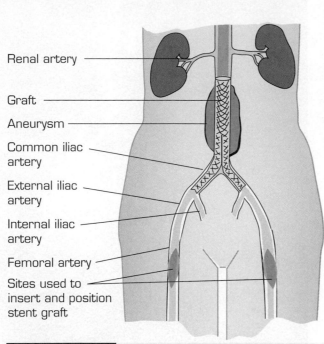

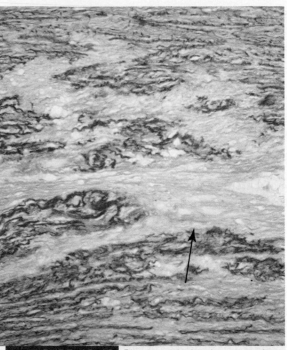

Renal artery

Graft

Aneurysm

Common iliac artery

External iliac artery

Internal iliac artery

Femoral artery

Sites used to insert and position stent graft

FIGURE 13-45 Endovascular graft to treat abdominal aortic aneurysm. The graft expands within the aorta, and the stent attachments fix graft to aorta proximally and iliac arteries distally.

FIGURE 13-46 Characteristic degenerative changes in the media of the aortic wall (called cystic medial necrosis) illustrated in the center of the photograph (*arrow*), which leads to loss of cohesion between the inner and outer layers of the aortic wall and predisposes to aortic dissection.

Dissecting aneurysm of the aorta
(an´ūr-izm)
A dissection of blood into the wall of the aorta secondary to degeneration of the arterial wall with an associated tear of the lining (intima) of the artery.

....

Aneurysm
(an´ūr-izm)
A dilatation of a structure, such as the aorta, a cerebral artery, or a part of the ventricular wall. See ventricular aneurysm.

After an intimal tear has developed, blood is forced into the aortic wall. The area of medial degeneration forms a cleavage plane that permits the blood to dissect within the media for a variable distance. This event, a **dissecting aneurysm of the aorta,** is associated with severe chest and back pain. The term dissecting refers to the splitting (dissection) of the media by the blood, and the somewhat misleading term **aneurysm** was applied because the affected part of the aorta appears wider than normal. The widening results from the hemorrhage within the aortic wall, but the lumen of the aorta is not dilated.

The intimal tear that starts the dissection is usually either in the ascending aorta just above the aortic valve or in the descending aorta just beyond the origin of the large arteries that arise from the aortic arch (FIGURE 13-47). If the tear is in the ascending aorta, the blood often dissects proximally as well as distally within the aortic wall, extending into the base of the aorta where the aortic valve attaches and the coronary arteries arise. The dissection may separate the aortic valve from its attachment to the deeper aortic wall so that it no longer functions properly, and severe aortic regurgitation develops. The origins of the coronary arteries may also be compressed by the hemorrhage in the wall, which compromises the blood supply to the heart muscle. A dissection in the ascending aorta is often fatal because the blood frequently ruptures through the outer wall of the aorta at the base of the heart, leading to extensive hemorrhage into the mediastinum or pericardial sac.

If the intimal tear is in the descending aorta, the blood dissects distally and may extend the entire length of the aorta. The blood in the aortic wall may also compress the origins of the large arteries that arise from the aorta, leading to impairment of blood flow to the kidneys, the intestines, or other vital organs. Sometimes the dissection may rupture back into the lumen of the aorta. If this occurs, blood flows not

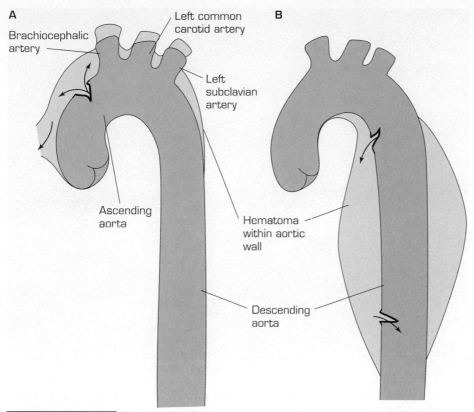

FIGURE 13-47 Sites of aortic dissection. **A**, Tear in ascending aorta causes both proximal and distal dissection. **B**, Tear in descending aorta may cause extensive distal dissection and may rupture back into lumen of aorta.

only through the lumen of the aorta, but also through the channel in the aortic wall created by the dissection, which communicates with the lumen of the aorta both proximally and distally (FIGURE 13-48).

Various surgical procedures have been devised to correct this condition.

Diseases of the Veins

The main diseases of veins are (1) venous thrombosis, (2) inflammation of veins, and (3) excessive dilatation and tortuosity of veins.

Venous thromboses occur most commonly in leg veins, but sometimes clots form within veins elsewhere in the body. Inflammation of a vein is called phlebitis (*phleb* = vein + *itis* = inflammation). If there is an associated thrombosis of the affected vein, the term thrombophlebitis is used. Dilated tortuous veins are called varices or varicose veins. (*Varix* is a Latin word meaning dilated vessel; the plural term is varices.) Varicosities occur most often in leg veins but may occur in other veins as well.

VENOUS THROMBOSIS AND THROMBOPHLEBITIS

Thrombus formation in deep leg veins is a frequent problem in postoperative patients and in those confined to bed, and it may be complicated by a pulmonary embolism, as described in the discussion on circulatory disturbances. The risk of leg vein thromboses in susceptible patients can be minimized by encouraging active

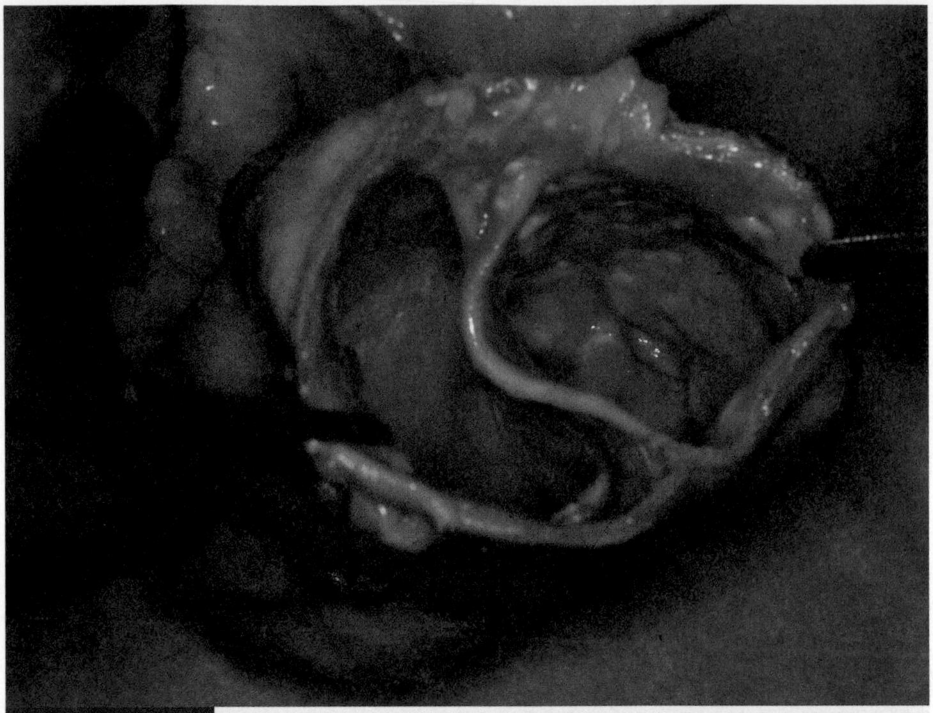

FIGURE 13-48 Cross section of aorta illustrating two channels ("double-barreled aorta") caused by dissecting aneurysm. The channel on the *right* of the photograph is true lumen of aorta. The channel on the *left* is the channel in the aortic wall created by the dissection.

leg exercises to improve venous blood flow and prevent venous stasis and by early ambulation.

Venous thrombosis and thrombophlebitis are treated by elevation of the leg, heat, and anticoagulant drugs. The anticoagulation stops the progression of the intravascular clotting process while the body's normal protective mechanisms remove the clot. The clot is dissolved by activation of the fibrinolytic mechanism and by ingrowth of connective tissue from the vein wall at the site where the clot adheres to the vein wall. Damage to the vein wall and its valves after thrombophlebitis may disturb venous return and predispose to later development of varicose veins.

VARICOSE VEINS OF THE LOWER EXTREMITIES

Two main groups of veins return blood from the lower limbs: the deep veins and the superficial veins. The deep veins carry most of the venous return. They accompany the major arteries and drain into the iliac veins, which in turn empty into the inferior vena cava. The superficial veins form a network of intercommunicating channels that travel just beneath the skin in the subcutaneous tissue and eventually drain into the deep veins. The largest superficial vein is the great saphenous vein, which extends up the medial surface of the leg from the ankle to the groin and drains into the more deeply placed femoral vein just below the groin. A second large superficial vein called the small saphenous vein ascends the back of the leg and drains into the deep venous system at the back of the knee. Both the superficial and deep veins contain cup-shaped valves, fashioned somewhat like the semilunar valves in the heart, which are interposed along the course of the veins. The arrangement of the valves is such that blood can flow upward in the veins but cannot flow in the reverse direction. The superficial and deep venous systems are also interconnected by short communicating branches that contain valves arranged so that blood normally flows only from superficial to deep veins and not in the reverse direction.

Blood is propelled upward within the deep veins by contraction of the leg and thigh muscles, which intermittently compress the veins and force the blood upward within the veins against gravity. The valves within the veins prevent retrograde flow. In contrast, the superficial veins are relatively unsupported, and venous return is much less efficient. Nevertheless, venous return through the superficial veins is normal provided that the veins do not become excessively dilated and the valves function properly to prevent retrograde flow and venous stasis.

Varicose veins result if the saphenous veins become dilated and their valves become incompetent. As a result, the blood tends to stagnate in the veins instead of flowing back normally to the heart, causing the veins to become elongated and tortuous. The condition tends to run in families, suggesting that the basic cause is a congenital weakness of the vein wall or its valves, which predisposes to the varicosities.

Varicose veins of the saphenous system may also develop if the deeper veins become blocked or if their valves become damaged by previous thrombophlebitis. As a result of damage to the deep veins, more of the venous return is shifted to the unsupported superficial veins, which are unable to cope with the increased flow and become varicose.

Complications of Varicose Veins

Complications result from stasis of blood in the veins, with poor nutrition of the tissues caused by chronic venous engorgement. The skin of the distal leg and ankle becomes thin and atrophic and quite susceptible to infection. Skin ulcers may develop and heal poorly. The dilated veins are easily injured and may rupture, leading to extravasation of blood and chronic discoloration of the skin. Stasis of blood in the veins also predisposes to repeated bouts of thrombophlebitis.

Treatment of Varicose Veins

Varicosities of the saphenous veins are treated by elastic stockings to support the veins and elevation of the legs whenever possible to promote more efficient venous return. Sometimes surgical removal of the varicose veins may be required. This is usually performed in conjunction with ligation of the communicating veins that interconnect the superficial and deep venous systems.

VARICOSE VEINS IN OTHER LOCATIONS

Dilated veins around the rectum are called **hemorrhoids** and are described in the discussion on the gastrointestinal tract in conjunction with disorders of the gastrointestinal tract. Varicose veins of the esophagus often occur in patients with a disease called **cirrhosis of the liver. Esophageal varices** may rupture and cause profuse life-threatening hemorrhage. Their pathogenesis and treatment are considered in the discussion on the liver and the biliary system. Varicose veins of the spermatic cord appear as a mass of vessels in the scrotum above the testicle. The condition is called a **varicocele** (*varix* = vein + *cele* = swelling). The varicosities usually do not cause symptoms but at times may cause mild scrotal discomfort. Rarely, they may impair fertility in some men. Usually no treatment is required.

Hemorrhoids
(hem'or-oyds)
Varicosities of anal and rectal veins.

Cirrhosis of the liver
(si-rō'sis)
A disease characterized by diffuse intrahepatic scarring and liver cell degeneration.

Esophageal varices
(var'i-sēz)
Dilated (varicose) veins of the esophagus, which are often present in patients with cirrhosis of the liver.

Varicocele
(var'-ik-kō-sēl)
Varicose veins within the spermatic cord that drain blood from the testis.

QUESTIONS FOR REVIEW

1. How do the heart valves function to provide unidirectional blood flow? What factors determine the level of the systolic and diastolic blood pressure?

2. What are the major causes of heart disease? What is the difference between rheumatic fever and rheumatic heart disease?

3. What is infective endocarditis? How does it arise? How is it prevented?

4. What is coronary heart disease? What are its manifestations? What is the difference between angina pectoris and myocardial infarction?

5. What is the effect of high blood pressure on the heart and the blood vessels?

6. What is heart failure? What is meant by the following terms: *forward failure, backward failure, acute heart failure, chronic heart failure, systolic heart failure, diastolic heart failure, and acute pulmonary edema*?

7. What is the usual cause of an aortic aneurysm? How is an aneurysm treated?

8. What is the difference between an arteriosclerotic aneurysm of the aorta and a dissecting aneurysm of the aorta?

9. What are the major complications of a large myocardial infarction?

10. What is meant by the following terms: *mitral valve prolapse, calcific aortic stenosis, atrial fibrillation,* and *ventricular fibrillation*?

11. What factors predispose to thrombus formation in leg veins? What are the major complications of venous thrombi?

12. What are varicose veins? What veins are commonly affected? What are the clinical manifestations?

SUPPLEMENTARY READINGS

Alpert, J. S., Thygesen, K., Antman, E., et al. 2000. Myocardial infarction redefined—a consensus document of The Joint European Society of Cardiology/American College of Cardiology Committee for the redefinition of myocardial infarction. *Journal of the American College of Cardiology* 36:959–69.

> ► Previously, a myocardial infarction was defined by a combination of two or three characteristics using standard World Health Organization criteria: typical symptoms, typical ECG pattern, and rise of cardiac enzymes. Now the very sensitive and specific cardiac troponin tests performed on patients with chest pain can detect very small foci of myocardial necrosis that are not large enough to cause the MB fraction of creatine kinase (CK-MB) to rise. Using the earlier criteria, these patients would have been considered to have severe unstable angina but now are diagnosed as having a small myocardial infarct.

Al Suwaidi, J., Berger, P. B., and Holmes, D. R., Jr. 2000. Coronary artery stents. *Journal of the American Medical Association* 284:1828–36.

> ► Intracoronary stents improve clinical outcome and are an essential component of catheter-based treatment of coronary artery disease.

Antman, E. M. 2002. Decision making with cardiac troponin tests. *The New England Journal of Medicine* 346:2079–82.

> ► Troponin tests are very sensitive and specific and can identify minor myocardial damage that is not sufficient to cause a rise in the cardiac specific fraction of creatine kinase. These observations have led to a reevaluation of the spectrum of coronary artery disease syndromes.

Beckett, N. S., Peters, R., Fletcher, A. E., et al. 2008. Treatment of hypertension in patients 80 years of age or older. *The New England Journal of Medicine* 358:1887–98.

> ► Reducing elevated blood pressure reduces the risk of strokes and also reduces death rate from cardiovascular disease even in very elderly patients.

Boden, W. E., O'Rourke, R. A., Teo, K. K., et al. 2007. Optimal medical therapy with or without PCI for stable coronary disease. *The New England Journal of Medicine* 356:1503–16.

▶ Insertion of stents to open narrowed coronary arteries, called percutaneous coronary intervention (PCI), is performed frequently as the initial treatment of patients with stable coronary artery disease along with standard medical therapy. A trial involving 2,287 patients with significant coronary artery disease and angina was undertaken in which the subjects were divided into two groups. PCI did not reduce the risk of death, myocardial infarction, or other cardiovascular events in patients with stable coronary artery disease when added to optimal medical therapy. Addition of elective PCI offers no advantage over medical treatment alone.

Bugiardini, R., and Bairey Merz, C. N. B. 2005. Angina with "normal" coronary arteries: A changing philosophy. *Journal of the American Medical Association* 293:477–84.

▶ Angina pectoris associated with apparently normal coronary arteries, or with nonobstructive coronary artery disease, is not a benign condition, as this condition occurs in about 10% of women and 6% of men. The various reasons that may explain this paradox are discussed, including the role of emotional stress.

Feldman, T., and Leon, M. B. 2007. Prospects for percutaneous valve therapies. *Circulation* 116:2866–77.

▶ A comprehensive discussion of percutaneous methods available or under active investigation that can be used to treat patients with valvular heart disease who are not good candidates for a standard surgical method of valve replacement. The percutaneous methodology is a "work in progress," as the valves and their methods of insertion are improved continuously based on clinical experience with the current percutaneous valves and their methods of replacement.

Ford, E. S., Ajani, U. A., Croft, J. B., et al. 2007. Explaining the decrease in U.S. deaths from coronary disease, 1980–2000. *The New England Journal of Medicine* 356:2388–98.

▶ Although coronary heart disease and its complications is a leading cause of death in the United States, great progress has been made in reducing mortality, which has declined about 50% in the last two decades. About half the mortality reduction resulted from better control of risk factors that promote coronary heart disease, such as lowering blood lipids, better control of hypertension, reduced smoking, and increased physical activity. The other half of the mortality reduction was related to improved methods for diagnosing and treating coronary heart disease and its complications.

Hagan, P. G., Nienaber, C. A., Isselbacher, E. M., et al. 2000. The International Registry of Acute Aortic Dissection (IRAD): New insights into an old disease. *Journal of the American Medical Association* 283:897–903.

▶ A review of the presentation, management, and outcomes of acute aortic dissection.

Hochman, J. S., and Steg, P. G. 2007. Does preventive PCI work? *The New England Journal of Medicine* 356:1572–74.

▶ PCI is effective in reducing angina in patients with coronary artery disease, and reduces mortality in patients who have an acute myocardial infarction or high-risk acute coronary syndromes accompanied by myocardial damage. These favorable outcomes have led to more widespread use of PCI to supplement medical therapy in an attempt to improve the long-term prognosis in patients with stable coronary artery disease. PCI offers no additional advantage over standard medical therapy for most patients with stable coronary artery disease.

Judge, D. P. 2009. Use of genetics in the clinical evaluation of cardiomyopathy. *Journal of the American Medical Association* 302:2471–76.

▶ Inherited forms of cardiomyopathy may be responsible for heart failure that is otherwise unexplained, and often the gene mutations can be identified by genetic tests. Screening of family members who may be at risk for an acquired form of cardiomyopathy may lead to earlier identification of affected family members, which in turn can lead to earlier treatment and a more favorable response to therapy.

Keeley, E. C., and Hillis, L. D. 2007. Primary PCI for myocardial infarction with ST-segment elevation. *The New England Journal of Medicine* 356:47–54.

▶ Plugging of a coronary artery by a thrombus cuts off the blood supply to the heart muscle in the distribution of the occluded vessel, which is soon followed by necrosis of the ischemic muscle. PCI is the preferred method of treatment. The site of the thrombosis is identified by angiography followed by insertion of a guide wire through the region blocked by the thrombus. Then a balloon catheter covered by a collapsed bare metal or drug-coated stent is directed over the guide wire and positioned at the site of the thrombus. Finally the balloon is inflated, which opens the artery and expands the stent to keep the artery open.

Kloner, R. A., and Rezkalla, S. H. 2003. Cocaine and the heart. *The New England Journal of Medicine* 348:487–88.

▶ A review of the mechanisms of action of cocaine on the cardiovascular system. The risk of myocardial infarction is highest within the first hour after cocaine use, and there is no clear relationship between the dose of cocaine and the occurrence of an acute myocardial infarction.

Lange, R. A., and Hillis, L. D. 2002. Reperfusion therapy in acute myocardial infarction. *The New England Journal of Medicine* 346:954–55.

▶ Restoration of blood flow through a blocked coronary artery reduces myocardial damage and improves survival. Thrombolytic therapy is effective but does not always completely dissolve the thrombus. Balloon angioplasty is more effective than thrombolytic therapy. The use of a stent along with antiplatelet drugs helps prevent restenosis of the dilated vessel.

Lederle, F. A. 2005. Endovascular repair of abdominal aortic aneurysm—Round two. *The New England Journal of Medicine* 352:2443–45.

▶ A review of the costs and benefits of the two procedures. The endovascular repair was associated with a lower postoperative mortality than the open surgical procedure, but the longer term follow-up revealed no survival advantage because there were late complications and deaths related to the endovascular repair. Long-term mortality data were similar for both procedures.

Le May, M. R., So, D. Y., Dionne, R., et al. 2008. A citywide protocol for primary PCI in ST-segment elevation myocardial infarction. *The New England Journal of Medicine* 358:231–40.

▶ A Canadian metropolitan community developed a protocol in which specially trained paramedics who were able to interpret an ST-elevation myocardial infarction responded to 911 calls. Patients in whom ST-segment myocardial infarction was demonstrated received a chewable aspirin tablet and sublingual nitroglycerine, and were transported directly to a cardiac care center for immediate angiogram and PCI. Overall in-hospital mortality was 4.7% compared with 5.7% mortality for patients not directly transferred to a coronary care center.

Mark, D. B., and Felker, G. M. 2004. B-type natriuretic peptide—A biomarker for all seasons? *The New England Journal of Medicine* 350:718–20.

▶ BNP is a useful diagnostic tool for evaluating a patient with acute dyspnea in an emergency department. If the BNP level is less than 100 pg per milliliter, the diagnosis of congestive heart failure is very unlikely. If the level is over 500 pg per milliliter, congestive cardiac failure is likely. Intermediate levels are not helpful.

Maron, B. J. 2002. Hypertrophic cardiomyopathy: A systematic review. *Journal of the American Medical Association* 287:1308–20.

▶ This disease is an important cause of disability, but the prognosis is not ominous and is compatible with normal longevity, which should provide reassurance to patients.

Mukamal, K. J., Conigrave, K. M., Mittleman, M. A., et al. 2003. Roles of drinking pattern and type of alcohol consumed in coronary heart disease in men. *The New England Journal of Medicine* 348:109–18.

▶ Consumption of alcohol at least three or four times per week reduces the risk of myocardial infarction, and the type of alcohol consumed (beer, red wine, or white wine, etc.) does not have any effect on the favorable result.

Otto, C. M., Kuusisto, J., Reichenbach, D. D., et al. 1994. Characterization of the early lesion of "degenerative" valvular aortic stenosis. *Circulation* 90:844–53.

▶ Mechanical stresses initiate structural changes in the valve followed by lipid deposition and infiltration of the valve leaflets by macrophages and T lymphocytes, similar to the changes in coronary atherosclerosis.

Pinto, D. S. 2010. A 43-year-old man with angina, elevated troponin, and lateral ST depression: Management of acute coronary syndromes. *Journal of the American Medical Association* 303:54–63.

▶ All patients with intermediate or high risk non-ST elevation myocardial infarction (NSTEMI) should have coronary angiography, and the cardiologist in consultation with the patient should determine the best way to proceed: (1) to open the coronary artery by angioplasty with stent placement (PCI), (2) to perform a coronary artery bypass graft (CABG), or (3) to continue with medical treatment. In general, patients with diffuse coronary artery disease have better results with CABG than PCI. The various types of antiplatelet and anticoagulant therapy associated with treatment are described and compared.

Roth, B. L. 2007. Drugs and valvular heart disease. *The New England Journal of Medicine* 356:6–9.

▶ Drugs that activate serotonin receptors in heart valves (agonists of 5-HT$_{2B}$ receptors, a subtype of serotonin receptors) stimulate mitosis and proliferation of valve connective tissue cells and collagen fibers, leading to valve thickening and impaired valve function. More recently, some drugs used to treat Parkinson's disease (pergolide and carbergoline) have been shown to cause heart valve damage by targeting the 5-HT$_{2B}$ serotonin receptors in heart valves.

Sacks, F. M., and Campos, H. 2010. Dietary therapy in hypertension. *The New England Journal of Medicine* 362:2102–12.

▶ In most cases, primary hypertension is a genetic disorder involving many individual genes which collectively regulate how the body deals with the dietary intake of sodium. Dietary treatment of hypertension includes a sodium intake restricted to 1.5 g per day along with maintaining or achieving a normal weight. A restricted alcohol intake is also recommended. No more than 2 alcoholic drinks per day for men of average size and 1 for women and smaller men. A trial of intensive dietary treatment is warranted for 6 months to achieve a goal of systolic blood pressure of less than 140 mm Hg and diastolic pressure less than 90 mm Hg before considering adding anti-hypertensive drugs.

Schade, R., Andersohn, F., Suissa, S., et al. 2007. Dopamine agonists and the risk of cardiac valve regurgitation. *The New England Journal of Medicine* 356:29–38.

▶ Ergot-derived dopamine agonists pergolide and cabergoline used to treat Parkinson's disease and restless leg syndrome may increase the risk of cardiac valve regurgitation. The drugs are potent agonists of the serotonin receptor (5-HT$_{2B}$) expressed on heart valves. Preferential activation of this receptor stimulates mitosis in cardiac valve cells leading to cell and connective fiber proliferation, which may impair valve function. The risk of valve dysfunction is high among subjects who have taken daily doses exceeding 3 mg for a period of 6 or more months. There was no increased risk with the use of other dopamine agonists.

Schermerhorn, M. L., O'Malley, A. J., Jhaveri, A., et al. 2008. Endovascular vs. open repair of abdominal aortic aneurysms in the medicare population. *The New England Journal of Medicine* 358:464–74.

▶ Endovascular repair compared with open repair is associated with a lower short-term rate of death and complications. Late additional procedures are required more often after endovascular repair, but there are also a comparable number of late procedures and hospitalizations after surgical procedures.

Shah, S. J., and Gheorghiade, M. 2008. Heart failure with preserved ejection fraction: Treat now by treating comorbidities. *Journal of the American Medical Association* 300:431–33.

▶ Half the patients with heart failure have a normal ejection fraction, and standard treatment for heart failure has had limited success. Most of these patients have other conditions that contribute to the heart failure, primarily coronary artery disease and hypertension.

Svilaas, T., Vlaar, P. J., van der Horst, I. C., et al. 2008. Thrombus aspiration during primary percutaneous coronary intervention. *The New England Journal of Medicine* 358:557–67.

▶ Primary PCI is effective in opening an infarct-related artery in patients with a ST-elevation myocardial infarction, but embolization of atheromatous debris and thrombus material plugs distal arterioles and reduces myocardial perfusion. Thrombus aspiration can be performed on most patients with ST-segment elevation myocardial infarction, which results in better reperfusion and better clinical outcomes than conventional PCI.

Thompson, R. W. 2002. Detection and management of small aortic aneurysms. *The New England Journal of Medicine* 346:1484–86.

▶ Routine physical examination cannot detect small aneurysms (between 4.0 to 5.4 cm diameter), but routine ultrasound screening of persons older than the age of 65 would detect almost all small aneurysms. Small aneurysms should be monitored periodically, and surgical repair is advisable if the aneurysm enlarges further or produces symptoms.

Thygesen, K., Alpert, J. S., and White, H. D. 2007. Universal definition of myocardial infarction. *Journal of the American College of Cardiology* 50:2173–95.

▶ A proposal to designate any degree of heart muscle damage as a myocardial infarction, with a discussion of diagnosis and treatment methods based on the degree of muscle necrosis. The authors believe that a change in the definition of a myocardial infarct will favorably influence the identification, prevention, and treatment of cardiovascular disease throughout the world.

Zanettini, R., Antonini, A., Gatto, G., et al. 2007. Valvular heart disease and the use of dopamine agonists for Parkinson's disease. *The New England Journal of Medicine* 356:39–46.

▶ Pergolide may cause fibrosis in valve leaflets and in the subvalvular tissues leading to stiffening, retraction, incomplete coaptation, and resulting valve regurgitation. Valve damage has been described following use of this drug to treat Parkinson's disease, and the drug has also been used in low dose to treat hyperprolactinemia. Drugs that mimic the effect of serotonin (serotonin agonist effect) on the serotonin receptor subtype 5-HT$_{2B}$ may damage heart valves by stimulating mitosis of inactive valve connective tissue cells (fibroblasts). Active fibroblast proliferation leads to an excess production of connective tissue (collagen) fibers, which thickens and deforms the heart valves.

Zile, M. R., Baicu, C. F., and Gaasch, W. H. 2004. Diastolic heart failure— Abnormalities in active relaxation and passive stiffness of the left ventricle. *The New England Journal of Medicine* 350:1953–9.

▶ Patients with heart failure and a normal ejection fraction had higher end diastolic pressures with lower end diastolic volumes than a control group, related to abnormal diastolic function.

OUTLINE SUMMARY

Cardiac Structure and Function

STRUCTURE OF THE HEART AND ITS CHAMBERS

Right heart circulates blood to lung.
Left heart circulates blood to peripheral tissues.

CARDIAC VALVES

AV valves attached to papillary muscles by chordae.
Cup-shaped semilunar valves.

BLOOD SUPPLY TO HEART

Left coronary artery:
Anterior descending: supplies anterior wall.
Circumflex: supplies lateral wall.
Right coronary artery: supplies posterior wall.

CONDUCTION SYSTEM

SA node.
AV node.
AV bundle, branches, and Purkinje fibers.

THE CARDIAC CYCLE

Blood fills ventricles passively during diastole.
Atrial contraction not essential for ventricular filling.
Only about 60% of ventricular blood ejected during systole (ejection fraction).

BLOOD VESSELS

Large elastic arteries stretch during systole and relax in diastole.
Arterioles lower pressure and regulate flow into capillaries.
Capillaries deliver nutrients and carry away waste products.

BLOOD PRESSURE

Systolic pressure: reflects force of ventricular contraction.
Diastolic pressure: measure of peripheral resistance.

THE ELECTROCARDIOGRAM (ECG)

Cardiac arrhythmias: diagnosis and treatment
Atrial and ventricular fibrillation.
Heart block.

Heart Disease as a Disturbance of Pump Function

CONGENITAL HEART DISEASE

Classification
Failure of fetal bypass channels to close normally.
Abnormal communication between cardiac chambers.
Abnormalities that impede blood flow through the cardiovascular system.
Abnormal division of truncus arteriosus:
Left-to-right blood shunts cause pulmonary hypertension and damage lungs.
Right-to-left blood shunts cause cyanosis, polycythemia, and clubbing of digits.
Treatment methods available for many patients.
Prevention: protect fetus from intrauterine injury.

VALVULAR HEART DISEASE

Rheumatic fever and rheumatic heart disease:
Rheumatic fever is a complication of beta-streptococcal infection and causes valvular damage.
Healing leads to valve scarring. Prevented by prompt treatment of beta-streptococcal infection.

Nonrheumatic aortic stenosis:
> *Bicuspid aortic valve: congenital malformation eventu-
> ally leads to valve thickening and scarring.*
> *Calcific aortic stenosis: degenerative change in el-
> derly individuals.*

MITRAL VALVE PROLAPSE
> *Valve stretches owing to degeneration of connective
> tissue and prolapses into left atrium.*
> *Chordae may rupture owing to stress.*
> *Predisposes to arrhythmia.*

SEROTONIN-RELATED HEART VALVE DAMAGE
High concentration of blood serotonin damages heart
valves.

Valve damage caused by drugs that activate serotonin
receptors, causing proliferation of connective tissue
in valves.

ANTIBIOTIC PROPHYLAXIS TO PREVENT ENDOCARDITIS
Transient bacteremia often follows dental or surgical
procedures.

Bacteria may implant on damaged heart valves and cause
endocarditis.

Antibiotic treatment for selected persons.

Prosthetic heart valves.

INFECTIVE ENDOCARDITIS
Subacute: organisms of low virulence implant on damaged
valves.

Acute: virulent organisms implant on normal valves and
may destroy valve. Intravenous drug abusers at
high risk.

Coronary Heart Disease

PATHOGENESIS OF ATHEROSCLEROSIS
Endothelial injury.

Lipids accumulate and precipitate.

Secondary fibrosis and calcification.

MAJOR RISK FACTORS
High blood lipids.

High blood pressure.

Cigarette smoking.

Diabetes.

MANIFESTATIONS
Angina pectoris.
> *Classification:*
>> *Stable angina: pain on exertion, subsides with
>> rest or medication.*
>> *Unstable angina: more frequent episodes,
>> last longer, poor response to rest or
>> medications.*
>> *Prinzmetal's angina: occurs at rest, caused by
>> coronary artery spasm.*

DIAGNOSIS
Angiography: detects extent of disease and localizes sites
of obstruction.

CORONARY DISEASE SYMPTOMS WITH NORMAL ANGIOGRAMS
Disease missed by angiography.

Coronary vasospasm.

Failure of arterioles to dilate normally.

TREATMENT
Medical treatment:
> *Drugs to reduce myocardial oxygen consumption and
> improve coronary circulation.*
> *Drugs to reduce myocardial irritability.*

Reduction of risk factors:
> *Cessation of smoking.*
> *Control of hypertension.*
> *Anti-coronary diet.*
> *Weight reduction where appropriate.*
> *Graduated exercises.*

Surgical treatment: myocardial revascularization.

Coronary angioplasty: balloon catheter smashes atheromatous plaque and dilates artery.

Severe myocardial ischemia and its complications:
a "heart attack."
> *Cardiac arrest: ventricular fibrillation or asystole.*

Myocardial Infarction

LOCATION: ALMOST ALWAYS LEFT VENTRICLE
Anterior wall: left anterior descending artery distribution.

Lateral wall: circumflex artery distribution.

Posterior wall: right coronary distribution.

Massive anterior and lateral wall: main left coronary
distribution.

MAJOR COMPLICATIONS
Arrhythmias.

Heart failure.

Intracardiac thrombi.

Cardiac rupture: a complication of transmural infarct.

SURVIVAL AFTER MYOCARDIAL INFARCTION
Depends on patient's age, size of infarct, presence of
complications.

Average survival: 95% of hospitalized patients.

Survival frequency does not reflect patients who die before entering the hospital or patients with small infarcts who do not consult physician.

DIAGNOSIS
History and physical: often inconclusive.

Electrocardiogram: can detect location and size of infarct.

Enzyme tests: enzymes leak from infarcted muscle.

TREATMENT OF CORONARY THROMBOSIS
Thrombolytic (clot-dissolving) therapy or angioplasty improves survival and salvages myocardium.

Bed rest advancing to graded activity.

Anti-arrhythmia drugs: to reduce myocardial irritability.

Treatment of complications:
> *Heart block: requires pacemaker.*
> *Heart failure: digitalis and diuretics.*
> *Long-term treatment with antiarrhythmia drugs
> (beta-blockers) and aspirin improves prognosis.*

COCAINE-INDUCED ARRHYTHMIAS/INFARCTS

Drug intensifies effects of sympathetic nerve impulses.
  Rapid heart rate: increases oxygen requirements.
  Myocardial irritability: predisposes to arrhythmias.
  Constricts blood vessels: raises blood pressure.
Drug may induce coronary artery spasm/severe ischemia/myocardial infarcts.
Fatal arrhythmias/myocardial infarcts may occur in persons with normal coronary arteries. Persons with coronary atherosclerosis are at even greater risk.

Blood Lipids and Coronary Heart Disease

NEUTRAL FAT: TRIGLYCERIDE

Composed of fatty acid combined with glycerol.
Fatty acids may be saturated, unsaturated, or polyunsaturated.

CHOLESTEROL

High levels associated with increased incidence of coronary heart disease.
Transport of cholesterol by lipoprotein.
  LDL cholesterol is atherogenic: "bad cholesterol."
  HDL cholesterol is protective: "good cholesterol."

ALTERATION OF BLOOD LIPIDS BY CHANGE IN DIET

Decrease cholesterol intake.
Decrease intake of saturated fats.
Derive carbohydrates from complex carbohydrates.
Reduce alcohol intake.

C-REACTIVE PROTEIN AS A CARDIOVASCULAR RISK FACTOR

A protein produced in response to inflammation or infection.
Sensitive CRP tests detect body's response to cells and lipids in unstable coronary artery plaques.
Test proposed as additional screening test to detect persons at risk of coronary artery disease.
The metabolic syndrome and cardiovascular disease:
  An obesity-related insulin resistance syndrome.
  Predisposes to cardiovascular disease and diabetes.
  Effective treatment may reduce risk.

HOMOCYSTEINE AND CARDIOVASCULAR DISEASE

Persons with very high homocysteine blood levels caused by a rare hereditary disease called homocysteinuria have early onset of severe atherosclerosis.
Persons with higher-than-normal homocysteine blood levels are at higher-than-normal risk of cardiovascular disease.
Deficiency of vitamin B_6, B_{12}, or folic acid can raise homocysteine blood concentration, which can be corrected by vitamin supplements, but treatment is harmful to coronary heart disease patients by promoting cell proliferation in coronary artery plaques.

TAKING ASPIRIN TO REDUCE CARDIOVASCULAR DISEASE RISK

Blood clots are initiated by platelets that adhere to roughened areas overlying an atherosclerotic plaque, which initiates an intravascular thrombosis.
Aspirin reduces risk by inactivating a platelet enzyme that is required for platelet aggregation.

Hypertension and Hypertensive Cardiovascular Disease

INCREASED PERIPHERAL RESISTANCE INCREASES WORK OF HEART

Vascular effects:
  Vessels wear out prematurely.
  Weakened arteries may rupture in brain causing cerebral hemorrhage.
Renal effects: narrowing of arterioles damages kidneys.

CAUSES AND TREATMENT

In most cases cause unknown.
Treatment by drugs that lower blood pressure.

ISOLATED SYSTOLIC HYPERTENSION

Affects older persons.
Rigid aorta unable to stretch to absorb the force of ejected blood.
Systolic pressure rises, but diastolic pressure is normal.
Treatment advisable despite normal diastolic pressure.

Primary Myocardial Disease

MYOCARDITIS

Usually viral; occasionally, other pathogens or hypersensitivity state.
Onset usually abrupt, with eventual complete recovery.

CARDIOMYOPATHY

Dilated cardiomyopathy:
  Heart enlarged and dilated.
  Cause uncertain, no specific treatment available.
Hypertrophic cardiomyopathy:
  Hereditary dominant transmission.
  Disorganized muscle fibers and greatly hypertrophied heart.
  Thick septum impinging on mitral valve leaflet may block outflow of blood from ventricle (idiopathic hypertrophic subaortic stenosis).
  Treated by drugs that slow heart and reduce force of contraction.
  Surgical resection of part of septum if medical management fails.

Heart Failure

DEFINITION

Heart no longer able to function efficiently:
  Acute heart failure: rapid progression.
  Chronic heart failure: slow onset and progression.
Pathogenesis:
  Forward failure: inadequate cardiac output leads to salt and water retention by kidneys.
  Backward failure: blood backs up in venous circulation.
Systolic and diastolic dysfunction in heart failure.
  Failing ventricle cannot eject adequate blood in systole: systolic heart failure.

Ventricle cannot fill adequately in diastole: diastolic heart failure.

Treatment:
Diuretics: promote salt and water excretion.
Digitalis: increases efficiency of cardiac contraction.
ACE inhibitors.
Natriuretic peptide (BNP).

Acute Pulmonary Edema

PATHOGENESIS

Temporary disproportion in output of blood from left and right ventricles.
Blood accumulates in lung.
Extravasation of fluid in alveoli.

Aneurysms

ARTERIOSCLEROTIC ANEURYSM

Arteriosclerosis damages wall, which dilates owing to high intraluminal pressure.
Aneurysm may rupture and cause profuse hemorrhage.
Treatment by replacement with nylon or Dacron graft.
Endovascular repair available for selected cases.

DISSECTING ANEURYSM OF THE AORTA

Splitting of layers of wall.
Blood dissects through intimal tear and may rupture back into lumen or externally.
Can be treated surgically.

Diseases of the Veins

VENOUS THROMBOSIS AND THROMBOPHLEBITIS

Deep veins of lower extremities most commonly affected.
Postoperative and bed patients predisposed.
Predisposing factors, pathogenesis, manifestations, and treatment covered in the discussion on circulatory disturbances.

VARICOSE VEINS OF LOWER EXTREMITIES

Usually a result of congenital weakness of vein wall or valves predisposing to varicosities.
May occur if deeper veins blocked or valves damaged by thrombophlebitis, diverting more blood flow to superficial veins.
Complications:
Stasis ulcers.
Rupture with bleeding.
Thrombophlebitis.
Treatment:
Medical: elastic stockings, elevation of limb.
Surgical: ligation and excision of varicosities.

VARICOSE VEINS IN OTHER LOCATIONS

Hemorrhoids: varicose veins of rectum (see the gastro-intestinal tract).
Esophageal varices: in patients with cirrhosis of liver (see the liver and the biliary system).
Varicocele: veins of spermatic cord. Usually asymptomatic, requiring no treatment.

The Hematopoietic and Lymphatic Systems

1 Describe the composition of the blood and enumerate its functions. Explain the functions of the lymphatic system.

2 Explain the principles by which anemias are classified and treated.

3 List and describe the usual causes of hypochromic microcytic anemia and macrocytic anemia. Explain how these anemias are treated.

4 List the usual causes of anemia as a result of bone marrow damage and anemia caused by accelerated blood destruction. Explain their treatment.

5 Describe the causes and effects of polycythemia and thrombocytopenia.

6 Describe the cause and clinical manifestations of infectious mononucleosis.

7 List the common causes of lymph node enlargement.

8 Explain the role of the spleen in protecting the body against infection. Describe the effects of a splenectomy on the body's defenses, and relate them to the management of the patient who has had a splenectomy.

The Hematopoietic System

COMPOSITION AND FUNCTION OF HUMAN BLOOD

Blood is essential to transporting oxygen and nutrients to the tissues; carbon dioxide and other waste products of cell metabolism to the excretory organs; and leukocytes, hormones, and antibodies to various locations in the body. The volume of blood, which varies with the size of the individual, is about five quarts in the average man. Almost half of the blood consists of cellular elements: red cells, white cells (leukocytes), and platelets suspended in a viscous fluid called blood plasma (FIGURE 14-1).

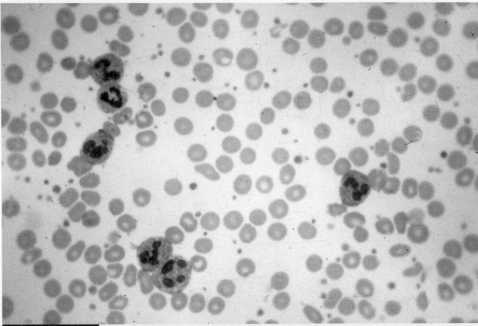

FIGURE 14-1 Stained blood film. Red cells appear as biconcave disks. Several neutrophils can be identified near the *center* of the photograph. Small dark structures are platelets (original magnification × 1,000).

All blood cells arise from precursor cells within the bone marrow called stem cells, which undergo further differentiation to form the red cells, white cells, and platelets circulating in the bloodstream. The numbers of circulating red cells, white cells, and platelets are so great that their numbers are expressed as the number per microliter (μl) of blood (1 ml = 1,000 μl). This same quantity can also be expressed as the number per cubic millimeter (mm^3) of blood. The terms are equivalent because 1 μl is the same as 1 mm^3.

Red cells, which are concerned primarily with oxygen transport, are the most numerous cells, averaging about 5 million per microliter of blood. A mature red cell is an extremely flexible biconcave disk measuring about 7 micrometers (microns) in cross-section diameter. Its biconcave configuration is responsible for its characteristic central pallor and more intensely stained periphery, as seen in a stained blood smear. The biconcave configuration also provides the red cell with a large surface area relative to its volume, which facilitates rapid uptake of oxygen as blood flows through the pulmonary capillaries, and a rapid release of oxygen to body cells as blood is delivered to the tissues. The red cell shape also contributes to its extreme flexibility, which allows red cells to squeeze through small blood capillaries less than half the diameter of the red cells. Red cells normally survive for about 4 months in the circulation.

Leukocytes are much less numerous, averaging about 7,000 per microliter. The following types of leukocytes are recognized:

1. Neutrophils
2. Eosinophils
3. Basophils
4. Monocytes
5. Lymphocytes

Although lymphocytes are produced chiefly in the lymph nodes and spleen, they are also manufactured in the bone marrow and elsewhere throughout the body where lymphoid tissue is present. Under normal circumstances, production of the other types of white cells is confined to the bone marrow. In contrast with the relatively long survival of red cells, most white cells have a short survival time within the circulation, varying from several hours to several days, and they must be replenished continually. Lymphocytes are an exception. Two populations of lymphocytes are present in the circulation, one surviving about the same length of time as most of the other leukocytes and another surviving for several years.

The proportions of the various leukocytes vary with the age of the individual. The most numerous in the adult are the **neutrophils**, constituting about 70% of the total circulating white cells. Neutrophils are actively phagocytic and predominate in acute inflammatory reactions. **Lymphocytes** are the next most common type of white cells in adults and are the predominant leukocytes in the blood of children. The lymphocytes in the peripheral blood constitute only a small fraction of the total lymphocytes, most being located in the lymph nodes, spleen, and other lymphoid tissues. Lymphocytes continually recirculate from the bloodstream into lymphoid tissues. Eventually, they leave the lymphoid tissue through the lymphatic channels and the thoracic duct, returning to the circulation and later becoming reestablished for a time in a different site of lymphoid tissue. Lymphocytes take part in cell-mediated and humoral defense reactions.

Small numbers of eosinophils, basophils, and monocytes also are normally present in the blood. **Eosinophils** are related in some manner to allergy. One of their functions appears to be phagocytosis and digestion of antigen–antibody complexes. Eosinophils increase in allergic diseases, in the presence of worm or other animal–parasite infections, and in a few other conditions. **Basophils** are similar to mast cells. Their granules contain histamine and an anticoagulant called **heparin**. **Monocytes** are actively phagocytic and increase in certain types of chronic infections. A monocyte–lymphocyte interaction is necessary in the initial phase of response to a foreign antigen; it also plays a role in the cell-mediated immune reaction.

Blood **platelets**, which are essential for normal blood coagulation, are much smaller than leukocytes. They represent bits of the cytoplasm of megakaryocytes, large precursor cells present in the bone marrow. Platelets have a short survival comparable to that of most leukocytes.

Normal Hematopoiesis

The bone marrow can be compared to a large manufacturing plant. It replenishes the blood cells that are continually being worn out and removed from the circulation. As with any manufacturing process, adequate quantities of raw materials are required. Moreover, the factory must be able to process these raw materials efficiently into finished products (the blood cells). The major raw materials necessary for hematopoiesis are protein, vitamin B_{12}, folic acid (one of the vitamin B group), and iron. Inadequate supplies of these substances will handicap the production of blood cells.

DEVELOPMENT, MATURATION, AND SURVIVAL OF RED CELLS

Red cells develop from large precursor cells in the bone marrow which are called **erythroblasts** (*erythro* = red + *blast* = a primitive cell). **Hemoglobin**, the oxygen-carrying protein that is formed by the developing red cells, is composed of four separate pieces called subunits, which in turn fit together to form a much larger aggregate called a tetramer (*tetra* = four). Each subunit consists of two parts: heme and globin.

Heme is a complex nitrogen-containing ring structure (called a porphyrin ring) containing an iron atom. Globin, which forms the largest part of each hemoglobin subunit, is a short, coiled protein (polypeptide) chain. Several types of globin chains,

Neutrophil (nū′trō-fil)
A leukocyte having a multilobed nucleus whose cytoplasm is filled with fine granules.

Lymphocyte (limf′ō-sīt)
A mononuclear blood cell produced in lymphoid tissue that takes part in cell-mediated and humoral immunity.

Eosinophil
(ē-ō-sin′o-fil)
A cell whose cytoplasm is filled with large, uniform granules that stain intensely red with acid dyes. See also basophil.

Basophil
A cell that contains numerous variable-sized granules that stain intensely purple with basic dyes. See also eosinophil.

Heparin
An anticoagulant obtained from the liver.

Monocyte (mon′ō-sīt)
A leukocyte having a kidney-shaped nucleus and light blue cytoplasm; a phagocytic cell that forms part of the reticulo-endothelial system.

Platelet
A component of the blood; a roughly circular or oval disk concerned with blood coagulation.

Erythroblast
(e-rith′rō-blast)
A precursor cell in the bone marrow that gives rise to red blood cells.

Hemoglobin
An oxygen transport protein within red cells composed of an iron-porphyrin complex (heme) combined with a protein chain (globin).

differing in their amino acid composition, are formed at varying times and in differing proportions in the fetus and in the adult. The chains are designated by Greek letters: alpha (α), beta (β), gamma (γ), delta (δ), and epsilon (ϵ).

Two different types of hemoglobin are found in the red cells of the normal adult. About 98% is called hemoglobin A or adult hemoglobin, in which two subunits of the tetramer contain alpha chains and two contain beta chains. The hemoglobin can also be designated by the shorthand notation $\alpha_2\beta_2$. (The chain is designated by the Greek letter and the number of subunits by the subscript.) The remaining 2% is called hemoglobin A_2, a tetramer composed of two alpha and two delta chains ($\alpha_2\delta_2$).

In the embryo and fetus, hemoglobin containing different globin chains is produced at various times in the course of prenatal development. Epsilon chain production predominates in the embryo but is soon superseded in the fetus by production of alpha and gamma globin chains. Beta chain production does not occur until relatively late in prenatal development. Consequently, the predominant hemoglobin in the fetus is a tetramer of alpha and gamma chains that is termed **fetal hemoglobin** (hemoglobin F). Fetal hemoglobin is able to take up and release oxygen more efficiently than adult hemoglobin when the oxygen partial pressure (PO_2) of the blood is low, an ability that is advantageous to the fetus because the PO_2 in fetal blood is lower than the PO_2 of adult blood. Late in pregnancy, fetal production of beta chains replaces gamma chains, and adult hemoglobin (hemoglobin A) begins to replace fetal hemoglobin in the red cells as the fetus prepares for life outside of the uterus.

The hemoglobin of a newborn infant contains both adult and fetal hemoglobin in approximately equal proportions. Normally, no significant fetal hemoglobin synthesis occurs after birth. As new red cells are produced by the infant to replace those containing fetal hemoglobin that have reached the end of their life span, the new "replacement" red cells contain essentially only hemoglobin A. Consequently, the concentration of hemoglobin A rises in the infant's blood as hemoglobin F falls. By about 6 months of age, the hemoglobin is almost entirely hemoglobin A, which functions normally in the circulation. Unfortunately, the gradual fall in hemoglobin F after birth is a disadvantage to an infant who is homozygous for the hemoglobin S gene (sickle hemoglobin gene) and is unable to make hemoglobin A, as is described later in this chapter in connection with the disease called sickle cell anemia.

The heme and globin components that make up normal hemoglobin A are synthesized separately within the erythroblast. The porphyrin ring is produced by the mitochondria. Then the iron, brought to the cell by a transport protein called transferrin, is inserted into the porphyrin ring to form heme. The globin chains are synthesized by groups of ribosomes (polyribosomes) in the cytoplasm and are joined to heme to form a hemoglobin subunit. Finally, the four subunits aggregate to form the complete hemoglobin tetramer.

The developing red cell accumulates increasing amounts of hemoglobin as it matures. When about 80% of its total hemoglobin has been synthesized, the nucleus is extruded. The cell is then discharged from the bone marrow into the circulation, where it completes its maturation and hemoglobin synthesis over the succeeding 24 hours. A newly formed red cell, which lacks a nucleus but still retains its mitochondria and other organelles for a short time, is called a **reticulocyte**. The name comes from its special staining characteristics. Certain stains precipitate the organelles within the cell cytoplasm, causing them to appear as a network (reticulum) of dark blue strands and granules. A reticulocyte is slightly larger than a mature red cell, and it also has a faint blue color because it contains less red-staining hemoglobin than a mature cell. These distinguishing features, which differentiate a reticulocyte from a mature red cell, are soon lost as the cell matures within the circulation.

The red cell, which derives its energy from the enzymatic breakdown of glucose, possesses enzyme systems that permit the cell to perform the diverse metabolic

Fetal hemoglobin
A type of hemoglobin containing two alpha and two gamma chains, which is able to take up and release oxygen at much lower PO_2 (oxygen partial pressure) than in adult hemoglobin.

Reticulocyte
*(rē-tik′ū-lō-sīt)
A young red cell that can be identified by special staining procedures.*

functions necessary for survival. Because the cell lacks a nucleus, it cannot synthesize new enzyme molecules to replace those that gradually wear out. As the cell ages, its enzyme systems gradually become depleted until eventually, after about 4 months, the cell is no longer able to function. The worn-out red cell is then removed by the mononuclear phagocyte system (reticuloendothelial system), primarily in the spleen, and its hemoglobin is degraded. The globin chains are broken down, and their component amino acids are used to make other proteins. The iron is extracted and saved to make new hemoglobin. The porphyrin ring, however, cannot be salvaged. It is degraded and is excreted by the liver as bile pigment.

REGULATION OF HEMATOPOIESIS

Red cell production is regulated by the oxygen content of the arterial blood. Decreased oxygen supply to the tissues stimulates erythropoiesis. However, low oxygen tension does not act directly on the bone marrow. The effect is mediated by the kidneys. Certain specialized cells in the kidneys elaborate a hormonelike erythrocyte-stimulating material called **erythropoietin.**

> **Erythropoietin**
> (er-ith-rō-poy′e-tin)
> *A humoral substance made by the kidneys that regulates hematopoiesis.*

The factors regulating the production of white blood cells and their delivery into the circulation are not well understood. Products of cell necrosis may cause the number of white blood cells in the peripheral blood to increase. Hormone secretion by the adrenals and some other endocrine glands also influences white cell production.

Oxygen Transport by Hemoglobin

The unique property of hemoglobin is its ability to enter into reversible combination with oxygen, which depends on the heme component of the hemoglobin molecule. For hemoglobin to transport and release oxygen effectively, the heme iron must be in the ferrous (Fe^{2+}) state, and its binding site must be available to pick up and release oxygen efficiently. In the lungs where the oxygen partial pressure is high, hemoglobin combines with oxygen to form oxyhemoglobin. In the tissues where oxygen partial pressure is much lower, the oxygen is released and reduced hemoglobin is formed. There are two important conditions that impair the ability of hemoglobin to transport oxygen: (1) oxidation of the heme iron to form a different type of hemoglobin called methemoglobin and (2) attachment of carbon monoxide to the heme iron to form carboxyhemoglobin.

METHEMOGLOBIN

If the iron in the heme of hemoglobin is oxidized from the normal ferrous (Fe^{+2}) to the ferric (Fe^{+3}) form by oxidizing agents, the hemoglobin is converted to methemoglobin and is no longer able to carry oxygen. Normally, a small amount of hemoglobin is oxidized to methemoglobin continuously but the concentration is less than 1% of the total hemoglobin because red cells have enzymes (*methemoglobin reductase*) that convert methemoglobin back to normal oxygen-carrying hemoglobin. Unfortunately, many different drugs and chemicals can oxidize hemoglobin to methemoglobin, including nitrates and nitrites in well water, some frequently used local anesthetics such as benzocaine contained in topical anesthetics, and several nonprescription drug products. Methemoglobin concentrations may rise significantly, which lowers the oxygen-carrying capacity of the blood. The higher the methemoglobin concentration, the greater is its effect on oxygen transport. Methemoglobin has a dark red-brown "chocolate" color. A 15–20% concentration in the blood changes the color of the skin, which may be confused with cyanosis caused by reduced hemoglobin. A concentration of 25–50% methemoglobin causes nonspecific symptoms related to the reduced oxygen delivered to the tissues, such as headache, confusion, and shortness of breath. Higher concentrations cause neurologic and cardiovascular symptoms, and a concentration of 70% is usually fatal. The preferred treatment of severe methemoglobinemia is methylene blue given intravenously. The compound increases the activity of the red cell methemoglobin reductase enzyme, which speeds the conversion of methemoglobin (Fe^{+3}) back to normal hemoglobin (Fe^{2+}), thereby restoring the oxygen-carrying capacity of the blood to normal.

CARBOXYHEMOGLOBIN

In the presence of adequate oxygen, carbon compounds are converted to carbon dioxide and water. However, incomplete combustion forms carbon monoxide, which is a potentially hazardous compound because it has over 200 times the ability to combine with hemoglobin than does oxygen. Consequently, carbon monoxide combines preferentially with hemoglobin to form carboxyhemoglobin, which blocks the ability of the hemoglobin to transport oxygen. Exposure of even a low concentration of carbon monoxide for a long time is harmful and may be fatal as progressively larger quantities of hemoglobin are converted to carboxyhemoglobin. If a person exposed to a sublethal concentration of carbon monoxide is removed from the source of the exposure, the carbon monoxide dissociates slowly from its combination with hemoglobin and the oxygen-carrying capacity of the blood slowly returns to normal.

Manifestations of exposure to carbon monoxide depend on the concentration to which the person has been exposed. A concentration of 3% or higher in a nonsmoker, and 10% or more in smokers (who have a higher concentration caused by the carbon monoxide in cigarette smoke) indicate significant exposure. Moreover, the carbon monoxide attaches not only to hemoglobin but also to cytochrome enzymes that perform essential metabolic functions. A high concentration of carboxyhemoglobin in the blood may lead to serious long-term cardiovascular and neurologic problems resulting from the exposure. An affected person should be removed from the source of exposure and given a high concentration of oxygen by mask to help replace the carbon monoxide with oxygen. If the affected person's blood carboxyhemoglobin concentration is very high, the oxygen should be given under increased pressure in a room where the atmospheric pressure can be raised above normal, which is called a hyperbaric chamber.

It is easier to prevent carbon monoxide poisoning than to treat it. Many communities now require carbon monoxide detectors in private homes to detect carbon monoxide, which calls attention to an undetected malfunction of the home heating system. Continued vigilance is also required to avoid accidental carbon monoxide exposure when working in areas where auto exhaust fumes are not well ventilated.

DIAGNOSTIC TESTS TO IDENTIFY METHEMOGLOBIN AND CARBOXYHEMOGLOBIN

An instrument called a co-oximeter, which measures the absorbency of light in the blood at four different wavelengths, can determine the concentration in the blood of reduced hemoglobin, oxyhemoglobin, carboxyhemoglobin, and methemoglobin as a guide to diagnosis and treatment. The results obtained also can help distinguish cyanosis caused by poor oxygenation of a person's blood from the somewhat similar appearing color of the skin caused by a high concentration of methemoglobin.

Anemia

Anemia literally means "without blood." Specifically, the term is used to refer to a decrease in red cells or to subnormal hemoglobin levels. Many classifications of anemia have been proposed, and two different methods of classification are widely used. One system, based on the factor responsible for the anemia, is an etiologic classification. A second system, based on the shape and appearance of the red blood cells (as determined by microscopic examination of a stained blood smear), is a morphologic classification.

Anemia (an-ē′mē-uh)
A decrease in hemoglobin or red cells or both.

ETIOLOGIC CLASSIFICATION OF ANEMIA

One simple classification of the anemias is based on the "bone marrow factory" concept (FIGURE 14-2). Anemia is classified as being caused by either inadequate production of red cells or an excessive loss of cells. Inadequate production, in turn, may result from an insufficiency of raw materials or from factors that render the factory inoperative and no longer able to deliver enough finished products into the circulation. Examples of the latter would be marrow damage or replacement of marrow by abnormal cells. Excessive loss of red cells may be caused either by external blood loss or by accelerated destruction of the cells (and hence shortened survival) in the circulation. TABLE 14-1 presents a classification of the various causes of anemia.

MORPHOLOGIC CLASSIFICATION OF ANEMIA

An anemia in which the cells are normal in size and appearance is called a normocytic anemia. If the cells are larger than normal, the anemia is called a macrocytic anemia. If the cells are smaller than normal, the anemia is called a microcytic anemia. Many times, microcytic cells also have a reduced hemoglobin content, appearing quite pale when examined under the microscope; here, the term hypochromic anemia is used. Often, the latter two terms are combined, and the anemia is called a hypochromic microcytic anemia. Classification of anemia on the basis of red cell appearance is useful because the appearance of the cells provides a clue to the etiology. Iron deficiency anemia is a hypochromic microcytic anemia. Anemia caused by vitamin B_{12} or folic acid deficiency is a macrocytic anemia. Most other types of anemia are normocytic.

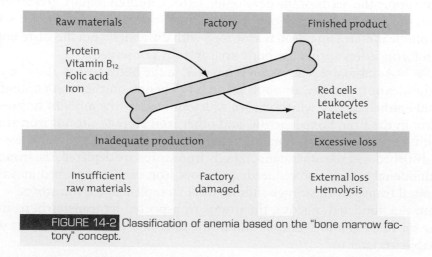

FIGURE 14-2 Classification of anemia based on the "bone marrow factory" concept.

TABLE 14-1

Etiologic classification of anemia

Inadequate production of red cells

Caused by inadequate "raw materials"
  Iron deficiency
  Vitamin B_{12} deficiency
  Folic acid deficiency
Caused by impaired function of bone marrow factory
  Anemia of chronic disease
  Bone marrow damaged or destroyed (aplastic anemia)
  Bone marrow replaced by foreign or abnormal cells (bone marrow replacement anemia)

Excessive loss of red cells

Caused by external blood loss (hemorrhage)
Caused by shortened survival of red cells in the circulation
  Defective red cells (hereditary hemolytic anemia)
    Abnormal red cell shape
    Abnormal hemoglobin within red cells
    Defective hemoglobin synthesis within red cells
    Deficient red cell enzymes
  "Hostile environment"
    Anti-red cell antibodies
    Mechanical trauma to circulating red cells

IRON METABOLISM AND HEMATOPOIESIS

The body contains about 4 g of iron, of which about 75% is contained in hemoglobin. Most of the rest is a reserve supply that is stored in the liver, bone marrow, and spleen combined with an iron-binding protein called apoferritin to form an iron–protein complex called ferritin. A small amount of iron also circulates in the blood bound to a protein called transferrin, which is the iron being transported from place to place in the body.

The usual diet of an adult contains from about 10 to 20 mg of iron, but men absorb merely 1 mg per day, and only slightly more iron is absorbed by women and children. Women need more iron to make up for menstrual losses because 1 ml of blood contains about 0.5 mg of iron. Additional iron is also required during pregnancy to supply the needs of the developing fetus. Children require greater amounts of iron in order to synthesize more hemoglobin during periods of growth when the blood volume is increasing. Iron is absorbed with difficulty from the gastrointestinal tract, and iron stores within the body are carefully conserved.

FIGURE 14-3 summarizes how iron is handled in the body. Iron is absorbed chiefly in the duodenum, and the amount absorbed depends on the iron content of the duodenal epithelial cells, which in turn is determined by the amount of iron stored as ferritin in the liver, bone marrow, and other iron storage sites. If iron stores are abundant, so also is the iron content of the intestinal epithelial cells, and less dietary iron is absorbed. On the other hand, if body iron stores are depleted, the iron content of the duodenal cells is also reduced, and more iron can be absorbed into the cells for eventual transport to storage sites in order to replenish ferritin stores.

From the duodenal mucosa, the iron is transported by transferrin to the bone marrow for hemoglobin synthesis and to the liver and other storage sites where it is available for later use.

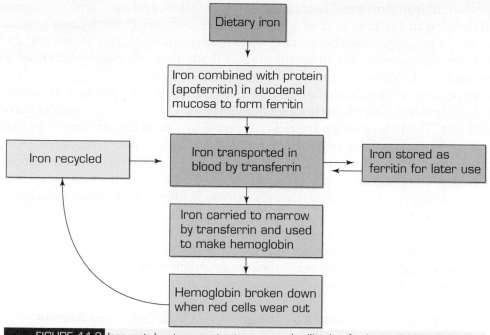

FIGURE 14-3 Iron uptake, transport, storage, and utilization for hemoglobin synthesis. Most of the iron used for hemoglobin synthesis is recycled from worn-out red cells. Chronic blood loss removes iron-containing cells from the circulation, and the iron contained in the red cells can no longer be recycled to make hemoglobin, which leads to iron deficiency anemia.

As red cells wear out and are destroyed, the iron from the hemoglobin is recycled, transported by transferrin back to the bone marrow, and used to make new hemoglobin. If sufficient recycled iron is not available for hemoglobin synthesis, additional iron is mobilized from storage sites.

IRON DEFICIENCY ANEMIA

Iron deficiency anemia is the most common anemia encountered in clinical practice. Iron forms an essential part of the hemoglobin molecule, and normal synthesis of hemoglobin requires adequate supplies of iron.

When red blood cells, which have a normal life span of about 4 months, become "senile," they are removed from the circulation. The iron from the destroyed cells is transported back to the bone marrow and is reused by the bone marrow to be incorporated into newly formed red cells. Iron deficiency anemia may result from either insufficient intake of iron in the diet or inadequate reutilization of the iron present in red cells.

Iron deficiency caused by inadequate dietary intake may occur in infants during periods of rapid growth. A normal, full-term infant has been provided with a reserve supply of iron that was transferred to the fetus from the mother during the last part of pregnancy. Consequently, the newborn infant generally has an adequate short-term supply of iron available for hematopoiesis during the neonatal period when the production of red cells accelerates to supply the needs of an increasing blood volume. A premature infant, however, may not get its full component of iron stores and may not have enough reserve to supply its postnatal needs. Even in full-term infants, the reserve supply of iron for hematopoiesis is limited and must be supplemented by iron from the diet. Breast milk contains very little iron, although the amount available is well absorbed. If the diet is not supplemented by cereals, fruits, vegetables, other foods containing iron, or some type of iron supplement, iron stores will become rapidly exhausted, and iron deficiency anemia will develop in the first year of life. For this reason, many physicians gradually add supplementary foods containing additional sources of iron to infants' diets. Occasionally, adolescents subsisting on an inadequate or poorly balanced diet develop iron deficiency anemia.

Most cases of iron deficiency anemia in adults result from a failure to recapture the iron present in red cells for hemoglobin synthesis. This failure is a result of chronic blood loss. The iron contained in red cells that is lost from the circulation by bleeding is no longer available to the body for the production of new red cells. Because each milliliter of blood contains 0.5 mg of iron, a loss of 500 ml of blood represents a loss of 250 mg of iron, which is equivalent to one-fourth of the body's entire iron reserves. Unless dietary intake of iron is extremely liberal, iron stores soon become exhausted, and iron deficiency anemia develops.

Iron deficiency anemia is a hypochromic microcytic anemia (FIGURE 14-4). The cells are pale because they contain less hemoglobin than normal. The cells are also abnormally small because the body apparently attempts to "scale down" the size of the cell to conform to the reduced hemoglobin content.

Laboratory Tests to Evaluate Iron Metabolism in Iron Deficiency Anemia

Various laboratory tests that measure iron stores, iron transport, and iron metabolism can be used as diagnostic tests in patients with suspected iron deficiency anemia. These include measurements of serum ferritin, serum iron, and serum iron-binding capacity.

A B

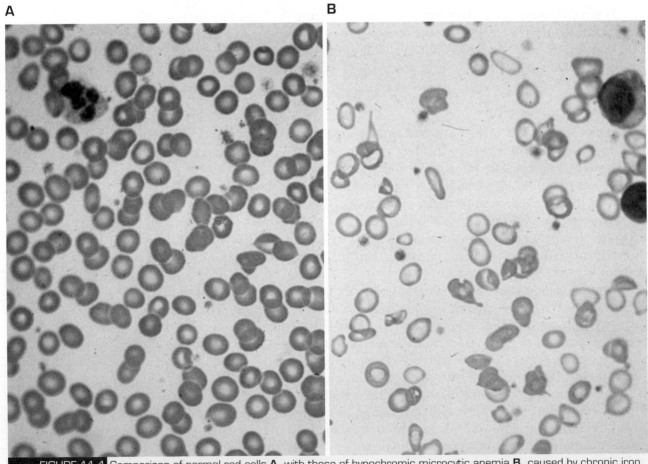

FIGURE 14-4 Comparison of normal red cells **A**, with those of hypochromic microcytic anemia **B**, caused by chronic iron deficiency (original magnification × 400).

A very small amount of ferritin (about 100 µg per liter) is normally present in blood serum, and this amount is proportional to the total amount of ferritin stored in the body. Consequently, measurement of serum ferritin can be used to estimate total body iron stores. One can also measure the amount of iron being transported by transferrin and can also determine the maximum amount of iron that can be carried when all of the iron-binding sites on transferrin are fully saturated with iron. When iron stores are normal, the concentration of iron in the serum is about 100 µg per 100 ml. Only about one-third of the maximum iron transport capacity is utilized, and the iron-binding protein is said to be about 30% saturated with iron.

In iron deficiency anemia, body iron stores are depleted and serum ferritin is low. Serum iron is also much lower than normal, but the amount of iron transport protein in the serum is much higher than normal, apparently reflecting the body's attempt to capture the meager iron available and transport it more efficiently. Consequently, the characteristic laboratory profile of iron deficiency anemia is low serum ferritin and serum iron, but a much higher than normal serum iron-binding protein with a much lower than normal percentage iron saturation.

Evaluation and Treatment of Iron Deficiency Anemia

A physician treating a patient with iron deficiency anemia is primarily concerned with learning the cause of the anemia and then directing therapy toward the cause rather than the symptoms. In an infant with a history of a very poor diet, the cause may be obvious. In an adult, the anemia is usually a result of blood loss, and the physician must always investigate to determine the source of the bleeding. Blood loss may be caused by a bleeding ulcer or an ulcerated carcinoma of the colon. In women, excessive menstrual bleeding is a common cause of iron deficiency anemia. Another sometimes overlooked cause of iron deficiency anemia in otherwise healthy young adults is too frequent blood donations. When the cause of the blood loss has been determined, proper treatment of the underlying cause can be instituted. In addition, the patient is given supplementary iron to replenish the body's depleted iron stores.

VITAMIN B$_{12}$ AND FOLIC ACID DEFICIENCY

Vitamin B$_{12}$ is found in meat, milk, liver, and other foods rich in animal protein, and some other foods that are fortified with vitamin B$_{12}$. Strict vegetarians who do not eat meat or dairy products must rely on vitamin B$_{12}$-fortified cereals or other nonprotein vitamin B$_{12}$-fortified foods as their source of the vitamin. Folic acid is widely distributed in nature, being found in abundance in green leafy vegetables as well as many foods of animal origin.

Vitamin B$_{12}$ and folic acid are required not only for normal hematopoiesis but also for normal maturation of many other types of cells. In the absence of either vitamin B$_{12}$ or folic acid, DNA synthesis is impaired, and the developing red cells in the bone marrow exhibit a characteristic disturbance of cell maturation. The impaired DNA synthesis inhibits cell division but has little effect on RNA and protein synthesis, which causes the developing red cells to become large abnormal cells that do not survive normally in the circulation. The developing red cells, which are larger than normal, are called **megaloblasts** (*megalos* = large). The abnormal red cell maturation is called megaloblastic erythropoiesis. The mature red cells derived from the abnormal maturation also are larger than normal. Therefore, the anemia is classified morphologically as a macrocytic anemia. The development of white cell precursors and megakaryocytes is also abnormal. Consequently, patients with megaloblastic anemia usually also have **leukopenia** and **thrombocytopenia** as well as a macrocytic anemia. Vitamin B$_{12}$, but not folic acid, is required to maintain the structural and

Megaloblast
(meg'al-ō-blast)
An abnormal red cell precursor resulting from vitamin B$_{12}$ or folic acid deficiency.

Leukopenia
(lōō-kō-pē'ni-uh)
An abnormally small number of leukocytes in the peripheral blood.

Thrombocytopenia
(throm'bō-sī-tō-pē'ny-yuh)
A deficiency of platelets.

functional integrity of the nervous system; thus, a deficiency of this vitamin also may be associated with pronounced neurologic disturbances.

Anemia as a Result of Folic Acid Deficiency

The body has very limited stores of folic acid, which rapidly become depleted if not replenished continually. As a result, folic acid–deficiency anemia is relatively common and may result from reduced dietary intake, impaired absorption, or increased folic acid requirements.

Deficiency caused by inadequate dietary intake is found in persons subsisting on inadequate diets and is encountered frequently in chronic alcoholics because of their typically deficient diet and, possibly, impaired absorption of folic acid compared with nondrinkers. Persons with chronic intestinal diseases may become folic acid deficient because of impaired ability to absorb the vitamin. Pregnant women also are at risk because pregnancy greatly increases folic acid requirements. Folic acid–deficiency anemia in pregnancy is uncommon because physicians routinely prescribe folic acid supplements to pregnant women.

Anemia as a Result of Vitamin B$_{12}$ Deficiency

Efficient absorption of vitamin B$_{12}$ ingested in food requires a substance called intrinsic factor, secreted by gastric mucosal cells along with hydrochloric acid and digestive enzymes. The intrinsic factor combines with the vitamin B$_{12}$, and the B$_{12}$–intrinsic-factor complex is absorbed from the distal small intestine. The absorbed vitamin is stored in the liver and made available to the bone marrow and other tissues as required for cell growth and maturation.

A common cause of vitamin B$_{12}$ deficiency is **pernicious anemia**. The basic defect in pernicious anemia is atrophy of the gastric mucosa, which sometimes develops in middle-aged and older individuals and is often associated with autoantibodies directed against gastric mucosal cells and intrinsic factor. The atrophic mucosa fails to secrete intrinsic factor, acid, and digestive enzymes, and consequently, vitamin B$_{12}$ is not absorbed. The vitamin B$_{12}$ deficiency causes impaired hematopoiesis as well as various neurologic disturbances.

Pernicious anemia is not the only cause of vitamin B$_{12}$ deficiency. Persons who have had most of their stomach surgically removed because of ulcer or gastric cancer or who have had a gastric bypass procedure to control obesity and its impact on the gastrointestinal tract may not be able to secrete enough intrinsic factor. Persons who have had a small bowel resection of the distal ilium, where the vitamin B$_{12}$–intrinsic factor complex is absorbed, may not be able to absorb enough vitamin to supply their needs, and an individual with chronic intestinal disease affecting the vitamin B$_{12}$–absorbing area (such as Crohn disease, which frequently involves the terminal ileum, described in the discussion on the gastrointestinal tract) also may be unable to absorb the vitamin adequately.

Pernicious anemia and other vitamin B$_{12}$ deficiencies are treated with intramuscular administration of vitamin B$_{12}$. Parenteral administration avoids the problem of poor absorption of the vitamin.

BONE MARROW SUPPRESSION, DAMAGE, OR INFILTRATION

Many conditions can depress bone marrow function. Chronic diseases of all types may impair hematopoiesis and lead to mild or moderate anemia, which is called the anemia of chronic disease. In this condition, iron and other "raw materials" supplied to the bone marrow are adequate, but they are not utilized efficiently to make red cells. White blood cell and platelet production are usually not disturbed. The most common cause of this type of anemia is chronic infection, but other chronic diseases and some malignant tumors also may be responsible.

Pernicious anemia
(per-ni'shus)
A macrocytic anemia caused by inability to absorb vitamin B$_{12}$ as a result of inadequate secretion of intrinsic factor by gastric mucosa.

The anemia of chronic disease usually causes only a relatively mild suppression of bone marrow function and improves when the disease that caused it is identified and treated. Chronic infections may respond to treatment, but unfortunately, it is often not possible to "cure" many of the other chronic diseases that lead to this type of anemia.

In contrast to the anemia of chronic disease, much more serious and sometimes irreversible damage to the bone marrow factory results from destruction of the bone marrow stem cells from which mature blood cells and platelets arise. This type of anemia is called aplastic anemia (*a* = without + *plasia* = growth), although this term is not strictly accurate because the stem cell damage leads to leukopenia and thrombocytopenia as well as anemia. The anemia is classified as a normocytic anemia because the red cells are normal in size and shape although inadequate in number. Many agents can cause aplastic anemia. Radiation, anticancer chemotherapy drugs, and various toxic chemicals may cause severe marrow damage. Other drugs, including some antibiotics, anti-inflammatory drugs, and anticonvulsant drugs, may damage marrow stem cells in susceptible individuals. In many cases, however, it is the body's own immune system that is responsible for the aplastic anemia, a manifestation of an autoimmune disease in which the body's own cytotoxic T lymphocytes attack and destroy the marrow stem cells.

Aplastic anemia is treated initially by blood and platelet transfusions to maintain an adequate volume of circulating blood cells while the cause of the bone marrow failure is being investigated. If the marrow damage is caused by a toxic drug or chemical and is not too severe, marrow function may recover; however, it is unlikely in severe aplastic anemia, and other methods of treatment are required to restore marrow function. Many patients respond to immunosuppressive agents that act against the destructive (cytotoxic) T lymphocytes responsible for stem cell destruction, such as the drug cyclosporine together with gamma globulin containing antilymphocyte antibodies. The discussion on neoplastic disease shows that bone marrow transplantation is also effective and can be performed in highly selected patients using the same methods used to treat patients with leukemia. A large volume of bone marrow is aspirated from the pelvic bones of a suitable donor and injected intravenously into the circulation of the recipient. The donor cells become established in the recipient's marrow and begin to produce blood cells. A marrow transplant is foreign tissue, however, and the recipient's own immune defenses must be suppressed, as discussed in immunity, hypersensitivity, allergy, and autoimmune diseases, to permit the transplanted bone marrow to survive.

An anemia similar to aplastic anemia involving white cells and platelets as well as red cells may also occur if bone marrow stem cells are crowded out and replaced by abnormal cells, such as leukemic cells or metastatic carcinoma. The term bone marrow replacement anemia is sometimes used to denote this type of anemia. Unfortunately, it may be difficult to restore marrow function after the marrow has been heavily infiltrated by leukemic cells or cancer cells, although adequate levels of hemoglobin and red cells can be maintained by blood transfusions.

ACUTE BLOOD LOSS

A normocytic anemia may result from an episode of acute blood loss, as from a massive hemorrhage from the uterus or gastrointestinal tract. Provided that iron stores are adequate, the lost blood is rapidly replaced by the bone marrow, and the newly formed red cells are normal. This is in contrast with the anemia of chronic blood loss, in which the red cells are hypochromic and microcytic because prolonged bleeding has depleted the body's iron stores.

ACCELERATED BLOOD DESTRUCTION

Normal red cells survive for about 4 months. Sometimes, however, their survival is considerably shortened, and anemia results because the regenerative capacity of the marrow is not sufficient to keep up with the accelerated destruction. This type of anemia is called a hemolytic anemia and may be a result of either defective red cells or a "hostile environment." Hemolytic anemias caused by defective red cells are called hereditary hemolytic anemias. Those resulting from damage to normal red cells by antibodies or other injurious agents are called acquired hemolytic anemias.

Hereditary Hemolytic Anemias

The genetically determined abnormalities of red cells that may shorten their survival fall into four major groups (TABLE 14-2):

1. Abnormally shaped cells
2. Abnormal hemoglobins
3. Defective hemoglobin synthesis
4. Enzyme deficiencies

TABLE 14-2

Inheritance and manifestations of some hereditary hemolytic anemias

Anemia	Inheritance	Characteristics of red cells	Manifestations
Hereditary spherocytosis	Dominant or recessive	Spherocytic	Mild-to-moderate chronic hemolytic anemia
Hereditary ovalocytosis	Dominant	Oval	Usually asymptomatic; may have mild anemia
Sickle cell anemia	Codominant	Normocytic; cells sickle under reduced oxygen tension	Marked anemia
Hemoglobin C disease	Codominant	Normocytic	Mild-to-moderate anemia
Sickle cell hemoglobin C disease	Codominant	Normocytic; cells sickle under reduced oxygen tension	Moderate anemia
Thalassemia minor	Dominant (heterozygous)	Hypochromic microcytic; total number of red cells usually increased	Mild anemia
Thalassemia major	Dominant (homozygous)	Hypochromic microcytic	Severe anemia; usually fatal in childhood
Glucose-6-phosphate dehydrogenase deficiency	X-linked recessive	Normocytic; enzyme-deficient cells	Episodes of acute hemolytic anemia precipitated by drugs or infections

Shape Abnormalities The most common abnormality of shape is called hereditary spherocytosis. There appear to be two distinct genetic forms. Most are transmitted as a Mendelian-dominant trait, but some follow a recessive-inherited pattern. In hereditary spherocytosis, the structural framework (cytoskeleton) of the red cell membrane is defective, which reduces its stability and flexibility. New red cells produced by the bone marrow and released into the circulation have a normal biconcave disk configuration, but bits of their unstable cell membranes become detached from the cells as the red cells squeeze through extremely small capillaries during their travel through the bloodstream, which progressively reduces the surface area of the red cell membranes. The red cells adapt to their reduced surface area relative to their cell volume by gradually changing from biconcave disks to spherical cells, which is the only way that the smaller cell membrane can surround the comparatively large volume of the red cell (FIGURE 14-5). Unfortunately, the spherical shape puts the red cells at a disadvantage that greatly shortens their survival in the bloodstream. As blood flows through the spleen, normal flexible disk-shaped red cells can "work their way" through the splenic pulp and into the thin-walled veins (sinusoids) that carry the blood out of the spleen, but spherocytes are not thin enough or flexible enough to get through the spleen. They become trapped in the spleen where they are destroyed by the phagocytic cells in the splenic pulp. The bone marrow increases red cell production to compensate for the shortened survival of the spherocytes, resulting in a chronic hemolytic anemia. Splenectomy cures the anemia by removing the main site of red cell destruction but has no effect on the basic red cell defect.

A somewhat similar condition, which is also transmitted as a Mendelian-dominant trait, is called hereditary ovalocytosis. As the name indicates, the red cells are oval rather than round. Most affected persons are not inconvenienced by the abnormality, but some have a mild hemolytic anemia that can be cured by splenectomy.

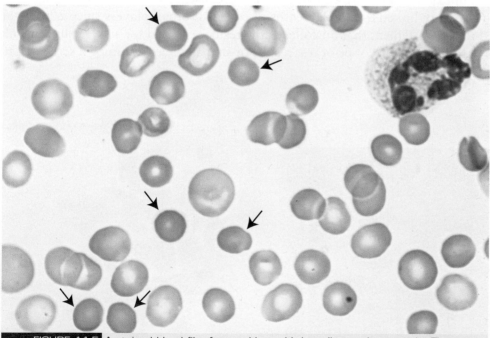

FIGURE 14-5 A stained blood film from subject with hereditary spherocytosis. The many small dark cells with little or no central pallor are spherocytes (*arrows*). The larger, more normal-appearing red cells are young red cells that have the same cell membrane defect but have not been circulating long enough to acquire a spherical shape. The relative large, faintly blue-staining red cell in the center of the field is a reticulocyte (original magnification × 400).

Abnormal Hemoglobins The arrangement of amino acids in the globin chains of hemoglobin is controlled by genes. If the gene is abnormal, the amino acids forming the globin chains will be altered, leading to the formation of an abnormal hemoglobin. Genes directing the synthesis of the various types of hemoglobin are codominant. If an abnormal gene is present, the abnormal hemoglobin appears in the red cells. Many different abnormal hemoglobins can be identified and characterized by various laboratory tests. Some of the abnormal hemoglobins function normally, but others have unusual properties that impair their function. Hemoglobin S (sickle hemoglobin) is one of the more important abnormal hemoglobins. Its formation results from a change in only a single amino acid in the beta chain of hemoglobin. When the oxygen tension of the blood falls, as in venous blood, the hemoglobin S molecules aggregate and form rigid fibers, a process somewhat like crystallization (FIGURE 14-6). The "crystallization" is largely reversible, and the hemoglobin becomes soluble again when the oxygen tension rises as the blood is oxygenated in the lungs. About 8% of the black population are heterozygous carriers of the sickle cell gene. Their erythrocytes contain both hemoglobin S and hemoglobin A. This condition is called sickle cell trait, and the hemoglobin S in their red cells can be demonstrated easily by a simple blood test. Persons with sickle cell trait usually do not experience any problems related to the sickle hemoglobin in their red cells unless they engage in vigorous activities at high altitude and the oxygen content of their blood falls to a very low level. However, even vigorous exercise or exertion at sea level may cause a similar drop in the oxygenation of arterial blood sufficient to cause the red cells to sickle, which may lead to sudden death caused by plugging of coronary arteries by clumps of sickled red cells. Exercise-related sudden death in persons with sickle cell trait was demonstrated in a classic article by Kark and associates related to sudden death among 2 million recruits during basic training in the U.S. Armed Forces from 1977 to 1981, which concluded that "recruits in basic training with the sickle cell trait have a substantially increased age-dependent risk of exercise-related sudden death unexplained by any known preexisting cause." More recently, sickle cell trait has also been linked to 9 of 21 deaths of college football players since 2000, which lead to a requirement that all college athletes be screened for sickle cell trait unless they provide a record of prior test results or sign a waiver declining a screening test.

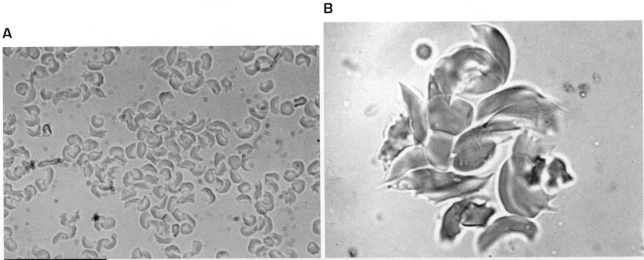

FIGURE 14-6 Distortion of red cells containing sickle hemoglobin when incubated under reduced oxygen tension. **A**, Overview of cells under low magnification (× 100). **B**, Higher magnification view (× 400) of red cell distortion caused by sickle hemoglobin.

The homozygous state is called sickle cell anemia and is a serious disease that results when both parents have the sickle cell trait and each transmits the sickle cell gene to the infant. The cells of affected individuals contain no hemoglobin A and become sickled within the capillaries where the oxygen partial pressure is lower than in arterial blood. The clumps of sickled red cells plug blood vessels, which obstruct blood flow, causing progressive damage to the heart, kidneys, spleen, and other organs resulting from the impaired circulation. Anemia develops because the sickle hemoglobin–containing cells have a shortened survival in the circulation. Consequently, the bone marrow must increase greatly its production of red cells, as demonstrated by an elevated peripheral blood reticulocyte count, in order to compensate for the shortened red cell survival.

Newborn infants with sickle cell anemia do not have problems initially because their red cells also contain a large amount of fetal hemoglobin, which "dilutes" the concentration of sickle hemoglobin in the red cells so that they function more like the red cells of a person with sickle cell trait. Symptoms usually do not appear until the infant is about 6 months old, when the red cells containing both fetal and sickle hemoglobin have been replaced by red cells containing almost entirely sickle hemoglobin. Some affected persons continue to produce some fetal hemoglobin, which can vary from about 5% to as much as 15% of the hemoglobin in their red cells, which reduces the concentration of sickle hemoglobin in their cells. These more fortunate individuals have less severe clinical manifestations than those who fail to produce significant fetal hemoglobin.

Although there is no cure for sickle cell anemia, advances in treatment have improved survival, and many affected persons now live 40–50 years. They are quite susceptible to infections and should receive pneumococcal vaccine and other immunizing agents to reduce their infection risk. The hyperactive bone marrow requires abundant folic acid to promote red cell production, and folic acid supplements are recommended to assure that supplies are adequate. Drugs such as hydroxyurea can be given to stimulate the bone marrow to produce fetal hemoglobin, which lowers the concentration of sickle hemoglobin in the red cells and thereby reduces the severity of the disease manifestations. The patient may also receive erythropoietin along with drugs to stimulate fetal hemoglobin production, which leads to an even greater rise in fetal hemoglobin.

Simple, readily available tests can detect sickle cell trait in affected individuals, and genetic counseling is recommended for couples who are at risk of having a child with sickle cell anemia. DNA analysis of fetal cells obtained by amniocentesis can determine whether the fetus carries the sickle cell gene and, if present, whether the fetus is homozygous or heterozygous for the gene.

Another common abnormal hemoglobin, called hemoglobin C, also is found predominantly in blacks. Heterozygous individuals, whose cells contain both hemoglobin A and hemoglobin C, are normal clinically. Persons homozygous for the hemoglobin C gene have a mild hemolytic anemia.

Some persons possess genes for two abnormal hemoglobins. This may occur, for example, if one parent carries the hemoglobin S gene and the other carries the hemoglobin C gene, and each parent transmits the abnormal gene. In this case, the red cells of the affected person contain both abnormal hemoglobins in approximately equal amounts, and a hemolytic anemia results.

Treatment of Sickle Cell Anemia by Bone Marrow Transplant

The same type of bone marrow transplantation procedure described in the discussion on neoplastic disease to treat leukemias and lymphomas, with its associated complications, is also used to treat sickle cell anemia, provided a suitable donor is available. However, many physicians have been reluctant to perform this procedure because destroying the patient's bone marrow in order to receive the transplant often is associated with serious life threatening complications. The risk of a bone marrow transplant-related fatality in order to treat a disease that is not life threatening is considered an excessive risk that is not in the patient's best interest.

Currently, a less intense procedure is being used to reduce the transplantation risk. Immunosuppressive drugs and low-dose radiation treatment are used to reduce the concentration of the patient's bone marrow cells and suppress to immune system but not completely destroy the patient's bone marrow. The less intense immune system suppression allows the transplanted marrow to grow in the bone marrow along with the patient's own bone marrow cells. The transplanted cells make normal red cells, and the patient's own red cells continue to make sickle cells, each in proportion to the concentrations of the patient's blood cells and transplanted normal cells in the bone marrow. Eventually, the immune system "learns" that both types of cells belong to the patient even though they are immunologically different. Less intense immunosuppression is needed, and sometimes, it can be discontinued completely.

Similar progress has been made toward inducing the immune system to tolerate a kidney transplant, as described in the section on the urinary system dealing with renal transplantation.

Defective Hemoglobin Synthesis   Sometimes, the globin chains of hemoglobin are normal, but their synthesis is defective. This genetically determined condition is called thalassemia and is transmitted as a Mendelian-dominant trait. The defective synthesis may be of either the alpha chains (alpha thalassemia) or the beta chains (beta thalassemia), but the latter defect is the more common and the more important clinically. This genetic abnormality is relatively common in persons of Greek and Italian ancestry. (The term thalassemia comes from the Greek word *thalassa*, meaning sea, and derives from the high incidence of the condition in persons who live in the regions surrounding the Mediterranean Sea.)

In the more common beta thalassemia, the production of beta chains is reduced; however, alpha chain production is not, and synthesis of the two types of chains is unbalanced. An excess of alpha chains accumulates and precipitates within the red cells, which shortens their survival. Because hemoglobin synthesis is reduced, the red cells appear hypochromic and microcytic, somewhat like the appearance of the cells in iron deficiency anemia. In thalassemia, however, the hypochromia is the result of deficient hemoglobin production because of inadequate beta chain synthesis, rather than deficient production caused by iron deficiency. Usually, the cells also contain an increased amount of hemoglobin A_2, which does not contain beta chains, to compensate in part for the reduced synthesis of hemoglobin A.

If a person is heterozygous for the thalassemia gene, the anemia is mild and the condition is called thalassemia minor. The red cells are hypochromic and microcytic, and usually there is a compensatory overproduction of red cells; thus, their numbers are greater than normal. The homozygous condition, which is called thalassemia major, occurs if both parents have thalassemia minor and each transmits the abnormal gene. The affected individual has a severe chronic hemolytic anemia that is usually fatal in childhood.

Red Cell Enzyme Deficiencies   Red cells derive energy by metabolizing glucose by a series of chemical reactions that are catalyzed by various enzyme systems. These same energy-producing reactions also indirectly help prevent oxidation of the hemoglobin, thereby protecting the hemoglobin from the potentially harmful effects of oxidizing drugs or other agents that can damage it. This protective function is compromised if certain red cell enzymes are deficient. Under such circumstances, exposing the red cells to an oxidizing agent causes denaturation and precipitation of the protein chains of hemoglobin, as well as the cell-membrane proteins.

One of the most common red cell enzyme defects is a deficiency of an enzyme called glucose-6-phosphate dehydrogenase. In this condition, which is transmitted as an X-linked recessive trait, the enzyme is unstable and does not function normally. (X-linked inheritance is considered in the discussion on chromosomes, genes, and cell division.) About 10% of black men are affected, and 30% of black women carry the abnormal gene on one of their X chromosomes. The abnormal gene occurs with high frequency in some white populations as well. The enzyme-deficient cells are highly susceptible to injury by drugs that do not affect normal red cells and to various bacterial and viral infections. More than 40 drugs are known to induce an acute hemolytic anemia in susceptible subjects, including such commonly used drugs as sulfonamides, aspirin, some diuretics, some antibiotics, and some vitamins. Hemolysis begins soon after exposure to the drug or infectious agent and continues for about a week. Considerable red cell destruction results, followed by red cell regeneration and return of red cell levels to normal in about 4 or 5 weeks.

Because the mutant gene is carried on the X chromosome, affected males do not produce any normal enzyme, and all of their red cells are subject to hemolysis. However, females who carry the mutant gene on one of their X chromosomes are also at risk of drug-induced hemolysis. However, because of random inactivation of one of the X chomosomes in the female, as described in the discussion on chromosomes, genes, and cell division, the red cells of the female contain two populations of red cells. Some are derived from red cell precursors in which the X chromosome containing the mutant gene is inactivated, and these cells will contain the normal enzyme. Other red cells will be derived from precursor cells in which the X chromosome containing the normal gene is inactivated, and these cells will contain a defective enzyme and will be susceptible to hemolysis. Usually the normal red cells and enzyme-deficient red cells are present in approximately equal proportions. Drug-induced hemolysis is less intense in a female carrier than in an affected male because the proportion of hemolysis-susceptible red cells in the female carrier is always less than that of an affected male, in whom all the red cells contain the defective enzyme.

Acquired Hemolytic Anemia

Sometimes, the red cells are normally formed but are unable to survive normally because they are released into a "hostile environment." For example, antibodies that attack and destroy the red cells may be present in the circulation. Some of the autoimmune diseases, such as lupus erythematosus, and some diseases of the lymphatic system may be associated with a hemolytic anemia caused by autoantibodies.

Some drugs also cause a hemolytic anemia by inducing formation of antibodies that damage red cells. Three different immunologic mechanisms have been identified. The most common mechanism results from the effect of the drug on the body's immune system. Certain drugs disrupt the immune system in some way, leading to the formation of an autoantibody directed against the red cell membrane. The autoantibody may persist for some time after the drug has been discontinued. Other mechanisms include formation of drug–protein complexes. In some cases, the drug combines with a plasma protein, forming a drug–protein complex that is antigenic and induces antibody formation. The antigen and antibody interact within the circulation, forming complexes that attach to the red cells and cause their destruction. In other cases, the drug binds to the red cell membrane, forming an antigenic drug–membrane complex. An antibody against the complex then forms, attacks the cell membrane, and damages the red cells.

In another type of acquired hemolytic anemia, red cells may be destroyed by mechanical trauma. Some diseases are characterized by significant enlargement of the spleen. Red cells passing through a greatly enlarged spleen may be subject to considerable mechanical trauma, accelerating their destruction. Occasionally, a hemolytic anemia may follow the insertion of an artificial heart valve. The red cells are injured by contact against some part of the artificial valve.

DIAGNOSTIC EVALUATION OF ANEMIA

After it is determined that a patient is anemic, the physician's function is to determine the cause so that proper, effective treatment can be instituted. A careful medical history and physical examination may provide important clues to the most likely cause. A complete blood count is essential in order to assess the degree of anemia and to determine whether leukopenia and thrombocytopenia also are present. Careful microscopic examination of a blood smear allows the physician to determine whether the anemia is hypochromic microcytic, normocytic, or macrocytic. This information helps identify the probable cause of the anemia. The rate of production of new red cells can be estimated by determining the percentage of reticulocytes in the circulation. This is called a reticulocyte count. An increased percentage of reticulocytes indicates rapid regeneration of red cells, as would be encountered after acute blood loss or hemolysis. In some patients, tests that measure iron stores, iron transport, and iron metabolism may be useful. In selected patients, examining the bone marrow provides very useful information. In this procedure, a small amount of bone marrow is removed from the pelvic bone, sternum, or other site and examined microscopically. Characteristic abnormalities in the maturation of the marrow cells are seen in pernicious anemia and in anemia caused by folic acid deficiency. Bone marrow examination also detects interference with bone marrow functions secondary to infiltration by leukemic cells or metastatic tumor. Aplastic anemia can generally be recognized by studying the bone marrow. Certain other tests are used when chronic blood loss from the gastrointestinal tract is suspected. Stools are examined for blood, and x-ray studies of the gastrointestinal tract are frequently performed to localize a site of bleeding. Other diagnostic procedures are performed in special circumstances.

Polycythemia

Polycythemia
(päl-ē-sī-thē′mē-yuh)
Increased number of red cells. May be caused by some types of chronic heart or lung disease (secondary polycythemia) *or to marrow erythroid hyperplasia of unknown causes* (primary polycythemia).

An increase of red cells and hemoglobin above normal levels is called **polycythemia**. Polycythemia usually is secondary to an underlying disease that produces decreased arterial oxygen saturation (secondary polycythemia), or less frequently it may represent a manifestation of a leukemialike overproduction of red cells for no apparent reason (primary polycythemia).

SECONDARY POLYCYTHEMIA

Any condition associated with a reduced amount of oxygen transported in the bloodstream (low arterial PO_2) leads to increased erythropoietin production and hence to increased numbers of circulating red cells. The condition may accompany pulmonary emphysema, pulmonary fibrosis, or some other type of chronic lung disease that impairs the oxygenation of the blood. Persons with types of congenital heart disease associated with shunting of unsaturated venous blood into the systemic circulation also develop secondary polycythemia. In these individuals, the amount of oxygen transported in the systemic circulation to supply the tissues is reduced (low arterial

PO_2) by the admixture of shunted venous blood, which is followed by a compensatory increase in red cell production. Rarely, polycythemia may be the result of a renal tumor. The polycythemia is caused by excess erythropoietin production by the tumor and subsides when the tumor is removed.

PRIMARY POLYCYTHEMIA

Primary polycythemia, also called polycythemia vera (true polycythemia), is a manifestation of a diffuse hyperplasia of the bone marrow of unknown etiology. It is characterized by overproduction not only of red cells but also of white blood cells and platelets. The disease has many features of a neoplastic process, and some patients with polycythemia vera eventually develop granulocytic leukemia.

COMPLICATIONS AND TREATMENT OF POLYCYTHEMIA

The symptoms of polycythemia are related to the increased blood volume and increased blood viscosity. Many patients with polycythemia develop thromboses because of the increased blood viscosity and elevated platelet levels. Polycythemia vera is usually treated by drugs that suppress the bone marrow overactivity. Secondary polycythemia is sometimes treated by periodic removal of excess blood.

Iron Overload: Hemochromatosis

Although iron is essential for normal hematopoiesis and has other essential functions in the body, an excess of iron in the body is harmful.

Iron is absorbed with difficulty and excreted with difficulty. Iron uptake is very closely controlled by the body, and there are no normal pathways that allow for excretion of iron in excess of the body's needs. Men excrete only about 1 mg of iron per day, which reflects primarily small losses of iron contained in the cells that are being lost from the skin, intestinal tract, and other sites that are replaced by new cells. Premenopausal women excrete slightly more because of menstrual losses, as each milliliter of red cells contains about 0.5 mg of iron.

Because iron excretory pathways are lacking, any excess iron entering the body cannot be eliminated, and the body becomes overloaded with iron, which accumulates in the body's tissues and organs. Eventually, this leads to organ damage followed by scarring, leading to permanent derangement in the functions of the affected organs.

The usual cause of iron overload is a genetic disease called **hemochromatosis,** which is transmitted as an autosomal recessive trait. The gene occurs in about 10% of the population, but the disease only occurs in homozygous carriers of the gene, who absorb an excessive amount of iron, which leads to excessive accumulation of iron in the body.

The manifestations of the disease take years to develop as iron accumulates in the body and causes organ damage. Patients with untreated hemochromatosis often have rather typical manifestations of iron accumulation: tan to brown skin caused by iron accumulation in the skin; diabetes caused by damage to the insulin-producing cells of the pancreas; diffuse scarring of the liver (cirrhosis), which interferes with blood flow through the liver, as discussed in abnormalities of blood coagulation; and heart failure caused by heart muscle damage and associated scarring, resulting from the iron deposits.

Hemochromatosis
(hemo-crow-mah-toe'-sis)
A genetic disease characterized by excessive iron absorption, leading to accumulation of excessive amounts of iron in the body, causing organ damage.

Early recognition and treatment prevents progression of the disease and arrests organ damage. Treatment consists of repeated withdrawal of blood (phlebotomy) to remove iron from the body, as each 500 ml of blood withdrawn removes 250 mg of iron. Phlebotomies are repeated until iron stores are depleted, and then periodic phlebotomies are continued for the rest of the patient's life.

The excessive iron absorption and storage characteristic of hemochromatosis can be identified by the same type of laboratory tests used to measure iron storage and transport in subjects with iron deficiency anemia: serum ferritin, serum iron, and serum iron binding capacity. When the body is overloaded with iron, serum ferritin is very high, reflecting the greatly increased iron stores that can be as much as 15–20 g or more instead of the normal amount of about 1 g. Serum iron is also much higher than normal and the iron-binding protein transferrin is completely loaded (saturated) with iron. These tests all point to increased uptake and storage of iron.

Since hemochromatosis is a common disease that is often not recognized in its early stages, many physicians recommend routine screening for this disease in order to prevent the late complications that arise from iron overload.

The following case illustrates the usefulness of screening studies for detecting this disease before irreparable organ damage occurs.

CASE 14-1

A 40-year-old healthy woman was seen in consultation by a physician because routine screening laboratory tests had detected elevated serum iron.

Physical examination was normal, as were routine blood and urine tests, but tests measuring iron stores and iron metabolism were all abnormal. Serum iron was much higher than normal (234 mg per 100 ml), and serum iron-binding protein was completely saturated with iron. Serum ferritin was 1,335 mg per liter, which is more than 10 times higher than normal. (Normal laboratory values for these tests were indicated in the section on iron deficiency anemia.)

A diagnosis of hemochromatosis was made, and treatment consisting of periodic phlebotomies was begun in order to remove the excess iron from her body.

Thrombocytopenia

Petechia
(pe-tē′kēy-uh)
A small pinpoint hemorrhage caused by decreased platelets, abnormal platelet function, or capillary defect.

Blood platelets are fragments of the cytoplasm of megakaryocytes that are released into the bloodstream. These small structures serve a hemostatic function, sealing small breaks in capillaries and interacting with plasma factors in the initial stages of blood clotting. A significant reduction in the numbers of platelets in the blood leads to numerous small, pinpoint hemorrhages from capillaries in the skin and mucous membranes, called **petechiae**, and to larger areas of hemorrhage, called ecchymoses. This type of skin and mucous membrane bleeding is called purpura, and the disease entity is called thrombocytopenic purpura. The number of platelets may be reduced by bone marrow disease, which impairs platelet production, or by accelerated destruction of platelets in the circulation.

Many cases of thrombocytopenic purpura develop when drugs, chemicals, or other substances damage the bone marrow. Others develop when the bone marrow is infiltrated by leukemic cells or metastatic carcinoma. These conditions are called secondary thrombocytopenic purpura because the purpura results from an underlying disease of the bone marrow.

Sometimes the bone marrow produces platelets normally, but the platelets are rapidly destroyed in the circulation. Autoantibodies directed against platelets can often be detected in the blood of affected individuals. Cases of this type, in which no underlying disease can be detected, are called primary thrombocytopenic purpura. Primary thrombocytopenic purpura is often encountered in children and subsides spontaneously within a short time. When the disease develops in adults, it tends to be more chronic, and it may not be necessary to treat a patient in whom the number of platelets in the bloodstream (platelet count) is only moderately reduced. However, treatment is essential if the platelet count is so low that the patient is at risk of severe life threatening bleeding, such as a cerebral hemorrhage. The initial treatment usually consists of drugs such as corticosteroid hormones that raise the platelet count by suppressing the function of the immune system, which is the source of the auto-antibodies that are destroying the platelets. Patients who do not respond to initial treatment are usually treated by removal of the spleen (splenectomy), the site where the antibody-coated platelets are removed from the circulation, and most patients respond to splenectomy. Other treatment methods are also available for selected patients who have failed to respond to corticosteroids and splenectomy.

The Lymphatic System

The lymphatic system consists of the lymph nodes and spleen, together with various organized masses of lymphoid tissue elsewhere throughout the body; these include the tonsils, the adenoids, the thymus, and the lymphoid aggregates in the intestinal mucosa, respiratory tract, and bone marrow. The primary function of the lymphatic system is to provide immunologic defenses against foreign material by means of cell-mediated and humoral defense mechanisms. The lymph nodes, which constitute a major part of the system, form an interconnected network linked by lymphatic channels.

Lymph nodes are small, bean-shaped structures that vary from a few millimeters to as much as 2 cm in diameter. They are interspersed along the course of lymphatic channels, where they act somewhat like filters. Frequently, they form groups at locations where many lymphatic channels converge, such as around the aorta and inferior vena cava, in the mesentery of the intestine, in the axillae (armpits) and groin, and at the base of the neck. Each node consists of a mass of lymphocytes supported by a meshwork of reticular fibers, which are scattered phagocytic cells of the mononuclear phagocyte system (reticuloendothelial system). As the lymph flows through the nodes, the phagocytic cells filter out and destroy any micro-organisms or other foreign materials that have gotten into the lymphatic channels. The lymphocytes and mononuclear phagocytes within the node also interact with the foreign material and initiate an immune response, as described in the discussion on immunity, hypersensitivity, allergy, and autoimmune diseases.

The spleen is specialized to filter blood rather than lymph. Much larger than lymph nodes, it is about the size of a man's fist and is located under the ribs in the left upper part of the abdomen. It consists of compact masses of lymphocytes and a network of sinusoids (capillaries having wide lumens of variable width) within a supporting framework composed of reticular fibers and numerous phagocytic cells. As the blood flows through the spleen, worn-out red cells are removed from the circulation by the phagocytic cells, and the iron that they contain is salvaged for reuse. Abnormal red cells—such as those that are damaged by disease, are abnormal in shape, or contain a large amount of an abnormal hemoglobin—also are destroyed by the splenic phagocytes, which accounts for their shortened survival in the circulation.

The thymus is a bilobed lymphoid organ overlying the base of the heart. It is a large structure during infancy and childhood but gradually undergoes atrophy in adolescence. Only a remnant persists in the adult. The thymus plays an essential role in the prenatal development of the lymphoid system and in the formation of the body's immunologic defense mechanisms.

DEVELOPMENT OF THE LYMPHATIC SYSTEM

The precursor cells of the lymphocytes are formed initially from stem cells in the bone marrow. In the fetus, some of these precursor cells migrate from the marrow into the thymus, where they undergo further maturation and develop into cells that are destined to form a specific type of lymphocyte called **T** (thymus-dependent) **lymphocytes**. Other lymphoid cells remain within the bone marrow, where they differentiate and develop into cells destined to form a second specific type of lymphocyte called **B** (bone marrow) **lymphocytes**. Before birth, the precursor cells of both T and B lymphocytes migrate into the spleen, lymph nodes, and other sites. Here they proliferate to form the masses of mature lymphocytes that populate the various lymphoid organs. Lymphocytes do not remain localized within the various lymphoid organs. They continually recirculate between the bloodstream and the various lymphoid organs. The functions of the various lymphoid cells and their role in immunity are considered in the discussion on immunity, hypersensitivity, allergy, and autoimmune diseases.

Diseases of the Lymphatic System

The principal diseases affecting the lymphatic system are infections and neoplasms.

INFLAMMATION OF THE LYMPH NODES (LYMPHADENITIS)

Lymph nodes draining an area of infection may become enlarged and tender, resulting from spread of infection through the lymphatic channels and acute inflammation in the node. This is called lymphadenitis.

INFECTIOUS MONONUCLEOSIS

Infectious mononucleosis is a relatively common viral disease. The virus belongs to the same family as the herpes virus that causes fever blisters. The virus has been named the **Epstein-Barr virus** (usually simply called EB virus). The disease is encountered most frequently in young adults and is transmitted by close contact, often by kissing. The virus causes an acute, debilitating, febrile illness associated with a diffuse hyperplasia of lymphoid tissue throughout the body. The lymphoid hyperplasia is manifested by a moderate increase of lymphocytes in the peripheral blood, enlargement and tenderness of lymph nodes, and some degree of splenic enlargement. The spleen, which normally weighs about 150 g and is well protected under the rib cage in the upper abdomen, may double or triple in size and extend several centimeters below the left costal margin. The lymphocytes circulating in the peripheral blood show rather distinctive morphologic abnormalities, and the diagnosis can generally be made by the pathologist from a careful examination of the blood smear. The lymphocytes are larger than normal, with abundant deep blue cytoplasm and an irregularly shaped nucleus (FIGURE 14-7). Enlargement and ulceration of lymphoid tissue in the throat is responsible for the sore throat often accompanying the disease.

The EB virus infects B lymphocytes, which proliferate actively during the first week of the infection. Then cytotoxic (CD8+) T lymphocytes and antibodies pro-

T lymphocyte
A type of lymphocyte associated with cell-mediated immunity.

B lymphocyte
A lymphocyte that differentiates into plasma cells and is associated with humoral immunity.

Epstein-Barr virus
A virus that causes infectious mononucleosis.

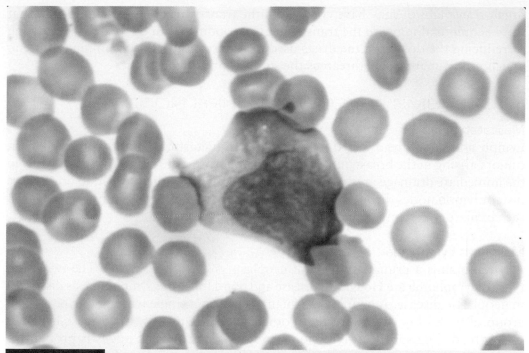

FIGURE 14-7 Large lymphocyte from subject with infectious mononucleosis, illustrating characteristic morphologic abnormalities, as described in text (original magnification × 1,000).

duced by plasma cells against the EB virus destroy the majority of the virus-infected cells, but some evade destruction and persist for life within the lymphatic system of the infected individual. The atypical lymphocytes seen in the blood are the activated cytotoxic T cells attacking the virus-infected cells. Many persons infected with EB virus never develop the clinical manifestations of infectious mononucleosis because the body's defenses destroy the virus-infected cells. Only a small proportion of infected persons develop the elevated temperature, sore throat, enlarged spleen, and enlarged lymph nodes that are characteristic of the disease.

The blood of patients with infectious mononucleosis frequently contains antibodies capable of clumping red cells taken from sheep. These are called heterophile antibodies. Antibodies against the EB virus can also be detected in the blood. The diagnosis of infectious mononucleosis can be established on the basis of the clinical features of the febrile illness in a young adult with lymphadenopathy, the characteristic appearance of the blood smear, and the presence of heterophile and EB virus antibodies in the patient's blood. Generally, the disease is self-limited, and no specific treatment is required; however, it may be several weeks before the patient feels well again. Young adults recovering from infectious mononucleosis should avoid contact sports such as basketball, as long as the spleen remains enlarged and extends below the ribs into the upper abdomen. Any athletic activities that expose the upper abdomen to possible trauma may rupture the enlarged spleen, which is a very serious injury. Individuals with an impaired or suppressed immune system, such as persons with AIDS or persons who have had a bone marrow or organ transplant and are receiving treatment to suppress the immune system, may face another problem. The surviving infected B cells, unrestrained by the nonfunctional immune system, may become activated and proliferate extensively, giving rise to a malignant B cell lymphoma. This condition is called post-transplantation lymphoproliferative disease when it follows an organ transplant. The EB virus–infected cells responsible for the proliferation could be the subject's own virus-containing lymphocytes that became activated when the immune system was deliberately suppressed to permit the organ transplant or may have come from the transplant donor's lymphocytes that were acquired along with the transplant. The condition can be treated by stopping or reducing the dosage of the drugs used to suppress the subject's immune system, which unfortunately also threatens the survival of the transplant.

NEOPLASMS AFFECTING LYMPH NODES

Metastatic Tumors

Lymph nodes may be affected by the spread of metastatic tumor from malignant tumors arising in the breast, lung, colon, or other sites. The nodes first affected lie in the immediate drainage area of the tumor. The tumor may then spread to other more distant lymph nodes through lymphatic channels and may eventually gain access to the circulatory system through the thoracic duct (FIGURE 14-8).

Malignant Lymphoma

A **lymphoma** is a primary malignant neoplasm of lymphoid tissue. The two main types of lymphoma are **Hodgkin's disease** and non-Hodgkin's lymphoma, as discussed in neoplastic disease. A lymphoma usually begins in a single lymph node or a small group of nodes but often spreads to other nodes; frequently, the disease becomes widespread. The spread of lymphoma to multiple groups of nodes is probably a consequence of the recirculation of lymphocytes within the lymphatic system.

Lymphocytic Leukemia

Leukemia may develop from lymphoid cells in the bone marrow or from lymphoid tissue elsewhere in the body. Leukemia is covered in the discussion on neoplastic disease.

Lymphoma
(limf-ō′muh)
A neoplasm of lymphoid cells.

Hodgkin's disease
One type of lymphoma.

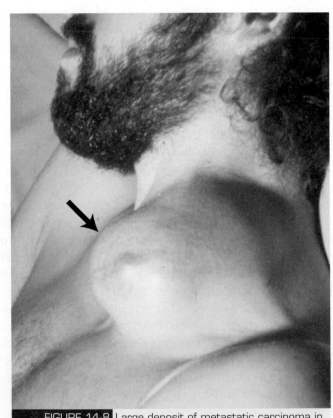

FIGURE 14-8 Large deposit of metastatic carcinoma in the supraclavicular lymph nodes of a young man with carcinoma of the testicle.

ALTERATION OF IMMUNE REACTIONS IN DISEASES OF THE LYMPHATIC SYSTEM

Because of the central role of the lymphatic system in immune reactions, many diseases affecting the lymphatic system diffusely, such as leukemias and lymphomas, are frequently associated with abnormal immune responses. These responses may be manifested either by production of autoantibodies directed against the red cells, white cells, or platelets of the affected individual or by a loss of normal cell-mediated and humoral defenses, leading to an increased susceptibility to infection.

THE ENLARGED LYMPH NODE AS A DIAGNOSTIC PROBLEM

The patient who visits a physician because one or more lymph nodes are enlarged may present a difficult diagnostic problem. Lymph node enlargement may be a manifestation of a localized infection in the area drained by the node. It may be caused by a systemic infection with initial manifestations in the node. It may be caused by metastatic tumor in the node, or it may be an early manifestation of leukemia or malignant lymphoma. Often, the cause of the lymphadenopathy can be determined by the physician from the clinical evaluation of the patient in conjunction with laboratory studies, including an examination of the peripheral blood. Sometimes the cause cannot be established, however, and the physician must perform a lymph node biopsy to determine the reason for the enlargement. The enlarged lymph node is surgically excised and submitted to the pathologist for microscopic examination and microbiologic studies. In difficult cases, more elaborate and sophisticated studies may be required. It is possible, for example, to determine whether a lymphocyte proliferation within a lymph node arose from a single abnormal lymphocyte that formed a clone of identical cells (a monoclonal proliferation), indicating a lymphoid neoplasm, or from many different lymphocytes that formed multiple clones of cells (a polyclonal proliferation), which is characteristic of a benign lymphocyte proliferation. Generally, the pathologist can make a specific diagnosis on the basis of such studies.

THE ROLE OF THE SPLEEN IN PROTECTION AGAINST SYSTEMIC INFECTION

The spleen is an efficient blood filtration system. Any bacteria or other foreign material that gains access to the bloodstream are promptly removed by the splenic phagocytes as the blood flows through the spleen. In addition, the spleen manufactures antibodies that facilitate prompt elimination of pathogenic organisms.

Sometimes it is necessary to remove the spleen. Splenectomy may be required to prevent fatal hemorrhage if the spleen has been lacerated in an automobile accident or other injury. Splenectomy is also frequently performed on patients with blood diseases characterized by excessive destruction of blood cells within the spleen, such as thrombocytopenic purpura and some types of hereditary hemolytic anemia.

Splenectomized persons are less able to eliminate bacteria that gain access to the bloodstream and do not produce antibodies as well as before removal of the spleen. Consequently, they are likely to develop serious bloodstream infections caused by pathogenic bacteria. These infections may respond poorly to antibiotics. To reduce this risk, splenectomized patients are often immunized with bacterial vaccines because high levels of antibacterial antibodies facilitate removal of bacteria from the circulation, and this can substitute for splenic function to some extent. Many physicians also recommend that a splenectomized individual either take antibiotics continuously or begin taking antibiotics at the first sign of a respiratory infection or other febrile illness.

QUESTIONS FOR REVIEW

1. What types of cells are found in the circulating blood, and what are their major functions?
2. What is anemia? What is the difference between an etiologic and a morphologic classification of anemia? Outline a simple etiologic classification of anemia.
3. What is an iron deficiency anemia? How does it arise? How is it treated? What is the morphologic appearance of the red cells?
4. What is the effect of vitamin B_{12} and folic acid on blood cell maturation? What type of anemia results from deficiency of these vitamins?
5. What is the difference between an aplastic anemia and a hemolytic anemia? What is the difference between polycythemia and thrombocytopenia? What is hemochromatosis? What are its manifestations? How is the condition diagnosed and treated?
6. What is the lymphatic system? How is it organized? What are the major cells of the lymphatic system? What are the major functions of the lymphatic system?
7. What is the EB virus? What is its relationship to infectious mononucleosis? What are the clinical manifestations of infectious mononucleosis? How is the disease treated? What are some possible complications of the infection?
8. A patient has an enlarged lymph node. What types of diseases could produce lymph node enlargement? How does the physician arrive at a diagnosis when the patient presents with enlarged lymph nodes?
9. What types of altered immune reaction are sometimes encountered in diseases of the lymphatic system?
10. What are the functions of the spleen? What are the adverse effects of splenectomy?

SUPPLEMENTARY READINGS

Bain, B. J. 2005. Diagnosis from the blood smear. *The New England Journal of Medicine* 353:498–507.

▶ Even in the "high-tech" era of medical practice, the blood smear remains a valuable diagnostic tool. Examination of a well-stained blood smear is essential whenever the results of a complete blood count indicate an abnormality. Methods are available to transmit photographs of atypical or abnormal blood smears to consultants for interpretation or second opinions.

Brittenham, G. M. 2011. Iron-chelating therapy for transfusional iron overload. *The New England Journal of Medicine* 364:146–56.

▶ Long-term treatment with red cell transfusions helps prevent strokes and other complications of sickle cell anemia but leads to iron overload because there are no normal pathways for excretion of excess iron from the body. The excess iron exceeds the storage capacity of the reticuloendothelial (mononuclear phagocyte) system and the transport capability of plasma transferrin. The iron becomes deposited in liver cells, cardiac muscle, the pituitary, pancreas, and other body tissues, where it causes progressive cell damage and organ dysfunction. The excess iron can be removed by an iron-removal drug (chelating agent), which forms a complex with excess iron in blood plasma and is excreted primarily by the kidneys. The chelating agent also forms complexes with iron in liver cells, which are excreted in the bile. One drug (deferoxamine) is poorly absorbed orally and must be given intravenously or subcutaneously. Another drug (deferasirox) can be given orally, is taken up by iron-filled liver cells, and the complexes are excreted in the bile. Ongoing chelation therapy is indicated for almost all patients requiring long-term transfusion treatment, and chelation treatment should begin as soon as patients have received between 10 and 20 red cell transfusions.

Friedrich, M. J. 2011. Advances reshaping sickle cell therapy. *Journal of the American Medical Association* 305:239–40.

► The first case of sickle cell anemia was recognized in a dental student 100 years ago by James Herrick and has become one of the best understood diseases at the genetic and cellular level. The most effective treatments are antibiotics, blood transfusions, hydroxyurea, and blood stem cell transplants. Sickle cell disease (SCD) was the first disease found to be caused by a single amino acid substitution of the β-globin chain of hemoglobin. This causes the hemoglobin molecules to link together, which deforms the affected red cells so that they clog small blood vessels, interrupting blood flow to the tissues. Despite the uniformity of the genetic hemoglobin defect, the severity of the disease can be quite variable and is related to the concentration of fetal hemoglobin in the affected cells, which contains two γ-globin subunits in place of two β-globin subunits. The fetal hemoglobin in the red cells inhibits the joining of the interconnection (polymerization) of sickle hemoglobin molecules. Soon, investigators began using the drug hydroxyurea, which is effective against tumors, to increase the fetal hemoglobin levels in the red cells in order to "dilute" the concentration of sickle hemoglobin in the red cells. Starting hydroxyurea in childhood is effective and appears safe, and levels of up to 20% fetal hemoglobin can be attained.

► Bone marrow transplantation can substitute a normal bone marrow from a compatible donor for the dysfunctional sickle cell marrow, but sometimes blood cells of both the donor and the recipient persist. When this occurs, recovery from the transplant occurs sooner and is associated with fewer complications. Less intense marrow suppression treatment prior to transplantation is becoming more popular and has fewer complications.

Hoagland, H. C. 1995. Myelodysplastic (preleukemia) syndromes: The bone marrow factory failure problem. *Mayo Clinic Proceedings* 70:673–6.

► A review article.

Kark, J. A., Posey, D. M., Schumacher, H. R., et al. 1987. Sickle-cell trait as a risk factor for sudden death in physical training. *The New England Journal of Medicine* 317:781–7.

► The association between sudden death and exertion is not widely appreciated. The prevalence of sickle cell trait is about 8% in the black population, and the incidence of sudden death related to exertion may be about 40 times higher than in the general population.

Likhite, V. V. 1976. Immunological impairment and susceptibility to infection after splenectomy. *Journal of the American Medical Association* 236:1376–7.

► Describes the adverse effects of splenectomy on phagocytosis of bacteria and on antibody formation.

Looker, A. C., Dallman, P. R., Carroll, M. D., et al. 1997. Prevalence of iron deficiency in the United States. *Journal of the American Medical Association* 277:973–6.

► Iron deficiency and iron deficiency anemia are still common in toddlers, adolescent girls, and women of childbearing age.

Pagano, J. S. 2002. Viruses and lymphomas. *The New England Journal of Medicine* 347:78–9.

► A survey of the viruses that cause various types of lymphoid neoplasms, emphasizing the role of EB virus in both B cell and T cell lymphomas.

Pietrangelo, A. 2004. Hereditary hemochromatosis—A new look at an old disease. *The New England Journal of Medicine* 350:2383–97.

▶ Several different gene mutations may cause hemochromatosis. The most common cause is a specific mutation of paired HFE genes, and transmission is an autosomal recessive trait; however, it is not possible to predict how the mutations will be expressed (gene penetrance) in a person homozygous for the mutant gene. Methods for detecting and evaluating hemochromatosis are described. Treatment depends on the manifestations of the disease in an affected person.

Schwartz, R. S. 2007. Immune thrombocytic purpura—from agony to agonist. *The New England Journal of Medicine* 357:2299–301.

▶ Current guidelines for management of immune thrombocytopenic purpura recommend no treatment as long as the blood platelet count is over 30,000 per microliter (normal range 150,000–450,000) because bleeding problems are unlikely to occur when the platelet count exceeds this level. Below this level, corticosteroid hormone treatment is usually started and is effective in many cases, but a sustained remission is not always possible. Splenectomy, which eliminates the major site of platelet destruction, is often effective in most patients. Other methods of treatment include suppressing the immune system by various combinations of drugs. Some newly developed drugs (called thrombopoietic agents) are being studied that can raise platelet counts by directly stimulating megakaryocytes, similar to the effects of a growth factor produced by the liver called thrombopoietin, which regulates platelet production.

Weaver, L. K. 2009. Clinical practice. Carbon monoxide poisoning. *The New England Journal of Medicine* 360:1217–25.

▶ An excellent article on the pathogenesis, manifestations, and treatment of this condition, which is often called the "silent killer." The advantages of administering oxygen under increased pressure in a hyperbaric chamber are described, although this facility may not be available in all communities.

OUTLINE SUMMARY

Composition and Function of Human Blood

COMPOSITION
Five quarts of blood in adult male.
Contains formed elements suspended in plasma.

NORMAL HEMATOPOIESIS
Marrow comparable to manufacturing plant.
Requires raw materials: iron, vitamin B_{12}, folic acid, and protein.
Erythropoiesis regulated by erythropoietin.
Oxygen transport hindered by formation of methemoglobin or carboxyhemoglobin.

Anemia

ETIOLOGIC CLASSIFICATION
Inadequate raw materials.
"Factory" damaged or inoperative.
Excessive loss of red cells.

MORPHOLOGIC CLASSIFICATION
Normocytic anemia: normal-sized cells.
Macrocytic anemia: larger than normal cells.
Hypochromic microcytic anemia: small cells with reduced hemoglobin content.

IRON METABOLISM AND HEMATOPOIESIS
Iron is absorbed from the duodenum, transported by transferrin, and stored as ferritin.
Iron uptake normally is regulated by content of iron in the body.
About 75% of body iron is contained in hemoglobin.
The iron from the hemoglobin in worn-out red cells that are removed from the circulation is recycled to make hemoglobin for newly produced red cells.

Iron Deficiency Anemia

PATHOGENESIS
Inadequate iron intake.
Depletion of iron stores: external blood loss.

TREATMENT
Establish cause and correct.
Supply supplementary iron.

Folic Acid Deficiency

PATHOGENESIS
As a result of inadequate diet or poor absorption caused by intestinal disease.
Occasionally occurs in pregnancy.

TREATMENT
Establish cause and correct.
Supply supplementary folic acid.

Vitamin B$_{12}$ Deficiency

MECHANISM OF VITAMIN B$_{12}$ ABSORPTION
Vitamin B$_{12}$ in food combines with intrinsic factor in gastric juice.
Vitamin B$_{12}$-intrinsic factor complex absorbed in ileum.
Pernicious anemia: lack of intrinsic factor.
Gastric resection/bypass: lack of intrinsic factor.
Distal small bowel resection or disease: impaired absorption of B$_{12}$-intrinsic factor complex.

TREATMENT
Supply vitamin B$_{12}$ intramuscularly.

Bone Marrow Suppression, Damage, or Infiltration

PATHOGENESIS
Anemia of chronic disease.
Marrow injured by drugs or chemicals.
Marrow infiltrated by tumor.
Marrow replaced by fibrous tissue.

TREATMENT
Blood transfusions.
No specific treatment in many cases.
Severe aplastic anemia treated by immunosuppressive agents or bone marrow transplant.

Acute Blood Loss or Accelerated Blood Destruction

ACUTE BLOOD LOSS
Usually the result of massive bleeding from gastrointestinal tract or uterus.
Lost blood regenerated if iron stores adequate.

HEMOLYTIC ANEMIA
Hereditary hemolytic anemia: genetic abnormality in red cells prevents normal survival.
  Shape abnormalities: hereditary spherocytosis and ovalocytosis.
  Abnormal hemoglobins: sickle cell anemia.
  Defective hemoglobin synthesis: thalassemia.
  Enzyme defects: glucose-6-phosphate dehydrogenase deficiency predisposes to episodes of acute hemolysis.

Acquired hemolytic anemia.
  Caused by antibodies.
  As a result of mechanical trauma: associated with marked splenomegaly or artificial heart valves.

Diagnostic Evaluation of Anemia

APPROACH
History and physical examination.
Complete blood count.
Morphologic classification of anemia: clue to etiology.
Reticulocyte count: measures red cell regeneration.
Bone marrow study: may be required to evaluate hematopoiesis.
Evaluation of blood loss from gastrointestinal tract:
  Stool examination.
  X-ray studies of gastrointestinal tract.
Other diagnostic procedures as indicated.

Polycythemia

SECONDARY POLYCYTHEMIA
Decreased arterial oxygen saturation leads to compensatory increase in red cells.
  Chronic lung disease.
  Some types of congenital heart disease.
  Increased erythropoietin production by renal tumor.

PRIMARY POLYCYTHEMIA
Diffuse marrow hyperplasia of unknown cause.
Overproduction of white cells, platelets, and red cells.
Some cases evolve into granulocytic leukemia.

COMPLICATIONS
As a result of increased blood viscosity.
Increased tendency to thromboses.

TREATMENT
Primary polycythemia treated by drugs that suppress marrow function.
Secondary polycythemia treated by periodic removal of excess blood.

Iron Overload: Hemochromatosis

A common genetic disease transmitted as a Mendelian recessive trait.
Body becomes overloaded with iron, leading to secondary organ damage.
Asymptomatic person can be identified by laboratory tests.
Treatment by phlebotomy prevents late complications of iron excess.

Thrombocytopenia

CLASSIFICATION
Secondary: as a result of marrow damage or infiltration.
Primary: usually associated with antiplatelet autoanti-bodies.

Structure and Function of the Lymphatic System

LYMPH NODES
Function as filters.
Grouped where lymph channels converge.
Clear foreign material from lymph.

SPLEEN
Specialized to filter blood.
Phagocytosis of worn-out red cells.

THYMUS
Located at base of heart.
Concerned with prenatal development of the lymphatic system.

DEVELOPMENT OF THE LYMPHATIC SYSTEM
T and B lymphocytes formed from precursors in bone marrow.
T lymphocyte precursors processed by thymus.
T and B lymphocytes populate spleen, lymph nodes, and other lymphoid tissues.

Diseases of the Lymphatic System

LYMPHADENITIS
Infection spreads to regional lymph nodes.
Nodes become enlarged and tender.

INFECTIOUS MONONUCLEOSIS
Caused by EB virus.
Causes enlargement and tenderness of nodes.
Virus infects B lymphocytes; T lymphocytes and antibodies destroy virus.
Excessive B cell proliferation in an immunocompromised person may cause B cell lymphoma.

NEOPLASMS
Metastatic carcinoma: tumor spreads from primary sites to regional nodes.
Malignant lymphoma: see discussion on neoplastic disease.
Lymphatic leukemia: see discussion on neoplastic disease.

Alteration of Immune Reactions in Diseases of the Lymphatic System

ABNORMAL IMMUNE RESPONSE
Autoantibodies formed against red cells, white cells, and platelets.
Loss of cell-mediated or humoral immunity or both.

The Enlarged Lymph Node as a Diagnostic Problem

DIAGNOSTIC POSSIBILITIES
Localized infection.
Systemic infection.
Lymphoma.
Metastatic tumor.

INVESTIGATION
Clinical evaluation.
Laboratory studies.
Lymph node biopsy.

The Role of the Spleen in Protection Against Systemic Infection

FUNCTIONS OF THE SPLEEN
Phagocytosis.
Antibody formation.

REASONS FOR SPLENECTOMY
Traumatic injury.
Patients with Hodgkin's disease prior to treatment.

EFFECTS OF SPLENECTOMY
Less efficient elimination of bacteria from bloodstream.
Impaired production of antibodies.
Predisposition to systemic bloodstream infection.

TREATMENT OF SPLENECTOMIZED PATIENTS
Immunize with antibacterial vaccines.
Antibiotic prophylaxis.

http://health.jbpub.com/humandisease/9e

Human Disease Online is a great source for supplementary human disease information for both students and instructors. Visit this website to find a variety of useful tools for learning, thinking, and teaching.

CHAPTER 15

The Respiratory System

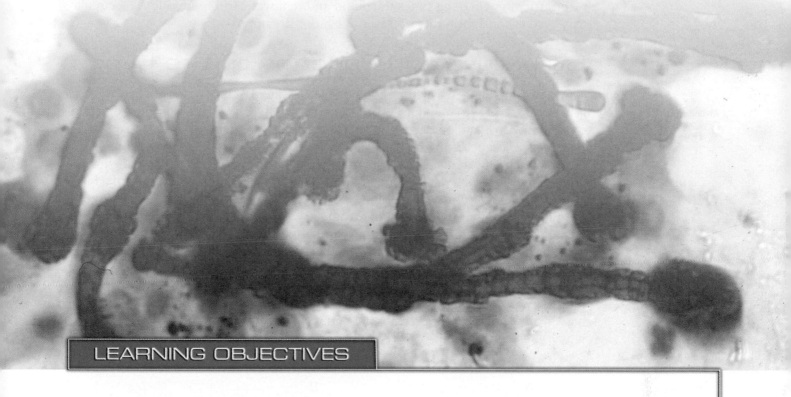

LEARNING OBJECTIVES

1 Explain the basic anatomic and physiologic principles of ventilation and gas exchange.

2 Describe the causes, clinical effects, complications, and treatment of pneumothorax and atelectasis.

3 Describe the histologic characteristics of a tuberculous infection. Explain the possible outcome of an infection. Describe methods of diagnosis and treatment.

4 Differentiate between bronchitis and bronchiectasis.

5 List the anatomic and physiologic derangements in chronic obstructive lung disease. Explain its pathogenesis. Describe the clinical manifestations and methods of treatment.

6 Describe the pathogenesis and manifestations of bronchial asthma and respiratory distress syndrome.

7 Explain the causes and effects of pulmonary fibrosis. Describe the special problems associated with asbestosis.

8 List the major types of lung carcinoma. Describe the clinical manifestations of lung carcinoma and explain the principles of treatment.

Oxygen Delivery: A Cooperative Effort

Normal life processes require that an adequate supply of oxygen be delivered to the tissues and that the waste products of cell metabolism be removed. These functions are carried out by a cooperative effort of the respiratory and circulatory systems. The respiratory system oxygenates the blood and removes carbon dioxide. The circulatory system transports these gases in the bloodstream.

Structure and Function of the Lungs

Alveolus (alvē'olus)
One of the terminal air sacs of the lung.

The lungs consist of two distinct components: a system of tubes whose chief function is to conduct air into and out of the lungs and the **alveoli** (singular, alveolus), where oxygen and carbon dioxide are exchanged between air and the pulmonary capillaries. Just as a tree branches progressively and ends in a foliage of leaves, so the conducting tubes branch repeatedly and terminate in clusters of pulmonary alveoli. The lung is divided into several large segments called lobes. Each lobe in turn consists of a large number of smaller units called lobules. The architecture and structural features of a normal lung can be studied to best advantage when the lung is inflated and air dried (FIGURE 15-1A). The individual lobes, fissures, and pleural surfaces are well defined. The poorly defined cobblestonelike pattern of the pleural surface defines the location of the individual lung lobules, which frequently are accentuated by carbon pigment deposited in the connective tissue that surrounds and circumscribes the individual lobules. When sections of normal air-dried lung are examined against an illuminated background, one can appreciate the spongelike, fine structure of a normal lung, which is essential for normal gas exchange (FIGURE 15-1B).

A   **B**

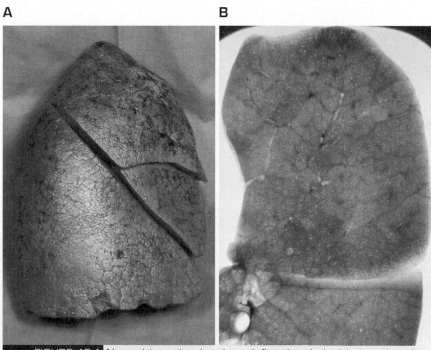

FIGURE 15-1 Normal lung that has been inflated and air dried so that the structure of the lobes and lobules can be visualized and the fine structure of the alveoli can be studied. **A**, External surface illustrating lobes and fissures. The faint cobblestonelike pattern of the pleural surface defines the individual lung lobules. **B**, A backlighted section of lung illustrating the fine, spongelike pattern produced by the respiratory units where gas exchange occurs.

BRONCHI, BRONCHIOLES, AND ALVEOLI

The largest conducting tubes are called **bronchi** (singular, bronchus). Tubes less than about 1 mm in diameter are called **bronchioles** (little bronchi), and the smallest bronchioles, which function only for conduction of air, are called terminal bronchioles. The tubes distal to the terminal bronchioles are called respiratory bronchioles because they have alveoli in their walls and not only transport air but also participate in gas exchange. Each terminal bronchiole gives rise to several respiratory bronchioles, which branch to form alveolar ducts. The alveolar ducts in turn subdivide into alveolar sacs, and multiple alveoli in turn open into each alveolar sac (FIGURE 15-2A AND B).

Each alveolus is a small air space surrounded by a thin wall, the alveolar septum, which consists of thin-walled capillaries supported by a few connective tissue fibers and lined by a layer of epithelial cells (FIGURE 15-2B). Each alveolus contains a relatively small volume of air surrounded by a large network of capillaries, conditions that promote rapid diffusion of oxygen and carbon dioxide between alveolar air and pulmonary capillaries as the blood flows through the lung. Any condition that enlarges the pulmonary alveoli or reduces the number of pulmonary capillaries impedes the efficiency of pulmonary ventilation.

Two types of cells line the alveoli. Most are flat squamous cells. A few are larger secretory cells that produce a lipid material called **surfactant**, which reduces surface tension. Surface tension is the attraction between molecules of a fluid that cause the fluid to aggregate into droplets instead of spreading as a thin film. The surface tension of the molecules in the fluid lining the alveoli would normally tend to pull the alveolar walls together. This effect would hinder expansion of the lungs during inspiration and would cause the alveoli to collapse during expiration because of the cohesive force of the water molecules. Surfactant acts somewhat like a detergent by lowering the surface tension of the fluid and thereby facilitating respiration.

The functional unit of the lung is called a **respiratory unit**. It is formed by the cluster of respiratory bronchioles, alveolar ducts and sacs, and alveoli derived from a single terminal bronchiole. A **lung lobule** consists of a small group of terminal bronchioles and the respiratory units that arise from them. Lobules are partially circumscribed by connective tissue septa and are easiest to identify just beneath the pleura, where the connective tissue septa defining the lobules can be easily seen (FIGURE 15-1A).

Respiration has two functions, corresponding to the two structural components of the lungs:

1. Ventilation, which concerns the movement of air into and out of the lungs
2. Gas exchange between alveolar air and pulmonary capillaries

Both ventilation and gas exchange must function normally if respiration is to be effective.

VENTILATION

Air is moved into and out of the lungs by the bellows action of the thoracic cage. During inspiration, the ribs become more horizontal because of the action of the intercostal muscles, and the diaphragm descends. Consequently, the volume of the thoracic cage increases. The lungs expand to fill the larger intrathoracic space, and air is drawn into the lungs through the trachea and bronchi. During expiration, the ribs become more vertical, and the diaphragm rises. The volume of the thoracic cage is reduced. The lungs, which conform to the size of the thorax, also decrease in volume, and air is expelled.

Bronchus
One of the large subdivisions of the trachea.

Bronchiole
(bron′ke-ōl)
One of the small terminal subdivisions of the branched bronchial tree.

Surfactant
(sur-fak′tant)
A lipid material secreted by alveolar lining cells that facilitates respiration by decreasing the surface tension of the fluid lining the pulmonary alveoli.

Respiratory unit
A functional unit of the lung consisting of a cluster of respiratory bronchioles, alveolar ducts, and alveoli derived from a single terminal bronchiole. Another term for acinus.

Lung lobule
A small group of terminal bronchioles and their subdivisions.

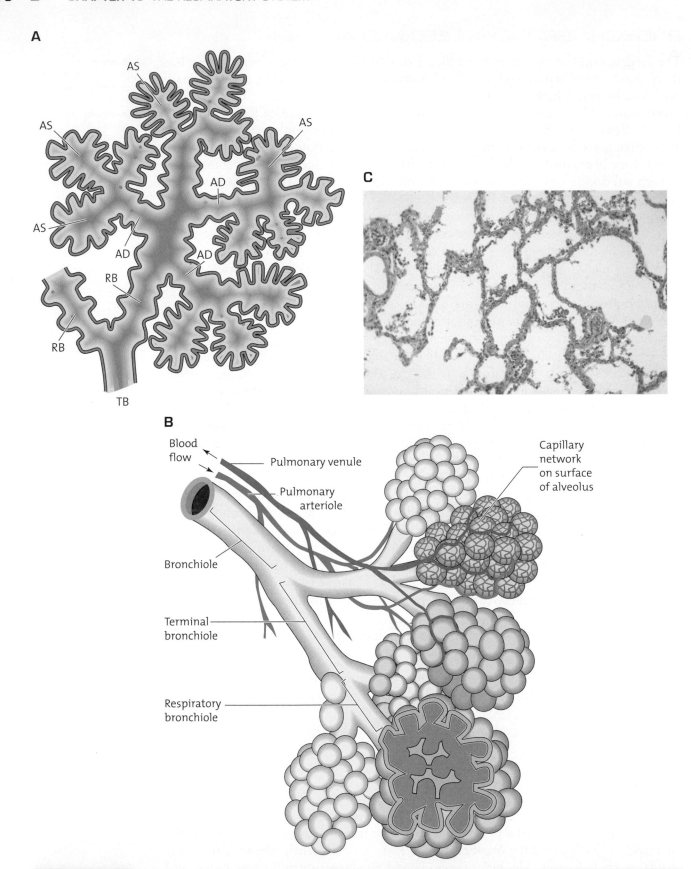

FIGURE 15-2 **A**, Structure of a respiratory unit. Representative terminal bronchiole are designated TB. Respiratory bronchiole (RB) has alveolar sacs projecting from the wall of the bronchiole. Alveolar ducts are designated AD, and alveolar sacs are designated AS. Multiple alveoli (not labeled) open into each alveolar sac. **B**, Structure of terminal air passages. The interior of one alveolar duct is illustrated in cutaway view. **C**, Histologic structure of the lung illustrating alveoli and thin alveolar septa containing pulmonary capillaries (original magnification × 100).

Normal respiratory movements require that respiratory muscles, innervation of the muscles, and mobility of the thoracic cage be normal. Ventilation is impaired if the nerve supply to the respiratory muscles is damaged by disease, as in poliomyelitis, or if the respiratory muscles undergo atrophy and degeneration, as in some uncommon types of muscle disease. Ventilation is also impaired if the thoracic cage is immobile. For example, a person buried in sand up to his neck will suffocate because he is unable to move his thoracic cage and therefore cannot move air into and out of his lungs.

GAS EXCHANGE

Oxygen and carbon dioxide, along with nitrogen and water vapor, are in the atmospheric air that we breathe, in the air within the pulmonary alveoli, and in the blood. At sea level, the atmospheric pressure exerted by the mixture of all the gases is 760 mm Hg. Each gas exerts a proportionate part of the total atmospheric pressure, depending on its concentration in the mixture of gases. For example, the concentration of oxygen in atmospheric air is 20%. Therefore, the pressure exerted by oxygen is 20% of the total pressure exerted by all the gases ($0.20 \times 760 = 152$ mm Hg). The part of the total atmospheric pressure exerted by a gas is called the partial pressure of the gas. Partial pressure is usually expressed by the letter "P" preceding the chemical symbol for the gas, as for example PO_2 152 mm Hg.

Gases diffuse between blood, tissues, and pulmonary alveoli because of differences in their partial pressures. Venous blood returning from the tissues is low in oxygen (PO_2 40 mm Hg) and high in carbon dioxide (PCO_2 47 mm Hg). This blood is pumped through the pulmonary capillaries, where it comes into contact with the air in the pulmonary alveoli. Alveolar air has a much higher concentration of oxygen (PO_2 105 mm Hg) but a lower concentration of carbon dioxide (PCO_2 35 mm Hg). Therefore, oxygen diffuses from alveolar air into pulmonary capillaries, and carbon dioxide diffuses from pulmonary capillaries into the aveoli. The situation is reversed in the tissues. The tissue oxygen concentration is much lower (PO_2 about 20 mm Hg), and the carbon dioxide concentration is much higher (PCO_2 about 60 mm Hg); so oxygen diffuses into the tissues from the blood, and carbon dioxide diffuses in the opposite direction.

Exchange of gases between alveolar air and pulmonary capillaries is accomplished by diffusion across the alveolar membrane. Efficient gas exchange requires (1) a large capillary surface area in contact with alveolar air, (2) unimpeded diffusion of gases across the alveolar membrane, (3) normal pulmonary blood flow, and (4) normal pulmonary alveoli. The spongy structure of the lungs, in which each tiny air sac is surrounded by a large network of capillaries, provides the large surface area required for efficient gas exchange (FIGURE 15-3A). Destruction of alveolar septa leads to coalescence of alveoli and a reduction in the size of the capillary network surrounding the alveoli, resulting in less efficient gas exchange (FIGURE 15-3B).

If the alveolar septa are thickened and scarred, the diffusion of gases across the thickened alveolar membranes is impeded (FIGURE 15-3C). Gas exchange is also impaired if pulmonary blood flow to a portion of the lung is obstructed, as might be caused by a pulmonary embolus obstructing a large pulmonary artery or by blockage of pulmonary capillaries by fat emboli or foreign material (FIGURE 15-3D). If the pulmonary alveoli become filled with fluid or inflammatory exudate, inspired air cannot enter the diseased alveoli, and pulmonary gas exchange is impeded (FIGURE 15-3E).

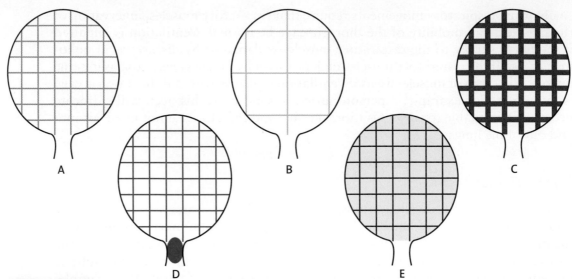

FIGURE 15-3 Types of structural and functional abnormalities that adversely affect pulmonary gas exchange. **A,** Normal alveoli and pulmonary blood flow. **B,** Destruction of alveolar septa, leading to coarsening of alveolar structure with corresponding reduction in size of pulmonary capillary bed. **C,** Fibrous thickening and scarring of alveolar septa, impeding diffusion of gasses across alveolar membrane. **D,** Obstruction of pulmonary blood flow to a part of the lung. **E,** Alveoli filled with fluid or inflammatory exudate.

PULMONARY FUNCTION TESTS

Vital capacity
The maximum volume of air that can be forcefully expelled after a maximum inspiration.

One-second forced expiratory volume (FEV₁)
The maximum volume of air that can be expelled from the lungs in 1 second.

Pulmonary function tests can be used to evaluate the efficiency of pulmonary ventilation and pulmonary gas exchange. Pulmonary ventilation is usually tested by measuring the volume of air that can be moved into and out of the lung under standard conditions. Two commonly used measurements are **vital capacity,** which measures the maximum volume of air that can be expelled after a deep inspiration, and the **one-second forced expiratory volume** (FEV_1), which measures the maximum volume of air that can be expelled in 1 second. If the bronchioles are narrowed by inflammation or spasm, impeding the movement of air out of the lungs, FEV_1 is often reduced. Specialized tests can measure the total volume of air in the lungs and the volume of air remaining in the lungs after a maximum expiration.

The concentrations of oxygen and carbon dioxide (O_2 and CO_2) in the patient's arterial blood can also be measured in order to determine the efficiency of gas exchange in the lungs. In chronic pulmonary disease, oxygenation of the blood is inefficient. Oxygen concentration is reduced, and arterial oxygen saturation is decreased correspondingly. Often, the arterial PCO_2 also is higher than normal because carbon dioxide is inefficiently eliminated by the lungs. Arterial blood for analysis is usually collected by inserting a small needle into the radial artery in the wrist and withdrawing a small amount of blood. One can also determine how effectively the lungs are oxygenating the blood (arterial oxygen saturation) using a device called a pulse oximeter. A fingertip is inserted into the device, which measures photoelectrically the changes in light absorption of the hemoglobin in the fingertip capillaries at various wavelengths during systole and diastole. Then the data are used to calculate automatically the oxygen saturation of the arterial blood, and the device promptly displays the result.

Pleura
(plŏŏr'äh)
The mesothelial covering of the lung (visceral pleura) and chest wall (parietal pleura).

THE PLEURAL CAVITY

The lungs are covered by a thin membrane called the **pleura,** which also extends over the internal surface of the chest wall. Because the lungs fill the thoracic cavity, the two pleural surfaces are in contact. The potential space between the lung and chest wall is the pleural cavity. Normally, the apposing pleural surfaces move smoothly over one another. In disease, however, the pleural surfaces may become roughened because of inflammation and may become adherent. Inflammatory exudate may accumulate in the pleural cavity and separate the two pleural surfaces.

Intrapleural and Intrapulmonary Pressures

The lungs are held in an expanded position within the pleural cavity because the pressure within the pleural cavity (intrapleural pressure) is less than the pressure of the air within the lungs (intrapulmonary pressure). The pressure differences develop when the thoracic cavity enlarges after birth. When respirations are initiated, the size of the thoracic cavity increases. The lungs become filled with air at atmospheric pressure and expand to fill the enlarged thoracic cavity, stretching the elastic tissue within the lungs. The tendency of the stretched lung to pull away from the chest wall and return to its original contracted state creates a slight vacuum within the pleural cavity. Because the intrapleural pressure is slightly less than atmospheric pressure, it is often called "negative pressure."

Pneumothorax

Because the intrapleural pressure is subatmospheric, air flows into the pleural space if the lung or chest wall is punctured. When this occurs, the subatmospheric ("negative") pressure that holds the lung in the expanded position is lost, and the lung collapses because the elastic tissue within the lung contracts. This condition, which is called a **pneumothorax** (*pneumo* = air), may follow any type of lung injury or pulmonary disease that allows air to escape from the lungs into the pleural space. It may also result from a stab wound or some other penetrating injury to the chest wall that permits atmospheric air to enter the pleural space (FIGURE 15-4).

Pneumothorax
(nōō-mō-thor′ax)
Accumulation of air in the pleural cavity.

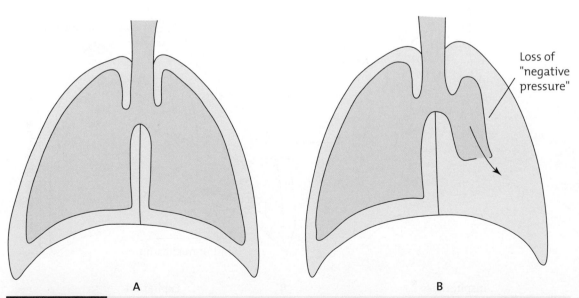

FIGURE 15-4 **A,** Normal relation of lung to chest wall. Pleural space is exaggerated, and surfaces are normally in contact. "Negative pressure" is primarily a result of the tendency of the stretched lung to pull away from the chest wall. **B,** Pneumothorax caused by a perforating injury of lung, allowing the air under atmospheric pressure to escape into the pleural cavity.

Loss of "negative pressure"

A

B

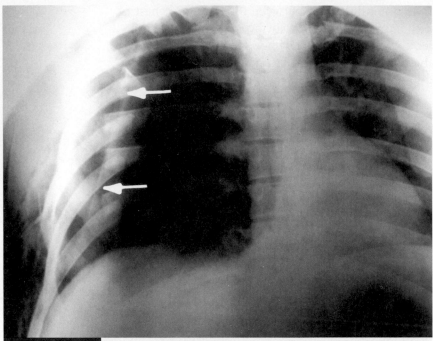

FIGURE 15-5 X-ray illustrating pneumothorax secondary to multiple rib fractures in which broken ends of fractured ribs have torn through the pleura and torn underlying lung. The *arrows* indicate the surface of lung that is no longer in contact with chest wall.

Occasionally, a pneumothorax occurs without apparent cause. This is called spontaneous pneumothorax. Most cases occur in young healthy persons, usually as a result of rupture of a small, air-filled, subpleural bleb at the apex of the lung.

The sudden escape of air into the pleural cavity that is associated with any type of pneumothorax usually causes chest pain and often some shortness of breath. The breath sounds, which normally can be heard with a stethoscope when the air moves in and out of the lung during respiration, are diminished on the affected side. A chest x-ray reveals partial or complete collapse of the lung and the presence of air in the pleural cavity (FIGURE 15-5).

The development of a positive (higher than atmospheric) pressure in the pleural cavity, called tension pneumothorax, may accompany any type of pneumothorax. This dangerous complication may occur if the lung has been perforated in such a way that the pleural tear acts as a one-way valve (FIGURE 15-6). In this circumstance, air flows through the perforation into the pleural cavity as the

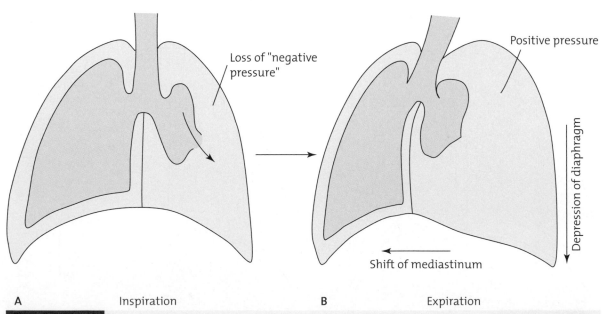

Loss of "negative pressure"

Positive pressure

Depression of diaphragm

Shift of mediastinum

A Inspiration

B Expiration

FIGURE 15-6 Pathogenesis of tension pneumothorax. **A**, Air enters the pleural cavity during inspiration as intrapleural pressure falls. **B**, Rising intrapleural pressure on expiration closes the pleural tear, trapping air within the pleural space. The diaphragm on affected side is displaced downward. The trachea and mediastinal structures are shifted away from side of pneumothorax and encroach on opposite pleural cavity.

intrapleural pressure falls on inspiration. On expiration, however, the intrapleural pressure rises and forces the edges of the pleural tear together, trapping the air within the pleural space. With each inspiration, more air enters the pleural cavity but cannot escape. Eventually, the pleural cavity becomes overdistended with air under pressure, and the affected lung collapses completely. As the pressure builds up in the pleural cavity, the heart and mediastinal structures are displaced away from the side of the pneumothorax and encroach on the opposite pleural cavity, impairing the expansion of the opposite lung (FIGURE 15-7). A tension pneumothorax can be fatal if it is not recognized and treated promptly by evacuating the trapped air to relieve the pressure.

A pneumothorax is usually treated by inserting a tube into the pleural cavity through an incision in the chest wall. The tube prevents accumulation of air in the pleural cavity and aids reexpansion of the lung. The tube is connected to an apparatus that permits the air to be expelled from the pleural cavity during expiration but prevents the air from being sucked back into the pleural cavity during inspiration. The tube is left in place until the tear in the lung heals and no more air escapes. Any air remaining in the pleural cavity is gradually reabsorbed into the bloodstream, and the lung reexpands as the air is absorbed. Sometimes a slight vacuum is applied to the tube in order to evacuate the air more rapidly and hasten reexpansion of the lung.

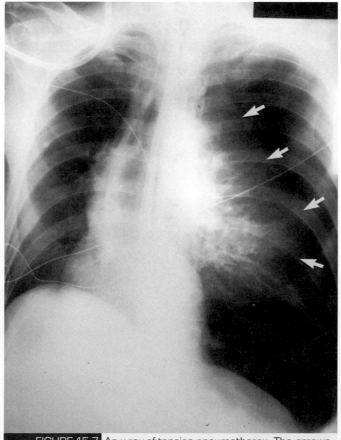

FIGURE 15-7 An x-ray of tension pneumothorax. The *arrows* indicate the surface of the collapsed lung. Note the low diaphragm on the affected side and displacement of mediastinal structures.

Atelectasis

Atelectasis
(ah-tel-ek´tuh-sis)
*Collapse of the lung,
either caused by
bronchial obstruction
(obstructive atelectasis)
or external compression
(compression atelectasis).*

Atelectasis literally means incomplete expansion of the lung (*ateles* = incomplete + *ectasia* = expansion). It refers to a collapse of parts of the lung. There are two types:

1. Obstructive atelectasis, which results from bronchial obstruction
2. Compression atelectasis, which results from external compression of the lung

OBSTRUCTIVE ATELECTASIS

Complete blockage of a bronchus by thick mucous secretions, by a tumor, or by an aspirated foreign object prevents air from entering or leaving the alveoli supplied by the blocked bronchus, and the air already present is gradually absorbed into the blood flowing through the lungs. As a result, the part of the lung supplied by the blocked bronchus gradually collapses as the air is absorbed. The volume of the affected pleural cavity also decreases correspondingly, causing the mediastinal structures to shift toward the side of the atelectasis and the diaphragm to elevate on the affected side (FIGURE 15-8). If the bronchial obstruction is relieved promptly, the lung reexpands normally. This is illustrated by the following unusual case of obstructive atelectasis, which was initially thought to be secondary to an obstructing lung carcinoma.

CASE 15-1

A 66-year-old man with a long history of heavy smoking and excessive alcohol consumption consulted his physician because of shortness of breath. He was found to have an atelectasis of the left lung (FIGURE 15-9). An obstructing carcinoma was suspected, and a bronchoscopic examination was performed. A soft rubber stopper was found obstructing the left main bronchus. The subject apparently had been chewing the stopper while intoxicated and had accidentally inhaled it. The stopper was removed. An x-ray taken the following day revealed that the lung had reexpanded completely.

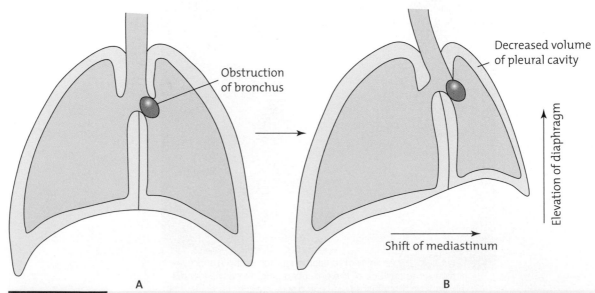

FIGURE 15-8 Atelectasis caused by bronchial obstruction. **A**, Blockage of bronchus prevents aeration of lung supplied by obstructed bronchus. **B**, Absorption of air causes collapse of the lung and a corresponding reduction in size of the pleural cavity. The diaphragm rises, and the mediastinum shifts toward the affected side.

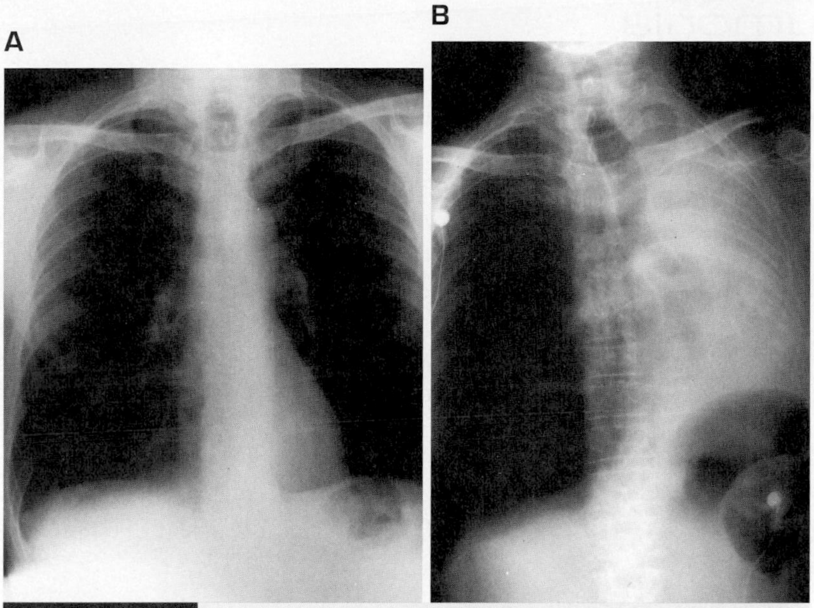

A

B

FIGURE 15-9 Complete atelectasis of the left lung caused by obstruction of left main bronchus (Case 15-1). **A**, Chest x-ray before development of atelectasis. **B**, Atelectasis of entire left lung. The collapsed lung appears dense because the air has been absorbed. The left half of diaphragm is elevated. Trachea and mediastinal structures are shifted toward the side of the collapse.

Atelectasis sometimes develops as a postoperative complication. Because of postoperative pain, the patient does not cough or breathe deeply, and mucous secretions accumulate in the bronchi (FIGURE 15-10). To prevent this problem, the physician encourages the postoperative patient to breathe deeply and cough frequently to keep the respiratory passages clear of secretions.

COMPRESSION ATELECTASIS

Compression atelectasis results when fluid, blood, or air accumulates in the pleural cavity, reducing its volume and thereby preventing full expansion of the lung.

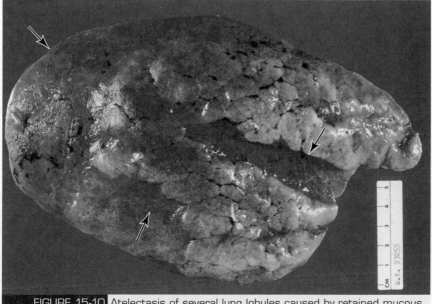

FIGURE 15-10 Atelectasis of several lung lobules caused by retained mucous secretions. Note the contrast between the pale normally aerated lung and the atelectatic areas (*arrows*), which appear dark and depressed.

Pneumonia

Pneumonia
(nōō-mōn yuh)
Inflammation of the lung.

Pneumonia is an inflammation of the lung characterized by the same type of vascular changes and exudation of fluid and cells as that of inflammation in any other location. However, the inflammatory process is influenced by the spongy character of the lungs. The inflammatory exudate spreads unimpeded through the lung, filling the alveoli, and the affected portions of lung becomes relatively solid (termed consolidation) (FIGURE 15-11A). The inflammatory exudate may reach the pleural surface in some areas, causing irritation and inflammation of the pleura; sometimes inflammatory exudate accumulates in the pleural space.

CLASSIFICATION OF PNEUMONIA

Pneumonia may be classified in several ways:

1. By etiology
2. By anatomic distribution of the inflammatory process
3. By predisposing factors that led to its development

The etiologic classification is the most important because it serves as a guide to treatment. Pneumonia may be caused by bacteria, chlamydiae, mycoplasmas, rickettsiae, viruses, or fungi. Whenever possible, the pneumonia is classified in greater detail by designating the exact organism responsible for the infection, such as the pneumococcus, staphylococcus, mycoplasma, or coronavirus.

The anatomic classification describes what part of the lung is involved (FIGURE 15-11). Lobar pneumonia refers to an infection of an entire lung lobe. Bronchopneumonia describes an infection involving only parts of one or more lobes (lung lobules) adjacent to the bronchi. Lobar pneumonia and bronchopneumonia are infections caused by pathogenic bacteria. A third anatomic classification is called interstitial pneumonia or primary atypical pneumonia and is usually caused by a virus or mycoplasma (*Mycoplasma pneumoniae*). This type of pulmonary infection involves the pulmonary alveolar septa rather than the alveoli, and the inflammatory cells infiltrating the septa are primarily lymphocytes, monocytes, and plasma cells rather than neutrophils.

Classification of pneumonia by predisposing factors is common. Any condition associated with poor lung ventilation and retention of bronchial secretions predisposes an individual to the development of pneumonia. Postoperative pneumonia is a pulmonary inflammation that develops in the

A

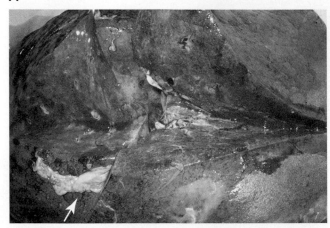

B

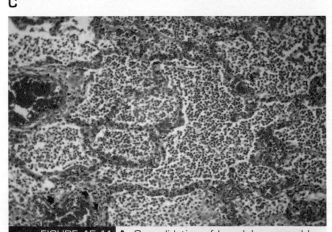

C

FIGURE 15-11 **A**, Consolidation of lung lobe caused by lobar pneumonia. The lung has been incised, and cut surfaces are exposed. An *arrow* indicates a deposit of fibrin on pleura. **B**, Bronchopneumonia. Inflammation involves lung lobules rather than an entire lobe. An *arrow* indicates most severely involved lobules. **C**, Histologic appearance of pneumonia. Alveoli are filled with neutrophils, and no air can enter the affected alveoli (original magnification × 100).

postsurgical patient who is unable to cough or breathe deeply because of pain; the resultant poor ventilation and retention of secretions predisposes to atelectasis of lung lobules, which is followed by secondary bacterial invasion leading to broncho-pneumonia. Aspiration pneumonia occurs when a foreign body, food, vomit, or other irritating substance is aspirated into the lung. Obstructive pneumonia develops in the lung distal to an area where a bronchus is narrowed or obstructed. Blockage of a bronchus by a tumor or foreign body leads to poor aeration and to retention of bronchial secretions in the obstructed part of the lung, which predisposes to infection.

CLINICAL FEATURES OF PNEUMONIA

The signs and symptoms of pneumonia are those of any systemic infection. The patient is ill and has an elevated temperature, and the number of white blood cells in the peripheral blood is frequently higher than normal. Bronchial inflammation is evident, manifested by cough and purulent sputum. If the inflammatory process involves the pleura, the patient experiences pain on respiration because the inflamed pleural surfaces rub against each other. The patient may also have symptoms related to partial loss of lung function caused by consolidation of part of the lung, resulting from the accumulation of inflammatory cells within the alveoli. Oxygenation of the blood is impaired, and the patient may become quite short of breath.

Pneumonia is treated by correcting any predisposing factors that contributed to the development of the pulmonary infection and administering appropriate antibiotic therapy.

Legionnaires' disease is a type of pneumonia caused by a gram-negative, rod-shaped bacterium called *Legionella pneumophila* that is widely distributed in the environment: in the soil and in freshwater ponds, lakes, and streams. The organism thrives in moist environments, such as air-conditioning ducts, shower heads, and humidifiers. People become infected by inhaling airborne organisms in aerosolized water droplets. The infection is not transmitted directly from person to person. The disease was first recognized in 1976 among people attending an American Legion convention in Philadelphia. After the infectious agent was identified, it was determined in retrospect that this same organism had in the past caused other outbreaks of pneumonia, but the infectious agent was not identified at the time. Clinically, the disease is characterized by the usual symptoms of a pulmonary infection, and the chest x-ray reveals evidence of pneumonia. The infection responds to appropriate antibiotics.

Legionnaires' disease
A type of pneumonia caused by an airborne bacterium called Legionella pneumophila.

SEVERE ACUTE RESPIRATORY SYNDROME (SARS)

This condition is a highly communicable serious pulmonary infection caused by an unusual coronavirus that has spread rapidly through several countries since it was first identified in late 2002. There are no effective antiviral drugs that can influence the course of the disease.

Coronaviruses are ribonucleic acid (RNA) viruses that received their name from the crownlike spikes projecting from the viruses as seen by electron microscopy (*corona* = crown). There are three major groups of coronaviruses that cause disease in animals and humans. Previously, most of the infections in humans caused by coronaviruses were common colds, not lower respiratory tract infections. The SARS-associated virus, however, is a unique virus that is not closely related to other known coronaviruses and is the first one known to cause severe disease in people. Precautions to prevent infection when dealing with patients include gloves, gowns, masks, and eye protection.

The illness begins with chills and fever, sometimes mild respiratory symptoms, and occasionally diarrhea. After 3–7 days, manifestations of lower respiratory tract infection appear: cough, shortness of breath, and evidence of pneumonia demonstrated by chest x-ray examination. The severity of the illness is quite variable. The lungs of severely affected patients show the characteristic features of the adult respiratory distress syndrome, and they require mechanical ventilation using an increased oxygen concentration to improve the diffusion of oxygen across the thickened edematous alveolar septa, as well as other measures to improve pulmonary function, as described in the section on the adult respiratory distress syndrome.

PNEUMOCYSTIS PNEUMONIA

Humans harbor *Pneumocystis jiroveci*, a small parasite of low pathogenicity now classified as a fungus, and many animals also harbor a similar parasite. The parasite does not affect normal persons but may cause serious pulmonary infections in susceptible individuals. Those at risk include adults whose immune defenses have been impaired by communicable disease, such as by AIDS, or by administration of immunosuppressive drugs, and premature infants in whom immune defenses are poorly developed.

The life cycle of the parasite is complex. The most easily recognized form is a round or cup-shaped cyst about the size of a red blood cell that cannot be identified by routine (hematoxylin and eosin) stains but can be demonstrated by means of special stains containing silver compounds. Within the cysts are small structures called sporozoites, which are released from the cyst and mature to form larger structures called trophozoites. Some trophozoites give rise to more cysts, repeating the cycle. Others attack and injure the cells lining the pulmonary alveoli, causing a mild inflammatory reaction within the alveolar septa, which leads to exudation of large amounts of protein-rich material that accumulates within the alveoli. The parasites, intermixed in the alveolar exudate but unstained by routine stains, appear as pale areas within the brightly stained exudate, imparting a foamy, "soap-bubble" appearance to the exudate. Special stains, however, demonstrate that the soap bubbles represent *Pneumocystis* cysts and may also reveal central clusters of sporozoites, which appear as dark dots within the centers of the cysts (FIGURE 15-12).

Clinically, pneumocystis pneumonia is characterized by progressive shortness of breath and cough in a person whose immunologic defenses are impaired and who is at high risk of developing the disease. Evidence of pulmonary consolidation caused by the alveolar exudate can be demonstrated by x-ray. The diagnosis of pneumocystis pneumonia is established by biopsy of lung tissue obtained by bronchoscopy. Histologic study of the biopsy material reveals the characteristic foamy alveolar exudate containing large numbers of parasites, as demonstrated by special stains. Often, the parasite also can be demonstrated in material aspirated from the bronchi by bronchoscopy. It is much more difficult to demonstrate the organisms in sputum because they are enmeshed in the alveolar exudate and do not escape from the alveoli. The infection is always very serious and is often life threatening because it affects persons whose ability to respond to infection is greatly impaired. Treatment consists of administering drugs that inhibit the growth of the organism.

Tuberculosis

Pulmonary tuberculosis is a special type of pneumonia caused by an acid-fast bacterium, the tubercle bacillus *Mycobacterium tuberculosis*. Because the tubercle bacillus has a capsule composed of waxes and fatty substances, it is more resistant to destruction than many other organisms. The body's response to the tubercle bacillus also differs from the usual acute inflammatory reaction. Monocytes accumulate around the bacteria; many of them fuse, forming rather characteristic large multinucleated

A

B

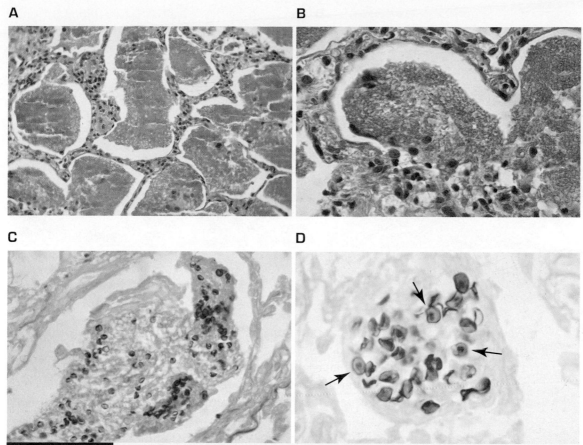

C

D

FIGURE 15-12 Pneumocystis pneumonia. **A**, Pulmonary alveoli filled with dense protein exudate (original magnification × 100). **B**, Higher magnification, illustrating the foamy "soap-bubble" appearance of the alveolar exudate. The clear areas in the alveolar exudate are *Pneumocystis* organisms that are not stained by routine stains (original magnification × 400). **C**, Demonstration of *Pneumocystis jiroveci* cysts within the alveolar exudate by means of silver-containing stains (original magnification × 400). **D**, High-magnification view of the organisms demonstrated by silver stains. Central dark dots within the cysts are clusters of sporozoites (original magnification × 1,000).

cells called giant cells. Lymphocytes and plasma cells also accumulate, and fibrous tissue proliferates around the central cluster of monocytes and giant cells. The central portion of the cellular aggregation usually becomes necrotic. This characteristic nodular mass of cells with central necrosis is called a granuloma, and the inflammatory process is called a granulomatous inflammation (FIGURE 15-13). The granulomatous response to the tubercle bacillus and the necrosis within the granulomas indicate the development of cell-mediated immunity against the organism, which is the primary immune defense against the tubercle bacillus.

COURSE OF A TUBERCULOUS INFECTION

The initial infection is acquired from organisms inhaled in airborne droplets that have been coughed or sneezed into the air by a person with active tuberculosis who is discharging organisms into the environment. The organisms lodge within the pulmonary alveoli, where they proceed to multiply. Initially, the organisms introduced into the lungs do not elicit a marked inflammatory reaction because they do not produce any toxins or destructive enzymes that damage the tissues. Macrophages phagocytose the bacteria but are unable to destroy them; they may even carry the organisms to other parts of the lung and into the regional lymph nodes. After several

A   B

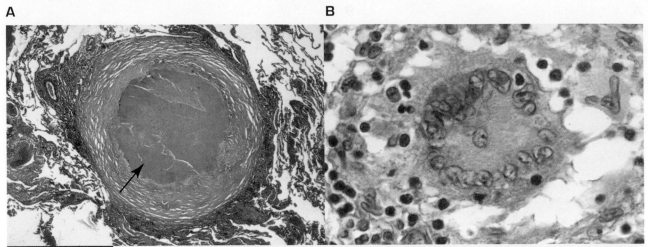

FIGURE 15-13 **A**, Granuloma as a result of tuberculosis. The central part (*arrow*) consists of necrotic tissue (original magnification × 40). **B**, Multinucleated giant cell characteristic of tuberculosis infection (original magnification × 400).

weeks, however, a cell-mediated immunity develops. Sensitized lymphocytes attract and activate macrophages, which acquire a greatly enhanced phagocytic and destructive capability. The activated macrophages attack and destroy many of the organisms, forming characteristic granulomas containing areas of necrosis and surrounded by a rim of fibrous tissue. In the majority of cases, the infection is arrested; the granulomas in the lung and regional lymph nodes heal with scarring, often followed by calcification of the granulomas. In most cases, the infection does not cause any symptoms, and the person may be unaware of the infection. Sometimes the granuloma in the lung is large enough to be identified in a chest x-ray (FIGURE 15-14), but often the area of infection is too small to be detected in an x-ray. The positive skin test (Mantoux test), which reveals a hypersensitivity to the proteins of the tubercle bacillus, may be the only evidence of recent infection.

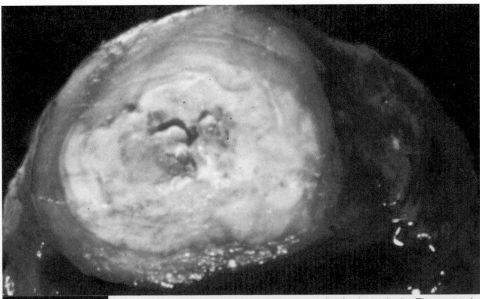

FIGURE 15-14 Old healed pulmonary granuloma as a result of tuberculosis. The central part consists of necrotic tissue containing calcium deposits surrounded by rim of dense fibrous tissue.

Cell-mediated immunity generally controls the infection, and the arrested infection may never cause any further problems. The healed granulomas, however, may contain small numbers of viable organisms, and the infection may become reactivated, leading to progressive pulmonary tuberculosis if the body's cell-mediated immunity declines.

Not all primary infections respond as favorably. If a large number of organisms are inhaled or if the body's defenses are inadequate, the inflammation will progress, causing more extensive destruction of lung tissue (FIGURE 15-15). Often, the granulomatous inflammatory process makes contact with a bronchus, and the necrotic inflammatory tissue is discharged into it. A cavity then forms within the lung, surrounded by granulomatous inflammatory tissue containing masses of tubercle bacilli (FIGURE 15-16). People who have active progressive tuberculosis with a tuberculous cavity can infect others because they discharge large numbers of tubercle bacilli in their sputum.

In a tuberculous infection of the lung, organisms are often carried in lymphatic channels from the lung into the peribronchial lymph nodes, leading to a tuberculous inflammation in the regional lymph nodes.

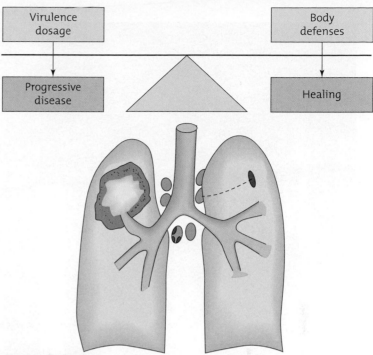

FIGURE 15-15 Possible outcome of a tuberculosis infection in relation to virulence and dosage of the organism and resistance of the body. The frequent involvement of the regional lymph nodes is indicated. *Left,* Progressive disease with formation of cavity within lung, caused by infection by a large number of organisms or inadequate body defenses. *Right,* Healing with scarring as a result of small numbers of organisms or a high degree of resistance to infection.

Many cases of active progressive pulmonary tuberculosis do not result from the initial infection. They develop in persons who have been infected at some time in the past and have developed a cell-mediated immunity directed against the organism. In the past, tuberculosis in previously infected persons was called reinfection tuberculosis because physicians believed that the active tuberculosis was caused by a new infection with the tubercle bacillus in a person who had been infected previously with the organism. Indeed, some cases of tuberculosis in previously infected persons are actually new infections. However, most cases of active tuberculosis in older patients result from a reactivation of an old infection rather than a new infection with the tubercle bacillus. It is well known that old tuberculous lesions that appear completely healed may harbor tubercle bacilli. If the resistance of the individual is lowered by AIDS or other debilitating diseases, by treatment with adrenal corticosteroids, or by other factors, an apparently healed focus of tuberculosis may flare up and lead to active progressive tuberculosis.

MILIARY TUBERCULOSIS AND TUBERCULOUS PNEUMONIA

Miliary tuberculosis and tuberculous pneumonia are two uncommon but extremely serious forms of tuberculosis. **Miliary tuberculosis** develops if a mass of tuberculous inflammatory tissue erodes into a large blood vessel, disseminating large numbers of organisms throughout the body through the bloodstream. The term miliary is derived

Miliary tuberculosis
(mi′lē-air-ē)
Multiple foci of tuberculosis throughout the body as a result of bloodstream dissemination of tubercle bacilli from a primary focus in the lung or peribronchial lymph nodes.

A   B

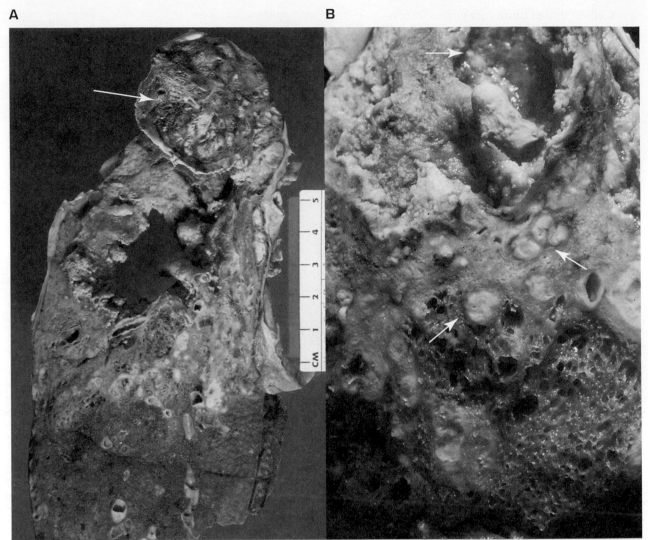

FIGURE 15-16 Far-advanced pulmonary tuberculosis. **A**, The upper lobe (*arrow*) has been completely destroyed by tuberculosis, and there is extensive tuberculosis in the lower lobe with a large cavity in the lung that communicates with a bronchus. Only the lower part of the lobe is free of disease (*extreme bottom* of photograph). **B**, A closer view of tuberculosis. A large cavity (*upper arrow*) surrounded by nodular and diffuse granulomatous inflammation. Several discrete granulomas (*lower arrows*) can be seen below the cavity.

from the resemblance of the multiple foci of disseminated tuberculosis (present in liver, spleen, kidney, and other tissues) to millet seeds. These foci are small white nodules from about 1 to 2 mm in diameter. Tuberculous pneumonia is an overwhelming infection characterized by extensive tuberculous consolidation of one or more lobes of the lung. Persons with AIDS and other immunocompromised persons are prone to this type of rapidly progressive infection.

EXTRAPULMONARY TUBERCULOSIS

Sometimes tuberculosis develops in the kidneys, bones, uterus, fallopian tubes, or other extrapulmonary location. The infection results from hematogenous spread of tubercle bacilli from a focus of tuberculosis in the lung. Sometimes, the secondary focus of infection may progress even though the pulmonary infection has healed, leading to an active extrapulmonary tuberculous infection without clinically apparent pulmonary tuberculosis.

DIAGNOSIS AND TREATMENT OF TUBERCULOSIS

Tuberculous infection is associated with the development of hypersensitivity to proteins in the tubercle bacillus, as discussed on immunity, hypersensitivity, allergy, and autoimmune diseases. A positive skin test (Mantoux test) indicates that the person was at one time infected with the tubercle bacillus; it does not necessarily indicate an active infection.

At present, many physicians recommend that persons who develop an infection with the tubercle bacillus, as manifested by conversion of a negative into a positive skin test reaction, be treated with antituberculosis drugs. Treatment is also recommended for patients with inactive tuberculosis who have an increased risk of developing a reactivation of an old, apparently healed tuberculous infection.

Unfortunately, the frequency of tuberculosis, which declined steadily from about 1950 to 1980, began to rise at an alarming rate in the United States, and a number of factors appear to be responsible for the increase. A large number of persons have immigrated to the United States from Asian, African, and Latin American countries, where the prevalence of tuberculosis is much higher. Many of these persons have been infected, although they do not have active tuberculosis. This group serves as a reservoir of infected persons in whom active tuberculosis can develop if immunity declines, which in turn may be followed by infection of other persons with whom they are in close contact. Social problems of poverty, drug abuse, alcoholism, and homelessness create conditions favoring transmission of tuberculosis from person to person. Many of these unfortunate persons with active tuberculosis do not receive adequate ongoing medical care; they may also not be motivated to complete the full course of treatment needed to arrest the disease. Failure to complete treatment leads to treatment failure, and premature cessation of treatment also promotes the emergence of drug-resistant strains of the organism.

DRUG-RESISTANT TUBERCULOSIS

Effective drug treatment of tuberculosis has transformed the infection from a potentially fatal chronic disease to one that could be treated effectively by a number of antibiotics and chemotherapeutic agents, but now drug-resistant tuberculosis (TB) is becoming a major problem. Tuberculosis caused by organisms resistant to at least two of the most commonly used antituberculosis drugs is designated multiple drug-resistant tuberculosis (MDR-TB), which is more difficult to treat. The course of treatment is more prolonged and the results of treatment are less satisfactory. Recently, the drug-resistance problem has become even more threatening. Some strains have become "super resistant." They no longer respond to a large number of antituberculosis drugs, and an infection by these organisms is designated extremely drug-resistant tuberculosis (XDR-TB). Were these strains to become widespread, tuberculosis would no longer be a potentially treatable infection. Instead, an XDR-TB infection would be a very serious disease having an outcome comparable to that of tuberculosis infections before antibiotic treatment had become available, and it is essential to prevent spread of this highly resistant strain. Persons with XDR-TB need to obtain treatment at a facility accustomed to dealing with these resistant organisms, and the patients' activities need to be restricted so they cannot spread the infection. The World Health Organization has become increasingly concerned about the spread of XDR-TB cases. Most have been concentrated in Eastern Europe, South Africa, and Asia, but cases are appearing in the United States, and control measures to prevent further spread are considered essential.

SPREAD OF TUBERCULOSIS

Tuberculosis remains a serious problem, and unrecognized cases such as that illustrated in Case 15-2 may expose many susceptible individuals. Infected individuals who take no precautions to prevent infecting others also may increase exposure, as illustrated by the case summarized in the Supplementary Readings article by Markel and others, which deals with extensively drug-resistant tuberculosis.

CASE 15-2

A 17-year-old female high school student developed a dry cough accompanied by weakness and fatigue, elevated temperature, chills, and a 15-lb weight loss. She had also recently noted that she became short of breath after climbing two flights of stairs. Previously, she had lived for a time with an uncle who had tuberculosis. Examination revealed extensive consolidation in the upper part of both lungs as a result of tuberculosis (FIGURE 15-17). Smears and cultures of sputum revealed tubercle bacilli. She was hospitalized and received a course of antituberculous drug therapy. Her school was contacted, and steps were taken to check other students with whom she had had contact for possible tuberculous infection. The infection slowly responded to therapy, and she was later released from the hospital to continue treatment as an outpatient.

Bronchiectasis
(bron-kē-ek'tuh-sis)
Dilatation of bronchi caused by weakening of their walls as a result of infection.

Bronchitis and Bronchiectasis

Acute inflammation of the tracheobronchial mucosa is common in many upper respiratory infections. The raw throat and cough associated with many respiratory infections are a result of the associated acute bronchitis. Chronic bronchitis also is common; often, it results from constant irritation of the respiratory mucosa by smoking cigarettes or breathing air containing large amounts of atmospheric pollution.

Sometimes the bronchial walls in parts of the lung become weakened as a result of severe inflammation or other factors, and the affected bronchi become markedly dilated. This condition is called **bronchiectasis** (*ectasis* = dilation). The distended bronchi tend to retain secretions. Consequently, patients with bronchiectasis frequently have a chronic cough associated with production of large amounts of purulent sputum. Often, they suffer repeated bouts of pulmonary infection. The only effective treatment of bronchiectasis is surgical resection of the affected segments of lung. Bronchiectasis can be recognized by means of a special type of radiologic examination called a bronchogram. The procedure consists of taking x-ray films after instilling a radiopaque oil into the trachea and bronchi. The oil covers the mucosa of the bronchi, and the abnormal bronchi can be recognized as dilated saccular or fusiform structures (FIGURE 15-18).

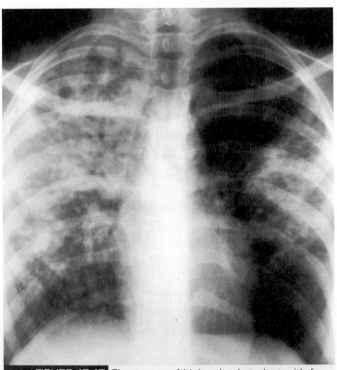

FIGURE 15-17 Chest x-ray of high school student with far-advanced pulmonary tuberculosis, illustrating extensive consolidation of both lungs (Case 15-2).

Chronic Obstructive Lung Disease

Pulmonary emphysema is a disease in which the air spaces distal to the terminal bronchioles are enlarged and their walls are destroyed. The disease is an important cause of disability and death, and its incidence is increasing at an alarming rate. In emphysema, the normally fine alveolar structure of the lung is destroyed, and large, cystic air spaces form throughout the lung (FIGURE 15-19). The destructive process usually begins in the upper lobes but eventually may affect all lobes of both lungs. Usually, there is an associated chronic inflammation of the terminal bronchioles. Emphysema and chronic bronchitis occur together so frequently that they are usually considered a single entity, designated chronic obstructive pulmonary disease (COPD). The chief clinical manifestations of any type of chronic pulmonary disease are dyspnea and cyanosis. Dyspnea is a sensation of shortness of breath. Cyanosis is a blue tinge of the skin and mucous membrane that results from an excessive amount of reduced hemoglobin in the blood. Reduced hemoglobin is dark purplish red, in contrast with normally oxygenated blood, which is bright red.

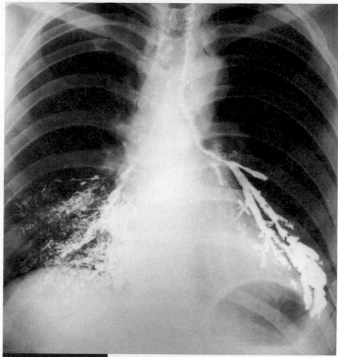

FIGURE 15-18 Chest x-ray illustrating bronchiectasis demonstrated by bronchogram. Right lower lobe bronchi (*left*) appear normal. Bronchi on the opposite side exhibit saclike and fusiform dilatation, as outlined by radiopaque contrast material within dilated bronchi.

The three main anatomic derangements in chronic obstructive pulmonary disease are (1) inflammation and narrowing of the terminal bronchioles, (2) dilatation and coalescence of pulmonary air spaces, and (3) loss of lung elasticity. These derangements in turn cause severe disturbances in pulmonary function.

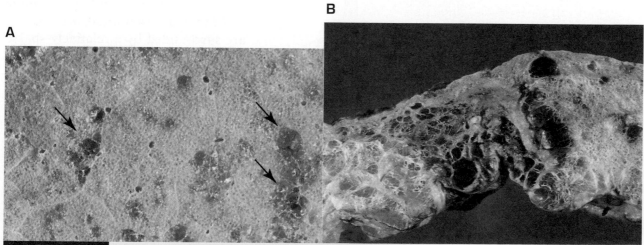

FIGURE 15-19 Sections of air-dried lung preparations illustrating the gross appearance of emphysema. **A**, Mild emphysema. Beginning breakdown of lung tissue to form cystic spaces (*arrows*). Most of the alveoli appear normal. **B**, Advanced emphysema with multiple confluent cystic spaces within lung. Very little normal lung tissue remains. The dark color is a result of accumulation of carbon pigment in the emphysematous lung from inhaling "dirty" air.

DERANGEMENTS OF PULMONARY STRUCTURE AND FUNCTION

Chronic inflammation of the bronchioles probably initiates the destructive process. Chronic inflammation causes swelling of the bronchial mucosa, which reduces the caliber of the bronchi and bronchioles and stimulates increased bronchial secretions. Because a tube's resistance to air flow varies with the fourth power of its diameter, a slight reduction in the caliber of the bronchioles greatly restricts the flow of air. Normally, the bronchi and bronchioles dilate slightly during inspiration and become smaller during expiration. Consequently, air can enter the lungs more readily than it can be expelled through the narrowed bronchioles; so air tends to become trapped in the lungs during expiration. The lungs cannot empty completely, and they become chronically overinflated. As a result, the amount of additional air that can be inspired when the subject takes a deep breath is much reduced, and the subject is unable to increase his or her ventilation adequately in response to increased demand.

The bronchiolar obstruction also disturbs pulmonary function by causing unequal air flow to various parts of the lung. Some alveoli are overventilated; others are inadequately supplied, reducing the overall efficiency of pulmonary ventilation. The excess air supplying the overventilated alveoli is "wasted" because more is provided than is needed to oxygenate completely the blood flowing through the surrounding pulmonary capillaries. Conversely, the blood flowing to the poorly ventilated alveoli does not become fully oxygenated. When it mixes with normally oxygenated blood flowing from other parts of the lungs, the oxygen content of the blood delivered to the tissues is reduced.

The destruction of the alveolar septa leads to enlargement of the air spaces and at the same time reduces the number of pulmonary capillaries available for gas exchange (FIGURE 15-20). Normally, there are about 400 million alveoli in both lungs, and the surface area of the pulmonary capillaries supplying the alveoli is about 30 times as great as the surface area of the body. Each alveolus contains a relatively small volume of air surrounded by a rich network of capillaries. This arrangement promotes optimal diffusion of gases between alveolar air and pulmonary capillaries. Diffusion of gases is much less efficient from large cystic spaces because the spaces contain a much larger volume of air than does a normal alveolus and are surrounded by a relatively sparse network of capillaries. Moreover, the movement of air into and out of the enlarged spaces is impeded by the bronchiolar obstruction.

Destruction of the alveolar septa also leads to loss of the elastic tissue in the septa that forms the structural framework of the lungs, and so the lungs no longer "recoil" normally after they have been stretched during inspiration. Expiration is no longer a passive process. The air must be actively forced out of the lungs by contraction of the intercostal muscles. Breathing requires more effort that in turn requires

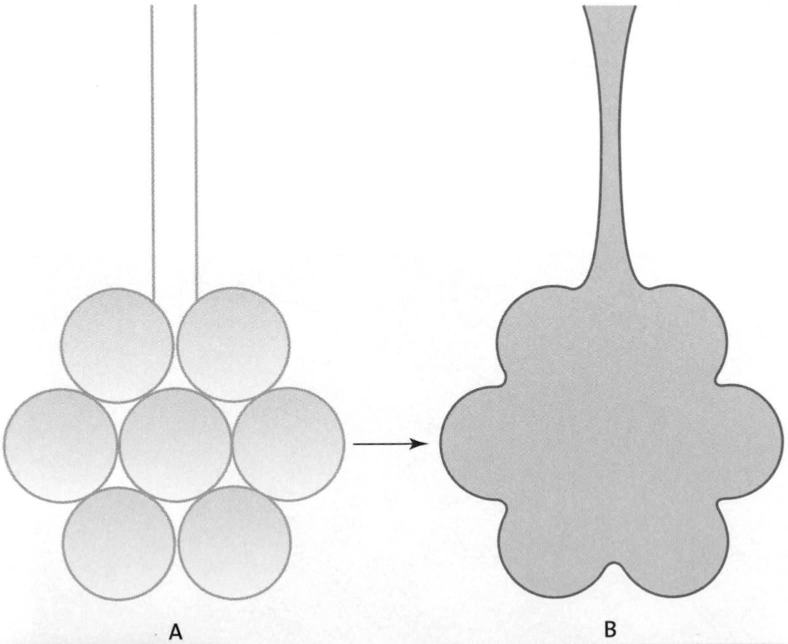

FIGURE 15-20 Derangement of pulmonary function, resulting from enlargement of air spaces and reduction of pulmonary capillary bed. **A**, Normal structure, illustrating schematically a cluster of alveoli surrounded by a rich capillary bed connected to normal bronchiole. **B**, Emphysema, illustrating coalescence of air spaces to form a large cystic space with greatly reduced capillary bed and narrowed bronchiole.

a greater oxygen consumption. The pressure required to actively force air out of the lungs during expiration also raises the intrapleural pressure and compresses the lungs, which causes further problems with pulmonary ventilation. The bronchi and bronchioles have lost their normal structural support because of loss of lung elasticity and tend to collapse during expiration, obstructing the outflow of air and trapping more air within the lungs.

The chief symptom of emphysema is shortness of breath. Initially, this is noted only on exertion, but later it may be present even at rest. The patient usually also has a chronic cough with purulent sputum, owing to the associated chronic bronchitis. Eventually, severely affected patients may die because they lack enough functionally normal lung tissue to sustain life or because of a superimposed pulmonary infection. Emphysema is also a frequent cause of respiratory acidosis, one of the common disturbances of acid–base balance. This is discussed in water, electrolyte, and acid–base balance.

PATHOGENESIS OF CHRONIC OBSTRUCTIVE PULMONARY DISEASE

Cigarette smoking and atmospheric air pollution appear to be the major factors responsible for the rising incidence of emphysema. Exactly how they exert their destructive effect on the lung is not completely understood. FIGURE 15-21 summarizes one concept of the pathogenesis of this serious and disabling disease. Smoking and air pollution are considered to expose the bronchial mucosa to chronic irritation, eventually producing chronic bronchitis associated with a chronic cough and increased bronchial secretions. The inflammatory swelling of the mucosa narrows the smaller bronchioles, increasing their resistance to expiration and causing air to be trapped within the lung.

The leukocytes that accumulate in the bronchioles and alveoli may also contribute to the lung damage by releasing proteolytic (protein-digesting) enzymes that attack the elastic fibers making up part of the lung's structural framework. Moreover, the mechanisms that inactivate the leukocyte enzymes are less efficient in the emphysematous lung.

Repeated bouts of coughing, with consequent extreme elevations in intrabronchial pressure, cause the alveolar septa to rupture, gradually converting the alveoli into large, cystic air spaces. The lungs become overdistended and lose their normal elasticity. The patient cannot expel air normally from the overdistended lungs because normal lung elasticity is lost and the bronchioles are obstructed; difficulty expectorating the excessive bronchial secretions also is apparent. Retention of secretions and poor drainage of secretions from the bronchi tend to perpetuate the chronic bronchitis, and a vicious circle is created. The diseased lungs are also more susceptible to infection because of

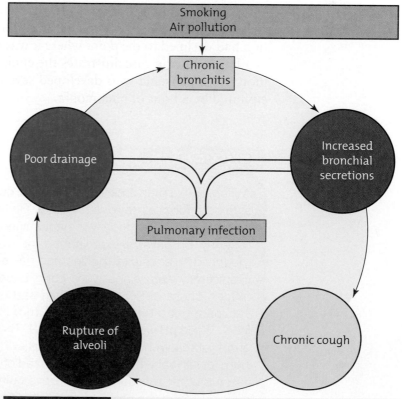

FIGURE 15-21 A concept of the pathogenesis of chronic obstructive pulmonary disease.

impaired pulmonary ventilation, bronchial inflammation, bronchiolar obstruction, and excessive bronchial secretions. Therefore, patients with emphysema frequently have repeated bouts of pneumonia, further damaging the lung tissue.

PREVENTION AND TREATMENT

For the most part, emphysema can be prevented by refraining from smoking and avoiding inhalation of other substances known to be injurious to the lungs. Atmospheric air pollution contributes to the increasing incidence of emphysema, and various measures are being undertaken to control this serious public health problem.

After emphysema has developed, the damaged lungs cannot be restored to normal. However, several measures can be employed to promote the drainage of bronchial secretions, to improve pulmonary ventilation, and to decrease the frequency of superimposed pulmonary infections. These measures, along with cessation of smoking, will retard or arrest further progression of the disease.

Surgical procedures called lung volume reduction surgery have also been investigated. These procedures excise the nonfunctional extremely emphysematous segments of the upper lobes, thereby reducing the size of the overinflated lungs so that the less severely involved lower lobes might be able to function more efficiently. A large recently completed U.S. government-sponsored clinical trial involving more than 1,000 patients (The National Emphysema Treatment Trial) compared the results of lung volume reduction surgery in one group of patients with medical treatment in a comparable group. In general, the overall mortality rates in both groups were similar, indicating that surgical treatment did not improve survival for most patients. One group, however, did benefit from surgery: patients who had a very limited capacity for exercise caused by the emphysema, in whom the emphysema was restricted to the upper lobes of the lungs. On the other hand, patients who did not meet these criteria had a higher mortality rate than medically treated patients and did not get any significant benefit from the surgical procedures. Unfortunately, even the initial benefit of surgery in the group who responded was of short duration, and 2 years later their pulmonary function had declined to the point where it was no better than it had been before surgery.

The following case illustrates the clinical features of a patient with chronic pulmonary emphysema who developed severe respiratory insufficiency that was precipitated by a bout of pneumonia.

CASE 15-3

A 70-year-old man entered the hospital because of severe, progressive shortness of breath for the previous 2 weeks. He had had chronic pulmonary emphysema for many years secondary to heavy cigarette smoking and had stopped smoking recently. On physical examination, he was very short of breath, and there was moderate cyanosis of the lips and nail beds. Lungs appeared overinflated, and respiratory excursions were poor. Laboratory studies revealed a low arterial oxygen content (PO_2 31 mm Hg) and oxygen saturation (53%), with elevated carbon dioxide tension (PCO_2 53 mm Hg) and plasma bicarbonate (40 mEq/liter). Blood pH was reduced to 7.29. These changes indicated severe pulmonary emphysema with respiratory acidosis. Chest x-ray revealed a pneumonia in the right lower lobe. Treatment consisted of supplementary oxygen, antibiotics, and various other measures to improve pulmonary function. The pneumonia slowly subsided, and the patient left the hospital 2 weeks later.

EMPHYSEMA AS A RESULT OF ALPHA1 ANTITRYPSIN DEFICIENCY

Blood and other body fluids contain a serum protein classified as an $alpha_1$ globulin that is capable of neutralizing trypsin and many other proteolytic (protein-digesting) enzymes such as fibrinolysins and thrombin. This specialized protein is called $alpha_1$ antitrypsin, and its concentration in the blood is genetically determined. Most individuals produce normal amounts of antitrypsin. Others are severely deficient, and a third group has subnormal levels of this protein.

Individuals with severe antitrypsin deficiency are prone to develop an unusual type of progressive pulmonary emphysema that usually becomes manifest in adolescence or early adulthood and tends to affect chiefly the lower lobes of the lungs. It is much less common than the usual type of emphysema described. Usually, there is no associated chronic bronchitis, so cough and excessive sputum production are absent. Persons with only moderately reduced antitrypsin levels do not develop severe emphysema at an early age but are quite susceptible to lung damage from cigarette smoking, atmospheric air pollution, or respiratory infections.

Low antitrypsin levels are correlated with lung disease because $alpha_1$ antitrypsin protects the lung from injury by leukocyte enzymes. Normally, polymorphonuclear leukocytes tend to accumulate in the pulmonary capillaries, and macrophages migrate from the bloodstream into the alveolar walls and pulmonary alveoli. Some of these leukocytes degenerate and release their proteolytic enzymes, but the enzymes are normally inactivated by antitrypsin so that they do not injure the alveolar septa. However, if antitrypsin is severely deficient, the leukocyte enzymes are not inactivated and can digest the connective tissues of the alveolar septa and terminal air passages, leading to pulmonary emphysema. The individual with a subnormal level of antitrypsin manifests an increased susceptibility to chronic pulmonary disease because pulmonary irritants (such as cigarette smoke and polluted air), and pulmonary infections cause leukocytes to accumulate within the lung. The liberated leukocyte enzymes are less efficiently neutralized than in normal individuals and may injure the lungs.

Bronchial Asthma

Bronchial asthma is a spasmodic contraction of the smooth muscle in the walls of the smaller bronchi and bronchioles. It is also associated with increased secretions by the bronchial mucous glands. Asthmatic attacks cause shortness of breath, and wheezing respirations occur caused by restricted movement of air through the tightly constricted air passages. The physiologic derangements in asthma result from narrowing of the bronchioles and are similar to those in patients with emphysema. Bronchiolar spasm exerts a greater effect on expiration than on inspiration because the caliber of the bronchioles varies with the phase of respiration. Consequently, air flow is impeded more on expiration than on inspiration, which leads to trapping of air within the lungs and overinflation of the lungs.

Many cases of asthma have an allergic basis. The attacks are precipitated by inhalation of dust, pollens, animal dander, or other allergens, which interact with mast cells coated with IgE antibody. This leads to release of chemical mediators that induce the bronchospasm. Acute attacks are treated by administering drugs such as epinephrine or theophylline, which relax the bronchospasm. Often, one can prevent attacks by administering drugs that block the release of mediators from mast cells. (Allergic diseases are considered in the discussion on immunity, hypersensitivity, allergy, and autoimmune diseases.)

Respiratory Distress Syndrome

RESPIRATORY DISTRESS SYNDROME OF NEWBORN INFANTS

The condition known as respiratory distress syndrome of newborn infants is characterized by progressive respiratory distress that occurs soon after birth, leading to serious problems in oxygenation of the blood. The condition occurs most often in premature infants, infants delivered by cesarean section, and infants born to mothers with diabetes. The basic cause is an inadequate quantity of surfactant in the lungs of the affected infants. As a result, the alveoli do not expand normally during inspiration and tend to collapse during expiration. The permeability of the pulmonary capillaries also is increased, and protein-rich fluid leaks from the pulmonary capillaries. The fluid, which is rich in fibrinogen, tends to clot and form adherent membranes that line the air passages. These membranes contribute to respiratory distress by impeding the diffusion of gases between the air passages and the pulmonary capillaries. The presence of these prominent acellular red-staining membranes lining the alveoli was the basis for the older name, hyaline membrane disease, which was given to this condition (FIGURE 15-22).

If delivery of a premature infant with immature lungs cannot be avoided, adrenal corticosteroid hormones administered to the mother within 24 hours of anticipated delivery will stimulate increased production of surfactant by the fetal lungs, thereby reducing the risk of respiratory distress syndrome. Infants who have developed respiratory distress syndrome after delivery are treated with supplementary oxygen and are also treated by instillation of a surfactant-type material that resembles natural surfactant. The material is instilled by means of a tube inserted into the infant's trachea (endotracheal tube), and the surfactant treatments are continued for several days

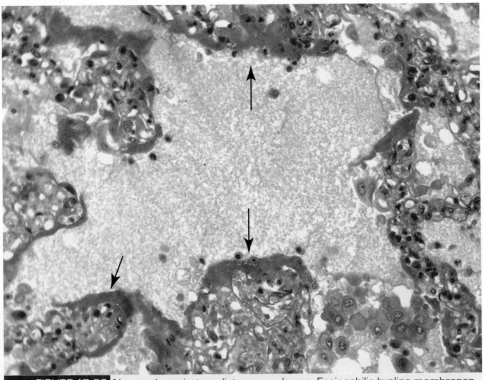

FIGURE 15-22 Neonatal respiratory distress syndrome. Eosinophilic hyaline membranes (*arrows*) composed of coagulated protein cover alveolar septa, impeding gas exchange between alveoli and pulmonary capillaries.

after delivery. TABLE 15-1 compares the respiratory distress syndrome in infants with a somewhat similar condition in adults, which has a different pathogenesis and method of treatment, although the histologic changes in both conditions are quite similar.

ADULT RESPIRATORY DISTRESS SYNDROME

The adult respiratory distress syndrome is often called by its initials ARDS, or sometimes by the term shock lung because shock is a major manifestation of the syndrome. The conditions causing this syndrome fall into two major groups. The first group contains many different conditions that cause shock with consequent fall in blood pressure and correspondingly reduced blood flow to the lungs. The shock may result from any type of severe injury (traumatic shock) or from a serious systemic infection (septic shock), and the pulmonary capillary and alveolar damage is an indirect result of the impaired pulmonary blood flow. The second group encompasses various conditions that directly damage the pulmonary capillaries and alveolar septa, including such conditions as aspiration of acid gastric contents, inhalation of irritant or toxic gasses, or lung damage caused by the SARS-associated coronavirus.

Whatever the predisposing cause of the alveolar damage, the pathophysiologic derangements are the same as in the neonatal respiratory distress syndrome: damage to alveolar capillaries and alveolar lining cells, impaired formation of surfactant, leakage of protein-rich fluid from the injured capillaries into the alveolar septa with formation of intra-alveolar hyaline membranes, and impaired diffusion of oxygen across the swollen, thickened alveolar septa.

Treatment is directed toward correcting the shock, treating the underlying condition that initiated the respiratory distress, and improving the oxygenation of the

TABLE 15-1

Comparison of neonatal and adult respiratory distress syndrome

	Neonatal	Adult
Groups affected	Premature infants	Adults who have sustained direct or indirect lung damage
	Delivery by cesarean section*	
	Infant born to diabetic mother**	
Pathogenesis	Inadequate surfactant	*Direct damage:* lung trauma, aspiration, irritant or toxic gasses
		Indirect damage: reduced pulmonary blood flow caused by shock or sepsis
		Associated condition: surfactant production reduced
Treatment	Corticosteroids to mother before delivery	Support circulation and respiration
	Endotracheal surfactant	Endotracheal tube and respirator
	Oxygen	Positive pressure oxygen

*Labor increases surfactant synthesis, which is lacking in cesarean delivery.
**High insulin blood level in the fetus of a mother with diabetes suppresses surfactant synthesis.

blood by means of a ventilator capable of delivering an increased concentration of oxygen to the lungs under slightly increased pressure, thereby facilitating diffusion of oxygen across the swollen alveolar septa.

Pulmonary Fibrosis

The lungs are continually exposed to a number of injurious substances, such as irritant gases discharged into the atmosphere and many kinds of airborne organic and inorganic particles. Severe pulmonary injury may lead to pulmonary fibrosis. Fibrous thickening of alveolar septa makes the lungs increasingly rigid, restricting normal respiratory excursions. Diffusion of oxygen and carbon dioxide between alveolar air and pulmonary capillaries also is hampered because of the increased thickness of the alveolar septa. Pulmonary fibrosis causes progressive respiratory disability similar to that encountered in pulmonary emphysema.

Some types of collagen diseases, characterized by injury to connective tissue, may have as their major manifestation injury to the connective tissue framework of the lung, leading to pulmonary fibrosis.

Certain occupational diseases are recognized as being caused by inhalation of injurious substances. The general term **pneumoconiosis** (*pneumo* = lung + *konis* = dust + *osis* = condition) is used to refer to lung injury produced by inhalation of injurious dust or other particulate material. The best known of the pneumoconioses are silicosis and asbestosis. **Silicosis** is a type of progressive nodular pulmonary fibrosis caused by inhalation of rock dust. **Asbestosis** is a diffuse pulmonary fibrosis caused by inhalation of asbestos fibers. Within the body, the fibers become coated with a protein having a high content of iron to form characteristic structures called asbestos bodies. Sometimes these can be identified in the sputum of patients with asbestosis (FIGURE 15-23). Inhalation of coal dust, cotton fibers, certain types of fungus spores, and many other substances attending certain occupations also may cause pulmonary fibrosis.

Pneumoconiosis
(nŏŏ′mō-kō-nēēiō′sis)
An occupational lung disease caused by inhalation of injurious substances such as rock dust.

Silicosis
(sil-ik-ō′sis)
A type of occupational lung disease caused by inhalation of rock dust.

Asbestosis
(as-bes-tō′sis)
A type of pneumoconiosis caused by inhalation of asbestos fibers.

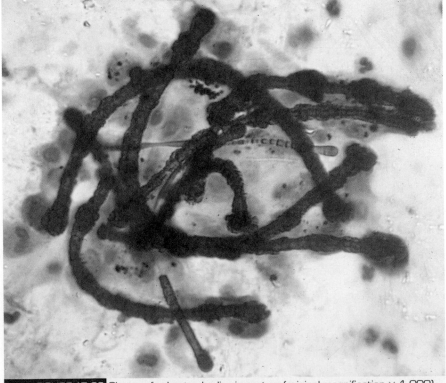

FIGURE 15-23 Cluster of asbestos bodies in sputum (original magnification × 1,000).

Patients with asbestosis have other problems as well because asbestos fibers appear to be carcinogenic. These patients have a higher incidence of lung carcinoma than the general population, and some develop an unusual type of malignant tumor arising from pleural mesothelial cells called a malignant mesothelioma.

Lung Carcinoma

Lung carcinoma is another important disease related to cigarette smoking. Lung carcinoma was once uncommon. Now lung cancer is the chief cause of cancer deaths, which kills 160,000 persons annually. It is a common malignant tumor in men, and the mortality in women caused by lung carcinoma now exceeds that of breast carcinoma. The tumor is uncommon in nonsmokers. Because the neoplasm usually arises from the bronchial mucosa, the term bronchogenic carcinoma is often used when referring to lung cancer. There are several different histologic types. Squamous cell carcinoma and adenocarcinoma are two of the more common (FIGURE 15-24). A third type composed of large, bizarre epithelial cells is called by the descriptive term large cell carcinoma. A fourth type is composed of small, irregular dark cells with scanty cytoplasm that look somewhat like lymphocytes. This type is called a small cell carcinoma and carries a very poor prognosis (FIGURE 15-25). Frequently, tumor cells can be identified in the sputum of patients with lung carcinoma (FIGURE 15-26).

Because of the rich lymphatic and vascular network in the lung, the neoplasm readily gains access to lymphatic channels and pulmonary blood vessels and soon spreads to regional lymph nodes and distant sites. Treatment usually consists of surgical resection of one or more lobes of the lung. Radiation therapy in combination with anticancer chemotherapy rather than surgery is used to treat small cell carcinoma and is also used to treat tumors that are too far advanced for surgical resection. Results of treatment are disappointing because the disease is often widespread by the time it is recognized.

Chest x-rays for lung carcinoma have not been very effective for reducing lung carcinoma mortality because, often, the detected tumor had already spread beyond the lungs and was no longer curable. In an attempt to improve lung cancer survival by early detection and prompt treatment of affected subjects, a lung screening trial was undertaken by the National Institutes of Health comparing the results of annual CT

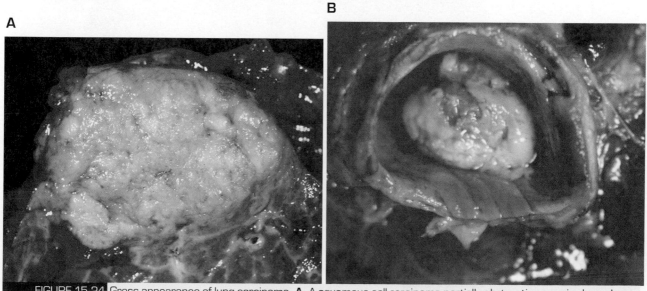

A

B

FIGURE 15-24 Gross appearance of lung carcinoma. **A**, A squamous cell carcinoma partially obstructing a major bronchus. **B**, An adenocarcinoma arising from smaller bronchus at the periphery of the lung.

A   B

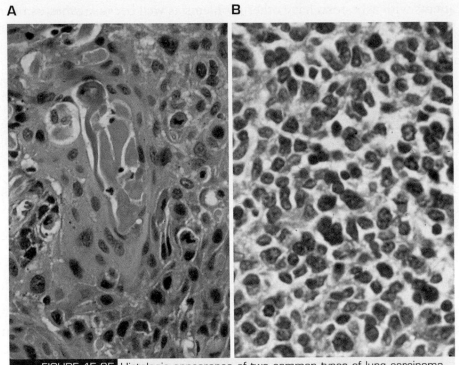

FIGURE 15-25 Histologic appearance of two common types of lung carcinoma. **A**, Moderately well-differentiated squamous cell carcinoma (original magnification × 200). **B**, Small cell carcinoma (original magnification × 200).

A   B

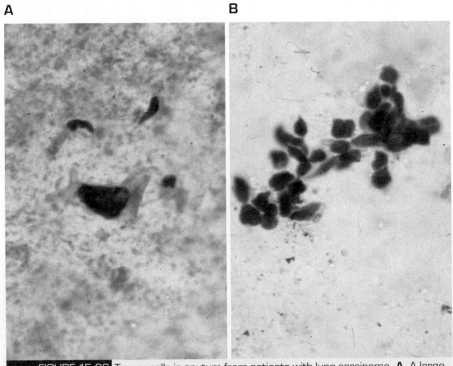

FIGURE 15-26 Tumor cells in sputum from patients with lung carcinoma. **A**, A large neoplastic squamous cell from a patient with squamous cell carcinoma of lung. **B**, A cluster of small, darkly stained cells from a patient with small cell carcinoma.

examinations for 3 years with routine chest x-ray examinations in 53,000 current and former smokers aged 55–74 years. Half the participants were screened by chest x-ray and half by CT. At the end of an 8-year follow-up, 364 CT-screened persons had died of lung carcinoma, compared with a significantly higher 442 deaths among the chest x-ray subjects. Presumably, the CT can pick up tumors earlier, which provides a better chance of survival. On the other hand, repeated CT procedures for screening are expensive and also expose the subject to significantly more radiation than chest x-ray exams. Many physicians believe that since 87% of lung cancers are caused by smoking, the longer term goal should be to eliminate the cause of most lung cancers by not smoking.

QUESTIONS FOR REVIEW

1. How do the lungs function? What is the difference between ventilation and gas exchange? How is pulmonary function disturbed if the alveolar septa are thickened and scarred?
2. What is pneumothorax? How does it develop? What is its effect on pulmonary function?
3. What is pneumonia? How is pneumonia classified? What are its major clinical features?
4. How does the tubercle bacillus differ in its staining reaction from other bacteria? What type of inflammatory reaction does it cause? What factors determine the outcome of a tuberculous infection? How does a cavity develop in lungs infected with tuberculosis? Is a person with a tuberculous cavity infectious to other persons? What is miliary tuberculosis?
5. A patient has tuberculosis of the kidney, but no evidence of pulmonary tuberculosis is detected by means of a chest x-ray. How did this happen?
6. What is meant by the term "inactive tuberculosis"? Under what circumstances may an old inactive tuberculous infection become activated? What type of patients are susceptible to reactivation of a tuberculous infection?
7. What is the difference between bronchitis and bronchiectasis?
8. What is pulmonary emphysema? What factors predispose to its development? How may it be prevented? What is the difference between pulmonary emphysema and pulmonary fibrosis?
9. What is the relationship between carcinoma of the lung and cigarette smoking? How is lung carcinoma treated?

SUPPLEMENTARY READINGS

Antonucci, G., Girardi, E., Raviglione, M. C., et al. 1995. Risk factors for tuberculosis in HIV-infected persons. A prospective study. The Gruppo Italiano di Studio Tubercolosis e AIDS (GISTA). *Journal of the American Medical Association* 274:143–8.
  ▶ TB is a big problem in HIV-infected persons and may progress rapidly. Methods for monitoring persons at risk are discussed.

Bach, P. B., Jett, J. R., Pastorino, U., et al. 2007. Computed tomography screening and lung cancer outcomes. *Journal of the American Medical Association* 297:953–61.
  ▶ Screening for lung cancer by computed tomography (CT) may detect cancers earlier but may not reduce the risk of advanced cancer or the lung cancer death rate.

Bernard, G. R., Luce, J. M., Sprung, C. L., et al. 1987. High-dose corticosteroids in patients with the adult respiratory distress syndrome. *The New England Journal of Medicine* 317:1565–70.

> ▶ High-dose corticosteroids are not beneficial in patients with ARDS as a result of sepsis, aspiration, or mixed causes.

Centers for Disease Control and Prevention. 1998. Recommendations for prevention and control of tuberculosis among foreign-born persons. *Morbidity and Mortality Weekly Report* (Supplement RR-16) 47:1–29.

> ▶ Most TB cases among foreign-born persons result from reactivation of previously acquired infections. The risk of reactivation is highest in the first years after U.S. arrival. Screening and preventive therapy are discussed.

Colditz, G. A., Brewer, T. F., Berkey, C. S., et al. 1994. Efficacy of BCG vaccine in the prevention of tuberculosis. Meta-analysis of the published literature. *Journal of the American Medical Association* 271:698–702.

> ▶ BCG vaccination reduces the risk of tuberculosis by about 50%.

Daley, C. L., Small, P. M., Schecter, G. F., et al. 1992. An outbreak of tuberculosis with accelerated progression among persons infected with the human immunodeficiency virus. *The New England Journal of Medicine* 326:231–5.

> ▶ HIV infection promotes rapid progression of tuberculosis.

Driver, C. R., Valway, S. E., Morgan, W. M., et al. 1994. Transmission of *Mycobacterium tuberculosis* associated with air travel. *Journal of the American Medical Association* 272:1031–5.

> ▶ A flight attendant became infected after exposure to a family member who died of tuberculosis. She did not receive prophylactic treatment and developed active tuberculosis 3 years later. She infected other airline crew members and may also have infected passengers before her disease was diagnosed and treated.

Dye, C. 2004. A booster for tuberculosis vaccines. *Journal of the American Medical Association* 291:2127–8.

> ▶ A large group of Alaska Eskimos who received BCG vaccination were followed for many years, and the vaccine appeared to be effective for as long as 60 years. BCG vaccination does provide some protection against infection.

Fraser, D. W., Tsai, T. R., Orenstein, W., et al. 1977. Legionnaires' disease: Description of an epidemic of pneumonia. *The New England Journal of Medicine* 297:1189–97.

> ▶ Describes the classic epidemic that occurred in Philadelphia in 1976.

Man, S. F., McAlister, F. A., Anthonisen, N. R., et al. 2003. Contemporary management of chronic obstructive pulmonary disease: Clinical applications. *Journal of the American Medical Association* 290:2313–6.

> ▶ Early evaluation and treatment are recommended for any patient suspected of having COPD. Principles of diagnosis and treatment are considered.

Markel, H., Gostin, L. O., and Fidler, D. P. 2007. Extensively drug-resistant tuberculosis: An isolation order, public health powers, and a global crisis. *Journal of the American Medical Association* 298:83–6.

> ▶ A very interesting article on extremely drug-resistant tuberculosis (XDR-TB) and its potential impact, including discussion of legal authority to quarantine in the United States and on travel restrictions when dealing with XDR-TB.

National Emphysema Treatment Trial Research Group. 2003. A randomized trial comparing lung-volume-reduction surgery with medical therapy for severe emphysema. *The New England Journal of Medicine* 348:2059–73.
▶ The definitive article analyzing the applications and limitations of this procedure.

Patel, J. D., Bach, P. B., and Kris, M. G. 2004. Lung cancer in US women: A contemporary epidemic. *Journal of the American Medical Association* 291:1763–8.
▶ As a result of increased smoking by women beginning in about 1930 and continuing to the present, lung cancer in women has increased by 600%, and lung cancer now causes as many deaths as all breast cancers and all gynecologic cancers combined. Women appear to be more susceptible than men to the carcinogenic properties of cigarette smoke.

Ryu, J. H., Colby, T. V., and Hartman, T. E. 1998. Idiopathic pulmonary fibrosis: Current concepts. *Mayo Clinic Proceedings* 73:1085–101.
▶ Pulmonary fibrosis results from many different causes, and proper classification allows more reliable prognosis and management.

Truong, D. H., Hedemark, L. L., Mickman, J. K., et al. 1997. Tuberculosis among Tibetan immigrants from India and Nepal in Minnesota, 1992–1995. *Journal of the American Medical Association* 277:735–8.
▶ Tuberculosis infection is nearly universal among Tibetans settling in Minnesota, and a single screening evaluation failed to detect most of the cases. Persons with a previous history of active TB require close follow-up even though sputum cultures are negative.

Voelker, R. 2007. Pattern of US tuberculosis cases shifting. *Journal of the American Medical Association* 297:685.
▶ Previously reported Centers for Disease Control and Prevention (CDC) data showed that from 1994 to 2004, TB cases among U.S.-born residents fell by 62%, while increasing in foreign-born persons to 54% of all U.S. cases. Twenty-four percent of the TB cases were in foreign-born persons who had been living in the United States for more than 5 years, and most of the cases resulted from reactivation of a latent infection that had been acquired in their country of origin many years ago. Tuberculin testing and treating of latent infections in foreign-born persons should be extended to include longer term foreign-born residents living in the United States.

OUTLINE SUMMARY

Structure and Function of the Lungs

THE STRUCTURE OF CONDUCTING TUBES AND ALVEOLI
Bronchi: larger conducting tubes.
Bronchioles: tubes less than 1 mm in diameter.
Respiratory bronchioles: bronchioles with alveoli in their walls.
Alveoli: small air sacs where gas exchange occurs.

VENTILATION
Air movement caused by movement of ribs and diaphragm.
Lungs change in volume in response to changes in size of thoracic cage.

GAS EXCHANGE
Gases diffuse owing to differences in partial pressures.
Efficient exchange in lungs requires large capillary surface area.

PULMONARY FUNCTION TESTS
Vital capacity: maximum volume of air expired after maximum inspiration.
One-second forced expiratory volume (FEV_1): maximum volume of air expelled in 1 second.
Arterial PO_2 and PCO_2 measure efficiency of gas exchange in lungs.
Pulse oximeter measures arterial oxygen saturation.

THE PLEURAL CAVITY
"Negative" intrapleural pressure is caused by the tendency of stretched lung to pull away from chest wall.
Release of vacuum in pleural cavity leads to collapse of lung.

Pneumothorax

PATHOGENESIS
Chest or lung injury permits air to escape into pleural cavity.
Spontaneous pneumothorax: no apparent cause.

MANIFESTATIONS
Subjective: chest pain and dyspnea.
Objective: air in pleural cavity demonstrated by x-ray and examination.
Tension pneumothorax: complication of pneumothorax when air can enter pleural cavity but cannot escape on expiration. Air under pressure displaces mediastinum and impairs expansion of opposite lung.

TREATMENT
Chest tube inserted in pleural cavity; vacuum sometimes applied.

Atelectasis

CLASSIFICATION
Obstructive: caused by bronchial obstruction.
Compression: caused by air or fluid in pleural cavity.

TREATMENT
Remove obstruction or material compressing lung.

Pneumonia

CLASSIFICATION
By etiologic agent.
By anatomic distribution of inflammation in lung.
By predisposing factors.

CLINICAL FEATURES
Manifestations of systemic infection.
Manifestations of lung inflammation: cough, chest pain.

Severe Acute Respiratory Syndrome (SARS)

A serious highly communicable pulmonary infection.
Caused by unique coronavirus.
Initial nonspecific manifestations followed by acute respiratory distress syndrome.
No antiviral therapy currently available.

Pneumocystis Pneumonia

Caused by protozoan parasite of low pathogenicity.
Affects immunocompromised persons.
Organisms injure alveoli, leading to exudation of protein-rich material into alveoli.
Cysts demonstrated by special stains.
Infection characterized by dyspnea, cough, pulmonary consolidation.
Diagnosis established by lung biopsy.
Treatment available, but infection has high mortality.

Tuberculosis

CHARACTERISTICS OF TUBERCULOSIS
A granulomatous inflammation characterized by necrosis and giant cells.

MANIFESTATIONS
Depends on dosage and resistance. May heal by scarring or progress to cavitation.

Miliary tuberculosis: dissemination of organisms by bloodstream.
Extrapulmonary tuberculosis: hematogenous dissemination from lungs to distant site.

DIAGNOSIS AND TREATMENT
Skin test: indicates previous exposure to organism.
Chest x-ray: indicates pulmonary infiltrate.
Culture: identifies organism in sputum.
Treatment by means of antibiotic and chemotherapeutic agents.

Bronchitis and Bronchiectasis

CLASSIFICATION
Acute bronchitis: common and self-limited.
Chronic bronchitis: secondary to chronic irritation.
Bronchiectasis: walls weakened by inflammation and dilate.

DIAGNOSIS AND TREATMENT
Acute bronchitis: self-limited.
Chronic bronchitis: cease irritation, as by cessation of smoking.
Bronchiectasis: bronchogram demonstrates dilation. Diseased areas resected.

Chronic Obstructive Lung Disease

DEFINITION
Combined emphysema and chronic bronchitis.

DERANGEMENTS OF STRUCTURE AND FUNCTION
Chronic inflammation of bronchioles leads to trapped air in lungs.
Nonuniform ventilation of alveoli reduces efficiency of ventilation.
Enlargement of air spaces and reduction of capillary bed reduces efficiency of gas exchange.
Loss of lung elasticity requires active expiratory effort.

PREVENTION AND TREATMENT OF EMPHYSEMA
Refrain from smoking and inhalation of injurious agents.
Treatment cannot restore damaged lung but can prevent further progression and may improve pulmonary function.

EMPHYSEMA AS A RESULT OF ALPHA$_1$ ANTITRYPSIN DEFICIENCY
Antitrypsin prevents lung damage from lysosomal enzymes released from leukocytes in lung.
Deficiency permits enzymes to damage lung tissue.

Bronchial Asthma

PATHOGENESIS
Spasmodic contraction of bronchial smooth muscle narrows air passages.

TREATMENT

Drugs that relax bronchospasm or prevent release of mediators from mast cells.

Many cases caused by allergy.

Neonatal Respiratory Distress Syndrome

PATHOGENESIS

Inadequate surfactant impedes normal lung expansion and promotes collapse.

Premature infants, infants born by cesarean section, and infants by diabetic mothers predisposed to syndrome.

TREATMENT

Administering of corticosteroids to mother may stimulate lung maturation in fetus. Intratracheal surfactant installation to treat affected infants.

Adult Respiratory Distress Syndrome

PATHOGENESIS

Systemic disease with shock and impaired lung perfusion.

Direct lung damage: trauma, gastric aspiration, inhalation of irritants or toxic gases.

DERANGEMENT

Damaged alveolar capillaries leak fluid and protein.

Impaired surfactant production from damaged alveolar lining cells.

Formation of hyaline membranes.

TREATMENT

Correct predisposing conditions.

Administer oxygen under positive pressure.

Pulmonary Fibrosis

PATHOGENESIS

Collagen diseases.

Pneumoconioses:

Silicosis.

Asbestosis (also predisposes to lung carcinoma and pleural mesothelioma).

Various other injurious substances inhaled in course of occupations.

TREATMENT

No specific treatment. Prevent occupational exposure.

Lung Carcinoma

PATHOGENESIS

A smoking-related neoplasm.

Mortality in women now exceeds breast carcinoma.

Arises from mucosa of bronchi and bronchioles.

CLASSIFICATION AND PROGNOSIS

Several histologic types, which differ in their prognosis.

Poor prognosis as a result of early spread to distant sites.

TREATMENT

Depends on histologic type. Generally by resection.

Small cell carcinoma treated by chemotherapy and radiation.

http://health.jbpub.com/humandisease/9e

Human Disease Online is a great source for supplementary human disease information for both students and instructors. Visit this website to find a variety of useful tools for learning, thinking, and teaching.

CHAPTER 16

The Breast

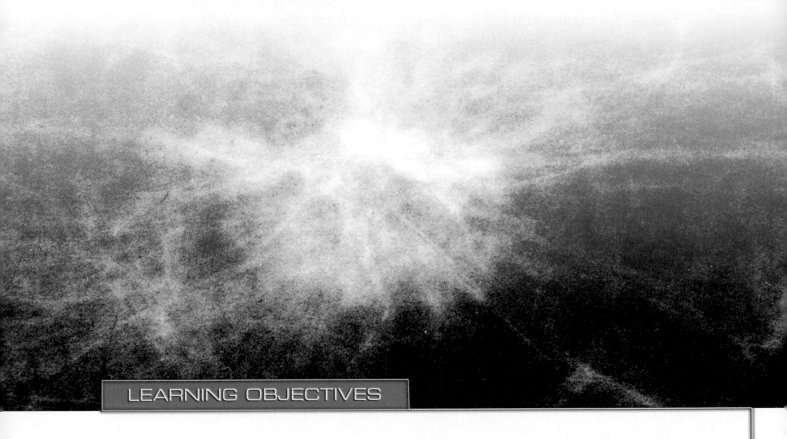

LEARNING OBJECTIVES

1 Describe the normal structure and physiology of the breast. List and define the common developmental abnormalities.

2 Explain the applications and limitations of mammography in the diagnosis and treatment of breast disease.

3 List the three common breast diseases that present as a lump in the breast, and explain how they are differentiated by the physician.

4 Describe the clinical manifestations of breast carcinoma. Explain the methods of diagnosis and treatment.

5 Explain the role of heredity in the pathogenesis of breast carcinoma.

Structure and Physiology of the Breast

The female breasts are each composed of about 20 lobes of glandular tissue embedded in fibrous and adipose tissue. Each lobe consists of clusters of glands, called lobules, connected by a series of branching ducts that converge to form large ducts that extend to the nipple. The breasts are modified sweat glands that have become specialized to secrete milk. Before puberty, breast tissue in both sexes consists only of branching ducts and fibrous tissue without glandular tissue or fat. In the female, they enlarge at puberty in response to estrogen and progesterone produced by the ovaries, whereas the unstimulated male breasts retain their prepubertal form. Postpubertal changes in the female include proliferation of glandular and fibrous tissue and accumulation of adipose tissue within the breasts. Variations in the size of the post-pubertal breasts of nonpregnant women are caused primarily by variations in the amount of fat and fibrous tissue in the breasts rather than to differences in the amount of glandular tissue.

The breasts are fixed to the chest wall by bands of fibrous tissue called suspensory ligaments, which extend from the skin of the breast to the connective tissue covering the muscles of the chest wall.

The breasts have an abundant blood supply and a rich lymphatic drainage. Lymphatic channels drain from each breast into groups of lymph nodes located in the armpit, or axilla (axillary lymph nodes), above the clavicle (supraclavicular lymph nodes), and beneath the sternum (mediastinal lymph nodes).

The breasts are extremely responsive to hormonal stimulation. Mild cyclic hyperplasia followed by involution of breast tissue occurs normally during the menstrual cycle. The glandular and ductal tissues of the breast become markedly hypertrophic under the hormonal stimulus of pregnancy and lactation, and the breast undergoes regression in the postpartum period. After menopause, sex-hormone levels decline, and the breasts gradually decrease in size. FIGURE 16-1 illustrates the histologic appearance of breast tissue under varying hormonal conditions.

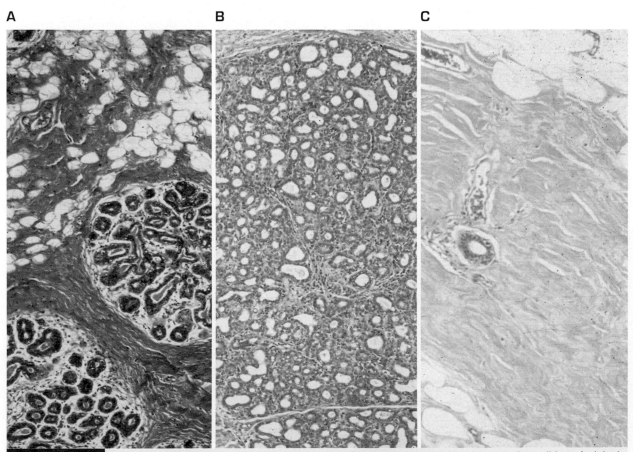

A   **B**   **C**

FIGURE 16-1 Photomicrographs illustrating the appearance of breasts under varying hormonal conditions (original magnification × 40). **A**, Normal nonpregnant breast. Two lobules of glandular tissue appear in the lower half of the photograph. **B**, Glandular hyperplasia in pregnancy. **C**, Postmenopausal atrophy.

Examination of the Breasts

MAMMOGRAMS

A **mammogram** is a special type of x-ray examination that allows the physician to visualize the internal structure of the breast and recognize abnormalities that may not be detected by clinical examination. In a mammogram, the fibrous and glandular tissue of the breast appear as interlacing white strands. The less dense fatty tissue, which transmits x-rays readily, appears dark (FIGURE 16-2). Cysts and tumors within the breast appear as dense white masses surrounded by the less dense dark tissue of the adjacent normal breast. Cysts and benign tumors appear well circumscribed, whereas malignant tumors often have irregular margins that indicate infiltration of the tumor into the surrounding breast tissue. These same criteria are used to distinguish between benign and malignant tumors on gross examination when a biopsy specimen is examined. Malignant tumors also frequently contain fine flecks of calcium that indicate calcification within the carcinoma. This is another feature suggestive of malignancy when seen on the mammogram.

The mammogram is most useful for examining the breasts of postmenopausal women because they contain more fat and less glandular tissue than the breasts of younger women. A dense tumor within a postmenopausal breast usually contrasts sharply with the less dense fatty tissue and is more easily identified. In contrast, a mammogram is less useful for examining the breasts of younger women, which appear much denser because they contain much more glandular and fibrous tissue. Consequently, it is more difficult to recognize a tumor in such a breast because there is less contrast between the tumor and the surrounding dense breast tissue.

Periodic mammograms are recommended for all women as a screening procedure. Mammograms can detect early breast cancers much sooner than they could be felt by physical examination of the breasts, and early detection followed by prompt treatment while a tumor is still small greatly increases the woman's chance of survival. The current recommendations are for an initial baseline mammogram at age 40, followed by repeat mammograms every 1 or 2 years until age 50, and yearly examinations thereafter. Mammography can pick up small tumors before they can be detected by breast examination, but the procedure has limitations and yields both false-positive and false-negative results. The procedure may not always identify a small carcinoma in the dense breast tissue of younger women, which obscures the tumor. Despite its limitations, the value of screening mammography appears to be well established because it has reduced breast cancer mortality about 20–30% in women aged 50–69 years, and slightly less in women age 40–49 years who have denser breast tissue and faster growing tumors.

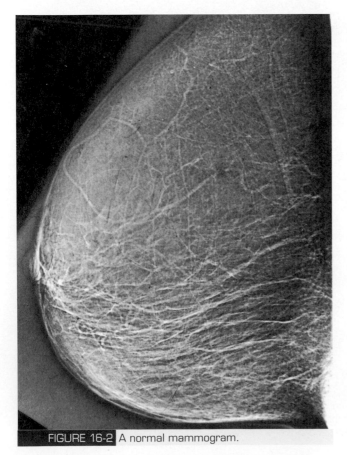

FIGURE 16-2 A normal mammogram.

MAGNETIC RESONANCE IMAGING

Magnetic resonance imaging (MRI) may be better than mammography for detecting a small carcinoma in dense breast tissue, which would be very difficult to identify in a mammogram. MRI may also be able to detect a localized area of increased blood flow in the breast, a feature often associated with a breast carcinoma. Therefore, MRI has been recommended as a supplementary procedure for screening women who are at high risk for breast carcinoma, such as women with a *BRCA1* or *BRCA2* gene mutation, and women in whom several family members have developed breast carcinoma. However, the extreme sensitivity of MRI is also a disadvantage because the procedure detects many nonsignificant benign changes in the breast, which must be investigated by breast biopsies and prove to be false-positive results.

A recent study also recommends that a woman with a carcinoma diagnosed in one breast should have an MRI as well as mammography of the other breast because she may also have a small undetected carcinoma in the opposite breast.

Abnormalities of Breast Development

ACCESSORY BREASTS AND NIPPLES

Embryologically, the breasts develop from columns of cells called mammary ridges, which extend along the anterior body wall from the armpits to the upper thighs (FIGURE 16-3). Most of the ridges disappear in the course of prenatal development except for the parts in the midthoracic region, which give rise to the breasts and nipples. Sometimes, persons have extra breasts or nipples. These are most commonly found in

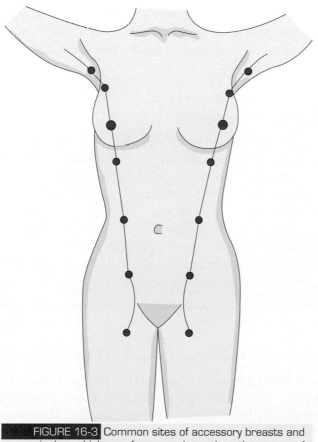

FIGURE 16-3 Common sites of accessory breasts and nipples, which may form anywhere along the course of the embryonic mammary ridges.

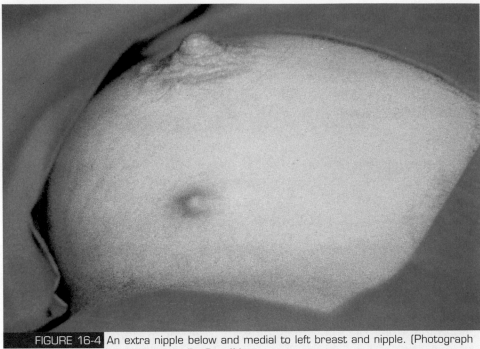

FIGURE 16-4 An extra nipple below and medial to left breast and nipple. (Photograph courtesy of Dr. Joel Kent Van De Graaff.)

the armpits or on the lower chest below and medial to the normal breasts, but they may appear anywhere along the course of the embryonic mammary ridges (FIGURE 16-4). Extra nipples and breast tissue may be a source of embarrassment to the subject, but usually, they do not cause other problems. Occasionally, however, accessory breast tissue may cause symptoms, as illustrated by the following case.

CASE 16-1

A 22-year-old woman visited a medical clinic for an examination and Pap smear. In the course of the examination, bilateral soft masses of tissue were palpated in both armpits. Each mass measured about 5 cm in diameter, and they became quite prominent when the subject raised her arms above her head. On further questioning, she stated the lumps had been present for some time. They often became tender just before the onset of her menstrual period, and the overlying skin sometimes became irritated by rubbing against her clothing. She was advised that the lumps were masses of extra breast tissue and could be removed surgically if they continued to cause problems.

UNEQUAL DEVELOPMENT OF THE BREASTS

The fully developed breasts are usually similar in size and shape but are not identical. Occasionally, one breast may fail to develop as much as its counterpart and may be significantly smaller than the opposite breast. Moreover, any condition that causes the breasts to enlarge may accentuate the disproportion. This possibility must be considered when prescribing medications, as illustrated by the following case.

> ┌─────────────────┐
> │ CASE 16-2   │
> └─────────────────┘
>
> A 20-year-old woman visited a medical clinic seeking contraceptive pills. Examination revealed that the left breast was much smaller than the right, which the subject masked by padding the left brassiere cup. The rest of the examination was normal. She was advised that contraceptive pills could be prescribed. However, because of the effect of the hormones contained in these pills on the glandular tissues of the breast, slight breast enlargement could result. Such enlargement might accentuate the difference in the size of the two breasts. The client decided not to use contraceptive pills and chose to be fitted with a diaphragm instead.

BREAST HYPERTROPHY

Sometimes, at puberty, one or both female breasts overrespond to hormonal stimulation and may enlarge excessively. True breast hypertrophy is primarily caused by overgrowth of fibrous tissue, not glandular tissue or fat. The subject may experience considerable back and shoulder discomfort caused by the excessive weight of the breasts. If symptoms are severe, the excessive breast tissue may be surgically resected, after which the breasts may be reconstructed so that they have a more normal size and shape.

GYNECOMASTIA

Occasionally, at puberty, the ductal and fibrous tissue of the adolescent male breast may begin to proliferate, forming a distinct nodule of breast tissue under the nipple. This condition, which is called **gynecomastia** (*gyne* = woman + *mastos* = breast), may affect one or both breasts. It appears to result from a temporary imbalance of male and female hormones that sometimes occurs in the male at puberty. Normally, the male secretes both male and female hormones, but male hormones predominate and "cancel out" the effects of the female hormones. Gynecomastia results when there is a temporary increase in estrogen relative to male hormones. The condition is not serious but may cause considerable emotional distress to the affected youth. Treatment usually consists of surgical removal of the excess breast tissue.

Gynecomastia
(gī-ne-ko-mas′ti-uh)
Excessive development of the male breast.

Benign Cystic Change in the Breast

Benign cystic change in breast tissue, often called benign cystic disease or benign fibrocystic disease, is a very common condition. It is characterized by focal areas of proliferation of glandular and fibrous tissue in the breast associated with localized dilatation of ducts, resulting in the formation of various-sized cysts within the breast. Cystic change appears to be caused by irregularities in the response of the breast tissue to the normal cyclic variations of each menstrual cycle. Clinically, a breast cyst may feel very firm and may appear to be a solid tumor. Ultrasound examination of the breast is often very helpful in distinguishing a cystic from a solid mass in the breast (FIGURE 16-5). Often, if the physician believes the mass to be a cyst rather than a solid tumor, an attempt is made to aspirate the cyst. A needle is introduced into the breast under local anesthesia. If a cyst is present, the fluid is aspirated and the mass disappears. If no fluid can be obtained, surgical excision is performed.

A

B

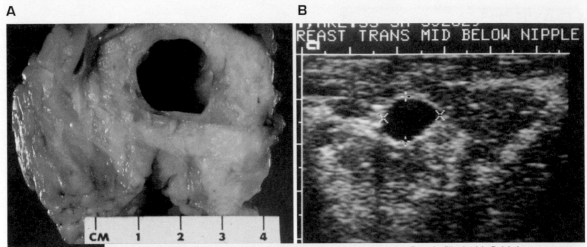

FIGURE 16-5 A benign cyst of the breast. **A**, A cyst viewed in cross section. Cyst is filled with fluid that escapes when the cyst is incised. **B**, An ultrasound examination of breast, revealing a breast cyst (*a dark area near the center of the photograph*).

Fibroadenoma

Fibroadenoma is a benign, well-circumscribed tumor of fibrous and glandular breast tissues that is seen most commonly in young women. It is readily cured by simple surgical excision (FIGURE 16-6).

Carcinoma of the Breast

Breast carcinoma occurs in both sexes. It is a rare tumor in men whose breast tissue is not subjected to stimulation by ovarian hormones, but is a very common tumor in women. There is some tendency for breast carcinoma to run in families, and a

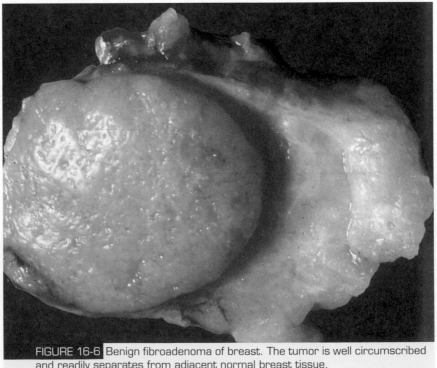

FIGURE 16-6 Benign fibroadenoma of breast. The tumor is well circumscribed and readily separates from adjacent normal breast tissue.

woman is at higher than normal risk if her mother or sister has had a breast carcinoma. Hormonal factors also influence the risk of breast carcinoma. Women who have never borne children or had their first child after age 30 are at increased risk, as are women who have had early onset of menses (menarche) or late menopause.

RISKS RELATED TO HORMONE TREATMENT

Hormones have been used for many years to treat menopausal symptoms. Treatment consists of either estrogen or estrogen along with a progestin (a synthetic compound with progesterone activity). Long-term hormone use does increase the risk of breast carcinoma, and the magnitude of the risk depends on what hormones are taken and how long they are used. Estrogen–progestin use poses the greatest risk. The definitive conclusions on breast carcinoma risk associated with hormone treatment came from a large study dealing with the risks and benefits of hormone therapy in healthy postmenopausal women (The Women's Health Initiative Randomized Controlled Clinical Trial), which was published in the *Journal of the American Medical Association* in 2002. The study concluded that hormone use increases breast carcinoma risk, increases the risk of heart attacks and strokes, and also increases the risk of leg vein thrombosis and pulmonary embolism. After the results of the Women's Health Initiative study were published, hormone used to treat menopausal symptoms declined 38% in the United States in 2002–2003 compared to previous years, as determined from the number of prescriptions written to treat menopausal symptoms. The decreased hormone use was followed by a 6.7% reduction in the incidence of breast carcinoma beginning in 2002, which continued the following year and then stabilized at the new lower level. The lower incidence occurred primarily in women age 50 and older and was most evident in women with estrogen receptor-positive tumors. The drop in breast carcinoma incidence was in sharp contrast to previous years in which breast carcinoma had been increasing about 0.5% per year, apparently related to long-term use of hormones to treat menopausal symptoms.

A more recent article in 2010 by Chlebowski and associates provided more follow-up data on a large number of women participating in the Women's Health Initiative clinical trial, which included 83% of the women who had enrolled in the original trial and continued to participate in the continuation of the original trial. The continuation group was matched with a comparable group who had not used hormones. The posthormone follow-up time increased the length of the clinical trial from 5.6 years in the original report to 11 years in the 2010 report, and the results were even more disturbing. Estrogen plus progestin increases the risk of breast carcinoma, and the tumors are more likely to have spread to the regional lymph nodes by the time they are recognized, which is associated with a less favorable prognosis and higher mortality. Women who took hormones also had a higher death rate from other conditions, primarily cardiovascular diseases. Currently, hormone treatment is only recommended to relieve menopause-related hot flashes and other disturbing menopausal symptoms, using only the lowest effective dose for as short a time as possible.

BREAST CARCINOMA SUSCEPTIBILITY GENES

A small proportion of breast carcinomas are hereditary and can be traced to inheritance of mutant breast cancer susceptibility genes. The two most important susceptibility genes have been designated as the *BRCA1* and *BRCA2* genes. The *BRCA1* gene is a very large gene, and a large number of different mutations have been described. A woman who inherits a mutant *BRCA1* gene has an 80% chance of developing breast carcinoma during her lifetime and an approximately 20–40% lifetime risk of ovarian carcinoma as well. A woman who inherits a mutant *BRCA2* gene also has an 80% lifetime risk of breast carcinoma, but the lifetime risk of ovarian carcinoma is about 10–20%, which is significantly lower than the ovarian carcinoma risk associated with a *BRCA1* mutation. (The role of tumor suppressor genes on cell functions and the effects of inherited mutations were considered in neoplastic disease discussion.) Because of the greatly increased cancer risk in *BRCA1* and *BRCA2* carriers, intensive screening tests every 6 months are recommended to identify and treat any newly detected carcinomas in this high-risk group. Unfortunately, early-stage carcinomas detected by screening tests do not guarantee a successful response to treatment. It is difficult to detect an ovarian carcinoma in its early stage, and many breast carcinomas in affected women are aggressive rapidly growing tumors that may already have spread by the time they are detected. Consequently, many high-risk women have chosen to have their fallopian tubes and ovaries removed or a bilateral mastectomy, and often, both procedures are performed to avoid the risk of both breast and ovarian carcinoma.

CLASSIFICATION OF BREAST CARCINOMA

Breast cancers are classified according to the site of origin, the presence or absence of invasion, and the degree of differentiation of the tumor cells. More than 90% of carcinomas arise from the epithelium of the ducts and are called ductal carcinomas. The rest arise from the lobules and are designated lobular carcinomas. Initially, a carcinoma remains confined for a time within the duct or lobule in which it arose and is called a noninfiltrating or in situ ductal or lobular carcinoma. Eventually, however, the tumor breaks through the ducts or lobules and extends into the adjacent breast tissue, becoming an invasive ductal or lobular carcinoma. Histologically, the degree of differentiation of the tumor also is specified. A well-differentiated carcinoma is composed of cells that resemble the epithelium of the ducts or lobules in which the tumor arose, whereas a poorly differentiated tumor is composed of bizarre cells in haphazard arrangement that appear immature and quite different from normal breast epithelial cells.

EVOLUTION OF BREAST CARCINOMA

In its early stages, a breast carcinoma is too small to be detected by breast examination but can often be demonstrated by mammography, sometimes as early as 2 years before it becomes large enough to form a palpable lump within the breast. Frequently, focal areas of necrosis occur within the proliferating tumor cells, and calcium salts diffuse from the bloodstream into the areas of necrosis (FIGURE 16-7).

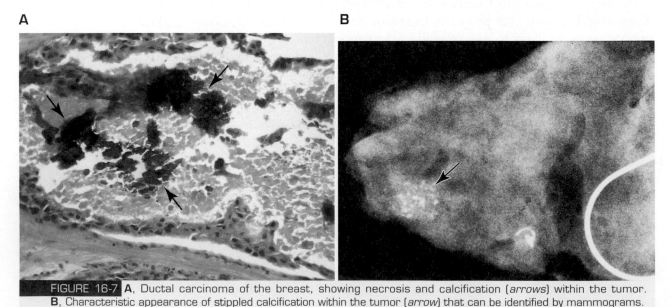

A

B

FIGURE 16-7 **A,** Ductal carcinoma of the breast, showing necrosis and calcification (*arrows*) within the tumor. **B,** Characteristic appearance of stippled calcification within the tumor (*arrow*) that can be identified by mammograms.

These small focal calcium deposits often can be identified in mammograms, which raises a suspicion of calcium deposits within a ductal carcinoma. Calcium deposits, however, are not conclusive evidence of breast carcinoma, as calcium deposits also can accumulate in some benign breast lesions.

As a breast tumor continues to grow, it infiltrates the breast tissues more extensively, and left untreated, eventually metastasizes to regional lymph nodes and distant sites. Early diagnosis allows prompt treatment and improves the cure rate. For this reason, all women are encouraged to examine their breasts regularly and to consult their physicians if an abnormality is detected. Routine screening mammograms also are highly recommended as noted earlier.

Many breast carcinomas induce fibrosis in the surrounding normal breast tissue that is being invaded by the tumor cells, as though the body were trying to defend itself by laying down fibrous tissue to contain the tumor. Consequently, many breast cancers are very firm and have a puckered, scarred appearance with irregular margins that blend into the surrounding breast tissue. This appearance is caused more by the proliferation of fibrous tissue in response to the tumor than to the tumor cells themselves. Nevertheless, this appearance is quite characteristic of many breast cancers and aids in identifying a carcinoma by mammography (FIGURE 16-8). Not all breast carcinomas have such a characteristic appearance. In many instances, the mammogram identifies only an abnormal or suspicious area within the breast that could be an early carcinoma but is not conclusive, and a biopsy is necessary to establish the exact diagnosis.

CLINICAL MANIFESTATIONS

The most common initial manifestation of breast carcinoma is a lump in the breast. It may be detected by the patient herself or by a routine mammogram. A more advanced carcinoma may cause secondary changes in the overlying skin or the nipple. The neoplasm may infiltrate the suspensory ligaments, exerting traction on the ligaments and causing them to shorten. Because the ligaments attach to the skin of the breast, shortening of the ligaments causes the overlying skin to retract as well (FIGURE 16-9). Consequently, skin or nipple retraction generally indicates the presence of an infiltrating carcinoma deeper within the breast (FIGURE 16-10).

If the tumor infiltrates and plugs the lymphatic vessels that drain lymph from the skin, the overlying skin will become edematous. (Lymphatic obstruction as a cause of edema is considered in circulatory disturbances discussion.) Skin edema produces a rather characteristic appearance in which the normal cutaneous hair follicles stand out sharply as multiple small depressions within the edematous skin. The appearance has been compared with the skin of an orange and is usually called the orange-peel sign (Figure 16-10A). Unfortunately, this finding indicates an advanced carcinoma that has already invaded lymphatic vessels and has probably also metastasized to regional lymph nodes. The likelihood of curing the cancer is much reduced at this stage.

If the patient delays in consulting her physician and a breast cancer is not treated, the tumor will eventually infiltrate the entire breast and will become fixed to the chest wall. The tumor will also metastasize widely. Although a far-advanced cancer often can be controlled for a time by various methods of treatment, there is no longer a possibility of cure.

TREATMENT

There are two ways to treat invasive breast carcinoma, and both methods achieve the same long-term results. One method of treatment is a surgical procedure

A

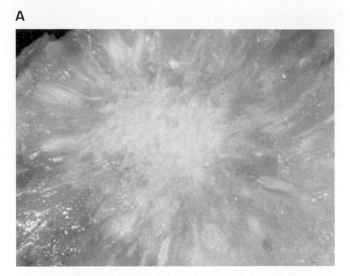

B

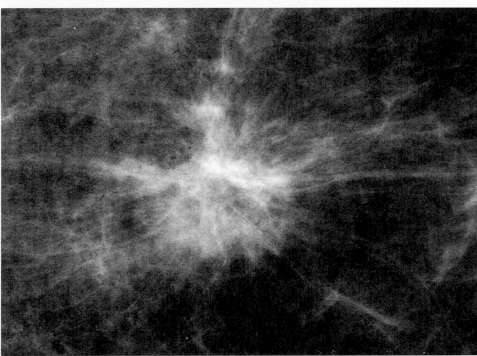

FIGURE 16-8 Breast carcinoma. **A**, Cross section of a breast biopsy. The tumor appears as firm, poorly circumscribed mass that infiltrates the surrounding fatty breast tissue. **B**, The appearance of breast carcinoma in a mammogram. The tumor appears as a white area with infiltrating margins. Note that the same criteria used to identify breast carcinoma on gross examination are used to recognize malignancy in the mammogram.

called modified radical mastectomy or total mastectomy with axillary lymph node dissection. As the names indicate, the procedure consists of resecting the entire breast along with the axillary tissues that contain the lymph nodes draining the breast but leaving the pectoral muscles overlying the chest wall. The mastectomy can be followed by a breast reconstruction using a saline or silicone-filled implant inserted under the major pectoral muscle or a more complex operation using tissues from the patient's abdomen or lower back. The reconstruction can be performed at the time of the mastectomy or several weeks later.

A second method of treatment consists of removing only part of the breast along with the tumor (partial mastectomy) or removing only the tumor along with a small amount of adjacent breast tissue (lumpectomy). In these procedures, axillary lymph nodes also are removed, as in a total mastectomy. A course of radiotherapy is then administered to the breast in order to eradicate any carcinoma remaining within the breast that was not removed by the surgical procedure. This treatment offers the advantage of preserving the breast but has the disadvantage of possible complications related to the radiotherapy.

Whichever method of treatment is selected, part of the tumor obtained at the time of the surgical procedure is tested for the presence of estrogen and progesterone receptors, and a test is also performed on the tumor cells to detect amplification of a gene called *HER-2*. These tests are described in the next section. In many cases, other specialized studies are also performed on the tumor cells, including determination of their nuclear DNA content and their growth rate, as determined by measuring the rate at which the tumor cells are synthesizing DNA. Determination of the hormone receptor status of the tumor has two purposes:

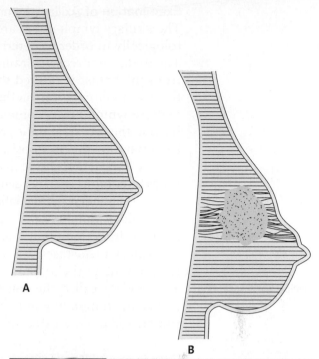

FIGURE 16-9 Mechanism of skin and nipple retraction in breast carcinoma. **A**, Normal breast. The horizontal lines represent suspensory ligaments extending from the chest wall to the skin. **B**, Tumor growing in the breast causes shortening of the suspensory ligaments, which leads to skin retraction.

1. To provide information on prognosis. Tumors containing hormone receptors are better differentiated than those lacking receptors, and patients with tumors containing hormone receptors have a more favorable clinical course.
2. As a guide to further treatment. Tumors containing hormone receptors respond to adjuvant therapy using drugs that block these receptors.

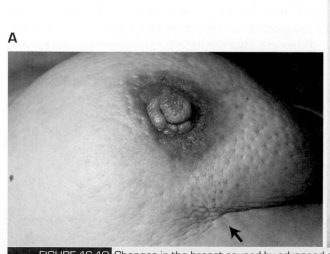

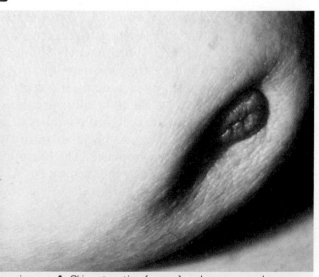

FIGURE 16-10 Changes in the breast caused by advanced carcinoma. **A**, Skin retraction (*arrow*) and orange-peel appearance of the skin. **B**, Nipple retraction.

Examination of Axillary Lymph Nodes: The Role of the Sentinel Node

The axillary lymph nodes are removed primarily so that they can be examined histologically in order to determine whether the tumor has spread beyond the breast. The nodes that receive drainage from the breast are interconnected, and the lymph from the breast is filtered through several lymph nodes before being returned to the venous circulation via the thoracic duct or right lymphatic duct. If one or more axillary lymph nodes contain metastatic carcinoma, the tumor already has spread beyond the breast, and the greater the number of involved axillary lymph nodes, the less favorable the prognosis.

Axillary lymph node dissection performed to guide further treatment may at times be complicated by edema of the arm resulting from disruption of the lymphatic drainage channels in the axilla and may also be associated with temporary limitation of shoulder mobility and axillary discomfort. Sometimes it is possible to avoid an axillary dissection while still obtaining information about the presence or absence of axillary metastases. Various procedures have been devised to identify the first lymph node in the axillary chain of nodes that receives drainage from the tumor. This node is called the **sentinel lymph node**. If the sentinel node does not contain metastatic tumor, it is very unlikely that any of the other axillary nodes will contain tumor, and a more extensive axillary dissection is avoided.

Sentinel lymph node
The lymph node in a group of lymph nodes that is located closest to a malignant tumor, which is examined to determine whether the tumor has spread to the node. If the sentinel node is not involved, additional lymph node dissection is not required.

Estrogen and Progesterone Receptors in Breast Carcinoma

A breast carcinoma is derived from cells whose growth and functions are influenced by various hormones: estrogen, progesterone, growth hormone, prolactin, and adrenal corticosteroids. Many breast tumors require these hormones for their continued growth and may undergo temporary regression if the body's hormonal balance is changed. The tumor cells of many breast carcinomas are stimulated by estrogen and progesterone and undergo regression if the hormone receptors on the tumor cells are blocked by drugs (called antiestrogen drugs) that prevent the tumor cells from responding to these hormones. Laboratory tests performed on the tumor cells can determine whether or not the tumor cells require these hormones by testing the cells for the presence of hormone receptor proteins in the cells. The protein that combines with estrogen is called estrogen receptor protein or simply estrogen receptor (ER). The higher the content of estrogen-binding protein, the greater the likelihood that the tumor will be inhibited by drugs that block estrogen receptors. A similar assay is used to determine the concentration of progesterone receptor protein, or simply progesterone receptor (PR). The presence of progesterone receptors in addition to estrogen receptors increases the likelihood of response to antiestrogen drugs. Approximately 60% of all breast tumors are estrogen-receptor positive, and most estrogen-receptor positive tumors are also positive for progesterone receptors. Tumors lacking these receptors do not respond to antiestrogen drugs.

FIGURE 16-11 illustrates how estrogen interacts with its receptor protein, and a similar mechanism applies to progesterone as well. In order for a cell to respond to estrogen, the hormone must enter the cell and combine with the estrogen receptors in the cytoplasm. The hormone–protein complex then moves into the nucleus and attaches to the nuclear DNA, where it stimulates the growth and other metabolic activities of the cell.

HER-2 Gene Amplification in Breast Carcinoma

The *HER-2* gene, located on chromosome 17, directs the production of growth factor receptors on the cell membrane. Soluble growth-promoting substances called growth factors (discussion on chromosomes, genes, and cell division) attach to the receptors, which stimulate the cell to proliferate.

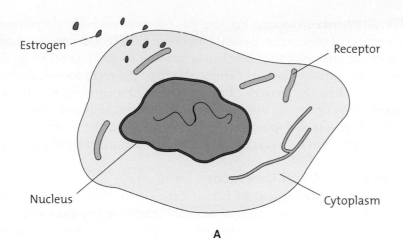

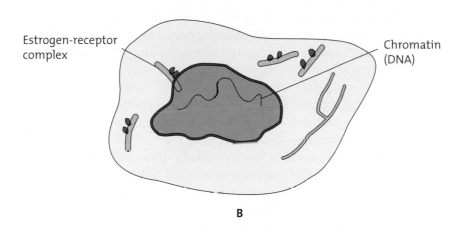

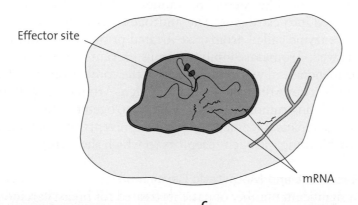

FIGURE 16-11 Action of estrogen receptor. **A**, Estrogen enters cytoplasm and binds to estrogen receptor protein. **B**, Estrogen receptor complex enters nucleus. **C**, Complex attaches to nuclear chromosome, activating mRNA synthesis. Messenger RNA directs protein synthesis on ribosomes in cytoplasm.

In about 25% of breast carcinomas, the tumor cells produce multiple copies of the *HER-2* gene, which is called gene amplification. As a result, the tumor cells produce a much greater than normal number of growth factor receptors that respond to growth factor stimulation, which speeds up the growth and multiplication of the tumor cells. These tumors are usually estrogen-receptor negative, grow very rapidly, and have a less favorable prognosis than other breast carcinomas. Laboratory tests can identify tumors in which the *HER-2* gene is amplified, and generally, this test is performed on all breast carcinomas because this information helps the physician select the proper method of treatment. Patients in whom the *HER-2* gene is amplified can be treated with an antibody that blocks the growth factor receptors on the tumor cells. Consequently, growth factors cannot attach to the receptors and stimulate the cells, which helps slow the growth of the tumor. When combined with other anti-cancer chemotherapy drugs, the antibody greatly reduces the breast cancer recurrence risk in women with *HER-2*–positive tumors. However, the combined antibody–chemotherapy treatment also increases the chemotherapy-related complications.

Adjuvant Therapy for Breast Carcinoma

In addition to surgical treatment of breast carcinoma, most patients also receive some type of adjuvant therapy in an attempt to eradicate any tumor cells that may have spread beyond the breast, thereby reducing the risk of recurrent or metastatic carcinoma. Many factors influence the selection of adjuvant therapy, including the size of the tumor, its differentiation and extent of infiltration, the results of various tests performed on the tumor cells, and the presence or absence of lymph node metastases.

The adjuvant therapy may consist of anticancer drugs (adjuvant chemotherapy) or antiestrogen drugs (adjuvant hormonal therapy), and often the patient receives both chemotherapy and hormonal therapy. Chemotherapy consists of administering two or three relative toxic anticancer drugs at monthly intervals for 4–6 months and is recommended for all women with invasive breast carcinoma. Hormonal therapy is reserved for patients with estrogen-receptor-positive tumors. Two types of drugs are available. One is tamoxifen or a similar drug taken daily for 5 years. Tamoxifen prevents estrogen from stimulating tumor cells by blocking the estrogen receptors to which estrogen must attach in order to stimulate tumor cells.

Aromatase inhibitor
(air-ō′-muh-tase)
A drug that inhibits the conversion of adrenal androgenic steroids to estrogens, used as post-resection adjuvant therapy to treat postmenopausal women with estrogen-positive breast carcinoma.

The other estrogen-blocking drugs are called **aromatase inhibitors**, which are also taken daily and are useful for treating postmenopausal women. Although their ovaries no longer produce estrogen, their adrenal glands produce small quantities of androgenic (testosteronelike) steroid hormones that circulate in the bloodstream and can be converted into estrogens. The androgen-to-estrogen conversion is accomplished by an enzyme called aromatase located primarily in adipose tissue but in other tissues as well. Aromatase inhibitor drugs prevent estrogen formation from androgens in postmenopausal women by blocking the conversion step. The action of aromatase inhibitors is quite different from tamoxifen. Aromatase inhibitors prevent estrogen from stimulating tumor cells by blocking estrogen formation from adrenal androgens in postmenopausal women. Tamoxifen prevents estrogen from stimulating tumor cells by blocking estrogen receptors to which the estrogen must attach.

Treatment of Recurrent and Metastatic Carcinoma

Unfortunately, a significant number of patients treated for breast carcinoma develop recurrent or metastatic carcinoma that may appear many years after the original tumor had been resected. The methods selected to treat patients with recurrent carcinoma depend on many factors, including the hormone receptor status of the tumor, the location of the metastases, the age of the patient, and the length of time that has elapsed between the initial treatment and the appearance of metastases. Although the tumor is no longer curable, treatment can control tumor growth, relieve symptoms, and improve the patient's quality of life.

Sarcoma of the Breast

Sarcoma of the breast is rare in comparison with breast carcinoma. It may raise from the fibrous tissue or blood vessels within the breast. Sarcomas often form large, bulky tumors that may metastasize widely. Treatment is by surgical resection of the involved breast.

A Lump in the Breast as a Diagnostic Problem

Many times, a physician faces the difficult problem presented by a patient who has a lump in her breast. It may have been detected either by the patient herself, by a routine mammogram, or by the physician in the course of a routine physical examination. The lump could be a benign cyst, a benign fibroadenoma, a carcinoma, or one of many other less common diseases of the breast. Certain clinical features may suggest to the physician the probability that the breast lesion is benign or malignant, and mammograms of the breast may provide helpful information. However, the only way to be certain is to perform an aspiration biopsy or needle biopsy of the mass or to excise the mass completely. This can be examined by a pathologist, who can make an exact diagnosis. If the lesion is benign, limited conservative treatment is all that is required. If the lesion proves to be malignant, the surgeon can perform a more extensive surgical operation.

QUESTIONS FOR REVIEW

1. What are the three common diseases of the breast that may be manifested as a lump in the breast? How are they distinguished from one another by a physician?
2. What is a mammogram? How is it used by a physician?
3. What are estrogen receptors in tumor cells? How is an estrogen receptor analysis used in management of patients with breast carcinoma?
4. What is gynecomastia?
5. What methods are used to treat breast carcinoma?
6. What is an aromatase inhibitor, and how is it used?

SUPPLEMENTARY READINGS

Berg, J. W., and Robbins, G. F. 1966. Factors influencing short and long term survival of breast cancer patients. *Surgery, Gynecology, & Obstetrics* 122:1311–6.
  ▶ A classic article on factors influencing prognosis. Information on late recurrences.

Chlebowski, R. T., Anderson, G. L., Gass, M., et al. 2010. Estrogen plus progestin and breast cancer incidence and mortality in postmenopausal women. *Journal of the American Medical Association* 304:1684–92.
  ▶ Estrogen plus progestin was associated with greater breast cancer incidence, and the cancers are more likely to have spread to the regional lymph nodes. Breast cancer mortality is also increased.

Cordeiro, P. G. 2008. Breast reconstruction after surgery for breast cancer. *The New England Journal of Medicine* 359:1590–601.
  ▶ A comprehensive, well-illustrated description of breast reconstruction, including a discussion of the types of implants. Approximately 178,500 women diagnosed with

breast carcinoma in 2008 have to decide how they want to be treated. Two-thirds will undergo a conservative resection of the tumor and associated follow-up treatment. One-third will choose a mastectomy. The major factor determining breast conservation surgery is the desire to retain the breast. The major factor determining mastectomy is fear of recurrent carcinoma in the treated breast. About 56,000 women underwent breast reconstruction in 2008. About 75% had breast implants, which are inserted underneath the pectoralis major and serratus anterior muscles. The outside shell of all implants is made of silicone, which can be filled either with a saline solution or with silicone.

Domcheck, S. M, Friebel, T. M., Singer, C. F., et al. 2010. Association of risk-reducing surgery in *BRCA1* or *BRCA2* mutation carriers with cancer risk and mortality. *Journal of the American Medical Association* 304:967–75.

▶ Risk-reducing mastectomy greatly reduces the risk of breast carcinoma. Risk-reducing removal of the fallopian tubes and ovaries (salpingo-oophorectomy) eliminated the risk of ovarian carcinoma and also reduced the risk of breast carcinoma because ovarian hormones were no longer stimulating breast tissue. Overall mortality from both breast and ovarian carcinoma were reduced by salpingo-oophorectomy.

Eisenhauler, E. A. 2001. From the molecule to the clinic—inhibiting *HER2* to treat breast cancer. *The New England Journal of Medicine* 344:841–2.

▶ A summary of the functions of *HER-2*, which is overexpressed in 25–30% of all breast cancers as a result of gene amplification and a review of the use of a monoclonal antibody to treat the neoplasm.

Elmore, J. G., Armstrong, K., Lehman, C. D., et al. 2005. Screening for breast cancer. *Journal of the American Medical Association* 293:1245–56.

▶ Screening mammograms are recommended for women aged 40 and older. They have reduced breast cancer mortality about 20–30% in women aged 50–69. The incidence is slightly less in women aged 40–49 who have denser breast tissue and faster growing tumors. In general, tumors detected by mammograms are smaller and better differentiated, but about 95% of women with abnormalities detected on a screening mammogram do not have breast cancer.

Fenton, J. J., Taplin, S. H., Carney, P .A., et al. 2007. Influence of computer-aided detection on performance of screening mammography. *The New England Journal of Medicine* 356:1399–409.

▶ Computer-aided detection does not increase the accuracy of the interpretation of screening mammograms and leads to increased numbers of biopsies. The detection rate of early invasive breast carcinoma was not improved by computer-aided mammography.

Fletcher, S. W., and Elmore, J. G. 2003. Clinical Practice. Mammographic screening for breast cancer. *The New England Journal of Medicine* 348:1672–80.

▶ An update on applications and limitations of mammography, including the problems associated with false-positive results. Many cases of ductal carcinoma in situ will never evolve into invasive breast cancer.

Lehman, C. D., Gatsonis, C., Kuhl, C. K., et al. 2007. MRI evaluation of the contralateral breast in women with recently diagnosed breast cancer. *The New England Journal of Medicine* 356:1295–303.

▶ Up to 10% of women with breast carcinoma also have an unsuspected carcinoma in the contralateral (opposite) breast. In a group of 969 women with a carcinoma in one breast, 3% had an unsuspected carcinoma in the opposite breast that appeared normal by clinical examination and mammography.

Meijers-Heijboer, H., van Geel, B., van Putten, W. L., et al. 2001. Breast cancer after prophylactic bilateral mastectomy in women with *BRCA1* and *BRCA2* mutation. *The New England Journal of Medicine* 345:159–64.

▶ Prophylactic mastectomy reduces the incidence of breast carcinoma. None of the 66 mastectomy patients developed cancer, but 8 of 63 patients followed by regular surveillance developed breast cancer.

Ravdin, P. M., Cronin, K. A., Howlader N., et al. 2007. The decrease in breast-cancer incidence in 2003 in the United States. *The New England Journal of Medicine* 356:1670–4.

▶ The age-adjusted incidence of breast carcinoma fell sharply (by 6.7%) beginning in 2002 and extending into 2003 and had begun to level off in 2004 as compared with the rate in 2002. The decrease was most marked in women age 50 or older and was most marked in women with estrogen receptor-positive tumors. The decrease most likely correlates with the decreased use or hormones to treat menopausal symptoms.

Rossouw, J. E., Prentice, R. L., Monson, J. E., et al. 2007. Postmenopausal hormone therapy and risk of cardiovascular disease by age and years since menopause. *Journal of the American Medical Association* 297:1465–77.

▶ The timing of beginning hormone therapy may influence its effect on cardiovascular disease. Initiating hormone treatment (HT) soon after onset of menopause reduced coronary heart disease (CHD) risk by retarding the accumulation of atheromatous plaque in coronary arteries. However, the risk increased if treatment was begun several years after the onset of menopause, presumably because the women were older, had more years to accumulate plaque, and had more advanced coronary artery disease. However, HT increased the risk of stroke regardless of the years since menopause.

Santen, R. J., and Mansel, R. B. 2005. Benign breast disorders. *The New England Journal of Medicine* 353:275–85.

▶ Describes pathogenesis of fibrocystic changes in breast and the various proliferative changes that increase breast cancer risk, as well as measures to reduce risk.

Shapiro, C. L., and Recht, A. 2001. Side effects of adjuvant treatment of breast cancer. *The New England Journal of Medicine* 344:1997–2008.

▶ Adjuvant chemotherapy, tamoxifen, or both are recommended for women with invasive breast cancers, regardless of whether axillary nodes are involved. Benefits are greatest in women under 50 years of age. Various adverse effects are described, including cardiovascular damage and second tumors related to treatment.

Writing Group for the Women's Health Initiative Investigators. 2002. Risks and benefits of estrogen plus progestin in healthy postmenopausal women: Principal results from the Women's Health Initiative randomized clinical trial. *Journal of the American Medical Association* 288:321–33.

▶ Hormone use increases breast carcinoma risk, risk of cardiovascular disease including heart attacks and strokes, and risk of leg vein thrombosis and pulmonary embolism.

OUTLINE SUMMARY

Structure and Physiology

STRUCTURE
Glands and branching ducts in fibrofatty tissue.
Fixed to chest wall by suspensory ligaments.
Abundant blood supply and lymphatic drainage.

PHYSIOLOGY
Responsive to hormonal stimulation.
Undergo cyclic changes.
Hypertrophy of glands in pregnancy.
Involution after menopause.

Examination of the Breasts

CLINICAL EXAMINATION
Inspection.
Palpation.
Examination of axillary tissues.

MAMMOGRAM
Application: may identify lesions not detected on clinical examination.
Limitation: less useful for examining dense breast tissue of younger women.

MAGNETIC RESONANCE IMAGING (MRI)
Useful to supplement mamogram in selected women with a high risk of breast carcinoma.

Abnormalities of Breast Development

ACCESSORY BREASTS AND NIPPLES
Breasts develop from mammary ridges extending from axillae to groins.
Extra breasts and nipples occur occasionally.

UNEQUAL DEVELOPMENT OF BREASTS
Breasts may not develop equally.
Disproportion accentuated if breasts enlarge.

BREAST HYPERTROPHY
Overgrowth of fibrous tissue.
Treated by surgical resection of excessive tissue.

GYNECOMASTIA
Enlargement of male breast.
Temporary hormonal imbalance at puberty.
Treated by surgical resection.

Benign Cystic Disease

PATHOGENESIS
Irregular cyclic response of breast to hormones.
May appear as solitary lump.

TREATMENT
Aspiration or surgical excision.

Fibroadenoma

APPEARANCE
Well-circumscribed tumor of glands and fibrous tissue.
Common in young women.

TREATMENT
Surgical excision.

Carcinoma of Breast

NATURE OF PROBLEM
Common malignant tumor in women.
Prone to late recurrence (see discussion on neoplastic disease).
Early diagnosis and treatment improves cure rate.

BREAST CARCINOMA RELATED TO HORMONE TREATMENT
Long-term estrogen–progestin use by postmenopausal women significantly increases breast carcinoma risk.
Use of estrogen without progestin only slightly increases risk.

BREAST CARCINOMA SUSCEPTIBILITY GENES
Mutant tumor suppressor genes transmitted by Mendelian inheritance patterns.
BRCA1 and *BRCA2* mutations increase both breast and ovarian cancer risk.

CLASSIFICATION AND EVOLUTION OF BREAST CARCINOMA
May arise from ducts (ductal carcinoma) or lobules (lobular carcinoma).
Initially in situ but eventually becomes invasive.
May metastasize to axillary lymph nodes and eventually spread throughout the body if untreated.

APPEARANCE OF CARCINOMA
Often has characteristic gross appearance.
Mammogram assists in diagnosis.

CLINICAL MANIFESTATIONS
Lump in breast.
Nipple or skin may be retracted owing to pull on suspensory ligaments.
Skin edema: caused by plugging of lymphatics.
Fixation of tumor to chest wall: late manifestation.

TREATMENT
Modified radical mastectomy or partial mastectomy/lumpectomy followed by breast radiation.
Examine axillary nodes for tumor as guide to prognosis and treatment.
Negative sentinel node avoids need for axillary dissection.

ESTROGEN RECEPTORS IN BREAST CANCER
Estrogen receptors (ER) in cytoplasm fix hormone, move to nucleus, and stimulate cell functions.

HER-2 GENE AMPLIFICATION
Indicates aggressive tumor.
Requires special treatment methods.

ADJUVANT THERAPY
Recommended for most patients.
Anticancer drug chemotherapy.
Antiestrogen drug (tamoxifen) for women with ER-positive tumors.
Aromatase inhibitor drugs useful in postmenopausal women with ER-positive tumors.

TREATMENT OF METASTATIC CARCINOMA
Chemotherapy, hormones, radiation control tumor growth, relieve symptoms, improve quality of life.

Sarcoma of the Breast
FREQUENCY
A rare tumor.
Often large and bulky.
Treated by surgical resection.

Lump in the Breast as a Diagnostic Problem
DIAGNOSTIC POSSIBILITIES
Cystic disease.
Fibroadenoma.
Carcinoma.
Other less common conditions.

DIAGNOSTIC APPROACH
Clinical evaluation.
Mammogram.
Biopsy.

The Female Reproductive System

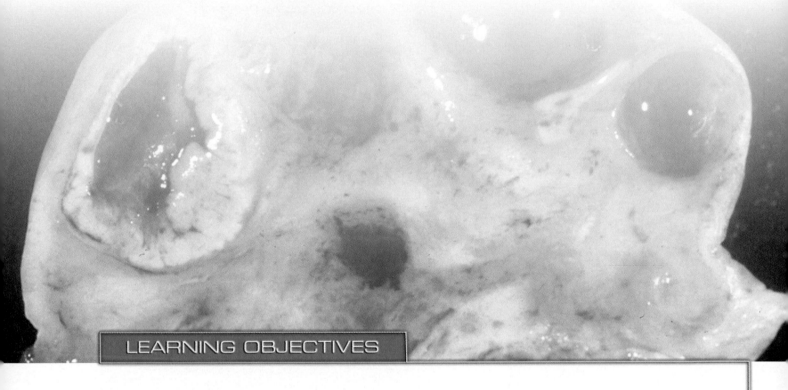

1 Describe the common infections of the genital tract and relate them to sexually transmitted diseases.

2 Describe the clinical manifestations and complications of endometriosis.

3 List the common causes of irregular uterine bleeding.

4 Describe the common diseases of the cervix, endometrium, myometrium, and vulva.

5 List the common cysts and tumors of the ovary.

6 Explain the pathogenesis, clinical manifestations, and treatment of toxic shock syndrome.

7 Categorize the common methods of artificial contraception, explain how they prevent conception, and describe their possible side effects.

Infections of the Female Genital Tract

Infections of the genital tract are common. Frequently involved sites are the vagina, the cervix, and the fallopian tubes. In addition, certain virus infections of the genital tract cause highly characteristic lesions called **condylomas**.

VAGINITIS

Vaginal infections are common. They frequently cause vaginal discharge, together with vulvovaginal itching and irritation. There are three major causes:

Condyloma
(kon-di-lō′ma)
A warty tumorlike overgrowth in the squamous epithelium of the anorectal or genital tract, caused by a virus that is spread by sexual contact.

1. The fungus *Candida albicans*
2. The protozoan parasite *Trichomonas vaginalis*
3. A small gram-negative bacterium called *Gardnerella (Haemophilus) vaginalis*, in conjunction with various anaerobic vaginal bacteria

Candida vaginitis is considered along with other fungal infections in the discussion on pathogenic micro-organisms. The protozoan parasite *Trichomonas vaginalis* is considered with the parasitic infections in the discussion on animal parasites. The third common type of vaginitis, often called nonspecific vaginitis, is usually associated with a profuse, foul-smelling vaginal discharge. Highly specific methods of treatment are available for each type of vaginitis.

CERVICITIS

Mild chronic inflammation of endocervical glands is very common in women who have had children. Cervicitis causes few symptoms and is of little clinical significance. More severe cervical inflammation may result from a gonococcal infection in communicable diseases or a chlamydial infection in diseases caused by pathogenic micro-organisms. Both infections are sexually transmitted and may be followed by the spread of the infection into the fallopian tubes and adjacent tissues.

SALPINGITIS AND PELVIC INFLAMMATORY DISEASE

Salpingitis means an inflammation of the fallopian tube (*salpinx* = tube). The more general term **pelvic inflammatory disease**, or simply PID, refers to any infection that affects the fallopian tubes and adjacent tissues. Sometimes the ovaries are infected along with the fallopian tubes. Most cases are secondary to the spread of a cervical gonorrheal or chlamydial infection through the uterus into the fallopian tubes and surrounding tissues. Less commonly, other pathogenic organisms are involved. An acute pelvic infection causes severe lower abdominal pain and tenderness, together with elevated temperature and leukocytosis.

Both gonorrheal and nongonorrheal salpingitis respond to appropriate antibiotic therapy; healing of the inflammation, however, may be associated with scarring and obstruction of the tubal lumen. Sterility may result if the tubal obstruction is bilateral (FIGURE 17-1). Sometimes, even if the tubes are not completely occluded, the scarring may delay the transport of a fertilized ovum through the tube and lead to implantation of the ovum in the fallopian tube rather than in the endometrial cavity. This condition is called an **ectopic pregnancy** and is considered in prenatal development and diseases associated with pregnancy.

CONDYLOMAS OF THE GENITAL TRACT

Condylomas, sometimes called venereal warts, are benign warty, tumorlike overgrowths of squamous epithelium caused by a virus called **human papillomavirus (HPV)** that is spread by sexual contact.

They vary in size from a few millimeters to more than 1 cm in diameter and are frequently multiple. Condylomas develop most often on the vulvar mucosa, on the mucosa of the cervix and vagina (FIGURE 17-2), around the vaginal opening, and around the anus (see discussion on pathogenic micro-organisms, Figure 6-8). Treatment consists of destroying the lesions, which may be accomplished by applying a strong chemical (podophyllin), by electrocoagulation, by freezing (cryocautery), or by surgical excision.

Salpingitis
Inflammation of the fallopian tubes.

Pelvic inflammatory disease (PID)
A general term for an infection affecting the fallopian tubes and adjacent pelvic organs.

Ectopic pregnancy
A pregnancy outside the endometrial cavity.

Condyloma
(kon-di-lō′ma)
A warty tumorlike overgrowth in the squamous epithelium of the anorectal or genital tract, caused by a virus that is spread by sexual contact.

Human papillomavirus (HPV)
(pap-i-lō′ma-vī-rus)
A virus that stimulates epithelial cell proliferation. Causes warts and genital tract condylomas.

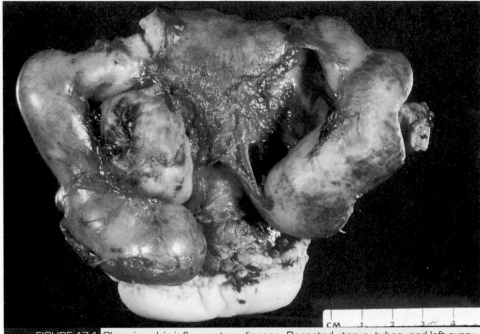

FIGURE 17-1 Chronic pelvic inflammatory disease. Resected uterus, tubes, and left ovary viewed from behind. Tubes are swollen, and fimbriated ends are occluded. There are numerous adhesions between tubes and uterus.

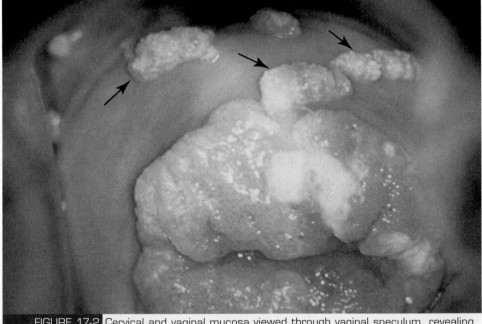

FIGURE 17-2 Cervical and vaginal mucosa viewed through vaginal speculum, revealing multiple condylomas (*arrows*) arising from mucosa.

Endometriosis

Endometriosis
(en-dō-mē trē-ō'sis)
Presence of endometrial tissue in abnormal locations, such as in the ovary or pelvis.

The term **endometriosis** refers to the presence of endometrium in any location outside the endometrial cavity (FIGURE 17-3). Ectopic deposits (*ecto* = outside) of endometrium may occasionally be encountered in the wall of the uterus (FIGURE 17-4), in the ovary (FIGURE 17-5), or elsewhere in the pelvis. Sometimes, endometrial tissue is found in the appendix or in the rectum. Endometriosis is a common problem, which occurs in

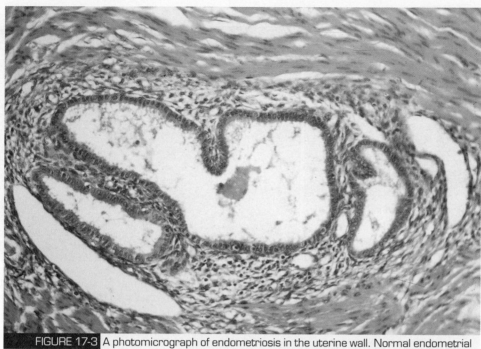

FIGURE 17-3 A photomicrograph of endometriosis in the uterine wall. Normal endometrial glands and stroma are surrounded by uterine muscle (original magnification × 100).

about 10–15% of women, and much more frequently in infertile women and in women with pelvic pain, irregular menses, or dysmenorrhea. Often, the condition appears to occur in families, and a woman is more likely to develop endometriosis if her mother had it. The reason that endometrial deposits occur in unusual locations is unknown, although many theories have been proposed. Some cases seem to be caused by reflux of bits of shed endometrium along with menstrual blood through the fallopian tubes into the peritoneal cavity during menstruation (retrograde menstruation), which then implant and grow in the pelvis. This does not provide a complete explanation,

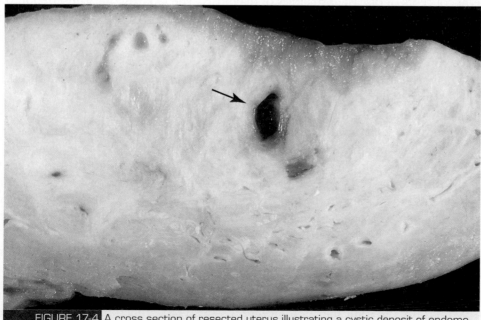

FIGURE 17-4 A cross section of resected uterus illustrating a cystic deposit of endometriosis filled with old blood located in the uterine wall (*arrow*).

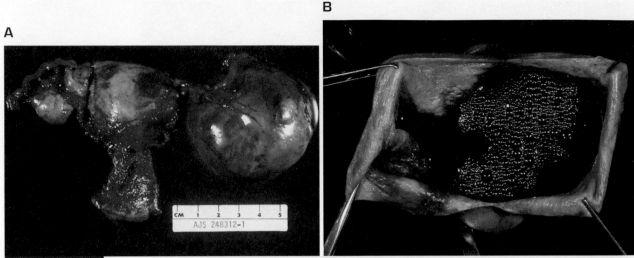

A

B

FIGURE 17-5 **A**, Endometriosis of the ovary. An accumulation of blood and debris within the ovarian endometriosis has led to formation of an endometrium-lined cyst filled with old blood and desquamated endometrial tissue within the right ovary (*right* side of photograph). **B**, Endometrial cyst opened, revealing cyst contents consisting of old blood and debris derived from the endometrium lining the cyst.

however, because retrograde menstruation is common, but implantation of menstrual endometrium carried through the tubes into the peritoneal cavity is infrequent.

Endometrial deposits respond to normal hormonal stimuli and therefore undergo cyclic menstrual desquamation and regeneration. Because the misplaced endometrial tissue does not communicate with the endometrial cavity, the "menstruating" tissue is not discharged through the vagina. Old blood and desquamated material are retained in the ectopic sites, leading to considerable scarring and causing crampy pain during menstrual periods. Obstruction of the fallopian tubes by scarring may cause sterility.

Diagnosis of endometriosis is usually established by visualizing the ectopic deposits within the pelvis with a lighted tubular instrument called a **laparoscope**, discussed on general concepts of disease: principles of diagnosis. The laparoscope is inserted into the abdominal cavity through a small incision in the umbilicus. Treatment consists of removing or destroying the deposits surgically or impeding the progression of endometriosis by administering drugs or hormones. Three methods of hormone treatment are commonly used:

Laparoscope

(lap′ -ă-rō-skōp)
A long tubular telescope-like instrument passed through the abdominal wall to examine structures within the peritoneal cavity.

1. Synthetic hormones having progesterone activity completely suppress the menstrual cycles.
2. Birth-control pills suppress ovulation, so the endometrium becomes thin and atrophic, and menstrual periods are very light. The endometriosis is similarly suppressed, retarding its progression and associated scarring.
3. Drugs are administered that suppress the output of gonadotropins from the pituitary gland. This in turn leads to a decline in ovarian function, similar to that occurring in the menopause. The deposits of endometriosis, deprived of cyclic estrogen–progesterone stimulation, undergo regression.

Cervical Polyps

Occasionally, benign polyps arise from the cervix. Usually, they are small and do not cause symptoms, but some may be quite large (FIGURE 17-6). Sometimes the tip of the polyp becomes eroded and causes bleeding. Treatment consists of surgically removing the polyp.

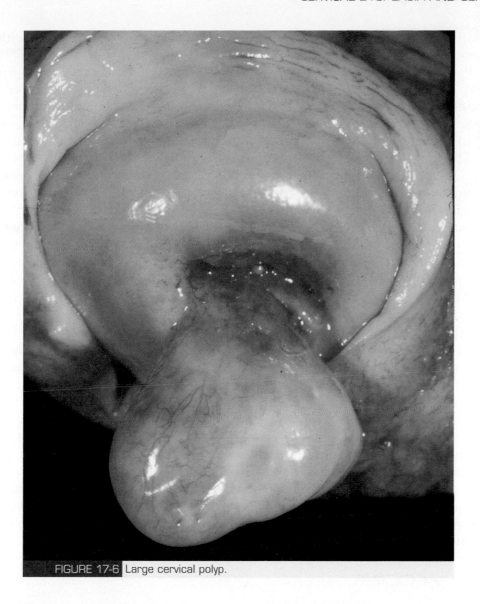

FIGURE 17-6 Large cervical polyp.

Cervical Dysplasia and Cervical Carcinoma

Abnormal growth and maturation of cervical squamous epithelium is called cervical dysplasia as discussed in cells and tissues: their structure and function in health and disease. Dysplastic changes range from mild disturbances of epithelial maturation to severe cellular abnormalities. Mild dysplasia may result from cervical inflammation or other causes and may regress spontaneously. Severe dysplasia usually does not regress and may progress to in situ carcinoma and eventually to invasive carcinoma after a variable period of time. Most physicians regard cervical dysplasia and in situ carcinoma as very closely related, constituting different stages in a progressive spectrum of epithelial abnormalities. Indeed, many physicians classify both dysplasia and in situ carcinoma under the general term cervical intraepithelial neoplasia, which is usually abbreviated CIN and is graded I, II, and III. In this terminology, mild dysplasia is called CIN I. Moderate dysplasia is termed CIN II. Severe dysplasia and in situ carcinoma are classified together and are designated CIN III. Another grading system called the Bethesda system (named from a city in Maryland) provides comparable information but supplements the CIN categories by adding a detailed classification of the cytologic changes observed in Pap smears together with an assessment of their significance.

Persons infected with some types of HPV, the same virus that causes genital condylomas, are at increased risk of developing cervical dysplasia and cervical carcinoma (FIGURE 17-7). The dysplasia–cancer-causing strains can infect the cervical epithelial cells, and the viral DNA becomes incorporated into the cell's DNA, which induces cell dysfunction leading to cervical dysplasia and cervical carcinoma.

There are more than 100 different types of HPV, and about 40 types can infect the genital tract; but only about 8 different types (called high-risk types) are considered to be carcinogenic (cancer causing). HPV genital tract infections are common. Many young sexually active women become infected, but over 90% of the infections resolve spontaneously within 6–12 months as the body's immune system responds to the infection and destroys the virus. Some women have repeated infections, and their immune systems eradicate the viruses, leaving no long-term harmful effects. Only the small proportion of women infected with a cancer-causing HPV type, who are unable to eliminate the virus, are at risk of cervical dysplasia and cervical carcinoma.

HPV testing of cervical material obtained when a routine Pap test is performed can be helpful when the cytologic changes in the Pap smear are inconclusive (classified as atypical squamous cells of undetermined significance in the Bethesda system). If the HPV test is negative, the cytologic changes are probably not significant, and no further studies are required. On the other hand, if the HPV test is positive, the patient may have cervical dysplasia, and further evaluation of the patient is required. Since a woman with cervical dysplasia or carcinoma will have a positive HPV test, some investigators have recommended substituting the HPV test for the Pap test as the primary screening test to detect these abnormalities; others have suggested routinely adding the HPV test to the Pap test for screening women. Currently, screening tests are available that can detect infection not only with HPV types 16 and 18, which are responsible for most cases of cervical dysplasia and carcinoma but also can detect infections with several other high risk but less hazardous HPV types.

HPV VACCINE

Two anti-HPV vaccines are available. Both are prepared from virus proteins and do not contain live virus. The first vaccine, which was licensed in 2006, provides

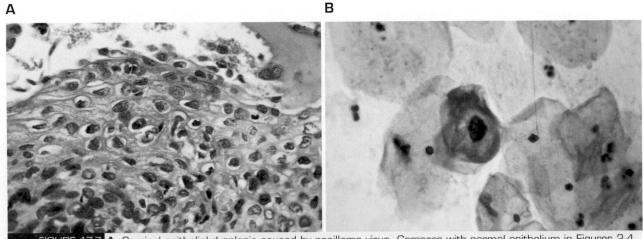

A   **B**

FIGURE 17-7 **A,** Cervical epithelial dysplasia caused by papilloma virus. Compare with normal epithelium in Figures 2-4 and 2-10A. **B,** Dysplastic epithelial cell identified in Papanicolaou smear (original magnification × 400).

immunity against four HPV types (6, 11, 16, and 18). Types 16 and 18 are called oncogenic (*onkos* = tumor + *genic* = causing) viruses because they are responsible for 70% of cases of cervical dysplasia and carcinoma. Types 6 and 11 are responsible for 90% of genital tract condylomas but are not considered to be oncogenic viruses. The second vaccine, licensed in 2009, only protects against the cancer-causing types 16 and 18. Unfortunately, the vaccines are not effective against any of the HPV types in the vaccine to which the subject has already been infected but will still provide protection from the other viruses in the vaccine. The vaccines are recommended primarily for girls 11–12 years old before they become sexually active because they are unlikely to have been infected with the HPV types covered by the vaccines and would get the most protection from the vaccines. HPV vaccine should not be considered an all-purpose "anticancer vaccine." Regular gynecologic care and Pap smears are still required because other carcinogenic viruses not covered by the vaccine may still cause papillomas, dysplasia, and cervical cancer.

Although the vaccines have been recommended for routine use, many physicians have reservations about the vaccines because of uncertainty about the possible adverse long-term effects, the duration of immunity, and concerns that other carcinogenic papilloma viruses are beginning to replace the HPV-16 and HPV-18 strains that have been suppressed by the vaccines.

DIAGNOSIS AND TREATMENT

The cellular abnormalities indicative of dysplasia or carcinoma develop first in the cells at the junction between the squamous epithelium covering the exterior of the cervix and the columnar epithelium lining the cervical canal. This region is called the squamocolumnar junction or transition zone and is usually located at the external opening (external os) of the cervix. Abnormal cells indicative of dysplasia or carcinoma can be identified by means of a Pap smear prepared from material obtained from around the external os and endocervical canal, as described in the discussion on neoplastic disease.

An abnormal Pap smear requires further evaluation, which is usually accomplished by means of a binocular magnifying instrument called a **colposcope**. This instrument provides the physician with a greatly magnified view of the cervix and endocervical canal. In cervical dysplasia and carcinoma, one can often identify characteristic abnormalities in the cervical epithelium and underlying blood vessels and can define the location and extent of the abnormal epithelium. Then multiple biopsy specimens are taken from the abnormal-appearing areas, and material is also obtained from the endocervical canal. Treatment depends on the results of the biopsies. Dysplasia and in situ carcinoma are usually treated by destruction of the abnormal epithelium by freezing (cryocautery), by laser light, by surgical excision of the abnormal area, or sometimes by removal of the uterus (hysterectomy). Invasive carcinoma is treated either by radiation or by resection of the uterus, fallopian tubes, ovaries, and adjacent tissues (radical hysterectomy).

Dysplasia and in situ carcinoma can be cured by proper treatment and carry an excellent prognosis. In situ carcinoma may remain localized within the epithelium of the cervix for as long as 10 years before eventually becoming invasive. After invasion has occurred, however, the neoplasm is much harder to treat, and the results are less satisfactory. The tumor may extend through the cervix into the adjacent tissues and may infiltrate the rectum and bladder. The ureters, which lie on each side of the cervix, may also be invaded and obstructed by the neoplasm. Metastatic spread to regional lymph nodes and distant sites also is common.

Colposcope
(kol'pos-kōp)
A binocular magnifying instrument used to view the cervix and endocervical canal.

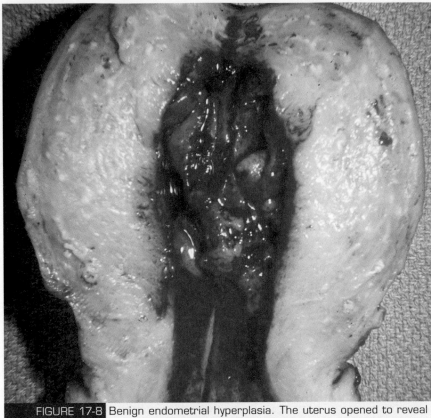

FIGURE 17-8 Benign endometrial hyperplasia. The uterus opened to reveal polypoid masses of hyperplastic endometrium filling endometrial cavity.

OTHER SITES OF HPV INFECTION

In addition to HPV-caused cervical cancer, HPV has also been identified in association with carcinoma of the vulva, penis, rectum, and oral cavity, where it may have been transmitted from a cervical infection.

Endometrial Hyperplasia, Polyps, and Carcinoma

Occasionally, the endometrium of the uterus may undergo benign hyperplasia, which is often associated with irregular uterine bleeding (FIGURE 17-8). Benign polyps in the endometrium are also common (FIGURE 17-9). Sometimes an endometrial polyp may cause uterine bleeding if the tip becomes inflamed or ulcerated. Endometrial adenocarcinoma has been increasing in frequency. This condition also is manifested by irregular uterine bleeding or postmenopausal bleeding. Endometrial carcinoma is often related to prolonged or excessive stimulation of the endometrium by estrogen.

Uterine Myomas

Myoma
(mī-ō′muh)
A benign smooth muscle tumor such as commonly develops in the uterus.

Benign, smooth muscle tumors called **myomas** arise in the wall of the uterus (FIGURE 17-10). They are frequently encountered and are said to occur in approximately 30% of women over 30 years of age. Occasionally, myomas may be responsible for excessive or irregular uterine bleeding or may produce symptoms related to pressure on the adjacent bladder or rectum (FIGURE 17-11). Hysterectomy is performed if the myomas are producing symptoms.

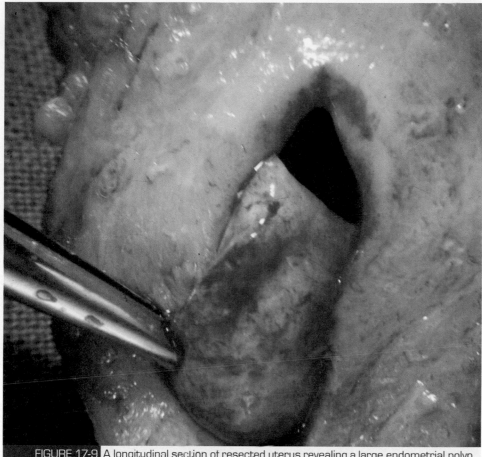

FIGURE 17-9 A longitudinal section of resected uterus revealing a large endometrial polyp (*held by forceps*) within the endometrial cavity.

Irregular Uterine Bleeding

Excessive or irregular uterine bleeding is a common gynecologic problem. Most cases in younger women result from a disturbance in the normal cyclic interaction of estrogen and progesterone on the endometrium. This is usually called dysfunctional uterine bleeding. In older women, bleeding can be the result of many causes.

DYSFUNCTIONAL UTERINE BLEEDING

Normally, the first half of the menstrual cycle is characterized by proliferation of endometrial glands and stroma under the influence of estrogen produced by the ovarian follicle. At about midcycle, ovulation occurs, and the follicle discharges its egg. Then the follicle becomes a corpus luteum, which produces both progesterone and estrogen. Under the influence of progesterone, the endometrium becomes a secretory phase in preparation for receiving a fertilized ovum. If no pregnancy occurs, the corpus luteum begins to decline, and estrogen–progesterone levels begin to drop. The secretory endometrium is deprived of its hormonal support and is shed along with a small amount of blood, constituting the menstrual flow, after which a new cycle begins.

Most cases of dysfunctional uterine bleeding occur because the follicle fails to mature to the point of ovulation and, consequently, no corpus luteum forms. As a result, the endometrium is subjected to continuous estrogen stimulation and responds by shedding in an irregular manner associated with irregular uterine bleeding, instead of shedding all at once as in a normal period. This condition is also called anovulatory

A

B

C

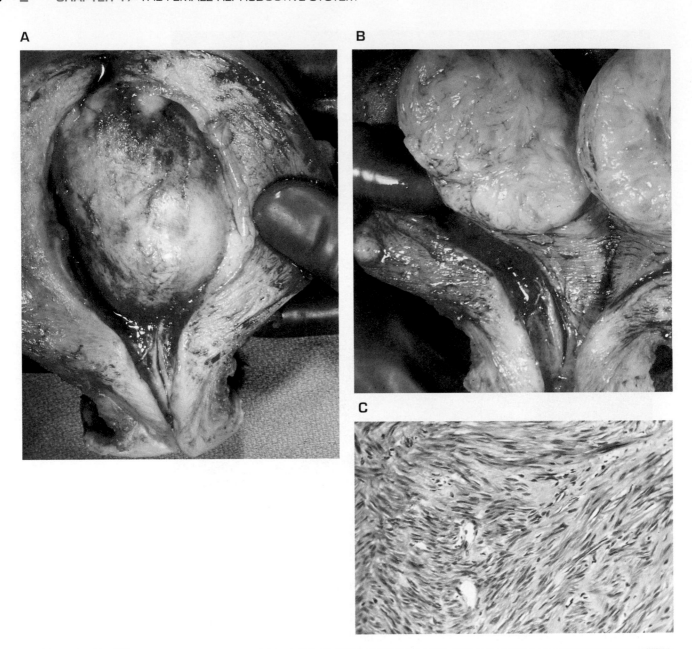

FIGURE 17-10 Uterine myoma. **A**, A uterus opened to reveal a large spherical myoma protruding into endometrial cavity. **B**, A cross section of myoma illustrating well-circumscribed tumor without evidence of necrosis, features suggesting a benign neoplasm. **C**, Histologic appearance, revealing interlacing bundles of mature smooth muscle cells that resemble the normal muscle cells from which the tumor arose (original magnification × 100).

bleeding (*ana* = without + ovulation). It tends to arise at both extremes of reproductive life: when normal menstrual cycles are being established at puberty and near menopause when ovarian function is declining. Less commonly, irregular bleeding is the result of continuous secretion of progesterone from a corpus luteum that fails to involute. This prolongs the secretory phase of the endometrium, which sometimes sheds irregularly.

Dysfunctional uterine bleeding is treated by administering hormones to restore the proliferative-secretory sequence in the endometrium that is characteristic of a normal menstrual cycle. In one common treatment, the patient is given a synthetic steroid hormone having progesterone activity. The hormone induces secretory changes in the endometrium and stops the bleeding. The hormone treatment is then stopped,

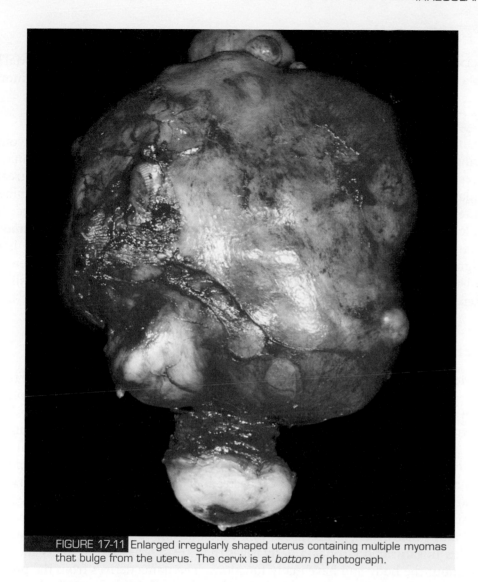

FIGURE 17-11 Enlarged irregularly shaped uterus containing multiple myomas that bulge from the uterus. The cervix is at *bottom* of photograph.

and the endometrium sheds as in a normal period. Frequently, the next cycle is normal and usually no further treatment is required. Multiple recurrent episodes of dysfunctional bleeding that lead to anemia resulting from excessive blood loss may require more aggressive treatment, as described in the following section.

ENDOMETRIAL ABLATION

Repeated episodes of excessive irregular uterine bleeding not caused by a treatable uterine disease can be managed by destroying the endometrium without removing the uterus. This procedure, called **endometrial ablation** (*ablatus* = taking away), can control heavy menstrual bleeding that has not responded to other treatments and is an option when the woman has completed childbearing and does not want to have a hysterectomy. A special instrument can be inserted into the uterus through the cervix, which destroys the endometrium by heat, freezing, or a high-frequency electric current, or a balloon or similar device can be placed in the endometrial cavity and filled with very hot water (185°F). After an ablation procedure, half the treated women no longer have menstrual periods, and the rest have very light menses.

Endometrial ablation
Permanent destruction of the endometrium by various methods to control excessive menstrual bleeding unresponsive to more conservative treatment.

OTHER CAUSES OF UTERINE BLEEDING

Other conditions that may cause endometrial bleeding include benign endometrial hyperplasia, endometrial and cervical polyps, uterine myomas, and uterine carcinoma.

DIAGNOSIS AND TREATMENT

Irregular bleeding is always a cause for concern when it occurs in an older woman nearing the end of her reproductive years or after the menopause because it may be the result of an endometrial carcinoma. Bleeding in older women is usually treated by dilating the cervix with various metal dilators and then scraping out the lining of the uterus with a long-handled scooplike instrument called a curette. This procedure is called dilatation and curettage or simply abbreviated **D & C.** The tissue removed is examined microscopically by the pathologist. If the endometrial tissue is not malignant, no further treatment is needed. If endometrial carcinoma is detected on histologic examination, further treatment is required. Usually this consists of hysterectomy, sometimes preceded by a course of radiation therapy.

D & C
Dilatation and curettage of the uterus. A scraping out of the uterine lining, often performed as a diagnostic or therapeutic procedure.

Dysmenorrhea

Dysmenorrhea means painful menstruation. There are two types: primary dysmenorrhea, in which the pelvic organs are normal, and secondary dysmenorrhea, which results from various diseases of the pelvic organs, such as endometriosis.

Primary dysmenorrhea is the more common type. The pain is crampy, begins just prior to menstruation, and lasts for 1 or 2 days after onset of the menstrual flow. Usually, menstrual periods are painless for the first year or two after onset of menses during adolescence because early menstrual cycles are usually anovulatory, and primary dysmenorrhea does not occur unless ovulation occurs. Dysmenorrhea does not usually become a problem until regular ovulatory menstrual cycles are established.

Crampy menstrual pain is caused by a class of compounds called **prostaglandins,** complex unsaturated fatty acid derivatives that are synthesized in many locations throughout the body and have many functions. The name derives from the prostate gland, where these substances were first identified. Prostaglandins are synthesized within the endometrium under the influence of progesterone produced by the ovary during the secretory phase of the cycle. When the endometrium breaks down during menstruation, the prostaglandins are released and diffused into the myometrium, where they cause the spasmodic myometrial contractions that are responsible for the crampy menstrual pain. Dysmenorrhea does not occur if cycles are anovulatory because no corpus luteum forms and no progesterone is produced to stimulate prostaglandin synthesis.

Treatment consists of aspirin or another anti-inflammatory drug, which is administered before the onset of menses. These drugs suppress the synthesis of prostaglandins within the endometrium. Primary dysmenorrhea can also be treated very effectively with oral contraceptive pills, which prevent dysmenorrhea by suppressing ovulation.

Dysmenorrhea
(dis-men-ō-rhē′uh)
Painful menstruation.

Prostaglandin
(pros-ta-glan′din)
A complex derivative of a fatty acid (prostanoic acid) that has widespread physiologic effects.

Cysts and Tumors of the Ovary

The ovary gives rise to a wide variety of cysts and tumors, and only the more common ones are considered here. Benign ovarian cysts are common. They arise either from ovarian follicles or from corpora lutea, as illustrated in FIGURE 17-12, that have failed to regress normally and instead become converted into fluid-filled cysts. Follicle cysts and corpus luteum cysts are often called functional cysts because they represent a

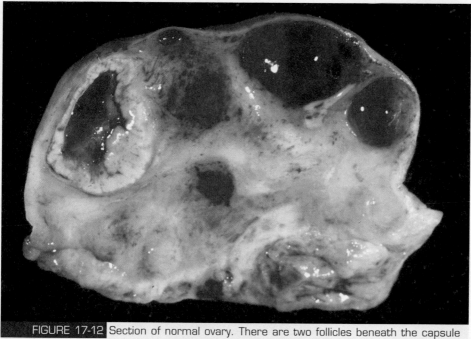

FIGURE 17-12 Section of normal ovary. There are two follicles beneath the capsule (*right side*) and a corpus luteum (*left side*).

derangement of the normal maturation and involution of a follicle or corpus luteum. Functional cysts do not usually become very large, and most regress spontaneously.

Endometrial deposits in the ovary may form cysts lined by endometrium and filled with old blood and debris. These are called **endometrial cysts** (Figure 17-5B).

True ovarian neoplasms may arise in one or both ovaries. They may be either benign or malignant, cystic or solid. Benign cystic teratomas, often called **dermoid cysts**, commonly develop in the ovary. These tumors arise from unfertilized ova that have undergone neoplastic change. They often contain skin, hair, teeth, bone, parts of gastrointestinal tract, thyroid, and other tissues growing in a jumbled fashion (FIGURE 17-13).

Endometrial cyst

(en-dō-mē′trē-ul)
An ovarian cyst lined by endometrium and filled with old blood and debris. A manifestation of endometriosis.

Dermoid cyst

(derm′oyd)
A common type of benign cystic teratoma that commonly arises in the ovary.

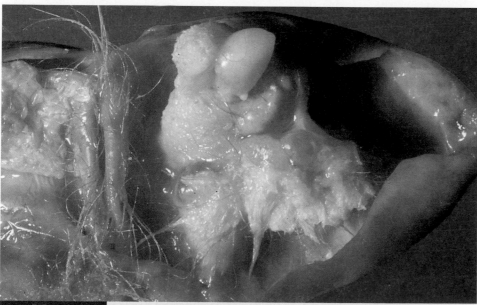

FIGURE 17-13 Opened dermoid cyst of ovary (benign cystic teratoma) with contents removed. The cyst contains a well-formed jawbone with two teeth (*center*). Note the hair arising from the skin that lines the cyst.

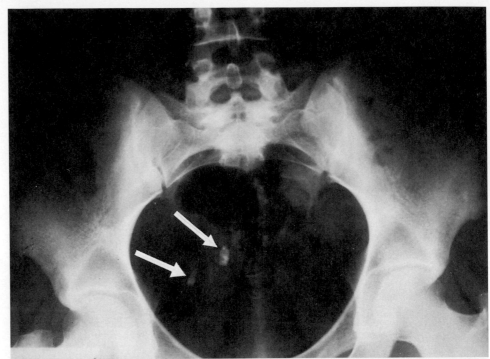

FIGURE 17-14 An x-ray of the pelvis illustrating teeth (*arrows*) contained within dermoid cyst.

Sometimes teeth and bone contained in dermoid cysts can be detected in x-ray films of the pelvis (FIGURE 17-14; see also discussion on neoplastic disease, Figure 10-15). A dermoid cyst apparently represents an attempt of an unfertilized ovum to realize its potential by producing diverse tissues like those in a fetus. In contrast with the frequency of benign ovarian teratomas, malignant teratomas of the ovary are quite rare.

Another group of ovarian tumors are those arising from the epithelial cells on the surface of the ovary, and the epithelium of the tumor cells may resemble the epithelium found in other parts of the genital tract. If the tumor epithelium resembles the cells lining the fallopian tube, the tumor is classified as a serous tumor. If the tumor epithelium resembles the mucus-secreting epithelium of the endocervix, it is called a mucinous tumor; if the tumor epithelium resembles endometrium, it is termed an endometrioid tumor. Many of the serous and mucinous tumors are cystic, and the term serous cystadenoma or serous cystadenocarcinoma is used. In many of these serous tumors, the neoplastic epithelium may extend onto the external surface of the tumor (FIGURE 17-15). When this occurs, small pieces of the projecting tumor may break off and implant elsewhere in the pelvis, peritoneal cavity, and omentum, where they continue to grow. Tumors manifesting this behavior may be difficult to remove completely.

A mucinous tumor is designated as either a mucinous cystadenoma or a mucinous cystadenocarcinoma. Most of the ovarian tumors with endometriumlike epithelium are malignant and are called endometrioid carcinomas. Another common ovarian tumor arises from the fibrous connective tissue cells of the ovary and is called a fibroma.

A few ovarian tumors produce sex hormones. One type arises from the estrogen-producing cells lining the follicles (granulosa cells) and the closely associated cells adjacent to the follicle cells (theca cells). These cells produce estrogen and so does a tumor arising from these cells, which is called a **granulosa cell tumor** or **granulosa-theca cell tumor**.

Granulosa cell tumor
(gran-u-lō′suh)
A tumor arising from granulosa cells, usually associated with excess production of estrogen.

Granulosa-theca cell tumor
An estrogen-producing ovarian tumor arising from the estrogen-producing granulose cell of an ovarian follicle.

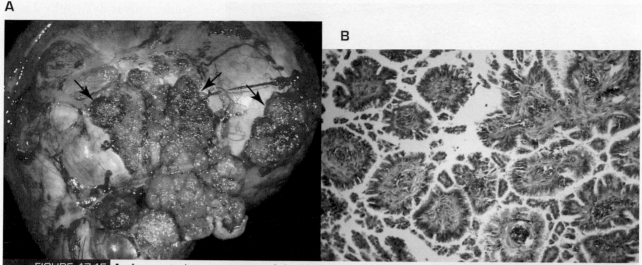

FIGURE 17-15 **A**, A resected serous tumor of the ovary measuring 10 cm in diameter. Several masses of tumor (*arrows*) project from the surface. **B**, Histologic appearance of the tumor, which forms papillary processes covered by well-differentiated epithelial cells (original magnification × 100).

The tumor may induce endometrial hyperplasia caused by excessive endometrial stimulation from the estrogen produced by the tumor. A granulosa cell tumor in a postmenopausal woman may induce irregular uterine bleeding. A few rare types of ovarian tumor produce male sex hormones instead of estrogen and may induce masculinization. Some ovarian tumors may become quite large, as illustrated by the following case.

CASE 17-1

A young woman who was 7 months pregnant had noted marked enlargement of the abdomen that she attributed to the pregnancy. Examination by her physician revealed a large cystic mass lying above and posterior to the pregnant uterus. At operation, a large benign cystic tumor of the ovary was encountered. It contained 15 liters of fluid and weighed 35 lbs (FIGURE 17-16). The day after the operation, the patient went into labor and delivered a premature infant who was transferred to the pediatric intensive care unit. Both mother and infant did well after the operation.

Diseases of the Vulva

VULVAR DYSTROPHY

The epithelium of the vulva may exhibit irregular areas of thickening and inflammation that appear as white patches. Histologically, the affected epithelium is heavily keratinized, and the epithelial cells show variable abnormalities of maturation. Clinically, the condition is associated with intense itching and tenderness of the affected areas. The descriptive term leukoplakia (*leuko* = white + *plakia* = patch) has often been applied to this lesion but has been discarded in favor of a newer term, vulvar dystrophy (*dys* = abnormal + *trophe* = growth). In some cases, vulvar dystrophy progresses gradually over a period of years into in situ carcinoma and eventually into invasive carcinoma. Consequently, many physicians consider vulvar dystrophy a pre-cancerous lesion. Various types of local treatment are frequently effective, but if significant pre-cancerous changes are present in the epithelium, the affected areas are generally removed surgically.

CARCINOMA OF THE VULVA

Vulvar carcinoma is occasionally found in both premenopausal and postmenopausal women, frequently arising in areas of vulvar dystrophy (FIGURE 17-17). Treatment consists of resection of the vulva (vulvectomy) along with the inguinal lymph nodes, which receive lymphatic drainage from the vulva.

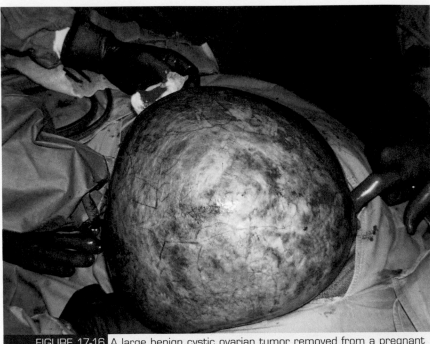

FIGURE 17-16 A large benign cystic ovarian tumor removed from a pregnant woman (Case 17-1). The tumor weighed 35 lbs.

Toxic Shock Syndrome

Toxic shock syndrome (TSS)
A symptom complex in menstruating women who use high-absorbency tampons, caused by a toxin produced by a staphylococcus that grows in the vagina.

Toxic shock syndrome (TSS) is a disease that was first recognized about 20 years ago in menstruating women who used high-absorbency tampons, but its frequency has declined as other menstrual products replaced them, although no tampon is entirely free from risk.

Clinically, the disease is characterized by elevated temperature, vomiting and diarrhea, muscular aches and pains, a fall in blood pressure (often to shock levels), and various other systemic manifestations. A characteristic feature of the disease is an erythematous (sunburnlike) skin rash that is followed by flaking and peeling of the affected skin (somewhat like the peeling that occurs after a severe sunburn).

The clinical manifestations of toxic shock syndrome are caused by a toxin produced by *Staphylococcus aureus* that grows in the vagina of the affected patients. The menstrual blood and secretions provide an excellent culture medium that fosters the growth of the staphylococci and the production of toxin. Tampons apparently promote the development of TSS in two ways. First, they prevent drainage of menstrual products from the vagina and thereby favor growth of staphylococci. Second, high-absorbency tampons may cause small superficial erosions of the vaginal mucosa, and absorption of toxins could occur rapidly through such injured areas.

Treatment of toxic shock syndrome consists of general supportive measures to sustain the patient until the effects of the toxin have worn off. There is no way to counteract or neutralize the toxin. Tampon use should be promptly discontinued. Antibiotics are often prescribed to eradicate the staphylococci, but the antibiotics do not shorten the course of the disease.

Rarely, toxic shock syndrome occurs in nonmenstruating women and in men. These cases are a result of staphylococcal infections in other parts of the body, such as the skin, kidneys, or bone, with liberation of toxins from the infected site into the circulation.

Contraception

Methods of contraception fall into two major groups: "natural" methods and artificial methods. Natural family planning methods attempt to prevent pregnancy by avoiding intercourse around the time of ovulation when pregnancy is more likely to occur. These methods have no side effects or medical complications but require a high degree of motivation and are generally less effective than artificial methods. In contrast, artificial methods act by preventing the union of sperm and egg, preventing ovulation, or preventing implantation of the fertilized ovum. Many of these methods are highly effective, but some have potentially serious side effects.

Diaphragms and condoms are mechanical devices that usually are used in conjunction with a spermicidal foam or jelly. They function by preventing the union of sperm and egg; they are highly effective when used correctly and have no serious side effects.

A vaginal contraceptive sponge functions much like a diaphragm. It is a soft, flat polyurethane disk with a central depression. The sponge contains a spermicide called nonoxynol-9. Inserted high in the vagina against the cervix before intercourse, the sponge blocks sperm from entering the cervix and the spermicide destroys any sperm that come in contact with the sponge. Contraceptive suppositories are another contraceptive method. The suppository is inserted in the vagina before intercourse, where it dissolves and releases a spermicide. Suppositories reduce the chance of conception but are less effective than the preceding methods because they are not used along with mechanical devices that cover the cervix.

Contraceptive pills, a very popular contraceptive method, consist of a synthetic estrogen combined with a compound having progesterone activity (progestin). "The pill" prevents ovulation by suppressing release of the pituitary gonadotropic hormones that regulate ovarian follicle growth, maturation, and ovulation and that cause changes in the cervical mucus and endometrial lining that also discourage pregnancy. When taken properly, contraceptive pills are almost 100% effective, but there are some side effects. The estrogen in the pill promotes increased synthesis of blood coagulation factors, predisposing to formation of blood clots within the circulatory system. Women who smoke cigarettes and women over 35 years of age are at especially high risk. Some women on the pill develop high blood pressure. The elevated pressure probably results from an increased synthesis of a blood protein (called angiotensinogen) induced by the estrogen in the pill, which interacts with renin produced by the kidney to yield angiotensin, a potent blood pressure–raising compound described in the urinary system. Women on the pill are closely observed for this complication, and the pill is discontinued if the blood pressure starts to rise.

For women who do not like to take pills, other methods are available for providing the same type of

Diaphragm
(di′ā-fram)
A partition separating one thing from another, applied to the dome-shaped partition between the thoracic and abdominal cavities. The term is also applied to a contraceptive device placed over the cervix prior to intercourse.

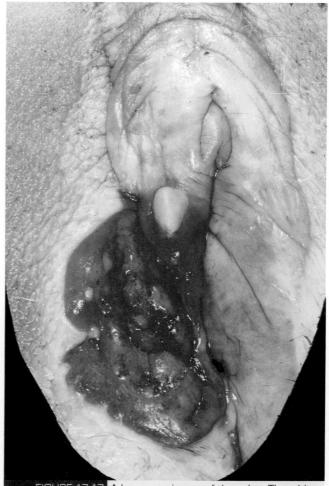

FIGURE 17-17 A large carcinoma of the vulva. The white appearance of the skin adjacent to the carcinoma is caused by preexisting vulvar dystrophy.

estrogen and progestin formulations used in contraceptive pills: either incorporated in a very small (54 mm diameter) ring that is inserted into the vagina, where the estrogen and progestin are slowly released from the ring and absorbed from the vagina into the bloodstream, or incorporated into an adhesive patch applied to the skin, where the estrogen and progestin are absorbed through the skin.

Another less frequently used type of contraceptive pill contains only progestin and may have fewer side effects than the combined estrogen–progesterone pill. The progestin acts by changing the character of the cervical mucus, which impedes sperm penetration, and changes the character of the endometrium so that a fertilized egg is unable to become implanted. The progestin may also suppress ovulation.

An **intrauterine device** (IUD) is a small, flexible plastic structure that is inserted into the uterine cavity by a physician or nurse practitioner (FIGURE 17-18). IUDs are used less frequently now by women in the United States and Canada, but worldwide they are used widely as an effective and relatively inexpensive contraceptive method that does not require much attention from the user. A string attached to the device extends through the cervix into the vagina. The string serves two purposes. The woman can assure herself that the device is still within the uterine cavity by feeling the string. It also facilitates removal of the IUD by the physician when it is no longer needed.

Intrauterine devices do not prevent conception but act by preventing implantation of the fertilized ovum. Most of the devices that were popular previously are no longer marketed because of concerns about lawsuits initiated by women who may have experienced complications from use of the devices. There are only two intrauterine contraceptive devices available currently. One is a T-shaped plastic device with copper wire wound around both the stem and the side arms. The effectiveness of copper-wound devices is related primarily to the contraceptive effect of the copper, which is released slowly within the endometrium as the copper wire gradually dissolves. Contraceptive effectiveness continues for about 10 years, after which the device must be replaced. The other IUD is also a T-shaped plastic device. A reservoir in the stem of the device contains a progesteronelike compound (progestin) that diffuses slowly

Intrauterine device (IUD)

A small plastic device inserted in the uterus to prevent pregnancy.

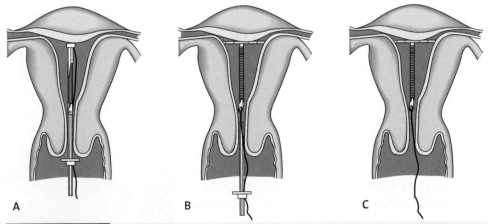

A   B   C

FIGURE 17-18 Technique of inserting intrauterine device. **A**, The device is retracted into the insertion tube, and the tube is introduced through the cervix to the fundus of the uterus. **B**, The tube is retracted, allowing the plastic device to resume its original configuration. **C**, The tube is withdrawn. A string attached to the IUD protrudes through the cervix into the vagina.

from the IUD. The device is effective for 5 years, and then must be replaced with a new one. Much of its effectiveness depends on the slow release of the progestin, which alters the endometrium, inhibiting implantation of the fertilized ovum.

Two major problems are associated with use of an IUD. The first is an increased incidence of uterine and tubal infections, which may be followed by tubal scarring and impaired fertility. Some women have developed serious chronic pelvic infections caused by anaerobic bacteria that sometimes infect a uterus containing an IUD. A second potential problem relates to tubal pregnancies. Because an IUD prevents implantation only within the uterus and does not prevent either ovulation or fertilization, implantation may occur within the tube.

If a woman becomes pregnant while wearing an IUD, the pregnancy may be in the tube rather than in the uterus. (Prenatal development and diseases associated with pregnancy discusses tubal pregnancy and the significance of previous tubal infection as a predisposing factor.)

Emergency Contraception

Many unintended pregnancies occur each year. Most result from failure to use effective contraception, but some result from failure of the method being used such as a broken condom, or from a sexual assault, and could be prevented by the use of emergency contraception. As described in the next chapter, sperm can survive in a woman's genital tract for as long as 5 or 6 days and still be able to fertilize an ovum. Therefore, intercourse several days before ovulation can still lead to a pregnancy. Even if an ovum is fertilized, it still takes about 1 week for the fertilized ovum to travel through the fallopian tube and implant within the uterus. The likelihood of pregnancy after unprotected intercourse can be greatly reduced by a postcoital (after intercourse) contraceptive. The best known contraceptive is a progestin-only 1.5 mg levonorgestrel pill (marketed as Plan B One-Step), which is available without a prescription and should be taken regardless of the cycle day when unprotected intercourse occurred. The progestin in the pills exerts several effects that prevent pregnancy. The progestin may inhibit ovulation, and it also impairs tubal motility, which slows transport of the ovum through the fallopian tube, effects that reduce the likelihood of conception. Finally, the progestin changes the endometrium so that it becomes unsuitable for implantation even if fertilization should occur, and the progestin-mediated change in the endometrium occurs before a fertilized ovum can complete its 7-day journey into the endometrium. When the pill is taken within 12 hours after unprotected intercourse, the pregnancy risk is less than 1% and is about 3% when taken within 72 hours, but some protection is still provided for as long as 5 days.

Recently, an emergency contraceptive used in Europe has become available in the United States, which requires a physician's prescription. The pill, which is marketed as ellaOne is a 30-mg tablet of ulipristal acetate, a synthetic steroid hormone related to mifepristone, which is used to perform abortions. Ulipristal acts by delaying or preventing ovulation and also changes the endometrium so that it becomes unsuitable for implantation, much like a progestin-only contraceptive. In contrast to Plan B, the pill is effective for as long as 5 days after unprotected intercourse, and its effectiveness does not decrease if there is a time delay between intercourse and the time that the pill is taken.

QUESTIONS FOR REVIEW

1. What parts of the female genital tract may be affected by gonorrheal infection? How does gonorrhea lead to sterility?
2. What is the difference between in situ and invasive cervical carcinoma? How is the Pap smear used in the diagnosis of carcinoma?
3. A patient consults her physician because of irregular uterine bleeding. What are some of the diseases of the genital tract that cause this bleeding?
4. What is endometriosis? What symptoms does it produce? What are some complications that may be associated with endometriosis?
5. What is a dermoid cyst?
6. What is toxic shock? How does tampon use predispose to this syndrome? What role do staphylococci play?
7. How do contraceptive pills and IUDs exert their contraceptive effects? What medical problems may be associated with their use?
8. What is vulvar dystrophy? What symptoms does it cause? What are its complications?

SUPPLEMENTARY READINGS

Boston Women's Health Book Collective. 2005. *Our bodies, ourselves for the new century*. New York: Simon & Schuster, Inc.
> Covers a wide range of subjects dealing with sexual anatomy, physiology, and pathology in a clear and concise manner. A useful reference.

Bulun, S. E. 2009. Endometriosis. *New England Journal of Medicine* 360:268–79.
> A comprehensive discussion of the factors contributing to the pelvic pain and disability associated with this condition, together with a description of treatment methods.

Davis, J. P., Chesney, P. J., Wand P. J., et al. 1980. Toxic-shock syndrome: Epidemiologic features, recurrence, risk factors, and prevention. *New England Journal of Medicine* 303:1429–35.
> A good review article.

Gostin, L. O., and DeAngelis, C. D. 2007. Mandatory HPV vaccination: Public health vs. private health. *Journal of the American Medical Association* 297:1921–3.
> An article cautioning against a mandatory vaccination requirement indicating that the vaccine will protect against an infection that can only come from sexual contact, but research has not shown how long the protection can last and whether or not there may be long-term harmful effects.

Haug, C. J. 2008. Human papillomavirus vaccination—reasons for caution. *New England Journal of Medicine* 359:861–2.
> Although the vaccine is very effective in reducing the incidence of cervical dysplasia caused by HPV-16 and HPV-18, the duration of the immunity is uncertain and the effect of HPV vaccination will not be apparent for decades. Suppression of the vaccine strains will favor the emergence of other carcinogenic HPV serotypes, as suggested by published reports that indicate a trend toward precancerous cervical lesions caused by carcinogenic HPV strains not covered by the vaccine. There are many unanswered questions about the vaccine, and we should concentrate on finding answers through research studies instead of basing important decisions on unproven assumptions.

Ho, G. Y. F., Bierman, R., Beardsley, L., et al. 1998. Natural history of cervicovaginal papillomavirus infection in young women. *New England Journal of Medicine* 338:423–8.

► 608 college women were examined every 6 months for 3 years by means of cervico-vaginal specimens for detection of HPV DNA, and results were correlated with age, ethnicity, number of sex partners, and types of sexual activity. The incidence of HPV infections during the period of observation was 43%, and the median duration of a new HPV infection was 8 months. Persistence of HPV infection for more than 6 months was more likely to occur in older women and in those infected with high-risk types as-sociated with cervical neoplasms. Abnormal Pap smears were more likely to occur in subjects with persisting HPV infections, especially those infected with high-risk types.

Lu, P., and Ory, S. J. 1995. Endometriosis: Current management. *Mayo Clinic Proceedings* 70:453–63.

► A review of the clinical features, theories of pathogenesis, and current methods of treatment.

Mandelblatt, J. S., Lawrence, W. F., Womack, S. M., et al. 2002. Benefits and costs of using HPV testing to screen for cervical cancer. *Journal of the American Medical Association* 287:2372–81.

► A HPV screening test in addition to a Pap test performed every 2 years is cost effective.

Muñoz, N., Bosch, F. X., de Sanjose, S., et al. 2003. Epidemiologic classification of human papillomavirus types associated with cervical cancer. *New England Journal of Medicine* 348:518–27.

► Cervical cancer is the most common cancer in women worldwide and is caused by the human papillomavirus. More than 80 HPV types have been identified, and about 40 can infect the genital tract. Fifteen HPV types are carcinogenic. Eight different types are responsible for 95% of carcinomas, with types 16 and 18 being the major viral carcinogens.

Olive, D. L. 2008. Gonadotropin-releasing hormone agonists for endometriosis. *New England Journal of Medicine* 359:1136–42.

► Gonadotropin-releasing hormones (GnRH) are peptides that are modifications of the normal GnRH molecule, which attach to normal GnRH receptor molecules and ac-tivate them, which leads to a marked initial release of gonadotropic hormones that have been produced previously and stored in the pituitary gland. However, the initial release is followed by reduced responsiveness (downregulation) of the GnRH recep-tors and a corresponding marked suppression of follicle stimulating hormone (FSH) and luteinizing hormone (LH). Estrogen and progesterone levels fall, which reduces their effect on the endometriosis and relieves symptoms.

Runowicz, C. D. 2007. Molecular screening for cervical cancer—time to give up Pap tests? *New England Journal of Medicine* 357:1650–3.

► The Pap test has been a very successful screening method for detecting cervical dys-plasia and carcinoma. However, the test is not very sensitive, so repeat screening tests must be performed at regular intervals in order to detect any cytologic abnormalities that were missed in an earlier examination. HPV testing has been proposed as the primary screening test for cervical cancer because it is more sensitive than the Pap test for detecting high-grade cervical dysplasia and carcinoma. However, although the HPV test is more sensitive than the Pap test, it is less specific, which means that the HPV test may produce a significant number of false-positive results in subjects who do not have a HPV infection. Two large studies confirm that the HPV test is more sensitive (but also more expensive) than the Pap test. If further studies confirm the HPV test advantage, efforts should be made to simplify the test, improve its specificity, reduce its cost, and determine the most effective way to use the test for cancer screening.

Shands, K. N., Schmid, G. P., Dan, B. B., et al. 1980. Toxic-shock syndrome in menstruating women: Association with tampon use and *staphylococcus aureus* and clinical features in 52 cases. *New England Journal of Medicine* 303:1436–42.

▶ A review of the subject.

Stoler, M. H. 2002. New Bethesda terminology and evidence-based management guidelines for cervical cytology findings (Editorial). *Journal of the American Medical Association* 287:2140–1.

▶ Half the women in whom the Pap test reveals atypical squamous cells of uncertain significance may have benign atypical changes in their cervical epithelium but do not have cervical dysplasia, but the other half of this group of women do have cervical dysplasia and require further evaluation and treatment. The HPV test helps separate the women in these two groups.

Westhoff, C. 2003. Clinical practice. Emergency contraception. *New England Journal of Medicine* 349:1830–5.

▶ Sperm can survive in the genital tract for 5–6 days and can fertilize an egg when ovulation occurs several days after unprotected intercourse. The preferred "morning after pill" is a progestin-only formulation that should be taken regardless of the cycle day when unprotected intercourse occurred.

Wright, T. C., Jr., Cox, J. T., Massad, L. S., et al. 2002. 2001 consensus guidelines for the management of women with cervical cytologic abnormalities. *Journal of the American Medical Association* 287:2120–9.

▶ Testing of women for human papillomavirus DNA in cytologic specimens is recommended as a supplementary test for most women in whom significant cytologic abnormalities are detected in a routine Pap smear.

Wright, T. C., Jr., and Schiffman, M. 2003. Adding a test for human papillomavirus DNA to cervical-cancer screening. *New England Journal of Medicine* 348: 489–90.

▶ In patients with atypical cells detected in a Pap test, a single test for human papillomavirus (HPV) DNA identified almost all women found to have severe cervical dysplasia and was more effective than a single colposcopic examination or two additional Pap tests.

OUTLINE SUMMARY

Infections of the Female Genital Tract

VAGINITIS

Manifestations: vaginal discharge, itching, and irritation.
Causes:
> *Candida albicans:* pathogenic micro-organisms.
> *Trichomonas vaginalis:* animal parasites.
> *Gardnerella (Hemophilus) vaginalis* in conjunction with anaerobic bacteria (nonspecific vaginitis).

CERVICITIS

Mild chronic inflammation: common and of little clinical significance.
More severe inflammation often caused by gonococci or *Chlamydia.* May spread to infect tubes and adjacent tissues (pelvic inflammatory disease).

SALPINGITIS AND PELVIC INFLAMMATORY DISEASE

Definitions:
> *Salpingitis: tubal infection.*
> *Pelvic inflammatory disease (PID): more general term referring to infection of tubes and adjacent tissues as well.*

Manifestations and complications:
> *Usually caused by gonococcal or chlamydial infection spreading from cervix.*
> *Causes lower abdominal pain and tenderness, elevated temperature, and leukocytosis.*

Tubal scarring following healing may cause sterility or predispose to ectopic pregnancy.

CONDYLOMAS OF THE GENITAL TRACT
Virus warts of genital tract.
Can be destroyed by chemicals, electrocoagulation, freezing (cryocautery), or excision.

Endometriosis
CLINICAL MANIFESTATIONS
Deposits of endometrium outside the normal location in the endometrial cavity.
Ectopic endometrium responds to hormonal stimuli; undergoes menstrual desquamation and regeneration.
Secondary scarring may obstruct fallopian tubes and cause infertility.

Cervical Polyps
POLYPS
Usually small.
Erosion of tip may cause bleeding.

Cervical Dysplasia and Cervical Carcinoma
CONCEPT OF CERVICAL INTRAEPITHELIAL NEOPLASIA
Varies from mild to severe.
Mild dysplasia may regress; severe dysplasia may progress to carcinoma.
Dysplasia and in situ carcinoma closely related.
Some HPV types are carcinogenic and predispose to cervical neoplasia.
HPV test may be useful supplement to Pap test when cytology is inconclusive.
HPV vaccine may prevent infection with some but not all carcinogenic papilloma viruses and does not replace regular gynecologic examinations.

DIAGNOSIS AND TREATMENT
Pap smear shows abnormal cells.
Colposcopy localizes abnormalities.
Biopsies establish diagnosis.
Treatment depends on extent of disease.
> *Dysplasia and in situ carcinoma treated by cryocautery, excision, or hysterectomy. Results are excellent.*
> *Invasive carcinoma treated by radiation or radical surgery. Results are less satisfactory.*

Endometrial Hyperplasia, Polyps, and Carcinoma
BENIGN HYPERPLASIA
May cause irregular uterine bleeding.

BENIGN POLYPS
Common lesion.
May bleed if tip eroded.

ENDOMETRIAL CARCINOMA
Estrogen use in menopause increases incidence.
Causes irregular uterine bleeding or postmenopausal bleeding.

Uterine Myomas
INCIDENCE AND MANIFESTATIONS
Very common: in approximately 30% of women over 30 years.
May cause uterine bleeding or pressure symptoms on bladder or rectum.
Treated by hysterectomy.

Irregular Uterine Bleeding
PATHOGENESIS
Dysfunctional uterine bleeding: caused by failure of ovulation.
Other causes: must rule out carcinoma in older women by dilatation and curettage.

Dysmenorrhea
PRIMARY DYSMENORRHEA
Onset about 1 or 2 years after menarche, when regular menstrual cycles established.
Prostaglandins synthesized under influence of progesterone during secretory phase of cycle are released from endometrium during menses and stimulate myometrial contractions causing pain.
Treated by prostaglandin inhibitors (aspirin or other anti-inflammatory drugs) or by birth-control pills, which suppress ovulation.

SECONDARY DYSMENORRHEA
As a result of disease of pelvic organs, such as endometriosis.
Treatment consists of correcting basic cause whenever possible.

Cysts and Tumors of the Ovary
CYSTS DERIVED FROM FOLLICLE OR CORPUS LUTEUM
Develop frequently.
Usually regress spontaneously.

ENDOMETRIAL CYSTS

DERMOID CYSTS
Contain various tissues.
Bone in dermoid may be identified.

CYSTADENOMA AND CYSTADENOCARCINOMA

GRANULOSA CELL TUMOR
Estrogen produced by tumor causes endometrial hyperplasia.
May cause postmenopausal bleeding.

MALE HORMONE-PRODUCING TUMORS

Diseases of the Vulva

VULVAR DYSTROPHY
Irregular white patches on vulvar skin (leukoplakia).
Intense itching.
May progress to carcinoma.
Local treatment usually effective.

CARCINOMA OF THE VULVA
Occasionally found in postmenopausal women.
Often preexisting vulvar dystrophy.
Treated by vulvectomy.

Toxic Shock Syndrome

INCIDENCE
Occurs most commonly in women using high-absorbency
  tampons.
No longer a problem with use of current menstrual
  products.

CLINICAL MANIFESTATIONS
Elevated temperature, vomiting, diarrhea.
Erythematous rash.

PATHOGENESIS
Toxin-producing *Staphylococcus* grows in vagina.
Menstrual blood is good culture medium.
Tampons hinder drainage and may injure vaginal mucosa.

TREATMENT
Supportive.
Discontinue tampon use.

Antibiotics to eradicate staphylococci.
Advise no further tampon use.

Contraception

NATURAL FAMILY PLANNING
Avoid intercourse around time of ovulation.
Less effective than artificial methods.

ARTIFICIAL CONTRACEPTION
Diaphragms and condoms: effective and no side effects.
Contraceptive pills: suppress ovulation but have side
  effects.
  Increased tendency to thromboembolic complications,
    especially in cigarette smokers.
  Hypertension develops in some patients.
Intrauterine contraceptive devices (IUDs): prevent
  implantation.
  Increased incidence of tubal infections.
  Increased incidence of tubal pregnancies.
  Emergency contraception used to prevent pregnancy
    after unprotected intercourse.
  Progestin-only pills effective.

Emergency Contraception
Postcoital contraception effective to prevent pregnancy
  resulting from sexual assault or from the failure of
  the contraceptive method being used.

---

http://health.jbpub.com/humandisease/9e

Human Disease Online is a great source for supplementary human disease information for both students and instructors. Visit this website to find a variety of useful tools for learning, thinking, and teaching.

Prenatal Development and Diseases Associated with Pregnancy

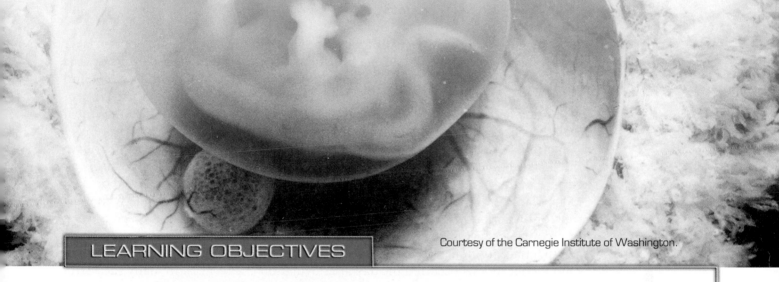

Courtesy of the Carnegie Institute of Washington.

1 Explain the processes of fertilization, implantation, and early development of the ovum, including the origin of the decidua, fetal membranes, and the placenta.

2 Describe how amnionic fluid is formed and eliminated. Identify the conditions leading to abnormal amounts of amnionic fluid.

3 Explain the causes and effects of spontaneous abortion and ectopic pregnancy.

4 Identify and explain the problems that may result if pregnancy occurs after failure of contraceptive pills or an intrauterine device.

5 Describe the mechanism and clinical manifestations of the problems associated with abnormal attachment of the placenta within the uterus and abnormal attachment of the umbilical cord.

6 Differentiate between identical and fraternal twins. Describe how zygosity can be determined from examination of the placenta.

7 List the disadvantages of a twin pregnancy.

8 Classify the types of gestational trophoblast disease. Explain their prognoses, and describe the methods of treatment.

9 Explain the pathogenesis, clinical manifestations, diagnostic criteria, and methods used to treat hemolytic disease of the newborn.

10 Understand the causes and effects of gestational diabetes and pregnancy-associated toxemia.

Fertilization and Prenatal Development

FERTILIZATION

The tadpolelike sperm consists of three parts: a head, a middle piece, and a tail (FIGURE 18-1A). The sperm head contains genetic material. It is partially covered by a thin, membranelike structure called the head cap, which contains enzymes that enable the sperm head to penetrate the ovum at the time of fertilization. The middle piece contains the enzymes that provide the energy required to propel the sperm, and the tail is the propulsive portion. Sperm can travel several millimeters per minute by their own propulsive efforts, but they are also passively transported by rhythmic contractions of the uterine muscles that aspirate them upward into the uterus and fallopian tubes.

The ovum is expelled from the follicle at ovulation. It is surrounded by a thin layer of acellular material called the **zona pellucida** to which are attached clusters of cells from the follicle that are called **granulosa cells** (FIGURE 18-1B). The ovum is swept into the fallopian tube by the beating of the cilia covering the tubal epithelium and is propelled down the tube by the peristaltic contractions of the smooth muscle in the tubal wall. Fertilization is possible when intercourse occurs reasonably close to the time of ovulation. However, the likelihood of a successful conception is related primarily to the survival time of the ovum, about 12–24 hours, rather than the sperm, which can survive in the genital tract and fertilize an ovum for as long as 6 days. Based on data from a large group of women who were trying to become pregnant and in whom the time of ovulation had been determined precisely, some conceptions occurred when intercourse occurred as early as 6 days before ovulation. The likelihood of a successful conception increased as intercourse occurred closer to the time of ovulation, but no conceptions occurred the day after ovulation (TABLE 18-1). In many successful conceptions, the sperm were already "lying in wait" for the ovum in the fallopian tube. When the ovum was ovulated and entered the fallopian tube, it was fertilized by the waiting sperm. The enzymes in the head cap of the sperm disperse the cluster

Zona pellucida
A layer of acellular material surrounding the ovum.

....

Granulosa cells
(gran-u-lō′suh)
Cells lining the ovarian follicles.

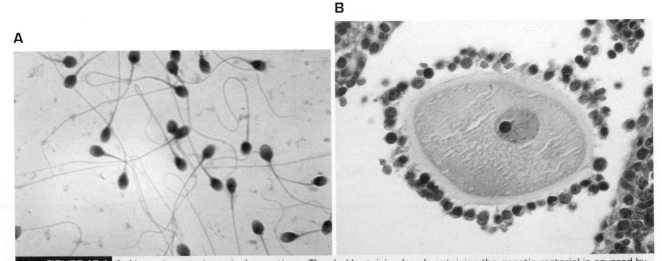

FIGURE 18-1 **A**, Normal sperm in vaginal secretions. The darkly staining head containing the genetic material is covered by a lightly staining head cap that contains the enzymes needed to penetrate the ovum during fertilization. The long narrow tail provides propulsion (original magnification × 1,000). **B**, Mature ovum with adherent granulosa cells. The nucleus is seen near the center of the cell. The homogeneous band surrounding the ovum is the *zona pellucida* (original magnification × 400).

TABLE 18-1

Conception rate based on day of intercourse

Day of intercourse	Percentage of conceptions
6 days before ovulation	8%
5 days before ovulation	10%
4 days before ovulation	16%
3 days before ovulation	no data
2 days before ovulation	28%
1 day before ovulation	32%
day of ovulation	36%
day after ovulation	none

Data from Wilcox, A.J. et al. Timing of sexual intercourse in relation to ovulation. Effects on the probability of conception, survival of the pregnancy, and sex of the baby. *N Engl J Med.* 1995 Dec 7;333(23):1517–21.

of granulosa cells and permit the sperm head to penetrate the zona pellucida. After the sperm has penetrated, the ovum completes its second meiotic division (oogenesis is described in the discussion on chromosomes, genes, and cell division). Sperm penetration causes the zona pellucida to become impermeable to penetration by other sperm, assuring that only one sperm can enter the egg. Fusion of the sperm head and egg nucleus (each containing 23 chromosomes) restores the genetic component of the cell to 46 chromosomes, and the fertilized ovum is now termed a **zygote**.

EARLY DEVELOPMENT OF THE FERTILIZED OVUM

As the fertilized ovum passes along the fallopian tube, it undergoes a series of mitotic divisions. The first cell division is completed about 30 hours after fertilization. Subsequent divisions occur in rapid succession and convert the zygote into a small, mulberry-shaped ball of cells called a **morula**, which is enclosed within the zona pellucida. The morula reaches the endometrial cavity by about the third day. Soon fluid begins to accumulate in the center of the morula, and a central cavity forms. At this stage of development, the structure is called a **blastocyst**. The cells of the blastocyst begin to differentiate into two different groups of cells: the **inner cell mass**, which will form the embryo, and a peripheral rim of cells, called the **trophoblast**, which will give rise to the fetal membranes and will contribute to the formation of the placenta.

The blastocyst lies free within the endometrial cavity for several days. Then the zona pellucida degenerates, exposing the trophoblast. The blastocyst begins to burrow into the endometrium by the end of the first week after fertilization and soon becomes completely embedded (FIGURE 18-2).

Soon after implantation, the inner cell mass becomes a flat structure called the **germ disk**, which differentiates into the three germ layers: ectoderm, mesoderm, and entoderm. Each of the layers will give rise to specific tissues and organs as described in the discussion on cells and tissues. A fluid-filled sac called the **amnionic sac** forms between the ectoderm of the germ disk and the surrounding trophoblast, and a second sac called the **yolk sac** forms on the opposite side of the germ disk. The interior of the blastocyst cavity then becomes lined by a layer of primitive connective tissue cells (**mesoderm**) that also covers the external surfaces of the amnionic sac and yolk sac. As soon as the blastocyst cavity acquires a connective tissue lining, it is called the chorionic cavity, and its wall is called the **chorion**. The entire sac with its enclosed amnion,

Zygote (zī′gōt)
The fertilized ovum.

Morula
A mulberry-shaped solid cluster of cells formed by division of the fertilized ovum.

Blastocyst
A stage of development of the fertilized ovum (zygote) in which a central cavity accumulates within the cluster of developing cells.

Inner cell mass
A group of cells that are derived from the fertilized ovum and are destined to form the embryo.

Trophoblast
Cell derived from the fertilized ovum that gives rise to the fetal membranes and contributes to the formation of the placenta.

Germ disk
A three-layered cluster of cells that will eventually give rise to an embryo.

Amnionic sac
(am-nē-on′ik)
The fluid-filled sac surrounding the embryo. One of the fetal membranes.

Yolk sac
A sac that is formed adjacent to the germ disk and that will form the gastrointestinal tract and other important structures in the embryo.

Mesoderm
(me′zō-derm)
The middle germ layer of the embryo, which gives rise to specific organs and tissues.

Chorion (kō′ri-on)
The layer of trophoblast and associated mesoderm that surrounds the developing embryo.

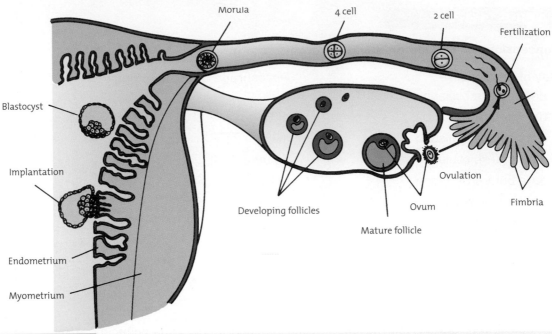

FIGURE 18-2 Summary of the maturation of the ovum, fertilization, and early development of the fertilized ovum.

Chorionic vesicle
The chorion with its villi and enclosed amnion, yolk sac, and developing embryo.

Chorionic villi
Fingerlike columns of cells extending from the chorion that anchor the chorionic vesicle in the endometrium.

Body stalk
The structure connecting the embryo to the chorion. Eventually develops into the umbilical cord.

yolk sac, and developing embryo is called the **chorionic vesicle**. Fingerlike columns of cells called **chorionic villi** extend from the chorion and anchor the chorionic vesicle in the endometrium (FIGURE 18-3).

The chorionic cavity continues to enlarge, and the chorionic vesicle increases in size and complexity. By the end of the second week after fertilization, the small germ disk with its surrounding amnion and yolk sac projects into the chorionic cavity, suspended from the wall of the chorion by a mass of connective tissue called the **body stalk** (FIGURE 18-4).

By the fourth week after fertilization, the organ systems begin to form, and the embryo, which had been flat, becomes cylindrical. The central part of the germ disk grows more rapidly than the periphery, owing to the beginning formation of the nervous system. As a result, the germ disk flexes and bulges into the amnionic

A **B**

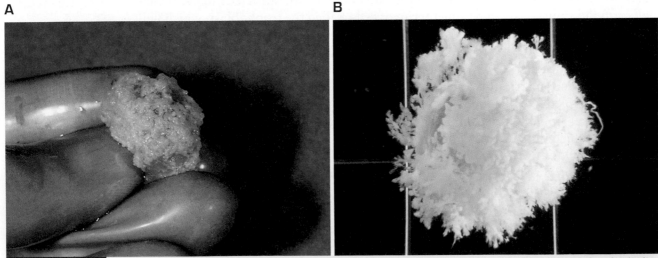

FIGURE 18-3 A, Spontaneously aborted chorionic vesicle about 6 weeks after conception. **B**, Closer view of a chorionic vesicle illustrating frondlike chorionic villi projecting from the chorion.

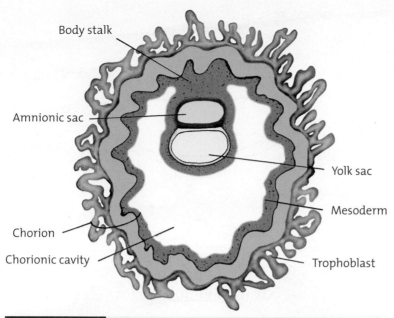

Body stalk

Amnionic sac

Chorion

Chorionic cavity

Yolk sac

Mesoderm

Trophoblast

FIGURE 18-4 Appearance of the chorionic vesicle at the end of the second week after ovulation, illustrating the relation of the germ disk to the amnion, chorion, body stalk, and chorionic cavity.

cavity. The amnionic sac, which is attached to the lateral margins of the germ disk, follows the changing contour of the embryo and is reflected around the embryo. Part of the yolk sac also becomes enfolded within the embryo when flexion occurs (FIGURE 18-5). The enclosed part will give rise to the intestinal tract and other important structures. The lateral margins of the germ disk also fuse in the midline to form the ventral (anterior) body wall. The fusion is incomplete in the middle of the body wall where the umbilical cord is attached, and part of the yolk sac that was not included within the embryo protrudes through the defect. It persists for a time but soon degenerates.

STAGES OF PRENATAL DEVELOPMENT

It is customary to subdivide prenatal development into three main periods:

1. The preembryonic period
2. The embryonic period
3. The fetal period

The first 3 weeks after fertilization are the preembryonic period. During this time, the blastocyst becomes implanted and the inner cell mass differentiates into the three germ layers that will eventually form specific tissues within the embryo.

The embryonic period extends from the third through the seventh week. This is the time when the developing organism begins to assume a human shape and is called an **embryo**. This is also the time when all the organ systems are formed. Consequently, it is a very critical period of development. At this stage, drugs ingested by the mother, radiation, some viral infections, and various other factors may disturb embryonic development and lead to congenital abnormalities, as described in the discussion on congenital and hereditary diseases.

The fetal period extends from the eighth week until the time of delivery. The developing organism is no longer called an embryo; the term **fetus** is now applied.

Embryo
(em′brē-ō)
The developing human organism from the third to the seventh weeks of gestation.

Fetus
The unborn offspring after 8 weeks' gestation.

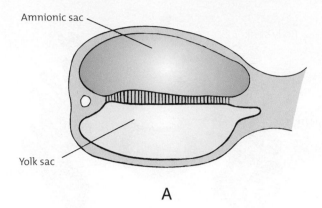

A

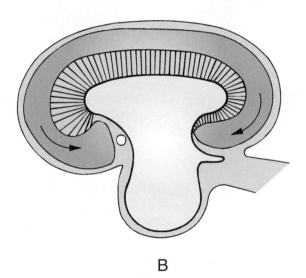

B

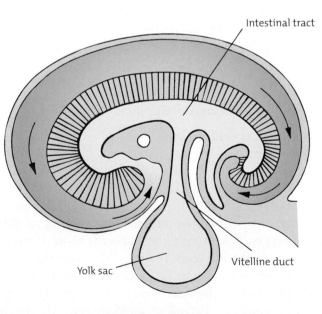

C

FIGURE 18-5 Changes in shape of the embryo resulting from more rapid growth of germ disk. **A**, The flat germ disk with the amnionic sac *above* and the yolk sac *below*. **B**, The embryo begins to bulge into amnionic sac. **C**, Flexion completed. Part of yolk sac is included in the body of the embryo and will form the intestinal tract. The embryo now has a cylindrical configuration. Part of the yolk sac remains connected to the embryo by a narrow vitelline duct.

As the fetus grows, it becomes larger and heavier, but there are no major changes in its basic structure comparable to those in the embryonic period. Initially, the fetal head is disproportionately large, and the body appears quite scrawny because subcutaneous fat has not yet been deposited (FIGURE 18-6). Shortly before delivery, subcutaneous fat begins to accumulate and the body begins to fill out. FIGURE 18-7 illustrates the progressive changes in the size of the fetus in relation to the duration of the gestation.

DURATION OF PREGNANCY

The total duration of pregnancy from fertilization to delivery is called the period of gestation. This is approximately 38 weeks when dated from the time of ovulation. Usually, however, the actual date of ovulation is not known, and the length of gestation is calculated from the beginning of the last normal menstrual period. Expressed in this way, the duration of pregnancy is 40 weeks because the first day of the calculation is actually about 2 weeks before the date of conception. The gestation calculated in this way may also be expressed as 280 days, as 10 lunar (28-day) months, or 9 calendar (31-day) months. Sometimes the 9 calendar months are subdivided into three periods called trimesters, each of 3 months' duration.

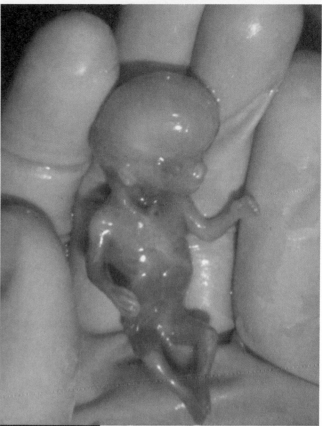

FIGURE 18-6 Small well-formed spontaneously aborted fetus near the end of the first trimester. At this stage, this fetus weighs only 10 g and measures 5 cm from head to buttocks. Its small size can be appreciated by comparing the fetus with the gloved hand that holds it.

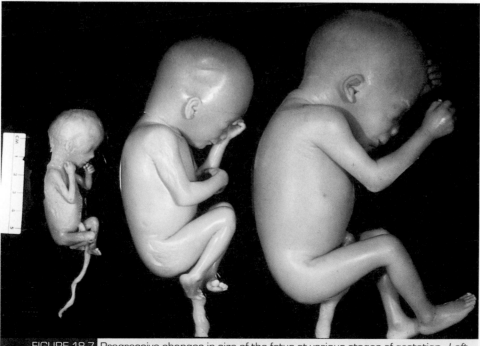

FIGURE 18-7 Progressive changes in size of the fetus at various stages of gestation. *Left,* Three and one-half months (32 g). *Center,* Four and one-half months (230 g). *Right,* Five and one-half months (420 g).

Decidua, Fetal Membranes, and Placenta

FIGURE 18-8 demonstrates the relationship of the embryo to the surrounding amnionic sac and chorion about 7 weeks after fertilization. FIGURE 18-9 diagrammatically illustrates these relationships in both early and late pregnancy.

THE DECIDUA

Decidua (de-sid'ū-ah)
The endometrium of pregnancy.

The endometrium of pregnancy is called the **decidua**. Special names are applied to the parts of the decidua in which the chorionic vesicle is embedded, as indicated in FIGURE 18-9. The part beneath the chorionic vesicle is called the decidua basalis. The part that is stretched over the vesicle is called the decidua capsularis, and the part that lines the rest of the endometrial cavity is called the decidua parietalis (*parietes* = wall). As the embryo and its surrounding amnionic sac continue to increase in size, the thin capsular decidua becomes stretched and thinned. Eventually, it fuses with the decidua parietalis on the opposite wall of the uterus.

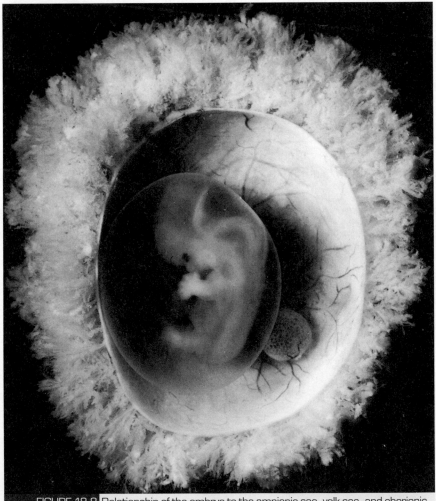

FIGURE 18-8 Relationship of the embryo to the amnionic sac, yolk sac, and chorionic cavity at about 7 weeks after conception. The chorionic sac has been bisected. At this stage, villi still arise from the entire periphery of the chorion, and the amnionic sac surrounding the embryo does not completely fill the chorionic cavity. The embryo is attached to the chorion by the umbilical cord (not shown in the photograph). The yolk sac is located to the right of the amnionic sac, between the amnionic sac and the chorion (photograph courtesy of the Carnegie Institution of Washington).

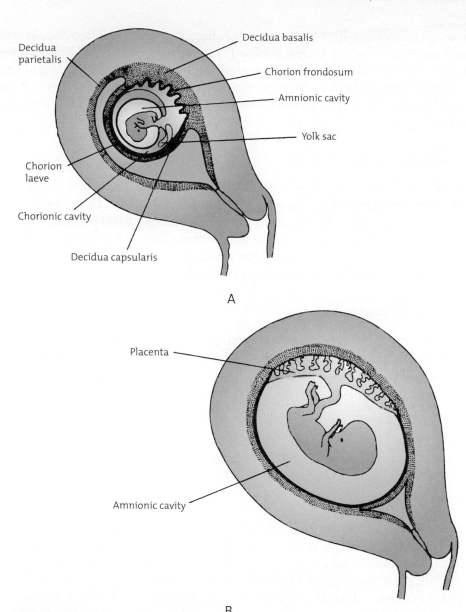

A

B

FIGURE 18-9 **A**, Relationship of the fetus to the decidua, fetal membranes, and chorion in early pregnancy. The part of the yolk sac not incorporated within the fetus lies between the amnionic sac and the chorion. **B**, Relationship in late pregnancy. The amnionic sac envelops the fetus and now completely fills the chorionic cavity. The amnionic membrane lies against the chorion. The decidua capsularis has fused with the chorion laeve and has become adherent to the decidua parietalis on the opposite wall of the uterus.

THE CHORION AND CHORIONIC VILLI

The chorion contains the fetal blood vessels that extend into the chorionic villi. At first, the chorionic villi arise from the entire periphery of the chorion, but soon the villi arising from the superficial part of the chorion become compressed by the decidua capsularis and atrophy. This part of the chorion, which is devoid of villi, is called the chorion laeve (*laeve* = smooth). In contrast, the villi arising from the deeper portion of the chorion adjacent to the decidua basalis proliferate actively. This part of the chorion is called the chorion frondosum because of the frondlike appearance of the villi. These villi project into the large blood-filled spaces within the decidua basalis through which the maternal blood flows. Some of the villi also function as anchoring villi, which attach the chorion to the basal decidua, as well as sending extensions into the maternal blood-filled spaces in the basal decidua. Blood vessels that form within the villi as they grow become connected with blood vessels in the chorion and the body stalk, as well as within the body of the embryo. As soon as the embryo's heart begins to beat, blood begins to flow through this developing network of vessels.

THE AMNIONIC SAC

The **amnionic sac** is enclosed within the chorion. At first the sac is much smaller than the chorionic cavity (see Figure 18-8), but the enlarging sac expands into the chorionic cavity. Eventually the amnionic sac completely fills the chorionic cavity and the amnionic membrane lies against the chorion. The sac functions as a buoyant, temperature-controlled environment that protects the fetus throughout pregnancy and assists in opening the cervix during childbirth.

THE YOLK SAC

In the human being, the yolk sac never contains yolk, but it performs other important functions. Part of the yolk sac becomes incorporated into the body of the embryo to form the intestinal tract. The part that is not included within the embryo persists for a time but eventually atrophies.

THE PLACENTA

The **placenta** is a flattened, disk-shaped structure weighing about 500 g. It has a dual origin, both fetal and maternal (FIGURE 18-10). The chorion and the villi are formed from the trophoblast, which is of fetal origin, and the decidua basalis in which the villi are anchored is derived from the endometrium. Incomplete partition of decidua extend into the villi and divide them into aggregates called cotyledons, which impart a vague cobblestone appearance to the maternal surface of the placenta. The amnion and chorion extend from the margins of the placenta to form the fluid-filled sac that encloses the fetus and that ruptures at the time of delivery. The fetus is connected to the placenta by the umbilical cord, which contains two arteries. On the surface of the placenta, the artery divides into multiple branches, each supplying an individual cotyledon. Blood returning from the cotyledons is collected into large veins on the surface of the placenta to form the umbilical vein, which returns the blood to the fetus.

Circulation of Blood in the Placenta

The placenta has a dual circulation of blood (FIGURE 18-11). The fetoplacental circulation delivers arterial blood low in oxygen from the fetus to the chorionic villi through the umbilical artery. It returns oxygenated blood to the fetus in the single umbilical vein. The uteroplacental circulation delivers oxygenated arterial blood from the mother into the large placental blood spaces that are located between the villi and are called the intervillous spaces. The blood spurts into the intervillous spaces from the many uterine arteries that penetrate the basal portion of the placenta. It flows back into the maternal circulation through veins that penetrate the basal part of the placenta. The arrangement of the two circulations in the placenta brings the maternal and fetal blood into close approximation. In this way, oxygen and nutrients can be exchanged between the maternal and fetal circulations, but there is no actual intermixing of fetal and maternal blood.

A

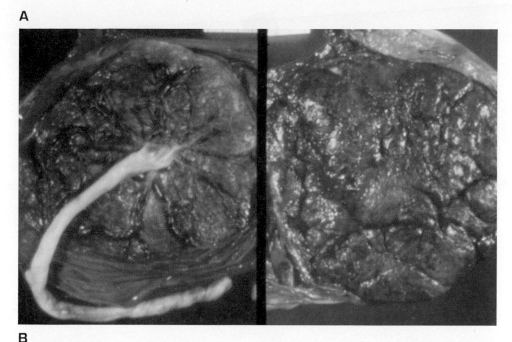

B

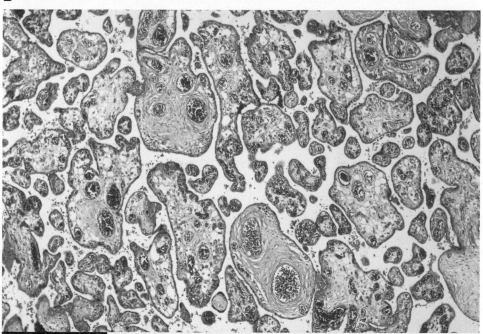

FIGURE 18-10 **A**, Normal placenta. The fetal surface on the *left* shows the umbilical cord and cord vessels that subdivide on placental surface to supply chorionic villi. The cobblestone appearance of the maternal surface of the placenta (*right* side of illustration) is caused by the cotyledons, which are clusters of villi separated by decidual partitions extending between the villi. **B**, Histologic section of placenta revealing chorionic villi viewed in cross section. Blood vessels in villi contain fetal cells. When the placenta is within the uterus, the spaces between the villi are filled with maternal blood (original magnification × 100).

Human placental lactogen (HPL)
(lak′tō-jen)
One of the hormones produced by the placenta that has properties similar to pituitary growth hormone.

Human chorionic gonadotropin (HCG)
(kōr-ē-on′ik gō-nadō -trō′pin)
A hormone made by the placenta in pregnancy having actions similar to pituitary gonadotropins. Same hormone is made by neoplastic cells in some types of malignant testicular tumors.

Endocrine Function of the Placenta

The placenta synthesizes two steroid hormones, estrogen and progesterone, and two protein hormones called **human placental lactogen** (HPL) and **human chorionic gonadotropin** (HCG). HPL stimulates maternal metabolic processes, and HCG is quite similar to the gonadotropic hormones produced by the pituitary gland. Tests that detect HCG are called pregnancy tests. The newer, very sensitive tests, which

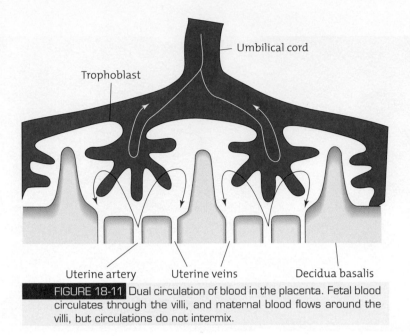

FIGURE 18-11 Dual circulation of blood in the placenta. Fetal blood circulates through the villi, and maternal blood flows around the villi, but circulations do not intermix.

are performed on blood or urine, become positive as early as 10–12 days after fertilization, even before the woman misses her first period.

Amnionic Fluid

Amnionic fluid is produced both by filtration and by excretion, and its quantity varies with the stage of pregnancy. During the early part of pregnancy, the amnionic fluid is formed chiefly by filtration of fluid into the amnionic sac from maternal blood as it passes through the uterus and from fetal blood passing through the placenta. Additional fluid diffuses directly through the fetal skin and from the fetal respiratory tract. Later, when the fetal kidneys begin to function in the last part of pregnancy, the fetus urinates into the amnionic fluid, and fetal urine becomes the major source of this fluid.

Both filtration and fetal urine continually add to the volume of fluid, but the additions are counterbalanced by losses of amnionic fluid into the fetal gastrointestinal tract. Normally, the fetus swallows as much as several hundred milliliters of fluid per day. This fluid is absorbed from the fetal intestinal tract into the fetal circulation, transferred across the placenta into the mother's circulation, and eventually excreted by the mother in her urine.

POLYHYDRAMNIOS AND OLIGOHYDRAMNIOS

Polyhydramnios is a condition in which the volume of amnionic fluid is markedly increased. There are two common causes:

1. A congenital maldevelopment of the fetal brain called **anencephaly** (in the discussion on the nervous system), which disturbs the normal swallowing mechanism, so that the fetus is unable to swallow amnionic fluid
2. A congenital obstruction of the fetal upper intestinal tract that blocks the entry of swallowed fluid into the small intestine where it can be absorbed

Oligohydramnios is a marked reduction in the volume of amnionic fluid. It occurs either because the fetal kidneys have failed to develop and no urine is formed or because a congenital obstruction blocks the urethra so that urine cannot be excreted.

Polyhydramnios
(pä-ē-hī-dram′nē-yus)
An excess of amnionic fluid.

Anencephaly
(an-en-seff′uh-lē)
A congenital malformation: absence of brain, cranial vault, and scalp as a result of defective closure of the neural tube.

Oligohydramnios
(ol-ig-ō-hī-dram′nē-yus)
An insufficient quantity of amnionic fluid.

Hormone-Related Conditions Associated with Pregnancy

Pregnancy affects almost all of the hormones produced by a woman's endocrine glands and by her placenta, which maintain the pregnancy and sustain the fetus, but some have undesirable effects on the pregnant woman.

NAUSEA AND VOMITING DURING EARLY PREGNANCY

This condition is related to the rapidly increasing levels of estrogen in early pregnancy; nausea and vomiting often occur in the morning (morning sickness) and usually subside by the end of the first trimester (first 3 months of pregnancy).

HYPEREMESIS GRAVIDARUM

This term literally means excessive vomiting of pregnancy, and probably has the same hormonal basis as morning sickness but is more prolonged and severe. Weight loss and dehydration may require treatment with intravenous fluids.

GESTATIONAL DIABETES

Effects of Hyperglycemia on Pregnancy

An elevated blood glucose concentration in the maternal blood (hyperglycemia), as occurs in diabetes (described in the discussion on the pancreas and diabetes mellitus), is harmful to the developing fetus. In early pregnancy when the organ systems are developing, the hyperglycemia may cause congenital malformations or even lead to fetal death. Later in the pregnancy, the extra glucose crossing the placenta into the fetal bloodstream causes the fetal pancreas to release more insulin, and the extra glucose is metabolized to promote fetal growth. As a result, the fetus becomes larger than average size and the larger fetal kidneys secrete more urine, which contributes to the volume of amnionic fluid and causes its volume to increase. Delivery of the oversized fetus may be more difficult, and a cesarean section may be required. After delivery, the infant's blood glucose may fall precipitously (hypoglycemia) because the newborn infant's pancreas has been accustomed to dealing with a much higher intrauterine blood glucose concentration and has not had time to compensate for the lower postdelivery blood glucose. The infant also faces neonatal respiratory distress problems caused by inadequate surfactant, as described in the discussion on the respiratory system. For these reasons, recognition and treatment of hyperglycemia in pregnancy are in the best interest of both the mother and her baby.

In all pregnancies during the second 3 months (second trimester) the high placental hormone levels cause the body to become less responsive to insulin (called insulin resistance), which tends to raise blood glucose, but usually the pregnant woman compensates by secreting more insulin, and the blood glucose remains normal.

Some women who were considered nondiabetic before becoming pregnant may not be able to produce enough insulin to maintain a normal glucose concentration during pregnancy because of the insulin resistance caused by the high hormone levels in pregnancy. The condition is called gestational diabetes because the blood glucose is likely to return to normal after the pregnancy, although women with gestational diabetes may be at higher risk of developing type 2 diabetes in later years.

Gestational diabetes occurs in about 2% of pregnancies and is much higher in older women, in obese women, and in women from ethnic groups having a high frequency of diabetes. It is important to identify pregnant women with gestational diabetes so that they can be treated by diet and additional insulin if necessary to maintain a normal blood glucose during pregnancy, which avoids the hazards of hyperglycemia on her fetus.

Prenatal patients should be evaluated on their initial visit for any risk factors—such as obesity, gestational diabetes in a previous pregnancy, a family history of diabetes, and any other factors that might predispose her to gestational diabetes—and some type of screening test should be performed. The usual screening test consists of 50 g of glucose solution given orally without regard to fasting status, and the concentration of glucose in the patient's blood is determined in a sample collected 1 hour later. If the result exceeds a predetermined concentration, more comprehensive studies are performed to confirm the diagnosis of gestational diabetes, and a course of treatment is begun.

Spontaneous Abortion ("Miscarriage")

Most spontaneous abortions occur early in pregnancy. The actual incidence is difficult to establish but is estimated to be from 10 to 20% of all pregnancies. Many spontaneous abortions are a result of chromosomal abnormalities or maldevelopment of the embryo that rendered it incapable of survival. Others result from defective implantation of the fertilized ovum within the endometrial cavity. In many cases, the cause of spontaneous abortion in early pregnancy cannot be determined.

Occasionally, intrauterine fetal death occurs late in pregnancy. This is generally caused by partial detachment of the placenta from the wall of the uterus, which is called placental abruption, or by obstruction of the blood supplied through the umbilical cord. Compression of the blood vessels in the umbilical cord, shutting off the blood supply to the fetus, may occur if the cord becomes knotted or wrapped tightly around the infant's neck or limbs (FIGURE 18-12). If the placenta becomes separated or the cord becomes obstructed, the fetus no longer receives oxygen and nutrients from the mother, and it dies. A dead fetus is usually expelled promptly, but occasionally, it is retained within the uterine cavity for several weeks or months.

Cocaine abuse in pregnancy also has been shown to cause intrauterine fetal death. Cocaine increases maternal heart rate, constricts arterioles, and raises blood pressure. The constriction of uterine arterioles reduces uterine blood flow and impairs oxygen supply to the fetus. In some patients, the high pressure within the uterine arterioles may cause one of the vessels to rupture. As a result, a large hemorrhage forms between the uterine wall and the placenta and partially separates

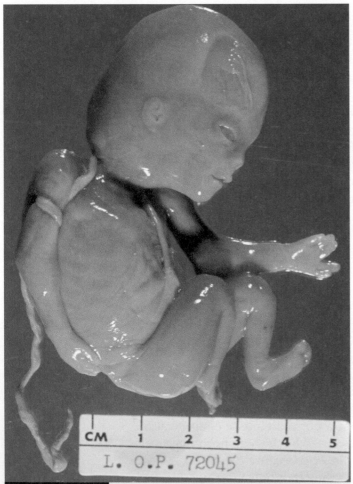

CM 1 2 3 4 5

L. O. P. 72045

FIGURE 18-12 Fetus spontaneously aborted late in pregnancy because of interruption of blood supply through the umbilical cord. The cord extended around back of neck and had become tightly wrapped around upper arm, shutting off circulation and leading to intrauterine death.

the placenta from the uterus (placental abruption), which severely compromises oxygenation of fetal blood.

If a dead fetus is retained for some time within the uterine cavity, products of degenerated fetal tissue diffuse into the maternal circulation. This material has thromboplastic activity and may induce a hemorrhagic disease in the mother because of depletion of maternal blood-coagulation factors that occurs when the coagulation mechanism is activated by the thromboplastic material. A retained dead fetus is one cause of the **disseminated intravascular coagulation syndrome**, which is discussed in the abnormalities of blood coagulation.

Ectopic Pregnancy

An ectopic pregnancy (*ecto* = outside) is the development of an embryo outside its normal location within the uterine cavity. Most ectopic pregnancies occur in the fallopian tubes, but on rare occasions a fertilized ovum develops in the ovary or abdominal cavity. Normally, fertilization occurs in the fallopian tube and the fertilized ovum then proceeds into the endometrial cavity, where implantation takes place at the end of the first week after fertilization. Implantation may take place in the fallopian tube, however, if transport of the ovum is delayed. Two factors predispose to this complication:

1. A previous infection in the fallopian tubes. Often this is followed by scarring and fusion of tubal folds, which retards the passage of the fertilized egg through the tube.
2. Failure of the muscular contractions of the tubal wall to propel the ovum through the tube.

Frequently, the conditions that predispose to a tubal pregnancy affect both fallopian tubes. Consequently, a woman who has had one tubal pregnancy is more likely to develop an ectopic pregnancy in the opposite tube.

CONSEQUENCES OF TUBAL PREGNANCY

An ectopic pregnancy in the fallopian tube gradually distends the tube. The embryo may develop normally for a time but rarely survives for more than a few months. The invading trophoblast erodes tubal blood vessels, causing bleeding into the lumen and wall of the tube and sometimes into the tissues surrounding it.

A woman with an ectopic pregnancy experiences signs and symptoms of early pregnancy and misses her expected menstrual period, as with a normal intrauterine pregnancy. She may also complain of some abdominal pain and tenderness caused by distention of the tube and irritation of the pelvic peritoneum caused by bleeding in the tube wall and adjacent tissues. She may also experience slight vaginal bleeding if blood leaks from the tubal implantation site, escapes into the uterus, and is discharged into the vagina.

Rupture of the tube can occur at any time (FIGURE 18-13). This catastrophe is accompanied by severe abdominal pain and profuse intra-abdominal bleeding caused by disruption of large tubal blood vessels at the site of rupture. If the patient is not treated promptly, tubal rupture may prove fatal because of the severe hemorrhage that occurs.

The following case illustrates some of the common clinical features encountered in a patient with a ruptured ectopic pregnancy.

Because of the potential life threatening risk of a ruptured tubal pregnancy, a physician always considers the possibility of a tubal pregnancy in any woman of reproductive age who exhibits any symptoms suggesting a tubal pregnancy. A pelvic examination reveals an area of tenderness adjacent to the uterus and may also reveal a fullness or mass caused by the swollen tube. A positive pregnancy test confirms the pregnancy, and an

Disseminated intravascular coagulation syndrome
A disturbance of blood coagulation as a result of activation of the coagulation mechanism and simultaneous clot lysis.

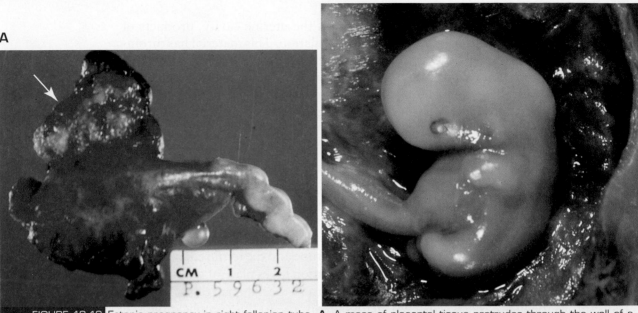

FIGURE 18-13 Ectopic pregnancy in right fallopian tube. **A**, A mass of placental tissue protrudes through the wall of a greatly distended fallopian tube (*arrow*). **B**, The embryo contained within the intact amnionic sac.

CASE 18-1

A 34-year-old woman consulted her physician because of recent onset of severe abdominal pain. Her last normal menstrual period had been 10 weeks earlier. For the previous 2 weeks, she had experienced mild abdominal pain and slight intermittent vaginal bleeding. On examination, she exhibited evidence of severe blood loss, and her abdomen was diffusely tender. A diagnosis of ruptured ectopic pregnancy was made, and an operation was performed immediately. A large amount of blood was found within the abdominal cavity as a result of a ruptured ectopic pregnancy in the midportion of the left fallopian tube. The ruptured tube was removed, and the severe blood loss was treated by four blood transfusions. The patient made a satisfactory recovery.

ultrasound examination demonstrates that the chorionic vesicle indicative of pregnancy is not within the uterus. If these findings indicate that a tubal pregnancy is likely, a laparoscopic examination is performed, which allows the physician to visualize the fallopian tubes and ovaries and to identify the unruptured pregnancy within the fallopian tube.

Although a ruptured tubal pregnancy is usually treated by resection of the torn fallopian tube along with the ectopic pregnancy, it is often possible to remove the ectopic pregnancy without resecting the tube if the tube has not yet ruptured. Sometimes the ectopic pregnancy can be dislodged from its tubal attachment by manipulating the tube and then expressing the ectopic pregnancy from the tube through the fimbriated end. Usually, it is necessary to incise the distended tube and evacuate the ectopic pregnancy.

A nonsurgical treatment has also been used successfully. A single oral dose of an antimetabolite drug called methotrexate destroys the tubal pregnancy, eliminating the need for a surgical procedure in which the tube is incised and the pregnancy is evacuated. Antimetabolite drugs destroy rapidly dividing cells by interrupting their metabolic processes and are used to treat patients with cancer, as described in the discussion on neoplastic disease.

Pregnancy Subsequent to Failure of Artificial Contraception

FAILURE OF CONTRACEPTIVE PILLS

Estrogen-progestin contraceptive pills are highly effective when used properly, but occasional pregnancies do occur, usually because of failure to take the pills regularly or at the proper time. If a woman becomes pregnant while taking oral contraceptives, the developing embryo is exposed to the synthetic estrogen and progestin compounds during the critical early stages of embryonic development. This exposure may lead to congenital malformations. The risk is low, but women must be advised of the possibility.

FAILURE OF AN INTRAUTERINE DEVICE

Intrauterine devices (IUDs) are no longer a popular method of contraception, and most of these devices are no longer marketed. Some women, however, are still using IUDs. In about 2% of women, an intrauterine device fails to prevent implantation and pregnancy occurs. This event may lead to serious and sometimes life threatening complications. The IUD predisposes to infection of the pregnant uterus that in some cases is followed without warning by a serious and sometimes fatal bloodstream infection (septicemia). Because of this hazard, the IUD should be removed as soon as the pregnancy is diagnosed. This can usually be accomplished without great difficulty if the string is visible. Often, the pregnancy continues normally after the IUD has been removed, but sometimes removal disturbs the implantation site and leads to spontaneous abortion. If the IUD cannot be removed or if the string has retracted inside the uterus, most physicians recommend that the pregnancy be terminated. If the woman decides to continue the pregnancy, she must be closely observed throughout her pregnancy because of the increased risk of serious infection.

Abnormal Attachment of the Umbilical Cord and Placenta

VELAMENTOUS INSERTION OF THE UMBILICAL CORD

Sometimes the umbilical cord vessels are not gathered together normally, and the cord attaches to the membranes attached to the placenta (fetal membranes) rather than to the placenta itself. When this occurs, the umbilical vessels must travel for a distance within the fetal membranes before reaching the placenta (FIGURE 18-14). This is called a **velamentous insertion of the umbilical cord** (*velum* = veil). The abnormality may be very hazardous to the fetus if the vessels are located in the membranes that extend over the cervix because these vessels may be compressed or ruptured in the course of labor or delivery. If one of the vessels ruptures, the circulation between the fetus and placenta is disrupted, and the fetus bleeds to death through the ruptured vessel. Because the maternal and fetal circulations are not interconnected, however, the flow of maternal blood through the intervillous space is not disturbed, and the mother does not suffer any adverse effects. Even if the vessels crossing the cervix do not rupture, they may be compressed by the fetal head during delivery, causing fetal death by shutting off the circulation through the umbilical vessels.

Velamentous insertion of umbilical cord
(vel′uh-men-tus)
Attachment of the umbilical cord to the fetal membranes rather than to the placenta.

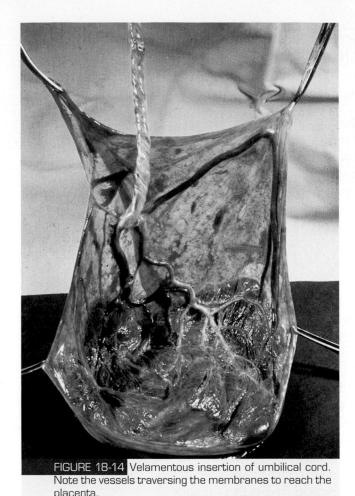

FIGURE 18-14 Velamentous insertion of umbilical cord. Note the vessels traversing the membranes to reach the placenta.

PLACENTA PREVIA

Normally, the placenta attaches high on the anterior or posterior uterine wall. If the placenta becomes attached in the lower part of the uterus, it may cover the cervix. This is called a **placenta previa** (FIGURE 18-15). The term literally means a placenta blocking the exit from the uterus (*pre* = before + *via* = pathway). A placenta that completely covers the cervix is called a central placenta previa. If only the edge of the placenta encroaches on the cervix, the abnormality is designated a partial placenta previa. The patient with a placenta previa experiences episodes of bleeding during the last part of pregnancy, as a consequence of partial separation of the placenta from the uterine wall. Normally, the lower part of the uterus undergoes gradual dilatation during the last part of pregnancy in preparation for childbirth. The abnormally located placenta is unable to stretch to conform to the contour of the expanding lower part of the uterus, and parts of the placenta therefore tear loose. The tearing disrupts the large uterine vessels that penetrate the basal part of the placenta to supply the intervillous spaces (see Figure 18-11). In contrast with a velamentous insertion of the cord, which places only the infant in jeopardy, placenta previa is hazardous to the mother as well. The mother may bleed to death if a large part of the placenta is

Placenta previa
(prē′vē-yuh)
Attachment of the placenta in the uterus such that it partially or completely covers the cervix.

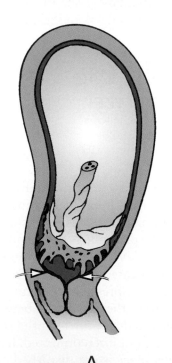
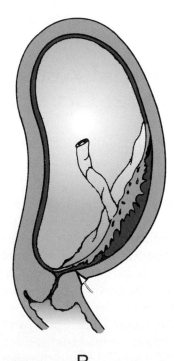

A   B

FIGURE 18-15 Types of placenta previa. **A**, Central placenta previa. **B**, Partial placenta previa. The *arrows* indicate the usual locations where the placenta tears from its attachment to the lower part of the uterus late in pregnancy.

torn from the uterine wall. Large areas of placental disruption may also prevent proper oxygenation of fetal blood passing through the placenta, leading to the death of the fetus.

Because the placenta blocks the cervix, vaginal delivery is not possible without the risk of severe hemorrhage and injury to the cervix. Delivery is generally accomplished by cesarean section.

Twins and Multiple Pregnancies

Normally, about 1% of all pregnancies are twins (approximately 1 in 100). Twins may be either identical (monozygotic) or fraternal (dizygotic). Approximately 0.01% of pregnancies (approximately 1 in 10,000) are triplets. Quadruplets, quintuplets, and sextuplets are rare. The incidence of all types of multiple pregnancies is much higher than normal when ovulation is induced by administration of gonadotropic hormones or other drugs.

FRATERNAL TWINS

Seventy percent of twins are fraternal and result from fertilization of two separate ova by two different sperm. Fraternal twins are no more alike than brothers and sisters, but they share a family resemblance because they are born of the same parents. Each fertilized ovum implants separately, and each twin forms its own placenta and fetal membranes. Frequently, the margins of the two placentas grow together and fuse, but each fetus remains enclosed within its own amnion and chorion. A fused placenta of this type is called a diamnionic dichorionic placenta.

IDENTICAL TWINS

Thirty percent of twins are identical and result from the splitting of a single fertilized ovum. Splitting may occur at various times after fertilization, as illustrated in FIGURE 18-16. In about 30% of monozygotic twin pregnancies, the fertilized ovum splits before the inner cell mass forms, which is on the third day after fertilization. Each half of the zygote implants separately, forms a complete embryo, and develops its own placenta. The two placentas may remain separate or may become fused to form a diamnionic dichorionic placenta in the same manner as that for fraternal twins.

More commonly (in almost 70% of monozygotic twin pregnancies), the inner cell mass divides after the blastocyst has formed but before implantation takes place. In this instance, each half of the inner cell mass forms a complete embryo and develops its own amnion and yolk sac, but both develop within a single chorionic cavity. This gives rise to a placenta called a diamnionic monochorionic placenta.

Rarely, the inner cell mass divides after the amnionic sac has already formed. When this occurs, the two embryos develop within a single amnionic cavity and form a monoamnionic monochorionic placenta. If the division of the inner cell mass is incomplete, conjoined (Siamese) twins are formed.

DETERMINATION OF ZYGOSITY OF TWINS FROM EXAMINATION OF PLACENTA

It is often desirable to know at the time of birth whether the twins are identical or fraternal. If they are of different sexes, they must be fraternal, but if they are the same sex, they could be either fraternal or identical. Sometimes, the zygosity of the twins can be determined by examining the placenta. If there are two separate placentas,

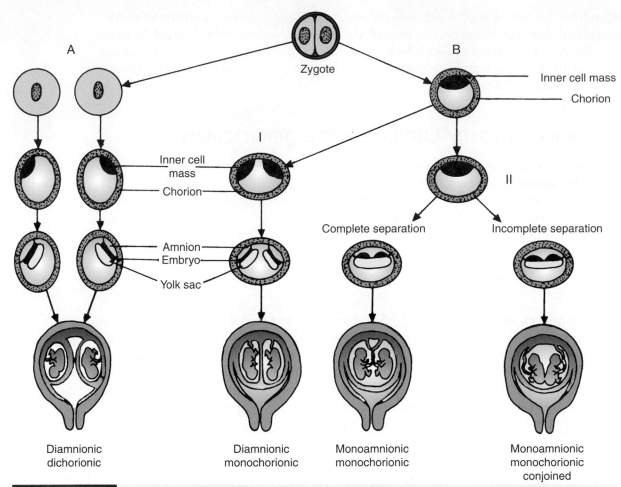

FIGURE 18-16 Stages at which formation of identical twins can occur, and types of placenta associated with each stage of twinning. **A**, Early splitting of fertilized ovum, forming two separate zygotes that develop and implant separately. **B** I, Inner cell mass splits, giving rise to two embryos within single chorionic cavity. **B** II, Later splitting of inner cell mass after the amnionic sac has formed. Complete separation of the inner cell mass gives rise to two embryos within a single amnionic sac. Incomplete separation gives rise to conjoined twins.

the twins must have implanted separately. A single placenta with two amnionic sacs, however, could be either a monochorionic placenta or a dichorionic placenta. It is possible to distinguish between these two types of placentas by gross and microscopic examination of the partition between the two amnionic sacs because the structure of the partition indicates how it was formed. FIGURE 18-17 compares the arrangement of fetal membranes of twins implanted separately (dichorionic placenta) with that of twins developing within a single chorionic cavity (monochorionic placenta). As the amnionic sacs gradually enlarge, the membranes eventually establish contact and form a midline partition between the two sacs (FIGURE 18-18). If the placenta is monochorionic, the dividing septum consists only of two amnions without intervening chorions; in a dichorionic placenta, four separate membranes can be identified in the partition: two outer amnions and two inner chorions (FIGURE 18-19). A diamnionic monochorionic placenta always indicates identical twins, as does the rare monoamnionic monochorionic placenta. If the placenta is diamnionic dichorionic or if there are two separate placentas, the twins could be either identical or fraternal. All fraternal twins have a diamnionic dichorionic placenta or separate placentas, but so do 30% of identical twins in whom the fertilized ovum split very soon after fertilization.

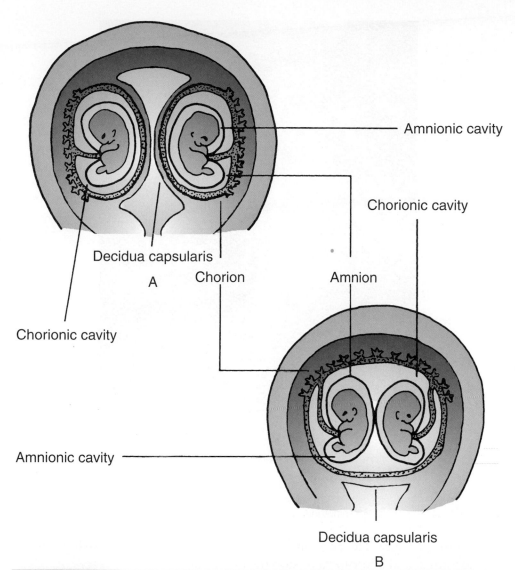

Amnionic cavity

Chorionic cavity

Decidua capsularis

A

Chorion

Amnion

Chorionic cavity

Amnionic cavity

Decidua capsularis

B

FIGURE 18-17 A comparison of the formation of the placentas and fetal membranes in twins. **A,** Separate implantations leading to the formation of a dichorionic placenta. **B,** Twins developing in a single chorionic cavity and forming a monochorionic placenta. A dichorionic placenta can be encountered in either fraternal or identical twins. A monochorionic placenta occurs only in identical twins.

TWIN TRANSFUSION SYNDROME

The placental circulations of identical twins are frequently joined by multiple vascular anastomoses (interconnecting blood vessels), and consequently, there is normally some intermixing of blood from the two fetuses in the placentas (FIGURE 18-20). Sometimes the placental anastomoses are such that an excess of blood from the fetoplacental circulation from one infant (called the donor twin) flows into the circulation of the second twin (called the recipient). If this occurs, the donor twin may become anemic and the recipient twin may become overloaded with blood (polycythemic). Some degree of twin-to-twin transfusion is relatively common and is reported in about 15% of all twin births. Minor differences in the blood volumes of the two twins can be tolerated, but large disproportions are harmful to both twins (FIGURE 18-21). The severe anemia may be fatal to the donor twin, and the circulation of the recipient twin may become so overloaded by the great excess of blood that the polycythemic twin dies of heart failure. None of the methods used to treat a severe twin-to-twin transfusion syndrome are ideal. As a last resort, an instrument can be inserted into the uterus to inspect the

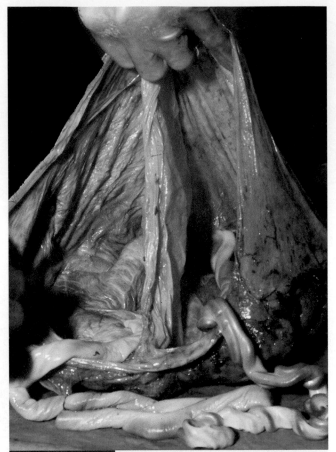

FIGURE 18-18 Partition between amnionic sacs in twin pregnancy. Examination of the partition may indicate the zygosity of the twins. Courtesy of the Carnegie Institute of Washington.

surface of the placenta. The anastomoses responsible for the twin-to-twin transfusion can be identified and interrupted to stop the blood transfer.

The less common identical twins formed from very early splitting of a fertilized ovum, as occurs in about 30% of identical twins, are not at risk of a twin transfusion syndrome. Each half of the fertilized ovum implants separately in the endometrium and each twin forms its own placenta, like the placenta of fraternal twins, so there is no possibility of interconnected placental circulations.

A   **B**

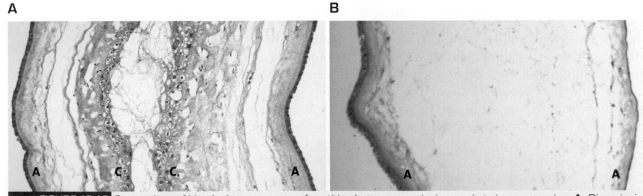

FIGURE 18-19 Comparison of histologic appearance of partition between amnionic sacs in twin pregnancies. **A**, Diamnionic dichorionic placenta, illustrating four layers—two outer layers of amnion (**A**) and two inner layers of chorion (**C**). **B**, Diamnionic monochorionic pregnancy of identical twins, illustrating only two layers of amnion (**A**) without chorions interposed between the two amnions.

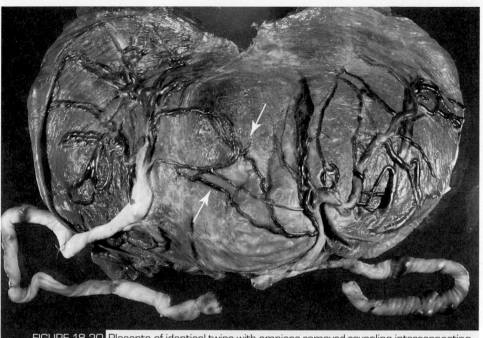

FIGURE 18-20 Placenta of identical twins with amnions removed revealing interconnecting blood vessels (*arrows*).

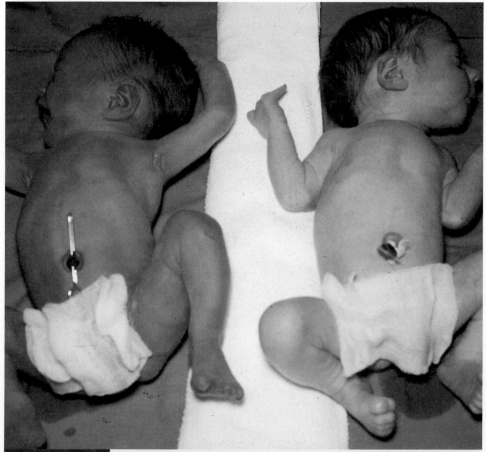

FIGURE 18-21 Identical twins exhibiting twin transfusion syndrome. The twin on the *right* in the photograph is pale and anemic. The twin on the *left* appears ruddy and contains an excess of blood. Both twins survived.

VANISHING TWINS AND BLIGHTED TWINS

Sometimes one twin of a twin pregnancy fails to develop and dies early in pregnancy. The actual incidence of twin pregnancies is significantly higher than indicated from data based on the delivery of two infants at term. Ultrasound studies of first trimester pregnancies reveals that many more pregnancies start out as twins than survive to term. The other twin that fails to survive may be a vanishing twin that is completely absorbed, leaving no trace, or may persist as a blighted twin, which is a degenerated embryo or fetus that is retained within the uterus until the surviving fetus is delivered at term. A blighted fetus associated with a triplet pregnancy is illustrated by the following case.

CASE 18-2

A 30-year-old woman delivered normal, well-formed female twins prematurely at 36 weeks' gestation. Examination of the placenta after delivery revealed a third amnionic sac containing a compressed degenerated fetus measuring 13 cm in length (FIGURE 18-22). The partition between the amnionic sacs consisted of double amnions and double chorions. In this triplet pregnancy, one fetus died at about 17 weeks' gestation and was retained within the uterus until the delivery of the two remaining infants at 36 weeks. Each fetus was enclosed within its own amnion and chorion. Consequently, the zygosity of the surviving twins could not be determined from examination of the placenta because a diamnionic dichorionic placenta can be associated with either identical or fraternal twins.

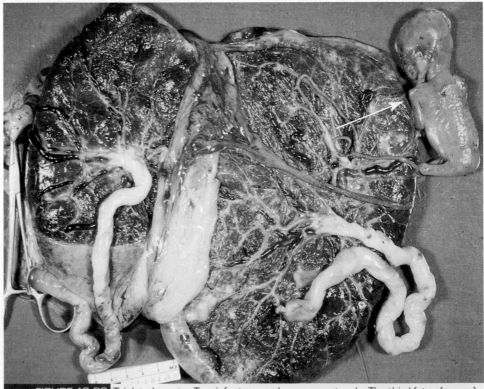

FIGURE 18-22 Triplet placenta. Two infants were born prematurely. The third fetus (*arrow*) died early in pregnancy and was retained within the uterus until delivery of the surviving twins (Case 18-2).

CONJOINED TWINS

Incomplete separation of the inner cell mass leads to a variable degree of union between two **conjoined twins**. The twins may be joined at the head, thorax, abdomen, or pelvis, the union being face to face, side to side, or back to back. The extent of union is variable but often quite considerable, and often the twins share common internal organs to such a degree that it is not possible to separate them surgically. The conjoined twins are generally equal in size and are often well formed except for their failure to separate.

The following case illustrates some of the clinical features associated with conjoined twins.

Conjoined twins
Identical twins that are joined to one another and often share organs in common. Siamese twins.

CASE 18-3

Conjoined twin girls were born to a 25-year-old woman at term. The infants lived only a few hours. Their combined weight was 8 lbs., 10 oz., and they were joined at the lower thorax and upper abdomen. A single umbilical cord supplied both fetuses, and there was a large defect in the lower abdominal wall covered with a thin membrane that ruptured during delivery (FIGURE 18-23). The infants shared a common heart but had separate great vessels entering and leaving the heart. They also shared a single liver but had separate gallbladders and biliary ducts. Each twin had a separate esophagus and stomach, but they shared a common pancreas and duodenum. The remainder of the small bowel and colon were separate. Other organs were separate and normally formed.

A   **B**

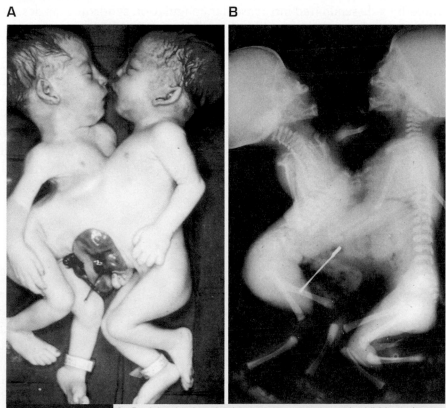

FIGURE 18-23 **A**, Conjoined twins sharing common organs and exhibiting a large congenital defect in the abdominal wall (Case 18-3). **B**, X-ray demonstrating extreme curvature of fetal spine. This resulted from twisting of the spine so that the twins, linked in face-to-face position, could fit within the confines of the crowded uterus.

DISADVANTAGES OF TWIN PREGNANCIES

Twins are at a disadvantage compared with singletons. Because they are overcrowded within the uterus, a twin is always smaller than a single infant at a comparable stage of gestation. Overdistention of the uterus frequently promotes premature onset of labor, leading to delivery of premature infants having a reduced chance of survival. Congenital malformations occur twice as often in twins as in singletons, and vascular anastomosis within the placental circulation may lead to a twin transfusion syndrome.

Preeclampsia and Eclampsia: Toxemia of Pregnancy

Preeclampsia
(prē-ēk-lamp-sē-a)
A pregnancy-related complication characterized by hypertension and proteinuria which usually occurs after the 20th week of gestation, thought to be caused by placental dysfunction.

Eclampsia
(ēk-lamp-sē-a)
One or more convulsions in a pregnant woman with preeclampsia.

Preeclampsia is a pregnancy-associated elevated blood pressure exceeding 140/90, accompanied by protein in the urine, which has its onset any time from the 20th week of gestation to the end of the pregnancy. It is more common in young girls and older women, in twin pregnancies, and in women who have had preeclampsia in a previous pregnancy. In severe cases, blood pressure exceeds 160/110 and may be associated with convulsions, which is called **eclampsia**, and the two conditions are grouped under the general term toxemia of pregnancy. The condition seems to be caused by inadequate blood flow to the placenta. The placental dysfunction leads to releases of substances that constrict blood vessels, raise blood pressure, and promote clumping of platelets with formation of intravascular thrombi in the kidneys (leading to proteinuria), in the placenta, and in other tissues. Extremely severe cases can lead to partial separation of the placenta from the uterine wall and also may be complicated by a disseminated intravascular coagulation syndrome, as described in the discussion on abnormalities of blood coagulation.

Mild cases can be managed by bed rest and close observation, delaying premature delivery as long as possible without endangering the mother's health. Severe cases are hazardous to both mother and fetus. Treatment consists of trying to control the hypertension and vascular damage until the fetus is mature enough to be delivered prematurely, even as early as 20 weeks' gestation but preferably delaying until 24 weeks' gestation if possible. A number of drugs are used to control the hypertension and hopefully prevent convulsions. The condition usually relents when the placenta (which appears to be the cause of the problem) is expelled after delivery.

Hydatidiform Mole and Choriocarcinoma

Gestational trophoblast disease
(jes-tay'-shun-ul tro'-fo-blast)
A general term for all diseases characterized by abnormal trophoblast proliferation. Includes both hydatidiform mole and choriocarcinoma.

Hydatidiform mole
(hī-da-tid'i-form mōl)
A neoplastic proliferation of trophoblast associated with formation of large cystic villi.

Sometimes, when a pregnancy does not develop normally, the embryo either fails to form or dies and is absorbed, but the trophoblastic cells covering the villi continue to grow at an excessive rate, and the proliferating trophoblast produces much greater amount of chorionic gonadotropins than are encountered in a normal pregnancy. Masses of abnormal proliferating trophoblastic tissue may invade the uterus, spread into the vagina, and even metastasize to distant sites. Three different degrees of abnormal trophoblastic activity are recognized, and the general term **gestational trophoblast disease** is used to encompass all three types:

1. The most common type, which occurs in about 80% of affected patients, is a relatively benign trophoblast proliferation called a **hydatidiform mole**.

2. A more aggressive and destructive proliferative process, which occurs in about 15% of patients, is called an **invasive mole**.

3. A malignant growth of trophoblastic tissue, which affects only a small percentage of patients, is called a **choriocarcinoma**. This aggressive trophoblastic neoplasm can metastasize widely and kill the patient unless controlled by proper treatment.

BENIGN HYDATIDIFORM MOLE

In a benign hydatidiform mole, the villi that are covered by proliferating trophoblast become converted into large cystic structures resembling masses of grapes (FIGURE 18-24). The unusual name given to this condition is derived from its gross appearance. A hydatid is a fluid-filled vesicle, and a mole is a shapeless mass of tissue.

Most hydatidiform moles result from fertilization of an abnormal ovum lacking chromosomes, apparently because the chromosomes have been lost from the ovum, have degenerated, or have been discarded. The abnormal ovum is fertilized by a single sperm bearing an X chromosome, which then duplicates its chromosomes so that there are 46 chromosomes in the fertilized egg, but they are all derived from the father and none come from the mother. No embryo develops, and the chorionic villi become cystic structures covered by actively proliferating trophoblastic tissue. This is the most common type of mole and is called a complete mole.

Less commonly a hydatidiform mole results from fertilization of a normal ovum by two sperm, resulting in a fertilized ovum containing three sets of chromosomes (69 chromosomes). An embryo forms but does not survive, and the trophoblastic tissue consists of a mixture of normal and cystic villi. This type of mole, which is less likely to exhibit aggressive behavior than is a complete mole, is called a partial mole.

A hydatidiform mole is a relatively common complication of pregnancy that occurs about once in 1,500 pregnancies in the United States and Canada, but is encountered 10 times more frequently in women from the Far East and Southeast Asia. Because of the increased volume of the placenta caused by the multiple cystic villi, the patient with a mole experiences an enlargement of the uterus that is much greater than would be expected in relationship to the duration of the pregnancy. Erosion of maternal blood vessels by the mole may cause irregular uterine bleeding. The

Invasive mole
An aggressive hydatidiform mole that invades the uterine wall.

Choriocarcinoma
(kōr′rē-ō-kär-sin-ō′muh)
A malignant proliferation of trophoblastic tissue.

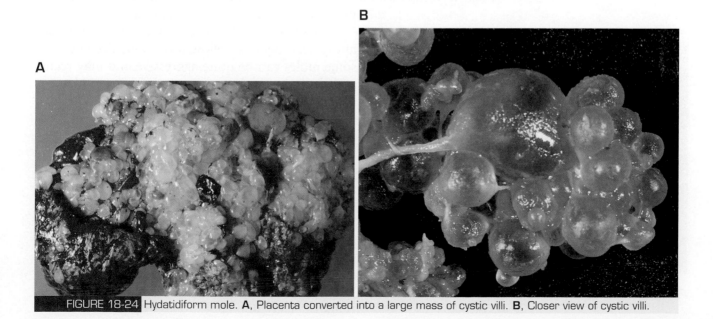

FIGURE 18-24 Hydatidiform mole. **A**, Placenta converted into a large mass of cystic villi. **B**, Closer view of cystic villi.

overdistension of the uterus caused by the mole may precipitate uterine contractions leading to expulsion of pieces of the mole. Diagnosis of a mole is based on the clinical features of the pregnancy, by identifying cystic villi covered by proliferating trophoblast that have been expelled from the uterus, or by ultrasound examination, which reveals a characteristic appearance caused by the cystic villi that fill the uterine cavity.

INVASIVE MOLE

An invasive mole resembles a complete hydatidiform mole but exhibits a much more marked trophoblastic proliferation and a much more aggressive behavior. The trophoblastic tissue may invade deeply into the uterine wall and cause considerable bleeding, but does not metastasize.

CHORIOCARCINOMA

This is the most aggressive form of gestational trophoblast disease and behaves like a malignant tumor. Masses of abnormal actively proliferating trophoblast may extend into the vagina and may metastasize to the lungs, brain, and other distant sites. Unless vigorously treated, the tumor may eventually kill the patient.

TREATMENT OF GESTATIONAL TROPHOBLAST DISEASE

Treatment of a mole consists of evacuating the uterus by curettage and then performing periodic determinations of the level of chorionic gonadotropins in the patient's blood to be certain all the abnormal tissue has been removed. After successful treatment, the chorionic gonadotropin level in the patient's blood should gradually fall to undetectable levels within about 8 weeks. If the level does not fall or if it starts to rise again after an initial fall, this means that the mole was incompletely removed or has recurred or become invasive, and further treatment is needed. Generally, the treatment consists of anticancer chemotherapy, although sometimes a hysterectomy is performed if the patient does not wish to have further pregnancies. A choriocarcinoma is usually treated vigorously by several courses of anticancer chemotherapy, and most patients can be cured by adequate treatment as illustrated by the metastatic choriocarcinoma (FIGURE 18-25) in a woman who was cured by chemotherapy. Subsequently, she became pregnant and delivered a normal infant.

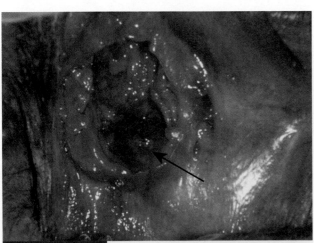

FIGURE 18-25 Metastatic choriocarcinoma in the posterior wall of the vagina (*arrow*). The patient had an excellent response to chemotherapy and later had a normal pregnancy and delivery.

A woman who has had a mole removed should always have periodic follow-up examinations because some moles can be quite aggressive and may recur, and choriocarcinoma may arise after incomplete removal of an invasive or incompletely removed mole. If a woman has had a mole removed and is being followed by periodic measurements of chorionic gonadotropins, she should not become pregnant for 1 year after the mole has been removed. The reason is because a pregnancy would complicate the interpretation of follow-up chorionic gonadotropin tests. The physician would be unable to determine whether the elevated chorionic gonadotropin was caused by recurrent gestational trophoblast disease, which requires anticancer chemotherapy, or a normal pregnancy.

The following three cases illustrate the wide range of behavior of gestational trophoblast disease.

Case Studies

CASE 18-4

HYDATIDIFORM MOLE A 20-year-old woman experienced episodes of bleeding during the early part of her pregnancy, and her uterus was greatly enlarged in relationship to the duration of her pregnancy. At about 6 months' gestation, she aborted a large hydatidiform mole, which was associated with considerable bleeding. She made an uncomplicated recovery. Follow-up examinations revealed fall of chorionic gonadotropins to undetectable levels and no recurrence of the mole.

CASE 18-5

INVASIVE MOLE A 32-year-old pregnant woman at 14 weeks' gestation consulted her physician because of vaginal bleeding. Her uterus was much larger than would be expected for a 14-week gestation. Soon afterward, she aborted a large hydatidiform mole, which was associated with considerable blood loss. After the mole had been expelled, however, the chorionic gonadotropins remained elevated, indicating that molar tissue was still present within the uterus. Curettage of the uterus was performed, which was associated with considerable bleeding, and revealed a large amount of molar tissue. A hysterectomy was performed, and examination of the resected uterus revealed that the mole had invaded deeply into the right lateral wall of the uterus. Subsequently, chorionic gonadotropins fell to undetectable levels, and she had no further difficulties.

CASE 18-6

CHORIOCARCINOMA A 50-year-old woman, whose pregnancy was complicated by irregular vaginal bleeding and marked enlargement of the uterus, aborted a large hydatidiform mole but did not return to her physician for follow-up examination. Two years later, she returned to her physician because of headaches, incoordination, difficulty in speaking, and other symptoms suggesting a brain tumor. Chest x-ray revealed multiple deposits of metastatic tumor through both lungs, and chorionic gonadotropins were elevated. These features, together with the history of a previous mole, suggested far-advanced widely disseminated choriocarcinoma that had developed from residual molar tissue retained within the uterus after the mole had been aborted 2 years previously. She lapsed into coma and died shortly after admission to the hospital. Autopsy revealed widespread choriocarcinoma in brain, lungs, liver, and kidneys.

Comment: These three cases illustrate the variability of the behavior of gestational trophoblastic disease and emphasize the importance of periodic follow-up examinations after evacuation of a mole. The first case illustrates the usual benign behavior of most moles. The second case illustrates the more aggressive behavior of an invasive mole. The third case, unfortunately, illustrates the behavior of a choriocarcinoma. As this third case illustrates, a choriocarcinoma may arise from abnormal trophoblastic tissue retained within the uterus after evacuation of a mole. This is an uncommon complication and occurs in only a small percentage of patients. Had the woman returned to her physician for follow-up examinations, the recurrent trophoblast proliferation could have been detected. Prompt treatment would probably have destroyed the abnormal trophoblast and prevented the fatal outcome. Prompt diagnosis and intensive chemotherapy treatment of a gestational choriocarcinoma, even though the tumor has already metastasized, are extremely successful (Figure 18-25). Many successfully treated patients have later become pregnant and delivered normal infants.

Hemolytic Disease of the Newborn (Erythroblastosis Fetalis)

Hemolytic disease of the newborn is a hemolytic anemia in the newborn infant resulting from sensitization of the mother to a "foreign" blood group antigen present in the red cells of the fetus but lacking in the maternal cells. Although most cases of severe hemolytic disease result from Rh incompatibility between an Rh-negative mother and her Rh-positive fetus, mother–fetus blood group incompatibility involving other blood group systems also may cause hemolytic disease. The mother reacts by forming antibodies directed against the fetal cells that cross the placenta and damage the fetal red cells, leading to a severe anemia in the affected fetus. The other name for this disease, erythroblastosis fetalis, comes from the large numbers of nucleated red blood cells (erythroblasts) in the blood of severely affected anemic infants.

The affected fetus attempts to "keep up" with the increased blood destruction caused by the antibody by increasing the rate of red cell production (compensatory hematopoiesis). The severity of the hemolytic disease depends on the intensity of the blood destruction in the infant.

The severely affected infant is extremely anemic and very edematous. This severe form of erythroblastosis is often called hydrops fetalis, the term hydrops referring to the severe edema in the affected infant (FIGURE 18-26). The edema is the result of heart failure and impaired hepatic plasma–protein synthesis, which are caused by the severe anemia. If the hemolytic process is less intense, the infant may be born alive but will be moderately or severely anemic. Infants with mild disease may appear normal at birth but become anemic and jaundiced soon afterward.

CHANGES IN HEMOGLOBIN AND BILIRUBIN AFTER DELIVERY

FIGURE 18-27 illustrates the typical changes in hemoglobin and bilirubin levels after delivery in an infant with hemolytic disease. Anemia invariably develops or increases in severity after delivery; jaundice also develops rapidly. The anemia is aggravated by a decline in the rate of compensatory hematopoiesis after delivery. In the uterus, hematopoiesis is stimulated by both the increased blood destruction and the low oxygen tension in the fetal blood. After delivery, respiration is established and the arterial oxygen tension in the infant's blood rises. Low intrauterine oxygen tension no longer stimulates hematopoiesis, and the rate of compensatory hematopoiesis declines. However, blood destruction continues at the same rate. The increasing severity of the anemia reflects the greater postnatal disproportion between blood production and blood destruction.

The accelerated blood destruction in hemolytic disease also causes jaundice. The high rate of red cell breakdown leads to production of large amounts of bile

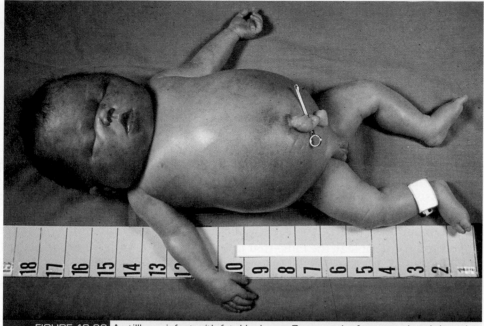

FIGURE 18-26 A stillborn infant with fetal hydrops. Because the fetus was head down in the uterus, the edema is more marked in the face than in the legs and feet. The abdomen is swollen because the liver and spleen are enlarged, and fluid has also accumulated in the peritoneal cavity.

pigment. Before delivery, the bile pigment crosses the placenta into the maternal circulation and is excreted by the mother. After delivery, the infant is called on to excrete the large amount of pigment formerly handled by the mother, but its liver is still relatively inefficient in conjugating and excreting bilirubin. As a result, the level of unconjugated bilirubin in the infant's blood rises rapidly. This condition is called hyperbilirubinemia (*hyper* = elevated + bilirubin + *heme* = blood) and is hazardous

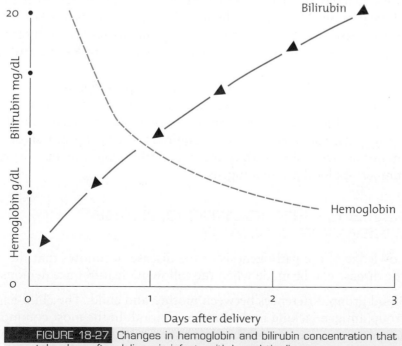

FIGURE 18-27 Changes in hemoglobin and bilirubin concentration that take place after delivery in infants with hemolytic disease.

to the infant. The high level of unconjugated bilirubin is toxic to the nervous system, where it causes bile staining and degeneration of basal ganglia (basal nuclei) and damage to other parts of the brain as well. This is a serious, preventable complication related to the hyperbilirubinemia, leaving the infant with cerebral palsy, mental retardation, and hearing loss. This condition is called kernicterus (*kern* = kernel, referring to brain basal nuclei + *icterus* = jaundice), also called bilirubin encephalopathy.

Rh HEMOLYTIC DISEASE

In order to understand the pathogenesis of Rh hemolytic disease and how to prevent it, a knowledge of the Rh system is helpful. The Rh system is a relatively complex system consisting of a series of allelic genes that determine multiple Rh antigens on the red cells. The Rh antigen most important clinically is an antigen named the D antigen in one terminology and the Rh_o antigen in another terminology. (The subscript "o" refers to original, meaning that it was the first Rh antigen recognized.) The presence of the D (Rh_o) antigen is considered to be determined by the allelic genes *D* and *d*, giving three possible genotypes: *DD*, *Dd*, and *dd*. For clinical purposes, persons whose red cells possess the D (Rh_o) antigen are considered Rh positive, regardless of the presence or absence of other Rh antigens, and persons lacking the D antigen (genotype *dd*) are considered Rh negative. An Rh-positive person may be either homozygous (*DD*) or heterozygous (*Dd*). Consequently, two heterozygous Rh-positive parents may have an Rh-negative child if each parent passes a *d* gene to the offspring. It is also possible for a heterozygous Rh-positive father and Rh-negative mother to have an Rh-negative child.

The first Rh-positive infant born to an Rh-negative mother is usually normal because a woman rarely forms Rh antibody during her first pregnancy. However, after the mother has been sensitized to Rh-positive fetal cells and has formed Rh antibody, Rh hemolytic disease will develop in any subsequent pregnancy in which the fetus is Rh positive.

Now Rh hemolytic disease rarely occurs because we usually can prevent the formation of Rh antibodies by an Rh-negative woman pregnant with an Rh-positive fetus, and we also have effective ways to treat any unfortunate newborn infants who have hemolytic disease. Although Rh hemolytic disease occurs infrequently, knowing about the disease and its effects on the fetus emphasizes how important it is to prevent the disease in susceptible Rh-positive infants born to Rh-negative mothers.

Hemolytic Disease as a Result of Other Blood Group Antigens

Hemolytic disease may occasionally result from sensitization of the mother to another antigen in the Rh system or from sensitization to an antigen in one of the other blood group systems. The essential feature required for the pathogenesis of hemolytic disease is maternal–fetal blood group incompatibility, and this may be caused by any of a number of blood group antigens.

DIAGNOSIS OF HEMOLYTIC DISEASE IN THE NEWBORN INFANT

From a knowledge of the pathogenesis of the disease, it follows that the diagnosis of hemolytic disease can be made when the following features are demonstrated.

1. Blood group differences between mother and child. The child has a blood group antigen lacking in the mother's blood. In the most common type of hemolytic disease, the mother lacks the D (Rh_o) antigen, which is present in the cells of the infant.

2. Sensitization of the mother to the "foreign" antigen in the infant's cells. Diagnosis requires demonstrating the presence of an antibody in the mother's blood directed against the "foreign" antigen. Usually this is anti-D (Rh_o).
3. Passage of antibody across the placenta into the infant's blood, with fixation of the antibody to the surface of the infant's cells. This is demonstrated by means of the direct Coombs test performed on the infant's blood. This test detects antibody–protein coating on the surface of the infant's red cells.
4. Evidence of increased destruction of the infant's cells. Determination of the hemoglobin and bilirubin levels in the infant's blood indicates the intensity of the hemolytic process.

Diagnosis of hemolytic disease is summarized in TABLE 18-2. When the foregoing criteria have been met, the diagnosis of hemolytic disease is established with certainty. In routine clinical practice, this information can be obtained promptly without great difficulty. Generally, blood typing of the mother and studies to determine the presence of antibodies are performed routinely during pregnancy by the physician, who generally knows before delivery whether the mother has been sensitized and is likely to deliver an affected infant. When the infant is born, a sample of blood from the umbilical cord (which is the infant's blood) is sent to the laboratory for a direct Coombs test and determination of blood type as well as hemoglobin and bilirubin levels. The Coombs test and blood typing indicate whether the infant is affected, and the hemoglobin and bilirubin levels indicate the severity of the hemolytic disease. The level of unconjugated serum bilirubin normally rises after delivery even in normal infants, usually reaching a peak of about 6 mg/dl or sometimes even higher within the first few days after delivery and then falls toward normal. In hemolytic disease, unconjugated bilirubin levels rise faster, and levels are often much higher than in a normal newborn infant. Levels exceeding 20 mg/dl are potentially hazardous, put the infant at risk of kernicterus, and require treatment to lower the serum bilirubin level.

TREATMENT OF HEMOLYTIC DISEASE

When hemolytic disease caused by Rh incompatibility was a more common problem than it is now, a commonly used treatment was **exchange transfusion**. The infant with hemolytic disease is in jeopardy because its body is saturated with passively transferred maternal antibody. The antibody is the cause of the hemolytic anemia

Exchange transfusion
Partial replacement of blood of infant with hemolytic disease by blood lacking the antigen responsible for hemolytic disease, as when transfusing Rh-negative blood to an Rh-positive infant. Performed to reduce intensity of hemolytic jaundice.

TABLE 18-2

Diagnosis of hemolytic disease

Characteristic feature	Means of recognition
Production of antigenic fetal cells	Maternal–fetal blood group differences; mother lacks antigen present in fetal cells
Maternal sensitization	Mother's blood contains antibody against antigenic cells
Transplacental passage of maternal antibody	Positive direct Coombs test on cord blood indicates antibodies attached to fetal cells
Increased blood destruction in newborn infant	Decreased hemoglobin in cord blood; elevated bilirubin

and jaundice, and several months are required before the antibody can be completely eliminated from the infant's circulation. The rationale of exchange transfusion is to provide the infant with a population of cells that will not be destroyed by the antibody. In the case of hemolytic disease caused by Rh incompatibility, a transfusion of Rh-negative blood is given. At the same time, exchange transfusion provides the infant with bilirubin-free plasma to replace the jaundiced plasma, thereby helping to prevent severe elevation of potentially toxic, unconjugated bilirubin. It should be emphasized that the exchange transfusion has no effect on the infant's own blood type. The transfused Rh-negative cells will be gradually eliminated and replaced by the infant's own Rh-positive cells. The purpose of the exchange transfusion is to tide the infant over an acute, life threatening situation. This is accomplished by decreasing the rate of red cell destruction through transfusion of cells not subject to hemolysis and by lowering the concentration of potentially toxic unconjugated bilirubin in the infant's plasma.

Exchange transfusion may be compared with replacing the contents of a barrel of salt water with fresh water without emptying and refilling the barrel. This can be accomplished by withdrawing a pail of salt water from the barrel and replacing it with an equal quantity of fresh water. If this is repeated many times, the salt concentration of the water in the barrel is gradually reduced until eventually the barrel is filled with virtually fresh water. An exchange transfusion is an application of the same principle. The usual method of exchange transfusion is to introduce a catheter into the umbilical vein. A small quantity of the infant's own blood is withdrawn and replaced with an equal quantity of blood lacking the sensitizing antigen (usually Rh-negative blood). The process of withdrawing a small quantity of blood and replacing it with an equal quantity of exchange blood is continued until about 500 ml of blood have been administered. At the conclusion of the exchange transfusion, about 85% of the infant's own cells will have been replaced by the transfused cells.

FLUORESCENT LIGHT THERAPY FOR HYPERBILIRUBINEMIA

The elevated level of unconjugated bilirubin that causes kernicterus can be reduced by exposing the unclothed jaundiced infant to fluorescent lights continuously for several days. The infant is turned frequently so that the skin receives maximum exposure to the fluorescent light. The eyes are covered to protect them from the bright light. The light exposure acts by converting the toxic unconjugated bilirubin into less toxic compounds that are not as hazardous to the infant. This procedure, called **photytherapy**, has reduced the need for exchange transfusions.

Photography
Fluorescent light treatment of jaundiced babies to reduce the concentration of unconjugated bilirubin in their blood.

PREVENTION OF Rh HEMOLYTIC DISEASE WITH Rh IMMUNE GLOBULIN

Postpartum Administration
As previously stated, the first Rh-positive infant born to an Rh-negative mother is usually normal because Rh antibodies are rarely formed during the first pregnancy. Although a few Rh-positive cells may periodically enter the mother's circulation during pregnancy, their numbers are not sufficient to induce sensitization. The greater numbers of Rh-positive cells required to sensitize the mother usually do not enter the maternal circulation until after delivery. When the placenta begins to separate from the uterus and is eventually expelled, the barrier separating the maternal and fetal circulations is disrupted, and some of the Rh-positive fetal cells within the villi may be expressed into the uterine blood vessels and may enter the mother's circulation

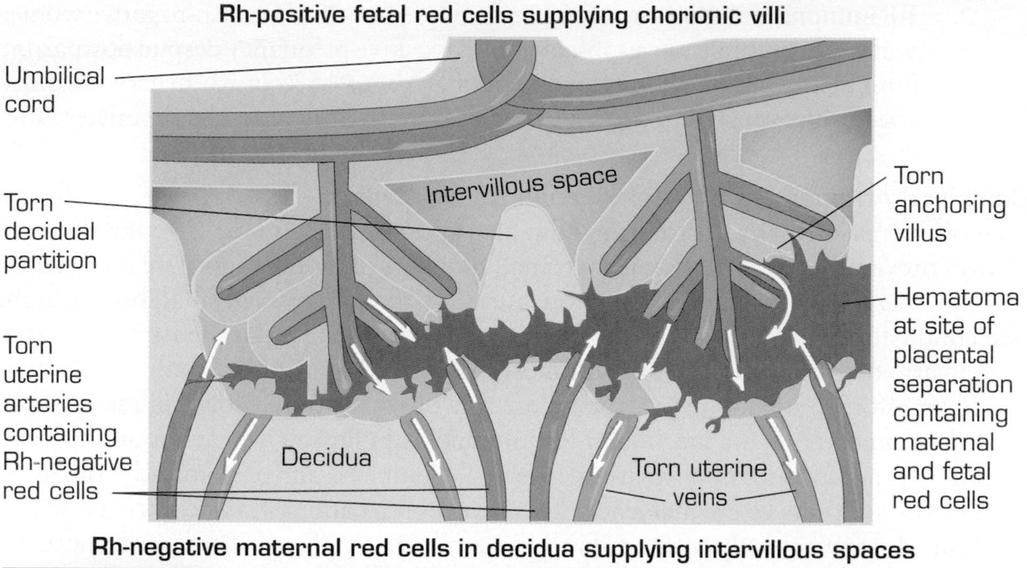

Rh-positive fetal red cells supplying chorionic villi

Rh-negative maternal red cells in decidua supplying intervillous spaces

FIGURE 18-28 Transfer of fetal Rh-positive red cells into maternal circulation during postpartum placental separation. Separation of the placenta disrupts basal decidua containing maternal blood vessels that supply blood to intervillous spaces and also disrupts blood vessels in villi anchoring placenta to basal decidua. Fetal and maternal red cells escaping from torn blood vessels form a collection of blood (hematoma) between the placenta and basal decidua. Uterine contractions that expel placenta compress hematoma and may force blood from hematoma (containing fetal red cells) into maternal circulation. The *arrows* indicate the direction of blood flow.

(FIGURE 18-28). In general, the larger the volume of fetal blood entering the mother's circulation, the greater the likelihood of sensitization to Rh antigen, and after sensitization has occurred, Rh hemolytic disease will develop in any subsequent pregnancy in which the fetus is Rh positive.

Rh immune globulin is a gamma globulin containing a high concentration of Rh antibody. When administered to an unsensitized Rh-negative mother within 72 hours after delivery of an Rh-positive fetus, it is extremely effective in preventing the formation of Rh antibody. The Rh antibody in the immune globulin coats the Rh antigen sites on the surface of any fetal red cells that have entered the mother's circulation, leading to rapid removal of the antibody-coated red cells so that they do not persist long enough to induce sensitization. Rh immune globulin is recommended for all Rh-negative mothers who have not already formed Rh antibodies and who have given birth to an Rh-positive infant. It is of no value if the mother has already formed antibodies. Unsensitized Rh-negative patients should also receive Rh immune globulin after an abortion or ectopic pregnancy because these conditions may also induce sensitization. The risk is low, however, if the gestation is less than 12 weeks.

The standard dose of Rh immune globulin is sufficient to "neutralize" and eliminate about 1 oz. of fetal blood. In the very uncommon situation in which a larger volume of fetal blood enters the maternal circulation, more Rh immune globulin is required. Special laboratory tests can detect and quantitate the volume of fetal blood in the mother's circulation, enabling the physician to determine how much additional Rh immune globulin to administer.

The incidence of Rh hemolytic disease has been greatly reduced by the routine use of Rh immune globulin, but the disease has not been completely eliminated. There are two reasons why the disease persists:

1. A very small number of Rh-negative women form Rh antibody in their first pregnancy, apparently because of prior contact with Rh antigen from an unrecognized abortion, transfusion of Rh-positive blood, or other cause.

2. Rh immune globulin is not 100% effective. About 1.5% of Rh-negative women will form antibodies in a subsequent Rh-positive pregnancy despite postpartum administration of Rh immune globulin. (About 15% of Rh-negative women would be expected to form antibodies if no treatment were administered.)

Combined Antepartum and Postpartum Administration

One of the reasons why postpartum administration of Rh immune globulin does not always prevent Rh sensitization is that small numbers of fetal Rh-positive red cells occasionally enter the mother's circulation late in pregnancy through small breaks in the placental villi. When this occurs, the antigenic fetal cells may induce sensitization prior to delivery, rendering postpartum administration of Rh immune globulin ineffective.

In an effort to further reduce the failure rate of Rh immune globulin, many physicians recommend that an injection of Rh immune globulin be given at about 28 weeks' gestation, in addition to the postpartum injection. Combined antepartum and postpartum administration reduces the incidence of sensitization to about 0.5% compared with a 1.5% incidence when only postpartum administration is employed. There are some drawbacks to this approach. When Rh immune globulin is used prior to delivery, it is given to all Rh-negative mothers, many of whom are carrying an Rh-negative fetus and do not need it. Only mothers with Rh-positive fetuses would receive the postpartum injection.

ABO HEMOLYTIC DISEASE

ABO hemolytic disease
A mild hemolytic disease in group A or B infants or group O mothers, as a result of maternal anti-A and anti-B antibodies.

With the decline in the frequency of Rh hemolytic disease, now most cases of hemolytic disease result from ABO blood group differences between the mother and infant. In this condition, called **ABO hemolytic disease**, the mother is group O (and has anti-A and anti-B antibodies in her serum), and the infant is either group A or group B. In most women, the A or B fetal antigens stimulate the maternal ABO antibodies, increasing their concentration and changing their character so that they are able to cross the placenta into the fetal circulation and attach to fetal cells. ABO hemolytic disease occurs in a first ABO-incompatible pregnancy because it is caused by preexisting anti-A and anti-B antibodies. This is quite different from Rh hemolytic disease in which a first pregnancy is required to provoke sensitization by transfer of Rh-positive fetal cells into the maternal bloodstream during placental separation after delivery, which is followed later by formation of Rh antibodies that complicate the next Rh-incompatible pregnancy.

Generally, ABO hemolytic disease is a much less severe disease than Rh hemolytic disease because A and B antigens on fetal cells are not as well developed as on adult cells, so the antibody does not fix as firmly to the fetal red cells and does not cause as much red cell membrane damage. In addition, A and B antigens are present not only on fetal red cells but also on other types of cells in fetal organs and tissues that absorb much of the anti-A or anti-B antibodies, leaving less available to fix to the red cells. As a result, fetal red cell destruction is less marked. The anemia is less pronounced, and blood transfusions are usually not required. However, the accelerated red cell destruction still generates an excessive amount of bile pigment, which the infant is unable to conjugate and excrete efficiently, and a high level of unconjugated bilirubin in the infant's blood can cause kernicterus. Consequently, hyperbilirubinemia caused by ABO hemolytic disease requires the same type of treatment as that used to control hyperbilirubinemia in Rh hemolytic disease. Generally, the elevated bilirubin responds well to fluorescent light phototherapy, and exchange transfusion usually is not required.

The following two cases illustrate hemolytic disease caused by ABO incompatibility with two different outcomes, which illustrate the importance of prompt and vigorous treatment of affected infants.

CASE 18-7

An ABO-incompatible pregnancy in which the hyperbilirubinemia was recognized promptly after the infant had left the hospital and responded well to fluorescent light therapy.

A normal full-term, 8-lb male infant was born without complications to a group O Rh-positive mother. The mother and baby did well after delivery and were discharged 2 days later. After returning home, the parents noted that the infant appeared jaundiced and brought him back to the hospital for further evaluation and treatment. When examined at the hospital, the baby did not appear ill but was moderately jaundiced, and the serum bilirubin was elevated. Laboratory tests revealed that the baby was group A Rh positive, and the Coombs test was positive, indicating that maternal anti-A antibodies were attached to the infant's red cells. Fluorescent light treatment was started, and serum bilirubin concentrations were monitored periodically. Bilirubin levels fluctuated from a maximum of 17.8 mg/dl to a low of 11.2 mg/dl in response to fluorescent light treatment. The infant was discharged after 4 days of fluorescent light treatment and had no further difficulties.

CASE 18-8

An ABO-incompatible pregnancy reported in the medical literature in which recognition and treatment of hyperbilirubinemia were delayed and kernicterus developed despite fluorescent light treatment and exchange transfusions.

A normal 6-lb male group A Rh-positive infant was delivered normally without complications to a group O Rh-positive mother and was discharged about 20 hours after delivery. A 2-week follow-up appointment was scheduled with a pediatric clinic. Nine days later, the parents called the clinic because the infant appeared very jaundiced, was lethargic, and was not eating well. A return appointment was scheduled, which revealed that the infant was very jaundiced, had lost weight, and was dehydrated. Serum bilirubin was 41.5 mg/dl, which was well above the maximum "safe" level of 20 mg/dl. Despite fluorescent light treatment and exchange transfusions, the infant developed severe permanent neurologic dysfunction characteristic of kernicterus.

QUESTIONS FOR REVIEW

1. Why do spontaneous abortions occur? What are the consequences of prolonged retention of a dead fetus within the uterine cavity?
2. What is an ectopic pregnancy? What factors predispose to development of an ectopic pregnancy in the fallopian tube? What are the consequences of a tubal pregnancy?

3. What is the difference between a hydatidiform mole and a choriocarcinoma?
4. What is hemolytic disease of the newborn? How does it affect the infant? How does it affect the mother? Why do severely affected infants become edematous?
5. In infants with hemolytic disease, why does jaundice increase after delivery? Why does anemia become more severe after delivery?
6. How does the physician make a diagnosis of hemolytic disease? How is the disease treated?
7. How does ABO hemolytic disease differ from Rh hemolytic disease?
8. What structures contribute to the formation of the placenta? What are the main functions of the placenta?
9. Describe some of the important abnormalities of the placenta and umbilical cord that may have an unfavorable effect on pregnancy.
10. What is the source of amnionic fluid? What factors regulate the total volume of amnionic fluid?
11. Why does a pregnancy test become positive? When does it become positive?
12. What are the possible causes and the significance of polyhydramnios? of oligohydramnios?

SUPPLEMENTARY READINGS

Biggio, J. R., Jr., Chapman, V., Neely, C., et al. 2010. Fetal anomalies in obese women: The contribution of diabetes. *Obstetrics and Gynecology* 115:290–6.

 ▶ A total of over 42,000 singleton pregnancies were evaluated over three time periods: 1991–1994, 1995–1999, and 2000–2004. Data were compiled on body mass index and major congenital abnormalities. During the study period, the prevalence of major congenital abnormalities increased from 0.43 to 0.84%. Obesity does not appear to cause the congenital abnormalities; however, obesity predisposes women to diabetes, which is responsible for the congenital abnormalities. Obese women should be screened for diabetes, preferably before conception, and those with diabetes should be treated before they become pregnant, which avoids hyperglycemia-associated fetal injury to the developing organ systems in early pregnancy.

Centers for Disease Control and Prevention. 2004. Availability of revised guidelines for identifying and managing jaundice in newborns. *Journal of the American Medical Association* 292:1678.

 ▶ Assess all infants before discharge from birth hospital. Measure serum bilirubin by chemical test or by transcutaneous bilirubin level. Schedule a follow-up visit within 3–5 days after birth when the bilirubin level is likely to be highest. Encourage breast-feeding at least 8–12 times per day (to promote rapid passage of bilirubin through the bowel to avoid reuptake of excreted bilirubin from bowel contents, which can greatly reduce risk of hyperbilirubinemia). Provide parents with written and oral information about the risks associated with hyperbilirubinemia (guidelines for parents are available online at http://www.cdc.gov/ncbddd/jaundice.htm).

Crowther, C. A., Hiller, J. E., Moss, J. R., et al. 2005. Effect of treatment of gestational diabetes mellitus on pregnancy outcomes. *New England Journal of Medicine* 352:2477–86.

 ▶ Women between 24 and 34 weeks' gestation were randomly assigned to two groups. One group received dietary advice, blood glucose monitoring, and insulin therapy (the intervention group); the other group received routine prenatal care. Both groups were monitored for serious perinatal complications, including fetal death, difficult delivery (shoulder dystocia), bone fractures, nerve palsy, admission to the neonatal care nursery, jaundice requiring phototherapy, induction of labor, and cesarean delivery.

▶ The infants of more women in the intervention group were admitted to the neonatal nursery, and the intervention group had a higher incidence if induction of labor than women in the routine care group, although the rates of cesarean delivery were similar in both groups. The rate of serious perinatal complications was lower among the infants of the 490 women in the intervention group, compared to the infants of the 510 women in the routine care group. A 3-month postpartum evaluation of the satisfaction and quality of life and frequency of postpartum depression was interpreted as improved health-related quality of life.

Dennery, P. A., Seidman, D. S., and Stevenson, D. K. 2001. Neonatal hyperbilirubinemia. *New England Journal of Medicine* 344:581–90.

▶ Discusses pathogenesis and treatment. A good diagram illustrating the pathways of heme breakdown and the formation of bilirubin. Newborn infants become jaundiced because the liver enzyme that conjugates bilirubin is less efficient, no bacterial flora have yet colonized the intestinal tract, which can break down excreted bilirubin into other compounds within the bowel, and intestinal peristalsis is less active, which allows the bilirubin to remain within the bowel instead of being excreted rapidly. Consequently, bilirubin derived from red cell breakdown is less efficiently conjugated with glucuronic acid and excreted into the intestinal tract, and sluggish peristalsis delays the excretion of the conjugated bilirubin. Intestinal enzymes split the glucuronic acid from the bilirubin, and some of the unconjugated bilirubin is reabsorbed, which adds to the level of bilirubin in the bloodstream. If the infant has experienced any birth trauma leading to bleeding, the extravasated blood is broken down and converted to additional bilirubin, which must be excreted. All of the factors that tend to raise unconjugated blood bilirubin play an even more important role in premature infants.

Eichenwald, E. C., and Stark, A. R. 2008. Management and outcomes of very low birth weight. *New England Journal of Medicine* 358:1700–11.

▶ About 12.5% of births occur before 37 weeks of gestation. Preterm infants who weigh 1,500 g or less are considered "very low" birth weight infants. Approximately 85% live long enough to be discharged from the hospital, but from 2 to 5% of the infants die from medical complications related to their prematurity.

▶ Infants weighing 1,000 g or less are considered "extremely low" birth weight infants. Those born in perinatal centers specialized in treating very premature infants do better than those transferred from another facility after birth, but they are still subject to a number of both short-term and long-term problems.

▶ Infants with a gestational age of 23–25 weeks or a birth weight of less than 500 g are at greatest risk of poor outcomes. Only about 39% survive to leave the hospital. Of the survivors, over 16% had evidence of severe brain injury, and about 75% required long-term supplementary oxygen therapy. Half of the surviving infants had neurologic disabilities that were often severe. Even infants with no disability were not normal. About one-third had an IQ of less than 85. Bronchopulmonary problems related to immaturity are common and difficult to manage.

The EXPRESS Group. 2009. One-year survival of extremely preterm infants after active perinatal care in Sweden. *Journal of the American Medical Association* 301:2225–33.

▶ During 2004–2007, 1-year survival of infants born alive at 22–26 weeks' gestation in Sweden was 70% and ranged from 9.8% at 22 weeks to 85% at 26 weeks.

The HAPO Study Cooperative Research Group. 2008. Hyperglycemia and adverse pregnancy incomes. *New England Journal of Medicine* 358:1991–2002.

▶ A total of 25,505 women at 15 centers in nine countries underwent glucose tolerance testing at 24 weeks' and 32 weeks' gestation in an attempt to determine whether maternal hyperglycemia less marked than in gestational diabetes is associated with increased risks of adverse pregnancy outcomes.

▶ As maternal blood glucose rises progressively, so does the birth weight of the babies and their blood glucose concentrations. There is a direct relationship between the maternal blood glucose and birth weight. Even maternal glucose levels lower than those diagnostic of gestational diabetes lead to higher birth weight babies with higher blood glucose concentrations, as manifested by increased cord blood serum C-peptide levels. Treatment guidelines for managing hyperglycemia during pregnancy should target lower glucose levels than those in current use.

Heffner, L. J. 2004. Advanced maternal age—how old is too old? *New England Journal of Medicine* 351:1927–9.

▶ Many women are having their first child at a much older age than in previous years. The number of first births in women aged 35–39 increased by 36% when compared with data 10 years previously and increased 70% in women aged 40–44. In 2002, 263 births were reported in women aged 50–55. Delaying conception creates problems. Fertility declines progressively after age 30, and older women have more difficulty becoming pregnant. They also have more difficulty in carrying the pregnancy to term because the frequency of spontaneous abortions rises as the woman ages, as does the incidence of chromosomal abnormalities in infants who survive to term. Older women are also more prone to develop hypertension and other pregnancy-related complications than younger women. The American Society for Reproductive Medicine is attempting to make women more aware of the risks related to delaying childbearing.

NIH Consensus Conference. 1995. Effect of corticosteroids for fetal maturation on perinatal outcomes. *Journal of the American Medical Association* 273:413–8.

▶ Administration of corticosteroids to mothers at risk of premature birth (24–34 weeks' gestation) improves infant survival by reducing neonatal respiratory distress syndrome.

Quintero, R. A., Dickinson, J. E., Morales, W. J., et al. 2003. Stage-based treatment of twin-twin transfusion syndrome. *American Journal of Obstetrics and Gynecology* 188:1333–40.

▶ Treatment should be based on stage of gestation and the changes resulting from the twin–twin transfusion. Endoscopic laser coagulation of artery-to-vein communications offers advantages over serial amniocentesis.

Senat, M. V., Deprest, J., Boulvain, M., et al. 2004. Endoscopic laser surgery versus serial amnioreduction for severe twin-to-twin transfusion syndrome. *New England Journal of Medicine* 341:136–44.

▶ Endoscopic laser coagulation of twin-to-twin anastomoses is more effective treatment than repeated amniocentesis to prevent hydramnios in the recipient twin.

Solomon, C. G., and Seely, E. W. 2004. Preeclampsia—searching for the cause. *New England Journal of Medicine* 350:641–2.

▶ A discussion of current concepts based on placental vascular insufficiency leading to systemic manifestations. Accurate classification is important in order not to misinterpret chronic hypertension without proteinuria in a pregnant woman as preeclampsia.

Stovall, T. G., Ling, F. W., and Gray, L. A. 1991. Single-dose methotrexate for treatment of ectopic pregnancy. *Obstetrics and Gynecology* 77:754–7.

▶ In selected cases, the ectopic pregnancy can be destroyed by administration of the antimetabolite methotrexate, rather than by laparoscopic salpingostomy or salpingectomy.

Stroup, M. 1977. Rh system. Genetics and function. *Mayo Clinic Proceedings* 52:141–4.

▶ Basic concepts of the genetics of the Rh system and the complexity of the Rh antigen.

Wilcox, A. J., Weinberg, C. R., and Baird, D. D. 1995. Timing of sexual intercourse in relation to ovulation. Effects on the probability of conception survival of the pregnancy, and sex of the baby. *New England Journal of Medicine* 333:1517–21.

▶ In a carefully studied group of women who were planning to become pregnant, the likelihood of conception from a single intercourse increased from 8% 6 days before ovulation to 36% on the day of ovulation. There were no pregnancies from intercourse on the day after ovulation and more than 6 days before ovulation.

Williams, W. W., Jr., Ecker, J. L., Thadhani, R. I., et al. 2005. Case records of the Massachusetts General Hospital. Case 38-2005. A 29-year-old pregnant woman with nephrotic syndrome and hypertension. *New England Journal of Medicine* 353:2590–600.

▶ A discussion of the management of preeclampsia in a patient who also has lupus. In mild preeclampsia, blood pressure is at least 140/90. In severe preeclampsia, blood pressure is at least 160/110 and is associated with systemic symptoms; treatment is to deliver the infant and the placenta, which is the cause of the preeclampsia. Delivery can be accomplished as early as 22–24 weeks' gestation; extremely premature infants have many problems and complications, but early delivery may be necessary to protect the mother's health. Delaying delivery to 24 weeks is preferable if possible without undue risk to the mother. The placenta showed vascular abnormalities, consistent with preeclampsia.

Woods, J. R., Jr., Plessinger, M. A., and Clark, K. E. 1987. Effects of cocaine on uterine blood flow and fetal oxygenation. *Journal of the American Medical Association* 257:957–61.

▶ Cocaine alters fetal oxygenation by reducing uterine blood flow and impairing oxygen transfer to the fetus.

OUTLINE SUMMARY

Fertilization and Prenatal Development

FERTILIZATION

Sperm contains genetic material and enzymes to penetrate egg.

Sperm has motility and is also transported by aspiration.

Ovum expelled, surrounded by zona pellucida and granulosa cells.

Union occurs in fallopian tube.

Only one sperm can enter egg.

EARLY DEVELOPMENT

Zygote develops into small ball of cells.

Fluid accumulates, and blastocyst forms.

Inner cell mass forms embryo.

Trophoblast forms placenta and membranes.

Implantation occurs at end of first week.

Amnionic sac, yolk sac, and germ disk form.

Germ disk rounds up to form tubular embryo by fourth week.

STAGES OF PRENATAL DEVELOPMENT

Preembryonic period: implantation and differentiation of blastocyst.

Embryonic period: third through seventh week.

Human shape develops and organ systems form, a critical period of development.

Fetal period: eighth week until term. Increase in size but no major changes.

DURATION OF PREGNANCY

Dated from conception: 38 weeks.

Dated from last menstrual period: 40 weeks.

Frequently expressed in trimesters.

Decidua, Fetal Membranes, and Placenta

DECIDUA
Decidua basalis: under chorionic vesicle.
Decidua capsularis: over chorionic vesicle.
Decidua parietalis: lines rest of uterus.

CHORION
Chorion laeve: superficial smooth chorion.
Chorion frondosum: bushy chorion that will form placental villi.

AMNIONIC SAC
Enclosed within chorion.
Forms protective environment for fetus.

YOLK SAC
Never contains yolk in human.
Forms intestinal tract and other structures.

PLACENTA
Provides oxygen and nutrition for fetus.
Fetus connected to placenta by umbilical cord.
Double circulation of blood in placenta.
> *Fetoplacental circulation: from fetus to villi.*
> *Uteroplacental circulation: maternal blood circulates around villi.*

No normal intercommunication between circulations.
Endocrine function of placenta:
> *Makes estrogen and progesterone.*
> *Makes HCG and HPL.*
> *Pregnancy tests detect HCG.*

Amnionic Fluid

FORMATION AND EXCRETION
Chiefly a filtration from maternal blood early in pregnancy.
Mostly fetal urine later in pregnancy.
Fetus swallows fluid, which is absorbed, transferred to maternal circulation, and excreted by mother.
Normally, balance maintained between secretion and excretion of fluid.

POLYHYDRAMNIOS
Fetus unable to swallow; thus, fluid accumulates in sac.
Congenital obstruction of fetal upper intestinal tract; thus, fluid cannot be absorbed from intestinal tract.

OLIGOHYDRAMNIOS
Fetal kidneys fail to develop: no urine formed.
Congenital obstruction of urethra: no urine escapes into amnionic fluid.

Hormone-Related Conditions Associated with Pregnancy

NAUSEA AND VOMITING OF EARLY PREGNANCY

HYPEREMESIS GRAVIDARUM

GESTATIONAL DIABETES
Hyperglycemia harmful to developing fetus.
Pregnancy hormones induce maternal insulin resistance.

Diabetes results from inability to increase insulin secretion to compensate for insulin resistance.
Identification by screening and treatment same as for nongestational diabetes.
Usually diabetes relents after delivery.

Spontaneous Abortion

INCIDENCE
Occurs in 10 to 20 percent of all pregnancies.
Early abortion often as a result of chromosomal abnormalities incompatible with survival, or defective implantation.
Late abortions usually caused by detachment of placenta or obstruction of blood supply through cord.
Cocaine abuse disturbs blood flow to placenta and may cause placental abruption and intrauterine fetal death.

COMPLICATIONS
Disseminated intravascular coagulation syndrome: see Chapter 12.

Ectopic Pregnancy

PREDISPOSING FACTORS OF TUBAL PREGNANCY
Previous tubal infection.
Disturbed tubal motility.
Frequently both fallopian tubes predisposed.

CONSEQUENCES
Tube ruptures within a few months.
May cause profuse bleeding from torn blood vessels.

Pregnancy Subsequent to Failure of Artificial Contraception

FAILURE OF CONTRACEPTIVE PILLS
Pills effective if used properly.
Synthetic estrogens, progestins in pills may induce congenital abnormalities in developing embryo.

FAILURE OF INTRAUTERINE DEVICE (IUD)
Predisposes to infection.
Remove IUD as soon as pregnancy diagnosed.
Advise patient of risks if IUD cannot be removed.

Abnormal Attachment of Umbilical Cord and Placenta

VELAMENTOUS INSERTION OF CORD
Cord attaches to membranes, and vessels must travel in membranes to reach placenta.
Vessels may tear or be compressed during labor; may be fatal to infant, but no effect on mother.

PLACENTA PREVIA
Central placenta previa: placenta covers entire cervix.
Partial placenta previa: margin of placenta covers cervix.
Causes episodes of bleeding late in pregnancy.
Hazardous to both mother and infant.
Cesarean section delivery required.

Twins and Multiple Pregnancies

TWIN TRANSFUSION SYNDROME

Vascular anastomoses connect placental circulations of identical twins.

One twin may receive excess blood while the other becomes anemic.

Minor disproportions in blood may be tolerated, but severe disproportions may be fatal to both twins.

VANISHING TWINS AND BLIGHTED TWINS

More twin conceptions than survivals to term.

One twin dies and is either completely absorbed (vanishing twin) or persists as a degenerated fetus (blighted twin).

CONJOINED (SIAMESE) TWINS

Variable union between identical twins.

Separation often not possible after birth.

DISADVANTAGES OF TWIN PREGNANCY

Twins smaller for gestational age.

Premature onset of labor.

Higher incidence of congenital malformations.

Twin transfusion syndrome.

Preeclampsia and Eclampsia: Toxemia of Pregnancy

Hydatidiform Mole and Choriocarcinoma

GESTATIONAL TROPHOBLAST DISEASE

Three categories: "benign" hydatidiform mole, invasive mole, and choriocarcinoma.

Moles related to abnormal fertilization of a defective ovum.

Villi form cystic structures.

Invasive mole invades uterine wall.

Moles treated by emptying the uterus. Chemotherapy if mole recurs.

Choriocarcinoma is malignant, consists of neoplastic trophoblast without villi, and is treated by anticancer chemotherapy.

Hemolytic Disease of the Newborn

PATHOGENESIS AND CLINICAL MANIFESTATIONS

Infant sensitizes mother to blood group antigen.

Maternal antibody damages fetal cells.

Infant increases blood production to compensate.

Variable severity.

Hydrops fetalis: severe anemia and edema.

Anemia and jaundice.

Mild disease with few symptoms.

CHANGES IN HEMOGLOBIN AND BILIRUBIN AFTER DELIVERY

Anemia increases because blood destruction continues and compensatory hematopoiesis declines.

Jaundice develops because of inefficient excretion of bilirubin by newborn infant's liver.

Severe jaundice causes brain damage (kernicterus).

Rh Hemolytic Disease

THE Rh SYSTEM

Determined by series of allelic genes.

Individual whose red cells contain D antigen is Rh positive.
May be homozygous or heterozygous.

Most cases of Rh hemolytic disease as a result of Rh-negative mother with Rh-positive infant.

Rarely occurs in first pregnancy.

DIAGNOSIS OF HEMOLYTIC DISEASE

Blood group differences between mother and infant (e.g., mother Rh negative and fetus Rh positive).

Mother has formed antibodies (e.g., anti-D).

Antibody coats infant's cells (positive direct Coombs test).

Evidence of increased blood destruction.

TREATMENT OF HEMOLYTIC DISEASE

Exchange transfusion.
Provides population of cells not attacked by maternal antibody.
Provides plasma low in bilirubin.
Does not change infant's blood type.

Fluorescent light therapy.
Converts unconjugated bilirubin into less toxic compound.
Reduces need for exchange transfusion.

Intrauterine fetal transfusion.
Used to salvage infants who would die prior to delivery.
Blood instilled into fetal peritoneal cavity or umbilical cord using special techniques.

PREVENTION OF Rh HEMOLYTIC DISEASE

Rh immune globulin administered to mother eliminates antigenic fetal cells.

Incidence of Rh hemolytic disease greatly reduced.

Not 100% effective.

Some physicians recommend injections late in pregnancy as well as after delivery to further reduce incidence of sensitization.

ABO HEMOLYTIC DISEASE

Fetal A or B antigens stimulate maternal ABO antibodies.

Causes mild hemolytic disease.

May be encountered in first pregnancy.

http://health.jbpub.com/humandisease/9e

Human Disease Online is a great source for supplementary human disease information for both students and instructors. Visit this website to find a variety of useful tools for learning, thinking, and teaching.

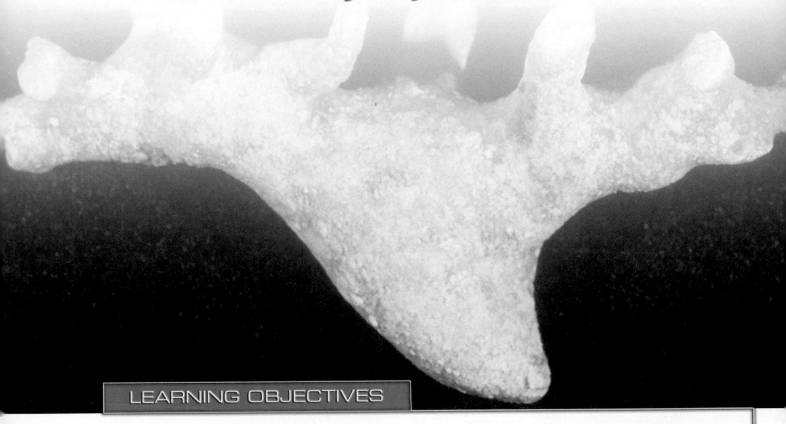

CHAPTER 19

The Urinary System

LEARNING OBJECTIVES

1 Describe the normal structures of the kidneys and their functions.

2 Explain the pathogenesis of glomerulonephritis, nephrosis, nephrosclerosis, and glomerulosclerosis. Describe the clinical manifestations of each of these disorders.

3 Describe the clinical manifestations and complications of urinary tract infections.

4 List the causes of renal tubular injury. Describe the manifestations of tubular injury and the treatments for each disorder.

5 Explain the mechanism for formation of urinary tract calculi. Describe the complications of stone formation. Explain the manifestations of urinary tract obstruction.

6 Differentiate the major forms of cystic disease of the kidney and their prognoses. Name the more common kinds of tumors affecting the urinary tract.

7 Describe the causes, clinical manifestations, and treatment of renal failure.

8 Describe the principles and techniques of hemodialysis.

Structure and Function of the Urinary System

The urinary system (FIGURE 19-1A) consists of

1. The kidneys, which produce the urine
2. An excretory duct system (renal calyces, renal pelves, and ureters) that transports the urine

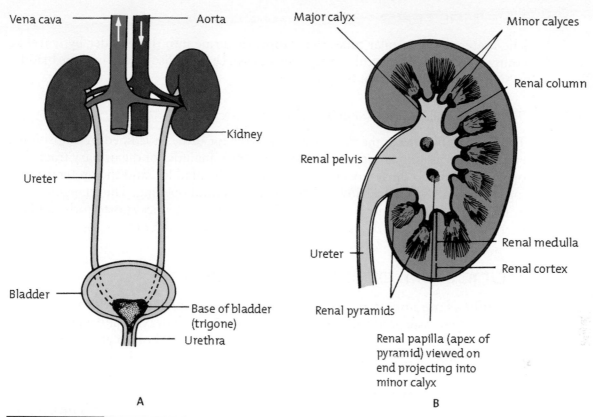

FIGURE 19-1 **A**, Components of the urinary system. **B**, Structure of the kidney in longitudinal section.

3. The bladder, where the urine is stored
4. The urethra, which conveys the urine from the bladder for excretion

THE KIDNEYS

The kidneys are paired, bean-shaped organs located along the back body wall below the diaphragm and adjacent to the vertebral column. Their structure is illustrated in FIGURE 19-1B. The region where the blood vessels enter and leave and where the ureter exits to descend to the bladder is called the hilus of the kidney. The expanded upper end of the ureter is the renal pelvis (plural, pelves). The pelvis divides into several large branches called the major calyces (singular, calyx), and these in turn subdivide to form the minor calyces. The renal substance is divided into an outer cortex and an inner medulla. The cone-shaped masses of renal tissue in the medulla that project into the minor calyces are called the renal pyramids, and the tip of each pyramid is called the renal papilla. Columns of cortical tissue that extend into the medulla between the pyramids are called the renal columns.

The calyces and pelves convey the urine into the ureters, which extend downward to enter the posterior wall of the bladder near its base, as illustrated in Figure 19-1A. Each ureter enters the bladder at an angle so that, when the bladder contracts, its muscular wall compresses the ureters as they run obliquely through it, somewhat like a one-way valve. This prevents backflow of urine into the ureters during voiding (urination). The ureteral openings in the bladder are also partially covered by folds of mucosa that help prevent retrograde flow of urine.

THE URETERS

The ureters are muscular tubes that propel the urine into the bladder by wavelike contractions of their muscular walls (**peristalsis**). Urine is discharged into the bladder in spurts. It does not drain by gravity.

THE BLADDER AND URETHRA

The urinary bladder is the distensible reservoir for urine. It is lined by transitional epithelium continuous with that which lines the remainder of the urinary tract. The opening of the urethra is located at the base of the bladder, and the ureteral openings are located on either side and behind the urethral opening. The triangular area at the base of the bladder bounded by the two ureteral orifices posteriorly, and the urethral orifice anteriorly, is called the trigone of the bladder (*tri* = three).

Function of the Kidneys

The kidneys are important excretory organs, functioning along with the lungs in excreting the waste products of food metabolism. Carbon dioxide and water are end-products of carbohydrate and fat metabolism. Protein metabolism produces urea, as well as various acids, which only the kidneys can excrete. The kidneys also play an important role in regulating mineral and water balance by excreting minerals and water that have been ingested in excess of the body's requirements and conserving minerals and water as required. It has been said that the internal environment of the body is determined not by what a person ingests but rather by what the kidneys retain.

The kidneys serve an endocrine function as well. Specialized cells in the kidneys elaborate a hormone called **erythropoietin**, which regulates red blood cell production in the bone marrow, and another humoral substance called **renin**, which takes part in the regulation of the blood pressure.

THE NEPHRON

The basic structural and functional unit of the kidney is the **nephron**, and there are about one million nephrons in each kidney. Each nephron consists of a glomerulus and a renal tubule. The glomerulus is a tuft of capillaries supplied by an afferent glomerular arteriole. The capillaries of the glomerulus then recombine into an efferent glomerular arteriole, which in turn breaks up into a network of capillaries that supplies the renal tubule. The site where the afferent arteriole enters the glomerulus and the efferent arteriole exits is called the vascular pole of the glomerulus.

The histologic structure of the glomerulus and related structures is illustrated schematically in FIGURE 19-2. The expanded proximal end of the tubule is called **Bowman's capsule**. The tuft of capillaries that make up the glomerulus is pushed into Bowman's capsule much as one would push a fist into a balloon. The layer of Bowman's capsule cells, which is pushed in (invaginated), becomes closely applied to the capillaries of the glomerulus and is called the visceral layer of Bowman's capsule or simply the glomerular epithelium. The cells of this layer have long, footlike cytoplasmic processes and are usually called podocytes (*podos* = foot) (Figure 19-2A). The outer layer of Bowman's capsule is called the parietal layer of Bowman's capsule, or simply the capsular epithelium. The space between the two layers, into which the urine filters, is called Bowman's space.

The capillary tuft is held together and supported by groups of highly specialized cells embedded in a basement membranelike material. The cells are located between the capillaries and are concentrated at the vascular pole of the glomerulus. Because of

Peristalsis
The wavelike contractions of the wall of the alimentary tract that propel contents through the bowel.

Erythropoietin
(er-ith-rō-poy′e-tin)
A humoral substance made by the kidneys that regulates hematopoiesis.

Renin (ren′in)
A humoral substance secreted by the kidneys in response to fall in blood pressure, blood volume, or sodium concentration.

Nephron (nef′răn)
The glomerulus and renal tubule.

Bowman's capsule
The cuplike expanded end of the nephron that surrounds the tuft of glomerular capillaries.

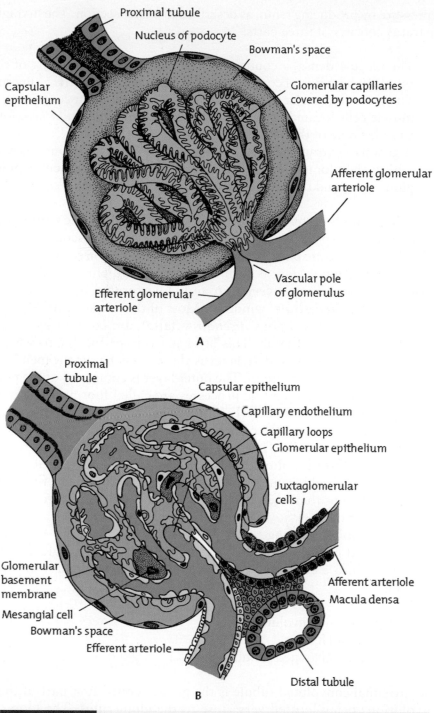

Proximal tubule

Nucleus of podocyte

Bowman's space

Capsular epithelium

Glomerular capillaries covered by podocytes

Afferent glomerular arteriole

Efferent glomerular arteriole

Vascular pole of glomerulus

A

Proximal tubule

Capsular epithelium

Capillary endothelium

Capillary loops

Glomerular epithelium

Juxtaglomerular cells

Afferent arteriole

Macula densa

Glomerular basement membrane

Mesangial cell

Bowman's space

Efferent arteriole

Distal tubule

B

FIGURE 19-2 The structure of the glomerulus and Bowman's capsule. **A**, Anterior half of Bowman's capsule removed to reveal capillary tuft covered by podocytes (schematic). **B**, Cross section through glomerulus to reveal structure of glomerular filter and juxtaglomerular apparatus.

Mesangial cell
(mes-an'jē-yul)
Modified connective-tissue cells at the vascular pole of the glomerulus that hold the capillary tuft together.

Juxtaglomerular apparatus
(jux'tu-glo-mãr'ū-lär)
A specialized group of cells at the vascular pole of the glomerulus that regulates blood flow through the glomerulus of the kidneys.

their location between the capillaries, they are called **mesangial cells** (*meso* = middle + *angio* = vessel). In addition to their support function, they are also contractile cells that play a role in regulating glomerular filtration by varying the caliber of the capillaries, and they are also phagocytic cells. Also located at the vascular pole is a specialized cluster of cells called the **juxtaglomerular apparatus** (*juxta* = near to), which regulates blood flow through the glomerulus. It also plays a role in regulating blood pressure by producing renin, as described in a later section. The juxtaglomerular apparatus consists of three parts:

1. The macula densa, a condensation of cells in the distal part of the renal tubule, where it is in contact with the vascular pole of the glomerulus
2. The juxtaglomerular cells, which are specialized renin-containing smooth muscle cells located in the wall of the afferent glomerular arteriole at the vascular pole of the glomerulus
3. A group of extraglomerular mesangial cells that are continuous with those within the glomerulus and interposed between the vascular pole of the glomerulus and the macula densa (Figure 19-2B)

Water and soluble material filter from the blood through the glomerular capillaries into Bowman's space. When visualized by electron microscopy, the membrane through which the filtrate passes can be seen to consist of three layers, as depicted in FIGURE 19-3. The inner layer is formed by the endothelium of the glomerular capillaries. The cytoplasm is very thin and is perforated by many small holes called fenestrations (*fenestra* = window). Most of the fenestrations are open, but some, called pseudofenestrations (*pseudo* = false), are covered by a thin membrane containing a central knob. This layer is freely permeable to water and to many large molecules. The middle layer is the porous basement membrane that supports the capillary endothelium. The outer layer is composed of the podocytes. Their highly branched cytoplasmic processes are called **foot processes**, and their terminal branches are called **pedicels** ("little feet"). The pedicels are attached to the basement membrane, and the pedicels of one cell interdigitate with others from the same cell or adjacent cells. The narrow spaces between adjacent interdigitating pedicels are called **filtration slits**. Each slit is covered by a thin membrane called a **filtration membrane** and is reinforced by a filamentous ridge. The filtration membranes are less porous than the other layers of the glomerular filter and perform much of the filtration.

The renal tubules are long tubes that measure as much as 4 cm in length. The proximal end of the tubule is invaginated by the glomerulus, and its distal end empties into a collecting tubule. The tubule is divided into three parts (FIGURE 19-4):

1. The proximal convoluted tubule
2. The loop of Henle
3. The distal convoluted tubule

The proximal convoluted tubule is the greatly coiled first part of the tubule, its convolutions being located very close to the glomerulus. The loop of Henle is a U-shaped segment composed of descending and ascending limbs joined by a short segment. The descending limb and proximal half of the ascending limb are lined by flat epithelial cells, forming the thin segment of Henle's loop. The distal part of the ascending limb, called the thick segment of Henle's loop, is lined by tall columnar epithelium similar to that lining the distal tubule. The loop descends from the cortex into the medulla and then bends back sharply, returning to the cortex close to the vascular pole of its own glomerulus, where it becomes continuous with the distal convoluted tubule. The distal convoluted tubule is much shorter than the proximal tubule. It empties into a collecting tubule, which passes through the medulla to drain into one of the minor calyces at the apex of a renal pyramid (renal papilla).

Foot processes
The highly branched cytoplasmic processes of the podocytes covering the glomerular capillaries of the kidneys.

Pedicel
(ped'i-cel)
One of the small terminal processes of the podocytes that cover the glomerular capillaries.

Filtration slits
The narrow spaces between the pedicels of the podocytes that cover the glomerular capillaries of the kidneys.

Filtration membrane
The thin membrane covering the filtration slit between pedicels of the podocytes that cover the glomerular capillaries of the kidneys.

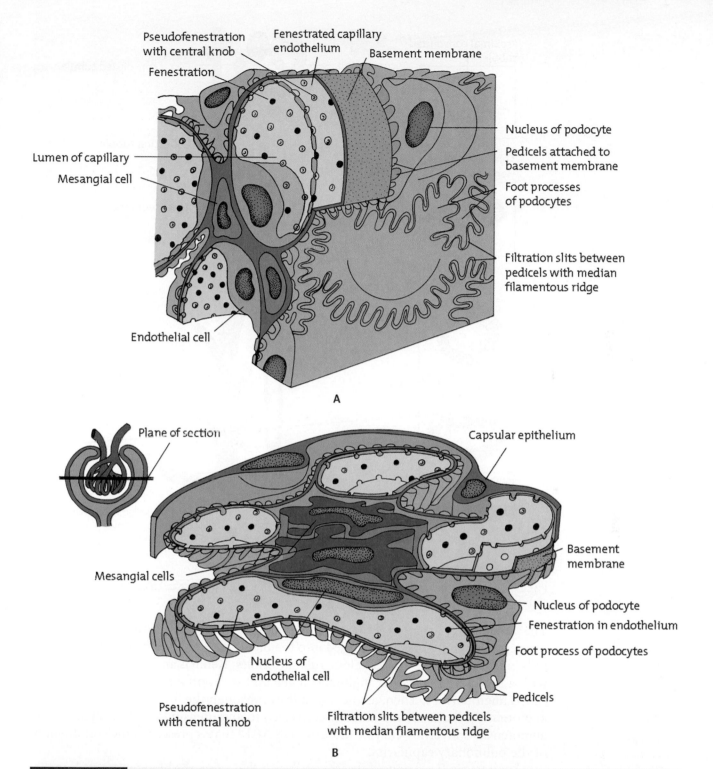

FIGURE 19-3 A schematic representation of fine structure of glomerular filter as visualized by electron microscopy. **A**, Segment of glomerular capillaries. **B**, Cross section through the center of the glomerulus, including part of Bowman's capsule.

The renal tubules selectively reabsorb water, minerals, and other substances that are to be conserved and excrete unwanted materials that are eliminated. Urine is the glomerular filtrate that remains after most of the water and important constituents have been reabsorbed by the renal tubules, and other substances excreted by the renal tubules have been added.

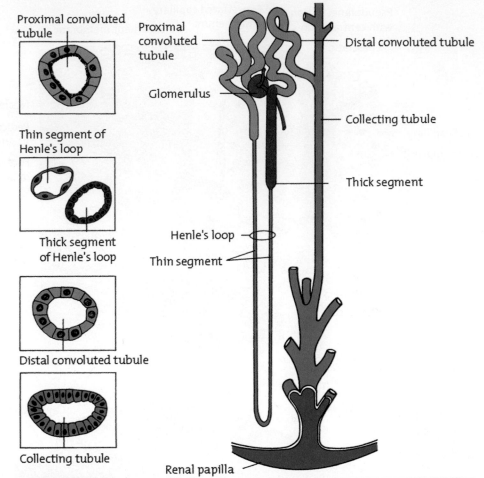

FIGURE 19-4 The structure of the renal tubule, illustrating its relationship to the glomerulus and the collecting tubule. The epithelium characteristic of each part of the renal tubule and the collecting tubule are also illustrated.

Renin (ren'in)
A humoral substance secreted by the kidneys in response to fall in blood pressure, blood volume, or sodium concentration.

Angiotensinogen
(an-jee-o-ten-sin'-o-gen)
A blood protein converted to angiotensin I by renin secreted by the kidneys. Part of the renin-angiotensin-aldosterone system.

Angiotensin
(an-jē-o-ten'sin)
A component of the renin-angiotensin-aldosterone system that raises blood pressure by constricting blood vessels and stimulating the adrenal grand to secrete aldosterone, which increases blood volume.

Angiotensin converting enzyme
An enzyme that converts angiotensin I to angiotensin II.

Aldosterone
A steroid hormone produced by the adrenal cortex that regulates the rate of sodium absorption from the renal tubules.

RENAL REGULATION OF BLOOD PRESSURE AND BLOOD VOLUME

The kidneys play a major role in regulating both the blood pressure and blood volume by secreting renin, which is released into the bloodstream from the juxtaglomerular cells in the walls of the afferent glomerular arterioles. **Renin** is an enzyme that interacts with a blood protein called **angiotensinogen** and splits off a short peptide fragment called **angiotensin I**. Then, as the blood flows through the lungs, the newly formed angiotensin I is almost immediately converted to **angiotensin II** by an enzyme called **angiotensin-converting enzyme** (abbreviated ACE) that is present in the endothelium of the pulmonary capillaries.

Angiotensin II is a powerful vasoconstrictor that raises the blood pressure by causing the peripheral arterioles to constrict. Angiotensin II also stimulates the adrenal cortex to secrete a steroid hormone called **aldosterone**, which increases reabsorption of sodium chloride and water by the kidneys. As a result, the blood volume is increased by the greater volume of salt and water entering the circulation, and the blood pressure rises because there is more fluid within the vascular system. Thus, renin regulates blood pressure both by controlling the degree of arteriolar vasoconstriction and by regulating the volume of fluid within the circulation. The system is self-regulating because renin secretion declines as blood pressure, volume, and sodium concentration are restored to normal (FIGURE 19-5).

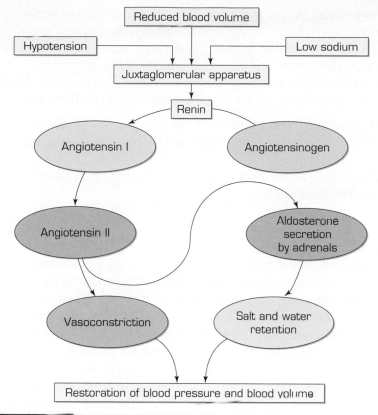

FIGURE 19-5 The role of the kidneys in regulation of blood pressure and blood volume, as described in the text.

REQUIREMENTS FOR NORMAL RENAL FUNCTION

The functions of the two kidneys reflect the sum of the functions of their individual nephrons. For a nephron to function normally, the following conditions must be satisfied:

1. There must be free flow of blood through the glomerular capillaries.
2. The glomerular filter must function normally. An adequate volume of filtrate must be produced, but the filter must restrict passage of blood cells and proteins.
3. The tubules must be able to selectively reabsorb important substances from the filtrate and to excrete other constituents into the filtrate.
4. The urine formed by the nephron must be able to flow freely from the kidney into the bladder and out of the urethra.

Derangement of any of these functions results in kidney disease.

Developmental Disturbances

The urinary system develops from several different components. The kidneys form from masses of primitive connective tissue (mesoderm) located along the back body wall of the embryo. The bladder develops as an offshoot of the lower end of the intestinal tract. The ureters, renal pelves, renal calyces (the urinary drainage system), and the renal collecting tubules derive from paired tubular structures called ureteric buds. Each bud grows upward from the developing bladder and connects with the kidney that is forming on the corresponding side. The kidneys begin their development within the pelvis. Later, as the embryo grows, the kidneys and their excretory ducts come to occupy a higher location, until eventually they ascend to reach their final positions in the upper lumbar region (FIGURE 19-6A).

Sometimes this developmental process is disturbed, and congenital malformations result. Three of the more common developmental abnormalities are:

1. Failure of one or both kidneys to develop, which is called renal agenesis
2. Formation of extra ureters and renal pelves, which are called duplications of the urinary tract
3. Malpositions of one or both kidneys, which is often associated with fusion of the two kidneys

Renal agenesis (*a* = without + *genesis* = formation) may affect one or both kidneys. Bilateral renal agenesis is uncommon. It often accompanies other congenital malformations and is incompatible with postnatal life. In contrast, unilateral renal agenesis (FIGURE 19-6B) is a relatively common condition that has an incidence of about one in a thousand persons, about the same frequency as cleft palate. When one kidney is absent, the other kidney enlarges and is able to carry out the functions of the missing kidney; so the affected person is usually not inconvenienced by the abnormality. The recognition of this condition, however, is of great importance to the clinician who is treating an individual with kidney disease because one can never assume that the patient has two kidneys. Before a surgeon performs a kidney operation, diagnostic studies must always be performed first in order to ascertain that the patient has two kidneys. Such precautions are essential to prevent inadvertent removal of a solitary kidney.

Duplications of the urinary tract may be unilateral or bilateral. Sometimes, a kidney has an extra renal pelvis and ureter that drains separately into the bladder (complete duplication). Sometimes, double ureters draining the kidney unite to form a single ureter just before entering the bladder (partial duplication). Duplications result from abnormal prenatal development of the ureteric buds. A complete duplication results when an extra ureteric bud develops and gives rise to a separate excretory system draining the kidney on the affected side. If the ureteric bud branches after it has formed, only the upper part of the excretory system is duplicated; the lower part of the ureter is not duplicated and enters the bladder normally (FIGURE 19-6C).

Abnormalities of position and fusion of the kidneys may occur if both kidneys remain in the pelvis where they began their development or if they ascend only part way (FIGURE 19-6D). Kidneys that fail to ascend normally are in very close approximation as they develop and may become fused. One of the more common fusion abnormalities is a union of the lower poles of the two kidneys to form a U-shaped mass of renal tissue called a horseshoe kidney (FIGURE 19-6E). In other cases, when the kidneys ascend abnormally, the upper pole of one kidney may become fused to the lower pole of the other (FIGURE 19-6F).

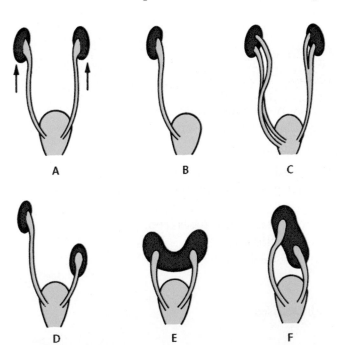

FIGURE 19-6 Common congenital abnormalities of kidneys and urinary tract. **A,** Normal ascent of kidneys. **B,** Unilateral renal agenesis. **C,** Various types of duplications of ureters and renal pelves resulting from formation of an extra ureteric bud (*left*) or premature splitting of a single ureteric bud (*right*). **D,** Failure of one kidney to ascend to normal position. **E,** Horseshoe kidney resulting from fusion of lower poles of kidneys. **F,** Fusion of the lower pole of one kidney to the upper pole of opposite kidney, which has failed to ascend normally.

Renal duplications, malpositions, and fusions often are of little clinical significance. At times, however, drainage of urine may be impeded by the abnormalities, causing the urine to stagnate and predisposing the patient to urinary infections. Another important developmental abnormality called congenital polycystic kidney disease is considered in the section on renal cysts.

Glomerulonephritis

Glomerulonephritis is an inflammation of the glomeruli caused by an antigen–antibody reaction within the glomerular capillaries. The interaction of antigen and antibody activates complement and liberates mediators that attract polymorphonuclear leukocytes. The actual glomerular injury is caused by destructive lysosomal enzymes that are released from the leukocytes that have accumulated within the glomeruli.

The antigen–antibody reaction within the glomeruli may take place in two ways. In most cases, the antigen and antibody interact within the circulation, forming small clumps called immune complexes. These are deposited in the walls of the glomerular capillaries as the blood filters through the glomeruli. Glomerulonephritis that occurs in this way is called immune-complex glomerulonephritis. Less commonly, the glomerular inflammation is caused by an autoantibody directed against the basement membranes of the glomerular capillaries. This type of glomerulonephritis is called antiglomerular basement membrane (anti-GBM) glomerulonephritis. FIGURE 19-7 illustrates the histologic appearance of these two types of glomerulonephritis compared with the appearance of a normal glomerulus.

Glomerulonephritis
(glo-mär′ū-lō-nef-rī′tis)
An inflammation of the glomeruli caused by either antigen–antibody complexes trapped in the glomeruli or by antiglomerular basement membrane antibodies.

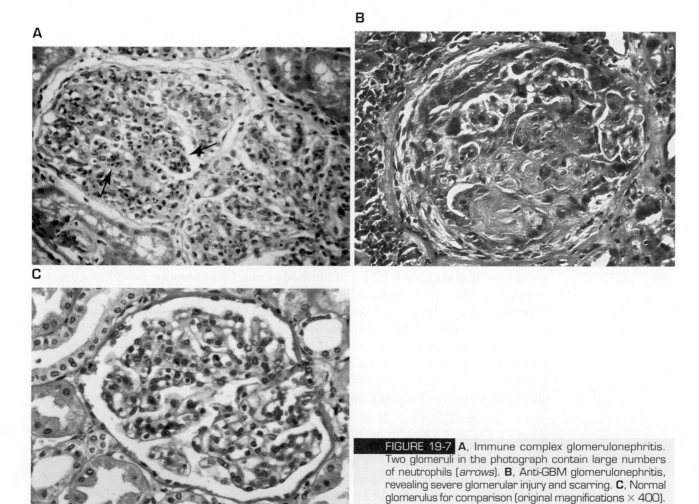

FIGURE 19-7 **A**, Immune complex glomerulonephritis. Two glomeruli in the photograph contain large numbers of neutrophils (*arrows*). **B**, Anti-GBM glomerulonephritis, revealing severe glomerular injury and scarring. **C**, Normal glomerulus for comparison (original magnifications × 400).

IMMUNE-COMPLEX GLOMERULONEPHRITIS

Immune-complex glomerulonephritis may develop as a complication about 2 weeks after infection by certain beta streptococci, the same type of organism that causes the familiar streptococcal sore throat. However, glomerular inflammation occurs only in a small percentage of patients with streptococcal infections. In affected subjects, the body responds to the streptococcal infection by forming antistreptococcal antibodies that interact in the bloodstream with soluble antigens from the streptococci to form immune complexes. Some of the antigen–antibody complexes are small enough to pass completely through the walls of the glomerular capillaries and be excreted in the urine. Larger complexes, however, pass through the endothelium and basement membranes of the glomerular capillaries but become trapped between the filtration slits of the glomerular epithelial cells, where they induce an inflammatory reaction.

Acute glomerulonephritis may at times follow other bacterial infections or viral infections. The mechanism of glomerular injury is similar to that of poststreptococcal glomerulonephritis. Immune complexes composed of a bacterial or viral antigen and its corresponding antibody interact in the circulation and are trapped in the glomeruli, where they produce inflammation and injury by activating complement and attracting leukocytes (Figure 19-7A).

The signs and symptoms of glomerulonephritis are related to the changes within the glomeruli. Many glomeruli are completely blocked by inflammation, and thus, less blood is filtered and less urine is excreted. As urinary output is reduced, waste products are retained and accumulate in the blood. Other glomeruli, damaged by lysosomal enzymes, are no longer able to function as efficient filters. Protein and red cells leak through the damaged glomerular capillary walls and are excreted in the urine. Frequently, masses of red cells and protein accumulate within the tubules and become molded to the shape of the renal tubules before finally being excreted. These structures, which are called urinary casts, are an important indication of glomerular injury.

In most cases, glomerulonephritis subsides spontaneously and the patient recovers completely without residual kidney damage. Occasionally, the disease is so severe that the patient requires dialysis treatment for renal insufficiency. In some patients, the glomerulonephritis never heals completely. The disease becomes chronic, progresses slowly, and eventually causes renal failure. Patients with chronic poststreptococcal glomerulonephritis who develop a streptococcal sore throat or other streptococcal infection may experience recurrent episodes of acute glomerulonephritis. This is analogous to the situation in rheumatic fever in which recurrent beta-streptococcal infections are sometimes followed by recurrent episodes of rheumatic fever.

Immune-complex glomerulonephritis may also occur in association with autoimmune diseases in which autoantibody-containing immune complexes become trapped in renal glomeruli, as in lupus erythematosus (discussion on immunity, hypersensitivity, allergy, and autoimmune diseases). Another relatively common type of immune-complex glomerulonephritis is associated with proliferation of mesangial cells and accumulation of immune complexes containing immunoglobulin A (IgA) within the cells. Because of the type of immunoglobulin associated with the disease, it is often called IgA nephropathy. Unfortunately, in many patients, this type of glomerulonephritis becomes chronic and slowly progressive.

ANTI-GBM GLOMERULONEPHRITIS

Glomerulonephritis caused by autoantibodies directed against glomerular basement membranes (anti-GBM glomerulonephritis) is a type of autoimmune disease. It is a relatively uncommon cause of acute glomerulonephritis. In some patients, the anti-GBM antibodies may also injure the basement membranes of the pulmonary capillaries and may cause intrapulmonary hemorrhage as well as acute glomerulonephritis.

It is possible to distinguish immune-complex glomerulonephritis from anti-GBM glomerulonephritis by special studies performed on kidney tissue obtained by renal biopsy. Immune-complex glomerulonephritis is characterized by large, irregular, lumpy deposits composed of antigen, antibody, and complement. These deposits form along the outer surface of the glomerular basement membranes, where the complexes have been trapped between the filtration slits of the glomerular epithelial cells. In contrast, anti-GBM nephritis is characterized by a relatively uniform layer of antibody and complement deposited along the inner surface of the glomerular basement membranes.

Case 19-1 illustrates the clinical features of glomerulonephritis that lead to renal failure and demonstrates the use of renal biopsy.

CASE 19-1

A 51-year-old man was admitted to the hospital because of cough, chest pain, and weight loss. Physical examination was essentially normal. The urine contained a moderate amount of protein and many red cells. Blood urea nitrogen was 87 mg/dl (normal range 10–20 mg/dl). Blood pH was reduced to 7.2 (normal range 7.35–7.45). Plasma bicarbonate was reduced to 15 mcq/L (normal range 24–28 meq/L). A renal biopsy revealed an active glomerulonephritis (Figure 19–7B). By means of special studies, immunoglobulins and complement were identified uniformly attached to the glomerular basement membranes. The lesion was interpreted as glomerulonephritis secondary to antiglomerular basement membrane antibodies. The patient was referred to another center for dialysis and further treatment.

Nephrotic Syndrome

The term **nephrotic syndrome** refers to a group of abnormalities characterized by a severe loss of protein in the urine. Urinary excretion of protein is so great that the body is unable to manufacture protein fast enough to keep up with the losses and the concentration of protein in the blood plasma falls. This, in turn, causes significant edema owing to the low plasma osmotic pressure (discussion on circulatory disturbances). Nephrotic syndrome may be produced by a number of different types of renal diseases. The basic cause is injury to the glomerulus that allows proteins to leak through the damaged basement membrane. Because the albumin molecule is much smaller than the globulin molecule, a disproportionately large amount of albumin is lost in the urine. The osmotic pressure of the plasma falls to such an extent that excessive amounts of fluid leak from the capillaries into the interstitial tissues and body cavities. Patients with the nephrotic syndrome have marked leg edema, and often fluid collects in the abdominal cavity (called **ascites**); sometimes; fluid also accumulates in the pleural cavities (called **hydrothorax**).

When the nephrotic syndrome occurs in children, it is usually caused by a relatively minimal abnormality in the foot processes of the glomerular epithelial cells. Nephrotic syndrome caused by this type of glomerular abnormality responds to corticosteroid therapy, and most children recover completely, as illustrated by Case 19-2.

Nephrotic syndrome
(nef-rä′tik sin′drōm)
A generalized edema resulting from excessive protein loss in the urine, caused by various types of renal disease.

Ascites
(a-si′tēz)
Accumulation of fluid in the abdominal cavity.

Hydrothorax
(hī-drō-thor′ax)
Accumulation of fluid in the pleural cavity.

CASE 19-2

A 6-year-old boy complained of abdominal discomfort. His mother noted that his face, abdomen, scrotum, and legs were very edematous. His urine contained large amounts of protein and a few casts. His serum protein and serum albumin were both much lower than normal. Additional studies of serum proteins by electrophoresis were also consistent with nephrotic syndrome. The child was hospitalized, placed on a low-sodium diet, and treated with adrenal corticosteroid hormones. The edema gradually subsided, and the corticosteroids were gradually discontinued. He was discharged after a 2-week hospitalization.

In contrast to the favorable outcome in children, the nephrotic syndrome in adults is usually a manifestation of progressive, more serious renal disease in which there are marked structural changes in the glomeruli. Some cases result from chronic progressive glomerulonephritis; others result from glomerular damage resulting from long-standing diabetes, as described later, or from a connective-tissue disease affecting the kidney, such as lupus erythematosus. Some other relatively uncommon types of kidney disease involving the glomeruli may also produce nephrotic syndrome.

Nephrosclerosis
Thickening and narrowing of the afferent glomerular arterioles as a result of disease.

Arteriolar Nephrosclerosis

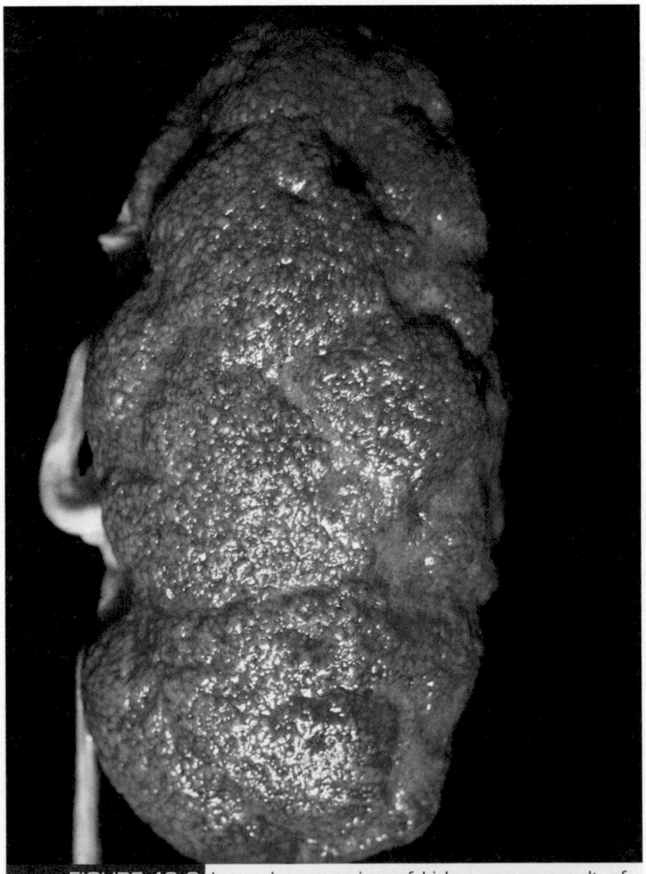

FIGURE 19-8 Irregular scarring of kidney as a result of nephrosclerosis.

Arteriolar nephrosclerosis (sometimes called simply **nephrosclerosis**) is a complication of severe hypertension. Because of the extreme elevation of the systemic blood pressure, the small arterioles and arteries throughout the body are called on to carry blood at a much higher pressure than normal. As a result, the blood vessels undergo severe degenerative changes characterized by thickening and narrowing of the lumens; this reduces blood flow through the narrowed arterioles. The name of the disease, which means literally "sclerosis of the arterioles of the nephrons," refers to these characteristic renal vascular changes. Glomerular filtration is reduced because the arterioles are greatly narrowed. The renal tubules, which are also supplied by the glomerular arterioles, also undergo degenerative changes. Eventually, the kidneys become shrunken and scarred as a result of reduction of their blood supply (FIGURE 19-8). Patients with severe nephrosclerosis may die from renal insufficiency, as well as from the effects of the severe hypertension.

Diabetic Nephropathy

Persons with long-standing diabetes mellitus often develop progressive renal damage. The glomerular

A   **B**

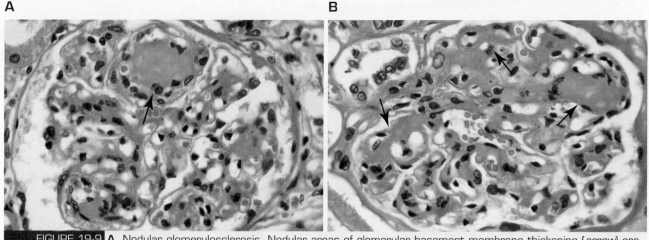

FIGURE 19-9 **A**, Nodular glomerulosclerosis. Nodular areas of glomerular basement membrane thickening (*arrow*) are characteristic of diabetes. **B**, Diffuse glomerulosclerosis. Diffuse glomerular basement membrane thickening (*arrows*) also occurs in diabetes, but it may also occur in other types of glomerular disease.

basement membranes exhibit characteristic nodular and diffuse thickening called **diabetic glomerulosclerosis** (FIGURE 19-9), which disturbs glomerular function. Usually there is also severe sclerosis of the glomerular arterioles, impairing the flow of blood to the glomeruli and tubules. Sometimes the general term **diabetic nephropathy** (*nephros* = kidney + *path* = disease) is used when referring to both the glomerular and the arteriolar lesions.

Clinically, the condition is characterized by progressive impairment of renal function that may eventually lead to renal failure. Protein leaks through the diseased glomeruli and is lost in the urine. In some patients, so much protein is lost that the nephrotic syndrome develops. There is no specific treatment that can arrest the progression of the disease. A renal transplant may be required if the patient develops renal failure. (Diabetes mellitus and its complications are considered in the pancreas and diabetes mellitus discussion.)

GOUT-ASSOCIATED NEPHROPATHY

Persons with gout, described in the discussion on the musculoskeletal system, have a higher than normal concentration of relatively insoluble uric acid in their blood and body fluids, which leads to periodic episodes of acute joint inflammation (gouty arthritis) caused by precipitation of uric acid as sodium urate crystals in their joints. Although the skeletal manifestations of gout are well known, gout also frequently affects the kidneys and urinary tract. Many patients develop kidney stones, described later in this chapter. Sodium urate crystals may also precipitate from the tubular filtrate within the Henle's loops and in the collecting tubules within the renal pyramids where the tubular filtrate is very concentrated. The precipitates obstruct and damage the renal tubules, which is followed by scarring and impaired renal function, a condition called **urate nephropathy** (FIGURE 19-10).

Infections of the Urinary Tract

Urinary tract infections are common and may be either acute or chronic. An infection that affects only the bladder is called **cystitis** (*cystis* = bladder). If the upper urinary tract is infected, the term is **pyelonephritis** (*pyelo* = pelvis + *nephros* = kidney + *itis*

Diabetic glomerulosclerosis
(glo-mēr′ū-lō-skler-rō′sis)
Diffuse and nodular thickening of glomerular basement membranes, a common occurrence in patients with long-standing diabetes mellitus.

Diabetic nephropathy
Kidney damage affecting primarily the kidney blood vessels (arterioles) and glomeruli caused by diabetes.

Urate nephropathy
(nĕf-rop′-uh-thē)
Kidney damage caused by precipitation of urate crystals within the kidney tubules of a person with gout.

Cystitis
(sis-tī′tis)
Inflammation of the bladder.

Pyelonephritis
(pī′el-ō-nef-rī′tis)
A bacterial infection of the kidney and renal pelvis.

B

A

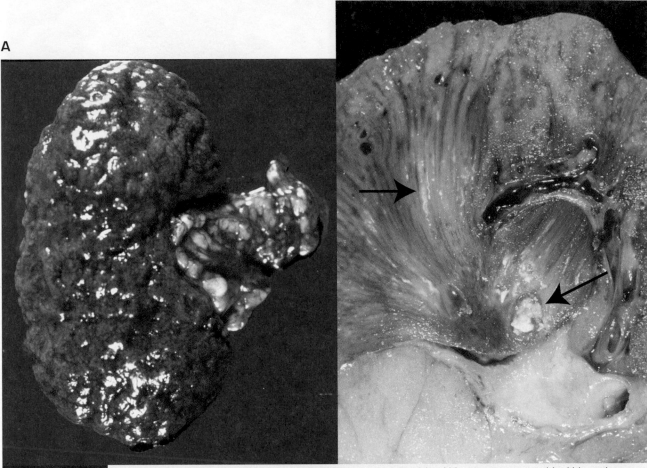

FIGURE 19-10 **A**, Urate nephropathy showing multiple depressed scars involving kidney cortex caused by kidney damage resulting from tubular obstruction by urate crystals. **B**, Section of kidney revealing white urate deposits within renal pyramid (*upper arrow*) and large urate deposit near tip of pyramid (*lower arrow*).

= inflammation). Most infections are caused by gram-negative intestinal bacteria. These organisms often contaminate the perianal and genital areas and gain access to the urinary tract by ascending the urethra.

Free urine flow, large urine volume, and complete emptying of the bladder protect against urinary tract infections because any bacteria that enter the bladder are soon flushed out during urination instead of being retained to multiply in the bladder urine. An acid urine is an additional defense against infection because most bacteria grow poorly in an acid environment. On the other hand, several conditions predispose to urinary tract infections:

1. Any condition that impairs free drainage of urine increases the likelihood of infection because stagnation of urine favors multiplication of any bacteria that enter the urinary tract.
2. Injury to the mucosa of the urinary tract, as by a kidney stone (calculus) or foreign body, disrupts the protective epithelium, permitting bacteria to invade the deeper tissues and set up an infection.
3. Introduction of a catheter or instrument into the bladder may carry bacteria into the urinary tract when the catheter or instrument is introduced and may also injure the bladder mucosa.

CYSTITIS

Cystitis is more common in women than in men, probably because the short female urethra allows infectious organisms to enter the bladder more easily. Young, sexually active women are especially predisposed because sexual intercourse promotes transfer of bacteria from the distal urethra into the bladder and may cause minor injury to the mucosa at the base of the bladder (trigone). Cystitis is also common in older men who cannot empty their bladders completely because of an enlarged prostate gland (discussion on the male reproductive system). The urine remaining in the bladder after voiding favors multiplication of bacteria and may lead to infection.

The manifestations of cystitis result from congestion and inflammation of the bladder (vesical) mucosa. The patient complains of burning pain on urination and a desire to urinate frequently. The urine contains many bacteria and leukocytes. Cystitis is not usually a serious problem and generally responds promptly to antibiotics. Sometimes, however, the infection may spread into the upper urinary tract to affect the renal pelvis and kidney.

PYELONEPHRITIS

Most cases of pyelonephritis are secondary to spread of infection from the bladder (ascending pyelonephritis), but occasionally, the organisms are carried to the kidneys through the bloodstream (hematogenous pyelonephritis). The symptoms of pyelonephritis are those of an acute infection, together with localized pain and tenderness over the affected kidney. Histologically, the infected portion of the kidney is infiltrated by masses of leukocytes and bacteria, and many of the renal tubules in the inflamed area are filled with leukocytes (FIGURE 19-11). Because cystitis and pyelonephritis are frequently associated, the patient also experiences urinary frequency and pain on urination; the urine contains many bacteria and leukocytes. Treatment is with appropriate antibiotics, together with measures directed at correcting any abnormalities in the lower urinary tract that may impede drainage of urine and predispose to infection.

Most episodes of pyelonephritis respond promptly to treatment. If part of the kidney is severely damaged by the infection, the injured area heals by scarring. The main danger of pyelonephritis lies in the tendency of the disease to become chronic and recurrent. With each subsequent attack, more kidney tissue may be destroyed and healed by scarring. After many episodes of infection, the kidneys may become markedly scarred and shrunken, until the patient eventually exhibits manifestations of renal insufficiency.

VESICOURETERAL REFLUX AND INFECTION

Normally, effective mechanisms prevent urine from flowing upward from the bladder into the ureters during urination. Sometimes, however, these

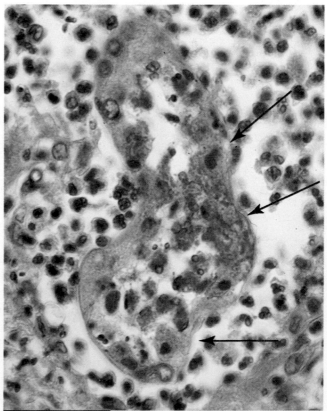

FIGURE 19-11 Acute pyelonephritis. The tubule in the center of field contains masses of bacteria that extend through wall of tubule (*middle arrow*.) Some tubule cells are necrotic (*upper and lower arrows*). Many neutrophils surround the tubules (original magnification × 400).

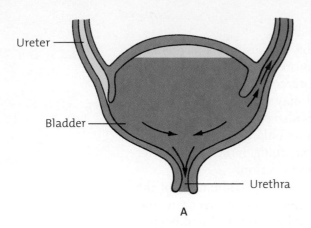

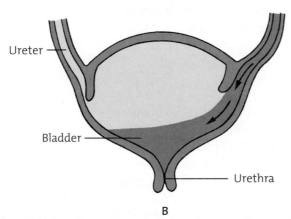

FIGURE 19-12 Vesicoureteral reflux. **A**, Urine is forced up one ureter during voiding (*right side* of illustration) because of defective function of the vesicoureteral valve. **B**, Urine flows back into bladder after voiding, which prevents complete emptying of bladder and predisposes to infection.

Vesicoureteral reflux
(ves′i-kō-ū r-ēt′er-al)
Retrograde flow of urine from the bladder into the ureter during voiding.

Calculus
A stone formed within the body, as in the kidney or gallbladder.

Gout
A disorder of nucleoprotein metabolism characterized by elevated uric acid and deposition of uric acid in and around joints.

Staghorn calculus
(kal′kū-lus)
A large renal calculus that has adopted the configuration of the renal pelvis and calyces where it formed.

Renal colic
Intense flank pain radiating into the groin, resulting from passage of a renal calculus into the ureter.

mechanisms are defective, permitting urine to flow retrograde (reflux) into one or both ureters when the bladder contracts during urination. This condition is called **vesicoureteral reflux**. It predisposes to urinary tract infection by preventing complete emptying of the bladder. The urine forced into the ureters during voiding flows back into the bladder at the completion of urination; so residual urine remains in the bladder (FIGURE 19-12). Bacteria also may be carried into the upper urinary tract by the reflux of urine; this predisposes to pyelonephritis.

Calculi

Stones may form anywhere in the urinary tract. They are usually called **calculi** (singular, calculus), which is a Latin word meaning "little stone" or "pebble." Most are composed either of uric acid or of a mixture of calcium salts. Three factors predispose to stone formation: increased concentration of salts in the urine, infection of the urinary tract, and urinary tract obstruction.

A greatly increased excretion of salts in the urine causes the urine to become supersaturated, and the salts may precipitate to form calculi, especially if the urine is concentrated. For example, in the disease called **gout** (discussion on the musculoskeletal system), excretion of uric acid is often greatly increased, which may cause uric acid to precipitate from the urine and form uric acid calculi. In conditions characterized by hyperfunction of the parathyroid glands, which regulate calcium metabolism (discussion on the endocrine glands), excessive calcium is excreted in the urine, often with the subsequent formation of urinary tract calculi composed of calcium salts.

Infection predisposes to calculi primarily by reducing the solubility of the salts in the urine. Clusters of bacteria also serve as sites where urinary salts may crystallize to form the stone.

Obstruction of the outflow of urine predisposes to stone formation by causing stagnation of urine, and urinary salts tend to precipitate out. Stagnation also predisposes to infection, which further increases the likelihood of stone formation.

Most calculi are small, but occasionally, they may gradually increase in size to form large branching structures that adopt the contour of the renal pelvis and calyces where they have formed. This kind of structure is called a **staghorn calculus** because it vaguely resembles the antlers of a male deer (FIGURE 19-13). Smaller stones sometimes pass into the ureter. The smooth muscle of the ureter contracts spasmodically to propel the stone along the ureter, causing **renal colic**—paroxysms of intense flank pain radiating into the groin. Frequently, the rough edges of the stone injure the lining of the ureter, causing red blood cells to appear in the urine. Many stones can be passed through the ureter and excreted in the urine, but some become impacted in the ureter and must be removed. A stone lodged in the distal ureter can usually be removed by inserting a cystoscope into the bladder and then passing a specially designed catheterlike instrument through the cystoscope into the ureter. The instrument is constructed to snare the stone, which is then pulled through the ureter into the bladder and extracted through the cystoscope. A stone lodged in the proximal ureter is usually broken into fragments by a procedure called **shock wave lithotripsy**, a procedure that can break into small fragments a large stone that is too big to pass through the ureter so that the smaller pieces can be excreted in the urine instead of requiring a surgical procedure to remove the stone. The usual method for fragmenting a calculus involves positioning the recumbent patient on a specially designed table. Above the table is x-ray equipment capable of visualizing the location of the stone within the kidney. Below the table is a device called a lithotriptor, which can generate electrically produced shock waves capable of fragmenting the stone. When the exact location of the stone has been determined by x-ray examination, the shock wave–generating equipment is focused very precisely on the kidney stone, and shock waves directed at the stone fragment the stone into fine particles that are excreted in the urine.

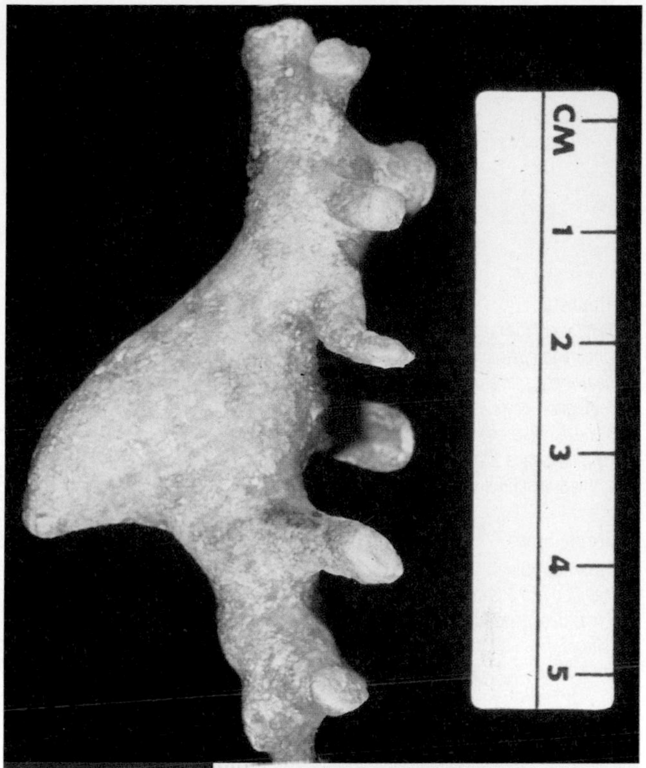

FIGURE 19-13 Large staghorn calculus of kidney.

Sometimes, stones form in the bladder. Usually, this stone formation is secondary to the combined effect of infection and stasis of urine, which decrease the solubility of dissolved salts in the urine. Sometimes bladder calculi can be removed through the bladder by means of a cystoscope. The stones are first broken up by an instrument passed through the cystoscope into the bladder and are then flushed out.

Shock wave lithotripsy
(lith-o-trip′sē)
A method for removing stones from the urinary tract by breaking them into small bits that can be excreted in the urine.

Foreign Bodies

It is not uncommon for people to insert various foreign bodies into the urethra and bladder either accidentally or as a means of sexual stimulation. Such objects must be removed because they may induce infection and may perforate the bladder wall. Frequently, the objects can be removed by means of a cystoscope passed into the bladder through the urethra. Sometimes, however, it is necessary to perform an operation in which the bladder is opened and the object is removed. The following two cases illustrate some of the clinical problems presented by intravesical (*intra =* within + *vesica =* bladder) foreign bodies (FIGURE 19-14).

CASE 19-3

An elderly woman was admitted to the hospital emergency room complaining of lower abdominal pain and burning on urination. An x-ray of the abdomen revealed a rectal thermometer lying horizontally within her bladder. A cystoscope was inserted into the bladder, and the thermometer was manipulated into a vertical position and then extracted through the urethra.

> ## CASE 19-4
>
> A 15-year-old boy inserted a long piece of stiff electrical wire into his bladder through his penis. The wire coiled within the bladder and could not be extracted. It was necessary to open the bladder and remove the wire through the bladder. Fortunately, neither the urethra nor the bladder were damaged by the wire, and the patient made an uneventful recovery.

Hydroureter
A dilatation of the ureter secondary to obstruction of the urinary drainage system, often associated with coexisting dilatation of the renal pelvis and calyces (hydronephrosis).

....

Hydronephrosis
(hydro-nef-rō′sis)
A dilatation of the urinary drainage tract proximal to the site of an obstruction.

Obstruction

In order for urine to be excreted normally, the urinary drainage system that transports the urine must permit free flow of urine. Obstruction or marked narrowing of the system at any point (stricture) causes the system proximal to the blockage to dilate progressively because of the pressure of the retained urine. Dilatation of the ureter is called **hydroureter**. Dilatation of the renal pelvis and calyces is called **hydronephrosis** (*hydro* = water + *nephros* = kidney + *osis* = condition) (FIGURE 19-15). The distention of the calyces and pelvis in turn causes progressive

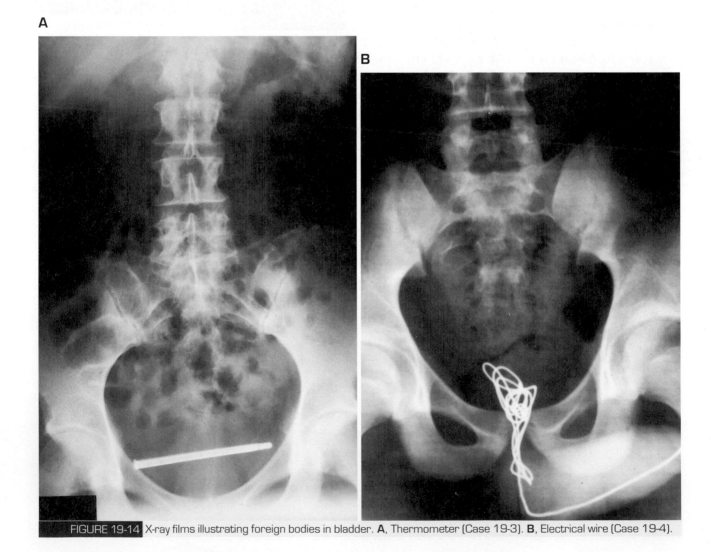

A

B

FIGURE 19-14 X-ray films illustrating foreign bodies in bladder. **A**, Thermometer (Case 19-3). **B**, Electrical wire (Case 19-4).

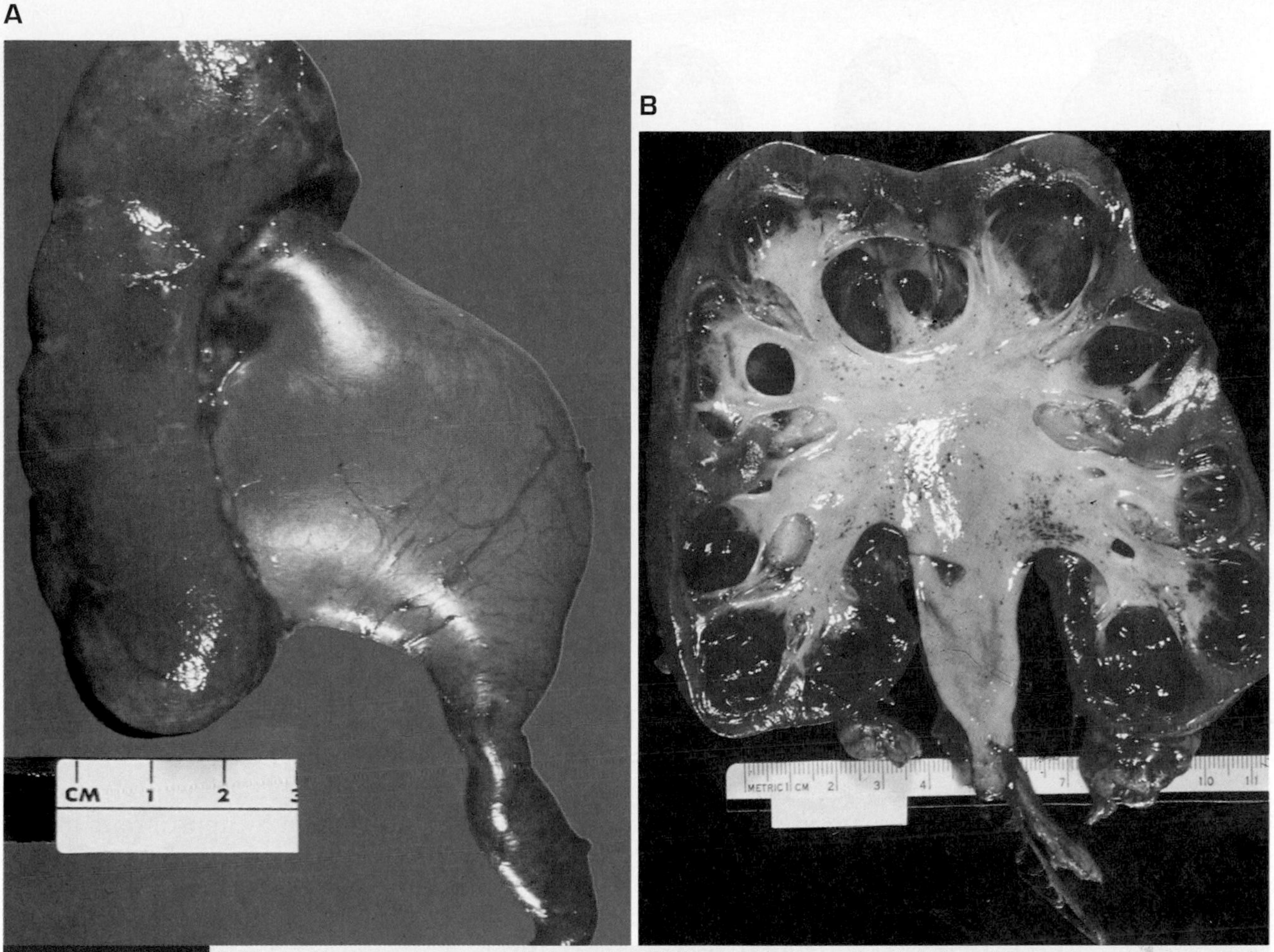

A

B

FIGURE 19-15 **A**, Marked hydronephrosis and hydroureter. **B**, Bisected hydronephrotic kidney, illustrating enlargement of calyces with atrophy of the renal parenchyma caused by the increased pressure exerted by the urine within the distended renal pelvis and calyces.

atrophy of the kidney on the affected side because of the high pressure of the urine within the obstructed drainage system. Eventually, if the obstruction is not relieved, the affected kidney is reduced to a thin shell of atrophic parenchyma covering the overdistended pelvis and calyces.

Which part of the drainage system is affected by the obstruction depends on the location of the block. Obstruction to the outflow of urine from the bladder, as by an enlarged prostate gland or stricture in the urethra, leads to bilateral hydronephrosis and hydroureter, as well as causing overdistention of the bladder (FIGURE 19-16A). Hydronephrosis and hydroureter are unilateral if the obstruction is located low in the ureter, as might be caused by an obstructing calculus impacted in the ureter or an obstructing tumor of the ureter (FIGURE 19-16B). If the obstruction is located at the junction of the renal pelvis and ureter, as might be caused by scarring of the ureter in this area, a unilateral hydronephrosis develops, but the ureter on the affected side is of normal caliber (FIGURE 19-16C).

Stagnation of urine secondary to obstruction of the drainage system may lead to further complications. Stagnation predisposes to infection and to stone formation caused by precipitation of urinary salts. A cycle may become established in which hydronephrosis leads to infection and urinary calculi; these in turn may increase the degree of urinary tract obstruction and cause further progression of the hydronephrosis.

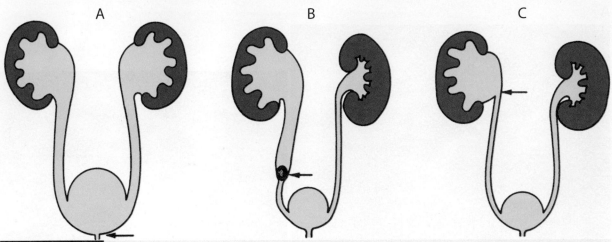

FIGURE 19-16 Possible locations and results of urinary tract obstruction. The *arrows* indicate sites of obstruction. **A**, Bilateral hydronephrosis and hydroureter with distention of the bladder caused by urethral obstruction. **B**, Unilateral hydroureter and hydronephrosis caused by obstruction of the distal ureter. **C**, Unilateral hydronephrosis caused by obstruction at the ureteropelvic junction.

Diagnosis of urinary tract obstruction is usually made by means of a pyelogram or by CT scan (procedures described in the discussion on general concepts of disease: principles of diagnosis). These procedures demonstrate the dilatation of the urinary tract. Treatment is directed toward relieving the obstruction by appropriate means before the kidneys are irreparably damaged.

Renal Tubular Injury

The blood supply to the renal tubules is derived from the efferent glomerular artery, and minor degrees of tubular injury are seen in many diseases affecting the renal glomeruli. Renal tubular injury in the absence of glomerular disease may be encountered in two situations: tubular necrosis as a result of impaired renal blood flow and tubular necrosis caused by toxic drugs and chemicals. Any condition associated with shock and marked drop in the blood pressure leads to impaired blood flow to the kidneys, which often causes degeneration and necrosis of renal tubules. Many drugs and chemicals that are ingested or absorbed by the body are excreted by the kidneys. Thus, they may cause direct toxic injury to the tubular epithelium.

Acute tubular necrosis causes severe impairment of renal function characterized by a marked decrease in urine output (oliguria) or complete suppression of urine formation (anuria). This condition is called acute renal failure. The reason why urine output is reduced is not well understood. Apparently, marked constriction of renal arterioles reduces blood flow to the kidneys and decreases glomerular filtration. Other factors also may contribute to the reduction of urine output. Many of the tubules are blocked by casts and necrotic debris. The damaged tubular epithelium also has lost its capacity for selective tubular reabsorption, and the glomerular filtrate diffuses back through the damaged tubular epithelium into the adjacent peritubular blood vessels. After a period of several weeks, tubular function is slowly restored by regeneration of the damaged epithelium, but several months may be required before renal function returns completely to normal. During the period of acute renal failure, waste products must be removed from the blood by means of dialysis (described in a later section) until tubular function has been restored.

Renal Cysts

SOLITARY CYSTS

Solitary cysts of the kidney are relatively common. They vary in diameter from a few millimeters to about 15 cm. They are not associated with impairment of renal function and are of no significance to the patient.

CONGENITAL POLYCYSTIC KIDNEY DISEASE

Although several different conditions are associated with the formation of kidney cysts, the most common and clinically most important of these conditions is congenital polycystic kidney disease. It is a very common hereditary disease transmitted as a Mendelian dominant trait that affects as many as 1 in 400 persons. Two different genes, designated *PKD1* and *PKD2* (for **P**olycystic **K**idney **D**isease), located on separate chromosomes are involved. About 85% of cases result from mutation of *PKD1*. In most of the others, the mutation involves *PKD2*, which is associated with later onset and slower progression of the disease. A few unfortunate persons have mutations of both *PKD1* and *PKD2*, which causes severe and rapidly progressive disease. The disease is characterized by disturbed proliferation of tubular epithelial cells, leading to the formation of cysts that become detached from the tubules. The epithelium lining the cysts secretes fluid that accumulates within the cysts and causes them to enlarge. As the cysts gradually increase in size, they cause progressive enlargement of both kidneys, where they compress and destroy adjacent renal tissue. Eventually, almost no normal kidney tissue remains, and renal failure supervenes (FIGURE 19-17). Sometimes small numbers of cysts also form in the liver, but usually they do not disturb liver function. Some affected persons also have small cystlike outpouchings extending from the cerebral arteries at the base of the brain, which are called congenital cerebral aneurysms. Because congenital cerebral aneurysms may rupture and cause a brain hemorrhage, some physicians have advocated routine magnetic resonance screening of all patients with autosomal dominant polycystic kidney disease, but the Mayo Clinic experience favors more limited screening only in a select group of polycystic kidney patients (see the reference by Torres and others in the list of Supplementary Readings). Congenital aneurysms and their complications are described in the discussion on the nervous system.

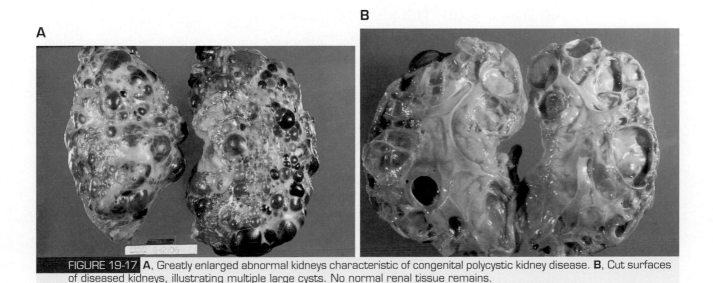

FIGURE 19-17 **A**, Greatly enlarged abnormal kidneys characteristic of congenital polycystic kidney disease. **B**, Cut surfaces of diseased kidneys, illustrating multiple large cysts. No normal renal tissue remains.

Because renal tissue is destroyed slowly, renal insufficiency does not usually occur until the patient reaches middle age, and some patients do not experience problems until they are in their 60s. Many persons with congenital polycystic kidney disease are free of symptoms until onset of renal failure, but some experience periodic urinary tract infections or episodes of bloody urine (hematuria) caused by bleeding into one of the enlarging cysts. Some patients also develop hypertension, which often accompanies renal failure.

Polycystic kidney disease can often be suspected by physical examination, which reveals the greatly enlarged kidneys. The diagnosis can be confirmed in several ways. Ultrasound examination or CT scan of the abdomen reveals the large cystic kidneys. An intravenous pyelogram (IVP) reveals the distortion of the pelves and calyces caused by the cysts. There is no specific treatment. When the kidneys fail, dialysis treatments or a kidney transplant may be required.

The following case illustrates some of the characteristic features of congenital polycystic kidney disease.

CASE 19-5

A 67-year-old man was admitted to the hospital after having sustained a severe heart attack. Marked enlargement of both kidneys was detected on physical examination, and there was also clinical and laboratory evidence of severe renal insufficiency. The patient had seven brothers and sisters, four of whom had died between the ages of 40 and 60 of renal failure as a result of congenital polycystic kidneys. The patient eventually died in the hospital of heart failure in conjunction with chronic renal failure. The autopsy revealed greatly enlarged polycystic kidneys. There were also a few cysts within the liver.

Tumors of the Urinary Tract

Tumors may arise from the epithelium of the renal tubules in the cortex of the kidney, from the transitional epithelium lining the urinary tract, or rarely from remnants of embryonic tissue within the kidney.

RENAL CORTICAL TUMORS

Benign tumors called renal cortical adenomas sometimes arise within the kidney. Usually, a benign adenoma is small, well circumscribed, located within the renal cortex, and can be removed by a limited resection. Some well-differentiated kidney carcinomas are also slowly growing, well-circumscribed tumors confined to the renal cortex, which can be removed along with adjacent normal kidney tissue without removing the entire kidney (partial nephrectomy). Unfortunately, less well-differentiated carcinomas are larger, grow more rapidly, extend into the renal medulla, and exhibit aggressive behavior (FIGURE 19-18). Often, the first manifestation of an aggressive carcinoma is blood in the urine (hematuria) as a result of ulceration of the epithelium of the pelvis or calyces caused by the growing tumor. Often, the tumor eventually invades the renal vein and gives rise to distant metastases. The tumor can be diagnosed by means of a pyelogram (discussion on general concepts of disease: principles of diagnosis), which reveals the distortion of the pelvis and calyces caused by the tumor, or by means of the CT scan, which demonstrates a mass within the kidney. Treatment is by resection of the kidney (nephrectomy).

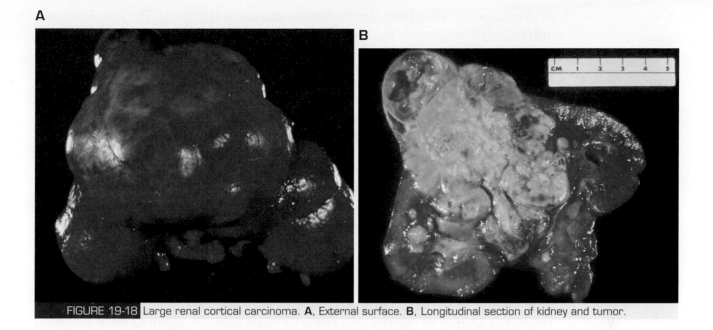

FIGURE 19-18 Large renal cortical carcinoma. **A**, External surface. **B**, Longitudinal section of kidney and tumor.

TRANSITIONAL CELL TUMORS

Almost all tumors arising from the transitional epithelium of the urinary tract are malignant and are called transitional cell carcinomas. Most arise from bladder epithelium, are of low-grade malignancy, and carry a good prognosis. The tumors are often quite vascular, and they tend to bleed; so hematuria may be the first manifestation of the neoplasm. Bladder tumors can be visualized by means of a cystoscope inserted into the bladder through the urethra and often can be resected by means of a similar type of instrument inserted through the urethra. Sometimes it is necessary to resect part of the bladder in order to remove the tumor completely.

NEPHROBLASTOMA (WILMS TUMOR)

An unusual highly malignant tumor composed of primitive cells sometimes arises in the kidney of infants and young children. Histologically, the tumor bears some resemblance to the structure of an embryonic kidney and is called a nephroblastoma or Wilms tumor. The neoplasm often metastasizes widely. Treatment is by nephrectomy followed by radiotherapy and anticancer chemotherapy.

Diagnostic Evaluation of Kidney and Urinary Tract Disease

A variety of methods are used to detect disease of the kidneys and urinary tract, to evaluate the degree to which renal function is disturbed, and to define the type of disease present.

URINALYSIS

The most widely used diagnostic test is an examination of the urine, which is called a **urinalysis**. The examination is useful for detecting whether urinary tract disease is present and for detecting other systemic diseases that alter renal function. The examination includes determinations of urine pH (acidity) and specific gravity (a measure

Urinalysis
(ur-in-al'i-sis)
A commonly performed chemical and microscopic analysis of the urine.

of urine concentration) and simple tests for glucose and protein. The urinalysis may also include tests for bile pigment, acetone, and other constituents that may appear in the urine in association with various diseases. A sample of the urine is also centrifuged, and the sediment is examined microscopically. If the urinalysis is normal, renal disease is unlikely. Alternatively, the presence of red cells and protein in the urine may indicate that damage to the glomerular filter has permitted these substances to leak into the glomerular filtrate or that bleeding is occurring somewhere in the urinary tract. Renal casts, which are collections of protein and cells molded into the shape of the kidney tubules, are an indication of glomerular disease. Leukocytes and bacteria in the urinary sediment indicate urinary tract infection.

Additional tests may be performed on the urine as indicated by the patient's clinical condition. If a urinary tract infection is suspected, for example, the urine is cultured for pathogenic bacteria and sensitivity tests are performed if bacteria are present.

CLEARANCE TESTS

Impairment of renal function can be recognized by measuring the concentration in the blood of various substances, such as urea and creatinine, which are waste products excreted by the kidneys. Elevated levels indicate impaired renal function, and the degree of elevation is a measure of the degree of impairment. Even before elevated levels of waste products are present in the blood, impaired renal function can be detected by means of renal function tests called **clearance tests**. Clearance tests provide a rough estimate of the degree of kidney damage, and periodic clearance tests can be used to follow the progress of renal disease. A gradual fall in the renal clearance of a substance means that renal function is declining.

Clearance tests measure the ability of the kidneys to remove various substances from the blood and excrete them in the urine. To determine the clearance of a substance, one calculates how much blood plasma must flow through the kidney each minute and be completely cleared of the substance in order to provide the quantity of the substance that appears in the urine within the same period of time. For example, if the concentration of a substance in the plasma is 1 mg per milliliter (mg/ml) and 50 mg of the substance is excreted in the urine in 1 minute, then 50 ml of blood must flow through the kidneys each minute and be cleared of the substance to obtain a urinary excretion of 50 mg per minute (mg/min).

Clearance is expressed in milliliters of plasma cleared of the constituent per minute and is expressed by the following formula:

$$\text{Clearance} = \frac{UV}{P}$$

where U is the concentration of the substance excreted in milligrams per milliliter of urine; V is the volume of urine excreted, expressed in milliliters per minute; and P is the concentration of the substance in the plasma expressed in milligrams per milliliter.

The most frequently used clearance test measures the clearance of the waste product **creatinine**, which is derived from the breakdown of a compound present in muscle, called phosphocreatine. In the original method used to determine creatinine clearance, the urine output is measured for a specific period of time and the average output per minute is calculated. The concentrations of creatinine in the urine and in the blood also are determined, and clearance is calculated by means of the standard formula. For example, if the urine output is 2 ml/min, the concentration of creatinine in the urine is 0.15 mg/ml, and the concentration of creatinine in the blood is 0.003 mg/ml, the creatinine clearance is

$$\frac{UV}{P} = \frac{0.15 \times 2}{0.003} = \frac{0.3}{0.003} = 100 \text{ ml/min}$$

Clearance test

(klēr′ans)
A test of renal function that measures the ability of kidneys to remove (clear) a substance from the blood and excrete it in the urine.

Creatinine

(krē-at′in-ēn)
A waste product derived from the breakdown of a compound present in muscle (phosphocreatine) that is excreted in the urine.

The test result, expressed as milliliters of plasma cleared of creatinine per minute, represents the glomerular filtration rate. Although simple in principle, the test is rather cumbersome in practice and also had some other disadvantages. Now the clearance is usually determined from a formula using the serum creatinine, along with the person's age, gender, and lean body weight, as illustrated in the formula:

$$\text{Creatinine clearance} = \frac{(140 - \text{age in years}) \times (\text{lean body weight in kilograms})}{72 \times \text{serum creatinine in mg/dl}}$$

For women, in whom the clearance is lower than in men, the result is multiplied by 0.85 to take into account the slightly lower clearance rate in women. The normal creatinine clearance is 85–105 ml per minute. It is not necessary to remember the formula or perform the calculations as long one understands what the test is measuring and its significance.

ADDITIONAL TECHNIQUES

Many other specialized procedures can be used to study the kidneys and urinary tract, including various x-ray examinations, ultrasound examinations, and cystoscopy. These examinations are described in the discussion on general concepts of disease: principles of diagnosis. Their specific diagnostic applications have also been considered in conjunction with the various renal and urinary tract diseases in which they provide useful information. X-ray examination of the abdomen, for example, can identify the size and location of the kidneys and can detect radiopaque calculi in the kidneys or urinary tract. CT scans and pyelograms can detect anatomic abnormalities within the kidneys, such as cysts and tumors, and many abnormalities of the urinary drainage system, such as hydronephrosis. Other specialized procedures using radioisotopes can measure renal blood flow and renal excretory function. Renal arteriograms, with the use of techniques similar to those used to study the coronary arteries, can determine the caliber of the renal arteries, can detect segmental areas of narrowing in the renal arteries, and can identify areas of increased vascularity within the kidney, which often occur when a tumor is present.

Sometimes the clinician cannot make an exact diagnosis concerning the type of renal disease without resorting to biopsy of the kidney. This can be accomplished without undue difficulty or serious risk to the patient by introducing a small biopsy needle through the skin of the flank directly into the substance of the kidney. A small bit of kidney tissue is removed for histologic study. Examination of the biopsy material by the pathologist often permits an exact diagnosis as to the nature and extent of the renal disease, which serves as a guide to proper treatment.

Renal Failure (Uremia)

Renal failure is an inability of the kidneys to adequately perform their normal regulatory and excretory functions. Function may decline rapidly, which is called acute renal failure, or slowly but progressively, which is called chronic renal failure.

ACUTE RENAL FAILURE

This condition results from necrosis of renal tubules caused by impairment of blood flow to the kidney or by the effects of toxic drugs that damage the kidney tubules, as described previously in the section dealing with renal tubular injury.

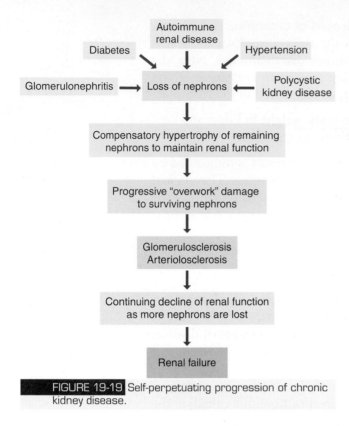

FIGURE 19-19 Self-perpetuating progression of chronic kidney disease.

CHRONIC RENAL FAILURE

In contrast to acute renal failure, this condition is a gradual deterioration of renal function resulting from chronic renal disease. Approximately 50–75% of all cases of chronic renal failure result from diabetes and hypertension. Chronic pyelonephritis, congenital polycystic renal disease, chronic glomerulonephritis, and autoimmune diseases involving the kidney account for most of the remainder.

A normal kidney contains about one million nephrons. In chronic renal failure, renal function declines as the population of nephrons decreases, although relatively normal renal function can be maintained until the number of functioning nephrons falls below 20–30% of normal. Unfortunately, all types of chronic renal disease tend to progress because of the way the surviving nephrons respond to the declining renal function (FIGURE 19-19). The surviving nephrons are forced to "work harder" in order to accomplish the functions previously performed by a full complement of nephrons. Each of the remaining nephrons receives a larger volume of blood to process at a higher than normal pressure. The high blood volumes and pressures damage the arterioles and glomerular capillaries, which leads to thickening of the walls of glomerular arterioles with narrowing of their lumens (arteriolosclerosis) along with glomerular capillary injury followed by scarring (glomerulosclerosis). The tubules are also damaged because the blood vessels that supply the glomeruli also supply the tubules. Consequently, a vicious cycle is created in which the reduced number of functioning nephrons indirectly damages the overworked surviving nephrons, many of which become scarred and cease to function. As more nephrons are lost, an additional burden is placed on those that still survive, which eventually causes many of them to fail. As this process continues, progressively more nephrons are lost at an increasing rate, until eventually renal function deteriorates to the point where the kidneys are no longer able to perform their regulatory and excretory functions. The patient experiences severe derangements of fluid, electrolyte, and acid–base balance. Various acids that would normally be excreted by the kidneys are retained, which disturbs the normal pH of body fluids, leading to a condition called metabolic acidosis described in the discussion on water, electrolyte, and acid–base balance. The failing kidneys cannot produce erythropoietin to stimulate bone marrow function, and the patient becomes anemic. Renal failure is sometimes called **uremia**. This term refers to the characteristic retention of urea in the blood when the kidneys fail. **Urea** is a normal by-product of protein metabolism and is excreted in the urine. It is not a toxic compound and is only one of many substances that accumulates in the blood when the kidneys fail. The amount of urea in the blood, however, correlates with the degree of retention of other waste products and with the clinical manifestations of deteriorating renal function. Therefore, measurement of the concentration of urea in the blood (blood urea nitrogen test or BUN) provides a rough estimate of the severity of the kidney failure. Another commonly used measure of renal functional impairment is the level of creatinine in the blood.

Uremia
(ur-ē′mi-yuh)
An excess of urea and other waste products in the blood, resulting from renal failure.

Urea
(ū-rē′yuh)
The nitrogen waste product derived from protein metabolism and excreted in the urine.

Symptoms of renal failure are nonspecific. They begin to appear when about 80% of renal function has been lost and are quite pronounced by the time renal function has fallen to 5% of normal. Symptoms include weakness, loss of appetite, nausea, and vomiting. Production of red cells by the bone marrow decreases because the failing kidneys cannot produce erythropoietin to stimulate bone marrow function, and the patient becomes moderately anemic. Waste products are not eliminated and increase to toxic levels. Excess salt and water are retained by the failing kidneys, resulting in weight gain as a result of retained fluid ("water weight"). The blood volume increases because of fluid retention, and the blood pressure also tends to rise as the intravascular volume increases. If untreated, the patient in chronic renal failure eventually lapses into coma, may have convulsions, and eventually dies.

The outlook for patients with renal failure has improved dramatically in recent years because of two effective methods of treatment:

1. Hemodialysis and peritoneal dialysis, which remove waste products from the patient's blood. Both methods are equally effective, and each has advantages and disadvantages. Every year, many new patients with advanced renal disease begin dialysis. Some will continue on dialysis indefinitely. Others will rely on dialysis until a kidney becomes available for transplantation.
2. Renal transplantation, using kidneys from living related donors or recently deceased persons (cadaver donors). Transplantation is the most desirable option; however, kidneys for transplantation are in very short supply.

HEMODIALYSIS

Hemodialysis substitutes for the functions of the kidneys. Waste products from the patient's blood diffuse across a semipermeable membrane into a solution (the dialysate) on the other side of the membrane. The rate of diffusion is determined by several factors: the concentration of the substances on the two sides of the membrane, the rate of blood flow and flow of the dialysate through the dialyzer, and the characteristics of the dialyzer membrane. Waste products, which are present in high concentrations in the patient's blood, diffuse from the blood into the dialysate because of differences in the concentration on the two sides of the membrane. Usually, the patient's blood is dialyzed by an "artificial kidney" machine. This type of hemodialysis is called extracorporeal hemodialysis (*extra* = outside + *corpus* = body) because the blood is transported outside the patient's body for dialysis in the artificial kidney and then returned by means of a system of tubes connected to the patient's circulatory system.

Hemodialysis is usually performed in an outpatient dialysis center 3 times per week for 3 or 4 hours during each dialysis session, but it can be performed at home with the assistance of a family member who has been given special training along with the patient. The patient's blood flows along one side of a synthetic semipermeable membrane that restricts the passage of blood cells and protein but permits the passage of water and small molecules. The dialysate flows on the other side of the membrane in a direction opposite to the flow of blood. This type of flow pattern, which is called countercurrent dialysis (*counter* = against + *current* = blood flow), promotes more efficient removal of waste products than when dialysate and blood flow in the same direction.

During dialysis, plastic tubes connect the patient's circulation to the dialyzer in the artificial kidney machine. One tube transmits blood to the dialyzer unit where the blood is cleansed and excess fluid is removed, and the other tube conveys the

Hemodialysis
(hēm-ō-dī-al′i-sis)
A dialysis procedure by which waste products are removed from the blood of patients in chronic renal failure, usually by means of an artificial kidney machine.

blood from the dialyzer back to the patient's circulation. Before dialysis begins, the clotting time of the patient's blood is prolonged by administration of heparin to prevent the blood from clotting as it flows through the dialyzer.

In order to perform hemodialysis on a regular basis, one of the patient's arteries and a large vein must be easily accessible so that the tubes that transport blood to and from the dialyzer unit can easily be connected to the patient's blood vessels. Although several methods have been devised to gain access to the patient's circulation, the preferred method consists of surgically interconnecting the radial artery in the wrist and an adjacent vein, forming an artificial communication called an arteriovenous fistula (FIGURE 19-20A). After the fistula has been created, arterial blood is short-circuited directly into the vein instead of flowing through the peripheral capillaries. The vein, which now receives blood directly under high pressure, becomes much larger and develops a thick wall.

After it has been determined that long-term dialysis will be needed, the arteriovenous fistula is created several months before the first dialysis treatment so that the vein has time to enlarge and thicken. When the vein has become suitable for use, dialysis treatments are begun. Two needles are inserted through the skin directly

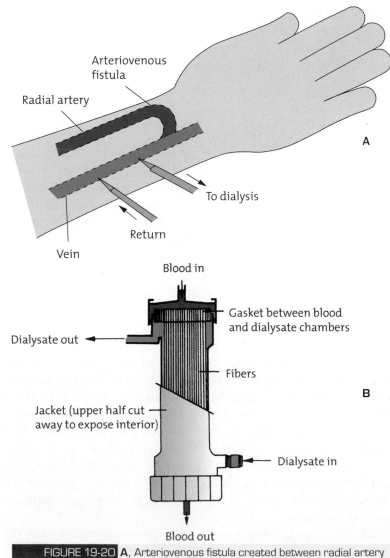

FIGURE 19-20 **A**, Arteriovenous fistula created between radial artery and adjacent vein. **B**, Hollow fiber dialyzer.

into the vein. One needle is attached to the tube that delivers blood to the dialyzer, and the second needle is attached to the tube that returns the blood to the patient (FIGURE 19-20A). Less commonly, other procedures are used to gain access to the patient's circulation for dialysis.

There are many types of artificial kidney machines. Many are quite compact, and portable units are available. Improvements in the design and operation of the machines are being made continually. The essential component of the artificial kidney machine is the dialyzer. Attached to it are the tubes that carry blood to and from the patient and the tubes that carry dialysate to and from the unit. A hollow fiber dialyzer, which is quite compact and efficient and is the most commonly used type, consists of a bundle of hollow synthetic fibers through which the blood passes. The dialysate circulates around the outside of the fibers in the opposite direction (FIGURE 19-20B).

PERITONEAL DIALYSIS

Peritoneal dialysis uses the patient's own peritoneum as the dialyzing membrane (FIGURE 19-21). In order to perform peritoneal dialysis, a large plastic tube must first be inserted into the patient's abdominal (peritoneal) cavity and fixed in position by

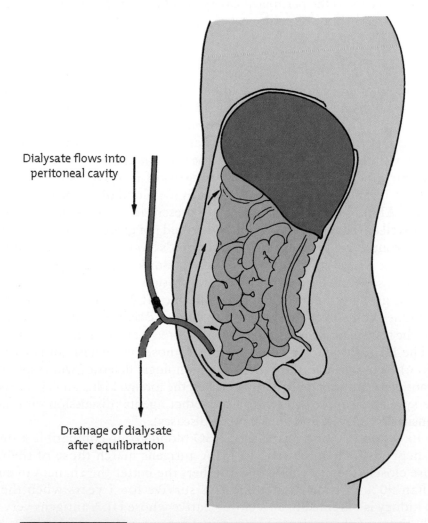

Dialysate flows into peritoneal cavity

Drainage of dialysate after equilibration

FIGURE 19-21 Principle of peritoneal dialysis. Dialysate fills peritoneal cavity. Waste products diffuse (*arrows*) from blood vessels beneath peritoneum into dialysate. Fluid is drained after equilibration.

suturing it to the skin. The dialysis procedure consists of instilling several liters of dialysis fluid through the tube into the peritoneal cavity and allowing the fluid to remain within the peritoneal cavity for a variable time. During this time, waste products diffuse across the peritoneum from the underlying blood vessels into the dialysis fluid that fills the peritoneal cavity. Dialysis fluid is then withdrawn and fresh fluid is instilled. Peritoneal dialysis can be performed by means of an automated system in which the machine automatically fills and drains the peritoneal cavity at night while the patient is asleep. Another similar method is called continuous ambulatory peritoneal dialysis. In this procedure, 2 liters of fluid remain within the peritoneal cavity all the time. The patient replaces the fluid with fresh dialysis fluid four or five times a day. Patients carry out their usual activities when they are not draining and refilling their peritoneal cavities.

Peritoneal dialysis is used less frequently than extracorporeal hemodialysis. Not all patients requiring dialysis are suitable candidates for peritoneal dialysis, but the procedure offers an advantage to patients who wish to continue working full time or part time, as they do not have to spend several daytime hours 3 days each week at a dialysis center, and many patients who choose peritoneal dialysis are quite satisfied with their choice. However, peritoneal dialysis has disadvantages. It is less efficient at removing waste products and carries some risk of peritonitis, which can result if bacteria gain access to the peritoneal cavity around the tube that extends from the skin surface directly into the peritoneal cavity.

RENAL TRANSPLANTATION

When the kidneys fail, a normal compatible kidney sometimes can be transplanted from a close relative, an unrelated volunteer donor, or a recently deceased person (cadaver donor). The best results are obtained from a living kidney donor.

In any kidney transplantation, the transplanted kidney must be matched as closely as possible with the donor in order to give the transplant the best chance of survival in the recipient. The ABO blood group antigens of the proposed donor must be compatible with the blood group antibodies in the blood of the proposed recipient because the ABO blood group antigens are present in body tissues (including the kidney) as well as red cells. For example, one could not give a kidney from a group A donor to a group O recipient because the recipient's blood contains anti-A and anti-B antibodies that would attack and destroy the donor kidney. The principles are the same as when selecting blood for a blood transfusion.

The next group of important antigens are the HLA antigens. Unless the transplanted kidney comes from an identical twin whose tissues contain identical HLA antigens, the transplant will invariably contain foreign HLA antigens that the patient lacks. (The HLA system is considered in chromosomes, genes, and cell devision discussion.) Consequently, the patient's immunologic defenses will respond to the foreign antigens and attempt to destroy (reject) the foreign kidney unless the patient's immune system is suppressed by drugs or other agents (discussion on immunity, hypersensitivity, allergy, and autoimmune diseases).

The likelihood that a transplanted ABO blood group compatible kidney will survive depends on how closely the HLA antigens match those of the patient. The more closely they resemble one another, the better the chances of survival. More than 90% of transplanted kidneys survive for 5 years when the transplanted kidney is obtained from a close relative whose HLA antigens very closely resemble those of the patient. The survival rate of cadaver transplants has improved greatly in recent years and now is almost as good as transplants from living related donors.

In the transplant operation, the transplanted kidney is usually placed in the iliac area outside the peritoneal cavity. The renal artery of the transplanted kidney is connected to the internal iliac (hypogastric) artery. The renal vein is connected to the iliac vein, and the ureter is connected to the bladder (FIGURE 19-22). In the great majority of patients, the transplant is successful and "takes over" for the patient's own nonfunctional kidneys. Some patients, however, reject the transplant despite intensive immunosuppressive therapy. Most rejections occur within the first few months after transplantation. Should this occur, the patient resumes dialysis treatments until another kidney suitable for transplantation becomes available.

Although a well-functioning transplanted kidney permits the patient to lead a relatively normal life, the patient with a renal transplant may have other problems. Immunosuppressive drugs may need to be continued indefinitely to prevent rejection of the foreign kidney, and adverse side effects sometimes result from these drugs. The immunosuppressed patient is also more susceptible to infection because the body's immune defenses have been weakened so that the transplant can survive. Occasionally, the disease that destroyed the patient's own kidneys, such as glomerulonephritis, also destroys the function of the transplanted kidney.

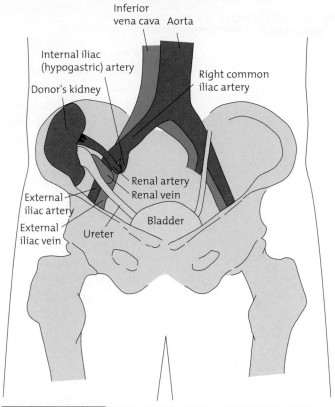

FIGURE 19-22 Method of kidney transplantation in an adult. A transplanted kidney is placed in the iliac region. Artery and vein of transplant are connected to patient's iliac artery and vein, and the ureter of the transplant is connected to the bladder.

Based on new studies on a selected group of transplant patients, in the future, it may not always be necessary to continuously suppress the immune system in order to prevent rejection of the transplant. These studies indicate that the immune system can be "taught" to recognize the foreign HLA antigens as part of the patient's own antigens. The key to success involves suppressing the patient's own immune system first before the kidney is transplanted, and then administering bone marrow from the proposed kidney donor into the circulation of the patient. The kidney donor blood cells become established in the patient's bone marrow because the weakened immune system is unable to reject the foreign blood cells. Eventually, the patient ends up with two different blood cell populations, the patient's own blood cells and the transplanted donor blood cells. As a result, the patient's immune system "learns" that the HLA antigens in both the donor blood cells and the patient's own blood cells must be the patient's own self-antigens. Consequently, continuous suppression of the immune system may no longer be required when the kidney from the donor whose blood cell HLA antigens have already been accepted by the patient's immune system. In some other dialysis patients, transplanted kidney cells can be manipulated so that they may no longer be recognized as foreign by the patient's immune system. In these initial studies, several patients have been followed for up to 5 years without requiring drugs to suppress the immune system, which is a remarkable accomplishment. Hopefully, continued progress at inducing the transplant cells and those of the recipient to live together in harmony will do much to simplify the life of the transplant recipient.

QUESTIONS FOR REVIEW

1. What is the difference between glomerulonephritis and pyelonephritis? What is the relationship between glomerulonephritis and beta-streptococcal infection? What factors predispose to urinary tract infection?
2. What is the difference between nephrotic syndrome and nephrosclerosis? Why does edema develop in a patient with nephrosis?
3. What are the common causes of urinary tract obstruction? What are its effects on the kidneys and lower urinary tract?
4. What conditions lead to renal tubular necrosis? What are its clinical manifestations?
5. What is uremia? What are its manifestations? How is it treated? What is the role of urea in producing the clinical manifestations of uremia?
6. What methods does the clinician use to establish a diagnosis of renal disease?
7. What is congenital polycystic kidney disease? What are its clinical manifestations? What is its pattern of inheritance? How is it treated?
8. What is the difference between acute and chronic renal failure?
9. What is the difference between hemodialysis and peritoneal dialysis? How is the patient's circulation connected to the artificial kidney for hemodialysis?
10. Why does a kidney transplant from a donor who is a close relative usually have a greater likelihood of survival than does a cadaver transplant?
11. How does diabetes affect the kidneys? What are the clinical manifestations? How does gout affect the kidneys?

SUPPLEMENTARY READINGS

Chertow, G. M. 2004. A 43-year-old woman with chronic renal insufficiency. *Journal of the American Medical Association* 291:1252–9.

▶ A case discussion dealing with the problems and treatment of a patient with chronic renal disease, based on the pathophysiology of renal failure.

Grantham, J. J. 2009. Clinical practice. Autosomal dominant polycystic kidney disease. *New England Journal of Medicine* 359:1477–85.

▶ An excellent article on the important concepts regarding this disease, including pathogenesis, genetics, associated conditions, complications, clinical manifestations, monitoring disease progression, and treatment.

Himmelfarb, J., and Ikizler, T. A. 2010. Hemodialysis. *New England Journal of Medicine* 363:1833–45.

▶ Patients with end-stage kidney disease often have significant cardiovascular complications such as hypertension, atherosclerosis, cardiac hypertrophy, and congestive cardiac failure related in part to loss of normal kidney function. Death rate among U.S. patients is approximately 20% per year after maintenance dialysis is begun. Arteriovenous shunts are preferred for obtaining vascular access, and hollow fiber dialyzers are recommended. The usual treatment time is about 4 hours and usual frequency is 3 times per week. More frequent dialysis and longer dialysis time reduce cardiovascular complications and improve survival.

Ibrahim, H. N., Foley, R., Tan, L., et al. 2009. Long-term consequences of kidney donation. *New England Journal of Medicine* 360:459–69.

▶ Survival and risk of end-stage renal disease (ESRD) in carefully screened kidney donors appears to be similar to those in the general population. However, the study has certain limitations. Only the donors who are still alive and could be contacted were able to participate in the study, which is less than 15% of the total donor population.

▶ Removal of a kidney is followed by a reduction in the glomerular filtration rate (GFR) of the remaining kidney to about 70% of the prenephrectomy value. There has been a concern that kidney donors who have a 50% loss of kidney tissue may experience "overwork" (hyperfiltration) damage to the remaining kidney in addition to the normal progressive loss of kidney function that occurs with age. ESRD occurred in 11 of 3698 kidney donors contacted who donated kidneys in the period from 1963 to 2007.

Meyer, T. W., and Hostetter, T. H. 2007. Uremia. *New England Journal of Medicine* 357:1316–25.

▶ Current concepts and discussion of the pathophysiology of chronic renal failure.

Mulley, A. G., Jr. 1986. Shock-wave lithotripsy: Assessing a slam-bang technology. *New England Journal of Medicine* 314:845–7.

▶ Lithotripsy is a well-engineered, highly selective application of brute force. Applications in fracturing gallstones are also described.

Rubin, H. R., Fink, N. E., Plantinga, L. C., et al. 2004. Patient ratings of dialysis care with peritoneal dialysis vs hemodialysis. *Journal of the American Medical Association* 291:697–703.

▶ New patients beginning dialysis must choose between hemodialysis and peritoneal dialysis. Although not all patients requiring dialysis are suitable candidates for peritoneal dialysis, those who chose peritoneal dialysis were more likely to be working full time or part time and were more satisfied with their care than were hemodialysis patients.

Starzl, T. E. 2008. Immunosuppressive therapy and tolerance of organ allografts. *New England Journal of Medicine* 358:407–11.

▶ The author reviews three landmark articles in the same issue of the January 24, 2008, *Journal* in which combined kidney and bone marrow stem cells induced formation of two cell populations that "tricked" the immune system into recognizing the antigens of both cell populations as normal antigens for the patients, so the immune system did not respond, and immunosuppression was not required to maintain the transplants. Details of the other cases reported are also provided.

Stevens, L. A., Coresh, J., Greene, T., et al. 2006. Assessing kidney function—measured and estimated glomerular filtration rate. *New England Journal of Medicine* 354:2743–83.

▶ Clearance calculated from serum and urine creatinine values overestimate the glomerular filtration rate because of tubular secretion of creatinine. The Cockcroft-Gault formula provides a reasonably good estimate. A reduction of GFR to less than 60 ml per minute (related to body surface area) defines chronic kidney disease.

Torres, V., Pirson, Y., and Wiebers, D. O. 2006. Cerebral aneurysms. *New England Journal of Medicine* 355:2703–4.

▶ In Mayo Clinic studies on patients with polycystic kidney disease, prospective screening detected intracranial aneurysms in 16% of 77 patients with a family history of intracranial aneurysms, and in 6% of patients without such a family history. All of the aneurysms were small (mean diameter 3.5 mm with range from 1–7 mm diameter). According to the International Study of Unruptured Intracranial Aneurysms, the expected rupture rate of such aneurysms is very low. Current Mayo Clinic indications for screening are limited to those who have a family history of an intracranial aneurysm, a previous rupture of an aneurysm, contemplated major elective surgery, a high-risk occupation where an aneurysm rupture would be a major catastrophe, or extreme patient anxiety about the possibility of rupture.

Structure and Function of Urinary Tract

KIDNEYS
Bean-shaped organs below diaphragm adjacent to vertebral column.
Divided into outer cortex and inner medulla.
Latter contains pyramids and renal columns.

EXCRETORY DUCT SYSTEM
Ureter conveys urine to bladder by peristalsis.
Pelvis: expanded upper end of ureter.
Major calyces: subdivisions of pelvis.
Minor calyces: subdivisions of major calyces into which renal papillae (apices of pyramids) discharge.

BLADDER
Stores urine.
Discharges urine into urethra during voiding.
Anatomic configuration of bladder and ureters normally prevents reflux of urine into ureters during voiding.

FUNCTION OF THE KIDNEYS
Excretory organ.
Regulates mineral and water balance.
Produces erythropoietin and renin.

THE NEPHRON
Composed of glomerulus and renal tubule.
Material filtered by three-layered glomerular filter.
Inner: fenestrated capillary endothelium.
Middle: basement membrane.
Outer: capillary epithelial cells (with foot processes and filtration slits).
Mesangial cells: contractile phagocytic cells that hold the capillary tuft together and regulate the caliber of the capillaries, which influences the filtration rate.

RENAL REGULATION OF BLOOD PRESSURE AND BLOOD VOLUME
Renin released in response to reduced blood volume, low blood pressure, or low sodium concentration.
Angiotensin II formed.
Functions as vasopressor.
Stimulates aldosterone secretion.

REQUIREMENTS FOR NORMAL RENAL FUNCTION
Free flow of blood through glomeruli.
Normal glomerular filter.
Normal tubular function.
Normal outflow of urine.

Developmental Disturbances

NORMAL DEVELOPMENT
Kidneys develop from mesoderm along back body wall of embryo.
Bladder derived from lower end of intestinal tract.
Excretory ducts (ureters, calyces, pelves) develop from ureteric buds that extend from bladder into developing kidneys.
Kidneys develop in pelvis and ascend to final position.

DEVELOPMENTAL ABNORMALITIES
Renal agenesis.
Bilateral: rare and associated with other congenital abnormalities. Usually incompatible with postnatal life.
Unilateral: relatively common and usually asymptomatic.
Duplications of the urinary tract.
As a result of abnormal development of ureteric buds.
Complete duplication: extra ureter and renal pelvis.
Incomplete duplication: only upper part of excretory system duplicated.
Malpositions.
Caused by failure of kidneys to ascend to normal position.
Kidneys may be fused.
Horseshoe kidney: fusion of lower poles.
Fusion of upper pole of one kidney to lower pole of other kidney.

Glomerulonephritis

IMMUNE-COMPLEX GLOMERULONEPHRITIS
Usually follows beta-streptococcal infection.
Circulating antigen–antibody complexes are filtered by glomeruli and incite inflammation.
Most patients recover completely.

ANTI-GBM GLOMERULONEPHRITIS
An autoimmune disease.
Autoantibodies directed against glomerular basement membranes.

Nephrotic Syndrome

CLINICAL FEATURES
Loss of protein in urine exceeds body's capacity to replenish plasma proteins.
Low plasma protein leads to edema and ascites.

PROGNOSIS
In children: minimal glomerular change, with complete recovery.
In adults: manifestation of more severe progressive renal disease.

Arteriolar Nephrosclerosis

PATHOGENESIS
Develops in hypertensive patients.
Renal arterioles undergo thickening.
Glomeruli and tubules undergo secondary degenerative changes.

Diabetic Nephropathy

PATHOGENESIS AND STRUCTURAL CHANGES
A complication of long-standing diabetes.
Nodular and diffuse thickening of glomerular basement membranes (glomerulosclerosis).
Usually coexisting nephrosclerosis.

MANIFESTATIONS
Impaired renal function.
Nephrotic syndrome may result from protein loss in urine.
May lead to renal failure.

Gout Nephropathy
PATHOGENESIS
Elevated blood uric acid leads to increased uric acid in tubular filtrate.
Urate may precipitate in Henle's loops and collecting tubules.
Tubular obstruction causes kidney damage.

MANIFESTATIONS
Impaired renal function
Common problem in poorly controlled gout.
May lead to renal failure.

Urinary Tract Infections
PATHOGENESIS
Usually caused by gram-negative bacteria ascending the urethra.
Free urine flow, large urine volume, complete emptying of bladder, and acid urine protect against infection.
Impaired drainage of urine, injury to mucosa of urinary tract, and introduction of catheters or instruments into bladder predispose to infection.

MANIFESTATIONS
Cystitis: bladder infection.
   Causes pain and burning on urination; bacteria and leukocytes in urine.
   Common in young, sexually active women and older men who are unable to empty their bladders completely owing to enlarged prostate.
   Usually responds promptly to antibiotics.
Pyelonephritis: infection of upper urinary tract.
   Usually ascending infection. May be hematogenous.
   Stagnation of urine or obstruction or both predispose.
   Usually responds to antibiotics.
   Some cases become chronic and may lead to kidney failure.

Role of Vesicoureteral Reflux in Urinary Tract Infections
Urine normally prevented from flowing retrograde into ureters during voiding.
Failure of mechanism allows bladder urine to reflux into ureter during voiding.
Urine forced into ureter flows back into the bladder after voiding, preventing complete emptying of bladder.
Reflux predisposes to urinary tract infection because of residual urine.

Urinary Tract Calculi
PREDISPOSING FACTORS
Increased concentration of salts in urine.
   Uric acid in gout.
   Calcium salts in hyperparathyroidism.
Infections: alter solubility of salts.
Urinary tract obstruction: promotes stasis and infection.

CLINICAL MANIFESTATIONS
Renal colic associated with passage of stone.
Obstruction of urinary tract causes hydronephrosis-hydroureter proximal to obstruction.
Predisposes to infection.

Foreign Bodies in the Urinary Tract
INCIDENCE AND MANIFESTATIONS
Usually inserted by patient.
May injure bladder.
Predispose to infection.

TREATMENT
Usually removed by cystoscopy.
Occasionally necessary to open bladder by surgical operation.

Obstruction of Urinary Tract
PATHOGENESIS
Blockage of urine outflow leads to progressive dilatation of urinary tract proximal to obstruction.
Eventually causes compression atrophy of kidneys.

MANIFESTATIONS
Hydroureter: dilatation of ureter.
Hydronephrosis: dilatation of pelvis and calyces.

COMMON CAUSES
Bilateral: obstruction of bladder neck by enlarged prostate or urethral stricture.
Unilateral: ureteral stricture, calculus, or tumor.

COMPLICATIONS
Stone formation.
Infection.

DIAGNOSIS AND TREATMENT
Pyelograms or CT scans or both demonstrate dilatation of drainage system.
Treat cause of obstruction.

Renal Tubular Injury
PATHOGENESIS
Caused by toxic chemicals.
As a result of reduced renal blood flow.

CLINICAL MANIFESTATIONS
Oliguria or anuria.
Tubular function gradually recovers.
Treated by dialysis until function returns.

Renal Cysts

SOLITARY CYSTS
Relatively common.
Usually asymptomatic.

CONGENITAL POLYCYSTIC KIDNEY DISEASE
Incidence one per thousand.
Mendelian dominant transmission.
Cysts enlarge and destroy renal function.
Onset of renal insufficiency in middle age or later.
May be complicated by infections or bleeding into cysts.
Relatively common cause of renal failure.

Tumors of the Urinary Tract

RENAL CORTICAL TUMORS
Arise from epithelium of renal tubules.
Adenomas small and asymptomatic.
Carcinomas more common.
> *May cause hematuria as first manifestation.*
> *Tumor may invade renal vein and metastasize through bloodstream.*
> *Treated by nephrectomy.*

TRANSITIONAL CELL TUMORS
Arise from transitional epithelium lining urinary tract.
Most are of low-grade malignancy and have good prognosis.
Hematuria may be first manifestation.
Diagnosis by cystoscopy.
Treated by resecting tumor.

WILMS TUMOR
Uncommon, highly malignant renal tumor of infants and children.
Treated by nephrectomy, radiotherapy, and chemotherapy.

Diagnostic Evaluation of Kidney and Urinary Tract Disease

URINALYSIS
Detects abnormalities in urine.
Widely used screening test.

URINE CULTURE AND SENSITIVITY TESTS
Where appropriate.

BLOOD CHEMISTRY TESTS
Measure retention of waste products normally excreted by kidneys.
Urea and creatinine commonly measured.
Degree of elevation correlates with degree of renal insufficiency and clinical condition.

CLEARANCE TESTS
Measure ability of kidneys to remove constituent from blood and excrete it in the urine.
Calculated by formula.
Creatinine clearance commonly used to monitor renal function.

X-RAY STUDIES
X-ray of abdomen: determines size and location of kidneys, radiopaque calculi.
Pyelograms: evaluate drainage system and distortion of calyces caused by renal cysts or tumors.
CT scan: detects renal cysts, tumors, hydronephrosis.
Arteriogram: detects abnormalities of renal blood flow, narrowing of renal arteries, increased renal vascularity associated with tumors.

ULTRASOUND EXAMINATION
Identifies cysts and tumors.

CYSTOSCOPY
Visualizes interior of bladder.

RENAL BIOPSY
Small biopsy of kidney obtained by needle inserted into kidney through flank.
Invasive procedure performed when nature of renal disease uncertain.
Histologic diagnosis serves as guide for proper treatment.

Renal Failure (Uremia)

CLASSIFICATION
Acute:
> *Caused by tubular necrosis from impaired renal blood flow or toxic drugs.*
> *Renal function returns when tubules regenerate.*
Chronic:
> *As a result of progressive chronic kidney disease.*
> *No recovery of renal function.*

MANIFESTATIONS
Nonspecific symptoms.
Anemia: as a result of reduced red cell production.
Toxic manifestations: caused by retained waste products.
Retention of salt and water.
Hypertension.

TREATMENT
Hemodialysis.
> *Patient's circulation connected to artificial kidney machine (dialyzer).*
> *Access to patient's circulation facilitated by creation of arteriovenous fistula between radial artery and adjacent vein.*
> *Blood cleansed and excess fluid removed.*
> *Several types of dialyzers used.*
> *Treatments last from 4 to 5 hours three times per week.*

Peritoneal Dialysis.
  Patient's own peritoneum used as dialyzing membrane.
  Indwelling tube placed in peritoneal cavity and fixed to skin.
  Dialysis fluid fills peritoneal cavity, is allowed to equilibrate, and is then drained. Cycles repeated.
  Less efficient than hemodialysis and carries risk of peritonitis.
Kidney transplantation.
  Kidney obtained from close relative, volunteer donor or recently deceased person (cadaver donor).
  Survival of ABO-compatible transplant depends on similarity of HLA antigens between donor and recipient.

http://health.jbpub.com/humandisease/9e

Human Disease Online is a great source for supplementary human disease information for both students and instructors. Visit this website to find a variety of useful tools for learning, thinking, and teaching.

The Male Reproductive System

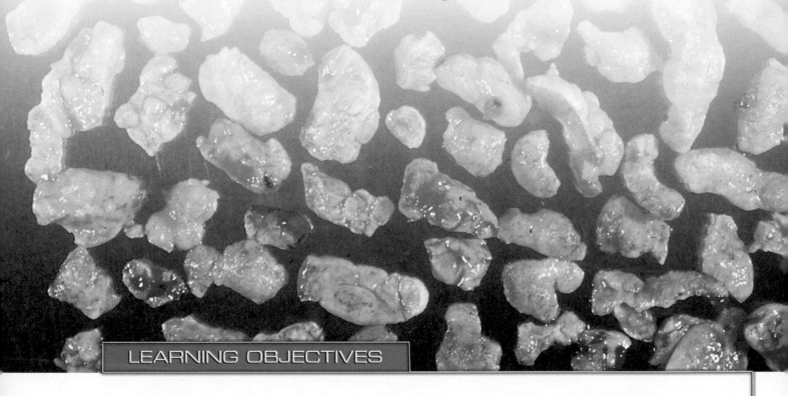

1 Differentiate between benign prostatic hyperplasia and prostatic carcinoma. Describe clinical manifestations and methods of treatment.

2 List the three most common types of testicular cancer. Describe their manifestations, and explain the methods of treatment.

3 Name the anatomic structures of the male reproductive system. Describe their functions as they relate to the diseases affecting them.

Structure and Function of the Male Reproductive Organs

The components of the male reproductive system are the penis, the prostate and certain accessory glands, the testes, and a duct system for transporting sperm from the testes to the urethra. The transport duct system begins as the epididymides (singular, epididymis), which are closely applied to the testes, and continues as the two vasa deferentia (singular, vas deferens). The two vasa deferentia extend upward in the spermatic cords, are joined by the seminal vesicles, and enter the prostatic urethra as the ejaculatory ducts. The urethra is divided into a long penile urethra and a short segment transversing the prostate gland called the prostatic urethra. It is conventional to speak of the distal penile urethra as the anterior urethra, and the prostatic urethra and adjacent proximal part of the penile urethra as the posterior urethra. FIGURE 20-1 illustrates the anatomy of the male reproductive system. A working knowledge of how these structures are interrelated is necessary in order to understand the spread of inflammatory disease in the male reproductive tract and the various complications that may result.

The prostate is a spherical gland about 5 cm in diameter that surrounds the urethra just below the base of the bladder (FIGURE 20-2A). It is composed of numerous branched glands arranged in two major groups intermixed with masses of smooth muscle and fibrous tissue (FIGURE 20-2B). The inner group of glands surrounds the urethra as it passes through the prostate, and the outer, or main group of glands, makes up the bulk of prostatic glandular tissue (FIGURE 20-2C). The prostate secretes a thin alkaline fluid containing a high concentration of an enzyme secreted by prostatic epithelial cells. The prostatic secretions are discharged into the urethra during ejaculation through very fine ducts that open near the orifices of the ejaculatory ducts. Secretions mix with sperm and the secretions of the seminal vesicles to form the seminal fluid.

The two testes (also called testicles), which originally developed within the abdomen, occupy separate compartments within the scrotum. In the fetus, the testes

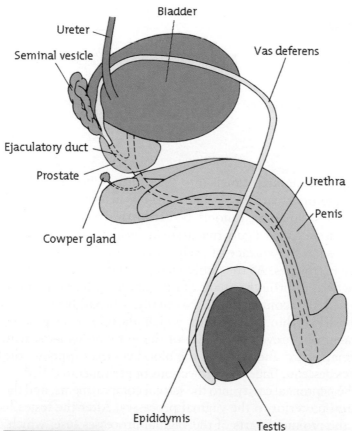

FIGURE 20-1 A side view of the male reproductive system. Seminal fluid consists of sperm mixed with secretions of seminal vesicles, prostate gland, and Cowper (bulbourethral) glands. The testes, excretory ducts, seminal vesicles, and Cowper glands are paired structures.

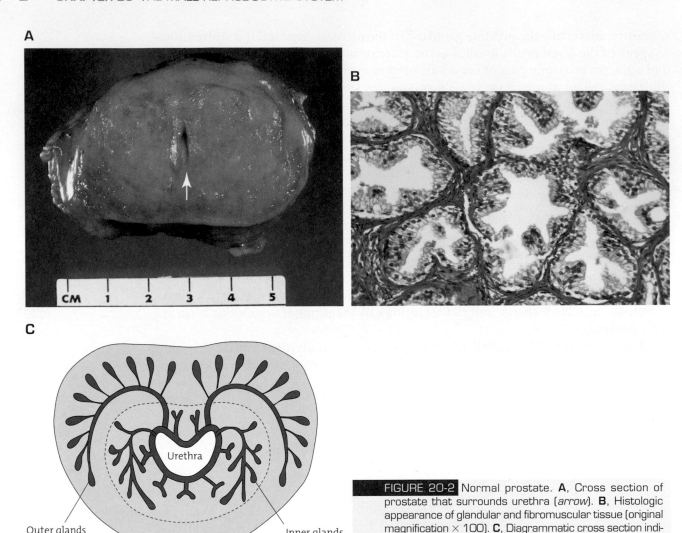

FIGURE 20-2 Normal prostate. **A**, Cross section of prostate that surrounds urethra (*arrow*). **B**, Histologic appearance of glandular and fibromuscular tissue (original magnification × 100). **C**, Diagrammatic cross section indicating arrangement of inner and outer groups of glands.

descend through the inguinal canals into the scrotum, bringing their blood vessels, nerves, and excretory ducts with them as the spermatic cords and usually have completed their descent about 1 month before birth. To guide descent of the testes, a band of fibrous tissue called a gubernaculum (a Latin word meaning rudder or guide) extends from the inferior surface of each testis through the inguinal canal into the scrotum where it attaches. As the gubernaculum shortens, it guides each testis into the scrotum, where a fibrous remnant of the gubernaculum remains to anchor each testis within its scrotal compartment. Normally, a broad band of connective tissue attaches each testis within the scrotum, which allows the testis some mobility, but the broad attachment prevents rotation of the testis on its axis, which would also twist the spermatic cord and obstruct the blood vessels supplying the testis.

As the testes descend, fingerlike projections of peritoneum called vaginal processes project from the peritoneal cavity into the scrotal compartments, and the testes descend into the scrotum posterior to the vaginal processes. After the testes have completed their descent, the proximal parts of the vaginal processes fuse, which obliterates the communications between the peritoneal cavity and the scrotum, but the distal part of each vaginal process persists as a small peritoneum-lined sac called the tunica vaginalis, which surrounds the anterior half of each testis (FIGURE 20-3). If the proximal part of a vaginal process does not fuse normally, the vaginal process remains as a communication between the peritoneal cavity and the scrotum, which may allow a loop of intestine to

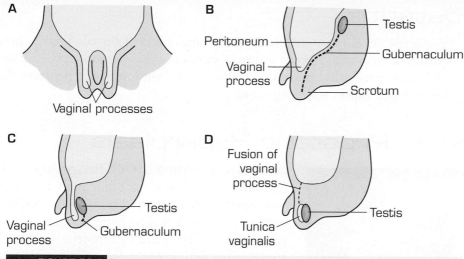

FIGURE 20-3 Descent of the testes. **A**, Anterior view, illustrating vaginal processes extending into scrotum. **B**, Lateral view prior to testicular descent, illustrating the gubernaculum extending from the testis into the scrotum posterior to the vaginal process. **C**, Testis descends into scrotum posterior to vaginal process. **D**, Proximal part of vaginal process obliterated; distal part persists as tunica vaginalis.

extend into the scrotum. This condition is called a congenital inguinal hernia. (Hernias are considered in the discussion on gastrointestinal tract.)

The testes, which are activated by gonadotropic hormones at puberty, have two major functions: production of sperm by sperm-producing cells called germ cells, which occurs within the testicular tubules, and production of the male hormone testosterone, which occurs in clusters of cells located between the tubules called interstitial cells or Leydig cells. The two types of cells have different temperature requirements. The testosterone-producing cells function at normal body temperature, as do most other cells. The sperm-producing germ cells require a temperature that is several degrees lower than body temperature, and the scrotum contains muscles that automatically raise or lower the testes, bringing the testes closer to the body if the scrotal temperature is too low or relaxing to move the testes away from the body if the scrotal temperature is too high. Maintaining a lower than normal scrotal temperature is very important because an elevated scrotal temperature impairs sperm production (spermatogenesis). Moreover, sperm-producing cells are damaged and eventually destroyed if the testes do not descend normally into the scrotum and are continually subjected to the higher intra-abdominal temperature.

Gonorrhea and Nongonococcal Urethritis

Gonorrhea is a relatively common disease. The gonococcus, spread by sexual contact, initially causes an acute inflammation of the anterior urethra. However, the inflammation may spread into the posterior urethra, prostate, seminal vesicles, and epididymides. The gonococcus also may cause an acute inflammation of the rectal mucosa. Occasionally, healing of the gonorrheal inflammation in the posterior urethra may be associated with considerable scarring, leading to narrowing of the urethra and thus to urinary tract obstruction. Inflammatory obstruction of the vasa deferentia may block sperm transport and lead to sterility. Nongonococcal urethritis, caused by chlamydia, causes an acute urethritis and clinically is very similar to gonorrhea. (Sexually transmitted diseases are considered in the discussion on communicable diseases.)

Prostatitis

Acute prostatitis develops when an acute inflammation of the bladder or urethra spreads into the prostate. It may follow a gonococcal infection of the posterior urethra. Chronic prostatitis is a mild chronic inflammation of the prostate that is quite common and causes few symptoms.

Benign Prostatic Hyperplasia

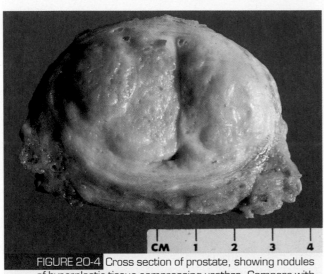

FIGURE 20-4 Cross section of prostate, showing nodules of hyperplastic tissue compressing urethra. Compare with Figure 20-2A.

Moderate enlargement of the prostate gland is relatively common in older men and usually involves the inner group of glands surrounding the urethra (FIGURE 20-4). The hyperplasia results from stimulation of the gland by a potent male sex hormone called dihydrotestosterone, which is formed in the prostate from testosterone by a prostatic enzyme called 5-alpha reductase. Prostatic enlargement is significant only if it obstructs the bladder neck, leading to incomplete emptying of the bladder, or causes complete urinary tract obstruction. An enlarged obstructing prostate causes difficulty in urinating and may lead to various other complications caused by urinary retention and stagnation of urine in the bladder, such as cystitis, pyelonephritis, hydronephrosis, and stone formation.

There are many ways to treat benign prostatic hyperplasia. These depend on various factors, such as the size of the gland, the severity of the urinary symptoms, the patient's age and health, and of course the patient's preference. Treatment options include

1. Oral medications to shrink the prostate using various drugs or drug combinations
2. Various outpatient procedures that destroy excess prostate tissue and reduce the size of the gland by using laser, microwave, or radio wave treatment, or by means of heat coagulation or freezing
3. Surgical resection of obstructing prostatic tissue

An obstructing prostate that prevents complete emptying of the bladder can be treated surgically. It is a very effective treatment and remains the "gold standard" against which all other treatments are compared, but it is an invasive procedure and is used less frequently than in previous years. The procedure relieves the urinary obstruction by "reaming out" the enlarged part of the gland that is encroaching on the urethra and blocking outflow of urine. This is usually accomplished by a procedure called a transurethral resection of the prostate (usually called simply TUR or TURP). A hollow tubular instrument is inserted through the penis into the urethra, and the site of the obstruction is visualized. Then, by means of a snarelike cutting instrument, pieces of the enlarged prostate are shaved off and removed (FIGURE 20-5). This procedure enlarges the urethral opening so that the patient can void normally. The resected tissue is examined histologically by the pathologist to establish the diagnosis of benign prostatic hyperplasia and exclude prostatic carcinoma as a cause of the obstruction (FIGURE 20-6). The lining of the urethra covering the enlarged prostate is removed along with the obstructing part of the gland, but the epithelial lining soon regenerates and the continuity of the urethral lining is restored.

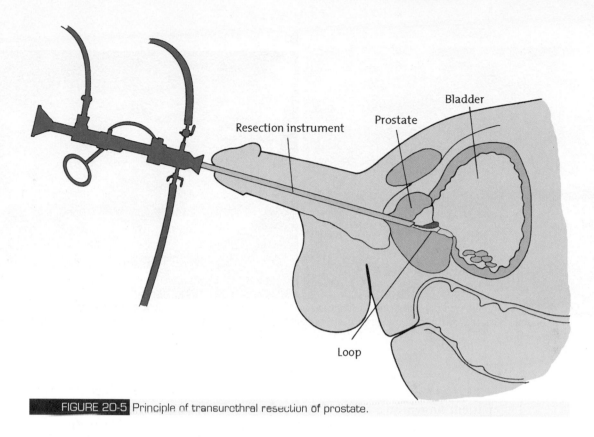

FIGURE 20-5 Principle of transurethral resection of prostate.

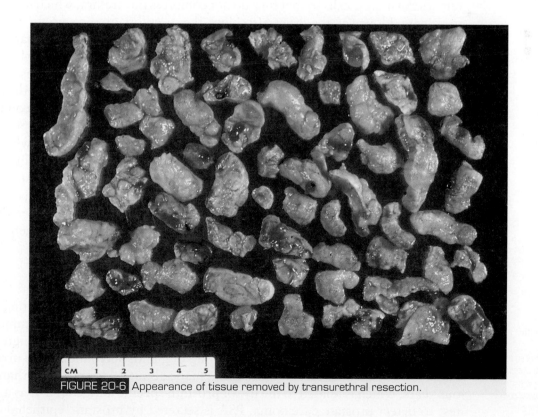

FIGURE 20-6 Appearance of tissue removed by transurethral resection.

A   B

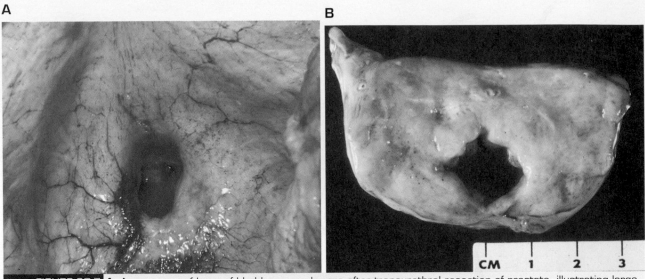

FIGURE 20-7 **A**, Appearance of base of bladder several years after transurethral resection of prostate, illustrating large urethral opening created by the resection. **B**, A cross section of the prostate, showing an enlarged opening. Compare with Figure 20-4.

FIGURE 20-7 illustrates the appearance of the base of the bladder and prostate in a patient on whom a transurethral resection had been performed several years earlier.

Two different types of oral medications are used to treat benign prostatic hyperplasia. One type is called alpha blockers. These drugs block transmission of the nerve impulses that cause contraction of the prostate and bladder neck smooth muscle cells, which relaxes the muscle cells so that they do not compress the urethra, which makes it easier to urinate. However, the drugs also block the receptors on the smooth muscle fibers that dilate the pupil, which interferes with the dilation of the pupil that is required for successful cataract surgery. Consequently, men with prostatic hyperplasia who are taking an alpha blocker to treat benign prostatic hyperplasia need to discontinue the drug for at least 2 weeks before cataract surgery. They should also advise their ophthalmologist because cataract surgery is more difficult and more prone to complications until the effects of the drug have subsided. The second type is called 5-alpha reductase inhibitors. One commonly used drug of this type is called finasteride, which inhibits the prostatic 5-alpha reductase enzyme that converts testosterone to dihydrotestosterone. As a result, the prostate is no longer stimulated by dihydrotestosterone, and it decreases in size. The use of both drugs given together is even more effective than either drug given separately. Whichever method of treatment is used, however, the patient must continue taking the oral medications in order to maintain their beneficial effects.

Carcinoma of the Prostate

Carcinoma of the prostate is the most common carcinoma in men, affecting primarily older men whose average age at the time of diagnosis is 68 years. The tumor usually originates in the outer group of prostatic glands, in contrast to benign prostatic hyperplasia, which involves the inner group of glands surrounding the urethra. The diagnosis of prostatic carcinoma is being made about 10 years earlier than in previous years, which is related to the use of **prostate-specific antigen (PSA)** as a screening test to detect prostate carcinoma. PSA is secreted by prostatic epithelial cells, and elevated levels appear in the blood of many patients with prostate cancer. The test is not specific for prostate carcinoma, however, because some patients with benign

Prostate-specific antigen
An antigen produced by prostatic epithelial cells that is often found in higher-than-normal concentrations in the blood of patients with prostatic cancer and other diseases of the prostate.

prostatic hyperplasia and other types of benign prostatic disease also may have higher-than-normal PSA levels. The diagnosis of prostatic carcinoma is established by needle biopsy of the prostate, in which a needle is inserted into a suspected abnormal area in the prostate through the rectum or perineum. Often, ultrasound examination is used to locate dense areas in the prostate, which assists in selecting the site for biopsy.

Patients in the early stages of prostate carcinoma may be completely free of symptoms, and the tumors are identified only by routine rectal examination as an area of irregularity or nodularity on the posterior surface of the prostate when palpated through the rectum by the examiner's finger. In other patients, the first manifestations may appear when the growing tumor partially obstructs the bladder neck, causing the same type of symptoms as in patients with benign prostatic hyperplasia. The tumor may eventually infiltrate the tissues surrounding the prostate and metastasize to the bones of the spine and pelvis.

Treatment depends on the degree of differentiation of the tumor, the age of the patient, and how far the tumor has spread at the time of diagnosis. A well-differentiated localized tumor in an elderly man may progress slowly and may not produce symptoms for as long as 10 years. Many patients in whom prostatic carcinoma is diagnosed fall into this group and may elect to be followed by their physician without any treatment unless the tumor appears to be progressing as determined by a progressive rise of PSA and other indications that the tumor is enlarging. However, it may be many years before this occurs, and the need for treatment may not even arise during the patient's lifetime. Depending on the patient's age and expected longevity, an elderly man may be more likely to die of some other disease before a well-differentiated tumor has progressed to the stage where more active treatment of the tumor would be required.

In contrast, a less well-differentiated tumor in a younger man requires more aggressive treatment. A small, localized prostatic carcinoma can be treated by removing the entire prostate and surrounding tissues. This procedure is called a radical prostatectomy (FIGURE 20-8). Although this operation may eradicate the tumor,

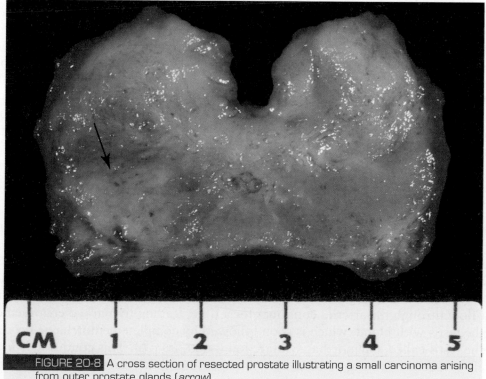

FIGURE 20-8 A cross section of resected prostate illustrating a small carcinoma arising from outer prostate glands (*arrow*).

it usually also disrupts the nerve supply to the penis, which leads to permanent inability to achieve an erection of the penis (impotence). In other cases, the tumor is treated by irradiation rather than surgery. Radical prostatectomy alone or combined with radiation therapy appears to improve survival in many patients. There is considerable controversy, however, about the effectiveness of radical surgery or radiation therapy in older men with localized well-differentiated carcinoma of the prostate. Many physicians believe that treatment does not improve survival in this group of patients, that the treatment causes more disability and complications than the tumor, and that a slowly growing prostatic carcinoma in an older man is best left alone.

When a prostatic carcinoma has advanced to the stage when it has spread beyond the prostate and has metastasized, it is often possible to induce regression of the tumor by altering the level of male sex hormones in the body. Most prostatic carcinomas are dependent on the male sex hormone for their continued growth. Therefore, many advanced prostatic tumors can be treated effectively by surgical removal of the testes, eliminating the source of the male sex hormone. Alternatively, drugs that suppress output of pituitary gonadotropic hormone can be administered, thereby inhibiting testicular testosterone secretion. Either castration or hormone treatment usually causes regression of the tumor.

Cryptorchidism

Sometimes the testis does not descend normally into the scrotum, a condition called either cryptorchidism (*crypto* = hidden + *orchis* = testis) or cryptorchism. Usually, an undescended testis is located within the abdominal cavity, but it sometimes may be within the inguinal canal. In some newborn infants, one or both testes have failed to descend into the scrotum, but testicular descent often will occur normally within about 6 months after birth. If the testes are not in the scrotum by the time the infant is 1 year old, the cryptorchid testis should be surgically brought into the scrotum because progressive damage to sperm-producing germ cells begins as early as 6 months after birth, and the longer the testis is retained within the abdomen, the more marked the germ cell damage. In contrast, the testosterone-producing interstitial cells are unaffected and will function normally at puberty when stimulated by gonadotropic hormones even though sperm production is no longer possible because the germ cells have been destroyed (FIGURE 20-9). An undescended testis also increases the long-term risk of testicular carcinoma, which is about 20 times more frequent in persons with an undescended testis than in the general population.

Testicular Torsion

If the fibrous tissue derived from the gubernaculum that attaches the testis to the scrotum is a relatively long and narrow band rather than a short broad attachment, the testis may undergo a rotary twist on its axis, which also twists the spermatic cord and interrupts the blood supply to the testis (FIGURE 20-10A). The thin-walled veins in the cord are compressed first, which impedes return of venous blood from the testis, but flow through the arteries continues for a time, leading to marked engorgement of the testis with blood, which is soon followed by complete hemorrhagic necrosis of the testis called a hemorrhagic infarction (FIGURE 20-10B). This condition is more likely to occur in young persons between age 10 and 25 years, but may occur at any age, and may even occur in the fetus during prenatal descent of the testis, as

A

B

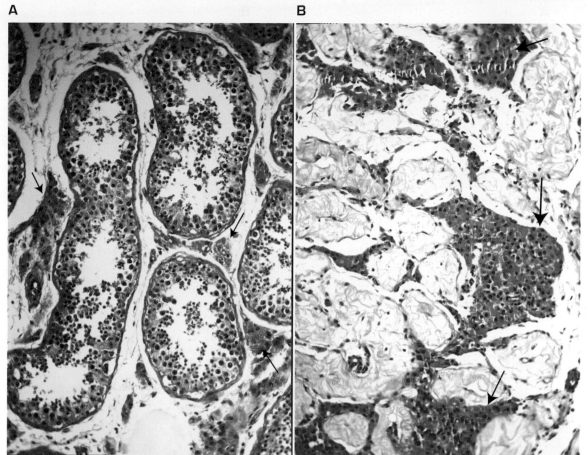

FIGURE 20-9 Photomicrographs comparing normal scrotal testis with intra-abdominal testis. **A**, Normal testis showing active spermatogenesis within testicular tubules. The clusters of cells between the tubules are interstitial cells (*arrows*). **B**, Intra-abdominal testis, showing marked atrophy and fibrosis of testicular tubules. The large clusters of cells between the hyaline atrophic tubules are interstitial cells, which function normally at body temperature. They appear quite prominent because of the marked tubular atrophy (original magnification × 160).

illustrated in Case 20-1. A testicular torsion is characterized by an acute onset of severe testicular pain associated with swelling of the involved testis and is an acute surgical emergency. If the torsion can be untwisted and the testis is properly anchored in the scrotum within a few hours after onset of the torsion, the testis probably can be salvaged, but the longer the delay, the less likely the possibility that the testis will survive. Because the abnormal mobility of the testis within the scrotum that caused the torsion is likely to be present in the other testis as well, generally, the other testis is surgically anchored in the scrotum so that it cannot undergo torsion.

CASE 20-1

A 6-lb. 10-oz. male infant was delivered at term to a 27-year-old mother after an uneventful labor and delivery. The infant appeared normal at birth except for a markedly enlarged right testicle that was adherent to the scrotal skin. The enlarged testicle was removed. Histologic examination revealed complete infarction of the testicle with associated inflammation and fibrous tissue proliferation in response to the testicular necrosis.

A

B

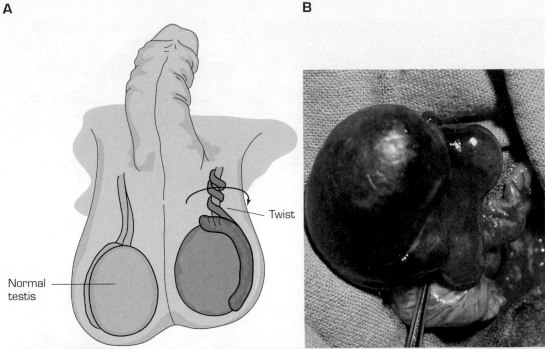

FIGURE 20-10 Cause and effect of testicular torsion. **A**, Rotary twist of testis also twists spermatic cord, interrupting blood supply to the testis. Normally, the epididymis is located along the posterior surface of the testis, but the torsion has rotated the testis and also rotated the epididymis anteriorly. **B**, Hemorrhagic infarction of testis caused by torsion.

Scrotal Abnormalities

HYDROCELE

Hydrocele
(hī′-drō-cēl)
An accumulation of excess fluid within the tunica vaginalis of the testis.

Normally the saclike tunica vaginalis contains only a very small amount of fluid (FIGURE 20-11A), but sometimes a much larger amount of fluid accumulates in the sac, which is called a **hydrocele** (*hydro* = water + *cele* = swelling). This is not a serious condition, and no treatment is required unless the hydrocele causes marked scrotal swelling and is uncomfortable (FIGURE 20-11B). The fluid can be aspirated as a temporary solution, but the fluid usually accumulates again. The long-term solution is surgical excision of the sac. When the physician examines a patient with a hydrocele, he or she usually also performs a careful examination of the testis and scrotum, which may be supplemented by an ultrasound examination in order to exclude the possibility of a testicular tumor or some other condition associated with the hydrocele.

VARICOCELE

The term varicocele (*varix* = dilated vein + *cele* = swelling) refers to varicose veins that develop within the spermatic cord veins that drain blood from the testis, caused by failure of the vein valves to function properly (FIGURE 20-11C). This is the same reason that varicose veins form in other locations, as described in the cardiovascular system. Normally functioning valves in the spermatic cord veins promote venous blood flow away from the testes and prevent backflow, but poorly functioning valves allow blood to pool in the veins, which become markedly dilated. Usually it is the veins draining the left testis that give rise to a varicocele because the venous drainage from the left half of the scrotum has a less direct route into the inferior vena cava and

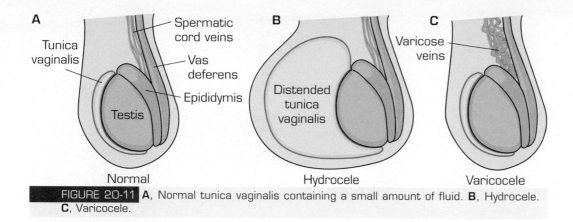

FIGURE 20-11 **A,** Normal tunica vaginalis containing a small amount of fluid. **B,** Hydrocele. **C,** Varicocele.

a slightly higher venous pressure than does the venous blood returning from the right half of the scrotum. When the scrotum is examined while the subject is standing, the scrotal varicose veins located above the testis are sometimes described as "feeling like a bag full of worms." When the subject lies down, blood drains easily from the veins, and the varicocele can no longer be felt. Generally, a varicocele does not cause symptoms. Occasionally, however, a varicocele may reduce fertility by impairing spermatogenesis, a result of the higher scrotal temperature caused by warm venous blood pooling in the varicose scrotal veins. A varicocele can be treated surgically if it causes scrotal discomfort or impairs fertility. Otherwise no treatment is required.

Erectile Dysfunction

PHYSIOLOGY OF PENILE ERECTION

The penis consists primarily of three cavernous bodies, which are cylinders of extremely vascular erectile tissue; two laterally placed corpora cavernosa; and the midline corpus spongiosum that surrounds the penile urethra. Each cylinder, surrounded by a thick fibrous tissue capsule, is composed of a spongy meshwork of endothelium-lined blood sinuses supported by trabeculae (partitions) composed of connective tissue and smooth muscle. The blood sinuses of the erectile tissue are supplied by arteries and drained by veins. Normally, the arteries are constricted so that very little blood flows into the cavernous bodies, and the vascular sinuses are collapsed. During sexual excitement, however, parasympathetic nerve impulses arising from the sacral part of the spinal cord release the neurotransmitter nitric oxide, which causes relaxation of the smooth muscle in the walls of the penile arteries and in the trabeculae between the sinuses. As a result, the penile arteries dilate, and the sinuses in the cavernous bodies expand. Blood pours under high pressure into the blood sinuses within the cavernous bodies. The greatly increased arterial blood flow and rising pressure within the blood sinuses compresses the draining veins, which retards outflow of blood from the penis and contributes to the engorgement of the blood sinuses. The penis rapidly becomes rigid and erect (FIGURE 20-12).

Erectile dysfunction is an inability to achieve and maintain a penile erection of sufficient rigidity to penetrate the vagina and maintain the erection during sexual intercourse. This is a relatively common problem that increases in frequency with advancing age. Penile erection is a complex process. First, sexual desire is required to initiate the physiologic events that increase blood flow to the penis. Second, the arteries supplying the cavernous bodies must dilate enough to deliver a large volume of blood to the penis. Third, the pressure of the blood within the cavernous bodies

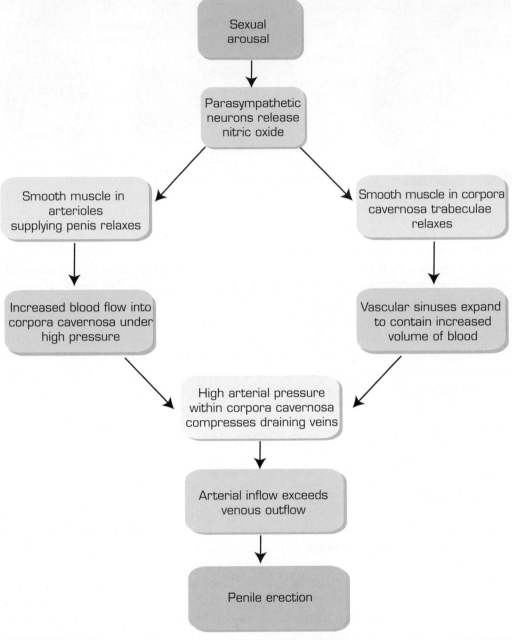

FIGURE 20-12 Physiology of penile erection.

must be sufficiently high to compress the draining veins. Blood must flow into the penis faster than it drains out, or an erection cannot be maintained.

CAUSES OF ERECTILE DYSFUNCTION

To achieve and sustain a penile erection, the sensory, motor, and autonomic nerve supply to the penis must be normal, and the blood vessels supplying the penis must be able to deliver an adequate volume of blood to the penis. Various factors may disturb these physiologic processes. These include

1. A low testosterone level, which inhibits sexual desire and arousal
2. Damage to the nerves supplying the penis resulting from radical prostate surgery or neurologic diseases

3. Impaired blood supply to the penis, resulting from arteriosclerosis of the blood vessels that deliver blood to the penis, as may occur in persons with systemic arteriosclerosis or long-standing, poorly controlled diabetes
4. Some drugs used to treat hypertension that target the autonomic nervous system, which also affects the autonomic nerves supplying the penis
5. Stress, emotional factors, and many chronic illnesses, which may impair the person's quality of life and also adversely affect sexual performance

TREATMENT

Many different medical and surgical procedures can be used to treat erectile dysfunction, depending the cause of the dysfunction and the individual's preference. One well-known treatment involves the use of drugs that inhibit an enzyme called phosphodiesterase in order to promote increased blood flow to the penis. Several phosphodiesterase drugs are available (sildenafil, vardenafil, tadanafil) that differ primarily in their duration of action. They are relatively safe drugs when used properly, but they have known side effects and rarely may be associated with serious complications. The best known of these drugs is sildenafil, better known by its trade name Viagra. The sequence of events involved in penile erection and the role of phosphodiesterase inhibitor drugs are as follows:

1. Sexual arousal stimulates parasympathetic neurons supplying the penis to release the neurotransmitter nitric oxide.
2. Nitric oxide diffuses into smooth muscle cells where it promotes the formation of a compound called cyclic guanosine monophosphate (cGMP), which in turn causes relaxation of the smooth muscle cells in the penile arteries and in the trabeculae within the corpora cavernosa. Blood under pressure fills the cavernous bodies, causing the penis to become rigid and erect.
3. Although cGMP is formed continuously as long as parasympathetic nerve impulses continue to release nitric oxide, the duration of action of the cGMP molecules is relatively brief because cGMP is broken down by a phosphodiesterase enzyme.
4. Phosphodiesterase inhibitor drugs such as sildenafil inhibit the enzyme, thereby prolonging the vasodilator effect of cGMP, which helps sustain the erection.

Carcinoma of the Testis

Testicular tumors are uncommon and usually develop in young men. Most arise from the germinal epithelium of the testicular tubules and are malignant. There are several different types. The type with the most favorable prognosis is called a **seminoma**. (This term is another exception to standard terminology. It means literally a tumor of semen-producing epithelium. In this case, the term refers to a malignant neoplasm, not a benign tumor.) Another type of testicular tumor is a malignant teratoma, which is composed of many different types of malignant tissues, as described in the discussion on neoplastic disease. Some other testicular tumors resemble placental trophoblastic tissue. One tumor of this type is called an **embryonal carcinoma**. Another is called a **choriocarcinoma**, which is the same kind of tumor that arises from trophoblastic tissue in the uterus, as described in prenatal development and diseases associated with pregnancy. Testicular cancers are treated by extensive surgical resection of the testicle, the spermatic cord, and sometimes the regional lymph nodes as well. In some cases, radiation and anticancer chemotherapy also are used.

The neoplastic cells of many testicular tumors produce **human chorionic gonadotropin (HCG)**, which is the same hormone made by the placenta in pregnancy.

Seminoma
(sem-in-ō′ma)
One type of malignant tumor of testis.

Embryonal carcinoma
A malignant testicular tumor in which the malignant cells have features resembling rapidly growing trophoblastic tissue.

Choriocarcinoma
(kōr′rē-ō-kär-sin-ō′muh)
A malignant proliferation of trophoblastic tissue.

Human chorionic gonadotropin (HCG)
(kōr-ē-on′ik gō-na-dō-trō′pin)
A hormone made by the placenta in pregnancy having actions similar to pituitary gonadotropins. Same hormone is made by neoplastic cells in some types of malignant testicular tumors.

Alpha fetoprotein
(al'fuh fē'tō-prō'tēn)
Protein produced by fetal liver early in gestation. Sometimes produced by tumor cells. Level is elevated in amnionic fluid when fetus has neural tube defect.

Consequently, a pregnancy test given to a man with testicular cancer may be positive. Some testicular tumors also produce another substance called **alpha fetoprotein** (AFP), which is a protein produced by the fetus early in prenatal development but not normally found in the adult. If a testicular carcinoma produces these substances, the concentrations fall after successful treatment of the tumor and rise again if the tumor recurs. Consequently, the physician can monitor the response of the testicular tumor to treatment by serial determinations of HCG and AFP, in the same way that carcinoembryonic antigen analyses are used to evaluate the response to treatment of other malignant tumors, as described in the neoplastic disease.

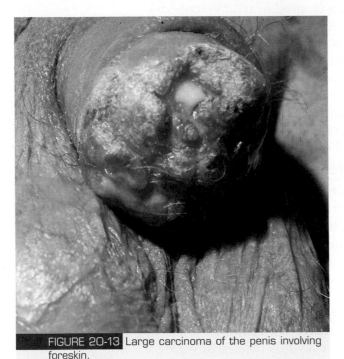

FIGURE 20-13 Large carcinoma of the penis involving foreskin.

Carcinoma of the Penis

Carcinoma of the penis is uncommon; it is almost never encountered in a circumcised male (FIGURE 20-13). It had been considered that the secretions that accumulate under the foreskin of the penis were carcinogenic, and that the accumulation was prevented by circumcision. However, other factors also may account for the low incidence of carcinoma in circumcised males. Carcinogenic strains of the papilloma virus, the same virus that appears related to cervical dysplasia and carcinoma in women, may play a major role in causing penile cancer. Probably the papilloma virus grows well beneath an intact foreskin but does not thrive if the foreskin has been removed.

Treatment usually consists of partial or complete resection of the penis.

QUESTIONS FOR REVIEW

1. What are the components of the male reproductive system?
2. What is benign prostatic hyperplasia? What are its clinical manifestations? How is it treated?
3. How does administration of female sex hormones affect prostatic carcinoma? What is the effect of castration on prostatic carcinoma?
4. A young man has a positive pregnancy test. Under what circumstances could this occur?
5. What factors predispose to the development of carcinoma of the penis? How may the disease be prevented?
6. What is cryptorchidism? What are the clinical manifestations? How is the condition treated? Why should it be treated?
7. What is a testicular torsion? What are its manifestations and complications? How is the condition treated?
8. A young man has an undescended testis within the abdomen. How does this affect testicular function? What complications may result from this condition?

SUPPLEMENTARY READINGS

Bell, C. M., Hatch, W. V., Fischer, H. D., et al. 2009. Association between tamsulosin and serious ophthalmic adverse events in older men following cataract surgery. *Journal of the American Medical Association* 301:1991–6.

▶ The alpha adrenergic blocker tamsulosin is frequently prescribed to treat benign prostatic hyperplasia, which increases the operative difficulty of cataract surgery because a widely dilated pupil is required for a successful complication-free operation. Tamsulosin also blocks the adrenergic receptors in the muscles that dilate the pupil, which interferes with the pupillary dilation required for successful cataract surgery and increases the risk of serious surgical complications. The tamsulosin-related problem is called the *floppy iris syndrome*.

▶ See also the editorial in the same issue.

Cooner, W. H., Mosley, B. R., Rutherford, C. L., Jr., et al. 1988. Clinical application of transrectal ultrasonography and prostate specific antigen in the search for prostate cancer. *Journal of Urology* 139:758–61.

Feldman, D. R., Bosl, G. J., Sheinfeld, J., et al. 2008. Medical treatment of advanced testicular cancer. *Journal of the American Medical Association* 299:672–84.

▶ Testicular carcinoma is a young man's disease and is the most common type of cancer diagnosed between the ages of 15 and 35 years. Classification and treatment of advanced testicular tumors are described, with tumors classified based on histologic features, sites of metastases, and degree of elevation of serum tumor markers. New, more aggressive treatment has improved the cure rate from 25% in the 1970s to nearly 80% now but was associated with significant toxic effects. Impaired fertility also occurred in patients who had a retroperitoneal lymph node dissection to supplement resection of the testis and chemotherapy. Disruption of the sympathetic retroperitoneal nerves concerned with emission and ejaculation was responsible for the infertility.

Fleming, C., Wasson, J. H., Albertsen, P. C., et al. 1993. A decision analysis of alternative treatment strategies for clinically localized prostate cancer. Prostate Patient Outcomes Research Team. *Journal of the American Medical Association* 269:2650–8.

▶ Radical prostatectomy and radiation therapy may benefit some men but appear harmful for patients older than 70 years.

Friedman, A. H. 2009. Tamsulosin and the intraoperative floppy iris syndrome. *Journal of the American Medical Association* 301:2044–5.

Javadpour, N. 1980. Germ cell tumors of the testis. *CA: A Cancer Journal for Clinicians* 30:242–55.

▶ A comprehensive review.

Johansson, J. E., Andrén, O., Andersson, S. O., et al. 2004. Natural history of early, localized prostate cancer. *Journal of the American Medical Association* 291: 2713–9.

▶ Two hundred ninety-one older men with early prostate carcinoma (diagnosed before the use of PSA testing) were followed without initial treatment for 21 years. During the first 15 years, the cancers progressed slowly but behaved more aggressively in the patients followed beyond 15 years, possibly related to dedifferentiation of the original tumor. A previous Swedish study has demonstrated that radical prostatectomy reduced cancer-related mortality by 50%, but many of the patients died of other conditions; so there was no change in overall mortality. In evaluating the survival advantage of radical prostatectomy on patients with early prostate carcinoma, it will be necessary to follow radical prostatectomy patients for a 15- to 20-year period.

Krahn, M. D., Mahoney, J. E., Eckman, M. H., et al. 1994. Screening for prostate cancer. A decision analytic view. *Journal of the American Medical Association* 272:773–80.

  ▶ Screening unselected men from ages 50 to 70 with prostate-specific antigen test and transrectal ultrasound did not improve health outcomes and increased costs dramatically.

Lu-Yao, G. L., McLerran, D., Wasson, J., et al. 1993. An assessment of radical prostatectomy. Time trends, geographic variation, and outcomes. The Prostate Patient Outcomes Research Team. *Journal of the American Medical Association* 269:2633–6.

  ▶ Radical prostatectomy carries a significant morbidity and mortality, especially in older men.

McVay, K. T. 2007. Clinical practice. Erectile dysfunction. *New England Journal of Medicine* 357:2472–81.

  ▶ A discussion of the pathophysiology of erectile dysfunction and its cause. Treatments are described.

Morgentaler, A. 2004. A 66-year-old man with sexual dysfunction. *Journal of the American Medical Association* 291:2994–3003.

  ▶ An excellent summary of the pathophysiology of erectile dysfunction together with the applications and limitations of various methods of treatment.

Persky, L. 1986. Carcinoma of the penis. *CA: A Cancer Journal for Clinicians* 36:258–73.

  ▶ Treatment consists of either partial or complete removal of the penis and may also require resection of groin and pelvic lymph nodes.

Pettersson, A., Richiardi, L., Nordenskjold, A., et al. 2007. Age at surgery for undescended testis and risk of testicular cancer. *New England Journal of Medicine* 356:1835–41.

  ▶ Cryptorchidism is associated with impaired fertility and is a risk factor for testicular cancer. From 5 to 10% of all men with testicular carcinoma have a history of cryptorchidism. Testes undescended at birth may descend spontaneously within the first few months after birth but are unlikely to descend spontaneously thereafter. Germ cell development rapidly deteriorates in an undescended testis. Surgical correction (orchiopexy) positions and fixes the testis in the scrotum and is performed on infants as young as 6 months old, both to preserve germ cell function and to reduce the risk of later development of testicular cancer. This study of 17,000 men surgically treated for cryptorchidism considered the age at which the procedures were performed. Treatment for undescended testis prior to puberty decreases the risk of testicular carcinoma but is less effective when performed after puberty.

Rhoden, E. L., and Morgentaler, A. 2004. Risks of testosterone-replacement therapy and recommendations for monitoring. *New England Journal of Medicine* 350:482–92.

  ▶ Testosterone replacement therapy is used to treat men with low testosterone levels, and it improves libido, bone density, muscle mass, and red cell production but also has some undesirable effects. Testosterone stimulates prostate growth and enlargement. Because many older men harbor small asymptomatic prostate carcinomas, the testosterone may also stimulate tumor growth as well. The administered testosterone also exerts a negative feedback effect on pituitary gonadotropin output in the endocrine glands which inhibits sperm production and impairs fertility. Some men also may experience breast tenderness and breast enlargement, possibly because some of the testosterone is converted to estrogen within the body. Men over 40 years of age should be evaluated to exclude occult prostate carcinoma before beginning treatment, and the level of prostate specific antigen (PSA) should be monitored periodically to assure that an undetected occult prostate carcinoma is not being activated by the testosterone treatment.

Stanford, J. L., Feng, Z., Hamilton, A. S., et al. 2000. Urinary and sexual function after radical prostatectomy for clinically localized prostate cancer: The Prostate Cancer Outcomes Study. *Journal of the American Medical Association* 283:354–60.

▶ In a large group of patients, 8.4% were incontinent, and 59.9% were impotent at 18 or more months after surgery. Despite the level of incontinence and sexual dysfunction, 75.5% of the men were satisfied with their treatment.

Thompson, I. M., and Klotz, L. 2010. Active surveillance for prostate cancer. *Journal of the American Medical Association* 304:2411–2.

▶ Sixty percent of men who are screened for prostate carcinoma are overdiagnosed and overtreated. Multiple biopsy specimen initiated by elevated PSA test results often reveal small well-differentiated tumors, and more than 90% of this group have either a radical prostatectomy or radiation therapy, which often has undesirable side effects that adversely affect their quality of life. Men can be followed by PSA tests and periodic prostate biopsies, with treatment reserved for men in whom PSA rises significantly or prostate biopsies reveal increased tumor grade. Up to 60% of men diagnosed with prostate carcinoma may not need treatment.

Walsh, P., DeWeese, T. L., and Eisenberger, M. A. 2007. Clinical practice. Localized prostate cancer. *New England Journal of Medicine* 357:2696–705.

▶ Patients with small well-differentiated tumors can be managed by observation without immediate treatment. Available evidence suggests that with careful monitoring every 6 months and biopsies at regular intervals, deferring treatment until there are signs of progression is unlikely to affect the likelihood of cure. The alternative options of surgery and radiation therapy along with their potential benefits and side effects should also be presented, and the patient can choose how he or she wants to proceed.

Zincke, H., Ote, D. C., Thulé, P. M., et al. 1987. Treatment options for patients with stage D1 (T0-3, N1-2, H0) adenocarcinoma of prostate. *Urology* 30:307–15.

▶ Describes results on 306 patients with advanced prostate cancer treated by prostatectomy followed by hormonal or radiation therapy or both. More than 87% 10-year survivals.

OUTLINE SUMMARY

Components of the Male Reproductive System

PENIS

TRANSPORT DUCTS

PROSTATE
Inner glands: may give rise to benign hyperplasia.
Outer glands: may give rise to carcinoma.

TESTES
Develop in abdomen and descend into scrotum.
Germ cells form sperm.
Interstitial cells form testosterone.

Gonorrhea and Nongonococcal Urethritis

GONORRHEA
A common disease spread by sexual contact.
May spread to posterior urethra and transport ducts.
Obstruction of vasa may cause sterility.

NONGONOCOCCAL URETHRITIS
Symptoms similar to gonorrhea.
Caused by *Chlamydia*.

Prostatitis

ACUTE PROSTATITIS
Spread of infection from bladder or urethra.
May be secondary to gonococcal infection.

CHRONIC PROSTATITIS
Mild chronic inflammation.
Causes few symptoms.

Benign Prostatic Hyperplasia

MANIFESTATIONS
Enlarged prostate obstructs outflow of urine.
Predisposes to infection, calculi, and hydronephrosis.

TREATMENT
Various medical and surgical treatments.
Transurethral resection is "gold standard."

Carcinoma of the Prostate

MANIFESTATIONS

Early case may be asymptomatic.

May obstruct bladder neck and cause symptoms of obstruction like benign prostatic hyperplasia.

Often metastasizes to pelvic and vertebral bone.

DIAGNOSIS

Rectal examination indicates abnormality.

Prostate-specific antigen or acid phosphatase or both often elevated.

Prostate biopsy, sometimes assisted by ultrasound examination of prostate.

TREATMENT

May not be required in elderly men with well-differentiated tumors.

Radical prostatectomy.

Radiation therapy.

Antiandrogen therapy if tumor no longer curable by surgery or radiation.

Cryptorchidism

CAUSE

Testis does not descend normally into scrotum.

Usually retained in abdominal cavity; sometimes in inguinal canal.

Germ cells required a lower than normal body temperature.

Interstitial cells function normally at body temperature.

MANIFESTATIONS AND TREATMENT

Germ cells destroyed at higher intra-abdominal temperature.

Interstitial cells function normally.

Undescended testis more prone to developing testicular cancer.

Surgically replace testis in scrotum.

Testicular Torsion

CAUSE

Abnormal attachment of testis in scrotum.

Predisposes to rotary twisting of testis and spermatic cord, shutting off blood supply to testis.

MANIFESTATIONS AND TREATMENT

Acute onset of testicular pain and swelling.

Leads to hemorrhagic infarction of testis unless promptly untwisted.

Scrotal Abnormalities

HYDROCELE

Excess fluid accumulates in tunica vaginalis.

Treated by aspiration or resection of tunica vaginalis.

VARICOCELE

Varicose veins in spermatic cord.

Usually the left side of scrotum involved.

May impair fertility.

No treatment required unless varicocele causes discomfort or impairs fertility.

Erectile Dysfunction

CAUSE AND MANIFESTATIONS

Inability to achieve and maintain a penile erection.

Many different causes that impair blood flow to penis.

TREATMENT

Many medical and surgical treatments available depending on the cause of dysfunction.

Phosphodiesterase inhibitor drugs effective but must be used with caution because of possible serious side effects.

Carcinoma of the Testis

CLASSIFICATION

Seminoma.

Malignant teratoma.

Embroyonal carcinoma and choriocarcinoma.

TREATMENT

Resection of testicle and associated structures.

Chemotherapy.

METHODS USED TO MONITOR RESPONSE TO THERAPY

Human chorionic gonadotropins (HCG).

Alpha fetoprotein (AFP).

Carcinoma of the Penis

MANIFESTATIONS AND PATHOGENESIS

Rare in circumcised male.

Secretions accumulating under foreskin may be carcinogenic.

Papilloma virus may play a role.

TREATMENT

Partial or complete amputation of penis.

Removal of inguinal lymph nodes also usually performed.

http://health.jbpub.com/humandisease/9e

Human Disease Online is a great source for supplementary human disease information for both students and instructors. Visit this website to find a variety of useful tools for learning, thinking, and teaching.

CHAPTER 21

The Liver and the Biliary System

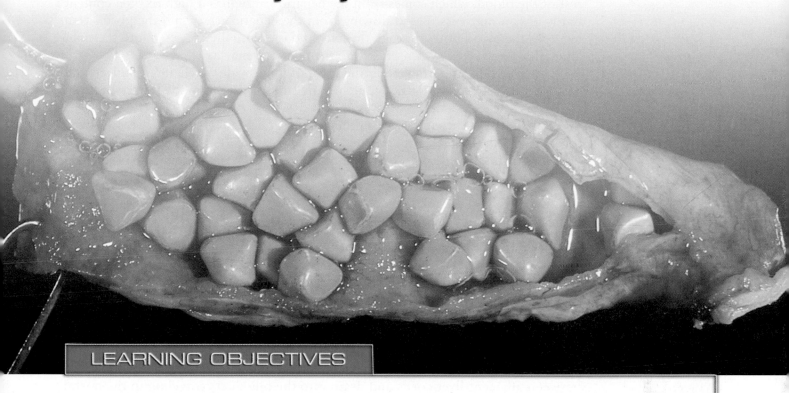

LEARNING OBJECTIVES

1 Describe the normal structure of the liver, and explain the functions of the liver as they relate to the major diseases of the liver.

2 List the major causes of liver injury, and describe their effects on hepatic function.

3 Compare the three major types of viral hepatitis in terms of their pathogenesis, incubation period, incidence of complications, and frequency of carriers. Explain the diagnostic tests used to identify each type of viral infection, and describe methods of prevention.

4 Explain the adverse effects of excess alcohol intake on liver structure and function.

5 Explain how gallstones are formed, and describe their causes and effects.

6 Compare the three major causes of jaundice.

Structure and Function of the Liver

The liver is the largest organ in the body. It has a roughly triangular shape and is located beneath the diaphragm in the upper abdomen (FIGURE 21-1). It is a complex organ with many functions. These are concerned mainly with the following:

1. Metabolism of ingested carbohydrates, protein, and fat delivered through the portal circulation
2. Synthesis of various substances, including plasma proteins and proteins taking part in blood clotting

3. Storage of vitamin B$_{12}$ and other materials
4. Detoxification and excretion of various substances

The liver has a double blood supply. About three quarters of the blood flow is provided by the portal vein, which drains the spleen and gastrointestinal tract. Portal blood is rich in nutrients absorbed from the intestines but low in oxygen content. The rest of the blood, which comes from the hepatic artery, has a high oxygen content but is low in nutrients. Blood flowing from the hepatic artery and the portal vein mixes as the blood flows through the liver and is eventually collected into the right and left hepatic veins, which drain into the inferior vena cava.

The liver cells are arranged in the form of long, wide plates interconnected at various angles to form a lattice. The hepatic sinusoids occupy the spaces between the plates (FIGURE 21-2A).

Branches of the hepatic artery, portal vein, bile ducts, and lymphatic vessels travel together within the liver and are called the **portal tracts** (FIGURE 21-2B). The terminal branches of both the hepatic artery and the portal vein discharge their blood into the hepatic sinusoids (FIGURE 21-2C). In histologic sections, the liver plates appear as cords surrounded on each side by sinusoids that converge toward the central veins. The portal tracts appear at the periphery. This anatomic configuration, which is called a **liver lobule**, is illustrated diagrammatically in FIGURE 21-3A.

Blood flow in the liver is from portal tracts through the sinusoids into central veins (FIGURE 21-3B). Consequently, the liver cells nearest the portal tracts receive the most oxygen and nutrients, and those nearest the central veins are much less well supplied. Because of their relatively poor nutritional state, the liver cells nearest the central veins are more vulnerable to injury from toxic agents or circulatory disturbances, as occurs in shock and heart failure, than are the cells nearer the portal tracts.

The small terminal bile channels are called **bile canaliculi**. They are located between adjacent liver cords and drain into the bile ducts traveling in the portal tracts. The direction of the bile flow is opposite that of the blood flow in the sinusoids (FIGURE 21-3B). The bile ducts gradually converge to form larger ducts,

Portal tract
Branch of hepatic artery, portal vein, and bile duct located at periphery of liver lobule.

Liver lobule
A histologic subdivision of the liver in which columns of liver cells converge toward a central vein and portal tracts are located at the periphery.

Bile canaliculus
(kan-al-ik′u-lus)
Small terminal bile channel located between liver cords.

A

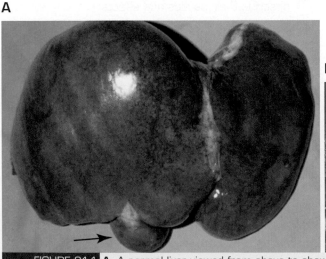

B

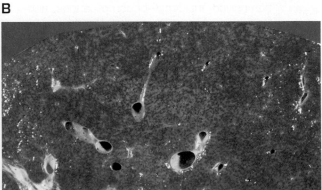

FIGURE 21-1 **A**, A normal liver viewed from above to show its superior and anterior surfaces. The gallbladder is located on the undersurface of the liver, and the fundus of the gallbladder projects slightly beyond the anterior edge of the liver (*arrow*). **B**, Section of liver illustrating the uniform appearance of the hepatic parenchyma and the large blood vessels (branches of the portal vein) transporting blood into the liver from the gastrointestinal tract.

A

B

C

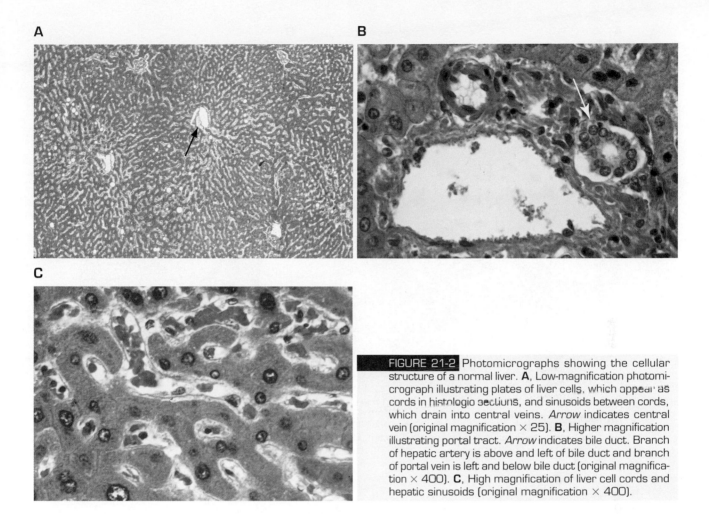

FIGURE 21-2 Photomicrographs showing the cellular structure of a normal liver. **A,** Low-magnification photomicrograph illustrating plates of liver cells, which appear as cords in histologic sections, and sinusoids between cords, which drain into central veins. *Arrow* indicates central vein (original magnification × 25). **B,** Higher magnification illustrating portal tract. *Arrow* indicates bile duct. Branch of hepatic artery is above and left of bile duct and branch of portal vein is left and below bile duct (original magnification × 400). **C,** High magnification of liver cell cords and hepatic sinusoids (original magnification × 400).

which finally unite as the large right and left hepatic ducts. The two hepatic ducts join to form the common hepatic duct. The gallbladder joins the common hepatic duct by means of the cystic duct to form the common bile duct that enters the duodenum.

Bile

FORMATION AND EXCRETION

Bile pigment is a product of the breakdown of red blood cells. Red cells normally survive for about 4 months. The worn-out erythrocytes are broken down by the mononuclear phagocytes (reticuloendothelial cells) throughout the body. The iron derived from the hemoglobin is conserved by the body and reused to synthesize new hemoglobin. The iron-free heme pigment forms **bilirubin**. Because the breakdown of red cells proceeds in mononuclear phagocytes throughout the body, small quantities of bile pigment are continually present in the blood. When the blood passes through the liver, the bilirubin is removed by the liver cells. Excretion is accomplished by combining the bilirubin with other substances, a process called conjugation, which requires certain specific enzymes. Most of the bilirubin is conjugated with glucuronic acid and excreted

Bilirubin
(bil-i-rū′bin)
One of the bile pigments derived from breakdown of hemoglobin.

A

B

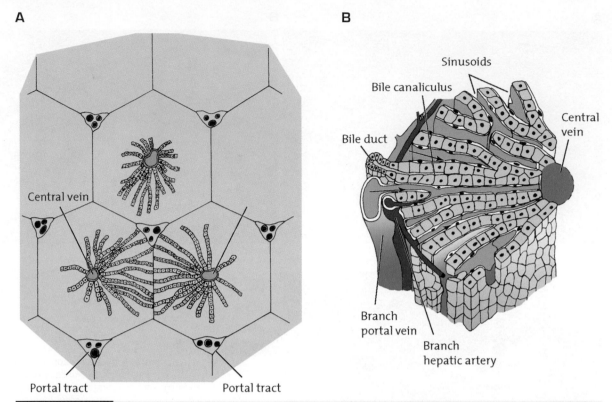

FIGURE 21-3 **A,** Concept of liver lobule, consisting of cords of cells radiating toward central vein with portal tracts at periphery. Lobules are outlined in diagram. **B,** Blood flow in sinusoids toward central vein; flow of bile toward portal tract.

Conjugated bilirubin
A more soluble form of bilirubin produced by the addition of two molecules of glucuronic acid to the bilirubin molecule.

Bile
A secretion of the liver containing bile salts, cholesterol, and other substances.

Cholesterol
(kō-les′ter-ol)
A complex compound (sterol) containing several ring structures.

Bile salts
Derivatives of bile acids present in bile that act as emulsifiers to promote fat digestion and absorption.

Lecithin (les′ith-in)
A phosphorus-containing lipid (phospholipid) having detergent properties similar to bile salts.

as bilirubin glucuronide. The **conjugated bilirubin** is much more soluble and less toxic than the unconjugated material. The bile pigment is excreted into the small bile channels between the liver cell cords; it is collected into large ducts at the periphery of the lobules that eventually unite to form the major bile ducts. FIGURE 21-4 summarizes the basic anatomy of the biliary duct system.

COMPOSITION AND PROPERTIES

Bile is an aqueous solution containing various dissolved substances excreted by the liver. In addition to conjugated bilirubin, it contains bile salts, lecithin, cholesterol, water, minerals, and other materials that have been detoxified by liver cells and excreted. **Cholesterol** is a lipid with a complex ring structure that is classified as a sterol. **Bile salts**, the major constituent of bile, are derivatives of cholesterol and certain amino acids. They function as detergents because of their molecular structure, which contains both a lipid-soluble (hydrophobic) and a water-soluble (hydrophilic) part. **Lecithin** is a phosphorous-containing lipid (phospholipid) that has detergent properties similar to bile salts. Bile is secreted continually and is concentrated and stored in the gallbladder. During digestion, the gallbladder contracts, squirting bile into the duodenum. Bile does not contain digestive enzymes but functions as a biologic detergent. Bile salts emulsify fat into small globules, increasing the surface area so that the fat can be acted on more readily by pancreatic enzymes. Digestion of fat is much less efficient in the absence of bile.

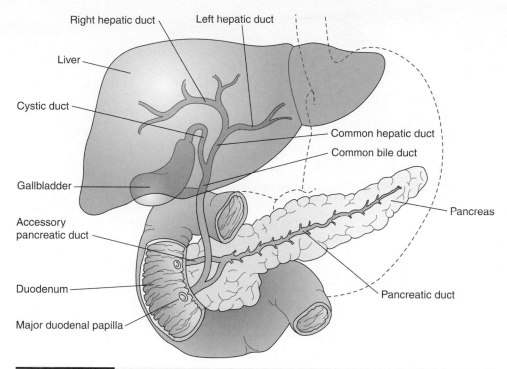

Right hepatic duct
Left hepatic duct
Liver
Cystic duct
Common hepatic duct
Common bile duct
Gallbladder
Accessory pancreatic duct
Pancreas
Duodenum
Pancreatic duct
Major duodenal papilla

FIGURE 21-4 Anatomy of the biliary duct system. Right and left hepatic ducts form the common hepatic duct, which is joined by the cystic duct to form the common bile duct, which opens into the duodenum along with the pancreatic duct through a common channel.

Causes and Effects of Liver Injury

The liver is vulnerable to injury by many agents. Histologically, liver injury may be manifested by necrosis of liver cells, by accumulation of fat within the liver cell cytoplasm, or by a combination of the two. Some injurious agents primarily cause cell necrosis, whereas others chiefly induce fatty change in liver cells.

The effect of hepatic injury depends on the extent of damage induced by the injurious agent. If liver injury is mild, the liver cells will completely recover, restoring liver function to normal. Fortunately, this is the usual outcome. If the injury is extremely severe, large amounts of liver tissue are completely destroyed, and not enough liver may remain to sustain life. If the patient does survive, healing of the severe injury may be associated with severe scarring (postnecrotic scarring), and liver function may never return to normal. Multiple episodes of relatively mild liver injury may have a cumulative effect, leading to scarring and permanent impairment of liver function. Similarly, any chronic or progressive injury may cause scarring and impairment of function.

Liver cell injury caused by drugs, chemicals, alcohol, or toxins can produce fatty change in liver cells rather than necrosis. FIGURE 21-5 diagrams the general causes and possible effects of various degrees of liver injury.

Clinically, the most common types of liver disease characterized by injury to liver cells are viral hepatitis, and liver cell injury associated with consuming excessive amounts of alcoholic beverages, which is called alcoholic liver disease. Chronic liver cell injury from any cause may in turn be followed by diffuse scarring throughout the liver, which is called cirrhosis of the liver.

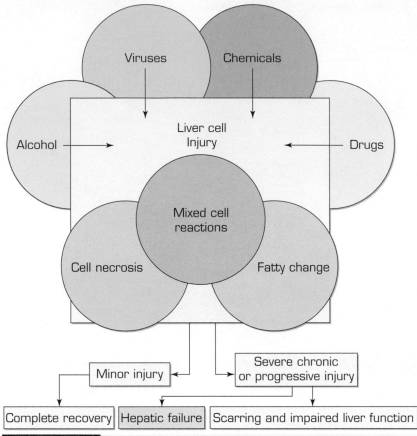

FIGURE 21-5 Summary of causes and effects of liver injury. Many agents can cause injury to liver cells, manifested either as fatty change, necrosis, or a combination of both. Mild injury is followed by complete recovery. Severe, chronic, or progressive injury may lead to hepatic failure or diffuse scarring with impaired hepatic function.

Viral Hepatitis

Within recent years, much new information has become available about the hepatitis viruses. The term viral hepatitis applies to several clinically similar infections. Two of these diseases, hepatitis *A* (formerly called infectious hepatitis) and hepatitis B (formerly called serum hepatitis), have been recognized as separate diseases since the early 1940s. Subsequently, a third type of viral hepatitis, originally designated non-A, non-B hepatitis, and later called hepatitis C, was recognized as a separate entity. These three types account for most cases of viral hepatitis. Two additional types of viral hepatitis also have been identified. One type, called hepatitis D or delta hepatitis, occurs in persons already infected with the hepatitis B virus. Another type, called hepatitis E, is found primarily in third world countries and is infrequently encountered in North America.

CLINICAL MANIFESTATIONS AND COURSE

Hepatitis
Inflammation of the liver.

Viral **hepatitis** is a type of liver injury, and the comments regarding the course and outcome of any liver injury also apply to viral hepatitis. All of the hepatitis viruses produce similar histologic changes in the liver that are characterized by diffuse inflammation throughout the liver lobules associated with liver cell swelling and necrosis of individual liver cells, as illustrated in FIGURE 21-6. The clinical manifestations of

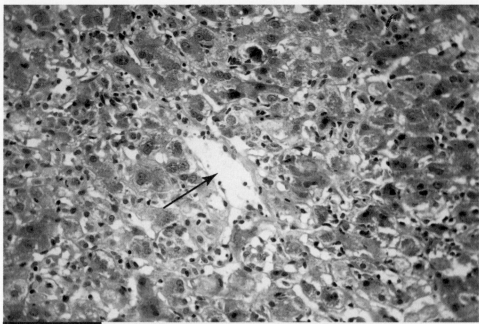

FIGURE 21-6 Acute viral hepatitis. Cords of liver cells extending from central vein (*arrow*) have lost their orderly arrangement and appear disrupted by swelling of liver cells, necrosis of individual cells, and scattered aggregates of inflammatory cells throughout the liver lobules (original magnification × 100).

viral hepatitis are quite variable and correlate with the degree of liver cell injury and associated inflammation. Some affected subjects experience loss of appetite, feel ill, become jaundiced, and laboratory tests are abnormal. Others become ill, and their laboratory tests are abnormal, but they never become jaundiced. This condition is called anicteric hepatitis (*ana* = without + *icterus* = jaundice). Still, others have few symptoms and do not seek medical attention, but laboratory tests reveal liver injury. Their infection, which could easily escape detection, is sometimes called subclinical hepatitis. Despite the absence of symptoms, these subjects can transmit the infection to others.

The outcome of viral hepatitis depends primarily on which virus caused the infection. Most cases of hepatitis caused by the hepatitis A virus (HAV) are quite mild, and patients recover completely without complications. An unfavorable outcome occurs in only a very small percentage of cases. In contrast, persons infected with hepatitis B virus (HBV) or the hepatitis C virus (HCV) may become chronic carriers of the virus and develop chronic progressive hepatitis that eventually leads to cirrhosis and liver failure. TABLE 21-1 summarizes the salient features of the three major types of viral hepatitis.

HEPATITIS A

Hepatitis A virus (HAV) is an RNA-containing virus measuring 27 nm (1 nanometer, abbreviated nm, equals 1 billionth of a meter). Hepatitis A has a relatively short incubation period that varies from 2 to 6 weeks. The virus is excreted in oropharyngeal (nose and throat) secretions and in the stools during the late-incubation period and for about 2 weeks after the onset of symptoms. Transmission is by direct person-to-person contact or by fecal contamination of food or water. Food- or water-borne infections frequently occur in epidemics. One epidemic of 107 cases, which occurred in a large city, was traced to a food-service employee who had

TABLE 21-1

Comparison of three major types of viral hepatitis

	Hepatitis A	Hepatitis B	Hepatitis C
Type of virus	RNA	DNA	RNA
Incubation period	2–6 weeks	6 weeks to 4 months	3–12 weeks
Method of transmission	Fecal–oral contaminated food or water	Blood or body fluids	Blood or body fluids
Antigen–antibody test results	Anti-HAV (confers immunity)	Infected persons are HBsAg positive and lack anti-HBs	HCV RNA in blood indicates virus in blood and active infection
		Immune persons lack HBsAg and have anti-HBs	Anti-HCV denotes infection (does not confer immunity)
Complications	No carriers or chronic liver disease	10% become chronic carriers and may develop chronic liver disease	75% become carriers and many develop chronic liver disease
Prevention of disease after exposure	Gamma globulin	Hepatitis B immune globulin	None available
Immunization available	Yes	Yes	No

contracted hepatitis A from her grandson and contaminated the food that she was preparing. In another epidemic, 240 persons developed hepatitis from eating raw oysters grown in virus-contaminated water.

The infection is self-limited, and there are no chronic carriers of the virus. Antibody to hepatitis A virus, which appears in the blood after recovery, provides immunity against hepatitis A virus but not against other hepatitis viruses. Hepatitis A is a common infection in the United States, and almost half the adult population has antibodies against the virus. If a susceptible person is exposed to hepatitis A, gamma globulin provides protection if administered within 14 days of exposure. An inactivated hepatitis A vaccine is available. It is recommended for immunizing persons who are at relatively high risk of becoming infected, such as healthcare workers who have frequent contact with infected persons and persons traveling in foreign countries where there is a high incidence of hepatitis A in the population. Currently, many physicians also recommend routine immunization of children living in states or communities where there is a high incidence of hepatitis A, which not only prevents childhood infections but also reduces the spread of hepatitis A from infected children to other members of the community.

HEPATITIS B

Hepatitis B virus (HBV) is a DNA-containing virus measuring 42 nm, which is somewhat larger than the hepatitis A virus. It is composed of an inner core and an outer

A   B

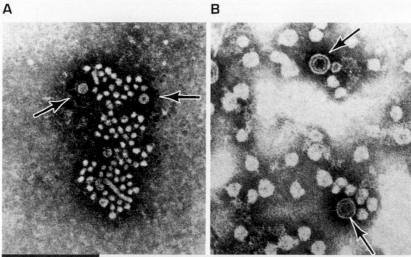

FIGURE 21-7 Electron photomicrographs of complete virus particles (*arrows*) and excess surface antigen in blood of patient with hepatitis B. **A**, original magnification × 130,000. **B**, Original magnification × 290,000 (from Dane, D. S., Cameron, C. H., and Briggs, M. 1970. Virus-like particles in serum of patients with Australia-antigen-associated hepatitis. *Lancet* 1:695–8. Used by permission).

coat. The core consists of a double strand of DNA and an enzyme (DNA polymerase) enclosed within a protein shell. The DNA strand and its inner protein shell together are called the **hepatitis B core antigen (HBcAg)**. The outer coat composed of lipid and protein is called the **hepatitis B surface antigen (HBsAg)**. The core antigen and surface antigen together form the complete virus particle, which is often called the Dane particle after the pathologist who first described it.

In contrast to hepatitis A, hepatitis B has a much longer incubation period, which varies from 6 weeks to 4 months. When an individual becomes infected, the virus invades the liver and multiplies within the hepatic cells. The core of the virus is produced in the nucleus, and the surface antigen is produced in the cytoplasm. For some unexplained reason, much more surface antigen is produced within the infected cells than is necessary to coat the virus particles, and the large excess is released into the bloodstream, where it can be detected by special laboratory tests (FIGURE 21-7). Such blood is called surface-antigen (HBsAg) positive. Although the laboratory tests detect only the surface antigen, HBsAg-positive blood is infectious because it also contains complete virus particles (FIGURE 21-7).

In the course of an infection, the surface antigen first appears during the incubation period and can be detected during the first few weeks of the infection. Normally, it does not persist in the blood for more than 2 or 3 weeks. Then antibodies begin to appear, both to the core of the virus (anti-HBc) and to the surface antigen (anti-HBs). Various other antigens and antibodies also appear in the blood of persons with HBV infection. One is a soluble protein called the e antigen (HBeAg), which appears along with HBsAg. The corresponding antibody, anti-HBe, often appears along with anti-HBs during recovery (FIGURE 21-8). Many people possess antibodies against the virus as a result of prior infection or as a result of immunization against the virus.

Most infected individuals eliminate the virus from the bloodstream in a few weeks and recover completely, but about 10% become chronic carriers of the virus. Some of the carriers develop chronic hepatitis, which causes progressive liver damage. About 1% of the US population are asymptomatic chronic carriers of the virus, and

Hepatitis B core antigen
The antigen contained in the core of the hepatitis B virus.

Hepatitis B surface antigen
The coating of the hepatitis B virus that is also found in great excess in the blood of infected patients.

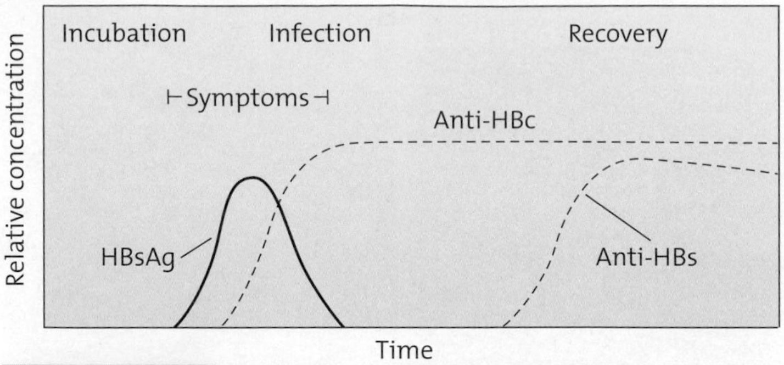

FIGURE 21-8 Acute HBV infection and recovery, illustrating serial changes of major antigens and antibodies used to aid in the diagnosis of HBV infection and monitor its course. Serial changes in HBeAg and anti-HBe are not shown. HBeAg rises along with HBsAg during active infection, and anti-HBe appears along with anti-HBc during recovery.

their blood is infectious. The carrier rate is much higher among drug abusers and male homosexuals. In the Vietnamese and some other population groups, the carrier rate may approach 20%.

Worldwide, more than 350 million people are infected with the hepatitis B virus, and about one million people each year die of the complications of the disease. Some antiviral drugs are available that can suppress viral multiplication and slow disease progression in persons who have active hepatitis and circulating virus in their bloodstream.

Hepatitis B virus is not excreted in the stool. Consequently, transmission does not occur by means of contaminated food or water. Most HBV infections result from contact with the blood or secretions of HBsAg-positive individuals. Drug abusers may transmit the virus by sharing needles and syringes. Physicians, dentists, nurses, laboratory personnel, and other health professionals may become infected from contact with blood of HBsAg-positive patients. Contaminated dental instruments or instruments used for ear piercing also may transmit HBV. Because HBV is also present in saliva, vaginal secretions, and seminal fluid, infection may also be spread by close family contacts or sexual contacts. An HBsAg-positive mother may transmit the virus to her newborn infant, who usually acquires the infection from maternal blood and vaginal secretions at the time of delivery. Unfortunately, infected infants are often unable to eliminate the virus and frequently become chronic carriers of the virus. Formerly, many cases followed blood transfusions; however, this is no longer true because all blood collected for transfusion is now tested routinely for HBsAg, and antigen-positive blood is not used for transfusion.

Hepatitis B immune globulin provides some protection if administered promptly after exposure to the virus and is given routinely to newborn infants born to HBsAg-positive mothers. A vaccine is available to immunize against HBV. The vaccine induces the formation of anti-HBs and provides a high degree of immunity against HBV infection. Universal vaccination is recommended, and HBV vaccination is included in vaccination schedules recommended for infants and children.

HEPATITIS C

The hepatitis C virus is an 80-nm RNA virus that is transmitted by infected blood and body fluids, as is HBV. There are six serologic types, which differ in their response to treatment. Type 1 is the most common type and, unfortunately, is the type most resistant to treatment. In many ways, HCV infection is an even more serious problem than HBV infection for several reasons:

1. HCV is a frequent cause of chronic hepatitis in the United States, accounting for almost half of the reported cases.
2. Most HCV-infected persons are unable to eliminate the virus and become chronic carriers. About 1 to 2% of the population are chronic carriers of the virus, and their blood and body fluids are infectious. Many of the chronic carriers will develop chronic hepatitis, which in turn is followed by cirrhosis in many of the infected persons.
3. There are no agents like gamma globulin that can protect an uninfected person who has been exposed to the virus, as by an accidental needle stick when drawing blood from an infected person.
4. There is no available immunizing agent that can be used to establish an active immunity against the virus, and none is likely to be developed in the foreseeable future.

HCV-infected persons may experience symptoms of hepatitis, as previously described, but many infected persons have few symptoms of infections, and some may not even know that they have become infected. Infected persons develop antibodies against HCV, but antibodies may not appear for several months after the infection. Viral RNA, a measure of virus particles in the circulation, is an indication of active infection, and the amount of viral RNA can be measured in the blood of infected persons to monitor the course of the infection.

In the past, many HCV infections followed blood transfusion of HCV-infected blood or use of blood products such as antihemophilic globulin prepared from infected blood. However, in 1992, a screening test to identify anti-HCV antibody became available as a diagnostic test for HCV infection. As soon as the test became available, it was used routinely by blood banks as a screening test. HCV-antibody–positive blood could be identified and not be used for transfusion. As a result, infections acquired by blood transfusion or use of blood products are no longer a problem.

Currently, most HCV infections are acquired from infected blood or body fluids in much the same ways that HBV and HIV infections are acquired. The Centers for Disease Control and Prevention, which monitors HBV infections, estimates that about 60% of HCV infections occur in injection drug users who share virus-contaminated needles. In 20% of cases, the infection was acquired by sexual contact, although HCV is not as easily transmitted by sexual practices as is HBV. About 10% of cases result from other types of blood and body fluid exposures, such as household contacts, infections associated with hemodialysis treatment, occupational exposures of healthcare workers, and virus transmission from mother to infant during childbirth. In another 10% of cases, the source of infection could not be determined.

Many people may have become infected by virus-contaminated blood or blood products before routine HCV blood testing procedures were available, but have no symptoms. Nevertheless, they are at risk of developing chronic hepatitis and its associated complications. Other persons in the past may have engaged in practices that put them at risk of becoming infected, such as injecting drugs, but they were unaware of the risks at the time. Most infected individuals cannot rid themselves of the virus and the HCV infection becomes chronic, although they may not have symptoms of active infection. Although an unfavorable outcome occurs in only a small percentage of infected persons, this is still a large number of people at risk of serious liver disease because HCV infection is so prevalent. Liver failure resulting from severe chronic liver disease caused by HCV is now the main indication for liver transplantation, and usually the virus also infects the transplanted liver just as it infected and destroyed the person's own liver.

Because of the serious late complications that can occur in some infected persons, the Centers for Disease Control and Prevention recommends that the following groups of high-risk individuals be tested for possible asymptomatic HCV infection:

1. Persons who have ever injected illegal drugs, even persons who injected drugs only once or a few times and do not consider themselves drug users.
2. Persons who received antihemophilic globulin or other clotting factor concentrates before 1987, when the manufacturing processes used were not adequate to eliminate the virus from the concentrates.
3. Persons who received blood transfusions before 1992, when screening blood for HCV was not available, or who had other contacts with blood before 1992, such as hemodialysis or organ transplants.
4. Health care personnel who had been exposed to blood or body fluids, as might have occurred following an accidental needle stick while drawing blood.
5. Children born to HCV-infected mothers because about 5% of infants born to infected mothers become infected.

Because of the potential late complications of HCV infection, all HCV-positive persons should be referred for further medical evaluation. Those who have chronic hepatitis, as demonstrated by abnormal liver function tests, viral RNA in their blood, and a liver biopsy demonstrating chronic inflammation in the liver, should be treated by drugs that inhibit viral multiplication. The preferred treatment is an antiviral compound called ribavirin combined with interferon or a modification of interferon (called pegylated interferon) that has a more prolonged antiviral action and appears to be more effective than interferon. Fortunately, treatment has improved recently with the addition of a protease inhibitor drug (boceprevir), which is given along with ribavirin and interferon. This new combination has improved greatly the response to treatment of type 1 HCV. It is hoped that other new drugs will follow to continue the progress being made against this disease.

HEPATITIS D (DELTA HEPATITIS)

This type of hepatitis is caused by a small defective RNA virus that can only infect persons who are already infected with the hepatitis B virus, either chronic carriers of HBV or those with an acute HBV infection. The delta virus is always associated with an HBV infection because the virus is unable to produce its own outer viral coat and can reproduce itself only by coating itself with HBsAg produced by HBV, thereby forming complete but hybrid virus particles composed of a delta virus core and an HBsAg outer layer. Delta hepatitis is less common than other types of viral hepatitis, and most cases in the United States are found among intravenous drug abusers who became infected by sharing contaminated needles.

HEPATITIS E

Hepatitis E is caused by an RNA virus that is transmitted by the fecal–oral route, like the hepatitis A virus; most of the cases are in third world countries, where outbreaks have been traced to contaminated water supplies. Only a few cases have been reported in North America, and the infected persons acquired the disease while traveling outside the United States. A diagnostic test has been developed to detect anti-HEV antibodies as an indication of HEV infection. Gamma globulin does not provide protection against HEV infection because gamma globulin preparations do not contain anti-HEV antibodies.

OTHER HEPATITIS VIRUSES

Other viruses may, at times, cause a mild hepatitis. These include the **Epstein-Barr (EB) virus,** which causes infectious mononucleosis (see the hematopoietic and lymphatic systems), and another somewhat similar virus called **cytomegalovirus,** which may also cause an infection resembling infectious mononucleosis.

HEPATITIS AMONG MALE HOMOSEXUALS

All types of viral hepatitis are common in male homosexuals and are transmitted by sexual contact. The hepatitis A virus is excreted in the stool of infected subjects and may also contaminate the anal–genital skin. Consequently, the virus is readily transmitted by anal–oral and oral–genital sexual activity. Hepatitis B virus, which is present in the blood and secretions of infected individuals, is transmitted among male homosexuals primarily by anal intercourse, and hepatitis C also may be transmitted in this way. Minor abrasions of the anal, rectal, and genital mucosa of sexual partners permits transfer of virus-infected blood and body fluids between partners.

The following case illustrates the usual clinical and laboratory features of viral hepatitis as a result of HBV infection:

CASE 21-1

A 22-year-old man was seen by a physician because of upper abdominal discomfort, nausea, loss of appetite, and jaundice. The patient had noted that his urine had become darker in color. He was homosexual and stated that a sexual partner had suffered a similar illness recently. Physical examination revealed a jaundiced young man with a slightly enlarged, tender liver. There were no findings to suggest chronic liver disease. Laboratory studies revealed a slight elevation of bilirubin and abnormalities of several liver function tests. Tests for hepatitis B surface antigen were positive. The patient was considered to have hepatitis B, probably contracted through sexual activities with a partner who either had active hepatitis or was a chronic carrier of the virus. The patient made an uneventful recovery. Hepatitis B surface antigen was no longer detected in the blood 3 weeks later, and antibody to hepatitis B surface antigen appeared during convalescence.

Fatty Liver

The liver performs many important functions related to the metabolism of food, including an important role in fat metabolism, and conditions that disturb liver functions can lead to accumulation of fat in liver cells. Fatty liver is a special type of liver injury (FIGURE 21-9). A number of injurious agents are capable of disrupting the metabolic processes within the liver cell, leading to an accumulation of fat globules within the liver cell cytoplasm (FIGURE 21-10). Diffuse fatty change within the liver can be demonstrated by ultrasound examination, by computed tomography (CT) scans, or by magnetic resonance imaging (MRI). Liver biopsy can determine whether there is any liver cell damage associated with the fatty change. In the United States, the most common cause of fatty liver is excessive alcohol ingestion, but a number of volatile solvents, drugs, chemicals, and some poisons can cause fat accumulation in liver cells. Obese persons and many persons with diabetes also accumulate excess fat in the liver unrelated to excess alcohol consumption. Usually, the affected persons

Epstein-Barr virus
A virus that causes infectious mononucleosis.

Cytomegalovirus
(sī-tō-meg′u-lō-vī-rus) One of the herpes viruses. Causes an infectious mononucleosislike syndrome in adults; may cause congenital malformation in fetus.

A

B

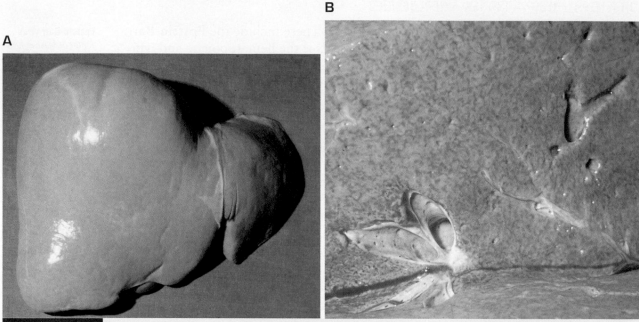

FIGURE 21-9 Fatty liver. **A**, The liver appears yellow because of a large amount of fat within liver cells, but otherwise appears normal. **B**, A section of liver that appears normal except for the yellow color caused by the fat.

Nonalcoholic fatty liver

Fatty liver without significant inflammation or scarring within the liver, which usually occurs in insulin-resistant obese subjects with lipid abnormalities.

Nonalcoholic steatohepatitis

Fat-associated liver damage associated with inflammation and scarring similar to the features seen in alcohol-related liver disease.

have a higher than normal blood glucose or diabetes caused by obesity, which causes the body cells to become less responsive to insulin. The fatty change in the liver cells is called **nonalcoholic fatty liver** to distinguish it from the fatty liver of alcoholic subjects. Usually, heavy fat infiltration impairs liver function and may cause mild liver injury, but the liver cell damage usually is reversible. However, prolonged and severe fatty infiltration can cause significant liver cell damage associated with inflammation and scarring similar to the liver cell damage encountered in alcoholic subjects. This condition is called **nonalcoholic steatohepatitis** (*steatos* = fat), which can progress to cirrhosis

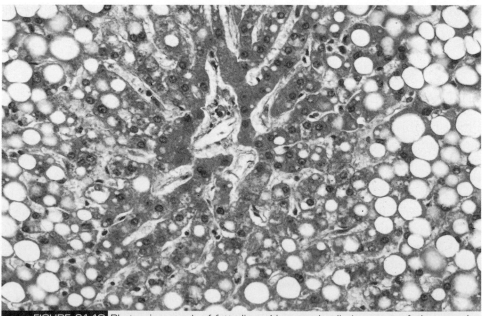

FIGURE 21-10 Photomicrograph of fatty liver. Liver cord cells in center of photograph appear relatively normal. Other cells contain large fat globules that appear as clear spherical vacuoles within liver cells in photograph (original magnification × 100).

and eventually to liver failure, like the similar condition that occurs in alcoholic liver disease. Unfortunately, nonalcoholic steatohepatitis and its complications are becoming more frequent because of the increasing obesity and diabetes in our population.

Fatty liver is also a characteristic feature of a condition called Reye's syndrome, which is described later in this chapter.

ALCOHOLIC LIVER DISEASE

The term alcoholic liver disease refers to a group of structural and functional changes in the liver resulting from excessive alcohol consumption. The severity of the liver injury and its rate of progression are determined not only by how much alcohol is consumed, but also how long the person has been drinking excessively.

It is convenient to subdivide alcoholic liver disease into three stages of progressively increasing severity: (1) alcoholic fatty liver, (2) alcoholic hepatitis, and (3) alcoholic cirrhosis.

Alcoholic Fatty Liver

This is the mildest form of alcoholic liver disease. If the subject stops drinking, the liver function gradually returns to normal, and the fat globules in the liver cells disappear as the liver cells process the accumulated fat.

Alcoholic Hepatitis

This is the next stage in the progressive liver injury caused by alcohol. Heavy alcohol intake not only promotes fatty change in liver cells, but causes other degenerative changes as well and may actually induce liver cell necrosis. A rather characteristic feature of severe alcoholic liver injury is the accumulation of irregularly shaped, pink deposits within the cytoplasm of the liver cells. These structures, which are called **Mallory bodies** or alcoholic hyalin, indicate that the cell has been irreparably damaged. Neutrophilic leukocytes also accumulate in response to the liver cell necrosis, and the injury is followed by progressive fibrous scarring throughout the liver. The term alcoholic hepatitis is used to refer to this type of liver injury, which is characterized not only by fatty change, but also by liver cell degeneration with Mallory bodies and leukocyte infiltration (FIGURE 21-11).

Mallory body
An irregular red-staining structure in the cytoplasm of injured liver cells, usually resulting from alcohol-induced liver injury.

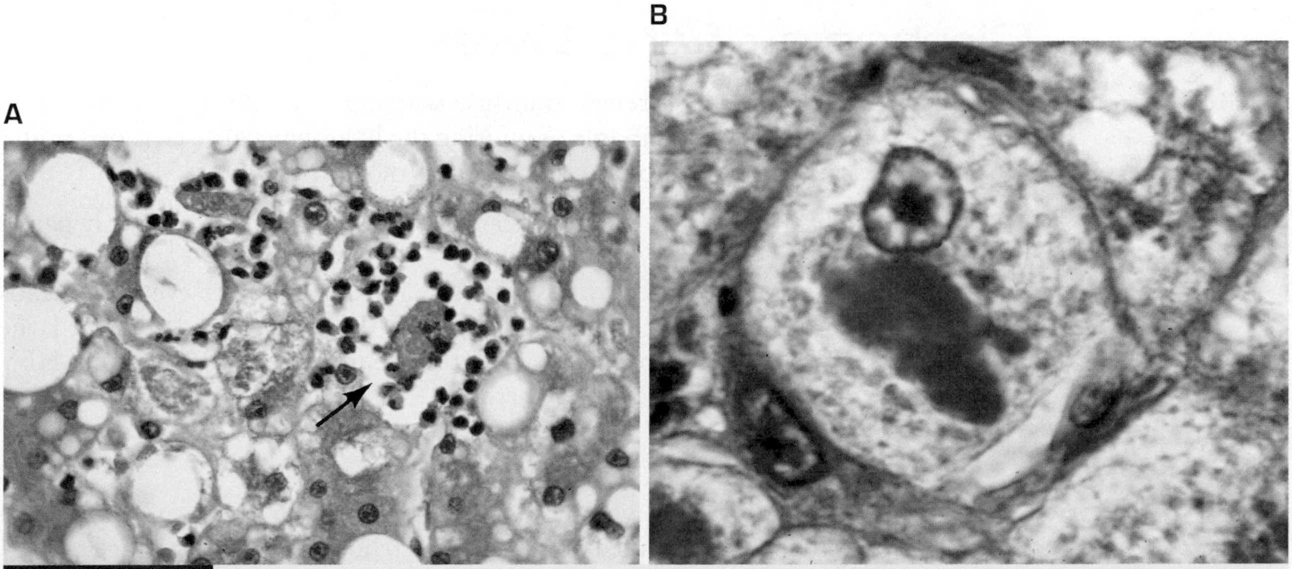

FIGURE 21-11 A photomicrograph illustrating hepatic cellular structure in alcoholic hepatitis. **A**, Many cells contain fat vacuoles. Others are swollen and contain Mallory bodies. One necrotic cell (*arrow*) is surrounded by cluster of neutrophils (original magnification × 400). **B**, A high-magnification photomicrograph of Mallory body in swollen liver cell (original magnification × 1,000).

In this case, the term "hepatitis" refers to the inflammatory cell infiltration secondary to liver cell necrosis and does not imply an infection, as in viral hepatitis.

Alcoholic Cirrhosis

This is the third and most advanced stage of alcoholic liver injury. It is characterized by diffuse scarring throughout the liver, which disturbs liver function and also impedes blood flow through the liver. Cirrhosis and its complications are described in the following section. In the United States, a large number of cases of cirrhosis are related to heavy alcohol ingestion and follow repeated episodes of alcoholic hepatitis. It is generally considered that a person must drink more than 1 pint of whiskey daily, or its equivalent in other alcoholic beverages, for 10 to 15 years in order to develop alcoholic cirrhosis. However, there is considerable individual variation in susceptibility to alcoholic liver injury. Occasionally, the disease develops more rapidly, and it has been seen in teenagers and young adults.

The following clinical summary illustrates the clinical features seen in a young man who died of severe alcoholic liver disease.

CASE 21-2

A 33-year-old man had been drinking heavily for many years and was in the habit of consuming about 1 qt. of liquor per day. Recently, he had noticed weakness and loss of appetite. The physical examination revealed that he was slightly jaundiced. His liver was enlarged, and there was moderate ascites. Laboratory studies revealed a reduced serum albumin and a moderate elevation of serum bilirubin.

Other tests of liver function were abnormal. The clinical impression was severe alcoholic liver disease. Despite intensive therapy, the patient's condition did not improve, and he eventually died of chronic liver failure. The autopsy revealed fatty change in liver cells and active alcoholic hepatitis with many Mallory bodies in the cytoplasm of the liver cells and the early stages of cirrhosis.

Cirrhosis of the Liver

Cirrhosis of the liver
(si-rō'sis)
A disease characterized by diffuse intrahepatic scarring and liver cell degeneration.

The term **cirrhosis of the liver** refers to diffuse scarring of the liver from any cause (FIGURE 21-12). Any substance capable of injuring the liver may cause cirrhosis under certain conditions. The two most common causes of cirrhosis are

1. Alcoholic liver disease, resulting from repeated episodes of alcoholic hepatitis followed by scarring.
2. Chronic hepatitis caused by HBV or HCV infections, which eventually leads to diffuse liver scarring. In many parts of Asia and Africa, where a large proportion of the population are chronic carriers of HBV, chronic HBV infection is the major cause of cirrhosis.

Less common causes of cirrhosis include

1. An episode of severe liver necrosis, such as after an attack of severe viral hepatitis (sometimes called posthepatitic cirrhosis or postnecrotic cirrhosis).
2. Various other drugs and chemicals that damage liver cells.
3. Various genetic diseases that directly or indirectly lead to liver damage such as hemochromatosis (discussion on the hematopoietic and lymphatic

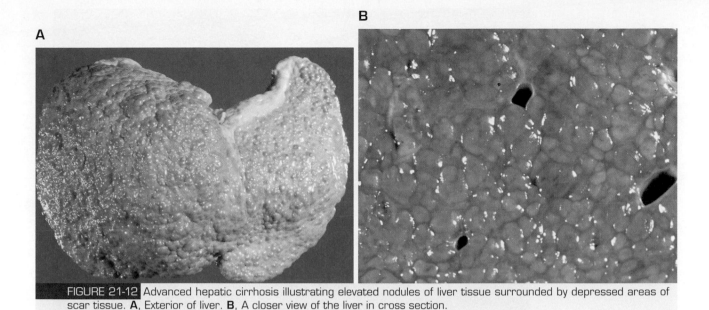

A

B

FIGURE 21-12 Advanced hepatic cirrhosis illustrating elevated nodules of liver tissue surrounded by depressed areas of scar tissue. **A**, Exterior of liver. **B**, A closer view of the liver in cross section.

systems) and alpha₁ antitrypsin deficiency, which also causes some types of pulmonary emphysema (discussion on the respiratory system).

4. Long-standing bile duct obstruction, which causes a special type of cirrhosis called **biliary cirrhosis.**

DERANGEMENTS OF LIVER STRUCTURE AND FUNCTION

In cirrhosis, the liver is converted into a mass of scar tissue containing nodules of degenerating and regenerating liver cells, proliferating bile ducts, and inflammatory cells (FIGURE 21-13). The normal architectural pattern of the liver is completely disorganized, and the intrahepatic branches of the hepatic artery and portal vein are constricted by scar tissue.

The two major functional disturbances in cirrhosis are impaired liver function and portal hypertension.

Impaired Liver Function

As a result of liver cell damage, scarring, and impairment of blood supply to the liver caused by scarring, the number of functioning liver cells is greatly reduced. Eventually, a patient with cirrhosis may die of liver failure. Clinical manifestations commonly found in men with advanced cirrhosis are testicular atrophy, loss of sex drive, and breast hypertrophy. These manifestations result from impaired liver function and appear to be the result of an excess of estrogen. Normally, men produce not only male sex hormone (testosterone), but small amounts of estrogen as well. The estrogen is normally inactivated by the liver and exerts little effect. The cirrhotic liver, however, is unable to accomplish this function efficiently; consequently, estrogen accumulates and produces these associated clinical manifestations.

Portal Hypertension

Normally, the portal vein blood passes through sinusoids into the hepatic veins and then into the inferior vena cava. In cirrhosis, venous return through the portal system is impaired, and the pressure in the portal vein rises because the blood flow is obstructed by scar tissue. The high pressure affects the portal capillaries, and this contributes to

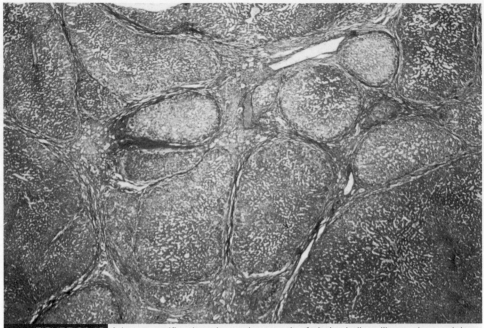

FIGURE 21-13 A low-magnification photomicrograph of cirrhotic liver illustrating nodules of liver cells circumscribed by dense scar tissue (blue-green stain). The normal architectural pattern is lost. The number of functioning liver cells is reduced and replaced by scar tissue, and the scar tissue disrupts blood flow through the liver. Compare with FIGURE 21-2 (original magnification × 25).

excessive leakage of fluid from the capillaries. Eventually, the abdomen becomes distended by fluids that accumulate within the abdominal cavity (ascites) (FIGURE 21-14).

A reduced concentration of albumin in the blood also contributes to ascites because albumin is crucial to maintaining the normal colloid osmotic pressure of the blood, which is the force that tends to hold fluid in the capillaries (discussion on circulatory disturbances). Albumin, which is produced by the liver, is reduced in

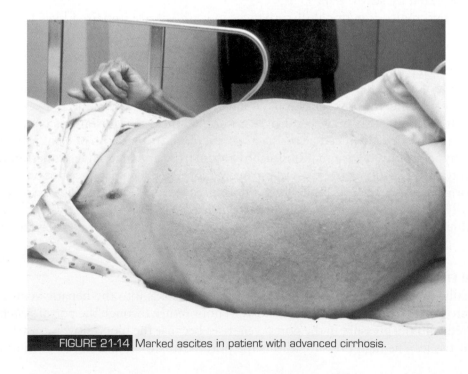

FIGURE 21-14 Marked ascites in patient with advanced cirrhosis.

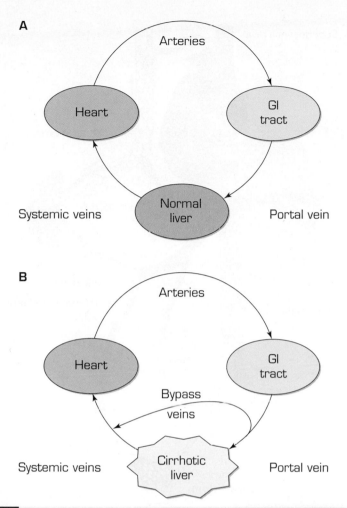

A

Arteries

Heart

GI tract

Normal liver

Systemic veins   Portal vein

B

Arteries

Heart

GI tract

Bypass veins

Cirrhotic liver

Systemic veins   Portal vein

FIGURE 21-15 A comparison of normal blood flow pathways with those in cirrhosis. **A**, Normal flow pattern. The heart pumps blood through the aorta to the gastrointestinal tract from which blood collects in portal vein and flows through hepatic sinusoids into hepatic veins, then into vena cava, and finally, back to heart to be repumped. **B**, The flow pattern in cirrhosis. Blood pumped to gastrointestinal tract is collected in portal vein; however, flow through hepatic sinusoids is interrupted by intrahepatic scarring, and portal vein pressure rises. Bypass channels shunt blood into superior or inferior vena cava in order to return blood to the heart. Bypass veins cannot handle increased blood flow under increased pressure and become dilated.

cirrhosis because the cirrhotic liver is unable to manufacture this protein in sufficient quantities; consequently, the colloid osmotic pressure of the blood is lower than normal, and fluid leaks from the portal capillary bed.

Because of the obstruction of portal venous return, a collateral circulation develops in an attempt to bypass the intrahepatic obstruction and deliver portal blood directly into the systemic circulation. Anastomoses develop where tributaries of portal and systemic veins are closely associated, and they shunt blood from the portal system of veins where the pressure is high into the veins of the systemic circulation where the pressure is much lower (FIGURE 21-15). The communications that are most important clinically are the anastomoses developing between veins around the stomach and spleen, which drain into the portal vein, and the esophageal veins that eventually drain into the superior vena cava by way of the intercostal veins and azygos veins (FIGURE 21-16). The esophageal veins are not equipped to handle the increased blood flow and high pressure. They become dilated and form varicose veins, which are called esophageal varices (plural of varix). Esophageal varices are thin-walled

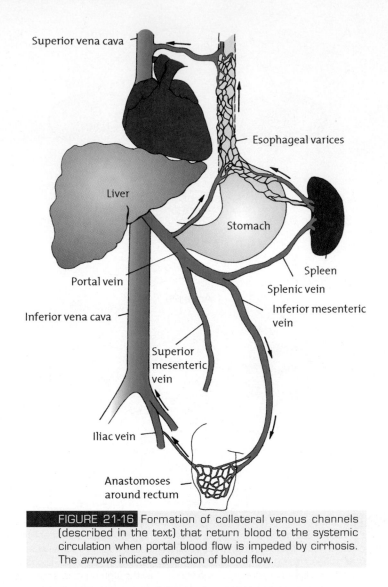

FIGURE 21-16 Formation of collateral venous channels (described in the text) that return blood to the systemic circulation when portal blood flow is impeded by cirrhosis. The *arrows* indicate direction of blood flow.

vessels covered by a thin layer of esophageal epithelium (FIGURE 21-17) and frequently rupture, leading to profuse and sometimes fatal hemorrhage.

Other anastomoses develop between branches of the portal vein and the veins draining the abdominal wall that eventually flow into either the superior or the inferior vena cava. Still, other anastomoses develop around the rectum between branches of the inferior mesenteric veins and the iliac veins, permitting blood to flow through the iliac veins into the inferior vena cava. The extent of the communications between the portal and systemic vein branches in patients with advanced cirrhosis is not always obvious. Special photographic techniques, however, can demonstrate the dilated veins extending in the subcutaneous tissues of the chest and abdominal wall that are shunting blood around the scarred liver (FIGURE 21-18).

The blood flow through the collateral channels reduces the engorgement of the abdominal organs that has resulted from overdistention of the portal circulation. The elevated portal pressure also declines somewhat but does not return to normal.

Hepatic Encephalopathy

Hepatic encephalopathy (*encephalon* = brain + *pathy* = disease) is a deterioration of brain function characterized by impaired consciousness, confusion, disorientation,

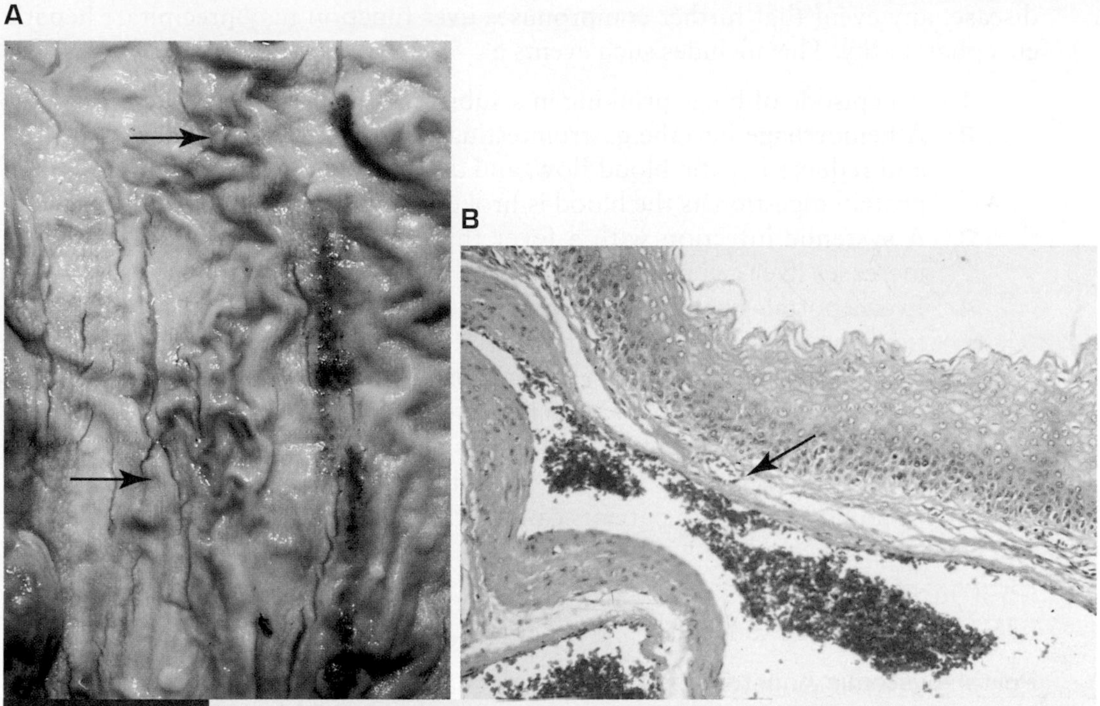

A

B

FIGURE 21-17 **A**, Mucosal surface of esophagus illustrating varices, which appear as tortuous elevations of the mucosa (*arrows*). **B**, A photomicrograph of a varix. The very thin vein wall (*arrow*) is covered only by a thin layer of esophageal squamous epithelium and is very susceptible to rupture (original magnification × 40).

and eventually coma. The condition results from toxic substances that accumulate in the bloodstream and are normally detoxified and excreted by the liver, a task that the cirrhotic liver is unable to accomplish efficiently. Not all of the toxic products have been identified, but many of them are products of protein digestion, especially ammonia, which comes from deamination of amino acids, and other products derived from bacterial decomposition of material in the colon. In a person with advanced liver

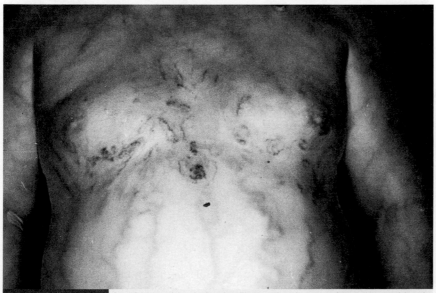

FIGURE 21-18 A subject with cirrhosis, illustrating large subcutaneous blood vessels that are part of the collateral circulation shunting blood around the cirrhotic liver, as demonstrated by an infrared-sensitive film technique.

disease, any event that further compromises liver function may precipitate hepatic encephalopathy. This includes such events as

1. An episode of binge drinking in a subject with alcoholic liver disease.
2. A hemorrhage into the gastrointestinal tract, which drops blood pressure and reduces hepatic blood flow, and also provides more toxic products of protein digestion as the blood is broken down within the intestinal tract.
3. A systemic infection with a fever that reduces hepatic blood flow and increases liver cell metabolism.
4. Even a portal–systemic vein bypass procedure, described in the following sections, which diverts some of the portal vein blood directly into the systemic circulation, may precipitate hepatic encephalopathy in some patients. The bypassed portal vein blood also bypasses whatever remaining detoxification function the diseased liver still possesses and delivers the bypassed blood and its toxins directly into the systemic venous circulation and then to the brain. Many bypass patients can tolerate the diversion, but some cannot.

PROCEDURES TO TREAT MANIFESTATIONS OF CIRRHOSIS

Portal–Systemic Anastomoses

If a patient has developed esophageal varices and is at risk of hemorrhage, it is possible to lower the pressure in the portal system by surgically connecting the splenic vein to the renal vein side-to-side (**splenorenal shunt**) or making a side-to-side connection between the portal vein and inferior vena cava (**portacaval shunt**). A shunt decompresses the portal system by permitting portal blood to flow directly into the inferior vena cava (FIGURE 21-19). Blood no longer is forced to circumvent the scarred

Splenorenal shunt

(splē′no-rē′nul)
Surgically created anastomosis between splenic vein and renal vein, performed to lower portal pressure in the treatment of esophageal varices.

. . . .

Portacaval shunt

(por′tuh-kay′vul)
Surgically created anastomosis between the portal vein and the vena cava, performed to lower portal pressure in the treatment of esophageal varices.

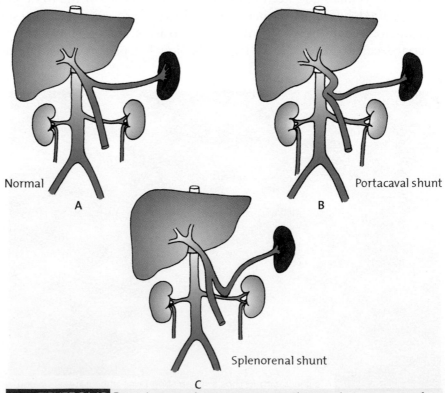

Normal

A

Portacaval shunt

B

Splenorenal shunt

C

FIGURE 21-19 Operative procedures to create portal–systemic anastomoses for treatment of esophageal varices. **A**, Normal anatomic relation. **B**, Portacaval shunt. **C**, Splenorenal shunt.

liver by collateral channels. The dilated esophageal veins decrease in size, and the risk of hemorrhage from varices is greatly reduced.

Intrahepatic Portosystemic Shunts

In selected patients, a nonsurgical portal–systemic communication can be accomplished by means of a procedure called a **transjugular intrahepatic portosystemic shunt,** which is often called simply the TIPS procedure. Under x-ray guidance, a catheter is introduced into the right internal jugular vein and passed retrograde into the inferior vena cava and then into one of the hepatic veins (which drain blood from the liver into the inferior vena cava). Then a guide wire is passed through the catheter, which penetrates the hepatic vein wall and passes through the liver tissue to connect with a large intrahepatic branch of the portal vein. The procedure creates a tract between portal vein and hepatic vein within the liver. The tract is dilated, and a device (called a stent) is inserted to keep the tract open. When the procedure has been completed, much of the portal blood flows directly from a portal vein branch directly into one of the hepatic veins and then into the inferior vena cava, without flowing through the hepatic sinusoids (FIGURE 21-20). As a result, the high pressure in the portal vein falls toward normal. The shunt may also improve the patient's ascites because the lower portal pressure resulting from the shunt lowers the venous pressure in the capillaries draining into the portal system, and less fluid is forced from the capillaries to accumulate in the abdominal cavity.

Transjugular intrahepatic portosystemic shunt
A nonsurgical method used to lower portal vein pressure in a person with cirrhosis by connecting an intrahepatic branch of the portal vein to a hepatic vein branch.

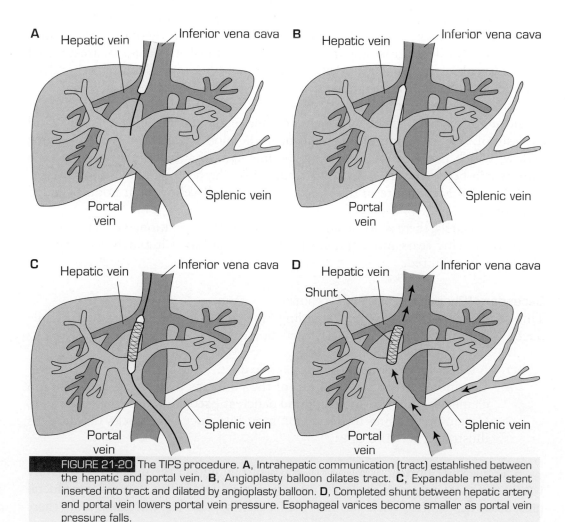

FIGURE 21-20 The TIPS procedure. **A,** Intrahepatic communication (tract) established between the hepatic and portal vein. **B,** Angioplasty balloon dilates tract. **C,** Expandable metal stent inserted into tract and dilated by angioplasty balloon. **D,** Completed shunt between hepatic artery and portal vein lowers portal vein pressure. Esophageal varices become smaller as portal vein pressure falls.

Obliteration of Varices by Sclerosing Solution

Another way to treat varices is to obliterate them by injecting them with a sclerosing solution. The procedure is performed by first visualizing the lining of the esophagus and the location of the varices by means of an esophagoscope. The sclerosing solution is then injected directly into the dilated veins and connective tissue around the vein. The solution, which is very irritating, causes an inflammation in and around the dilated veins, which is followed by scarring and eventual obliteration of the varices. Multiple injections over a period of several months are usually required.

BILIARY CIRRHOSIS

Biliary cirrhosis
Diffuse liver cell damage and scarring with distortion of liver cell structure and function (cirrhosis) caused by obstruction of bile ducts.

In some types of cirrhosis, the primary target of the liver damage is the epithelium of the bile ducts rather than the functional cells (hepatocytes) of the liver lobules. This type of cirrhosis is called **biliary cirrhosis** to distinguish it from the more common type of cirrhosis in which liver cell injury involves primarily the hepatocytes. There are two main types of biliary cirrhosis. The first, which is called primary biliary cirrhosis, is an autoimmune disease that targets the small intrahepatic bile ducts. The second, called secondary biliary cirrhosis or obstructive biliary cirrhosis, results from long-standing obstruction of the large extrahepatic bile ducts.

Primary Biliary Cirrhosis

This is a slowly progressive chronic disease characterized by inflammation and destruction of the small intrahepatic bile ducts. Bile excretion is disrupted and is followed by scarring, which begins in the portal tracts and eventually spreads into the liver lobules. The disease appears to be caused by autoantibodies that are directed against bile duct epithelial cells. Antinuclear autoantibodies and antimitochondrial antibodies can usually be demonstrated in the blood of affected patients.

Because excretion of bile is impeded, products accumulate in the blood that are normally excreted in the bile, including bile pigment (bilirubin), bile salts, and cholesterol. Accumulation of bile pigment in the blood causes the skin to become yellow, which is called jaundice, and the bile salts that accumulate irritate the skin, which becomes very itchy. As a result of the high blood cholesterol, masses of cholesterol accumulate in the skin and form small yellow skin nodules called xanthomas.

Unfortunately, there is no effective treatment for this condition, which progresses slowly over many years and eventually leads to liver failure. Ultimately, a liver transplant may be required.

Secondary (Obstructive) Biliary Cirrhosis

This condition is caused by long-standing blockage of the large extrahepatic bile ducts. Common causes of bile duct obstruction are

1. A gallstone blocking the common bile duct.
2. Carcinoma arising in the head of the pancreas that blocks the common channel transporting both bile and pancreatic secretions into the duodenum.
3. Carcinoma arising from the common bile duct that blocks the duct, as illustrated in FIGURE 21-21.

The bile duct obstruction leads to stasis of bile within the ducts. The pressure within the ducts rises, and the larger ducts become dilated. The elevated intraductal pressure is transmitted back into the smaller intrahepatic bile ducts and from there

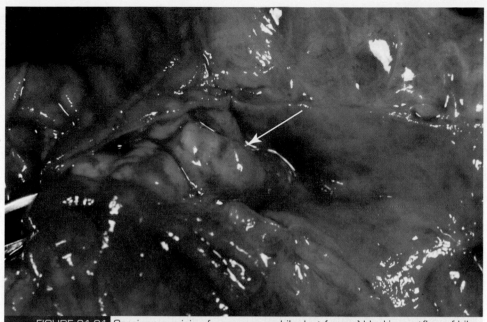

FIGURE 21-21 Carcinoma arising from common bile duct (*arrow*) blocking outflow of bile into duodenum. Common bile duct has been opened and is distended, a result of the increased pressure of the bile within the common duct caused by the duct obstruction.

into the small bile channels (bile canaliculi) that carry bile from the liver lobules into the bile ducts within the portal tracts at the periphery of the lobules. The elevated intraductal pressure and bile stasis damage the intrahepatic bile ducts, which is followed by portal tract inflammation and scarring.

The clinical manifestations of the extrahepatic bile duct obstruction are much the same as those caused by primary biliary cirrhosis. Treatment consists of various surgical procedures to unblock the obstructed bile duct. If this is not possible, some type of surgical procedure is used to bypass the obstruction and reestablish bile flow into the duodenum.

Reye's Syndrome

Reye's syndrome (rhymes with "eye") is a relatively uncommon acute illness that develops in infants and children after a mild viral infection and is characterized by both marked swelling of the brain with neurologic dysfunction and accumulation of fat within the cytoplasm of liver cells associated with impaired liver function. Clinically, the illness manifests as a sudden onset of vomiting and impaired consciousness, which may progress to delirium and coma. Laboratory tests reveal the disturbed liver function that is related to the accumulation of fat in the liver cells, and some patients become jaundiced. In severely affected patients, the mortality rate is about 25%, and some of the survivors may be left with neurologic abnormalities or psychiatric disturbances. There is no specific treatment.

Current evidence suggests that Reye's syndrome is related in some way to acetylsalicylic acid (aspirin) given to treat the fever and discomfort associated with the viral infection. The aspirin may increase the injurious effects of the virus or interact with the virus to cause the liver and brain injury. Therefore, acetaminophen (for example, Tylenol) is recommended to treat symptoms of viral infections in infants and children.

Cholelithiasis

The formation of stones within the gallbladder is called **cholelithiasis** (*chole* = bile + *lith* = stone). Gallstones are very common and are estimated to develop in about 20% of the population. Most gallstones are composed entirely or predominantly of cholesterol, and they form because the bile contains more cholesterol than can be held in solution by the available bile salts and lecithin (FIGURE 21-22).

FACTORS AFFECTING THE SOLUBILITY OF CHOLESTEROL IN BILE

Because cholesterol is a lipid, it is not soluble in an aqueous solution such as bile but is brought into solution by bile salts and lecithin, which aggregate in clusters called **micelles**. In a micelle, the lipid-soluble (hydrophobic) parts of the bile salt molecules are oriented toward the center of the cluster, and the opposite water-soluble (hydrophilic) ends face outward. Cholesterol becomes soluble by dissolving in the hydrophobic center of the micelles, and the cholesterol-containing micelles dissolve in the bile because the peripheral hydrophilic parts of the bile salt molecules are water soluble. Lecithin participates in the formation of the micelles by fitting between the molecules of the bile salts (FIGURE 21-23).

Approximately seven molecules of bile salts interspersed between lecithin molecules in a micelle are required to dissolve one molecule of cholesterol. Consequently, the solubility of cholesterol in bile depends not only on its cholesterol content, but also on its content of bile salts and lecithin, because these substances are needed to hold the cholesterol in solution. Cholesterol remains soluble provided its concentration is not excessive in relationship to the amounts of available bile salts and lecithin. If there is an excess of cholesterol relative to bile salts and lecithin, the bile becomes supersaturated with cholesterol and cholesterol crystals may precipitate. On the other hand, if there is an excess of bile salts and lecithin relative to cholesterol, more cholesterol can dissolve in the bile. These relationships can be conceptualized by a board on a fulcrum, one end of the board being weighted by cholesterol and

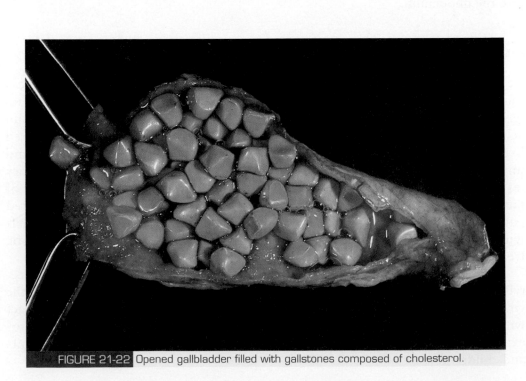

FIGURE 21-22 Opened gallbladder filled with gallstones composed of cholesterol.

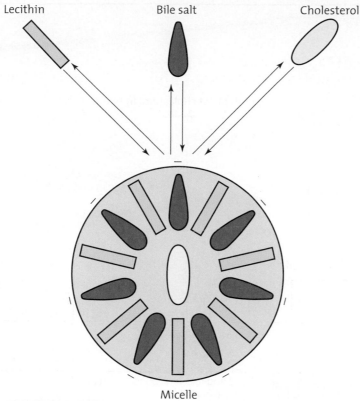

Lecithin   Bile salt   Cholesterol

Micelle

FIGURE 21-23 The manner in which cholesterol dissolves in micelles composed of bile salts and lecithin. If the bile salt concentration is insufficient relative to that of cholesterol, cholesterol will precipitate and form gallstones.

the other end by bile salts and lecithin. Variations in the "weight" on either end of the board cause corresponding changes in the solubility of the cholesterol in the bile (FIGURE 21-24).

Whenever bile contains a relative excess of cholesterol, it becomes supersaturated with cholesterol, and under proper conditions, the cholesterol may precipitate to form the beginnings of gallstones. This situation may arise because of an increased excretion of cholesterol in the bile, a reduced excretion of bile salts and lecithin, or a combination of both factors. As long as the bile remains supersaturated, cholesterol crystals continue to accumulate around those that have already precipitated, and the gallstones slowly increase in size. Eventually, the gallbladder may become filled with gallstones, the end stage of a process that began several years earlier.

Some people are known to have an increased risk of forming gallstones. The incidence of gallstones is

1. Higher in women than in men.
2. Higher in women who have borne several children than in childless women.
3. Twice as high in women who use contraceptive pills as in women who use other types of contraception.
4. Higher in obese women than in women of normal weight.

The incidence of gallstones is higher in these groups because their bile is more highly saturated with cholesterol. The incidence is higher in women than in men because estrogen promotes increased excretion of cholesterol in the bile while decreasing excretion of bile salts. The correlation of gallstones with multiple pregnancies

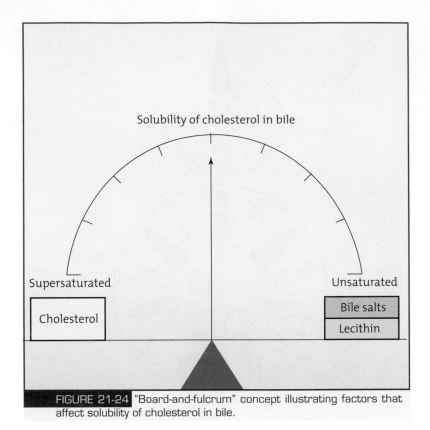

FIGURE 21-24 "Board-and-fulcrum" concept illustrating factors that affect solubility of cholesterol in bile.

is related to the high estrogen levels associated with pregnancy. (Estrogen levels are much higher in pregnancy than in the nonpregnant state because large amounts of estrogen are produced by the placenta.) Contraceptive pills predispose to cholelithiasis because they contain synthetic estrogens that, like natural estrogens, increase the saturation of gallbladder bile. Obesity predisposes to gallstones because extremely overweight persons have a higher blood cholesterol and excrete more cholesterol in their bile than do persons of normal weight.

Less commonly, gallstones form as a result of infection of the gallbladder. Infection predisposes to gallstones by reducing the solubility of cholesterol and other constituents in the bile.

COMPLICATIONS OF GALLSTONES

Gallstones that remain in the gallbladder do not cause symptoms. Unfortunately, gallstones are sometimes extruded into the cystic duct or common bile duct when the gallbladder contracts after a fatty meal, and they may become impacted within the biliary ducts. This event causes severe abdominal pain called **biliary colic**. The pain results from spasm of the smooth muscle in the ducts combined with forceful contractions of the gallbladder that attempt to propel the stone through the ducts. Sometimes a stone can be passed through the ducts into the duodenum, but often it becomes impacted. If the stone lodges in the cystic duct, bile can neither enter nor leave the gallbladder, but flow of bile from the liver into the duodenum is not disturbed even though storage of bile in the gallbladder is no longer possible. If the gallbladder is the site of a chronic infection, the impaction of the stone may precipitate a flare-up of the infection in the gallbladder called **cholecystitis** (FIGURE 21-25). If there is no underlying gallbladder infection, the bile trapped within the gallbladder by the impacted stone is gradually absorbed into the bloodstream, and eventually the contents

Biliary colic
Abdominal pain that results when a gallstone enters the biliary duct system.

Cholecystitis
(ko'lē-sis-tī'-tis)
An inflammation of the gallbladder.

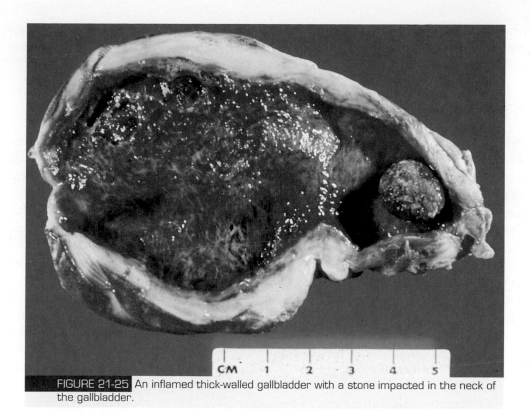

FIGURE 21-25 An inflamed thick-walled gallbladder with a stone impacted in the neck of the gallbladder.

of the gallbladder consist only of mucus that has been secreted by the epithelial cells lining the gallbladder.

If the stone blocks the common duct, bile can no longer be excreted into the duodenum, and it accumulates in the bloodstream. This condition is called obstructive jaundice.

TREATMENT OF GALLSTONES

The standard treatment of gallstones producing symptoms is surgical removal of the diseased gallbladder. In the past, it was necessary to perform a major surgical operation to remove the gallbladder. Now, most cholecystectomies can be performed by means of a laparoscopic procedure through a very small incision in the abdomen. It is possible, however, to dissolve cholesterol gallstones in some carefully selected patients who want to avoid a surgical procedure. This is accomplished by administering a bile salt (either ursodeoxycholic acid or chenodeoxycholic acid or a combination of both), which decreases the amount of cholesterol excreted in the bile. As the cholesterol content of the bile decreases, the bile becomes more unsaturated with cholesterol, and more cholesterol can be dissolved in the bile. As a result, the cholesterol contained within the gallstones becomes soluble in the unsaturated bile, and the gallstones slowly dissolve. Unfortunately, even if the stones are dissolved successfully, new stones often form within the gallbladder after the treatment is discontinued.

Cholecystitis

Inflammation of the gallbladder is called **cholecystitis** (*chole* = bile + *cyst* = bladder + *itis* = inflammation). It is a relatively common disease. Chronic cholecystitis appears to predispose an individual to develop gallstones. As previously described,

Cholecystitis
(ko'lē-sis-tī'-tis)
An inflammation of the gallbladder.

impaction of a gallstone in the neck of the gallbladder or the cystic duct may precipitate an acute cholecystitis if the gallbladder is the site of a preexisting chronic inflammation.

Tumors of the Liver and Gallbladder

Adenoma
A benign tumor arising from glands.

Primary tumors of the liver and gallbladder are uncommon. Benign hepatic **adenomas** develop occasionally in women taking contraceptive pills, but we do not know why the pills predispose to tumors in some women. Primary carcinoma of the liver is quite rare in the United States and Canada but is a common malignant tumor in Asian and African countries. The current evidence indicates that chronic carriers of the hepatitis B virus (HBV) not only have a relatively high incidence of chronic liver disease, but also carry an increased risk of developing a primary liver carcinoma, suggesting that chronic HBV infection predisposes both to liver injury and to liver cancer. The frequency of primary liver cancer in Asia and Africa is probably related to the high incidence of chronic HBV carriers in these populations. Failure of the body's immune defenses to destroy the infected liver cells and eliminate the virus leads to a smoldering chronic infection that may eventually lead to cirrhosis and predisposes to liver cancer. Patients with chronic HCV infections also are at risk of cirrhosis and liver cancer (FIGURES 21-26 AND 21-27).

In contrast to the infrequency of primary liver cancer in developed countries, the liver is a common site of metastatic carcinoma (FIGURE 21-28). Carcinoma arising in the gastrointestinal tract may spread to the liver, bits of tumor being carried to the liver in the portal venous blood. Tumors from the breast, lung, and other sites also often spread to the liver. The tumor cells are carried in the blood delivered to the liver by the hepatic artery. Sometimes, enlargement of the liver

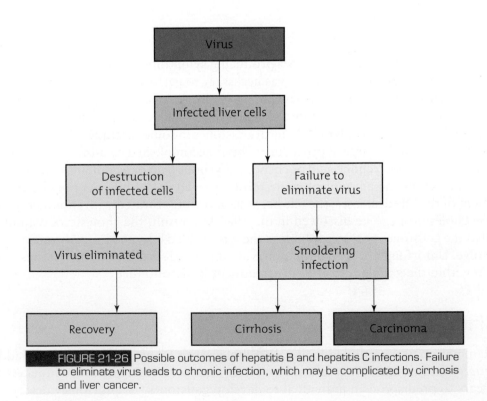

FIGURE 21-26 Possible outcomes of hepatitis B and hepatitis C infections. Failure to eliminate virus leads to chronic infection, which may be complicated by cirrhosis and liver cancer.

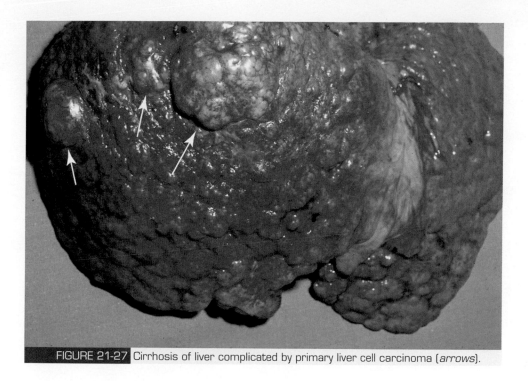

FIGURE 21-27 Cirrhosis of liver complicated by primary liver cell carcinoma (*arrows*).

as the result of metastatic carcinoma may be the first sign of a malignant tumor that originated in some other part of the body. Various diagnostic procedures can be used to identify tumors in the liver. The computed tomographic (CT) scan described in the discussion on general concepts of disease: principles of diagnosis is a very effective means of detecting cysts and tumors in the liver (FIGURE 21-29).

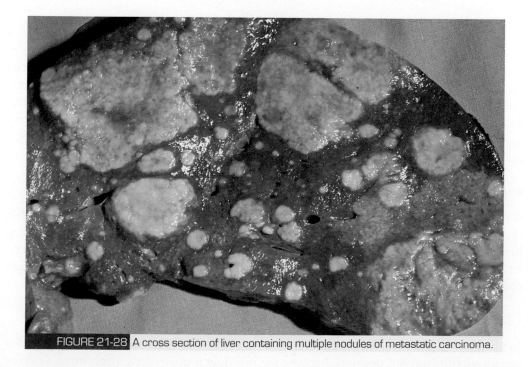

FIGURE 21-28 A cross section of liver containing multiple nodules of metastatic carcinoma.

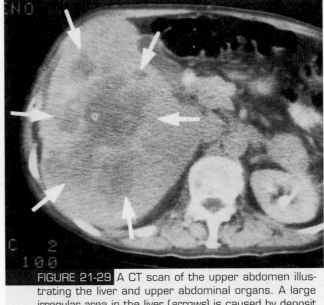

FIGURE 21-29 A CT scan of the upper abdomen illustrating the liver and upper abdominal organs. A large irregular area in the liver (*arrows*) is caused by deposit of metastatic carcinoma.

Jaundice

Jaundice
(jawn′dis)
Yellow color of the skin that results from accumulation of bile pigment within the blood.

Jaundice is a yellow discoloration of the skin and the sclerae (whites of the eyes) that results from accumulation of bile pigment (bilirubin) in the tissues and body fluids. This accumulation can have several causes. Bile pigment is derived from the breakdown of red cells, as described elsewhere in this text. The pigment is extracted from the blood by the liver cells, conjugated, and excreted into the biliary ducts. It is convenient to classify jaundice on the basis of the disturbance responsible for the retention of bile pigment. On this basis, jaundice is classified as hemolytic, hepatocellular, or obstructive. Jaundice can usually be classified correctly on the basis of certain laboratory tests in conjunction with the clinical features.

HEMOLYTIC JAUNDICE

In conditions associated with accelerated breakdown of red cells, excessive bile pigment is delivered to the liver, beyond the liver's ability to conjugate and excrete the pigment. Therefore, unconjugated bile pigment accumulates in the blood. Hemolytic jaundice is sometimes seen in adults with hemolytic anemia, but it is encountered most frequently in newborn infants with hemolytic disease as a result of blood group incompatibility between mother and infant (discussion on prenatal development and diseases associated with pregnancy).

HEPATOCELLULAR JAUNDICE

If the liver is severely damaged, as in hepatitis or cirrhosis, conjugation of bilirubin is impaired. Moreover, the excretion of conjugated bilirubin is extremely hampered because of injury to liver cells and disruption of small bile channels that lie between liver cell cords. As a result, conjugated bilirubin leaks back into the blood through the ruptured intrahepatic bile channels.

OBSTRUCTIVE JAUNDICE

In obstructive jaundice, the extraction and conjugation of bilirubin by liver cells are not impaired, but jaundice develops because the bile duct is obstructed, preventing delivery of bile into the duodenum. Often, the obstruction is caused by an impacted stone in the common duct. Carcinoma of the head of the pancreas is another common cause of common bile duct obstruction. As indicated in Figure 21-4, the common duct passes very close to the head of the pancreas as it enters the duodenum. Therefore, a pancreatic tumor frequently compresses and invades the common duct. As previously described, long-standing common bile duct obstruction leads to obstructive biliary cirrhosis.

Biopsy of the Liver

Many times, the exact cause and extent of liver disease in a given patient is difficult to determine. In such cases, a biopsy of the liver can be performed by inserting a needle through the skin directly into the liver and extracting a small bit of liver tissue. This can be examined microscopically by the pathologist, and generally, an exact diagnosis of the nature and severity of the liver disease can be made. This information can provide a basis for proper treatment.

QUESTIONS FOR REVIEW

1. What are some of the principal functions of the liver? How does the blood supply to the liver differ from that to the other organs? Why does severe liver disease cause disturbances in blood clotting?

2. What is the difference between hemoglobin and bilirubin? How does conjugated bilirubin differ from unconjugated bilirubin? What is the difference between bilirubin and bile? What role does bile play in digestion?

3. What are the possible causes and effects of liver injury (see Figure 21-5)? What is the usual outcome of a liver injury?

4. What is viral hepatitis? What are its major symptoms? How is hepatitis transmitted?

5. What is the difference between hepatitis A and hepatitis B? What is anicteric hepatitis? What is subclinical hepatitis?

6. What effect does alcohol have on the liver? What types of liver disease are associated with excessive alcohol ingestion?

7. What is cirrhosis? What liver diseases may lead to cirrhosis? Why does portal hypertension develop in patients with cirrhosis? Why does ascites develop in patients with cirrhosis? Why do esophageal varices develop?

8. What is jaundice? How is jaundice classified? Under what circumstances do gallstones cause jaundice?

9. What factors predispose to the development of gallstones?

10. What is the difference between viral hepatitis and alcoholic hepatitis?

SUPPLEMENTARY READINGS

Angulo, P. 2002. Nonalcoholic fatty liver disease. *The New England Journal of Medicine* 346:1221–31.

▶ Nonalcoholic fatty liver disease affects from 20 to 24% of the population and also occurs in 57–74% of obese subjects. Pathogenesis of the disease is described. Most affected persons have no symptoms of liver disease, but laboratory tests reveal abnormal liver function tests. Diffuse fatty change within the liver can be demonstrated by ultrasound examination, by computed tomography (CT) scans, or by magnetic resonance imaging (MRI). Liver biopsy can assess the extent of the liver cell damage caused by the fatty change. Advanced liver cell damage with associated scarring and inflammation cannot be differentiated from alcohol-related liver disease.

Bleich, H. L., and Boro, E. S. 1977. Metabolic and hepatic effects of alcohol. *The New England Journal of Medicine* 296:612–6.

► Describes the metabolism of alcohol by the liver and effects of alcohol on carbohydrate, protein, and fat metabolism. Describes alcohol-related disorders.

Centers for Disease Control and Prevention. 1993. Hepatitis E among U.S. travelers. *Morbidity and Mortality Weekly Report* 42:1–4.

► Hepatitis E outbreaks in third world countries are related to contaminated water supplies. Although the infection is not established in the United States, a few cases have been reported, and cases of hepatitis E may become more frequent among residents of states at the US–Mexico border. Gamma globulin does not contain anti-HEV antibodies; thus, gamma globulin does not provide protection against infection.

Galperin, C., and Gershwin, E. 1997. Immunopathogenesis of gastrointestinal and hepatobiliary diseases. *Journal of the American Medical Association* 278:1946–55.

► Discusses viral hepatitis, autoimmune hepatitis, and primary biliary cirrhosis.

Gross, J. B., Jr. 1998. Clinician's guide to hepatitis C. *Mayo Clinic Proceedings* 73:355–60.

► A review article dealing with epidemiology, diagnosis, prognosis, and treatment.

Hoofnagel, J. H., and Seeff, L. B. 2006. Peginterferon and ribavirin for chronic hepatitis C. *New England Journal of Medicine* 355:2444–51.

► Hepatitis C is often silent, and most infected patients have few symptoms of infection. Persisting infection leads to cirrhosis in 20–30% of infected patients, and from 1–4% of patients with cirrhosis also develop hepatocellular carcinoma each year. Liver cell injury in infected patients results from activation of the immune system in which natural killer cells and cytotoxic T cells attempt to eliminate the virus-infected liver cells. Hepatitis C progresses more rapidly in HIV-infected persons. Treatment is recommended for all subjects with detectable hepatitis C viral RNA in their bloodstream, elevation of serum enzyme levels indicating liver damage, and a positive liver biopsy indicating the characteristics and the severity of the liver cell injury. A 48-week course of treatment consists of weekly subcutaneous injection of pegylated interferon (a long-acting interferon produced by attaching polyethylene glycol to the interferon molecule) and twice daily oral doses of ribavirin. Unfortunately, the course of therapy has a high rate of side effects.

Jensen, D. M. 2011. A new era of hepatitis C therapy begins. *The New England Journal of Medicine* 364:1272–74.

► Boceprevir inhibits the protease complex of type 1 HCV when given along with interferon and ribavirin but has no significant effect against other HCV types. Side effects include anemia and neutropenia.

Kaplan, M. M., and Gershwin, M. E. 2005. Primary biliary cirrhosis. *The New England Journal of Medicine* 353:1261–73.

► Long-term outcome of this autoimmune disease has improved in recent years. Autoimmune damage to the liver appears to be related to antibodies directed against a bacterial or viral antigen that cross-reacts with similar antigens within liver cell mitochondria, and such antibodies are considered diagnostic of the disease. Treatment with a bile acid (ursodeoxycholic acid) appears promising.

Krawitt, E. L. 2006. Autoimmune hepatitis. *The New England Journal of Medicine* 354:54–66.
 ▶ Another autoimmune disease that appears to be caused by antibodies formed as a result of a viral infection in which antiviral antibodies cross-react with similar antigens in liver cells. Has many features similar to primary biliary cirrhosis, and the two conditions may be related.

Lauer, G. M., and Walker, B. 2001. Hepatitis C virus infection. *The New England Journal of Medicine* 345:41–52.
 ▶ A review of the current status of the disease and methods of treatment. In the United States, 1.8% of the population is positive for HCV antibodies, and 75% of seropositive persons have circulating virus in their bloodstream, indicating active HCV infection.

Navarro, V. J., and Senior, J. R. 2006. Drug-related hepatotoxicity. *New England Journal of Medicine* 354:731–39.
 ▶ Describes and classifies hepatotoxic drugs based on their clinical presentation and approaches to treatment. Acetaminophen is a commonly encountered hepatotoxin.

Poordad, F., McCone, J., Jr., Bacon, B. R., et al. 2011. Boceprevir for untreated chronic HCV genotype 1 infection. *The New England Journal of Medicine* 364:1195–206.
 ▶ Boceprivir is a potent protease inhibitor of HCV type 1 in conjunction with ribavirin and interferon is effective against type 1 HCV in whom previous treatment has been ineffective.

Scott, J. D., and Gretch, D. R. 2007. Molecular diagnostics of hepatitis C virus infection: A systematic review. *Journal of the American Medical Association* 297:724–32.
 ▶ Hepatitis C is a serious disease and is not always detected because many infected persons do not have symptoms of infection, anti-HCV antibodies may not be detected in their blood, and liver function tests indicating liver injury may not be abnormal. The conclusive test of infection is a nucleic acid test to identify viral RNA (HCV RNA) in the blood of the infected person. The test can also be used to monitor changes in the amount of circulating viral RNA in response to treatment. There are six different strains of virus designated genotypes 1 through 6, which respond differently to treatment, and genotype identification helps the physician select the type and duration of treatment.

Seef, L. B., et al. 2000. 45-year follow-up of hepatitis C virus infection in healthy young adults. *Annals of Internal Medicine* 132:105–11.
 ▶ The rate of HCV infection was determined from reexamination of frozen serum specimens collected from military recruits between 1948 and 1954 and revealed 0.1% infection rate in whites and 1.8% infection rate in African Americans. A 45-year follow-up revealed that liver disease occurred in 11.8% of HCV-positive persons and 2.4% of HCV-negative persons. One HCV-positive person died of liver disease. Healthy HCV-positive persons are at low risk of progressing to end-stage chronic liver disease.

Steffen, R., Kane, M. A., Shapiro, C. N., et al. 1994. Epidemiology and prevention of hepatitis A in travelers. *Journal of the American Medical Association* 272:885–89.
 ▶ Hepatitis A vaccine (or gamma globulin if vaccine not available) is recommended for all nonimmune travelers visiting developing countries.

Zemel, G., Katzen, B. T., Becker, G. J., et al. 1991. Percutaneous transjugular portosystemic shunt. *Journal of the American Medical Association* 266:390–93.
 ▶ An intrahepatic shunt between a branch of the hepatic and portal veins can decompress the portal venous pressure effectively.

OUTLINE SUMMARY

Structure and Function of the Liver

IMPORTANT FEATURES
Complex metabolic functions.
Double blood supply from hepatic artery and portal vein.
Liver lobule is basic structural unit.
Branches of hepatic artery, portal vein, and bile duct travel in portal tracts.
Blood flow in lobule is from portal tract to central vein.
Bile flow in canaliculi is from central vein toward portal tract.

Bile

FORMATION AND EXCRETION OF BILIRUBIN
Bile pigment derived from breakdown of red blood cells in reticuloendothelial system.
Conjugation and excretion by liver.

COMPOSITION AND PROPERTIES
Contains bile pigment, cholesterol, bile salts, lecithin, and other materials.
Functions as biologic detergent: no digestive enzymes.

Causes and Effects of Liver Injury

MANIFESTATIONS
Cell necrosis.
Fatty change.
Mixed necrosis and fatty change.

CLINICAL EFFECTS
Mild injury with complete recovery.
Severe injury with hepatic failure.
Chronic or progressive injury causes scarring with impaired liver function.

COMMON TYPES OF LIVER INJURY
Viral hepatitis.
Fatty liver.
Alcoholic liver disease.
Cirrhosis.

Viral Hepatitis

CLINICAL MANIFESTATIONS AND COURSE
One third become sick and jaundiced.
One third become sick but not jaundiced.
One third asymptomatic but liver function abnormal.

HEPATITIS A
RNA virus.
Short incubation period.
Virus in secretions and stools during early phases.
Transmitted by direct contact or contaminated food or water.

Self-limited, low mortality, no carriers.
Gamma globulin provides protection.
Immunization available.

HEPATITIS B
DNA virus.
Long incubation.
Large amount of surface antigen produced by virus can be detected in blood of carriers and infected persons.
Ten percent of infected persons become chronic carriers of virus.
High carrier rate in some populations.
Transmitted by blood or secretions of infected persons.
Gamma globulin provides some protection.
Immunizing vaccine provides protection against infection.

HEPATITIS C
Transmitted like hepatitis B.
Incubation period intermediate between HAV and HBV.
Many persons become chronic carriers.
No immunization available.
Gamma globulin does not provide protection.

HEPATITIS D (DELTA HEPATITIS)
Virus only infects persons with acute or chronic HBV infection.
Delta virus unable to produce own virus coat and uses HBsAg produced by HBV.

HEPATITIS E

OTHER HEPATITIS VIRUSES
Epstein-Barr (EB) virus.
Cytomegalovirus.

HEPATITIS AMONG MALE HOMOSEXUALS
Spread by sexual practices.

ALCOHOLIC LIVER DISEASE

Fatty Liver

PATHOGENESIS
Fat accumulates in liver cells owing to liver injury.
Common in heavy drinkers and alcoholics.
Sometimes caused by other chemicals and solvents.
Impaired liver function but injury reversible.
May also occur in obese subjects with insulin resistance and other manifestations of metabolic syndrome.

Alcoholic Liver Disease

MANIFESTATIONS
Three stages of progressively increasing severity.
Related to amount and duration of alcohol consumption.
Fatty liver: cells accumulate fat.
Alcoholic hepatitis: cell necrosis with Mallory bodies and inflammation.
Cirrhosis: diffuse scarring throughout liver.

Cirrhosis of the Liver

DEFINITION

Scarring in liver from any cause.

Repeated bouts of alcoholic hepatitis.

Massive liver necrosis.

Repeated episodes of liver injury.

Associated derangements of liver cell regeneration and liver function.

MANIFESTATIONS

Impaired liver function.

Portal hypertension.

Bypass routes connect systemic-portal venous systems.

Risk of fatal hemorrhage from esophageal varices.

PROCEDURES TO TREAT CIRRHOSIS

Portal–systemic anastomoses to control varices.

Splenorenal shunt.

Portacaval shunt.

Intrahepatic portosystemic shunt.

BILIARY CIRRHOSIS

Primary

An autoimmune disease attacking small intrahepatic bile ducts.

No specific treatment. May lead to liver failure and require liver transplant.

Secondary

Obstruction of large extrahepatic bile ducts.

Treated by relieving duct obstruction or bypassing obstruction.

Reye's Syndrome

PATHOGENESIS

Probably related to combined effect of viral illness and aspirin.

Acetaminophen recommended rather than aspirin to reduce risk.

CHARACTERISTICS

Affects primarily infants and children.

Fatty liver with liver dysfunction.

Cerebral edema with neurologic dysfunction.

No specific treatment available.

Cholelithiasis

FACTORS AFFECTING SOLUBILITY OF CHOLESTEROL IN BILE

Cholesterol insoluble in aqueous solution.

Dissolved in micelles composed of bile salts and lecithin.

Solubility of cholesterol depends on ratio of cholesterol to bile salts and lecithin.

Supersaturated bile promotes calculi.

COMPLICATIONS OF GALLSTONES

Asymptomatic in gallbladder.

Biliary colic results if stone extruded into ducts.

Common duct obstruction: obstructive jaundice.

Cystic duct obstruction: no jaundice, but acute cholecystitis may occur if preexisting infection of gallbladder.

TREATMENT OF GALLSTONES

Cholecystectomy.

Chenodeoxycholic acid dissolves gallstones.

Cholecystitis

Chronic infection common.

Gallstones may predispose to infection.

Impaction of stone in neck of gallbladder may precipitate acute cholecystitis.

Tumors of the Liver and Gallbladder

INCIDENCE

Benign adenomas uncommon: occur in women taking oral contraceptives.

Primary carcinoma uncommon: occurs in patients with cirrhosis.

Metastatic carcinoma common.

Spread from gastrointestinal tract, breast, lung, or other sites.

CT scan aids in recognition.

Jaundice

CLASSIFICATION

Hemolytic: excessive red cell breakdown.

Hepatocellular: liver cell injury.

Obstructive: common duct obstruction by tumor or stone.

Biopsy of the Liver

INDICATIONS AND METHOD

Indicated when cause of liver disease undetermined after clinical and laboratory evaluation.

Needle inserted through skin directly into liver.

Biopsy specimen examined histologically by pathologist.

http://health.jbpub.com/humandisease/9e

Human Disease Online is a great source for supplementary human disease information for both students and instructors. Visit this website to find a variety of useful tools for learning, thinking, and teaching.

CHAPTER 22

The Pancreas and Diabetes Mellitus

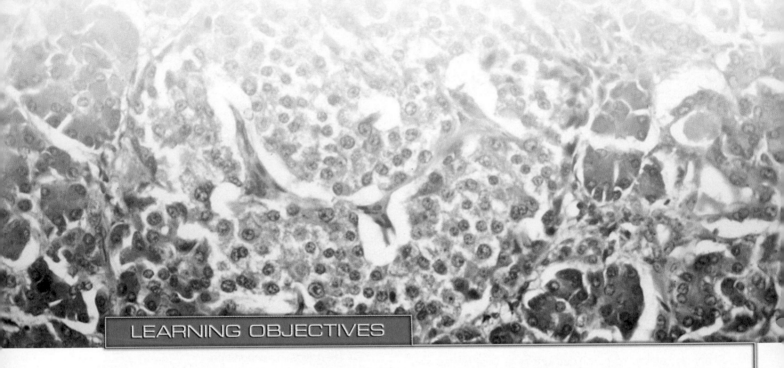

LEARNING OBJECTIVES

1 Describe the pathogenesis and treatment of acute pancreatitis.

2 Describe the pathogenesis, manifestations, complications, and prognosis of pancreatic cystic fibrosis.

3 Differentiate between the two principal types of diabetes mellitus with respect to pathogenesis, incidence, manifestations, complications, and treatment.

Structure and Function of the Pancreas

The pancreas is actually two glands in one: a digestive gland and an endocrine gland. The exocrine tissue of the pancreas, which is concerned solely with digestion, secretes an alkaline pancreatic juice rich in digestive enzymes into the duodenum through the pancreatic duct. The powerful digestive enzymes break down proteins (trypsin and chymotrypsin), carbohydrates (amylase), and fats (lipase). The protein-digesting (proteolytic) enzymes are secreted in an inactive form and are activated after they are discharged into the duodenum. The endocrine tissue of the pancreas consists of multiple small clusters of cells scattered throughout the gland called the pancreatic islets or **islets of Langerhans,** which discharge their secretions directly into the bloodstream. Each islet is composed of several different types of cells. The three main types are alpha cells, beta cells, and delta cells. Alpha cells secrete a hormone called glucagon. The more numerous beta cells secrete insulin in response to a rise in blood glucose after eating, which restores blood glucose to normal. Both glucagon and insulin regulate the level of glucose in the blood but have opposing effects. Glucagon raises blood glucose; insulin lowers it. Delta cells produce a hormone called somatostatin, which inhibits secretion of both glucagon and insulin. Three other relatively rare cell types also have been described, and they produce hormones concerned primarily with regulating gastrointestinal functions. FIGURE 22-1 shows the anatomy and cellular structure of the pancreas.

Islets of Langerhans
(län′ger-hänz)
Cluster of endocrine cells in the pancreas.

Pancreatitis

ACUTE PANCREATITIS

Acute pancreatitis is caused by escape of pancreatic juice from the ducts into the substance of the pancreas, which leads to destruction of pancreatic acinar and islet tissue by activated pancreatic enzymes, accompanied by acute inflammation of the affected pancreatic tissue. Some of the enzymes leak from the damaged tissue into the bloodstream, where elevated levels of amylase and lipase can be detected by appropriate laboratory tests. The clinical manifestations of acute pancreatitis depend on how much pancreatic tissue has been damaged. Mild episodes are accompanied by abdominal pain together with elevated pancreatic enzymes detected by blood tests; however, the pain subsides, and the patient recovers. Patients with severe acute pancreatitis have marked abdominal pain and tenderness, and they are seriously ill. The activated pancreatic enzymes not only destroy much of the pancreas but also damage pancreatic blood vessels, which lead to marked hemorrhage in the damaged tissues. This condition is often called **acute hemorrhagic pancreatitis** (FIGURE 22-2).

Acute hemorrhagic pancreatitis
Severe pancreatic inflammation with necrosis of pancreatic ducts and release of pancreatic enzymes that damage the pancreas

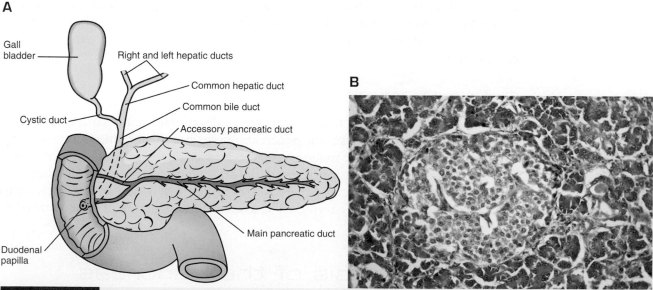

A
Gall bladder
Right and left hepatic ducts
Common hepatic duct
Common bile duct
Cystic duct
Accessory pancreatic duct
Main pancreatic duct
Duodenal papilla

B

FIGURE 22-1 **A,** Duct system of pancreas. The main pancreatic duct usually joins the common bile duct to form a common channel that enters the duodenum by a single opening at the apex of a nipplelike projection called the duodenal papilla (ampulla of Vater). A much smaller accessory pancreatic duct, illustrated in the diagram, is frequently present and opens into the duodenum by a separate opening proximal to the duodenal papilla. **B,** A photomicrograph of pancreatic islet surrounded by exocrine pancreatic tissue.

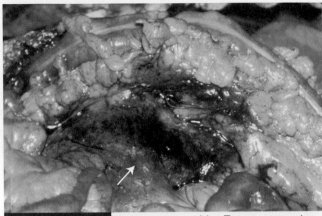

FIGURE 22-2 Acute pancreatitis. Transverse colon (*upper part of photograph*) has been elevated to reveal pancreas (*arrow*), which is inflamed and contains large areas of hemorrhage.

The pathogenesis of acute pancreatitis usually involves active secretion of pancreatic juice while the pancreatic duct is obstructed at its entrance into the duodenum. The buildup of obstructed secretions greatly increases the pressure within the duct system, causing the ducts to rupture and the pancreatic juice to escape. Two factors predispose to acute pancreatitis: disease of the gallbladder and excessive alcohol consumption.

Pancreatitis often develops in patients with gallstones because in most individuals, the common bile duct and common pancreatic duct usually enter the duodenum through a common channel (the ampulla of Vater). If a stone becomes impacted in the ampulla, it can obstruct the pancreatic duct and precipitate pancreatitis.

Patients who drink excessive amounts of alcohol also are prone to pancreatitis. Alcohol is a potent stimulus of pancreatic secretions, and it may also induce edema and spasm of the pancreatic sphincter in the ampulla of Vater. Pancreatitis develops because alcohol-induced hypersecretion combined with sphincter spasm leads to high intraductal pressure, followed by duct necrosis and escape of pancreatic juice.

CHRONIC PANCREATITIS

Chronic pancreatitis results from repeated episodes of mild acute pancreatitis. Each bout of pancreatitis destroys some pancreatic tissue but the inflammation subsides, and the damaged pancreatic tissue is replaced by scar tissue. Eventually, as progressively more pancreatic tissue is destroyed, the affected person has difficulty digesting and absorbing nutrients because there is not enough surviving pancreatic tissue to produce adequate digestive enzymes. The associated destruction of pancreatic islets may also lead to diabetes.

Cystic Fibrosis of the Pancreas

Cystic fibrosis is a relatively common, serious hereditary disease that is transmitted as an autosomal recessive trait and first becomes manifest in infancy and childhood. The disease has an incidence of about 1 per 3,000 whites but is quite rare in blacks and other races. The abnormal gene involved in the disease results from a mutation of a normal gene called the *CFTR* gene, which stands for cystic fibrosis transmembrane conductance regulator, a rather formidable term meaning that the gene regulates the movement of salt and water in and out of epithelial cells by means of ion channels located on the cell membranes. The gene has been localized to the long arm of chromosome 7, and a very large number of *CFTR* gene mutations have been identified. Tests have been developed to identify carriers of the more common gene mutations that are responsible for most cases of cystic fibrosis. The functions of the defective gene also appear to be modified by other genes that influence expression of the gene and the manifestations of the disease. In some individuals, the disease is relatively mild and compatible with survival into adolescence or adult life. Others, with more severe disease, die in childhood. Modern therapy has improved survival, but nevertheless, the average (median) life expectancy is only about 35 years.

As a result of the gene mutation, there is defective transport across cell membranes of chloride, sodium, and the water molecules in which they are dissolved. Electrolyte and water secretion is deficient in the mucus secreted by the epithelial cells of the pancreas, bile ducts, mucosa of respiratory tract, and other mucus-secreting cells throughout the body. As a result, the mucus becomes abnormally thick and tends to coagulate, forming dense plugs that obstruct the pancreatic ducts, bronchi and bronchioles, and bile ducts.

The most characteristic structural abnormalities are usually in the pancreas. Mucous plugs in the small pancreatic ducts block the secretion of pancreatic juice, which accumulates under increased pressure within the obstructed ducts. Eventually, the ducts become cystically dilated. The pancreatic secretory cells, unable to discharge their secretions into the duodenum, undergo atrophy and are replaced by fibrous tissue, but the pancreatic islets are unaffected because they discharge their hormones directly into the bloodstream. Eventually, the pancreas becomes converted into a mass of cystically dilated ducts surrounded by dense fibrous tissue (FIGURE 22-3). The name of the disease derives from these characteristic structural abnormalities.

In the lungs, the small bronchi and bronchioles become obstructed by the thick mucous secretions of the epithelial cells lining the respiratory tract. Bronchial obstruction predisposes to pulmonary infection, leading to bronchitis, bronchiectasis, and repeated bouts of pneumonia in the lung distal to the blocked bronchi. Eventually, the lungs are severely damaged by the repeated infections.

The function of sweat glands also is abnormal in cystic fibrosis. The sweat glands are unable to conserve sodium and chloride, and the sweat of affected individuals contains an excessively high salt concentration. This biochemical abnormality has served as the basis of a diagnostic test for cystic fibrosis called a sweat test. A small quantity of sweat is collected, and the sodium and chloride concentrations are determined. The salt concentration of the sweat is low in normal persons and high in persons with cystic fibrosis.

Many cystic fibrosis patients need to take capsules containing pancreatic enzymes in order to digest and absorb food properly because their own pancreas has been destroyed by the disease. Various types of treatment are also used to preserve as much pulmonary function as possible. Pulmonary infections caused by antibiotic-resistant bacteria are a serious problem and are difficult to deal with. Lungs so severely damaged by repeated infections that they can no longer function effectively can be treated by lung transplants.

The discovery of the *CFTR* gene and its defective counterpart have stimulated active research efforts that have led recently to the development of a drug that improved *CFTR* gene function, as demonstrated by more efficient chloride transport

A

B

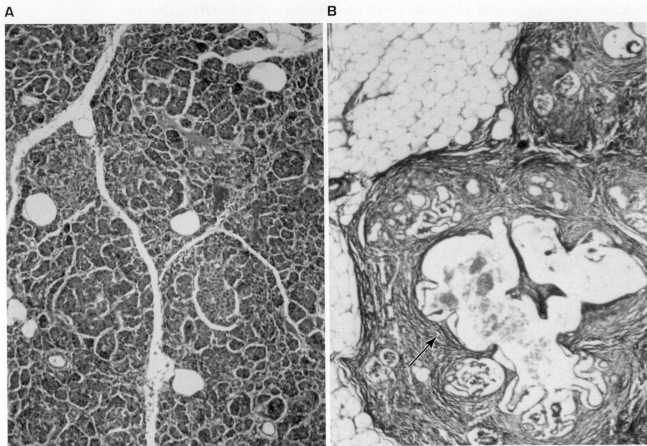

FIGURE 22-3 Low magnification photomicrographs comparing normal pancreas (**A**) with pancreas of patient with cystic fibrosis (**B**). Duct in center of field (*arrow*) exhibits cystic dilatation. Most of pancreatic glandular tissue has undergone atrophy and has been replaced by fibrous tissue (original magnification × 25).

across the cell membrane, which was associated with improved pulmonary function. These encouraging results have stimulated further pharmacologic studies designed to correct the biochemical disturbances resulting from the genetic defects responsible for cystic fibrosis.

Diabetes Mellitus

Diabetes mellitus is a very common and important metabolic disease that results either because the pancreatic islets are incapable of secreting sufficient insulin or because the insulin is not being utilized efficiently. One of its major manifestations is an elevated level of glucose in the blood, which is called **hyperglycemia** (*hyper* = excess + *glyc* = sweet + *heme* = blood). A normal fasting blood glucose concentration is considered to be 60–100 mg per 100 ml of plasma, abbreviated 60–100 mg/dl. A diagnosis of diabetes requires a fasting glucose of 126 mg/dl or higher, which must be confirmed by repeat testing, or a glucose concentration over 200 mg/dl determined by an oral glucose tolerance test. Recently, another test called a **glycated hemoglobin test** also called the **hemoglobin A$_{1C}$ test** is also acceptable, but with some reservations described later in this section.

Diabetes is divided into two major groups, depending on whether the diabetes results primarily from insulin deficiency, which is called type 1 diabetes, or from an inadequate response to insulin, which is called type 2 diabetes. Previously, type 1 diabetes was called insulin-dependent diabetes or juvenile-onset diabetes because it

Diabetes mellitus
(dī-u-bē′tēz mel′lit-is)
A metabolic disease characterized by hyperglycemia and caused by insufficient insulin secretion or inefficient utilization of insulin.

Hyperglycemia
(hī-per-glī-sē′mi-uh)
Excessively high blood glucose concentration.

Glycated hemoglobin test (Hemoglobin A$_{1C}$ test)
A test that measures the amount of glucose permanently attached to hemoglobin, which is higher than normal in many persons with diabetes.

TABLE 22-1

Comparison of two major types of diabetes mellitus

	Type 1	Type 2
Usual age of onset	Childhood Young adulthood	Middle age or later
Body build	Normal	Overweight
Plasma insulin	Absent or low	Normal or high
Complications	Ketoacidosis	Hyperosmolar coma
Response to insulin	Normal	Reduced
Response to oral antidiabetic drugs	Unresponsive	Responsive

resulted from insulin deficiency and often occurred in children and teenagers. Type 2 diabetes was called non-insulin–dependent diabetes or adult-onset diabetes because the islets produced insulin and the diabetes typically occurred in older adults. The two types of diabetes are not restricted to the age groups implied by this terminology, however, and these terms are used less frequently now.

TABLE 22-1 compares the major features of the two types.

TYPE 1 DIABETES MELLITUS

Type 1 diabetes is an autoimmune disease in which cytotoxic and delayed hypersensitivity T lymphocytes attack and destroy the pancreatic islets, assisted by anto-antibodies directed against islet cells. The rate at which islets are destroyed by the immune system and the rate at which insulin secretion declines vary among affected subjects. In some, islet cell destruction proceeds rapidly, and in others, the destruction occurs more slowly. In some cases, onset of diabetes follows a viral infection, suggesting that the virus may have induced the disease by injuring or destroying the islets. Type 1 diabetes occurs primarily in children and young adults, and affected subjects are prone to develop a condition called **diabetic ketosis** caused by a lack of insulin. There is a hereditary predisposition to type 1 diabetes. Persons who inherit certain HLA-D types are at increased risk of acquiring this type of diabetes. (HLA types and predisposition to disease were considered in the discussion on chromosomes, genes, and cell division.)

TYPE 2 DIABETES MELLITUS

Type 2 diabetes is by far the more common type and is a more complex metabolic defect. The pancreatic islets secrete normal or increased amounts of insulin, but the tissues are relatively insensitive to the action of insulin and are unable to respond appropriately. (Inadequate response to insulin is called *insulin resistance*.) The condition develops most frequently in older overweight and obese adults. The reason for the impaired response to insulin is not completely understood, but it seems to be related in some way to obesity because weight reduction restores insulin responsiveness and frequently controls the diabetes. Ketosis does not usually occur as a complication of type 2 diabetes, but affected persons may develop another complication called **hyperosmolar coma**, which results from the marked hyperglycemia.

Diabetic ketosis
A disturbance of the body's acid–base balance (acidosis) caused by an inability to utilize glucose, which requires the body to use fat as an energy source. Fat metabolism generates excessive amounts of acid ketone bodies, which disrupts the normal alkalinity of body fluids.

Hyperosmolar coma
(hī-per-oz-mō'lär)
Coma resulting from neurologic dysfunction caused by hyperosmolarity of body fluids as a consequence of severe hyperglycemia.

Although insulin resistance plays an important role in the pathogenesis of type 2 diabetes, islet cell function is not completely normal either because the pancreas is unable to increase insulin output sufficiently to compensate for the insulin resistance.

Type 2 diabetes is a hereditary disease in which genetic factors play an even greater role than in type 1 diabetes, although in most cases we do not know the exact mode of inheritance or the genes that predispose to this type of diabetes. Children of parents who have type 2 diabetes are at significant risk of also eventually becoming diabetic. In some population groups, such as the Pima Indians of Arizona, as many as 40% of adults are diabetic.

PREDIABETES

Prediabetes
Higher than normal blood glucose but not high enough to establish diagnosis of diabetes.

In many people who eventually develop diabetes, blood glucose is higher than normal but not high enough to establish a diagnosis of diabetes. This condition was called impaired carbohydrate tolerance, later renamed **prediabetes**, to indicate that the number of insulin-producing beta cells is beginning to decline, and a further loss of islet cell function can lead to more marked hyperglycemia characteristic of diabetes. Often, a further reduction of functioning beta cells can be prevented or at least slowed by measures that make less demand on the pancreatic beta cells so that they do not have to "work as hard" to produce the amount of insulin required to return an elevated blood glucose to normal. Reducing the demands on the pancreas can be accomplished by weight loss if overweight, which reduces the insulin resistance of body cells so that less insulin is required; by moderate exercise, which uses the glucose as an energy source as it is being absorbed so less insulin is required; and by healthy eating habits emphasizing more slowly absorbed complex carbohydrates over sugar-rich foods that are absorbed quickly and raise blood glucose rapidly. All these measures help preserve beta cell function and promote more efficient utilization of glucose so that blood glucose does not rise as high after eating.

α-glucosidase
(glu-ko-si-das)
inhibitor
Inhibitor of an enzyme required to break down a glucose-containing disaccharide so glucose can be absorbed from the small intestine.

If diet and weight reduction are unable to lower postprandial (after eating) glucose elevations adequately, a drug can be added to improve glucose tolerance, which is called pharmacologic treatment. A frequently used type of glucose-lowering drug acts by inhibiting the absorption of glucose. Drugs of this type are called α-**glucosidase inhibitors** because they inhibit an enzyme required to absorb glucose from the small intestine. During the initial stages of carbohydrate digestion, complex carbohydrates are broken down into disaccharides, but only monosaccharides such as glucose and fructose can be absorbed and transported into the bloodstream. Breakdown of the disaccharides into glucose and other monosaccharides so they can be absorbed into the bloodstream is accomplished by an enzyme called α-**glucosidase** present on the absorbing surface (brush border) of intestinal epithelial cells, which breaks down disaccharides into glucose and other monosaccharides for absorption and transport into the bloodstream. An α-glucosidase inhibitor drug interferes with the disaccharide breakdown by inhibiting the α-glucosidase enzyme. Consequently, less glucose is available for absorption, which can help prevent progression to diabetes by reducing the glucose load presented to the overworked pancreatic beta cells. The effectiveness of this approach was demonstrated by a recent study involved two large groups of persons with prediabetes. One group was treated by weight reduction and diet; the other group received in addition an α-glucosidase inhibitor. After 2 years of observation, only 3.6% of the subjects receiving an α-glucosidase inhibitor had progressed to type 2 diabetes, in contrast to 9.6% of the other group who developed diabetes. Other drugs can also prevent progression of impaired carbohydrate tolerance to type 2 diabetes by reducing the demands on the less efficiently functioning pancreas. The same drugs used also to treat persons who have already developed type 2 diabetes are useful to slow the progression of prediabetes to diabetes.

PREGNANCY-ASSOCIATED DIABETES

As described in prenatal development and diseases associated with pregnancy, the high levels of placental hormones in pregnancy cause the pregnant woman to become less responsive to insulin (develop insulin resistance) but most women can compensate by secreting more insulin, and the blood glucose does not rise excessively. However, some women are unable to secrete enough additional insulin, and they develop pregnancy-related diabetes caused by their insulin resistance. The condition is called **gestational diabetes**, and is treated by diet along with supplementary insulin if necessary because hyperglycemia is harmful to the developing fetus. Although blood glucose returns to normal after delivery, a woman who has demonstrated significant insulin resistance during pregnancy is at risk of developing permanent diabetes in later years. Pregnancy-related diabetes serves as a "wake-up call" to begin taking steps that may avoid later permanent hyperglycemia: eating a healthy diet, controlling her weight, being active, and exercising moderately. A program of this type helps maintain normal blood glucose without promoting excessive insulin secretion, which helps preserve pancreatic beta cell function.

Gestational diabetes
Elevated blood glucose caused by insulin resistance resulting from elevated hormones related to the pregnancy. Blood glucose returns to normal postpartum, but woman has increased risk of diabetes later in life.

DIABETES AND THE METABOLIC SYNDROME

The term metabolic syndrome, also called the insulin resistance syndrome, is a group of conditions that often are identified in persons with impaired glucose tolerance or type 2 diabetes, and which can progress to diabetes-associated complications as well as cardiovascular disease and its complications. The metabolic syndrome components include

1. Obesity, especially when much of the excess fat accumulates in the abdomen
2. Insulin resistance, characterized by high normal or elevated blood glucose
3. Blood lipid abnormalities that predispose to cardiovascular disease (described in the discussion on the cardiovascular system), which is called dyslipidemia
4. Hypertension

Overweight people with excess abdominal fat, as indicated by their waist circumference (over 40 in. in men or 35 in. in women), should be screened for the other conditions associated with the syndrome by measuring blood pressure, blood glucose, and blood lipids. If other metabolic syndrome-associated abnormalities are detected, treatment to correct or improve the associated conditions can be undertaken.

ACTIONS OF INSULIN

Insulin has multiple effects that influence not only carbohydrate metabolism, but protein and fat metabolism as well. The chief sites of insulin action are on liver cells, muscle, and adipose tissue (fat). Insulin promotes entry of glucose into cells and favors utilization of glucose as a source of energy. In muscle and liver cells, it promotes storage of glucose as **glycogen**. In adipose tissue, insulin favors the conversion of glucose into fat (triglyceride) and storage of the newly formed triglyceride within the fat cells. Insulin also promotes entry of amino acids into the cells and stimulates protein synthesis. The main stimulus for insulin release is elevation of the level of glucose in the blood, as occurs after a meal.

Glycogen (glī′kō-jen)
A storage form of glucose present chiefly in liver and muscle.

FAT METABOLISM AND FORMATION OF KETONE BODIES

Fatty acid
A long, straight-chain carbon compound that contains a terminal carboxyl group, which enters into the formation of a triglyceride.

Acetyl coenzyme A
(acetyl-CoA)
A combination of a two-carbon acetate fragment with a complex organic compound called coenzyme A.

Ketone bodies
Various derivatives of acetyl-CoA, resulting from excessive mobilization of fat as an energy source.

Hyperglycemia
(hī-per-glī-sē′mi-ah)
Excessively high blood glucose concentration.

When fat is metabolized as a source of energy, it is split first into **fatty acids** and glycerol. The fatty acids are broken down into two carbon fragments, which are combined with a large carrier molecule called coenzyme A (CoA). The combination is called **acetyl coenzyme A** or acetyl-CoA. Some of the acetyl-CoA molecules are normally converted by the liver into compounds called **ketone bodies**: acetoacetic acid, beta-hydroxybutyric acid, and acetone. Acetoacetic acid is formed by condensation of two acetyl-CoA molecules, with loss of coenzyme A. Beta-hydroxybutyric acid is formed by the addition of a hydrogen atom to an oxygen atom, which becomes converted into a hydroxyl (OH) group. The term beta designates the carbon atom to which the hydroxyl group is attached. The first carbon after the carboxyl (COOH) group is called the alpha carbon, and the second is the beta carbon. Acetone is formed by removal of the carboxyl group of acetoacetic acid (FIGURE 22-4).

BIOCHEMICAL DISTURBANCES IN DIABETES

In diabetes mellitus, glucose is absorbed normally. However, because of lack of insulin or insulin insensitivity, it is not used normally for energy and is not stored normally as glycogen. Consequently, it accumulates in the bloodstream, resulting in a high level of blood glucose (hyperglycemia). The excessive glucose "spills over" in the urine and is excreted. Because glucose must be excreted in the urine in solution, the body loses excessive amounts of water and electrolytes along with the glucose. This may lead to disturbance in water balance and acid–base balance. (Water and electrolyte balance is discussed in water, electrolyte, and acid–base balance.)

Protein synthesis is also compromised, and body protein is broken down into amino acids. The liver converts these amino acids into glucose, augmenting the hyperglycemia and leading to additional losses of glucose, water, and electrolytes in the urine.

Diabetic Ketoacidosis

The person with type 1 diabetes, lacking insulin, is unable to use carbohydrates because insulin is required to promote entry of glucose into the cells where the glucose can be metabolized to yield energy. So the body turns to fat as an energy source.

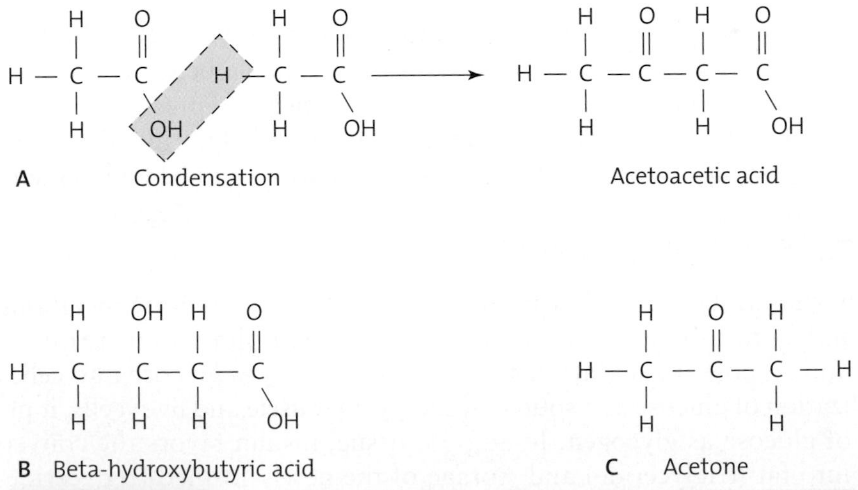

FIGURE 22-4 Structure of ketone bodies. **A**, Condensation of two acetyl-CoA molecules (illustrated as acetic acid) to form acetoacetic acid. **B**, Beta-hydroxybutyric acid, which is formed by reduction of keto group to form a hydroxyl group. **C**, Acetone formed by decarboxylation of acetoacetic acid.

Body fat is split into long-chain fatty acid molecules and glycerol. The fatty acids are broken down by enzymes into two carbon (acetyl) fragments, which are joined to coenzyme A to form acetyl coenzyme A (acetyl-CoA), but the acetyl-CoA molecules are produced in such large quantities that they cannot be oxidized efficiently to yield energy. Many of the acetyl CoA molecules condense to form ketone bodies, which can be used as an energy source, but so many ketone bodies are produced that the body cannot deal effectively with the excess. This condition is called **ketosis**. The ketone bodies accumulate in the blood and are excreted in the urine, carrying with them more water and electrolytes. The acid-ketone bodies can be buffered to some extent by the bicarbonate buffer systems in the bloodstream. If the diabetes is extremely severe, however, so many ketone bodies may be produced that the buffer systems cannot maintain a normal blood pH, and diabetic acidosis develops. The term ketoacidosis is often used for this type of acidosis because of its relationship to overproduction of ketone bodies. Severe acidosis may lead to coma because acidosis has an adverse effect on cerebral function.

Ketosis
An excess of ketone bodies in the blood resulting from utilization of fat as the primary source of energy.

All these effects can be reversed by supplying insulin, which promotes normal utilization of glucose and storage of glycogen. The disturbances of fat and protein metabolism also are reversed by the action of insulin. FIGURE 22-5 summarizes the major metabolic disturbances in type 1 diabetes.

The following case illustrates the clinical and biochemical disturbances in severe diabetic ketoacidosis.

CASE 22-1

A middle-aged woman with diabetes became unconscious while babysitting and was brought to the hospital by ambulance. Her temperature was moderately elevated. Respirations were rapid and deep. Blood pressure was normal. The patient was comatose but responded to painful stimuli. The skin was warm and dry. The remainder of the physical signs were normal. The patient's urine contained large amounts of glucose and a small amount of albumin. There was a strongly positive reaction for acetone and other ketone bodies. Blood glucose was 865 mg/dl (normal range 60–100 mg/dl). Other laboratory studies revealed a low blood pH and reduced plasma bicarbonate of 8 mEq/liter (normal range 24–28 mEq/liter). The patient was considered to have severe diabetic acidosis probably precipitated by a respiratory infection. She received intensive treatment with intravenous fluids, insulin, and antibiotics. Her condition gradually improved. The following day she was conscious and oriented and was able to take fluids orally. She continued to improve and was eventually discharged from the hospital on a diabetic diet and supplementary insulin therapy.

Hyperosmolar Hyperglycemic Nonketotic Coma

Persons with type 2 diabetes mellitus may become comatose as a result of the extreme hyperosmolarity of body fluids that results from severe hyperglycemia in the absence of ketosis. (Osmotic pressure and osmolarity are considered in the discussion on cells and tissues in connection with movement of materials into and out of cells.)

Although individuals with type 2 diabetes exhibit a reduced responsiveness to insulin, much less insulin is required to inhibit fat mobilization than is needed to promote entry of glucose into cells. In these subjects, the response to insulin is usually sufficient to prevent ketosis but inadequate to prevent hyperglycemia. Consequently,

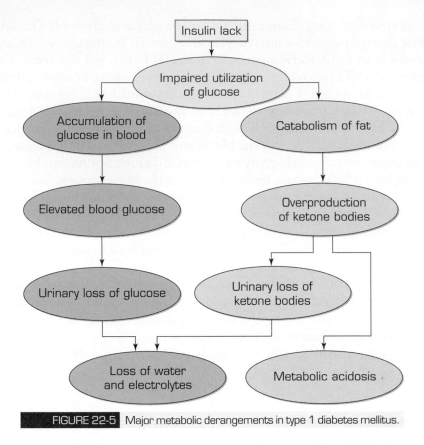

FIGURE 22-5 | Major metabolic derangements in type 1 diabetes mellitus.

blood glucose rises, often to levels that are from 10 to 20 times normal. The extreme hyperglycemia causes the osmolarity of the body fluids to rise significantly, and water moves by osmosis from the cells into the more concentrated extracellular fluids. The cells become dehydrated, which disturbs the function of neurons and causes coma. Treatment consists of supplying insulin to reduce the hyperglycemia and administering hypotonic fluids to help reduce the hyperosmolarity of the body fluids, as illustrated by the following case.

CASE 22-2

A 52-year-old woman who was not previously known to be diabetic had experienced increased urinary output and thirst for the previous 2 weeks and had consumed large quantities of sugar-containing soft drinks. She became progressively more confused and eventually lapsed into coma. She was found by a neighbor and was brought to the hospital by ambulance. On admission, she was comatose and dehydrated. Her respiratory rate was not increased. Blood pressure was normal. The urine contained a large amount of glucose but no ketone bodies. Blood pH and bicarbonate were normal. Blood glucose was 1,750 mg/dl (normal range 60–100 mg/dl), and the osmolarity of the plasma was 396 mOsm/liter (normal range 280–295 mOsm/liter). A diagnosis of hyperosmolar nonketotic coma was made, and she was treated with large volumes of hypotonic (0.45%) saline solution and with insulin. Her condition gradually improved over the succeeding several days. Her blood glucose gradually fell toward normal and eventually reached 150 mg/dl on the fourth day. Plasma osmolarity also returned to normal as the elevated blood glucose declined.

MONITORING CONTROL OF DIABETES

The current goal of treatment is to achieve control of blood glucose that is as close as possible to normal, as close control of hyperglycemia reduces the long-term complications caused by diabetes. Tests used to monitor control of diabetes include

1. Frequent periodic measurements of blood glucose.
2. Measurement of a compound in the blood called **glycated hemoglobin** (also called hemoglobin A_{1C} and often abbreviated as HbA_{1C}) as an index of long-term control of hyperglycemia.
3. Urine tests for glucose used to be performed frequently to monitor blood glucose indirectly by detecting glucose spilling into the urine when blood glucose was too high, but are not used very often now because they have been replaced by frequent blood glucose tests. However, urine tests are still used in special situations, such as to check for ketone bodies as an indication of diabetic ketosis in persons with type 1 diabetes.

Glycated hemoglobin
Hemoglobin to which glucose molecules have become permanently attached. Concentration is related to concentration of glucose in the blood.

Blood tests can be performed by the diabetic at home or at work. Blood testing products permit diabetics to monitor their own blood glucose at frequent intervals. A drop of blood is drawn by a sterile disposable lancet, collected on a specially treated strip of paper, and inserted into an instrument that displays the glucose concentration. Simple urine test strips are also available that can be dipped into a urine specimen and record a color change that is proportional to the amount of glucose in the urine.

The glycated hemoglobin test is a more complex test that must be done by a medical laboratory but is only necessary every 3–6 months. The test monitors how well the blood glucose is being controlled by treatment. Normally, a small amount of blood glucose becomes permanently attached to hemoglobin. This glucose–hemoglobin combination is called glycated hemoglobin, and its concentration is directly proportional to the average blood glucose concentration over the preceding 6–12 weeks, unlike the blood glucose test, which only indicates the concentration of blood glucose at the time the sample was collected. In normal persons, up to 6% of hemoglobin is glycated. In persons with very poorly controlled diabetes, the concentration may be much higher than normal. A value exceeding 6.5% indicates abnormally high blood glucose over the previous several weeks. Diabetics in whom blood glucose levels have been closely controlled can achieve glycated hemoglobin levels that are close to normal. Higher levels indicate less satisfactory control of blood glucose and indicate a need for more intensive treatment. In general, the better the long-term control of blood glucose, as indicated by a close to normal glycated hemoglobin value, the less likely the development of long-term late diabetic complications.

Currently, the glycated hemoglobin test is recommended by the American Diabetes Association as a diagnostic test for diabetes in nonpregnant adults. However, confirmation by blood glucose test results is recommended because the glycated hemoglobin test has some limitations and the results do not always correlate with blood glucose tests. To obtain a reliable glycated hemoglobin test result, the hemoglobin concentration must be normal and the hemoglobin must be hemoglobin A. The test will not be reliable if the hemoglobin is an abnormal hemoglobin, such as hemoglobin S or hemoglobin C, if the subject is anemic, or if the survival of the subject's red cells is shorter than normal.

TREATMENT OF DIABETES

Type 1 diabetics require insulin, and the dose should be adjusted in order to control the level of blood glucose as closely as possible because this appears to reduce late complications. Most type 1 diabetics require several insulin injections spaced throughout the day in order to maintain blood glucose within reasonably normal limits. Frequent measurements of blood glucose permit better regulation of insulin dosage and improve control of the diabetes.

Insulin pumps are sometimes useful for type 1 diabetics who are difficult to treat because of their need for frequent insulin injections. An insulin pump is a small battery-operated device that can be attached to the patient's belt. A short length of tubing extends from the pump to a fine (27 gauge) needle that is inserted into the subcutaneous tissue of the abdominal wall and secured with tape. The pump is programmed to deliver a small constant infusion of insulin, supplemented by larger doses just before meals, simulating the release of insulin by the pancreas. Despite the convenience, use of an insulin pump requires very close medical supervision because complications can arise from pump malfunction or infections at the site of needle placement. Many other devices are available to simplify insulin injections, and many different insulin preparations having different durations of activity are available. Human insulin produced by genetic engineering has almost completely replaced insulin from animal sources.

Type 1 diabetic patients are treated with insulin. Insulin dose, type of insulin used, and times of administration are adjusted to maintain blood glucose within a reasonably normal range.

Type 2 diabetic patients can often be managed by diet and weight reduction alone. If they do not respond adequately, oral hypoglycemic drugs are added. Several groups of drugs called oral hypoglycemic agents are available to treat type 2 diabetes. The four major groups are (1) sulfonurea drugs, (2) biguanide drugs, (3) α-glucosidase inhibitors, and (4) thiazolidinedione drugs. Sulfonurea drugs stimulate the pancreas to release insulin, which lowers blood glucose by stimulating the pancreas to work harder, even though the islets are already having difficulty supplying enough insulin. Biguanides do not stimulate insulin secretion. Instead they lower blood glucose by inhibiting the production of glucose from other nutrients primarily in the liver, which is called gluconeogenesis (*gluco* + glucose + *neo* = new + *genesis* = formation). The drug is not metabolized in the body and is excreted in the urine. α-Glucosidase inhibitor drugs lower blood glucose by inhibiting the enzyme that breaks down disaccharides into monosaccharides, a step required in order to absorb glucose from the small intestine. Thiazolidinedione drugs decrease insulin resistance so the secreted insulin is more effective. If diet, weight reduction, and hypoglycemic drugs do not control the hyperglycemia, insulin is used to regulate blood glucose in the same way that it is used in type 1 diabetes.

COMPLICATIONS OF DIABETES

Diabetics are liable to develop a number of complications that can be reduced to some extent by proper adherence to diet and other prescribed treatments. They have an increased susceptibility to infection, apparently related to the high levels of blood glucose. Pathogenic bacteria seem to grow more readily in the presence of elevated blood glucose levels. They may develop diabetic coma, as a result either of ketoacidosis or of the greatly increased osmolarity of body fluids resulting from hyperglycemia. They have a greater incidence of arteriosclerosis and its associated vascular complications such as strokes, heart attacks, and gangrene of the legs and feet as a result of poor circulation. The vascular problems probably result both from abnormalities in fat metabolism associated with diabetes and from the elevated blood lipids frequently found in diabetics. They are also subject to other late complications, which increase in frequency with the duration of the disease. The small blood vessels supplying the retina of the eye often undergo degenerative changes, which may eventually lead to blindness in some subjects. The glomerular arterioles and capillaries within the kidneys also undergo degenerative changes, which impair renal function and may result in renal failure (discussed in the section on the urinary system). The peripheral nerves may undergo degenerative changes, called peripheral neuritis, which cause pain and disturbed sensation in the extremities.

How high glucose leads to organ damage is not completely understood, but the organ damage is related either directly or indirectly to the hyperglycemia. One concept proposes that the hyperglycemia causes the proteins in the retina, peripheral nerves, and capillary basement membranes to undergo the same type of glycation as hemoglobin, and that the glycated proteins undergo further interactions with other cell components, leading eventually to the blood vessel and organ damage characteristic of long-standing poorly controlled diabetes.

OTHER CAUSES OF HYPERGLYCEMIA

Other conditions at times may lead to impaired glucose utilization and hyperglycemia, but they are much less common than true diabetes mellitus. These conditions include the following:

1. Chronic pancreatic disease, in which the hyperglycemia results from damage or destruction of pancreatic islets
2. Endocrine diseases associated with overproduction of pituitary or adrenal hormones because these hormones act in various ways to raise blood glucose
3. Ingestion of many different drugs, such as diuretics or antihypertensive drugs, in which glucose utilization is impaired as a side effect of the drug
4. A few rare hereditary diseases in which carbohydrate metabolism is disturbed

Hypoglycemia

The normal pancreas continually monitors the blood glucose and automatically adjusts its output of insulin to maintain the blood glucose level within the normal range. The type 1 diabetic patient, however, must adjust the dose of insulin to match the amount of carbohydrate to be metabolized. If there is insufficient insulin, the blood glucose is too high. If there is too much insulin, the blood glucose is too low, a condition called **hypoglycemia** (*hypo* = under). Two conditions predispose to hypoglycemia in a diabetic patient taking insulin. The first is a reduced intake of food, such as skipping a meal; blood glucose falls because carbohydrate intake is insufficient in relation to the amount of insulin injected. The second condition is increased activity, such as vigorous exercise, which lowers blood glucose by increasing glucose utilization. As a result, there is a relative excess of insulin. Too much insulin causes a precipitous drop in the level of glucose in the blood and initiates a chain of events called an insulin reaction or insulin shock. The adrenal medulla responds to the hypoglycemia by discharging epinephrine (adrenaline), which tends to raise blood glucose by converting liver glycogen into glucose. Epinephrine exerts widespread systemic effects as well: rapid heart rate, rise in blood pressure, constriction of cutaneous blood vessels causing the skin to appear pale, stimulation of sweat glands causing a cold sweat, and stimulation of the nervous system leading to increased excitability, anxiousness, hyperactive reflexes, and tremors.

Neurologic manifestations appear if the blood glucose continues to fall because the nervous system requires glucose to carry out its metabolic processes and begins to malfunction when deprived of its energy source. The subject becomes confused, loses consciousness, may have convulsions, and soon lapses into a deep coma. Prolonged severe hypoglycemia may cause permanent brain damage.

If the patient is still conscious and able to swallow, the insulin reaction can be stopped by ingesting a quick-acting carbohydrate, such as a piece of candy or a

Hypoglycemia
(hī-pō-glī-sē′mē-ah)
Lower than normal concentration of glucose in the blood.

TABLE 22-2

Differentiation of insulin shock from ketoacidosis and hyperosmolar coma

Diagnostic feature	Insulin shock	Ketoacidosis	Hyperosmolar coma
Food intake	May be insufficient	Normal or excessive	Normal or excessive
Insulin	Excessive	Insufficient	Normal or increased
Onset of symptoms	Rapid	Gradual (several days)	Gradual (several days)
Skin	Cold sweat, pale	Dry and flushed	Dry and flushed
Respirations	Normal or shallow	Slow and deep	Usually normal
Reflexes	Hyperactive	Depressed	Normal
Heart rate	Rapid	Rapid	Usually normal
Blood pressure	Normal or slightly elevated	Low	Usually normal
Glucose in urine	Absent	Large amount	Large amount
Blood glucose	Very low	High	Extremely high
Blood bicarbonate and pH	Normal	Low	Normal
Acetone in blood and urine	Absent	Present	Absent

glucose tablet. The diabetic patient should always have a quick-acting carbohydrate available for such emergencies. If the patient is unconscious, an injection of glucagon can be given; this raises blood glucose by mobilizing glucose from liver glycogen. A concentrated glucose solution may also be given intravenously.

TABLE 22-2 compares the clinical manifestations of insulin shock with those of diabetic ketoacidosis and hyperosmolar nonketotic coma, two other conditions to which the diabetic patient is predisposed.

Severe hypoglycemic reactions can also be caused by oral hypoglycemic drugs. Rarely, nondiabetic persons with emotional problems may deliberately ingest oral hypoglycemic drugs or inject themselves with insulin. They then consult a physician or enter a hospital emergency room with manifestations of severe hypoglycemia. If the possibility of self-induced hypoglycemia is suspected, special laboratory tests can determine the level of insulin in the blood. Tests can also determine whether the insulin in the patient's blood was secreted by the patient's own pancreas or is the type of insulin that is used by diabetic patients.

Tumors of the Pancreas

Carcinoma of the pancreas is relatively common and develops most often in the head of the pancreas. In this location, the neoplasm blocks the common bile duct, resulting in obstructive jaundice. Carcinoma elsewhere in the pancreas is usually far advanced when first detected and produces no specific symptoms.

Sometimes, benign tumors arise from the islet cells and produce symptoms as a result of overproduction of hormones. Beta cells give rise to insulin-secreting tumors that cause episodes of severe hypoglycemia similar to those experienced by a diabetic who receives too much insulin.

QUESTIONS FOR REVIEW

1. What is the difference between acute and chronic pancreatitis?
2. What are the major metabolic disturbances in type 1 diabetes? How does insulin correct these disturbances?
3. What are the major complications of diabetes?
4. Which type of diabetes can be treated by diet alone?
5. What is meant by the following terms: *sweat test, hyperosmolar nonketotic hyperglycemic coma, ketoacidosis,* and *ketone bodies?*
6. What is cystic fibrosis of the pancreas? What are its clinical manifestations? What is its pattern of inheritance?
7. What is hypoglycemia? What are its clinical manifestations? How is it treated?
8. What are the major differences between diabetic ketoacidosis and insulin shock?
9. What is gestation diabetes? Why does it occur?

SUPPLEMENTARY READINGS

Abrahamson, M. J. 2007. A 74-year-old woman with diabetes. *Journal of the American Medical Association* 297:196–204.

▶ A case-based discussion emphasizing that the metabolic disorder affects over 20 million people in the United States, of which 90% have type 2 diabetes. The basic disturbance is insulin resistance associated with impaired beta cell insulin production. In most persons who develop diabetes, the insulin resistance progresses for many years before type 2 diabetes finally results. Treatment with oral medications that stimulate insulin secretion by beta cells is effective, but supplementary insulin is needed by many patients to control the hyperglycemia. Oral drugs that act by promoting insulin secretion may hasten the failure of beta cell function.

American Diabetes Association. 2000. Type 2 diabetes in children and adolescents. *Pediatrics* 105:671–80.

▶ A review of current concepts. Type 2 diabetes is becoming more frequent in this age group, related primarily to obesity. Children with type 2 diabetes usually have a family history of diabetes, and those of non-European ancestry are disproportionately represented.

Beckman, J. A., Creager, M. A., and Libby, P. 2002. Diabetes and atherosclerosis: Epidemiology, pathophysiology, and management. *Journal of the American Medical Association* 287:2570–81.

▶ The prevalence of type 2 diabetes in children and in the developing nations is rising substantially. Most patients with diabetes die of the complications of atherosclerosis.

Bode, B. W., Sabbah, H., and Davidson, P. C. 2001. What's ahead in glucose monitoring? New techniques hold promise for improved ease and accuracy. *Postgraduate Medicine* 109:41–9.

▶ A review of the technologic advances in glucose monitoring, including easy-to-use meters and development of continuous glucose monitoring systems.

Boyle, M. P. 2007. Adult cystic fibrosis. *Journal of the American Medical Association* 298:1787–93.

▶ New methods of treatment and emphasis on nutritional support have greatly increased the survival of patients with cystic fibrosis and have also documented a number of mild cases that survive into middle age. The article describes principles of diagnosis and treatment, and describes the various complications resulting from the disease. The author suggests that the disease should be considered in adult patients presenting with any one of three conditions: bronchiectasis, chronic sinusitis with nasal polyps, or infertility in males. The value of the sweat test for screening is emphasized. The effectiveness of current treatment is illustrated by a 52-year-old man with cystic fibrosis who had few health or activity-limiting problems until his 40s.

Callery, M. P., and Freedman, S. D. 2008. A 21-year-old man with chronic pancreatitis. *Journal of the American Medical Association* 299:2589–94.

▶ Evaluation and treatment of chronic pancreatitis are considered based on the case history of a young man with pancreatitis having its onset at age 11 and recurring periodically. Causes and methods of treatment are discussed, including a rather limited role of surgical treatment. Some uncommon cases are caused by gene mutations, one of which is a different mutation of the same gene responsible for cystic fibrosis. Pancreatitis may also be a manifestation of an autoimmune disease targeting pancreatic tissue.

Ludwig, D. S., and Ebbeling, C. B. 2001. Type 2 diabetes mellitus in children: Primary care and public health considerations. *Journal of the American Medical Association* 286:1427–30.

▶ In prior years, type 2 diabetes occurred primarily in older overweight adults, and type 1 diabetes occurred in children and young adults. Now as many as half the new cases of diabetes in children are classified as type 2, which is related to the increasing prevalence of overweight children. Insulin resistance related to overweight causes the pancreas to secrete more insulin, eventually leading to failure of beta cell function. Many factors have contributed to childhood obesity and its most serious complication, which is type 2 diabetes.

McMahon, G. T., and Arky, R. A. 2007. Inhaled insulin for diabetes mellitus. *New England Journal of Medicine* 356:497–502.

▶ A review of the applications and limitations of a method for using insulin that does not require subcutaneous injection. A dry powder form of insulin was developed that can be inhaled using a specially designed inhaler to deliver the insulin into the pulmonary alveoli. However, there were several problems and potential complications associated with its use. It was not well received by diabetic patients, and the manufacturer discontinued the preparation, which is no longer available.

Mokdad, A. H., Bowman, B. A., Ford, E. S., et al. 2001. The continuing epidemic of obesity and diabetes in the United States. *Journal of the American Medical Association* 286:1195–200.

▶ As body mass index rises, so does the prevalence of type 2 diabetes.

Rosenbloom, A. L., Young, R. S., Joe, J. R., et al. 1999. The emerging epidemic of type 2 diabetes in youth. *Diabetes Care* 22:345–53.

▶ A review of the problem. Nonautoimmune forms of youth-onset diabetes are becoming more prevalent as rate of obesity in children and adolescents accelerates.

Rubinow, K. B., and Hirsch, I. B. 2011. Reexamining metrics for glucose control. *Journal of the American Medical Association* 305:1132–3.

► Glycated hemoglobin has assumed greater importance recently because a higher than normal concentration predicts vascular complications in persons with both type 1 and type 2 diabetes and has been promoted as the primary diagnostic test for diabetes and for making treatment decisions in diabetic patients. However, the test can be very unreliable and can provide misleading results because it is influenced by many factors, many of which are often encountered in ethnic groups prone to diabetes. For an individual patient, these limitations limit its usefulness for diagnosing diabetes, assessing the care of the diabetic patient and predicting diabetes-associated complications.

Weir, G. C. 1995. Which comes first in non-insulin-dependent diabetes mellitus: Insulin resistance or beta-cell failure? Both come first (Editorial). *Journal of the American Medical Association* 273:1878–9.

► This type of diabetes results from a mix of genetic and environmental factors that vary among different racial and ethnic groups.

Welsh, M. J. 2010. Targeting the basic defect in cystic fibrosis. *New England Journal of Medicine* 363:2056–57.

► The favorable results of this study indicate that drugs targeting the functions of *CFTR* can improve gene function and the patient's clinical condition.

Yoon, J. W., Austin, M., Onodera T., et al. 1979. Isolation of a virus from the pancreas of a child with diabetic ketoacidosis. *New England Journal of Medicine* 300:1173–9.

► A detailed investigative study.

OUTLINE SUMMARY

Structure and Function of the Pancreas

EXOCRINE FUNCTION
Secretes digestive enzymes.

ENDOCRINE FUNCTION
Islet alpha cells secrete glucagon: raise blood glucose.
Islet beta cells secrete insulin: lower blood glucose.
Islet delta cells secrete somatostatin, which inhibits insulin and glucagon secretion.

Pancreatitis

ACUTE PANCREATITIS
Pancreatic juice escapes from ducts and digests pancreas.
Serious illness with high mortality.

CHRONIC PANCREATITIS
Mild inflammation leading to progressive destruction of pancreatic tissue.

Cystic Fibrosis of the Pancreas

INCIDENCE
One in 3,000 whites, transmitted as autosomal recessive.
Rare in blacks and other races.

PATHOGENESIS
Responsible gene identified.
Tests available to identify carrier.
Cell dysfunction leads to thick mucus that plugs ducts.
Obstruction of pancreatic ducts causes atrophy and fibrosis of pancreas.
Obstruction of bronchi causes lung injury.
Obstruction of biliary ducts causes liver scarring.

SWEAT TEST IN CYSTIC FIBROSIS
Sweat gland function abnormal.
High concentration of sodium and chloride in sweat is basis of diagnostic test.

Diabetes Mellitus

TYPE 1 DIABETES
As a result of damage or destruction of islets.
Insulin secretion reduced or absent.
Develops chiefly in children and young adults.
Ketosis prone.

TYPE 2 DIABETES
More common type.
Insulin secretion normal or increased.
Tissues insensitive to insulin.
Not associated with ketosis.

PREDIABETES

Higher than normal glucose but not high enough to diagnose diabetes.

Progression to diabetes can be slowed or possibly prevented by diet, and exercise.

Some drugs are useful.

PREGNANCY-ASSOCIATED DIABETES

Hormones in pregnancy cause insulin resistance.

Some women unable to secrete enough insulin to compensate, and glucose rises.

Treatment by diet and insulin if needed.

Glucose returns to normal postpartum.

Increased long-term risk of permanent diabetes.

DIABETES AND THE METABOLIC SYNDROME

A group of conditions associated with insulin resistance.

Includes obesity, insulin resistance, abnormal blood lipids, and hypertension.

Screen overweight persons with abdominal obesity by checking blood pressure, blood glucose, and blood lipids.

Treat associated conditions when appropriate.

FAT METABOLISM AND FORMATION OF KETONE BODIES

Catabolism of fat yields acetate fragments (acetyl-CoA).

Converted by liver into ketone bodies.

BIOCHEMICAL DISTURBANCES IN DIABETES

Glucose absorbed but not utilized normally and accumulates in blood.

Excreted in urine with water and electrolytes.

Protein catabolism yields more glucose.

Ketoacidosis in type 1 diabetics.

Hyperosmolar nonketotic coma in type 2 diabetics.

> *Amount of insulin sufficient to prevent ketosis but not enough to prevent hyperglycemia.*
> *Hyperosmolarity of extracellular fluid as a result of hyperglycemia causes cellular dehydration.*

COMPLICATIONS OF DIABETES

Increased susceptibility to infection.

Diabetic coma.

Ketoacidosis.

Hyperosmolar coma.

Arteriosclerosis.

Blindness.

Renal failure.

Peripheral neuritis.

TREATMENT

Diet.

Insulin required for type 1 diabetes.

Oral hypoglycemic drugs or insulin for type 2 diabetes not controlled adequately by diet alone.

Hypoglycemia

PATHOGENESIS AND MANIFESTATIONS IN TYPE 1 DIABETIC SUBJECTS

Excessive insulin in relation to food intake.

As glucose falls, epinephrine is released by adrenal medulla, which mobilizes glucose from hepatic glycogen and exerts widespread systemic effects.

Neurologic manifestations occur because neurons are deprived of glucose, which is required for normal function.

Prolonged hypoglycemia causes permanent brain damage.

TREATMENT

Give oral carbohydrate if subject is conscious and able to swallow.

Inject glucagon or intravenous glucose solution if subject is unconscious.

OTHER CAUSES OF HYPOGLYCEMIA

Oral hypoglycemic drugs in type 2 diabetic patients.

Self-administration of oral hypoglycemic drugs or insulin by emotionally disturbed persons.

Rarely, islet cell tumor of pancreas.

Tumors of the Pancreas

CARCINOMA OF PANCREAS

Usually develops in head of pancreas.

Blockage of common bile duct causes obstructive jaundice.

ISLET CELL TUMORS

Beta cell tumors produce hyperinsulinism.

CHAPTER 23

The Gastrointestinal Tract

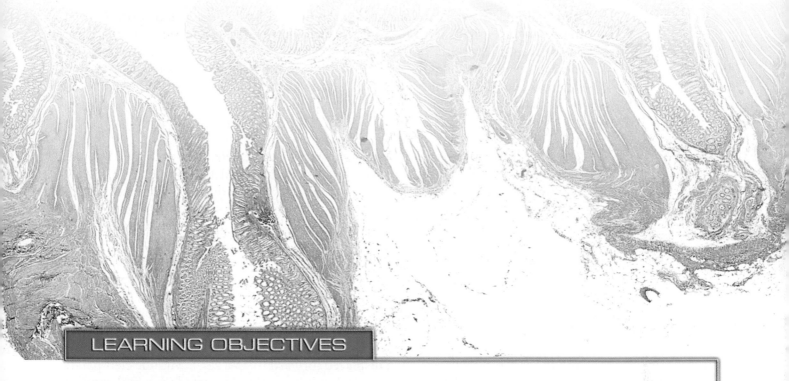

LEARNING OBJECTIVES

1 Identify the major types of cleft lip and cleft palate deformity.

2 Explain the pathogenesis of dental caries and periodontal disease, and describe prevention and treatment.

3 Name the common congenital abnormalities of the gastrointestinal tract. Describe their clinical manifestations, and explain the methods of diagnosis and treatment.

4 Name and describe the three most common lesions of the esophagus that lead to esophageal obstruction.

5 Explain the pathogenesis of peptic ulcer. Describe the three major complications of peptic ulcer and their treatment. Name the methods of treatment.

6 Describe the common types of chronic and acute enteritis and their clinical manifestations.

7 Differentiate between appendicitis and Meckel diverticulitis in terms of pathogenesis, clinical manifestations, and treatment.

8 Describe the pathogenesis of diverticulitis, and explain the role of diet in the development of lesion.

9 Name the causes, clinical manifestations, and complications of intestinal obstruction, carcinoma of the colon, and diverticulosis of the colon. Explain their treatment.

10 Understand the major eating disturbances and their effects.

Structure and Functions

The gastrointestinal tract, which is concerned with the digestion and absorption of food, comprises the oral cavity and related parts of the face, the esophagus, the stomach, the small and large intestines, and the anus.

Cleft Lip and Cleft Palate

Embryologically, the face and palate are formed by coalescence of proliferating masses of cells that merge to form the facial structures and to separate the nasal cavity from the mouth. In the upper part of the face, the areas of coalescence are located on either side of the midline in a line that passes through the upper lip and jaw and extends into each nostril. The palate is formed by two shelflike masses of tissue that grow medially and fuse in the midline to close the communication between nose and mouth. If these developmental processes are disturbed, defects may result in the upper lip and jaw (**cleft lip**) or in the palate (**cleft palate**).

Cleft lip and palate are common abnormalities that frequently occur in combination. The incidence of these abnormalities is about 1 per 1,000 births.

Both cleft lip and cleft palate follow a multifactorial pattern of inheritance, as discussed in congenital and hereditary diseases. The incidence is significantly higher among the children of parents who have previously given birth to an infant with a cleft lip or palate and among the children of parents who themselves have a cleft lip or palate.

Cleft lip may be unilateral or bilateral and may range in severity from a relatively minor defect in the mucosa of the lip to a large cleft extending deeply into the upper jaw. In the most severe deformity, the cleft extends completely through the upper jaw into the floor of the nose (complete cleft) and may also extend posteriorly into the palate (FIGURE 23-1). Large bilateral clefts extending into the palate completely separate the hard palate from the midline tissue that forms part of the upper jaw, and the separated tissue is often displaced forward (FIGURE 23-2). Midline cleft palate may occur as an isolated abnormality, but it is usually associated with unilateral or bilateral cleft lip. FIGURE 23-3 illustrates the various types of cleft lip and palate that are encountered clinically.

TREATMENT

Although cleft lip and palate frequently occur together, they are corrected surgically at different times. Generally, cleft lip is repaired very soon after birth. Repair of

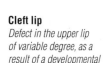

Cleft lip
Defect in the upper lip of variable degree, as a result of a developmental disturbance.

Cleft palate
Defect in hard palate allowing communication between oral cavity and nasal cavity, as a result of a developmental disturbance.

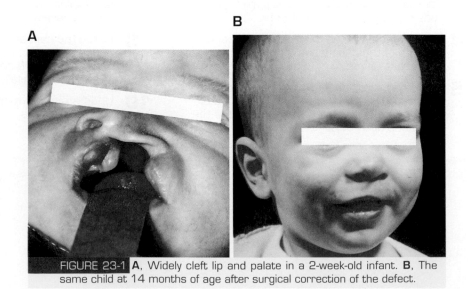

FIGURE 23-1 **A**, Widely cleft lip and palate in a 2-week-old infant. **B**, The same child at 14 months of age after surgical correction of the defect.

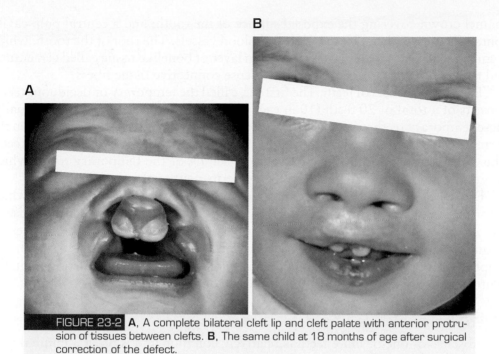

FIGURE 23-2 **A**, A complete bilateral cleft lip and cleft palate with anterior protrusion of tissues between clefts. **B**, The same child at 18 months of age after surgical correction of the defect.

cleft palate is generally deferred until the child is between 1 and 2 years old. After the cleft palate is repaired, speech therapy is begun in early childhood to correct the nasal quality that often results from abnormal palatal function.

Abnormalities of Tooth Development

The teeth are specialized structures developed in the tissues of the jaws. Each tooth consists of a solid portion called **dentine**, which forms the bulk of the tooth; an

Dentine
(den'tēn)
Bony structure of the tooth.

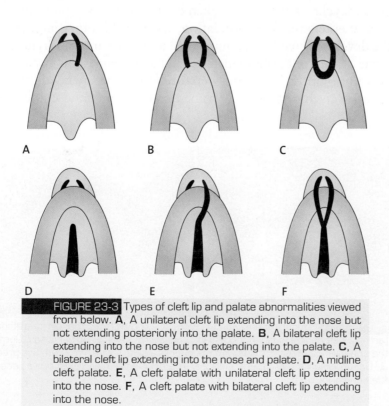

FIGURE 23-3 Types of cleft lip and palate abnormalities viewed from below. **A**, A unilateral cleft lip extending into the nose but not extending posteriorly into the palate. **B**, A bilateral cleft lip extending into the nose but not extending into the palate. **C**, A bilateral cleft lip extending into the nose and palate. **D**, A midline cleft palate. **E**, A cleft palate with unilateral cleft lip extending into the nose. **F**, A cleft palate with bilateral cleft lip extending into the nose.

enamel crown covering the exposed surface of the tooth; and a central pulp cavity containing nerve fibers, lymphatics, and blood vessels. The root of the tooth, which is embedded in the jaw, is covered by a thin layer of bonelike tissue called cementum, and the tooth is anchored in the jaw by dense connective tissue fibers.

There are two sets of teeth. The first set, called the temporary or deciduous teeth, consists of a total of 20 teeth (10 in each jaw) that erupt in childhood. Eventually, these temporary teeth are replaced by a second, permanent set of 32 teeth. When the permanent teeth begin to grow, they press against the roots of the temporary teeth. This causes resorption of the roots and loosening of the temporary teeth, which eventually fall out and are replaced by the permanent teeth.

Each deciduous and permanent tooth develops from a separate tooth bud, which is composed of two parts: one that forms the crown and a second that gives rise to the remainder of the tooth. The deciduous teeth are formed before birth and erupt during childhood. The permanent teeth do not begin to develop until after birth and erupt at various times in late childhood and adolescence. Calcium is deposited in the dentine and enamel of the tooth as it is being formed.

MISSING TEETH AND EXTRA TEETH

The absence of one or more teeth is relatively common and is often a familial trait that follows a multifactorial pattern of inheritance (FIGURE 23-4). It results from failure of one or more tooth buds to develop. Sometimes an extra tooth bud forms, resulting in an extra tooth.

ABNORMALITIES OF TOOTH ENAMEL CAUSED BY TETRACYCLINE

Enamel forms within the developing teeth at specific times. If the antibiotic tetracycline is administered while enamel is being formed in the teeth, the antibiotic is deposited with calcium in the enamel and causes permanent yellow-gray to brown discoloration in the crowns. The antibiotic may also disturb the formation of the enamel. If a tetracycline antibiotic is taken by a pregnant woman, the drug crosses the placenta and enters the fetal circulation, where it becomes incorporated in the enamel of the developing teeth. If administered to infants and children, tetracycline is deposited in the crowns of the permanent teeth that are undergoing enamel formation at the time the antibiotic is ingested. Therefore, it is recommended that tetracycline antibiotics not be given to pregnant women or to infants and children during the

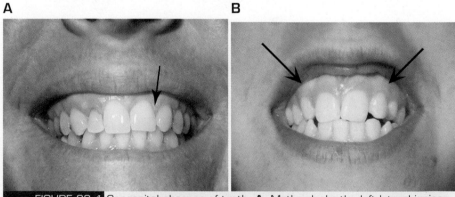

A   **B**

FIGURE 23-4 Congenital absence of teeth. **A**, Mother lacks the left lateral incisor (*arrow*). Left canine (cuspid) tooth is located lateral to left central incisor. Compare the appearance of the left side with the opposite side in which all teeth are present. **B**, Daughter lacks both lateral incisors. The canine teeth (*arrows*) are adjacent to the central incisors.

time when enamel is forming in the developing permanent teeth. This period extends through infancy and childhood to about the age of 8 years.

Dental Caries and Its Complications

The oral cavity contains a diverse collection of both aerobic and anaerobic bacteria. Masses of these bacteria intermixed with bacterial products and proteins from saliva form aggregates called **dental plaque** that adhere to the teeth and predispose to tooth decay.

    Caries, the term for tooth decay, is a Latin word meaning dry rot. The condition is a decalcification of the tooth structure caused by mouth bacteria acting on bits of retained food material, such as sugar and highly refined, starchy foods. Bacterial fermentation liberates organic acids that erode the covering enamel, exposing the underlying dentine, which is attacked by the acids and invaded by mouth bacteria. The loss of tooth structure that results from the combined acid and bacterial action is called a dental **cavity**. The affected area appears discolored and is quite soft when probed with a dental instrument. Dental x-rays reveal the cavity as an area of decreased density in the affected tooth.

    If the cavity is not treated and continues to enlarge, the decay eventually reaches the dental pulp. The bacteria invade the pulp and incite an inflammation that causes the throbbing pain characteristic of a toothache. Unchecked, the infection may spread to the apex of the tooth root, which is embedded in the jawbone, and from there spread to the bone surrounding the dental root. The result may be an abscess surrounding the apex of the tooth, which is called a periapical abscess (*peri* = around).

PREVENTION AND TREATMENT

The incidence of tooth decay can be reduced by proper mouth hygiene, including frequent brushing of the teeth and use of dental floss to remove food particles that promote bacterial growth. Fluoride added to water supplies and toothpaste helps to prevent cavities by promoting formation of a more acid-resistant tooth structure that resists decay. Dental caries is treated by removing the decayed area and packing the defect with some type of dental filling material. After infection of the pulp and dental root has occurred, more extensive treatment is required. Antibiotics may be needed if there is an acute infection or abscess at the apex of the tooth. After the infection is under control, the entire pulp cavity must be cleaned out and packed with dental filling material, a procedure called a root canal treatment. Sometimes the tooth cannot be salvaged and must be extracted.

Periodontal Disease

Masses of bacteria and debris accumulating around the base of the teeth may incite an inflammation. Initially, the inflammation affects only the gums surrounding the roots of the teeth, which is called gingivitis (*gingiva* = gum). Later, the inflammation extends between the teeth and the adjacent gums, leading to the formation of small pockets of infection between the teeth and gums. This condition is called periodontal disease (*peri* = around + *dens* = tooth). If pus is discharged from the margins of the infected gums, the descriptive term pyorrhea (*pyo* = pus + *rhea* = flow) is often used. The infection may spread into the tooth sockets that anchor the teeth in the jawbone, causing the teeth to loosen and eventually fall out. Various methods of treatment to the gums and teeth may control or arrest the condition, which is an important cause of loss of teeth.

Dental plaque
Masses of bacteria, bacterial products, and salivary proteins adherent to teeth, which predisposes to tooth decay.

Caries
(ka′rēz)
Tooth decay.

Cavity (dental)
A loss of tooth structure caused by the combined action of mouth bacteria and organic acids derived from bacterial fermentation of retained food particles.

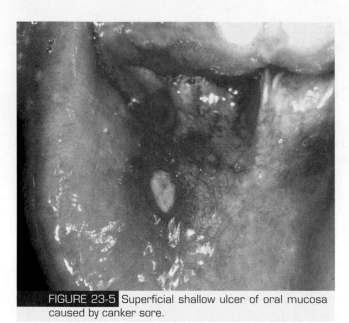

FIGURE 23-5 Superficial shallow ulcer of oral mucosa caused by canker sore.

Stomatitis
(stō-mäh-tī′tis)
Inflammation of the oral cavity.

Inflammation of the Oral Cavity

An inflammation of the oral cavity is called **stomatitis** (*stoma* = mouth). It may be caused by a number of irritants and infectious agents. Common irritants are alcohol, tobacco, and hot or spicy foods. Infectious agents include the herpes virus and some other viruses, the fungus *Candida albicans* (which also causes vaginal infections), and certain bacteria that cause a type of infection called trench mouth or Vincent infection.

Canker sores are another relatively common inflammatory disease involving the oral cavity. A canker sore appears as a small painful superficial ulcer of the oral mucosa surrounded by a narrow zone of inflammation that appears as a red border surrounding the ulcer (FIGURE 23-5). We do not know what causes canker sores, and there is no specific treatment for this condition, although various measures can reduce the discomfort caused by the ulcers.

Tumors of the Oral Cavity

Carcinoma of the oral cavity, which may arise from the squamous epithelium of the lips, cheek, tongue, palate, or back of the throat, is relatively common (FIGURE 23-6). It is treated by surgical resection or by radiation therapy.

Diseases of the Esophagus

The esophagus is a muscular tube extending from the pharynx to the stomach with sphincters at both upper and lower ends. The upper sphincter relaxes to allow passage of swallowed food, which is propelled down the esophagus by rhythmic peristaltic contractions. The lower esophageal sphincter (called the gastroesophageal or cardiac sphincter) relaxes when the food reaches the lower end of the esophagus and allows the food to pass into the stomach. Some of the more important conditions affecting the esophagus include the following:

1. Failure of the lower (cardiac) sphincter to function properly
2. Tears in the lining of the esophagus from retching and vomiting
3. Esophageal obstruction as a result of carcinoma, food impaction, or stricture

Symptoms of esophageal disease include difficulty in swallowing (dysphagia) together with

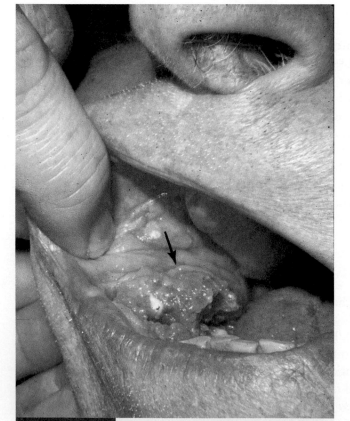

FIGURE 23-6 Squamous cell carcinoma of oral mucosa (*arrow*), which appears as an irregular overgrowth of tissue arising from the mucosa of the cheek.

variable degrees of substernal discomfort or pain. Complete obstruction of the esophagus leads to inability to swallow, which is often associated with regurgitation of food into the trachea, causing episodes of choking and coughing.

CARDIAC SPHINCTER DYSFUNCTION

The two major disturbances of cardiac sphincter function are failure of the cardiac sphincter to open properly, which is called cardiospasm, and inability of the sphincter to remain closed properly, which is called an incompetent cardiac sphincter, and leads to a condition called reflux esophagitis.

Cardiospasm

Sometimes the cardiac sphincter fails to open properly, caused by a malfunction of the nerve plexuses in the esophagus that control its functions. As a result, food cannot pass normally into the stomach, and the smooth muscle in the wall of the esophagus must contract more vigorously to force the food past the constricted sphincter. Eventually the esophageal muscle undergoes marked hypertrophy, and the esophagus becomes dilated proximal to the constricted sphincter because of food retention. Treatment consists of periodic stretching of the sphincter by means of an instrument introduced into the esophagus or by surgically cutting the muscle fibers in the constricted area. An alternative treatment in selected cases consists of injecting botulinum toxin into the sphincter through an esophagoscope. The toxin blocks the transmission of nerve impulses from the nerve plexuses to the muscle fibers for several months, which relaxes the sphincter and relieves the patient's symptoms.

Incompetent Cardiac Sphincter and Its Complications

In this relatively common condition, acid gastric juice leaks back into the esophagus through the improperly closed incompetent lower esophageal sphincter. The squamous epithelial lining of the esophagus, which was not "designed" to tolerate high-acid secretions, becomes irritated and inflamed, which is called **reflux esophagitis**. In some patients, the squamous mucosal lining may actually become ulcerated and scarred. Sometimes the squamous lining responds to the acidity by undergoing a change (metaplasia) into a more acid-resistant columnar gastric type mucosa. This condition, which is called Barrett esophagus after the person who first described it, may lead to additional problems. Unfortunately, the metaplastic columnar epithelium is frequently abnormal and poses an increased risk of developing adenocarcinoma arising in the abnormal columnar epithelium. Treatment of reflux esophagitis consists of avoiding lying down soon after eating because the recumbent position promotes reflux, sleeping with the head of the bed elevated to minimize reflux, and avoiding alcoholic beverages because alcohol not only stimulates gastric acid secretion but also tends to relax the lower esophageal sphincter, which facilitates reflux. Drugs that reduce secretion of gastric acid and antacids that neutralize gastric acid are helpful.

Reflux esophagitis
Inflammation of the lining of the esophagus caused by reflux of acidic gastric secretions through an incompetent lower gastroesophageal sphincter.

GASTRIC MUCOSAL TEARS

Retching and vomiting may cause tears in the mucosa of the gastroesophageal junction where the esophagus passes through the diaphragm or in the lining of the distal esophagus, and these tears can bleed profusely (FIGURE 23-7). The repetitive, intermittent, vigorous contractions of the abdominal muscles associated with vomiting raise intra-abdominal pressure and forcefully jam the upper part (cardia) of the stomach against the opening in the diaphragm through which the esophagus passes, causing tears in the mucosa. The additional stresses resulting from vigorous contractions of the muscular walls of the stomach and esophagus associated with vomiting probably place

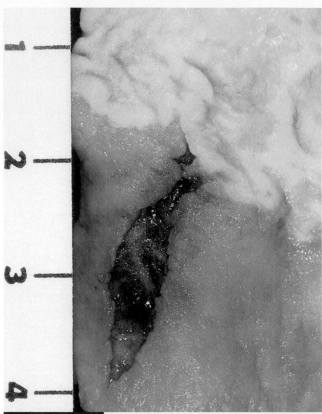

FIGURE 23-7 Gastric mucosal tear caused by retching and vomiting. The opaque mucosa in the upper part of the photograph is the normal stratified squamomus mucosa of the esophagus. The 2 cm long tear extends distally from the gastroesophageal junction and caused a fatal gastric hemorrhage.

additional stress on the mucosa, which also plays a role in causing the laceration. This vomiting-related complication most often follows the retching and vomiting related to excess alcohol intake but may follow vomiting from any cause, including self-induced vomiting to control weight.

ESOPHAGEAL OBSTRUCTION

Carcinoma of the Esophagus

Carcinoma may arise anywhere in the esophagus, either from the squamous epithelium or from the columnar epithelium associated with Barrett esophagus. The tumor gradually narrows the lumen of the esophagus, frequently infiltrates the surrounding tissues, and may invade the trachea. Necrosis of the tumor extending between the esophagus and trachea may lead to the formation of an abnormal communication between these two structures called a tracheoesophageal fistula (*fistula* = tube).

Food Impaction

Obstruction of the esophagus may be caused by impaction of poorly chewed meat in the distal part of the esophagus. This is sometimes encountered in persons who are unable to chew their food properly because they have poor teeth or improperly fitting dentures or who have poor eating habits.

Stricture

A stricture is a narrowing caused by scar tissue. Reflux esophagitis with ulceration and scarring may lead to a stricture. Esophageal scarring may also result from accidentally or deliberately swallowing a corrosive chemical that causes necrosis and inflammation. Severe scarring eventually follows. A common cause of esophageal stricture in children is accidental swallowing of commercial lye solutions (used for cleaning clogged drains).

Gastritis

Inflammation of the stomach is called gastritis, and the inflammation may be either acute or chronic. Many patients with gastritis have few symptoms, but some experience abdominal discomfort and nausea.

ACUTE GASTRITIS

In most cases, acute gastritis is a self-limited inflammation of short duration. However, at times, the acute inflammation may be quite severe and may be complicated by ulceration of the mucosa with bleeding from the ulcerated areas. Patients in whom the acute gastritis is associated with mucosal ulceration often have more pronounced symptoms, and the ulcerated areas may bleed profusely.

There are many causes of acute gastritis, but most are caused by nonsteroidal anti-inflammatory drugs such as aspirin, ibuprofen, and naproxen. These drugs are widely used to treat symptoms of arthritis and related musculoskeletal pain problems. The drugs act by inhibiting an enzyme called cyclooxygenase that is required for the synthesis of prostaglandins, which are potent mediators as discussed in inflammation and repair. Prostaglandins, however, are produced by many different cells and have many different functions.

Those produced by gastric epithelial cells help protect the stomach from the damaging effects of gastric acid by promoting the secretion not only of sodium bicarbonate to counteract the acid but also of mucin to coat and protect the stomach lining. Nonsteroidal anti-inflammatory drugs reduce inflammation by inhibiting the synthesis of prostaglandin mediators of inflammation, but they also inhibit the synthesis of the prostaglandins that help protect the gastric mucosa. Consequently, the mucosa becomes more vulnerable to injury from acidic gastric juice, which may lead to acute inflammation of the mucosa and may even be followed by mucosal ulceration with bleeding.

There are actually two forms of cyclooxygenase. One form (abbreviated COX-1) promotes the synthesis of the prostaglandins that protect the gastric mucosa. The other form (abbreviated COX-2) is involved in the synthesis of the prostaglandins that function as mediators of inflammation, which are responsible for the joint and muscle inflammation in patients with musculoskeletal problems. Many nonsteroidal anti-inflammatory drugs inhibit both forms of the enzyme, which suppresses inflammation by inhibiting COX-2, but puts the gastric mucosa at risk by also inhibiting COX-1. Some nonsteroidal anti-inflammatory drugs are more selective. They are called COX-2 inhibitors because they inhibit primarily the COX-2 enzyme that promotes inflammation, but have much less effect on the COX-1 enzyme that helps protect the gastric mucosa. Unfortunately, patients treated with COX-2 inhibitors had a higher risk of heart attacks and strokes than did a comparable group treated with less selective nonsteroidal anti-inflammatory drugs. Now most physicians favor limiting the use of COX-2 inhibitors unless their benefits outweigh the possible cardiovascular risks.

Excess ingestion of alcoholic beverages is another common cause of acute gastritis because the alcohol is a gastric irritant and also stimulates gastric acid secretion.

CHRONIC GASTRITIS AND ITS COMPLICATIONS: THE ROLE OF *HELICOBACTER PYLORI*

Many cases of chronic gastritis are related to growth (colonization) of a small, curved, gram-negative organism called *Helicobacter pylori* on the surface of the gastric mucosa. This unique organism grows in the layer of mucus covering the epithelial cells lining the stomach, where it can be identified by special bacterial stains, by culture, or by other specialized tests. The organism produces an enzyme called urease that decomposes urea, a normal by-product of protein metabolism that is present in small amounts in blood and body fluids. Decomposition of urea yields ammonia, a substance that neutralizes the gastric acid and allows the organism to flourish in an acid environment that would destroy other bacteria. *Helicobacter* also produces enzymes that can break down the layer of protective mucus that covers the epithelial surface. Presumably, the chronic gastritis is caused by the ammonia and other products produced by the organism that damage the gastric mucosa of susceptible persons.

Colonization of the gastric mucosa by *Helicobacter pylori* is very common, and not all persons who harbor the organism have chronic gastritis. Moreover, many persons harbor the organism, and the frequency of bacterial colonization increases with age. About 30% of persons younger than 30 years of age are colonized by *Helicobacter pylori*. By age 50, the proportion increases to about 50% and may be as high as 65% in persons older than age 65. The organism is spread from person-to-person in households by close contacts. The spread of the organisms appears to be by mouth-to-mouth contact and also by the fecal–oral route because the organism has been cultured from both dental plaque material and from fecal material.

There are also some uncommon but important long-term harmful effects of *Helicobacter* infection. Chronic gastritis caused by this organism slightly increases the risk of two different gastric tumors: gastric carcinoma and malignant lymphoma arising from lymphocytes in the gastric mucosa (called mucosa-associated lymphoid tissue). The gastric carcinoma risk occurs because the gastritis often leads to atrophy of the gastric mucosa and causes the gastric epithelium to change into an abnormal intestinal-type epithelium (a process called intestinal metaplasia). It is these cellular changes in the gastric mucosa that predispose to gastric carcinoma. The lymphoma risk probably results because the gastritis overstimulates the mucosa-associated lymphoid tissue, which may lead to unregulated growth of lympho-cytes that eventually progresses to gastric lymphoma.

Acute Gastroenteritis

An inflammation involving the intestine as well as the stomach is called a gastroen-teritis, and most are acute infections. Many different infectious organisms may cause acute gastroenteritis, but most cases are caused by RNA viruses. The condition is characterized by an abrupt onset of nausea, vomiting, abdominal cramps, and profuse diarrhea, which may affect only a few persons or may occur as an epidemic affecting large numbers of persons. Usually, the illness subsides spontaneously within a few days and no specific treatment is required, although severely affected persons may require intravenous fluids to replace depleted body fluids and electrolytes resulting from the diarrhea.

Norovirus
An extremely infectious RNA virus easily spread from person to person and by contaminated food or water

Some viruses (rotaviruses, astroviruses, and enteroviruses) affect primarily in-fants and young children and do not spread widely in the community. In contrast, another virus called a **norovirus** is more likely to infect adults and older children and may spread as an epidemic to infect many people. Previously, the virus was called Norwalk virus because it was identified first at a school in Norwalk, Ohio, where it infected half the students in the school, and then spread to infect teachers, family members, and other adults in the community. The virus is an extremely infectious RNA virus easily spread from person-to-person by hand-to-hand transmission, or by virus-contaminated food or water. The virus is resistant to inactivation by freez-ing, heating, and by many disinfectants, and only a few virus particles are enough to cause an infection. Although norovirus infections may occur sporadically and spread only to family members, epidemics may occur when large groups of persons are in close contact, as in schools, military bases, summer camps, cruise ships, nursing homes, hospitals, and restaurants. It is estimated that about 90% of cases of acute gastroenteritis are caused by the norovirus. There are many strains of norovirus, and a recent infection may provide some temporary immunity against the strain that caused the infection, but does not protect against other strains of the virus.

Peptic Ulcer

Peptic ulcer is a chronic ulcer that usually involves the distal stomach or proximal duodenum (FIGURE 23-8). The ulcer results from digestion of the mucosa by acid gastric juice. Persons who secrete large volumes of acidic gastric juice are prone to ulcers.

The initial event is probably a small, superficial erosion of the gastric or duode-nal mucosa. Gastric acid and pepsin begin to digest the deeper tissues, which have

A B

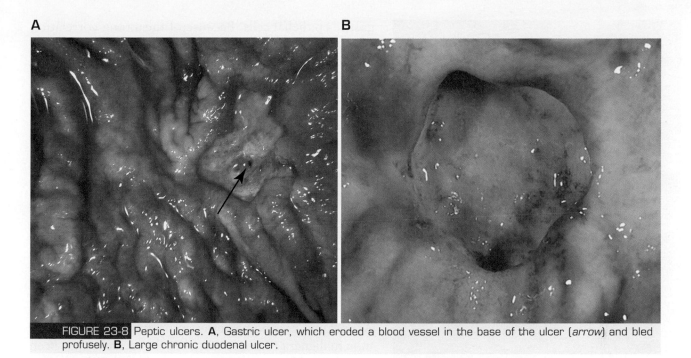

FIGURE 23-8 Peptic ulcers. **A**, Gastric ulcer, which eroded a blood vessel in the base of the ulcer (*arrow*) and bled profusely. **B**, Large chronic duodenal ulcer.

been denuded of covering epithelium. Attempts at healing in the presence of continuing digestion eventually lead to considerable scarring at the base of the ulcer. Clinically, ulcers produce pain that is usually relieved by ingestion of food or antacids that neutralize the gastric acid.

Helicobacter pylori, the same organism that is associated with chronic gastritis, also plays an important role in the pathogenesis of both gastric and duodenal ulcers. Presumably, the organism injures the mucosa and initiates the mucosal erosion that eventually develops into a chronic ulcer. The role of *Helicobacter* in causing a gastric ulcer is understandable because this is the same organism that causes the mucosal damage leading to chronic gastritis. Its role in causing duodenal ulcers is more difficult to explain because the organism characteristically colonizes gastric mucosa, not duodenal mucosa. Some investigators have speculated that there are small areas of gastric epithelial cells in the duodenum where the organism can grow and damage the duodenal mucosa, making it more susceptible to ulceration. An alternative explanation postulates that the organism does not damage the duodenal mucosa directly, but does so indirectly because the *Helicobacter*-induced gastritis causes the gastric mucosa to secrete excess acid, and it is the hyperacidity that causes the duodenal ulcers. According to this concept, the mucosal damage caused by the gastritis disturbs various functions of gastric mucosal cells that regulate gastric acid secretion and causes the mucosa to secrete excess acid which leads to the duodenal ulceration.

Peptic ulcer has complications: hemorrhage (bleeding), perforation, and obstruction. An ulcer that erodes into a large blood vessel may cause severe hemorrhage. An ulcer may also erode completely through the wall of the stomach or duodenum, causing a perforation of the wall through which gastric and duodenal contents leak into the peritoneal cavity, resulting in a generalized inflammation of the peritoneum, the membrane that lines the abdominal cavity and covers the exterior of the abdominal organs. The inflammation is called peritonitis. Sometimes the scarring that follows healing of a gastric ulcer may be so severe as to cause obstruction of the outlet of the stomach, called the pylorus, preventing the stomach from emptying properly.

Peptic ulcer is generally treated by antacids, which neutralize the excess gastric acid and promote healing of the ulcer, or by drugs that block the secretion of acid by the

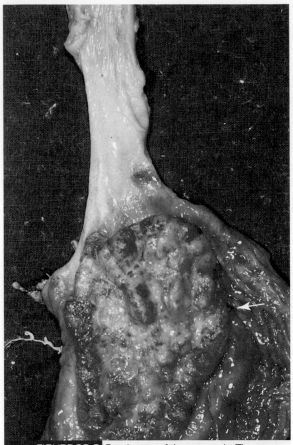

FIGURE 23-9 Carcinoma of the stomach. The stomach has been opened revealing a large ulcerated neoplasm arising from gastric mucosa (*arrow*) and extending upward to gastroesophageal junction. Esophagus is seen in upper part of photograph.

gastric epithelial cells. Because of the strong correlation between *Helicobacter pylori* and peptic ulcers, patients with ulcers who are colonized by this organism are often treated not only with drugs to neutralize gastric acid or suppress its secretion, but also with antibiotics and other medications to eradicate *Helicobacter pylori*. A large number of laboratory tests are available to identify the presence of *Helicobacter* in the gastric mucosa. Combined antacid and antimicrobial therapy in patients who are colonized by *Helicobacter* leads to faster healing of the ulcers and fewer recurrences than antacid treatment alone.

Surgical treatment is sometimes required if medical therapy fails to heal the ulcer or if complications develop.

Carcinoma of the Stomach

At one time, carcinoma of the stomach was the most common malignant tumor in men, but the incidence has been decreasing. The initial symptom may be only vague upper abdominal discomfort. Sometimes the first manifestation is an iron deficiency anemia, the result of chronic blood loss from the ulcerated surface of the tumor. Gastric carcinoma is treated by resection of a large part of the stomach together with the surrounding tissues and draining lymph nodes (FIGURE 23-9). Unfortunately, a gastric carcinoma is often far advanced by the time it causes symptoms; consequently, long-term survival of patients with stomach carcinoma is relatively poor. Sometimes, gastric carcinoma may produce symptoms similar to those of a benign peptic ulcer. At times, it may be difficult for the physician to determine whether a patient has a benign peptic ulcer of the stomach or an ulcerated gastric carcinoma. The distinction can usually be made by gastroscopy, an examination in which a flexible gastroscope is passed into the stomach so that the physician can visualize the lesion and take biopsy specimens from various areas.

Inflammatory Disease of the Intestine

Enteritis
(en-ter-ī′tis)
Inflammation of the intestine.

Colitis
(kō-lī′tis)
Inflammation of the colon, such as chronic ulcerative colitis.

The intestine may be the site of both acute and chronic inflammation. The term **enteritis** (*enteron* = bowel) is used to describe inflammation of any part of the intestinal tract. The term **colitis** denotes inflammation restricted to the colon, and the general term bowel inflammation refers to any part of the intestinal tract, either small intestine, colon, or both.

ACUTE ENTERITIS

Acute intestinal infections are usually caused by known pathogens or their toxins, as described in the discussions on pathogenic micro-organisms and animal parasites. They are generally of short duration and may subside without specific treatment, or may respond to appropriate antibiotics or other agents. Clinical manifestations include nausea, vomiting, abdominal discomfort, and passage of many loose stools. In severe infections, the bowel mucosa may be ulcerated, and the diarrheal stools may be bloody.

CHRONIC ENTERITIS

Chronic enteritis is less common and more difficult to treat. The two important types of chronic enteritis are Crohn disease and chronic ulcerative colitis. Often, the two diseases are grouped together under the general term chronic inflammatory bowel disease. Both diseases tend to be chronic, with periodic flare-ups manifested by cramplike abdominal pain and diarrhea, followed by periods when the disease is inactive. During periods of activity, the affected persons may also have systemic manifestations, including joint inflammation, eye inflammation, and various types of skin nodules and skin infections. Although the diseases have many similarities, there are also significant differences between them.

These two diseases appear to be autoimmune diseases as described in the discussion on immunity, hypersensetivity, allergy, and autoimmune diseases, and recent studies have provided further insight into their pathogenesis. Several factors working together appear to trigger the autoimmune response that leads to these diseases:

1. The ability of the immune system to regulate the immune response, which is genetically determined, is impaired in affected persons.
2. In contrast to normal bowel epithelium, which prevents the normal bacterial flora in the bowel from invading the bowel wall, the intestinal epithelium of persons with chronic enteritis is less able to resist invasion by intestinal bacteria, which is called defective epithelial barrier function.
3. Because barrier function is defective, intestinal bacteria can penetrate the epithelium and extend into the deeper tissues. The bacteria are recognized as foreign antigens by the immune system, which generates an intense cell-mediated immune response to destroy the bacteria.
4. The activated T lymphocytes and their destructive cytokines are responsible for the intestinal inflammation and necrosis in persons with chronic enteritis. However, we do not know whether the inflammatory reaction that damages the bowel is directed against intestinal bacteria that get into the intestinal wall periodically because epithelial barrier function is defective, or is an autoimmune response directed against the patient's own cells because they contain some of the same antigenic determinants (cross-reacting antigens) as those possessed by the intestinal bacteria to which the immune system has responded.

Crohn Disease

Crohn disease is a chronic inflammation and ulceration of the bowel mucosa with marked thickening and scarring of the bowel wall (FIGURE 23-10). The distal ileum is a frequently involved site. The inflammation often affects scattered areas of the small bowel, leaving normal intervening segments of bowel (called "skip areas") between the areas of severe disease. Occasionally, affected persons have such severe thickening and scarring of an involved segment of bowel that the lumen becomes greatly narrowed or even completely blocked, which impedes passage of bowel contents. Crohn disease was originally called regional ileitis because the inflammatory process is often localized to the distal ileum, but now we know that the disease is not restricted to the ileum. Other parts of the small intestine may also be involved, and the disease may involve the colon as well.

Chronic Ulcerative Colitis

In contrast to Crohn disease, chronic ulcerative colitis targets the colon, not the small intestine. The inflammation is limited to the mucosa, and the bowel wall is not thickened as in Crohn disease. Frequently, the disease begins in the rectal mucosa

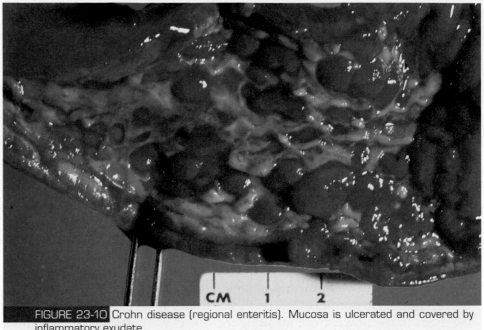

FIGURE 23-10 Crohn disease (regional enteritis). Mucosa is ulcerated and covered by inflammatory exudate.

but may spread progressively until eventually the entire colon is involved. In severe cases, the ulcerated mucosa may bleed profusely, leading to bloody diarrhea, and at times the inflammatory process becomes so extensive that it leads to a perforation of the colon with escape of bowel contents into the peritoneal cavity. Affected persons with long-standing disease also may develop carcinoma arising in the diseased regions of the colon or rectum.

Treament of Chronic Enteritis

Treatment of inflammatory bowel disease involves symptomatic and supportive measures, including antibiotics and corticosteroid hormones to control disease symptoms during flare-ups, and immunosuppressive drugs. Eventually, surgical resection of severely diseased bowel segments may be required in many patients. Persons with severe and extensive chronic ulcerative colitis may require total removal of the entire colon and rectum, both to control the disease and also to eliminate the risk of colon carcinoma, which is prone to occur in patients with long-standing chronic disease.

ANTIBIOTIC-ASSOCIATED COLITIS

Some persons taking broad-spectrum antibiotics develop mild diarrhea. Others, unfortunately, develop severe bloody diarrhea with abdominal pain, fever, and other systemic manifestations, which may be life threatening. In the mild cases, the intestinal mucosa is slightly inflamed. In the more severely affected persons, there are multiple ulcerations of the colonic mucosa, and the ulcerated areas are covered by masses of fibrin and inflammatory cells.

The broad-spectrum antibiotics cause the colitis by changing the intestinal bacterial flora. Most of the normal flora is destroyed by the broad-spectrum antibiotic. This allows overgrowth of an anaerobic spore-forming intestinal bacterium called *Clostridium difficile* (pronounced dif-fís-sill) that is not inhibited by the antibiotic. The organism produces two toxins that cause the intestinal inflammation and necrosis.

The diagnosis of antibiotic-associated colitis is established by detection of the bacterial toxin in the stool and by identification of the organism in stool cultures. Treatment consists of stopping the antibiotic, and in severe cases, giving a drug that inhibits anaerobic bacteria (metronidazole) or an antibiotic (vancomycin), which inhibits growth of the organism. Treatment should not include drugs that reduce the diarrhea by inhibiting intestinal motility. Such drugs prolong the illness by allowing the injurious clostridial toxins to remain in the intestine instead of being eliminated rapidly in the diarrheal stools.

Unfortunately, *C. difficile* has acquired increased virulence. Previously useful antibiotics have become less effective, and the infection may recur within 60 days after apparently successful treatment. Consequently, the incidence of the infection has more than doubled since the original cases were reported, which makes the infection the most common cause of bacterial diarrhea in the United States. Some patients have multiple recurrences of infection over several months or years, which can spread to infect other hospitalized patients. Current treatment is directed to restoring the normal bacterial population in the colon in order to discourage growth of *C. difficile* and to treat recurrences with an antibiotic that is least likely to be followed by a recurrent infection. One promising method to supplement antibiotics and reduce recurrences consists of administration of a single infusion of antibodies directed against toxins A and B, which reduces recurrences. Other studies are underway to find new antibiotics and other methods of treatment that may be able to achieve a more permanent cure of the infection.

APPENDICITIS

Appendicitis is the most common inflammatory lesion of the bowel. In many animals, the portion of the bowel represented in humans by the appendix is a large, wide caliber intestinal segment, similar in appearance to the remainder of the colon. In humans, this segment of bowel is reduced in both size and caliber to the extent that it is a vestigial structure.

The high incidence of acute appendicitis is due primarily to the narrow caliber of the appendix, the base of which often becomes plugged by firm bits of fecal material. Because of the obstruction, the secretions normally produced by the epithelial cells lining the appendix drain poorly from the area distal to the blockage. The accumulated secretions create pressure within the appendiceal lumen. This compresses the blood vessels in the mucosa, impairing its viability (FIGURE 23-11). Bacteria normally present in the appendix and colon invade the devitalized wall, causing an acute inflammation.

Clinically, appendicitis is characterized by generalized abdominal pain that soon becomes localized to the right lower part (quadrant) of the abdomen. Examination of the abdomen reveals localized tenderness over the appendix when pressure is applied

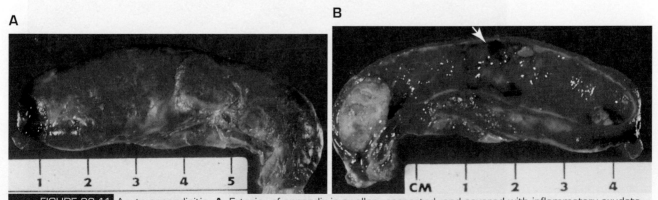

A

B

FIGURE 23-11 Acute appendicitis. **A**, Exterior of appendix is swollen, congested, and covered with inflammatory exudate. **B**, Appendix bisected to reveal interior. Pus within lumen has been removed. Mucosa is congested and ulcerated (*arrow*). The base of the appendix (*left side* of photograph) is plugged by a firm mass of fecal material.

to the abdomen by the fingers of the examiner. Often, the patient also experiences pain when the pressure is released suddenly (rebound tenderness). In addition, there is usually reflex contraction of the abdominal muscles (abdominal rigidity) in response to the underlying inflammation. Laboratory tests reveal that the number of polymorphonuclear leukocytes in the blood also is increased as a result of the infection. Sometimes it may be difficult to distinguish appendicitis from other conditions with similar manifestations, such as acute gastroenteritis or a gynecologic problem in a young woman such as a fallopian tube infection (salpingitis) or ruptured ovarian cyst. When the diagnosis is uncertain, other diagnostic studies such as ultrasound or CT examination, or even a laparoscopy, may help establish the correct diagnosis and lead to appropriate treatment.

Mild cases of appendicitis may heal spontaneously. More severe inflammation may lead to rupture of the appendix and peritonitis. For this reason, it is essential to identify appendicitis and remove the appendix in any patient in whom appendicitis is suspected.

MECKEL DIVERTICULUM

During embryonic development, the small intestine is connected for a time to the yolk sac of the embryo by means of a narrow tubular channel called the vitelline duct (*vitellus* = yolk). Normally, the duct disappears along with the yolk sac, and no trace persists in the adult. In about 2% of persons, however, a remnant of the vitelline duct persists as a small tubular outpouching from the distal ileum about 12–18 in proximal to the cecum. This structure is called a Meckel diverticulum (FIGURE 23-12). Normally, a Meckel diverticulum has the same type of epithelial lining as that lining the small intestine, but sometimes part of the epithelial lining consists of acid-secreting gastric mucosa. Most Meckel diverticula are asymptomatic, but sometimes the diverticulum becomes infected, causing the same symptoms and complications as an acute appendicitis. If a Meckel diverticulum contains misplaced (ectopic) gastric mucosa, the acidic "gastric juice" secreted by the diverticulum may cause a peptic ulcer of the diverticulum, which may be complicated by bleeding or perforation, as may occur with peptic ulcers in the stomach or duodenum. Whenever an operation is performed for a suspected appendicitis or other gastrointestinal problem, the surgeon

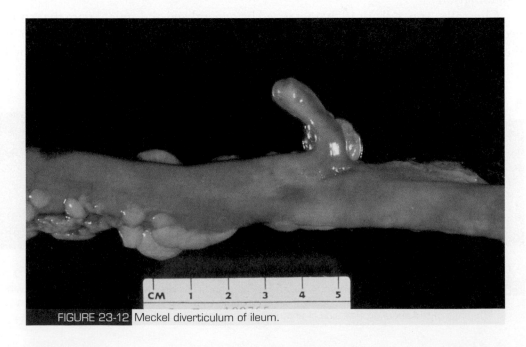

FIGURE 23-12 Meckel diverticulum of ileum.

always checks to see whether the patient's symptoms are caused by an inflammation or other problem in an unsuspected Meckel diverticulum.

Foreign Bodies

Accidentally swallowed foreign objects that are small and have a relatively uniform shape without sharp edges that can penetrate the bowel mucosa, such as a detached dental tooth crown, a coin, or a closed safety pin can pass through the colon without complication and can be recovered in the feces to confirm that the object has traveled safely through the bowel. However, an object with a sharp point, such as the accidentally swallowed canapé toothpick from a club sandwich, may become stuck by its tip in the intestinal mucosa and penetrate the bowel, as described in Case 23-1. A larger rigid object may be able to get through the small bowel but may be unable to pass through the ileocecal valve into the colon and may injure the bowel, as described in Case 23-2.

CASE 23-1

A late middle-aged man consulted a physician because of abdominal discomfort and cramps for several days. Examination of the abdomen revealed a localized area of tenderness but no evidence of peritonitis. An x-ray examination of the colon revealed a narrow irregular area in the colon of uncertain nature, and an exploratory operation was performed to determine its cause. The abnormality was caused by a large canapé toothpick that had perforated the colon with some associated inflammation in the colon surrounding the perforation site but no significant leakage of bowel contents into the peritoneal cavity (FIGURE 23-13). The toothpick was removed, and the site of the perforation was closed. The patient made an uneventful recovery.

Toothpick perforations of the bowel may occur when the person eating a canapé sandwich has dentures, which may interfere with oral sensation, or the subject has been drinking alcoholic beverages and is not paying attention to the food being consumed. Usually, the end of the toothpick projecting from the three-layer canapé sandwich has some identifying cellophane attached to the end of the toothpick, which designates its location. Toothpicks should be removed before starting to eat the sandwich.

A   B

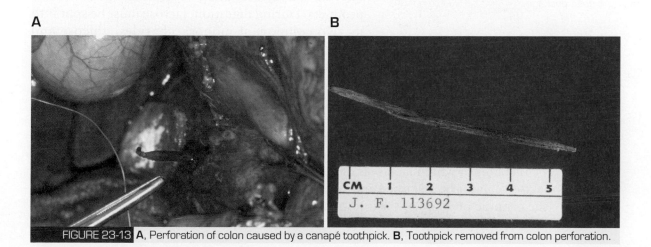

FIGURE 23-13 **A**, Perforation of colon caused by a canapé toothpick. **B**, Toothpick removed from colon perforation.

CASE 23-2

A 68-year-old diabetic nursing home resident was accustomed to leaving the nursing home on passes. When she was away from the nursing home, she was allowed to take her medications with her. One was a 25-mg tablet of thioridazine (Mellaril) provided in a unit dose package composed of a rigid foil-covered cardboard base fixed to a plastic cover with a central elevation (blister) that contains the pill. The blister pack is opened to obtain the pill by pulling the base away from the plastic cover. In the nursing home, the medications are dispensed by a nurse but opened by the patient when away from the nursing home.

A few days after she returned from the home pass, she began to experience abdominal pain and her abdomen became distended. She was hospitalized, and an operation was performed. Instead of opening the unit dose blister pack to obtain the pill, she had apparently become confused and ingested the entire unit dose package containing the pill, which had traveled through the upper gastro-intestinal tract but was too big to pass through the ileocecal valve into the colon despite vigorous small bowel peristalsis. There were two parallel perforations of her ileum caused by the rigid edges of the unit dose package with an edge protruding through one of the perforations (FIGURE 23-14). The involved segment of ileum was excised, and the bowel segments were reconnected.

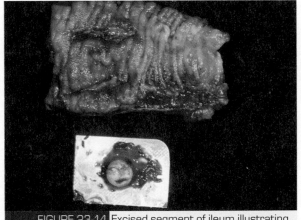

FIGURE 23-14 Excised segment of ileum illustrating two linear ulcerations and the pill contained in the intact unit dose package.

Disturbances of Bowel Function

FOOD INTOLERANCE

Some patients manifest crampy abdominal pain, abdominal distention, flatulence (excessive gas in the intestinal tract), and frequent loose stools as a result of food intolerance. The two most common types are

1. Lactose intolerance
2. Intolerance to the wheat protein gluten

Lactose Intolerance

Lactose is a disaccharide found in milk and dairy products. During digestion, lactose must be split into its two component monosaccharides, glucose and galactose, before it can be absorbed. This process is accomplished by an enzyme called lactase, which is present on the mucosal surface of the epithelial cells in the small intestine. The enzyme is abundant in infants and young children. In many populations, however, the concentration of lactase gradually declines to very low levels during adolescence and early adult life. The enzyme is deficient in about 20% of adult whites, 70% of American blacks, 90% of American Indians, and almost all Asians.

Persons in whom lactase is deficient are unable to digest lactose. Consequently, lactose cannot be absorbed and remains within the intestinal lumen, where it raises the osmotic pressure of the intestinal contents. Because of the high intraluminal osmotic pressure, fluid is retained within the intestinal tract instead of being absorbed normally, leading to abdominal discomfort, cramps, and diarrhea. Some of the unabsorbed lactose is fermented by bacteria in the colon, yielding lactic acid and other organic acids that further raise the intraluminal osmotic pressure and contribute to the person's discomfort. The symptoms are related to ingestion of dairy products and abate promptly when intake of dairy products is reduced or discontinued.

Gluten Intolerance

Gluten is a general term, which refers to a group of similar proteins found in wheat, rye, oats, and barley; it is the gluten in wheat flour that is responsible for imparting the elasticity to bread dough. Some persons have a hereditary predisposition to become sensitive to the protein in gluten called gliadin, and they form antigliadin antibodies and activated gliadin-sensitized T cells, which causes atrophy of the intestinal villi in the duodenum and proximal jejunum (FIGURE 23-15). As a result, digestion and absorption of fats and other nutrients is impaired. Several different names have been applied to this condition. The most descriptive term is **gluten enteropathy,** but the condition is also known as celiac disease or celiac sprue. Clinically, the condition is characterized by passage of frequent large, bulky stools containing much unabsorbed fat, associated with weight loss and vitamin deficiencies as a result of the impaired intestinal absorption.

Diagnosis is made on the basis of the clinical features and is confirmed if biopsy of the small intestinal mucosa reveals atrophy of the intestinal villi. The specimen for biopsy is obtained by a flexible biopsy device with a small capsule on the end that is swallowed by the patient. The device is positioned in the upper jejunum and is manipulated so that a small bit of intestinal mucosa enters the capsule. Then the capsule is closed, cutting off and retaining a piece of mucosa.

Treatment by a gluten-free diet promptly cures the condition, and the intestinal villi return to normal in about 3–4 months.

Gluten enteropathy
Damage to intestinal villi caused by ingesting gluten-containing foods by persons sensitive to a protein in gluten; characterized by passage of large bulky stools containing a large amount of poorly absorbed fat.

IRRITABLE BOWEL SYNDROME

Some patients exhibit episodes of crampy abdominal discomfort, loud gurgling bowel sounds, and disturbed bowel function. Frequent loose stools sometimes alternate

A　　　　　　　　　　　　　　　　　　**B**

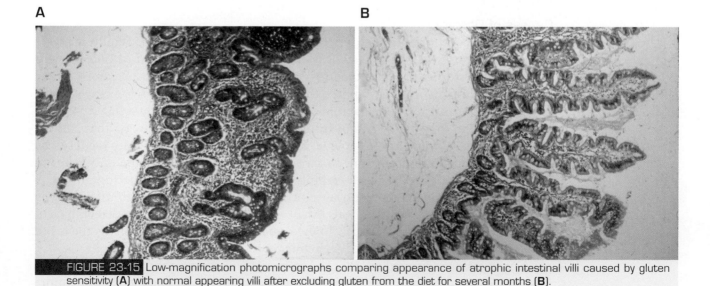

FIGURE 23-15 Low-magnification photomicrographs comparing appearance of atrophic intestinal villi caused by gluten sensitivity (**A**) with normal appearing villi after excluding gluten from the diet for several months (**B**).

with periods of constipation, and excessive amounts of mucus are secreted by the colonic mucosal glands. These manifestations are frequently quite distressing to the affected individual, but no structural or biochemical abnormalities can be identified to account for the functional disturbances. This condition is often called the irritable bowel syndrome. Other terms for this very common condition are spastic colitis and mucous colitis.

The diagnosis of irritable bowel syndrome is one of exclusion. The physician must rule out infections as a result of pathogenic bacteria and intestinal parasites, food intolerance, and various types of chronic enteritis such as Crohn disease and chronic ulcerative colitis.

Treatment consists of measures that reduce emotional tension and improve intestinal motility. Sometimes, substances that increase the bulk of the stool provide relief of symptoms.

INTESTINAL INFECTIONS IN HOMOSEXUAL MEN

Some homosexual men suffer from intestinal complaints that are caused by various combinations of pathogenic micro-organisms, such as *Shigella* and *Salmonella* and intestinal animal parasites such as *Entamoeba histolytica* and *Giardia*. Spread of the enteric infection is by anal–oral sexual practices that transfer the intestinal pathogens from the infected individual to his sexual partner. In some cases, the intestinal complaints may be misinterpreted as an irritable bowel syndrome if adequate diagnostic studies are not undertaken. Specific methods of treatment are available to cure these infections.

Eating Disorders

Eating disorders are conditions in which food intake is inappropriate and harmful because it leads to serious health consequences. Excessive food intake leading to obesity, which has many harmful effects on health, is the most prevalent disorder. However, abnormal eating habits associated with anorexia nervosa, bulimia nervosa, and binge eating disorders also pose serious health problems for the affected persons.

OBESITY

Causes of Obesity

Fat is the storage form of energy. Any caloric intake that exceeds requirements is stored as adipose tissue and weight is gained. Each excess pound of body weight represents the storage of approximately 3,500 calories. Weight is lost if caloric intake is reduced below the amount required for normal metabolic processes. Many genetic, environmental, and hormonal factors play a role in regulating body weight by affecting appetite and food intake and by influencing the metabolic pathways that convert food into energy or into adipose tissue. It is sometimes said that obesity is caused by an endocrine gland malfunction. In rare instances, hypothyroidism contributes to obesity by reducing the body's metabolic rate. Adrenal cortical hyperfunction may be associated with increased deposition of fat and an abnormal distribution of body fat. These are uncommon situations. Most obese individuals have no detectable endocrine or metabolic disturbances. In the vast majority of cases, obesity is the result of overeating and can be "cured" by reducing food intake.

Current data indicate that 60% of Americans are overweight. Half of the persons in this overweight group are classified as obese, which is defined as 20% or more over ideal body weight, or a body mass index of 30 or more. (Body mass index is a calculated value based on weight in kilograms divided by the square of height in meters.) Moreover, the prevalence of obesity has increased about 8% in the last decade. About 6% of women and 3% of men are more than 100% over their ideal body weight, which is called morbid obesity.

Health Consequences of Obesity

Overweight persons have a higher incidence of diabetes, hypertension, cardiovascular disease, and several other diseases than do persons of normal weight. Therefore, being significantly overweight is undesirable, and extreme obesity is a major health hazard. Obese persons have a mortality rate almost twice that of normal individuals. The excess fat is harmful to the cardiovascular system in three ways:

1. Blood volume and cardiac output must increase to nourish the excess adipose tissue, which overworks the heart.
2. Obese persons are prone to develop high blood pressure, which places a further strain on the heart and blood vessels.
3. Blood lipids are often elevated, which predisposes to arteriosclerosis of the coronary arteries.

Other systems also are adversely affected. Large masses of adipose tissue may impair normal pulmonary ventilation, producing various types of respiratory difficulty and increased susceptibility to pulmonary infection. An otherwise relatively minor respiratory illness may, in an obese person, be a catastrophe because of the increased demands placed upon already overtaxed cardiovascular and respiratory systems.

The high incidence of diabetes in obese persons is the result of an impaired ability to utilize insulin efficiently, as described in the discussion on pancreas and diabetes mellitus. Musculoskeletal disabilities are frequent because the excess weight places undue stress on the bones, joints, and ligaments. Finally, the obese individual is at a serious disadvantage if an operation is required. The operative procedure carries a higher risk, and postoperative complications are more frequent. Any surgical procedure is technically much more difficult in an obese person, and wound healing is delayed. The adipose tissue, which has a relatively poor blood supply, heals poorly and is also quite vulnerable to infection, resulting in an increased incidence of postoperative wound infections.

Another ominous effect of obesity also has been well documented. In obese persons, the death rate from cancer is 52% higher in men and 62% higher in women than are comparable death rates in men and women of normal weight. It has been estimated that 90,000 deaths from cancer could be prevented each year in the United States if men and women could maintain normal weight. The reasons for the higher mortality rate caused by obesity are probably related to higher levels of steroid hormones, insulin, and tumor-promoting growth factors in obese persons compared to persons of normal weight.

Treatment of Obesity

Most overweight persons are too heavy because they are eating too much and are not active enough. Obesity virtually always results from overeating and can be abolished by reducing food intake and becoming more active. Even small weight losses can bring significant health benefits. However, the results of treatment of obesity by dieting have been surprisingly poor because obese individuals are either unable or unwilling to reduce their caloric intake.

Because of the limited success of treating obesity by diet, various other measures have been proposed. Drugs that suppress appetite have been used, but many of these drugs have undesirable side effects.

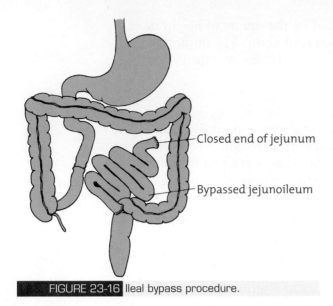

Closed end of jejunum

Bypassed jejunoileum

FIGURE 23-16 Ileal bypass procedure.

Ileal bypass
A surgical procedure performed on the small intestine to promote weight loss.

Gastric bypass
An operation to treat massive obesity in which the capacity of the stomach is reduced.

As a last resort, massive obesity is sometimes treated by various surgical operations. One of the first weight-reduction operations was called an **ileal bypass**. In this procedure, the ileum was divided about 18 cm proximal to the ileocecal valve, and the jejunum was divided about 30 cm distal to the duodenojejunal junction. Then the proximal jejunum and distal ileum were sutured together, bypassing the remaining part of the small intestine. The proximal (jejunal) end of the bypassed segment was closed. The distal end was connected to an opening made in the sigmoid colon, which permitted intestinal secretions to drain from the bypassed segment into the colon (FIGURE 23-16). Weight was lost because absorption of nutrients from the greatly shortened small intestine was very poor, which had the same effect as restricting food intake. Unfortunately, this drastic procedure was associated with so many late complications resulting from inadequate absorption of nutrients that it had to be abandoned. Other similar procedures were developed in which weight loss was achieved primarily by preventing absorption of nutrients, but also reduced the capacity of the stomach. Rapid weight loss was achieved but gave rise to the same problems related to impaired absorption of nutrients as the procedure it replaced, and its use is limited to special situations.

The current surgical procedures produce weight loss primarily by restricting the capacity of the stomach without resorting to drastic restriction of nutrient absorption in the small intestine. They can be performed using standard surgical incisions or by laparoscopy using small abdominal incisions (described in the general concepts of disease) and are often grouped together under the general term of "stomach stapling operations." The best known and most widely used of these procedures is called the Roux-en-Y gastric bypass, named after the man who devised it (Roux) and the Y-shaped connection made between the small bowel loops in the procedure.

In a **gastric bypass**, a line of staples is placed across the upper part of the stomach. This divides the stomach into two compartments, a very small upper compartment having a volume of only about 15 ml, and a much larger lower compartment that is continuous with the duodenum. Then the jejunum is divided. The distal cut end is anastomosed (connected) to the gastric pouch, and the proximal cut end is connected by means of a second anastomosis to the jejunum distal to the anastomosis between the jejunum and gastric pouch (FIGURE 23-17). When the procedure is completed, food from the gastric pouch empties directly into the jejunum. The main part of the stomach no longer receives food. Gastric secretions can drain into the duodenum normally, but the secretions enter the jejunum distal ("downstream") to the segment of jejunum receiving the contents from the gastric pouch.

Gastric bypass induces weight loss because the upper compartment of the stomach is so small that it soon becomes overdistended with food when the individual starts to eat. The subject feels "stuffed" and has to stop eating. Weight is lost by enforced reduction of food intake, but absorption of nutrients is also impeded to some extent because gastric contents are shunted into the distal jejunum, bypassing absorption from the proximal part of the small intestine. Unfortunately, gastric bypass procedures may lead to late complications in many patients: anemia caused by poor absorption of iron and vitamin B_{12} and weakening of bones (osteoporosis) as a result of inadequate calcium intake and absorption.

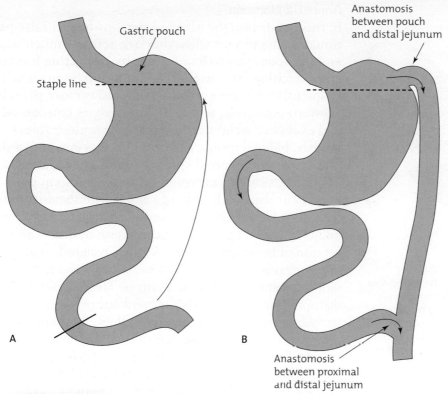

FIGURE 23-17 Gastric bypass. **A**, The upper *dashed line* indicates location of gastric staples placed to create gastric pouch. The lower *solid line* indicates the site where the jejunum is divided. The *arrow* indicates how the distal segment of jejunum is moved for anastomosis with gastric pouch. **B**, Completed bypass illustrating proximal and distal anastomoses. The *arrows* indicate the direction of movement of gastrointestinal contents, as described in text.

Adjustable gastric banding is another laparoscopic procedure to control food intake by placing an inflatable saline-filled adjustable gastric band around the upper part of the stomach. The band compresses the stomach to form a small upper gastric pouch that is almost completely separated from the rest of the stomach except for a very small channel that allows food in the upper gastric pouch to empty slowly into the lower part of the stomach. The amount of compression applied to the inflatable band, which controls the rate of gastric emptying, can be adjusted by adding or removing saline through a port placed under the skin of the abdomen. The procedure has the advantage of not requiring a "major redesign" of the gastrointestinal tract, but banding does not lead to as much weight loss as a gastric bypass (FIGURE 23-18).

Adjustable gastric banding
A method for treating obesity by applying an adjustable gastric band to the stomach in order to reduce its capacity, thereby promoting weight loss.

ANOREXIA NERVOSA AND BULIMIA NERVOSA

These two conditions are characterized by profound eating disturbances. Although they are characterized as separate disorders, there is considerable overlap between the two conditions. A more recently recognized condition called binge eating disorder, which occurs in older overweight and obese persons, is probably best considered as a variation of bulimia. Any of these conditions can lead to extreme malnutrition caused by inadequate nutrients, along with associated vitamin and mineral deficiencies. These conditions can lead to serious health consequences, which can be fatal if not adequately treated.

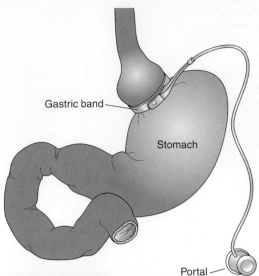

Gastric band

Stomach

Portal

FIGURE 23-18 Principle of the adjustable gastric banding procedure. Adjustable band filled with saline limits capacity of stomach by constricting outflow from stomach above the band. Rate of gastric emptying can be regulated by adding or removing saline from the band.

Anorexia Nervosa

In this condition, the affected persons have a false perception of being too fat when they are actually much too thin, and they continue to lose weight by restricting food intake and exercising excessively. The condition occurs much more frequently in women than in men and is more prevalent in Western countries, where a slim body is considered ideal and excessive weight is thought to be undesirable. Fashion models, ballet dancers, and other groups in whom a slender body is required, are disproportionately represented.

Often, anorexia nervosa begins in adolescent girls during puberty as their bodies change along with the distribution of their body fat, which is perceived as getting fat from overeating and is followed by dieting and exercise to deal with the perception of being overweight. As their weight loss accelerates, other measures may be taken to reduce weight, such as self-induced vomiting or taking laxatives. The excessive weight loss disrupts many of the body's physiologic processes. Menstrual periods cease, thyroid function declines, fluid and electrolyte disturbances develop, and bones become fragile from loss of calcium (osteoporosis). Extreme emaciation is a life threatening condition that may lead to death if the condition is not treated.

Severe anorexia nervosa is difficult to treat; both the medical and psychological problems associated with the condition must be dealt with. Medical treatment requires correcting the physiologic disturbances caused by the fasting, which may require intravenous fluids and whatever other methods are needed to restore health. Psychologic treatment requires the assistance of a psychiatrist or clinical psychologist experienced in dealing with eating disorders. The affected person needs to acquire a more realistic perception of her (or his) own body, needs to understand what may have led to the eating problem, and needs to learn how to adjust eating habits to prevent a recurrence of the condition.

Bulimia Nervosa

This condition is another method of weight control that is characterized by repeated episodes of binge eating (rapidly eating an excessively large amount of food) followed by purging (self-induced vomiting) to counteract the effects of the bingeing and is followed by guilt and remorse at the inability to control the binge–purge behavior. The purging may be supplemented by taking laxatives to decrease food absorption by promoting rapid passage of digested food through the small intestine. The condition occurs most often in young women. Their body weight may fluctuate in relation to their binge–purge behavior but they do not become emaciated. Their friends and relatives usually are not aware of their problem because they look normal and carefully conceal their binge–purge behavior.

Bulimia nervosa carries with it some serious health problems. Repeated self-induced vomiting leads to dental problems caused by the corrosive effect of the gastric acid on the tooth enamel. The repeated loss of excess gastric juice may lead to metabolic alkalosis and electrolyte disturbances, as discussed in water, electrolyte, and acid–base balance. One of the most serious effects of self-induced vomiting is a tear in the mucosa of the stomach near the gastroesophageal junction, which can bleed profusely and may be fatal, as illustrated in FIGURE 23-7.

Treatment involves the same medical and psychological approaches used to deal with anorexia nervosa.

BINGE-EATING DISORDER

The condition called a binge eating disorder is characterized by binge eating without compensatory purging to restrict the excess calories contributed by the binge eating, and leads to weight gain. The condition occurs in overweight and obese older adults, with both genders represented in roughly equal proportions. The binge eating complicates the problems of the obese person who is trying to lose weight, and it is estimated that up 20% of persons in weight loss programs may have a binge eating problem. The same approach used to motivate a person to lose weight also applies when dealing with the additional problem posed by the binge eating.

Chronic Malnutrition: Its Causes and Effects

CAUSES OF MALNUTRITION

Malnutrition results when the intake of nutrients is insufficient to supply the body's needs either because there is insufficient food available or the food is not being used efficiently. In developing countries, inadequate food to supply the population may result from crop failure, a natural disaster such as a flood or a drought, poor food distribution, an unstable government, or other causes that impact on food production or delivery. Often, infants and children are disproportionately affected because they have a greater need for nutrients to sustain their rapid growth rate during infancy and childhood.

In modern industrialized countries, many cases of chronic malnutrition are caused by diseases that impair food intake, digestion, or absorption or by conditions that increase nutrient and protein requirements, such as an acute illness, a severe burn, or a major surgical procedure. Other persons at risk are persons living in poverty, the elderly, persons who consume alcohol in excess, drug abusers, persons with AIDS or advanced cancer, and persons with the eating disorders. Treatment consists of supplying adequate nutrients together with vitamins and minerals before the malnutrition-induced organ damage has progressed to such a degree that response to treatment is unlikely to be successful.

IDENTIFYING PERSONS AT RISK

Malnutrition in children may be a manifestation of parental neglect, which should be investigated. Malnutrition in adults should be suspected when an adult has lost weight and whose food intake or absorption have decreased for any reason or whose nutrient requirements have increased significantly as a result of disease. Prevention and early detection of malnutrition in high-risk patients facilitates early treatment. More advanced and severe malnutrition takes longer to correct.

EVALUATION AND TREATMENT

Nutritional deficiencies often involve not only inadequate food nutrients but also multiple vitamin and mineral deficiencies. Weight loss of 5–10% of normal body weight usually can be tolerated but as weight loss increases, so do the manifestations of inadequate nutrition and protein deficiency. Extreme emaciation is a life threatening condition, and loss of over 30% of body weight may be fatal.

When evaluating a malnourished subject, the initial clinical evaluation should be supplemented by laboratory tests to assess the extent of organ and tissue damage, including determination of serum albumin as an index of protein deficiency. Medical treatment requires correcting any fluid and electrolyte disturbances and other physiologic disturbances caused by the deficiencies, followed by slowly increasing calorie and protein intake, preferably by oral feeding. Appropriate vitamin and mineral supplements are also provided, along with whatever additional measures are necessary to restore health.

ALCOHOL: ITS ROLE IN MALNUTRITION

Drinking modest amounts of alcoholic beverages is considered acceptable in many cultures and even provides some health benefits by favorably influencing blood lipids. Although not classified as a nutrient, alcohol provides 7 calories per gram, which is almost as many calories as in fat. So alcohol can be categorized as a "high-calorie nonnutrient." Excess alcohol intake can cause serious problems. Rapidly drinking large amounts of alcohol in a short period can be lethal, as documented by many reports of fatal alcohol intoxication, resulting from binge drinking among high school and college students. Chronic alcohol use has its own set of potential problems. It may lead to dependence on alcohol, which can progress to alcohol addiction in susceptible individuals. Alcoholism is a common cause of malnutrition because the alcohol is substituting nonnutritive "empty calories" from alcohol for calories from food, which supply the nutrients, vitamins, and minerals that the body needs. Many of the harmful results of chronic alcoholism are related not only to the organ damage caused by excess alcohol, such as alcoholic liver disease and its complications described in the discussion on the liver and biliary system, but also from the associated vitamin deficiencies that accompany an inadequate diet.

Diverticulosis and Diverticulitis of the Colon

Outpouchings of the mucosa of the colon often project through weak areas in the muscular wall of the large intestine. These outpouchings are called diverticula (singular, **diverticulum**), and the condition is called **diverticulosis** (FIGURES 23-19, 23-20, AND 23-21). This is an acquired condition, in contrast to a Meckel diverticulum, which

Diverticulum
(dī-vur-tik'u-lum)
An outpouching from an organ, as from the mucosa of the colon, which projects through the muscular wall.

Diverticulosis
(dī-vur-tik-u-lō'sis)
A condition characterized by an outpouching of the colonic mucosa through weak areas in the muscular wall.

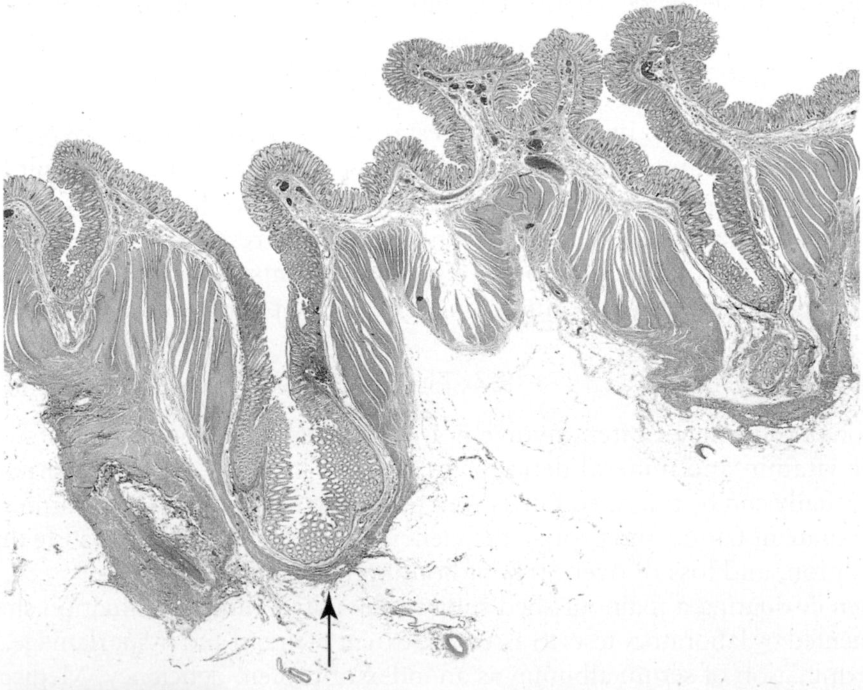

FIGURE 23-19 A low-magnification photomicrograph of colon illustrating diverticula. Mucosa of the colon (*upper part* of photograph) protrudes through muscular wall (*arrow*) into the serosa of colon (original magnification × 10).

A

B

C

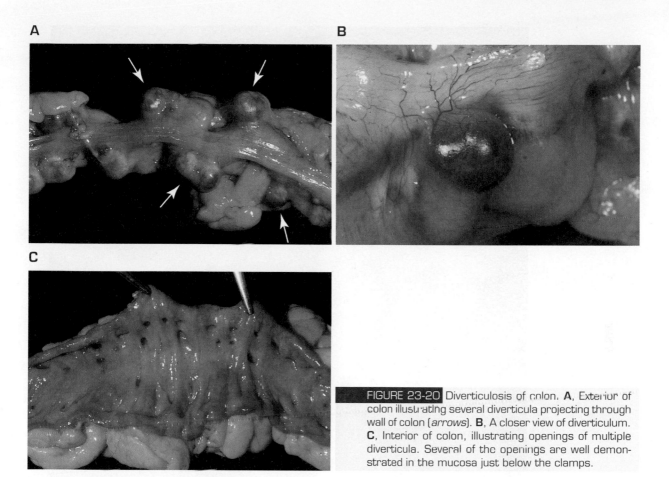

FIGURE 23-20 Diverticulosis of colon. **A**, Exterior of colon illustrating several diverticula projecting through wall of colon (*arrows*). **B**, A closer view of diverticulum. **C**, Interior of colon, illustrating openings of multiple diverticula. Several of the openings are well demonstrated in the mucosa just below the clamps.

is a congenital abnormality (see FIGURE 23-12). Diverticula, which usually occur in the distal colon, are encountered with increasing frequency in older patients. Highly refined, low-residue diets predispose to diverticula because stools are small and hard, and high intraluminal pressure must be generated by peristalsis to propel the stool through the colon. This high intracolonic pressure forces the mucosa through weak areas in the muscular wall. In contrast, people who subsist on high-residue diets have large, bulky stools that can be propelled through the colon easily at low intraluminal pressures, and diverticula occur infrequently among them.

Most diverticula are asymptomatic, but occasionally problems arise. Bits of fecal material may become trapped within these pouches and incite an inflammatory reaction called **diverticulitis**. The inflammation may be followed by considerable scarring. Occasionally, perforation of a diverticulum may occur, leading to an abscess in the pelvis. Sometimes blood vessels in the mucosa of the diverticulum may become ulcerated by abrasion from the fecal material, resulting in bleeding. Diverticula attended by such complications as infections, perforation, or bleeding are often treated by surgical resection of the affected segment of bowel.

Diverticulitis
(dī-vur-tik-u-lī'tis)
An inflammation of a diverticulum.

Intestinal Obstruction

If the normal passage of intestinal contents through the bowel is blocked, the patient is said to have an intestinal obstruction. The site of the blockage may be either the small intestine (high intestinal obstruction) or the colon (low intestinal obstruction). Bowel obstruction is always serious. The severity of the symptoms depends on the location of the obstruction, its completeness, and whether there is interference with the blood supply to the blocked segment of bowel.

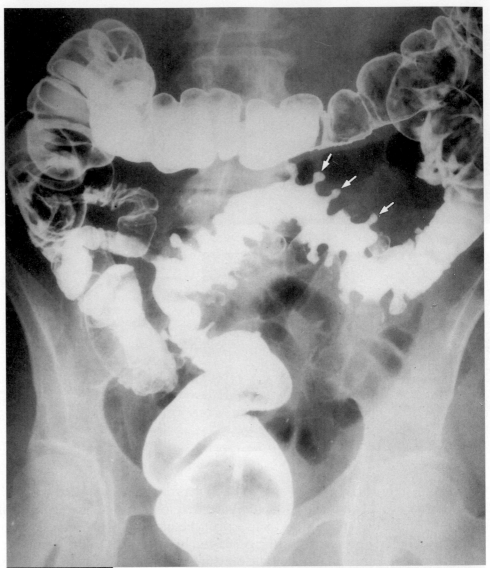

FIGURE 23-21 Diverticula of colon demonstrated by injection of barium contrast material into colon (barium enema). Diverticula filled with contrast material appear as projections from the mucosa (*arrows*).

Obstruction of the small intestine causes severe, crampy pain as a result of vigorous peristalsis, reflecting the attempt of the intestine to force bowel contents past the site of obstruction. This is associated with vomiting of copious amounts of gastric and upper intestinal secretions, resulting in loss of large quantities of water and electrolytes. As a consequence, the patient becomes dehydrated and develops pronounced fluid and electrolyte disturbances.

Symptoms are much less acute when the distal colon is obstructed. There may be mild, crampy abdominal pain and moderate distention of the abdomen. However, vomiting with associated loss of fluid and electrolytes is not as serious a problem as in high intestinal obstruction. Disturbances of fluid and electrolytes do not develop as rapidly.

The common causes of intestinal obstruction are as follows:

1. Intestinal adhesions
2. Hernia
3. Tumor
4. Volvulus
5. Intussusception

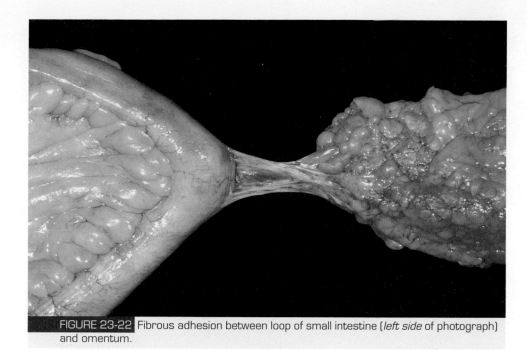

FIGURE 23-22 Fibrous adhesion between loop of small intestine (*left side* of photograph) and omentum.

Adhesions
(ad-hē'shuns)
Bands of fibrous tissue that form subsequent to an inflammation, and bind adjacent tissues together.

Hernia
(her'nē-yuh)
A protrusion of a loop of bowel through a narrow opening, usually in the abdominal wall.

ADHESIONS

Adhesive bands of connective tissue (**adhesions**) may form within the abdominal cavity after surgery (FIGURE 23-22). Sometimes a loop of bowel becomes kinked, compressed, or twisted by an adhesive band, causing obstruction proximal to the site of the adhesion.

HERNIA

A **hernia** is a protrusion of a loop of bowel through a small opening, usually in the abdominal wall. The herniated loop pushes the peritoneum ahead of it, forming the hernia sac. Inguinal hernia is quite common in men (FIGURE 23-23). A loop of small bowel protrudes through a weak area in the inguinal ring and may descend downward into the scrotum. Umbilical and femoral hernias occur in both sexes. In an umbilical hernia, the loop of bowel protrudes into the umbilicus through a defect in the abdominal wall (FIGURE 23-24). In a femoral hernia, a loop of intestine extends under the inguinal ligament along the course of the femoral vessels into the groin. If a herniated loop of bowel can be pushed back into the abdominal cavity, the hernia is said to be reducible. Occasionally, a herniated loop becomes stuck and cannot be reduced. This is called an incarcerated hernia. Sometimes the loop of bowel is so tightly constricted by the margins of the defect that allowed the herniation that the blood supply to the herniated bowel is obstructed, causing necrosis of the protruding segment of bowel. This is called a strangulated hernia and requires prompt surgical intervention.

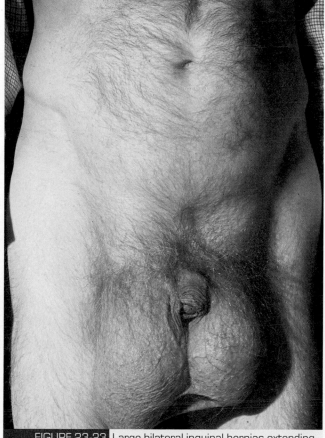

FIGURE 23-23 Large bilateral inguinal hernias extending into the scrotum.

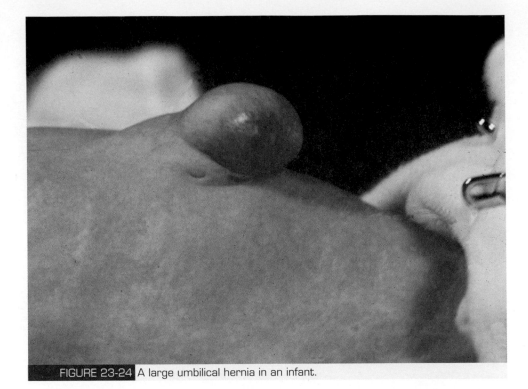

FIGURE 23-24 A large umbilical hernia in an infant.

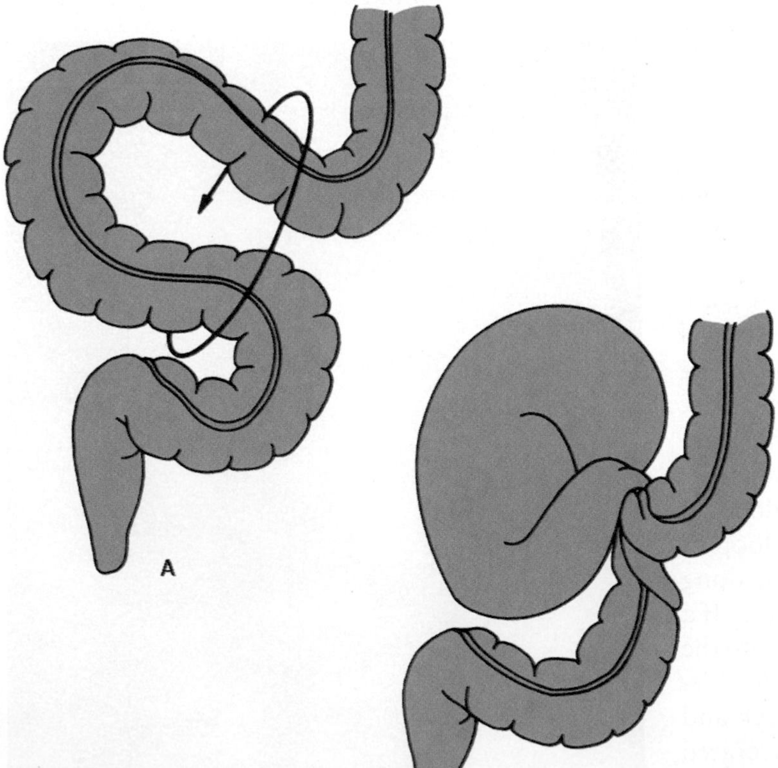

Volvulus

(vol'vū-lus)

A rotary twisting of the intestine on its mesentery, with obstruction of the blood supply to the twisted segment.

....

Intussusception

(in'tus-us-cep'shun)

A telescoping of one segment of bowel into an adjacent segment.

FIGURE 23-25 Pathogenesis of volvulus. **A**, Rotary twist of sigmoid colon on its mesentery. **B**, Obstruction of colon and interruption of its blood supply caused by volvulus.

VOLVULUS AND INTUSSUSCEPTION

A **volvulus** is a rotary twisting of the bowel on the fold of peritoneum that suspends the bowel from the posterior wall of the abdomen, which is called the mesentery of the bowel. The blood supply to the twisted segment also is impaired because the blood vessels supplying the bowel travel in the mesentery, and they are compressed when the bowel and mesentery become twisted. The sigmoid colon is the usual site (FIGURE 23-25).

An **intussusception** is a telescoping of one segment of bowel into an adjacent segment. This is a common cause of intestinal obstruction in children and usually results from vigorous peristalsis that telescopes the terminal ileum into the proximal colon through the ileocecal valve (FIGURE 23-26). In adults, the condition is usually secondary to a benign tumor of the bowel that is supported by a narrow stalk. A tumor of this type is often called a pedunculated tumor, the name being derived from the stalk (pedicle) that supports it (*pediculus* = little foot). As the tumor is propelled by a peristaltic wave, the base of the tumor exerts traction on the bowel wall at its site of attachment, causing the proximal segment of bowel to be pulled into the distal segment (FIGURES 23-27 AND 23-28).

Carcinoma of the colon may obstruct the distal colon and is a common cause of low intestinal obstruction.

Mesenteric Thrombosis

The blood supply to the gastrointestinal tract is derived from several large arteries arising from the aorta. The blood supply to most of the bowel is provided by the superior mesenteric artery. This vessel supplies blood to the entire small intestine and the proximal half of the colon. The arteries supplying the gastrointestinal tract may develop arteriosclerotic changes and become occluded by thrombosis in the same way as may other arteries. Thrombosis of the superior mesenteric artery leads to an extensive infarction of most of the bowel.

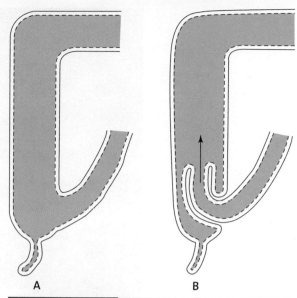

FIGURE 23-26 Pathogenesis of ileocecal intussusception. **A**, Normal anatomic relationships. **B**, Vigorous peristalsis carries distal ileum into cecum. *Dashed line* indicates mucosa.

Tumors of the Bowel

Tumors of the small intestine are uncommon, whereas benign pedunculated polyps of the colon occur quite frequently. Usually they do not cause symptoms, but occasionally the tip of the polyp may become eroded and cause bleeding. Often, a polyp can be removed by inserting a flexible instrument called a colonoscope into the bowel through the rectum and cutting the narrow stalk.

Carcinoma of the colon is a common tumor that may arise anywhere in the large intestine or rectum. Carcinoma arising in the cecum and right half of the colon generally does not cause obstruction of the bowel because the caliber of this portion of the colon is large and the bowel contents are relatively soft. However, the tumor often becomes ulcerated and bleeds, leading to chronic iron deficiency anemia. The patient with a carcinoma of the right half of the colon may consult a physician because of weakness and fatigue caused by the anemia, without experiencing any symptoms referable to the intestinal tract.

Carcinoma of the distal portion of the colon, which has a much smaller caliber than the proximal colon, often causes partial obstruction of the bowel and leads to symptoms of lower intestinal obstruction (FIGURES 23-29 AND 23-30).

Imperforate anus
(im-per'for-āt)
Congenital absence of anal opening, often associated with absence of distal rectum as well.

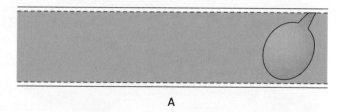

A

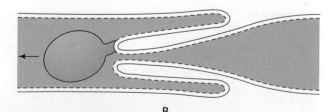

B

FIGURE 23-27 Pathogenesis of intussusception caused by tumor. **A**, Pedunculated tumor protrudes into lumen of bowel. **B**, Peristalsis propels tumor and produces traction on its base causing proximal segment of bowel to be telescoped into distal segment. *Dashed line* indicates mucosa.

Imperforate Anus

Imperforate anus is an uncommon congenital abnormality in which the colon fails to acquire a normal anal opening (FIGURE 23-31). There are two major types. In one type, the rectum and anus are normally formed and extend to the level of the skin, but no anal orifice is present. Often, a small tract (fistula) extends

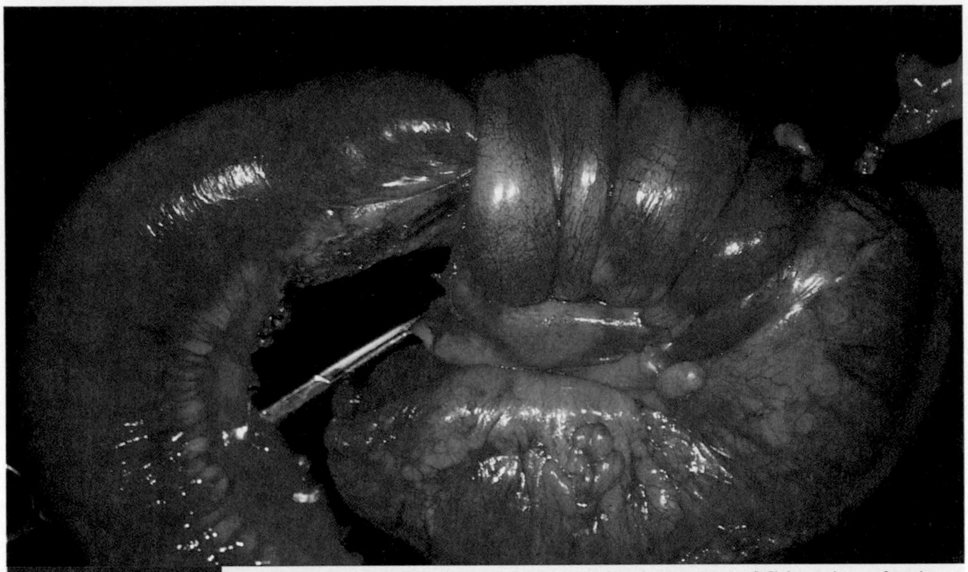

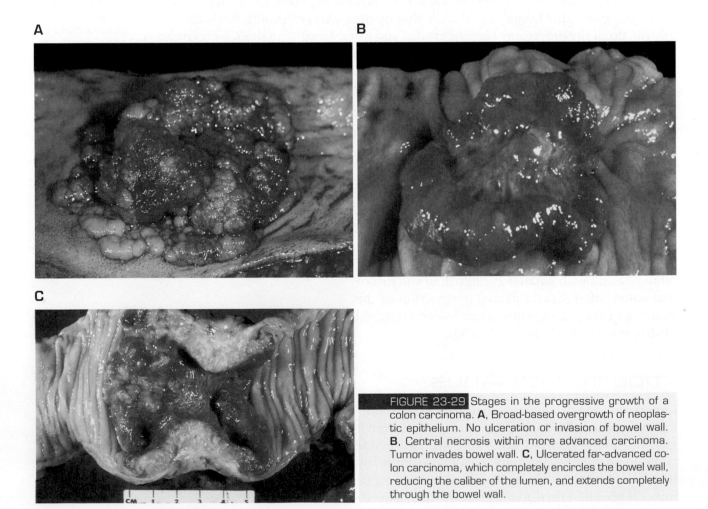

FIGURE 23-28 Intussusception of colon as a result of colon tumor. Midportion of colon is swollen because of telescoping of the proximal segment (*left side* of photograph) into distal segment (*right side* of photograph).

A

B

C

FIGURE 23-29 Stages in the progressive growth of a colon carcinoma. **A**, Broad-based overgrowth of neoplastic epithelium. No ulceration or invasion of bowel wall. **B**, Central necrosis within more advanced carcinoma. Tumor invades bowel wall. **C**, Ulcerated far-advanced colon carcinoma, which completely encircles the bowel wall, reducing the caliber of the lumen, and extends completely through the bowel wall.

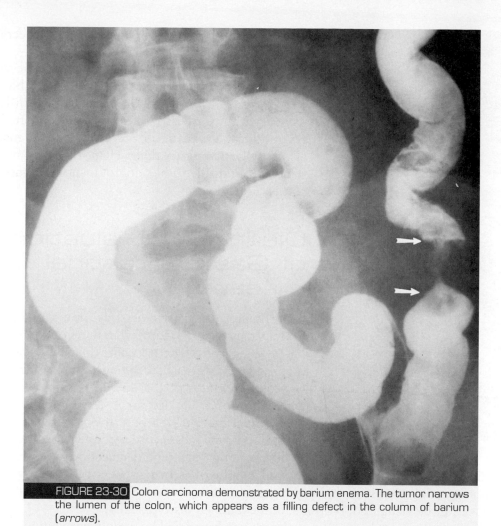

FIGURE 23-30 Colon carcinoma demonstrated by barium enema. The tumor narrows the lumen of the colon, which appears as a filling defect in the column of barium (*arrows*).

Hemorrhoids
(hem′or-oyds)
Varicosities of anal and rectal veins.

from the blind end of the anal canal to terminate in the urethra, in the vagina, or on the surface of the skin. Usually, this type of imperforate anus can be easily treated by excising the tissue covering the anal opening. In the second type of imperforate anus, the entire distal rectum fails to develop, and often there are associated abnormalities of the urogenital tract and skeletal system. Surgical repair of this type of abnormality is much more difficult, and results are less satisfactory.

Hemorrhoids

Hemorrhoids are varicosities of the venous plexus that drains the rectum and anus (FIGURE 23-32). Constipation and increased straining during bowel movements predispose to their development. Internal hemorrhoids, which involve the veins of the lower rectum, may become eroded and bleed, may become thrombosed, or may prolapse through the anus. External hemorrhoids involve the veins of the anal canal and perianal skin. They sometimes become

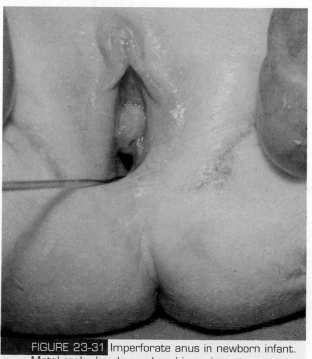

FIGURE 23-31 Imperforate anus in newborn infant. Metal probe has been placed in vagina.

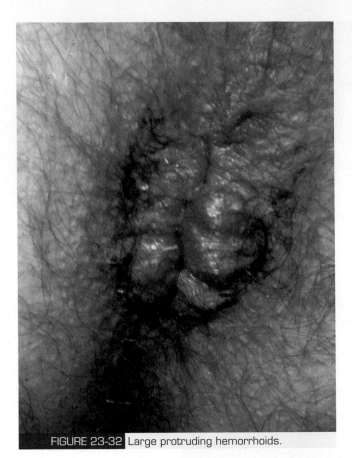

FIGURE 23-32 Large protruding hemorrhoids.

thrombosed, which causes considerable anorectal discomfort.

Symptoms of hemorrhoids can often be relieved by a high-fiber diet rich in fruits and vegetables, which promotes large, bulky stools that can be passed without excessive straining. Stool softeners and local application of rectal ointments may also provide temporary relief. Hemorrhoids can be removed surgically if they do not respond to more conservative therapy.

Diagnostic Evaluation of Gastrointestinal Disease

Unfortunately, the gastrointestinal tract cannot be examined as easily as many other parts of the body. However, it is possible to visualize the interior of the esophagus, the stomach, the duodenum, and the entire colon by endoscopic procedures using specially designed instruments that are inserted into the gastrointestinal tract either through the oral cavity or the anus. Endoscopy is described in the general concepts of disease in the section on diagnostic procedures.

Endoscopic procedures are generally employed if the patient experiences symptoms suggesting disease of the esophagus, stomach, or colon. Abnormal areas in the mucosa can be visualized, biopsied, and examined histologically.

Areas that cannot be visualized directly can be studied by radiologic examination. Examination of the upper gastrointestinal tract is accomplished by having the patient ingest a radiopaque material (contrast medium), allowing the clinician to visualize the transport of the material through the intestinal tract by x-ray studies. Any areas where the motility of the bowel appears abnormal, indicating disease, can be seen on the film. This technique also allows the clinician to visualize the contours of the gastrointestinal mucosa and thereby to identify the location and extent of disease affecting the bowel mucosa, such as ulcer, stricture, tumor, or an area of chronic inflammation. The colon can be studied in a similar manner by instilling radiopaque material into the bowel through the anus in order to outline the contours of the large intestine. This type of study is called a barium enema (see FIGURES 23-19 AND 23-30).

QUESTIONS FOR REVIEW

1. What is a cleft palate? What is its usual mode of inheritance? How is it treated?
2. What factors affect the development of dental caries? What complications may result from dental caries? What are the causes and possible effects of periodontal disease?
3. What are some of the major causes of esophageal obstruction? What symptoms does esophageal obstruction produce?
4. What is peptic ulcer? In what parts of the gastrointestinal tract are peptic ulcers encountered? What factors contribute to the development of peptic ulcers? What are the complications of a peptic ulcer?

5. What is the difference between Crohn disease and chronic ulcerative colitis? Diverticulosis and diverticulitis?
6. What is a Meckel diverticulum? Where is it located? What clinical manifestations can it produce?
7. What is intestinal obstruction? What symptoms does it produce? What are some of the common causes of intestinal obstruction?
8. What is the pathogenesis of acute appendicitis?
9. What symptoms and physical findings are likely to be encountered in a patient with a carcinoma of the colon? Why?
10. What is an intussusception? How is it caused? What is the difference between volvulus and intussusception?

SUPPLEMENTARY READINGS

Allen, J. J. 1995. Molecular biology of colorectal cancer: A clinician's view. *Perspectives in Colon and Rectal Surgery* 8:181–202.
▶ An excellent review article on genes related to cancer development, the "multiple hit" concept of cell deregulation, and the hereditary types of colon cancer.

Blaser, M. J. 1999. Where does *Helicobacter pylori* come from and why is it going away? *Journal of the American Medical Association* 282:2260–2.
▶ *H. pylori* infects only primates, and there is no reservoir in nature. The organism can be identified in dental plaque and in stool specimens. Very large numbers of organisms are present in the vomit of infected persons and in the air in the vicinity of the vomitus. Fewer persons are colonized by the organism as a result of better sanitation and less close family contacts, which reduces the person-to-person spread of the organism.

Brolin, R. E. 2002. Bariatric surgery and long-term control of morbid obesity. *Journal of the American Medical Association* 288:2793–6.
▶ Describes the magnitude of the "obesity epidemic" and the applications and limitations of various surgical procedures used to treat morbid obesity. Includes description of gastric banding and another procedure somewhat similar to the ileal bypass procedure.

Calle, E., Rodriguez, C., Walker-Thurmond, K., and Thun, M. J. 2003. Overweight, obesity, and mortality from cancer in a prospectively studied cohort of U.S. adults. *The New England Journal of Medicine* 348:1625–38.
▶ In a 16-year prospective study of more than 900,000 U.S. adults, increased body weight is associated with increased death rates for all cancers combined and for cancers at multiple specific sites.

Christakis, N. A., and Fowler, J. H. 2007. The spread of obesity in a large social network over 32 years. *The New England Journal of Medicine* 357:370–9.
▶ Evaluation of a densely connected social network of 12,067 people assessed repeatedly from 1971 to 2003 as part of the Framingham Heart Study revealed that obesity spreads within social groups, especially among close friends, siblings, and spouses, strongly suggesting that the spread of obesity among spouses, brothers and sisters, close friends, and associates may be influenced by developing shared ideas and concepts about the acceptability of overeating, weight gain, and obesity. For example, a person's chance of becoming obese increased by 57% if he or she had a close friend who was obese. Among brothers and sisters,

if one became obese, the other had a 42% chance of a similar fate, and if one spouse became obese, the other spouse had a 37% chance of also becoming obese.

Crowley, L. V., Sean, J., and Wullin, G. 1984. Late effects of gastric bypass for obesity. *American Journal of Gastroenterology* 79:850–60.

▶ Many patients developed iron and vitamin B_{12} deficiencies and osteoporosis as late complications of gastric bypass. Hematopoietic complications usually can be prevented and are relatively easy to treat, but musculoskeletal complications are more difficult to prevent and treat.

Cummings, D. E., and Flum, D. R. 2008. Gastrointestinal surgery as a treatment for diabetes. *Journal of the American Medical Association* 299:341–3.

▶ Obese patients with diabetes who had laparoscopic adjustable gastric banding procedures to treat their diabetes lost weight, and 73% had remission of their diabetes. Patients who had a Roux-en-Y gastric bypass procedure sustained a greater response than gastric banding patients. It appears likely that the gastric bypass increases insulin sensitivity but also improves beta cell function.

DeMaria, E. J. 2007. Bariatric surgery for morbid obesity. *The New England Journal of Medicine* 356:2176–83.

▶ A discussion of the applications and limitations of the various types of surgical procedures available to reduce food intake by reducing the size of the stomach and/or impairing absorption of nutrients from the small intestine. Some of the newer laparoscopic procedures are described.

Dolin, R. 2007. Noroviruses—challenges to control. *The New England Journal of Medicine* 351: 1072–3.

▶ Noroviruses are the most common cause of nonbacterial gastroenteritis. Transmission is mainly by fecal–oral route. Infections may occur sporadically but may affect large groups of persons in close contact, as in cruise ships, schools, recreational areas, military facilities, and so forth. The viruses are highly infectious and resistant to inactivation. As little as 10 virus particles may cause an infection. No specific treatment is available.

DuPont, H. L. 2011. The search for effective treatment of *Clostridium difficile* infection. *The New England Journal of Medicine* 364:473–5.

▶ A review of the current treatment problems and need for better therapy.

Eckel, R. 2008. Clinical practice. Nonsurgical management of obesity in adults. *The New England Journal of Medicine* 358:1941–50.

▶ Nonsurgical treatment is described for obese patients whose body mass index is not high enough to be considered for bariatric surgery. Patients should be encouraged to set realistic goals, record food intake, and record their weight at least weekly. Applications and limitations of weight loss drugs are considered.

Fontaine, K. R., Redden, D. T., Wang, C., et al. 2003. Years of life lost due to obesity. *Journal of the American Medical Association* 289:187–93.

▶ Obesity greatly shortens life expectancy, especially among younger adults.

Glass, R. I., Parashar, U. D., and Estes, M. K. 2009. Norovirus gastroenteritis. *The New England Journal of Medicine* 361:1776–85.

▶ Noroviruses are the leading cause of gastroenteritis epidemics and also an important cause of sporadic gastroenteritis in children as well as adults. The virus is usually spread by the fecal–oral route, but may also be transmitted by person-to-person contact, as well as by particles of clothing, towels, and other fomites. Exposure to only a small number of virus particles is sufficient to cause an infection, and the infected person may begin to shed virus capable of infecting other persons when the infected subject is still asymptomatic. Moreover, the infected person, such as a food handler or restaurant employee, may continue to shed virus long after recovery from the norovirus infection, which may expose many other people. The virus can survive a wide range of temperatures from freezing to 60°C and can persist on the surfaces of household items, as well as in water and on foods. Repeated infections may occur because there are so many strains of norovirus that recovery from one infection provides very little cross protection against infection by another strain of the virus. There are no agents effective against the virus. Only symptomatic and supportive treatment of infected persons is available.

Hossain, P., Kawar, B., and El Nahas, M. E. 2007. Obesity and diabetes in the developing world—a growing challenge. *The New England Journal of Medicine* 356:213–5.

▶ The rates of obesity have tripled in developing countries that have adopted a Western lifestyle characterized by decreased physical activity and overconsumption of cheap high-calorie foods, and affects children as well as adults. Type 2 diabetes, cardiovascular disease, and some cancers have followed the obesity epidemic. These problems are severe in middle-income countries of Eastern Europe, Latin America, and Asia, but are rare in developing countries that continue to observe their traditional lifestyle. The obesity, diabetes, hypertension triad also targets the kidneys, leading to development of diabetic nephropathy in one-third of persons with diabetes, and its incidence has increased greatly in Asia, where diabetic nephropathy is the most common cause of end-stage renal disease in 9 of 10 Asian countries.

Kenchaiah, S., Evans, J. C., Levy, D., et al. 2002. Obesity and the risk of heart failure. *The New England Journal of Medicine* 347:305–13.

▶ Approximately 11% of cases of heart failure among men and 14% among women can be attributed to obesity. Efforts to promote optimal body weight may reduce the risk of heart failure.

The Longitudinal Assessment of Bariatric Surgery (LABS) consortium. 2009. Perioperative safety in the longitudinal assessment of bariatric surgery. *The New England Journal of Medicine* 361:445–54.

▶ Bariatric surgery is recommended as a weight control procedure in obese subjects with a body mass index (BMI) of 40 or more who do not have major coexisting obesity-related medical conditions and is also appropriate for obese subjects with a BMI of at least 35 when there are obesity-related coexisting medical problems. In this study, weight loss procedures were performed on 4,776 subjects by experienced bariatric surgeons in bariatric surgery centers. More than half of the group had coexisting medical conditions. A Roux-en-Y gastric bypass was performed on 3,412 subjects, with 87.2% performed as a laparoscopic procedure. Mortality in this group was 0.3%. Complications were considered to be death, deep vein thrombosis, pulmonary embolism, need for a subsequent operation for complications related to the initial surgery, or failure to be discharged by 30 days after surgery. The complication rate was 4.1% in the laparoscopy treatment group and 7.8% in the group treated by an open surgical procedure. Adjustable gastric banding was performed on 1,198 patients, and the complication rate was 1.0%; 166 patients underwent other rarely performed procedures that were not included in the analysis.

▶ In most patients, the Roux-en-Y procedure lowers blood glucose before any weight loss occurs; this effect apparently is caused by release of peptides from the intestinal mucosa that lower blood glucose and may also enhance weight loss. Obesity is a major cause of illness and death, and bariatric surgery is the only approach that consistently results in significant sustained weight loss. The short-term risks of surgery should be considered in relation to the long-term health benefits of the weight loss.

McColl, K. E. 2010. Clinical practice. *Helicobacter pylori* infection. *The New England Journal of Medicine* 362:1597–604.

▶ *Helicobacter pylori* lead to the development of both gastric and duodenal ulcers. The gastric ulcers begin with chronic gastritis caused by the organism, which is associated with stimulation of the gastric-secreting mucosal cells leading to increased secretion of acid gastric juice. Duodenal ulcers result from the excessive gastric acid secretion.

Nishioka, N. S., and Lauwers, G. 2006. Case records of the Massachusetts General Hospital. Case 10-2006. A 66-year-old woman with Barrett's esophagus with high-grade dysplasia. *The New England Journal of Medicine* 354:1403–9.

▶ Partial resection of the esophagus has many complications and less aggressive treatment is preferred. Affected area of dysplasia can be replaced by normal squamous epithelium by various methods, which are described and discussed.

O'Brien, P. E., Sawyer, S. M., Laurie, C., et al. 2010. Laparoscopic adjustable gastric banding in severely obese adolescents: A randomized trial. *Journal of the American Medical Association* 303:519–26.

▶ Fifty adolescents aged 15–18 having a body mass index (BMI) over 35 and obesity-related medical complications were randomly divided into two groups. Half were assigned to a program of diet, exercise, and lifestyle modification; the other half had a laparoscopic adjustable gastric banding procedure; and both groups were followed for 2 years. The goal was to achieve at least a 50% reduction of the excess weight. The lifestyle modification group achieved a 13.2% loss of excess weight, compared with a 78.8% reduction of excess weight in the gastric banding group, and also achieved greater improvement in obesity-related complications. However, long-term follow-up by trained health professionals is required to sustain the improvement obtained by the procedure.

Paulson, E. K., Kalady, M. F., and Pappas, T. N. 2003. Clinical practice. Suspected appendicitis. *The New England Journal of Medicine* 348:236–42.

▶ The three signs most predictive of appendicitis are right lower quadrant pain, abdominal rigidity, and migration of pain from the epigastrium to the right lower quadrant. Diagnosis in women is more difficult because of other conditions related to ovarian or tubal disease. Abdominal CT or ultrasound study is helpful for evaluating confusing cases.

Pratt, J. S., Cummings, S., Vineberg, D. A., et al. 2004. Case records of the Massachusetts General Hospital. Weekly clinicopathological exercises. Case 25-2004. A 49-year-old woman with severe obesity, diabetes, and hypertension. *The New England Journal of Medicine* 351:696–705.

▶ This article describes the evaluation and management of a typical patient with severe obesity being considered for bariatric (weight loss) surgery. Medical, nutritional, psychological, and surgical evaluations are described, and various surgical procedures are considered. The major obesity-related complications resolve as normal weight is restored. Diabetes improves as weight is lost and may resolve completely if the obesity-related type 2 diabetes has been present for less than 5 years. Gastric bypass patients require supplementary vitamin B_{12}, iron, calcium, and vitamin D, as absorption of these substances is impaired as a result of the bypass.

Service, G. J., Thompson, G. B., Service, J., et al. 2005. Hyperinsulinemic hypoglycemia with nesidioblastosis after gastric-bypass surgery. *The New England Journal of Medicine* 353:249–54.

▶ Gastric bypass ameliorates obesity-related complications, and diabetes improves rapidly even before there has been significant weight loss, apparently because the bypass of nutrients into the distal jejunum induces the release of intestinal hormones that stimulate pancreatic islets to increase insulin secretion. In some bypass patients, the prolonged islet stimulation causes hyperplasia of islets (called nesidioblastosis) and excessive insulin secretion, which leads to hypoglycemia (see also the editorial by Cummings in the same issue, pages 300–301).

Sharma, P. 2009. Clinical practice. Barrett's esophagus. *The New England Journal of Medicine* 361:2548–56.

▶ This condition is prone to occur in persons with gastroesophageal reflux and often leads to epithelial dysplasia that may progress to esophageal carcinoma. Various methods are available to eradicate the abnormal epithelium without resorting to a radical esophageal resection.

Suerbaum, S., and Michetti, P. 2002. *Helicobacter pylori* infection. *The New England Journal of Medicine* 347:1175–86.

▶ A current review article with an extensive bibliography.

Uemura, N., Okamota, S., Yamamoto, S., et al. 2001. *Helicobacter pylori* infection and the development of gastric cancer. *The New England Journal of Medicine* 345:784–9.

▶ Gastric cancer develops in persons with *Helicobacter pylori* infection but not in uninfected persons. Persons with gastritis associated with marked gastric atrophy and intestinal metaplasia are at risk.

OUTLINE SUMMARY

Face and Oral Cavity

CLEFT LIP AND PALATE

Face and palate formed by coalescence of cell masses.
Maldevelopment leads to defects in lip, jaw, and palate.
Multifactorial inheritance pattern.
Treatment by surgical correction of defect.

ABNORMALITIES OF TOOTH DEVELOPMENT

Missing teeth common. Multifactorial inheritance pattern.
Tetracycline stains enamel of developing teeth and may cause abnormal tooth development.
Do not give to pregnant women.
Do not give to children younger than 8 years of age.

DENTAL CARIES (TOOTH DECAY) AND ITS COMPLICATIONS

Organic acids produced by bacterial fermentation of retained food particles erode enamel.
Combined acid and bacterial action destroy tooth structure, forming cavity.
Spread of bacteria to pulp cavity causes pulp infection and toothache.
Infection may affect apex of tooth and bone in which tooth embedded.
Treatment:
Cavities treated by removing decay and filling the defect.
Pulp infection and infection in bone at apex of tooth may require antibiotics, root canal treatment, or occasionally tooth extraction.

PERIODONTAL DISEASE

An infection between roots of teeth and gums.
Spread of infection into tooth sockets may cause teeth to loosen and eventually fall out.
Various local dental treatments may control or arrest condition.

Inflammation of the Oral Cavity

STOMATITIS

Caused by various irritants.

Tumors of the Oral Cavity

CARCINOMA

Arises from squamous epithelium of oral cavity.
Treated by resection or radiation.

Diseases of the Esophagus

CARDIAC SPHINCTER DYSFUNCTION

Cardiospasm: sphincter fails to open and obstructs food transport.
Incompetent sphincter.
Reflux of acid gastric juice causes inflammation, ulceration, scarring (reflux esophagitis).
Glandular metaplasia of squamous epithelium (Barrett esophagus) carries increased risk of esophageal cancer.

MUCOSAL TEARS

Retching and vomiting lacerates mucosa, which may bleed profusely.

CARCINOMA OF ESOPHAGUS

Squamous cell carcinoma gradually narrows lumen.
May invade trachea and cause fistula.

FOOD IMPACTION

Poorly chewed meat may block esophagus.
Occurs in persons unable to chew properly.

STRICTURE

Esophagus narrowed by scar.
Ingestion of corrosive chemicals causes inflammation
that heals by scarring.

Gastritis and Gastroenteritis

ACUTE

Often caused by nonsteroidal anti-inflammatory drugs or
alcohol.
Acute gastroenteritis usually caused by norovirus.

CHRONIC

Often associated with *Helicobacter pylori* colonization of
mucosa.

Peptic Ulcer

PATHOGENESIS

Increased acid secretions and digestive enzymes erode
gastric mucosa.
Helicobacter pylori plays role in pathogenesis.

COMPLICATIONS

Bleeding.
Perforation.
Pyloric obstruction by scarring.

TREATMENT

Administer drugs to block acid secretion or neutralize acid.
Antibiotic therapy if ulcer associated with *H. pylori*.
Surgery may be required for ulcer complications.

Carcinoma of Stomach

MANIFESTATIONS AND TREATMENT

Upper abdominal discomfort.
Iron deficiency anemia from chronic blood loss.
Diagnosis established by biopsy of tumor by means of
gastroscopy.
Treated by gastric resection.

Inflammatory Disease of the Intestine

ACUTE ENTERITIS

Common and self-limited.
Caused by many different organisms and bacterial toxins.

CHRONIC ENTERITIS

Crohn disease (regional enteritis).
Chronic inflammation with scarring affects distal ileum.
Treatment by resection.
Chronic ulcerative colitis.
Recurrent chronic inflammation of colon and rectum.
Various forms of medical treatment.
Often requires resection of colon.

COMPLICATIONS OF CHRONIC ENTERITIS

Nutritional disturbances from chronic diarrhea.
Bleeding.
Obstruction by scarring.
Perforation.

ANTIBIOTIC-ASSOCIATED COLITIS

Broad-spectrum antibiotics eliminate normal intestinal
bacterial flora. Anaerobic *Clostridium difficile* not inhibited by broad-spectrum antibiotic.
Organism no longer held in check by normal intestinal
flora.
Organism proliferates and produces toxins that injure
colonic mucosa.
Severe cases treated with antibiotics directed against
Clostridium difficile.

Appendicitis

PATHOGENESIS AND TREATMENT

Narrow caliber of appendix favors obstruction at base.
Accumulation of secretions raises intraluminal pressure,
impairing viability of wall.
Intestinal bacteria invade wall.
Inflamed appendix may perforate and cause peritonitis.
Appendectomy performed in all suspected cases.

Meckel Diverticulum

PATHOGENESIS

Embryonic remnant of vitelline duct.
Appears as tubular outpouching from distal ileum.

MANIFESTATIONS AND TREATMENT

Usually asymptomatic.
Inflammation of diverticulum causes symptoms similar
to appendicitis.

Foreign Bodies

Most objects with smooth edges pass through bowel
without difficulty.
Objects with sharp edges may perforate bowel.
Bowel injury may result.

Disturbances of Bowel Function Caused by Food Intolerance

LACTOSE INTOLERANCE

Many adults unable to digest lactose caused by lactase
deficiency.
Unabsorbed lactose raises osmotic pressure of bowel
contents, leading to retention of fluid in intestinal
lumen associated with cramps and diarrhea.
Symptoms abate when dairy products discontinued.

GLUTEN INTOLERANCE

Hypersensitivity to wheat protein leads to impaired intestinal absorption and atrophy of intestinal villi.
Diagnosis established by small bowel biopsy.

Treatment by gluten-free diet relieves symptoms and villi return to normal.

Irritable Bowel Syndrome

PATHOGENESIS AND MANIFESTATIONS

Disturbed bowel function without structural or biochemical abnormalities.

A diagnosis of exclusion.

Symptomatic treatment relieves symptoms.

Symptomatic treatment may also improve intestinal motility.

Intestinal Infections in Homosexual Men

PATHOGENESIS AND MANIFESTATIONS

Intestinal complaints among homosexual men caused by bacterial–parasitic infections spread by sexual practices.

May be misinterpreted as irritable bowel syndrome.

Specific treatment given after diagnostic studies completed.

Eating Disorders

OBESITY

Calorie intake exceeds requirement.

Major health consequences.

Cardiovascular disease.

Musculoskeletal problems.

Impaired pulmonary function.

Operation carries high risk.

Higher death rate from cancer.

Treatment.

Medical management often ineffective.

Surgical treatment: gastric bypass or adjustable gastric banding.

ANOREXIA NERVOSA AND BULIMIA NERVOSA

Anorexia nervosa.

False perception of being fat despite marked weight loss.

Food intake restricted to lose weight.

Self-induced vomiting and laxatives may be used to promote weight loss.

Organ system abnormalities occur related to food restriction.

Requires psychiatric–medical treatment by persons experienced in dealing with eating disorders.

Bulimia nervosa.

Binge eating followed by self-induced vomiting.

Usually weight maintained. Family and friends may not be aware of behavior.

Risk of gastric mucosa tears from retching and vomiting.

Dental problems and metabolic alkalosis from vomiting-induced loss of gastric acid.

Treatment similar to treatment of anorexia nervosa.

BINGE EATING DISORDERS

Characterized by binge eating without self-induced vomiting leading to weight gain.

Affects older adults and complicates problems of person trying to lose weight.

Treatment requires patient motivation, as when dealing with overeating problems.

CHRONIC MALNUTRITION

In developing countries caused by inadequate food or poor distribution.

In industrialized countries usually caused by diseases that impair food utilization.

Identify and treat persons at risk.

Diverticulosis and Diverticulitis of Colon

PATHOGENESIS

Outpouching of colonic mucosa through weak areas in wall.

Chronic constipation and low-residue diet predisposes.

COMPLICATIONS

Inflammation.

Bleeding.

TREATMENT

Asymptomatic diverticula do not require treatment.

Surgical resection of affected bowel if complications occur.

Intestinal Obstruction

HIGH INTESTINAL OBSTRUCTION

Crampy pain and vomiting.

Severe water and electrolyte disturbances develop rapidly.

LOW INTESTINAL OBSTRUCTION

Mild crampy pain and distention.

Water and electrolyte disturbances not a major problem.

CAUSES

Adhesions: from previous surgery.

Hernia: protrusion of bowel through weak area in abdominal wall.

Volvulus: rotary twisting of sigmoid colon on its mesentery.

Intussusception: telescoping of one segment of bowel into adjacent segment.

As a result of vigorous peristalsis.

Caused by pedunculated tumor.

Mesenteric Thrombosis

PATHOGENESIS

Superior mesenteric artery supplies small bowel and proximal half of colon.

Artery may become blocked by thrombus, embolus, or atheroma.

Obstruction of artery causes extensive bowel infarction.

Tumors of Bowel

SMALL INTESTINE

Small-bowel tumors are uncommon.

COLON
Benign polyps.
Carcinoma.
> *Left half of colon: tumors often obstruct colon.*
> *Right half of colon: usually causes chronic blood loss but does not obstruct.*

Imperforate Anus
MANIFESTATIONS AND TREATMENT
Congenitally absent anal opening, sometimes with absent distal rectum as well.
Can be corrected surgically.

Hemorrhoids
PATHOGENESIS
Varicose veins of hemorrhoidal venous plexus.
Constipation predisposes.

CLASSIFICATION
Internal hemorrhoids: may bleed or prolapse or become thrombosed.

External hemorrhoids: may become thrombosed.
TREATMENT
Conservative treatment preferred.
Can be treated surgically if not responsive to conservative therapy.

Diagnostic Evaluation of Gastrointestinal Tract Disease
DIAGNOSTIC METHODS
Endoscopy: tube inserted to visualize interior of gastrointestinal tract. Biopsies performed if indicated.
X-ray studies.

Water, Electrolyte, and Acid-Base Balance

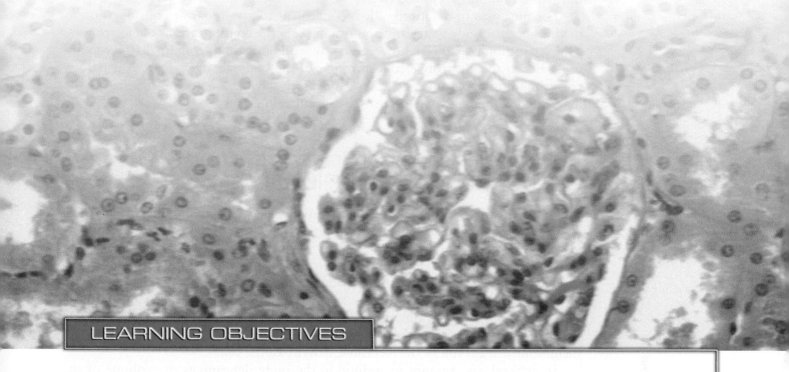

1 Explain the basic concepts relating to the regulation of the concentration of electrolytes in the body. List the major ions in the intracellular and extracellular water, and define units of concentration.

2 Describe the common disturbances of water balance and their pathogenesis.

3 Explain the physiologic mechanisms concerned with the control of pH.

4 Describe the pathogenesis of the four common disturbances of acid–base balance and the body's compensatory mechanisms.

5 Define the role of the kidneys and the lungs in the regulation of acid–base balance.

Body Water and Electrolytes

About 70% of the body consists of water. Most is within cells as intracellular water. The remainder, called extracellular water, is within the interstitial tissues surrounding the cells and in the blood plasma. The body water contains dissolved mineral salts (**electrolytes**) that dissociate in solution, yielding positively charged ions (**cations**) and negatively charged ions (**anions**). The body fluids are electrically neutral, and the sum of the positively charged ions in solution is always balanced by the sum of the negatively charged ions. In disease, the concentrations of the individual ions may vary, but electrical neutrality is always maintained.

Electrolyte
(ē-lek′trō-līt)
A compound that in solution dissociates into positive and negative ions.

Cation (kat′ī-on)
An ion that carries a positive charge.

Anion (an′ī-on)
An ion carrying a negative charge.

To help remember the distribution of water and contained electrolytes within the body, it may be convenient to use the "rule of thirds." Approximately two-thirds of the body weight is water, and two-thirds of the water is within the cells. The remaining one-third is extracellular, and most of the extracellular fluid is in the tissues surrounding the cells (interstitial fluid). The rest is in the blood and lymph within vessels in the interstitial tissues. The water content of a woman's body is about 10% lower than a man's body of comparable size because a woman has more body fat, which contains very little water.

For purposes of description, it is convenient to give separate consideration to disturbances of body water and abnormalities in the concentrations of electrolytes. This separation is artificial, however, because all body fluids contain dissolved mineral salts. If the electrolyte concentration of the body changes, there is usually a corresponding change in body water. Conversely, changes in body water are usually associated with changes in electrolyte concentrations.

Interrelations of Intracellular and Extracellular Fluid

Fluid and electrolytes diffuse freely between the intravascular and interstitial fluids. However, the capillaries are impermeable to protein, so the interstitial fluid contains very little protein.

The fluid within the cells is separated from the interstitial fluid by the cell membrane, which is freely permeable to water but relatively impermeable to sodium and potassium ions. The principal extracellular ions are sodium (Na^+) and chloride (Cl^-), whereas the principal intracellular ions are potassium (K^+) and phosphate (PO_4^{3-}). The differences in the concentration of the ions on different sides of the cell membrane are a result of the metabolic activity of the cell.

In general, the amount of sodium in the body determines the volume of the extracellular fluid because this is the chief extracellular cation, and the amount of potassium in the body determines the volume of the intracellular fluid because this is the chief intracellular cation.

Units and Concentration of Electrolytes

In dealing with disturbances of electrolytes, the clinician is concerned primarily with concentrations of the various ions and with the interrelation of positively and negatively charged ions with one another, rather than with the actual number of milligrams or grams of the various salts dissolved in the plasma. Therefore, the concentrations of electrolytes are expressed in units that define their ability to combine with other ions.

The quantity that expresses "combining weight" is termed the equivalent weight. An equivalent weight is the molecular weight of a substance in grams divided by its valence. When one equivalent weight of a substance is dissolved in a solution to make 1 liter, the concentration is one equivalent per liter. For a monovalent substance, this is the same as a one molar solution, expressed as one mole per liter.

As an example, the equivalent weight of sodium chloride is determined by adding 23 g (atomic weight of sodium) to 35.5 g (atomic weight of chloride) and dividing by the valence (which is one), to equal 58.5 g of sodium chloride, the equivalent weight.

In body fluids, the concentrations of electrolytes are low and are usually expressed in milliequivalents per liter (abbreviated mEq/liter) rather than in equivalents, although some physicians prefer to express concentrations of monovalent ions in millimoles per liter (abbreviated mmol/liter), which is the same as mEq/liter, when dealing with monovalent ions. A milliequivalent is 1/1,000 of an equivalent. Concentrations of ions expressed in milliequivalents have equal combining properties, even though their equivalent weights are not equal. For example, a milliequivalent of bicarbonate ion is equal in electrical and ionic characteristics to a milliequivalent of chloride ion, even though the molecular weight of bicarbonate is greater than that of chloride.

Regulation of Body Fluid and Electrolyte Concentration

The amount of water and electrolytes in the body represents a balance between the amounts ingested in food and fluids and the amounts excreted in the urine, through the gastrointestinal tract, in perspiration, and as water vapor excreted by the lungs. The kidneys are important in controlling the concentration of body water and electrolytes. Under the influence of adrenal cortical and posterior pituitary hormones, the kidneys regulate the internal environment of the body by selectively excreting or retaining water and electrolytes as required to maintain a uniform composition of the body fluids.

Disturbances of Water Balance

DEHYDRATION

The most common disturbance of water balance is dehydration, which may be caused by inadequate water intake or excess water loss. Most cases of dehydration seen in medical practice result from excessive loss of fluid from the gastrointestinal tract as a consequence of vomiting or diarrhea. Fluid intake is usually decreased, contributing to the dehydration. Occasionally, comatose or debilitated patients become dehydrated because of inadequate intake of fluid.

OVERHYDRATION

Overhydration is less common than dehydration. Sometimes overhydration results from administering too much fluid intravenously, but may also occur when a person with impaired renal function drinks a large amount of fluid, which the kidneys are unable to excrete efficiently. Drinking a large amount of water may also change the concentration of the electrolytes in the extracellular fluid, even in a person with normal renal function. As the ingested water is absorbed into the circulation, the water increases the volume of the extracellular fluid, which lowers its sodium ion concentration (hyponatremia) as the fluid becomes more dilute. Marked hyponatremia may have serious and sometimes life-threatening consequences. This condition may occur in an infant who is given water to supplement formula feedings or when the infant's formula is prepared with too much water and is too dilute. Infants under 6 months of age are at greatest risk, as their kidneys are relatively immature and they are less able to excrete the excess water. Another group at risk includes athletes engaging in strenuous sports, such as marathon runners, who consume excessive amounts of water while exercising in order to prevent dehydration. Their renal function also may be compromised during vigorous exercise because renal blood flow falls and urine output declines as blood is diverted from the kidneys to actively exercising muscles.

Disturbances of Electrolyte Balance

In general, the same conditions that produce disturbances of water balance also disturb the electrolyte composition of the body fluids. Most electrolyte disturbances result from depletion of body electrolytes. Depletions of sodium and potassium generally occur together, often because of loss of electrolytes along with water from the gastrointestinal tract as a result of vomiting or diarrhea. Large amounts of sodium and potassium may also be lost in the urine as a result of prolonged use of diuretics. Diuretics are substances that promote excretion of salts and water by the kidneys by impairing reabsorption of these substances from the glomerular filtrate; they are often administered to patients with heart failure, cirrhosis of the liver, and some types of kidney diseases. Loss of large amounts of electrolytes may also accompany excessive excretion of water in the urine in uncontrolled diabetes, as a result of the diuretic effect of the excreted glucose (discussion on the pancreas and diabetes mellitus), or in renal tubular disease, in which the regenerating renal tubules are unable to conserve electrolytes and water (discussion on the urinary system).

Acid–Base Balance

The body may be considered an acid-producing machine that generates large amounts of organic and inorganic acids in consequence of normal metabolic processes. It produces various nonvolatile acids such as sulfuric, phosphoric, and uric acid in the breakdown of proteins. It forms ketone bodies in the oxidation of fat (discussion on the pancreas and diabetes mellitus) and produces lactic acid from breakdown of glucose when oxygen supplies are insufficient. Large amounts of carbon dioxide also are formed as by-products of intracellular metabolic processes, and some of the carbon dioxide dissolves in body fluids to form carbonic acid.

Despite the large amounts of acid produced, the body fluids remain slightly alkaline, and their pH is maintained within the narrow range of 7.38–7.42. The body is able to maintain the alkalinity of body fluids because it has three regulatory mechanisms that neutralize and eliminate the acids as rapidly as they are formed:

1. The buffer systems of the blood
2. The lungs, which regulate the carbonic acid concentration
3. The kidneys, which control bicarbonate concentration

BUFFERS

The buffer systems of the blood are the first line of defense against change in pH. In a general sense, a buffer is anything that cushions a blow or absorbs an impact. Chemically, a buffer may be defined as a weak acid and a salt of the acid or as a weak base and its salt. Buffers minimize change in hydrogen ion concentration by converting strong (completely ionized) acids and bases into weaker (less completely dissociated) acids and bases.

The major buffer system of the blood is the sodium bicarbonate–carbonic acid system. This system is of major importance because both components of the buffer system are present in large amounts, and the concentration of each component can be regulated by the body. The concentration of carbonic acid (dissolved carbon dioxide) is controlled by the lungs, and the concentration of bicarbonate is controlled by the kidneys. Although the bicarbonate–carbonic acid buffer system is not the only buffer system of the body, the system is in equilibrium with the other buffer systems. Therefore, measurement of the components of this system provides an overall evaluation of the acid–base status of the patient.

RESPIRATORY CONTROL OF CARBONIC ACID

Carbonic acid represents physically dissolved carbon dioxide in plasma. This is in equilibrium with the carbon dioxide in the pulmonary alveoli. (The concentration of a gas is expressed in terms of its partial pressure; it is also common to speak of the partial pressure as the tension of the gas.) Hyperventilation lowers the alveolar carbon dioxide partial pressure (PCO_2) and leads to a rapid decrease in the concentration of carbon dioxide and carbonic acid in the plasma. Decreased or inadequate pulmonary ventilation results in elevation of alveolar PCO_2, which in turn raises plasma carbon dioxide and carbonic acid.

CONTROL OF BICARBONATE CONCENTRATION

The kidneys regulate bicarbonate concentration in the plasma by selectively reabsorbing filtered bicarbonate as necessary to meet the body's requirements. In addition, the kidneys can manufacture bicarbonate to replace the amounts lost in buffering acids produced as a consequence of normal metabolic processes. These two bicarbonate-regulating functions depend on the secretion of hydrogen ions by the renal tubules in exchange for sodium ions, which are simultaneously reabsorbed from the tubular filtrate into the circulation as illustrated in FIGURE 24-1. Under the influence of the enzyme carbonic anhydrase, carbonic acid (H_2CO_3) is formed from carbon dioxide (CO_2) and water (H_2O) within the tubular epithelial cells and dissociates into hydrogen (H^+) and bicarbonate (HCO_3^-) ions. The hydrogen

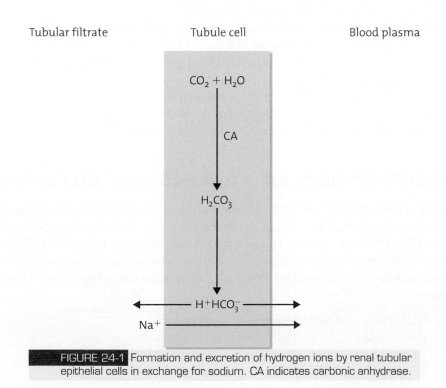

FIGURE 24-1 Formation and excretion of hydrogen ions by renal tubular epithelial cells in exchange for sodium. CA indicates carbonic anhydrase.

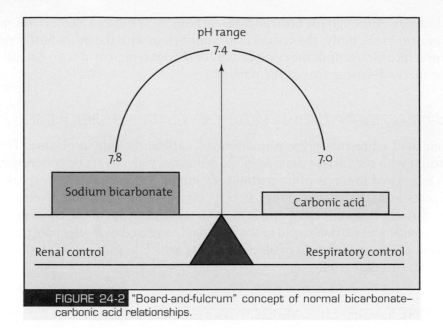

FIGURE 24-2 "Board-and-fulcrum" concept of normal bicarbonate–carbonic acid relationships.

ions enter the tubular filtrate in exchange for sodium ions (Na^+). The bicarbonate ions enter the bloodstream along with the sodium ions that have been absorbed from the filtrate.

RELATIONSHIP BETWEEN pH AND RATIO OF BUFFER COMPONENTS

In any buffer system, the pH depends on the ratio of the two components and not on the absolute quantities of the components. For the bicarbonate–carbonic acid buffer system, at normal body pH of 7.4, the normal ratio consists of 20 parts of sodium bicarbonate and 1 part of carbonic acid.

Another way of visualizing the bicarbonate–carbonic acid relationship is to think of a board on a fulcrum. One side of the board is weighted by 20 parts of sodium bicarbonate, and the other side is weighted by 1 part of carbonic acid. The fulcrum is placed so that the board is exactly in balance, corresponding to a body pH of 7.4. Variations in the "weight" of either the sodium bicarbonate or the carbonic acid can be visualized as unbalancing the board, resulting in a shift of pH to a new level, either higher or lower than the normal value (FIGURE 24-2).

Disturbances of Acid–Base Balance

A disturbance in which blood pH is shifted to the acid side of the physiologic range is called **acidosis**. It may be caused by an excess of carbonic acid or by a reduced amount of bicarbonate. A shift in the opposite direction is termed **alkalosis**. This shift may be the result of a decrease in carbonic acid or to an excess of bicarbonate. These possibilities allow classification of acid–base disturbances into four large categories:

1. Metabolic acidosis (decrease in bicarbonate)
2. Respiratory acidosis (increase in carbonic acid)
3. Metabolic alkalosis (increase in bicarbonate)
4. Respiratory alkalosis (decrease in carbonic acid)

Acidosis
A disturbance in the acid–base balance of the body in which body fluids have a lower pH than normal.

Alkalosis
A disturbance in the body's acid–base balance in which the pH of the extracellular fluids is shifted toward the alkaline side of normal.

The term metabolic is applied when the disturbance lies primarily in the bicarbonate member of the buffer pair. The term respiratory indicates that the primary disturbance lies in the carbonic acid component of the buffer.

The various forms of acid–base disturbance are compared in TABLE 24-1.

COMPENSATORY MECHANISMS RESPONDING TO DISTURBANCES IN pH

If the acid–base disturbance shifts the pH outside of the physiologic range, various control measures are activated to resist the change in pH. Compensatory mechanisms attempt to preserve the normal 20:1 ratio of bicarbonate to carbonic acid and thereby return the pH to physiologic range. For example, if the concentration of carbonic acid rises, there is a compensatory increase in bicarbonate that tends to restore the ratio of the two constituents and maintain pH in the physiologic range. Conversely, if there is a decrease in bicarbonate, compensation involves a decrease in the concentration of carbonic acid to maintain a relatively normal ratio. The body's major concern is maintaining a normal ratio of constituents to maintain a physiologic pH, even though this is accomplished by changing the absolute concentrations of the members of the buffer pair. Compensation is accomplished by both renal and respiratory methods.

TABLE 24-1

Comparison of common acid–base disturbances

Disturbance	Primary abnormality	Compensation	Usual causes
Metabolic acidosis	Excess endogenous acid depletes bicarbonate	Hyperventilation lowers PCO_2; kidney excretes more hydrogen ions and forms more bicarbonate	Renal failure; ketosis; overproduction of lactic acid
Respiratory acidosis	Inefficient excretion of carbon dioxide by lungs	Formation of additional bicarbonate by kidneys	Chronic pulmonary disease
Metabolic alkalosis	Excess plasma bicarbonate	None	Loss of gastric juice; chloride depletion; excess corticosteroid hormones; ingestion of excessive bicarbonate or other antacids
Respiratory alkalosis	Hyperventilation lowers PCO_2	Increased excretion of bicarbonate by kidneys	Severe anxiety with hyperventilation; stimulation of respiratory center by drugs; central nervous system disease

If one member of the buffer pair is disturbed by disease, the compensation is achieved by the other member of the buffer pair. For example, if the primary disturbance is in the bicarbonate, the compensation involves a change in carbonic acid, which is controlled by the lungs. Conversely, if the primary disturbance is in carbonic acid, the compensation involves a change in bicarbonate, which is controlled by the kidneys. The compensations are the body's attempt to minimize the extent of the pH change resulting from a disease-related change affecting one member of the buffer pair by changing the other member. This provides a short-term solution to the acid–base disturbance. The long-term correction of an acid–base balance derangement involves treating successfully the underlying disease that caused the pH disturbance, which may not always be possible.

For the student attempting to grasp the fundamentals of the major disturbances in acid–base balance, the "board-and-fulcrum" concept shown in FIGURE 24-2 is frequently helpful. The "weight" of carbonic acid is controlled by respiration, and the "weight" of bicarbonate is controlled by renal excretion or conservation of bicarbonate. The student should consider two things: (1) the nature of the primary disturbance and how it will "unbalance" the board and (2) the steps that the body should take to bring the board back into balance. These are the compensatory mechanisms, and they generally consist of "adding weight" or "subtracting weight" from the other member of the board. Admittedly, this is a mechanical oversimplification of a complex process, but it is a helpful learning device.

The two most common clinical disturbances of acid–base balance are metabolic acidosis and respiratory acidosis.

METABOLIC ACIDOSIS

Metabolic acidosis, a common problem in medical practice, occurs when the amount of acid generated exceeds the body's buffering capacity. The concentration of bicarbonate in the plasma falls because it is consumed in neutralizing the excess acid (FIGURE 24-3A). Three of the more common conditions leading to metabolic acidosis are:

1. Renal failure (uremia)
2. Ketosis (overproduction of ketone bodies)
3. Lactic acidosis (excessive production of lactic acid)

Uremia
(ur-ē′mi-yuh)
An excess of urea and other waste products in the blood, resulting from renal failure.

Ketosis
(kē-tō′sis)
An excess of ketone bodies (acetoacetic acid, beta-hydroxybutyric acid, and acetone) in the blood resulting from utilization of fat as the primary source of energy.

Uremia is the end stage of many different types of kidney disease, as described in the discussion on congenital and hereditary diseases. Metabolic acidosis occurs because the failing kidneys are unable to excrete efficiently the various acid waste products that are produced by the body's normal metabolic processes. **Ketosis** results from overproduction of the acid ketone bodies acetoacetic acid and beta-hydroxybutyric acid, which are derived from the metabolism of fat.

Ketosis commonly occurs in untreated type 1 diabetes because the body is unable to use carbohydrate efficiently and is forced to rely on fat as a major energy source (discussion on the pancreas and diabetes mellitus). Ketosis may also occur in any condition in which carbohydrate intake is inadequate, as in starvation, or if persistent vomiting prevents the retention of nutrients. In such cases, the body has to metabolize adipose tissue because carbohydrate is not available as an energy source. Some diets, called ketogenic diets, are actually designed to produce ketosis. They contain a large amount of fat, limited carbohydrates, and moderate protein. Ketogenic diets can be used to treat some types of epilepsy and have also been used to promote weight loss.

Lactic acidosis occurs in a number of different conditions, such as shock or severe heart failure in which the tissues receive an inadequate supply of oxygen. The lactic acid is formed from the breakdown of glucose in the presence of an insufficient oxygen supply.

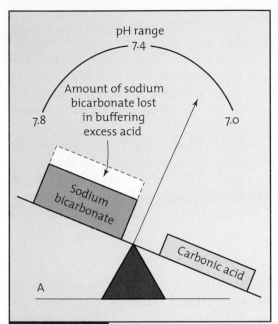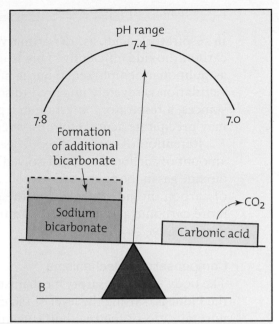

FIGURE 24-3 **A**, Derangement of acid–base balance in metabolic acidosis. **B**, Compensation by reduction of carbonic acid and formation of additional bicarbonate.

Compensatory Mechanisms

Compensation for metabolic acidosis is accomplished by both the lungs and the kidneys (FIGURE 24-3B). The acidosis stimulates the respiratory center in the brain stem, leading to an increase in both the rate and the depth of respiration. The hyperventilation reduces the partial pressure of carbon dioxide (PCO_2) in the alveoli, which in turn leads to a reduction in the amount of dissolved carbon dioxide and carbonic acid in the plasma. The decline in carbonic acid tends to restore the bicarbonate–carbonic acid ratio and pH toward normal. If renal function is not impaired, the kidneys also produce more bicarbonate to replenish the depleted supplies and at the same time excrete more hydrogen ions.

The following case illustrates a severe metabolic acidosis secondary to renal insufficiency. Case studies dealing with other diseases that cause metabolic acidosis are considered in the urinary system and the pancreas and diabetes mellitus discussion.

CASE 24-1

A 65-year-old woman consulted her physician because of discomfort in the lower back. Physical examination revealed moderate enlargement of both kidneys. Laboratory studies revealed a small amount of albumin in the urine and a moderate degree of anemia. Urea nitrogen was 57 mg/dl, a moderate elevation (normal range 10–20 mg/dl). A pyelogram revealed bilateral polycystic kidneys. The patient declined further treatment but was readmitted 6 months later because of further deterioration of her condition. She was more anemic, and the blood urea nitrogen had risen to 148 mg/dl. Blood pH was reduced to 7.2 (normal range 7.38–7.42). Plasma bicarbonate was also reduced to 10 mEq/liter. The PCO_2 was 30 mm Hg, a slight decrease that was secondary to hyperventilation. The patient was considered to be in terminal renal failure with marked metabolic acidosis. Despite intensive therapy, her condition did not improve, and she died in the hospital a few days later.

RESPIRATORY ACIDOSIS

In respiratory acidosis, the primary abnormality is failure of the lungs to excrete carbon dioxide efficiently. This is usually secondary to chronic lung disease such as pulmonary emphysema, but it may occur in any situation in which pulmonary ventilation is severely impaired (discussion on the respiratory system). In many instances, a respiratory infection in a patient with an underlying chronic lung disease may precipitate acute respiratory acidosis.

Retention of carbon dioxide leads to a rise in the alveolar PCO_2. Because the amount of carbon dioxide dissolved in the plasma is in equilibrium with the carbon dioxide gas in the pulmonary alveoli, a rise in alveolar PCO_2 also increases the amount of carbon dioxide dissolved in the plasma. As more carbon dioxide is dissolved, more carbonic acid is formed and the pH shifts to the acid side of the physiologic range (FIGURE 24-4A).

Compensatory Mechanisms

The body's compensatory mechanism is the formation of additional bicarbonate by the kidneys, raising the level of bicarbonate in the plasma. This tends to restore the normal ratio of the two buffer components, thereby shifting the pH back toward the physiologic range (FIGURE 24-4B).

The following case illustrates an example of respiratory acidosis precipitated by a right lower-lobe pneumonia in an emphysematous patient.

CASE 24-2

A 64-year-old man had noted progressive chronic cough and shortness of breath on exertion and repeated bouts of respiratory infection. He had become so short of breath that he was no longer able to climb stairs or do any kind of work around the house. Chest x-ray revealed hyperinflation of the lungs, compatible with pulmonary emphysema, and pulmonary function studies also showed marked impairment. Physical examination revealed a severely dyspneic man who was also slightly cyanotic. Scattered wheezes were heard throughout both lungs with a stethoscope. The temperature was slightly elevated. Chest x-ray revealed pulmonary emphysema and an area of consolidation in the right lower lobe of the lung representing a superimposed pneumonia. Arterial blood oxygen saturation was reduced; partial pressure of carbon dioxide was increased (PCO_2 50 mm Hg), and blood pH was reduced (pH 7.30). The patient was treated with antibiotic therapy and supplementary oxygen. He eventually recovered from the pneumonia and was able to leave the hospital.

METABOLIC ALKALOSIS

Metabolic alkalosis is characterized by an increase in the concentration of plasma bicarbonate relative to the concentration of carbonic acid, which shifts the pH to the alkaline side of the physiologic range. The main causes of the metabolic alkalosis are as follows:

1. Loss of acid gastric juice or neutralization of gastric juice by antacids
2. Chloride depletion
3. Excess adrenal corticosteroid hormones

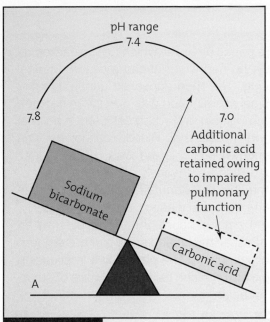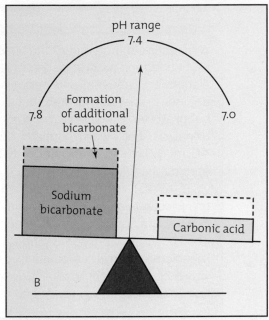

FIGURE 24-4 **A**, Derangement of acid–base balance in respiratory acidosis. **B**, Compensation by formation of additional bicarbonate.

Loss of Acid Gastric Juice or Neutralization by Antacids

Excessive amounts of gastric juice may be lost by prolonged vomiting. Sometimes it is necessary to keep the stomach empty by continuous aspiration of gastric contents by means of a tube inserted through the nose into the stomach (nasogastric tube). In both situations, the loss of gastric juice causes loss of hydrogen ions. Alkalosis results because of the way that hydrochloric acid (HCl) is formed in the stomach. Within the gastric epithelial cells, carbon dioxide (CO_2) and water (H_2O) combine under the influence of the enzyme carbonic anhydrase to form carbonic acid (H_2CO_3), which dissociates into hydrogen (H^+) and bicarbonate (HCO_3^-). The hydrogen ion (H^+) is secreted along with the chloride ion (Cl^-) to form hydrochloric acid, and the remaining bicarbonate ion is absorbed into the blood plasma.

Normally, most of the acid secreted by the stomach is neutralized in the duodenum by alkaline pancreatic juice that is rich in bicarbonate ions. Consequently, the amount of bicarbonate decomposed in the duodenum when gastric juice is neutralized is equivalent to the amount of bicarbonate that is absorbed when acid was being secreted; therefore, there is no net increase in the plasma bicarbonate concentration (FIGURE 24-5A). However, if gastric juice is lost by vomiting or by continuous aspiration of gastric juice, the bicarbonate absorbed when acid is secreted is not "cancelled out" by loss of an equivalent amount of bicarbonate to neutralize acid in the duodenum. Consequently, the concentration of bicarbonate in the plasma rises and alkalosis occurs (FIGURE 24-5B).

Excessive use of antacids may also cause metabolic alkalosis by neutralizing gastric acid, which has the same effect as loss of gastric juice by vomiting or continuous aspiration of gastric juice. Ingesting sodium bicarbonate as an antacid to neutralize gastric acid has the same effect as any other antacid. In addition, any sodium bicarbonate ingested that exceeds the amount required to neutralize the gastric acid will be absorbed, contributing further to the metabolic alkalosis.

The following case illustrates an example of marked metabolic alkalosis related to a chronic stomach ulcer treated by antacids and complicated by vomiting of gastric juice.

CASE 24-3

A 45-year-old man had a long history of a peptic ulcer for which he took antacids as needed for gastric distress. Recently, he had experienced more abdominal discomfort, nausea, and periodic vomiting. The man appeared uncomfortable and somewhat dehydrated, but the physical examination was otherwise normal. Laboratory studies revealed a normal hemoglobin and white cells and a normal urinalysis, but blood chemistry studies were abnormal. Blood bicarbonate was 48 mEq/liter (normal range, 22–29 mEq/liter), chloride was 82 mEq/liter (normal range, 98–105 mEq/liter), and blood pH was 7.48 (normal range, 7.35–7.45). A tube was inserted into the stomach, and a large volume of gastric juice was aspirated, indicating that the stomach was not emptying properly. X-ray examination of the stomach using a small amount of barium revealed an obstruction at the pylorus, apparently from scar tissue and spasm of the smooth muscle at the pylorus caused by the chronic ulcer. The physician's impression was marked metabolic alkalosis resulting from vomiting related to pyloric obstruction, associated with prolonged use of antacids.

Chloride Depletion

Chloride depletion results from loss of gastrointestinal secretions caused by severe vomiting or diarrhea. It may also follow administration of some diuretics. Chloride and bicarbonate are the two chief anions in the plasma, and their concentrations vary inversely. When the plasma chloride falls, plasma bicarbonate rises so that the total concentration of anions in the extracellular fluids remains relatively constant.

Excess Adrenal Corticosteroids

An excess secretion of adrenal corticosteroids that regulate salt and water metabolism (mineralocorticoids) often causes not only metabolic alkalosis, but potassium depletion as well. A major site of action of corticosteroids is the distal renal tubule, where the hormone promotes absorption of sodium in exchange for potassium, which is secreted into the tubular filtrate. An excess of mineralocorticoids increases absorption of sodium in exchange for potassium in the distal tubules, leading to excessive potassium loss and depletion of body potassium. As potassium deficiency develops, less potassium is available for exchange, and much of the sodium must be absorbed from the distal tubules in exchange for hydrogen ions rather than potassium ions. (The secretion rates of hydrogen and potassium ions vary inversely.) Each hydrogen ion secreted by the renal tubules is associated with the formation of a bicarbonate ion that diffuses into the plasma, as previously described (see FIGURE 24-1). Consequently, plasma bicarbonate rises when hydrogen ions are secreted in excess and metabolic alkalosis results.

Compensatory Mechanisms in Metabolic Alkalosis

Compensatory measures in metabolic alkalosis are quite inefficient. Respiratory compensation is extremely limited. If pulmonary ventilation were decreased enough to raise alveolar carbon dioxide tension, oxygenation of the blood would be inadequate. Bicarbonate excretion by the kidneys is inefficient in the presence of potassium deficiency, which frequently coexists with metabolic alkalosis. When intracellular potassium is depleted, sodium reabsorption from the distal tubule occurs primarily in exchange for hydrogen ions. The increased secretion of hydrogen ions leads to the formation of additional bicarbonate ions, which diffuse into the circulation and raise the concentration of bicarbonate in the plasma. As a result, the potassium-depleted kidney not only is unable to compensate for the alkalosis, but actually accentuates it by forming excess bicarbonate. Successful treatment of metabolic alkalosis generally requires simultaneous correction of the potassium deficiency.

RESPIRATORY ALKALOSIS

Respiratory alkalosis is a result of hyperventilation, which lowers the alveolar PCO_2. This in turn leads to a corresponding decrease in the amount of dissolved carbon dioxide and carbonic acid in the plasma. As a result, there is a relative excess of bicarbonate, and the blood pH tends to rise (FIGURE 24-6A). The hyperventilation that initiates this disturbance may result from stimulation of the respiratory center by drugs or may result from disease of the nervous system. Sometimes, the hyperventilation is the result of an emotional disturbance such as severe anxiety. The temporary discomfort experienced by a vacationer traveling from sea level to a high altitude is caused in part by a mild respiratory alkalosis resulting from the hyperventilation induced by the lower PO_2 in the atmospheric air at high altitude. Fortunately, the body gradually learns to adapt and the initial discomfort gradually subsides.

Compensatory Mechanisms

Compensation is achieved by increased excretion of bicarbonate by the kidneys, which lowers the plasma bicarbonate and tends to restore the ratio of the buffer components toward normal (FIGURE 24-6B).

DIAGNOSTIC EVALUATION OF ACID–BASE BALANCE

In evaluating the acid–base status of a patient, the clinician frequently determines the concentration of the bicarbonate in the plasma as an index of the patient's overall status. This is supplemented in many cases by the determination of

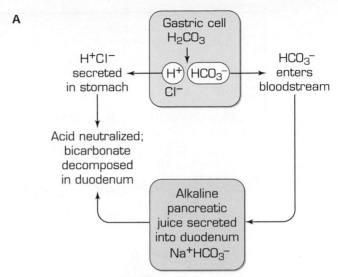

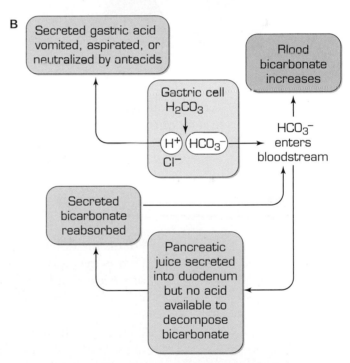

FIGURE 24-5 Metabolic alkalosis caused by loss or neutralization of gastric juice by antacids. **A,** Normal secretion of hydrochloric acid (HCl). Each H^+ secreted into the stomach with Cl^- to form HCl is associated with secretion of a HCO_3^- into the bloodstream. Each secreted H^+ is neutralized by a HCO_3^- in alkaline pancreatic juice secreted into the duodenum, so there is no net increase of bicarbonate in the bloodstream related to the acid secretion. **B,** In metabolic alkalosis, secreted H^+ in HCl is aspirated, lost by vomiting, or neutralized by antacids, and HCO_3^- (formed when H^+ is secreted as HCl) is released into the bloodstream; however, the HCO_3^- in pancreatic secretions released into the duodenum is not neutralized, and HCO_3^- in the pancreatic secretions is absorbed from the duodenum into the bloodstream. The HCO_3^- concentration in the bloodstream rises.

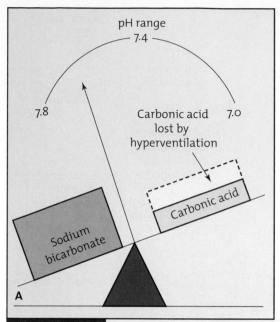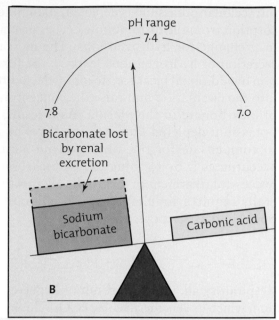

FIGURE 24-6 **A,** Derangement of acid–base balance in respiratory alkalosis. **B,** Compensation by excretion of bicarbonate.

the blood pH and the determination of the carbonic acid in the plasma. The clinical state of the patient, as evaluated by the clinician, together with these various laboratory tests, generally permits a determination of the patient's acid–base status and serves as a guide for effective treatment.

QUESTIONS FOR REVIEW

1. What is the difference between intracellular fluid and extracellular fluid?
2. What is meant by the following terms: *milliequivalent*, *diuretic*, *carbonic anhydrase*, and *buffer*?
3. What is metabolic acidosis? How does it arise? What are the body's compensatory mechanisms?
4. What is respiratory acidosis? How does it arise? What are the body's compensatory mechanisms?
5. What is metabolic alkalosis? How does it arise? What are the body's compensatory mechanisms?
6. What is respiratory alkalosis? How does it arise? What are the body's compensatory mechanisms?

SUPPLEMENTARY READINGS

Almond, C. S., Shin, A. Y., Fortescue, E. B., et al. 2005. Hyponatremia among runners in the Boston marathon. *The New England Journal of Medicine* 352:1550–6.
▶ Four hundred eighty-eight participants in the 2002 Boston marathon provided a blood sample at the conclusion of the marathon and a completed questionnaire describing their fluid consumption and urine output during the race. Thirteen percent had a significant hyponatremia; three persons had a severe, potentially life-threatening hyponatremia to less than 120 mmol/liter. Many hyponatremic runners drank more than 3 liters during the race, which diluted their body fluids and led to the hyponatremia.

Excess fluid intake should be avoided during strenuous exercise because the kidneys may be unable to excrete the excess water efficiently.

See also the accompanying editorial in the same issue: Levine, B. J., and Thompson, P. D. 2005. Marathon maladies. *The New England Journal of Medicine* 352:1516–7.

Beers, M. H., Fletcher, A. J., Jones, T. V., et al. 2003. *The Merck manual of medical information. Second home edition.* New York: Pocket Books, a division of Simon & Schuster, Inc.
▶ A very well-known medical reference based on the version produced for physicians. The material is very clearly written and concise.

Centers for Disease Control and Prevention. 1994. Hyponatremic seizures among infants fed with commercial bottled drinking water—Wisconsin, 1993. *Morbidity and Mortality Weekly Report* 43:641–3.
▶ Several cases of severe water intoxication with hyponatremia are described in infants caused by supplementing infant formula with commercial bottled drinking water or when infant formula was diluted with water. Infants experienced irritability, drowsiness, and convulsions. Water should not be given to infants less than 6 months old.

Cohen, R. D., and Woods, H. F. 1983. Lactic acidosis revisited. *Diabetes* 32:181–91.
▶ Reviews sites of production of lactic acid, pathophysiology, and treatment.

Dale, D. C., and Federman, D. D., eds. 1999. *Scientific american medicine.* New York: Scientific American, Inc.
▶ Updated monthly.

Davenport, H. W. 1974. *The ABC of acid–base chemistry*, 6th ed. Chicago: University of Chicago Press.
▶ The classic monograph on this subject.

Guyton, A. C., and Hall, J. E. 1997. *Human physiology and mechanisms of disease*, 6th ed. Philadelphia: W. B. Saunders Company.
▶ A comprehensive clinically oriented treatment of fluid and electrolyte disturbances.

Lowenstein, J. 1993. *Acid and basics: A guide to understanding acid–base disorders.* New York: Oxford University Press.
▶ A concise treatment of acid–base disorders.

Narins, R. G., Jones, E. R., Stom, M. C., et al. 1982. Diagnostic strategies in disorders of fluid, electrolyte and acid–base homeostasis. *American Journal of Medicine* 72:496–520.
▶ Discusses pathophysiology and biochemistry of acid–base and fluid-electrolyte disturbances.

Schrier, R. W., ed. 1997. *Renal and electrolyte disorders*, 5th ed. Philadelphia: W. B. Saunders Company.
▶ A comprehensive text.

Silverthorn, D. U. 1998. *Human physiology: An integrated approach.* Saddle River, N.J.: Prentice-Hall, Inc.
▶ A user-friendly section on fluid and electrolyte balance.

Tierney, L. M., McPhee, S. J., and Papadakis, M. A. 2006. *Current medical diagnosis & treatment*, 45th ed. New York: Lang Medical Books/McGraw-Hill.
▶ Good section on fluids, electrolytes, and acid–base balance.

Walsh, P. C., ed. 1998. *Campbell's urology*, 7th ed. Philadelphia: W. B. Saunders Company.
▶ A comprehensive textbook with good sections on urologic aspects of acid–base and electrolyte disturbances.

OUTLINE SUMMARY

Interrelations of Intracellular and Extracellular Fluid

BASIC CONCEPTS
Intracellular water is 70% of total body water.
Water contains dissolved electrolytes.
Sum of positive ions balanced by negative ions.
Disturbances of body water are associated with corresponding changes in electrolytes.
Fluids and electrolytes diffuse readily but capillaries are impermeable to protein.
Sodium (Na^+) and chloride (Cl^-) are chief extracellular ions; potassium (K^+) and phosphate (PO_4^{3-}) are principal intracellular ions.

UNITS OF CONCENTRATION
Molecular weight of substance in grams divided by valence dissolved in 1 liter equals one equivalent per liter (1 Eq/liter).
Units usually expressed in milliequivalents per liter (1,000 mEq = 1 Eq).

Regulation of Body Fluid and Electrolyte Concentration

PHYSIOLOGIC CONCEPTS
Amount of water and electrolytes in body is balance between amount ingested and amount excreted.
Kidneys are major excretory organs.

DISTURBANCES OF WATER BALANCE
Dehydration.
   Inadequate intake: comatose or debilitated patients.
   Excess water loss: vomiting or diarrhea.
Overhydration.
   Excessive fluid intake when renal function impaired.
   Excessive administration of intravenous fluids.

DISTURBANCES OF ELECTROLYTE BALANCE
Depletion of electrolytes.
   Vomiting or diarrhea.
Excessive use of diuretics.
Excessive diuresis in diabetic acidosis.
Renal tubular disease.

Acid–Base Balance

PHYSIOLOGIC CONCEPTS
Body produces large amounts of acid.
Regulatory mechanisms maintain pH.
   Blood buffers: resist pH change.
   Lungs: control carbonic acid concentration.
   Kidneys: control bicarbonate concentration.

DISTURBANCES OF ACID–BASE BALANCE
Metabolic acidosis.
   Excess acid neutralized by bicarbonate, and bicarbonate concentration falls (uremia, ketosis, lactic acidosis).
   Compensation by hyperventilation (lowers PCO_2) and increased production of bicarbonate by kidneys.
Respiratory acidosis.
Respiratory insufficiency leads to retention of CO_2 and rise in carbonic acid (H_2CO_3).
   Compensation by increased production of bicarbonate by kidneys.
Metabolic alkalosis.
   Increased concentration of bicarbonate as a result of various causes (loss of gastric juice, chloride depletion, excess corticosteroids, excess antacids).
   Frequently coexisting potassium deficiency.
   Compensation inefficient, and requires correction of coexisting potassium deficiency.
Respiratory alkalosis.
   Hyperventilation lowers PCO_2, and H_2CO_3 falls.
   Compensation by excretion of bicarbonate by kidneys.

EVALUATION OF ACID–BASE BALANCE BY THE CLINICIAN
Clinical evaluation.
Laboratory studies: pH, PCO_2, bicarbonate.

http://health.jbpub.com/humandisease/9e

Human Disease Online is a great source for supplementary human disease information for both students and instructors. Visit this website to find a variety of useful tools for learning, thinking, and teaching.

CHAPTER 25

The Endocrine Glands

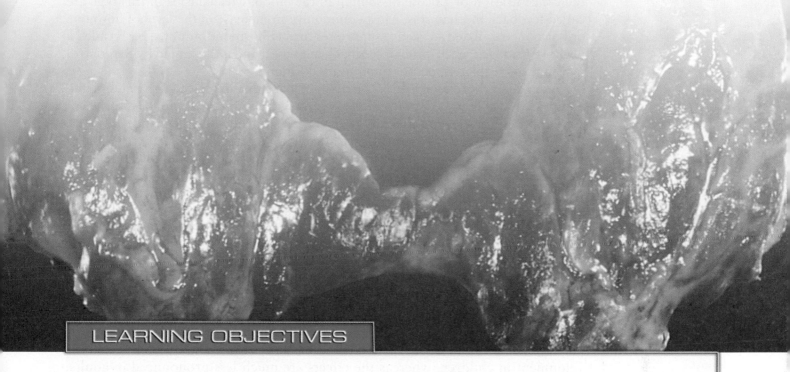

LEARNING OBJECTIVES

1 Explain the normal physiologic functions of the pituitary hormones. Name the common endocrine disturbances, and describe the methods of treating each disturbance.

2 Describe the major disturbances of thyroid function and their clinical manifestations, and explain the methods of treatment.

3 Explain the normal physiologic functions of the adrenal cortex and medulla. Name the common endocrine disturbances resulting from dysfunction, and describe methods of treatment.

4 Define the causes and effects of parathyroid dysfunction, and describe the methods of treatment.

5 Understand the concept of ectopic hormone production by nonendocrine tumors.

6 Explain how stress affects the endocrine system.

Endocrine Functions and Dysfunctions

Endocrine glands liberate their secretions directly into the bloodstream and exert a regulatory effect on various metabolic functions.

The major endocrine glands are the pituitary, thyroid, and parathyroid glands; the adrenal cortex and medulla; the pancreatic islets; and the ovaries and the testes. However, these glands are not the only sites of hormone production. Many groups of specialized cells throughout the body also secrete hormones. Renin and erythropoietin are secreted by the kidneys; the hormones gastrin, secretin, and cholecystokinin are produced by the mucosa of the gastrointestinal tract. By convention, these hormones are considered along with the organs with which they are associated and are not generally regarded as part of the endocrine system.

The amount of hormone synthesized and released into the circulation by an endocrine gland may be regulated directly, by the level of hormone circulating in the blood, or indirectly, by the level of a substance under hormonal control, such as the concentration of glucose or sodium in the blood. Mechanisms of this type are called feedback mechanisms. Most commonly, an increase in the level of hormone or hormone-regulated substance suppresses further hormone output. This is called a negative feedback mechanism or feedback inhibition and is illustrated by the control mechanisms regulating output of pituitary hormones.

A disorder of an endocrine gland may consist of either hypersecretion of the gland, manifested as overactivity of the target organ regulated by the gland, or insufficient secretion, resulting in underactivity of the organ controlled by the gland.

The clinical effects of a disturbance of endocrine gland function are determined by the degree of dysfunction of the gland and by the age and sex of the affected individual. All degrees of glandular dysfunction may be encountered, ranging from barely detectable variations from normal to extreme hypofunction or hyperfunction.

The age of the person when the endocrine disturbance becomes manifest has a pronounced effect on the clinical features. Some endocrine glands, such as the thyroid gland, affect growth and development as well as metabolic processes; therefore, disturbed function in a child will produce a somewhat different clinical picture than will a similar disturbance in an adult.

The sex of the individual also influences the effect of disturbed endocrine function. Many hormones are concerned with the development and maintenance of sexual function and secondary sexual characteristics, and several endocrine glands produce sex hormones. Some endocrine disturbances cause alteration in sexual development in children, whereas the effects are much less pronounced in adults. Overproduction of an inappropriate sex hormone in some endocrine diseases causes masculinization (virilization) of the female or feminization of the male; conversely, overproduction of a sex hormone appropriate to the sex of the individual has little clinical effect.

The Pituitary Gland

Eosinophil
A cell whose cytoplasm is filled with large, uniform granules that stain intensely red with acid dyes. See also basophil.

Basophil (bas′ophil)
A cell that contains numerous variable-sized granules that stain intensely purple with basic dyes. See also eosinophil.

Chromophobe cells
(krō′-mo-fō b)
Anterior lobe pituitary epithelial cells containing sparse poorly stained granules. See also eosinophil and basophil.

The pituitary gland is a small, pea-shaped gland suspended by a narrow stalk from the hypothalamus at the base of the brain. The gland is located within a small depression within the sphenoid bone called the pituitary fossa or sella turcica and is located just behind the optic chiasm. The gland is composed of an anterior lobe and a posterior lobe. Many mammals also have an intermediate lobe located between the anterior and posterior lobes, which produces melanin-stimulating hormone (MSH). However, in humans, the intermediate lobe and its MSH functions have been incorporated into the anterior lobe, and the intermediate lobe is no longer present as a distinct structure.

The anterior lobe is composed of cords of epithelial cells containing hormones that are synthesized and stored within this lobe. It has been conventional to classify anterior-lobe cells on the basis of the staining reaction of their cytoplasmic granules, using routine staining methods. Three cell types were recognized: **eosinophils**, which contain bright-red–staining cytoplasmic granules; **basophils**, which have abundant blue-staining granules in their cytoplasm; and **chromophobe cells**, which contain sparse, poorly stained granules. Newer, more specialized staining methods, however, have identified five different cell types, each producing its own specific hormones. Currently, these cells are more commonly designated by the hormones that they produce rather than by the staining reactions of their granules.

The anterior lobe is connected to the hypothalamus by a special system of blood vessels called a portal system, which begins as capillaries in the hypothalamus and extends down the pituitary stalk to terminate as capillaries around the cells of the anterior lobe. Release of the hormones stored within the cells of the anterior lobe is regulated by hormonal substances called releasing hormones, which are synthesized in the hypothalamus and carried to the cells of the anterior lobe in the blood flowing through the portal system. Usually, a hypothalamic releasing hormone activates a single gland, but some releasing hormones exert an effect on more than one gland. Other hypothalamic hormones inhibit rather than stimulate specific glands, and the hormone response of the target gland reflects the net effect of the interaction between releasing and inhibiting hormones (TABLE 25-1).

The posterior lobe consists of a meshwork of nerve fibers intermixed with modified neuroglial cells. It is connected to the hypothalamus by bundles of nerve fibers extending through the pituitary stalk rather than by the portal circulation. The hormones in the posterior lobe are synthesized within the hypothalamus and are then transmitted down the nerve axons in the pituitary stalk to the posterior lobe, where they are stored. They are then released from the posterior lobe in response to nerve impulses transmitted from the hypothalamus down the pituitary stalk.

The **hypothalamus**, which controls release of hormones from both the anterior and posterior lobes, is in turn under the control of higher cortical centers; consequently, pituitary secretion is to some extent influenced by emotional stimuli such as anxiety, rage, and fear and is also influenced by sensory impulses that enter the nervous system and are in turn relayed to the hypothalamus.

Hypothalamus
Portion of the brain stem that forms the floor of the third ventricle. It contains clusters of nerve cells that regulate various body functions.

TABLE 25-1

Hypothalamic hormones and their targets

Hypothalamic hormone	Response of pituitary and target gland
Thyrotropin-releasing hormone (TRH)	1. Stimulates release of thyroid-stimulating hormone (TSH), which in turn stimulates production and release of thyroid hormone. 2. Stimulates prolactin production and release.
Corticotropin-releasing hormone (CRH)	Stimulates release of adrenocorticotropic hormone (ACTH), which in turn stimulates production and release of adrenal cortical hormones.
Gonadotropin-releasing hormone (GnRH)	Stimulates follicle-stimulating hormone (FSH) and luteinizing hormone (LH), which in turn affect gonadal function.
Growth hormone releasing hormone (GHRH)	Stimulates synthesis of growth hormone, which in turn promotes production of growth factors that promote general tissue growth.
Prolactin inhibitory hormone (Dopamine)	1. Inhibits prolactin release from pituitary gland. 2. Inhibits FSH and LH.
Somatostatin	1. Inhibits secretion and release of growth hormone, which in turn inhibits growth factors that promote general tissue growth. 2. Inhibits TSH.

PITUITARY HORMONES

The pituitary gland secretes a total of nine separate hormones, which have multiple functions. Six are produced by the anterior lobe. Four of these hormones, which regulate other endocrine glands as indicated by their names and abbreviations, are called tropic hormones.

1. Growth hormone
2. Prolactin
3. Thyroid-stimulating hormone (TSH)
4. Adrenocorticotropic hormone (ACTH)
5. Melanin-stimulating hormone (MSH)
6. Follicle-stimulating hormone (FSH)
7. Luteinizing hormone (LH)

The posterior lobe produces two hormones: antidiuretic hormone (ADH) and oxytocin.

Anterior-Lobe Hormones

Growth hormone, also called somatotropin, has multiple actions, all concerned with general tissue growth. Growth hormone exerts its growth-promoting effects on tissues indirectly by stimulating the liver to produce a peptide called somatomedin (*soma* = body + *medin* = mediator of growth), also called insulinlike growth factor. The growth factor enters the circulation and travels throughout the body where it promotes growth of the skeletal system and internal organs. **Prolactin** stimulates the secretion of milk by the breast that has been previously stimulated by estrogen and progesterone. **Thyroid-stimulating hormone** (**TSH**), also called thyrotropin, stimulates the thyroid gland to secrete thyroid hormone. **Adrenocorticotrophic hormone** (**ACTH**), also called corticotropin, stimulates the adrenal cortex to manufacture and secrete adrenocortical hormones. It exerts its main effect on the adrenal hormones that control carbohydrate metabolism (glucocorticoids). ACTH is produced from a large precursor molecule, which gives rise not only to ACTH but also to **melanin-stimulating hormone** (**MSH**) and some other products that also have MSH activity as a "by-product" of ACTH synthesis. MSH causes darkening of the skin by stimulating melanocytes, but normally not enough is produced to have any significant effect when output of ACTH is normal. **Follicle-stimulating hormone** (**FSH**) and **luteinizing hormone** (**LH**) are called gonadotropic hormones. They regulate the growth and development of the gonads (ovaries and testes) and control the output of sex hormones that are responsible for the development of male and female secondary sex characteristics.

Posterior-Lobe Hormones

Antidiuretic hormone (**ADH**) causes the cells of the renal collecting tubules to become more permeable to water so that more water is absorbed and a concentrated urine is excreted. Secretion of ADH is regulated by receptors in the hypothalamus that respond to variations in the osmolarity of the extracellular fluid. If the osmolarity rises, the hypothalamic neurons send impulses to the posterior lobe to stimulate release of ADH. Water is retained instead of being excreted, which dilutes the extracellular fluid and lowers its osmolarity. Conversely, if the extracellular fluids become too dilute, the hypothalamus directs the pituitary to decrease its output of ADH. More water is excreted in the urine, which causes the osmolarity of the body fluids to rise.

Oxytocin stimulates the contraction of the pregnant uterus and causes ejection of milk from the lactating breast. Oxytocin is secreted in response to stimulation of the nipples during nursing. The sensory nerve impulses are transmitted to the hypothalamus, and the hypothalamic neurons in turn send impulses to the posterior lobe that cause the release of oxytocin.

PHYSIOLOGIC CONTROL OF PITUITARY HORMONE SECRETION

The level of the various trophic hormones elaborated by the pituitary is regulated by the level of circulating hormone produced by the target gland (FIGURE 25-1). Cells in the hypothalamus measure the level of the various hormones in the blood and liberate various releasing and inhibiting hormones that control the release of pituitary hormones into the circulation. Generally, hormones produced by the hypothalamus and pituitary gland are released in pulses, rather than as a continuous output. Many hormone levels also may vary over a 24-hour period (called a diurnal variation), usually with the highest levels in the early morning followed by a gradual fall throughout the day. When the concentration of the hormone falls below a certain level, releasing hormones are elaborated. They travel by the portal venous system to the pituitary gland, causing release of the tropic hormone. This, in turn, affects the target organ. The level of the hormone elaborated by the target organ rises until it reaches the upper range of normal. At this point, the high level of circulating hormone "shuts off" further elaboration of tropic hormone. This mechanism maintains a relatively

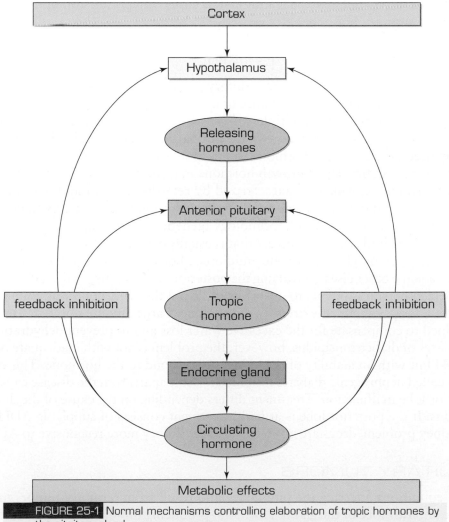

FIGURE 25-1 Normal mechanisms controlling elaboration of tropic hormones by the pituitary gland.

steady hormone output from the target organ and prevents wide fluctuations in hormonal level that might disrupt the smooth functioning of the body's hormone-regulated organ systems.

Prolactin secretion is regulated by a somewhat different mechanism from that of the other pituitary hormones. With other hormones, the main effect of hypothalamic releasing hormones is to stimulate secretion. For prolactin, however, the principal control is by an inhibitory hormone called **prolactin inhibitory factor** (PIF). Secretion of prolactin would continue unabated if it were not continuously suppressed. If PIF output falls for any reason, prolactin secretion rises.

We know now that PIF is a chemical mediator called **dopamine**, which suppresses prolactin output by inhibiting prolactin-secreting anterior lobe cells. If dopamine output falls for any reason, prolactin secretion rises. Therefore, a drug that alters the concentration of dopamine in the hypothalamus or blocks dopamine receptors also changes the output of prolactin, which is controlled by dopamine. Release of prolactin is also affected by stimuli from the nipples during nursing. The stimuli are relayed to the hypothalamus, which responds by releasing less dopamine (PIF), and prolactin secretion increases.

Although dopamine is the major regulator of prolactin secretion, thyrotropin-releasing hormone (TRH), which stimulates release of TSH by the pituitary, also directly stimulates release of prolactin as well.

Abnormalities in the secretion of tropic hormones may involve either single or multiple hormones and may be manifested as either a hypofunction or an overproduction of pituitary hormone.

PITUITARY HYPOFUNCTION

Sometimes the anterior lobe of the pituitary gland is destroyed by a tumor or undergoes necrosis owing to a disturbance of its blood supply. In this condition, called **panhypopituitarism** (*pan* = multiple + *hypo* = decrease), the anterior lobe fails to secrete any hormones. The functions of the thyroid gland, adrenal glands, and gonads are impaired because tropic hormone stimulation is lost.

An isolated deficiency of growth hormone in a child leads to a condition called pituitary dwarfism, which is characterized by retarded growth and development. Normal growth and development can be restored by administering growth hormone produced by recombinant DNA technology (genetic engineering).

Diabetes insipidus is a rare disease that is usually caused by failure of the posterior lobe of the pituitary gland to secrete antidiuretic hormone (ADH) because of injury, tumor, or some other disease involving the posterior lobe. Because of the lack of ADH, the affected person is unable to absorb water from the renal collecting tubules and excretes a large volume of extremely dilute urine. Large amounts of water must be consumed to compensate for the excessive water loss and to prevent dehydration. In some cases of diabetes insipidus, however, the problem is not with inadequate output of ADH but with an inability of the kidneys to respond to the hormone. This condition is called nephrogenic diabetes insipidus to set it apart from the disease caused by posterior lobe malfunction. Treatment differs depending on the cause of the diabetes insipidus. If the posterior lobe is at fault, treatment consists of supplying ADH. If it is a kidney problem, drugs are given to make the kidney more responsive to ADH.

PITUITARY TUMORS

Many conditions affecting the pituitary gland result from pituitary tumors involving the anterior lobe of the gland. Hormone-producing tumors are called functional tumors, and the clinical manifestations of a functioning tumor are determined by

---

Prolactin inhibitory factor (PIF)
Hypothalamic hormone that suppresses release of prolactin from the anterior lobe of the pituitary.

Dopamine
(dō'puh-mēn)
Chemical mediator released by hypothalamic neurons.

Panhypopituitarism
Failure of secretion of all anterior lobe pituitary hormones.

Diabetes insipidus
(dī-u-bē'tēz in-sip'id-us)
A condition resulting from a deficiency of antidiuretic hormone, characterized by excretion of a large volume of very dilute urine.

what hormone it makes, how much hormone it produces, the size of the tumor, and the age of the subject. The two most common functional pituitary tumors are those that produce growth hormone and those that produce prolactin. Generally, each type of tumor produces a characteristic clinical syndrome. Tumors that do not produce hormones are called nonfunctional tumors. Although no hormones are produced, a nonfunctional tumor may cause problems because of its location, which is close to the optic chiasm, optic nerves, and other vital structures at the base of the brain. An enlarging tumor may erode the pituitary fossa, encroach on the optic chiasm, and may disrupt the hormone-producing functions of adjacent normal anterior lobe cells that are compressed by the expanding tumor.

Treatment of a pituitary tumor is determined by the type of tumor, the hormones that it produces, and the size of the tumor. A small prolactin-secreting adenoma may respond well to drugs that shrink the tumor, and some drugs can be used to suppress the secretion of growth hormone produced by a functional tumor. In most cases, however, the usual treatment of a pituitary tumor is surgical removal of the tumor, occasionally followed by radiation treatment in selected patients.

Because a pituitary tumor is so difficult to approach through the cranial cavity, it is usually resected through the nasal cavity and sphenoid sinus, a procedure called a transsphenoidal resection (FIGURE 25-2). The standard transsphenoidal method for resecting all types of pituitary tumors, used for many years, involves entering the nasal cavity through an incision under the upper lip and removing part of the nasal septum. Then the sphenoid sinus is entered, and the anterior part of the pituitary fossa (sella turcica) is opened to expose the pituitary tumor, which is resected. Finally, the nasal septum is replaced after the tumor has been removed. Recently, modifications to the standard procedure have been developed, such as making the initial surgical incision within the nose instead of under the upper lip and removing only a small posterior part of the nasal septum to enter the sphenoid sinus. Each modification has both advantages and disadvantages when compared with the standard procedure, and the surgeon selects the procedure that is most appropriate for the individual patient.

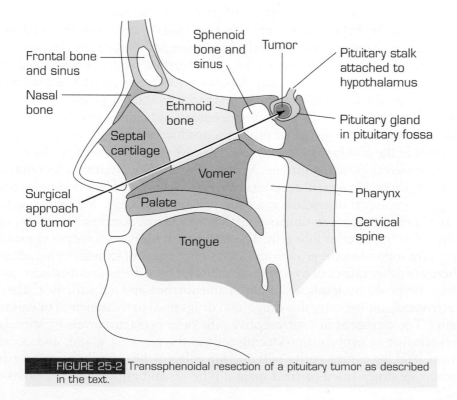

FIGURE 25-2 Transsphenoidal resection of a pituitary tumor as described in the text.

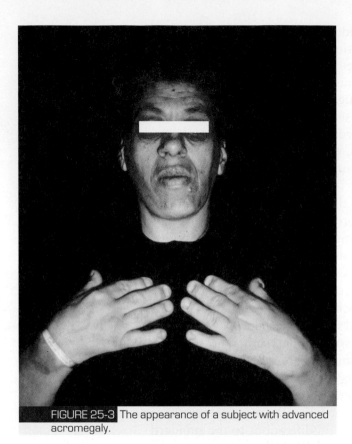

FIGURE 25-3 The appearance of a subject with advanced acromegaly.

OVERPRODUCTION OF GROWTH HORMONE

Overproduction of growth hormone in children and adolescents, whose epiphyses have not yet fused, causes excessive growth in the length of bones, and the subject becomes too tall. This condition is called pituitary gigantism. Some associated coarsening of the facial features usually occurs in response to the effect of growth hormone on the structure of the facial bones.

In adults, excessive growth hormone causes **acromegaly**. Because the epiphyses have fused, there can be no growth in height, but the growth hormone produces thickening and coarsening of bones and generalized enlargement of the viscera. Affected individuals have coarse facial features, large prominent jaws, and large spadelike hands, but they are no taller than normal (FIGURE 25-3). The term acromegaly (*acron* = extremity + *megas* = large) describes one prominent feature of the disease.

In addition to the hormonal effects, manifestations related to the size and location of the tumor may also occur. Treatment consists of transsphenoidal resection of the tumor, sometimes supplemented by radiation therapy.

Acromegaly
(ak′ro-meg′al-ē)
A condition resulting from excessive secretion of growth hormone in the adult.

Galactorrhea
(gā-lak-tō-rē′yuh)
Secretion of milk by breast not associated with pregnancy or normal lactation.

Amenorrhea
(äh-men-ō-rē′äh)
Absence of menses.

Dopamine agonist
(do′-pă-mēn ag′-on-ist)
A drug such as bromocriptine that combines with cell dopamine receptors and causes the same cell response that would be produced by dopamine, such as inhibition of prolactin secretion.

OVERPRODUCTION OF PROLACTIN

In a nonpregnant woman, excess secretion of prolactin may cause spontaneous secretion of milk from the breasts (**galactorrhea**) and cessation of menstrual periods (**amenorrhea**). Galactorrhea results from the effect of the hormone on breast tissue. Amenorrhea occurs because high levels of prolactin also inhibit secretion of pituitary gonadotropins FSH and LH, which in turn leads to cessation of ovulation and menstrual cycles. This is sometimes called the amenorrhea-galactorrhea syndrome.

The various causes of the amenorrhea galactorrhea syndrome described in this section are summarized in (FIGURE 25-4). A prolactin-secreting pituitary adenoma is an important cause and should be considered first as the most likely possibility. Sometimes the tumor is quite small (called a microadenoma) and causes few symptoms other than those related to the increased prolactin production. Larger tumors may cause enlargement of the pituitary fossa and visual disturbances like those produced by adenomas that secrete growth hormone. A prolactin-secreting pituitary adenoma can be removed surgically, but a small adenoma can often be inhibited by a **dopamine agonist** drug (*agon* = competitor), which is a drug that functions like dopamine, such as a drug called bromocriptine or similar drug that attaches to dopamine receptors on the prolactin-secreting anterior lobe cells. The attachment suppresses output of prolactin, which in turn suppresses the growth and secretion of the prolactin-secreting adenoma.

There are other causes of hyperprolactinemia. Some drugs and medications may at times raise prolactin levels, resulting in amenorrhea and galactorrhea. These include estrogens, antihypertensive drugs, and drugs used to treat mental or emotional problems. The estrogens in contraceptive pills raise prolactin levels by stimulating the proliferation of prolactin-producing cells in the pituitary gland, and occasionally, women taking contraceptive pills develop galactorrhea. Antihypertensive drugs, phenothiazine drugs (used to treat mental illness), and antidepressant drugs raise

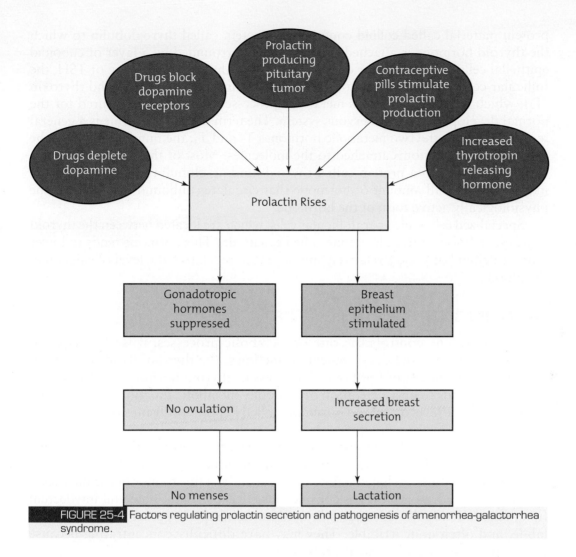

FIGURE 25-4 Factors regulating prolactin secretion and pathogenesis of amenorrhea-galactorrhea syndrome.

prolactin levels by depleting dopamine or blocking dopamine receptors in the hypothalamus. Consequently, less PIF is secreted and prolactin rises. Prolactin levels also rise in hypothyroidism, which is related indirectly to reduced thyroid hormone secretion. The hypothalamus detects the low hormone output and secretes more thyrotropin-releasing hormone (TRH), which "tells" the pituitary to produce more thyroid-stimulating hormone (TSH) in an attempt to raise thyroid hormone output. It is the elevated TRH that increases prolactin secretion because TRH not only stimulates pituitary TSH secretion, but also directly stimulates the pituitary to secrete more prolactin.

The Thyroid Gland

The thyroid gland consists of two lateral lobes connected by a narrow isthmus (FIGURE 25-5A). It is located in the neck overlying the upper part of the trachea and is regulated by pituitary thyroid-stimulating hormone (TSH). The four parathyroid glands are located on its posterior surface.

Histologically, the thyroid gland is composed of multiple minute spherical vesicles called thyroid follicles. Each follicle consists of a central mass of eosinophilic

Colloid
An eosinophilic protein material present within the thyroid follicles.

....

Thyroglobulin
A protein within the colloid of the thyroid follicles to which the thyroid hormone is attached.

....

Calcitonin
A hormone that lowers blood calcium, produced by the interfollicular cells of the thyroid gland.

protein material called **colloid** containing a protein called **thyroglobulin** to which the thyroid hormone is attached. The colloid is surrounded by a layer of cuboidal epithelial cells called follicular cells (FIGURE 25-5B). Under the influence of TSH, the follicular cells synthesize two hormones called triiodothyronine (T_3) and thyroxin (T_4), which regulate the body's metabolic processes and are also required for the normal development of the nervous system. The term thyroid hormone is a general term referring to the two metabolic hormones T_3 and T_4; the numbers indicate the number of iodine atoms attached to the molecules. Most of the thyroid hormone circulates bound to a protein called thyroid-binding globulin and is biologically inactive. The small amount of hormone that circulates unbound to protein is the physiologically active form of the hormone.

Specialized cells called parafollicular cells, which are located between the thyroid follicles, elaborate a third hormone called **calcitonin**. This hormone tends to lower blood calcium but plays a relatively minor part in regulating the level of calcium in the blood.

ACTIONS OF THYROID HORMONE

Thyroid hormone controls the rate of metabolic processes; it is also required for normal growth and development. Sometimes, the thyroid gland secretes an inappropriate amount of hormone. An excess of thyroid hormone, called hyperthyroidism, leads to an acceleration of all bodily metabolic functions. Conversely, a decrease in the level of thyroid hormone, called hypothyroidism, slows metabolic processes.

Clinically, some of the most pronounced effects of excess thyroid hormone are manifested in the cardiovascular and neuromuscular systems. The heart rate is accelerated. Reflexes are hyperactive, and frequently, a fine tremor of the muscles is apparent. The hormone also has conspicuous effects on emotional and intellectual functions. Individuals with excess thyroid hormone are hyperactive, emotionally labile, and often quite irritable. They may have difficulty concentrating because mental processes are accelerated excessively.

The effects of thyroid hypofunction are the reverse of those in hyperthyroidism. The hypothyroid individual is slow and lethargic. Bodily metabolic functions are

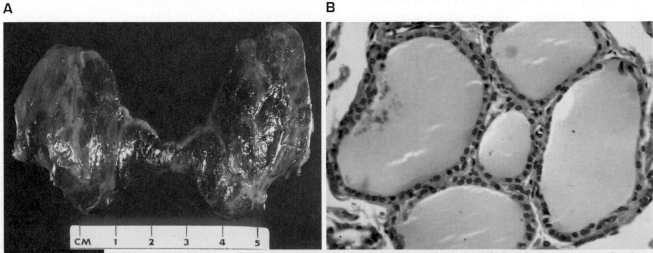

A   **B**

FIGURE 25-5 **A**, Normal thyroid gland, illustrating two lateral lobes connected by narrow isthmus. **B**, High-magnification photomicrograph of normal thyroid follicles, illustrating central masses of colloid surrounded by follicular epithelial cells (original magnification × 400).

subnormal. Reflexes and speech are slow and sluggish. TABLE 25-2 summarizes the major clinical effects resulting from abnormal levels of thyroid hormone.

GOITER

An enlargement of the thyroid gland is called a **goiter**. The gland may be uniformly enlarged, called a diffuse goiter, or multiple nodules of proliferating thyroid tissue may form a nodular goiter. An enlarged gland that produces an excessive amount of hormone and causes symptoms of hyperthyroidism is called a toxic goiter. A goiter that does not secrete excess thyroid hormone is called a nontoxic goiter.

Goiter (goy′ter)
Any enlargement of the thyroid gland.

Nontoxic Goiter

The basic cause of both nodular and diffuse nontoxic goiter is an inadequate secretion of thyroid hormone. The reduced hormone output causes the hypothalamus to elaborate releasing hormone, which in turn stimulates the pituitary to liberate more TSH (FIGURE 25-6). As a result, the gland enlarges in order to produce more hormone.

Three major factors predispose to the development of a nontoxic goiter:

1. Iodine deficiency
2. Deficiency of enzymes required for synthesis of thyroid hormone or ingestion of substances that interfere with the function of these enzymes
3. Increased hormone requirements

Iodine Deficiency   If iodine is deficient in the diet, not enough will be available to produce adequate hormone for the needs of the individual. The enlargement of the gland in response to TSH stimulation is an attempt to extract the meager amount of iodine from the blood more efficiently to make enough hormone. Iodine deficiency is rarely a cause of goiter in the United States because table salt, bread, and many other foods are fortified with iodine. Consequently, the average American diet actually contains abundant iodine.

TABLE 25-2

Comparison of major effects of hyperthyroidism and hypothyroidism

	Hyperthyroidism	Hypothyroidism
Cardiovascular effects	Rapid pulse, increased cardiac output	Slow pulse, reduced cardiac output
Metabolic effects	Increased metabolism, skin hot and flushed, weight loss	Decreased metabolism, cold skin, weight gain
Neuromuscular effects	Tremor, hyperactive reflexes	Weakness, lassitude, sluggish reflexes
Mental, emotional effects	Restlessness, irritability, emotional lability	Mental processes sluggish and retarded, personality placid and phlegmatic
Gastrointestinal effects	Diarrhea	Constipation
General somatic effects	Warm, moist skin	Cold, dry skin

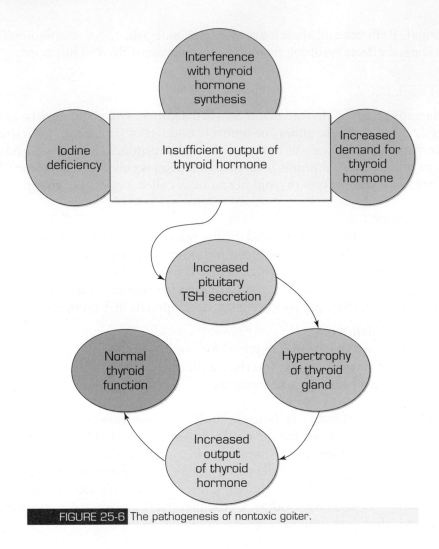

FIGURE 25-6 The pathogenesis of nontoxic goiter.

Enzyme Deficiency or Impaired Enzyme Function Goiter more commonly results from a mild deficiency in a glandular enzyme that is required for hormone synthesis; the enzyme-deficient gland is unable to produce sufficient hormone without enlarging. Less commonly, the enzymes are present in normal amounts, but their functions are impaired by ingestion of drugs or other substances that interfere with the action of the enzymes. Even some "natural" foods, such as cabbage and turnips, contain small amounts of substances that interfere with thyroid-hormone synthesis, but these foods are not usually eaten in quantities sufficient to cause difficulty.

Increased Hormone Requirements Normally, the need for thyroid hormone increases in puberty, during pregnancy, and under conditions of stress. In some individuals, the thyroid gland may be able to produce adequate hormone under normal circumstances but may be unable to increase its output in response to increased requirements without enlarging.

Whenever hormone output is inadequate, no matter what the cause, more TSH is released in order to step up hormone production. Because hormone requirements often fluctuate, a gland may undergo successive alternating periods of enlargement and reduction in size. At first, the gland enlarges uniformly in response to TSH stimulation, and it returns to its original size when increased hormone output is no longer required. Eventually, however, the gland may respond in an irregular manner

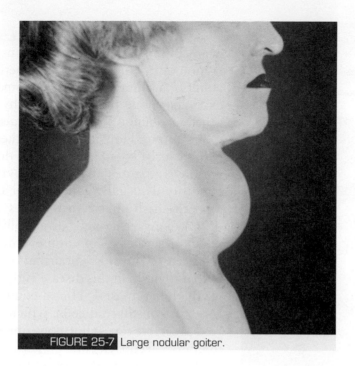

FIGURE 25-7 Large nodular goiter.

to TSH stimulation. If this occurs, the enlargement of the gland is not uniform and a nodular goiter results (FIGURE 25-7).

Treatment of Nontoxic Goiter Because a nontoxic goiter results from excessive stimulation of the thyroid gland by TSH, it is usually treated by administration of thyroid hormone, which suppresses TSH output by the negative feedback mechanism. Treatment usually causes the enlarged gland to shrink because it is no longer being stimulated by TSH. A large nodular goiter may have to be removed surgically if it compresses the trachea, interferes with respiration, or obstructs the neck veins returning blood to the heart. FIGURE 25-8 shows a large nodular goiter obstructing the venous drainage of the head, neck, and chest.

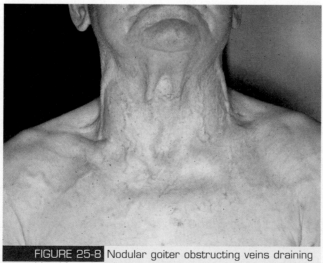

FIGURE 25-8 Nodular goiter obstructing veins draining blood from head, neck, and chest. Note the large dilated veins in the skin of the neck and chest. Treated by thyroidectomy.

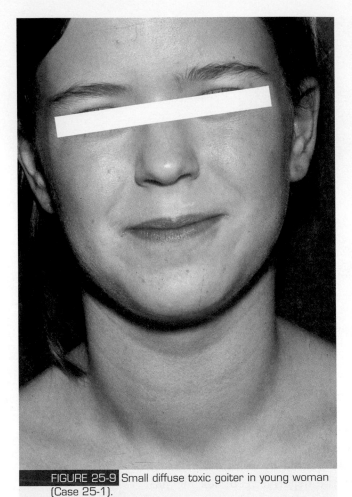

FIGURE 25-9 Small diffuse toxic goiter in young woman (Case 25-1).

Graves disease
An autoimmune thyroid disease in which autoantibodies resembling thyroid-stimulating hormone stimulate an excessive output of thyroid hormone, causing hyperthyroidism.

Exophthalmic goiter
(ex-āf-thal′-mik)
Another term for Graves disease, named for the protrusion of the eyes seen in many patients with this disease.

HYPERTHYROIDISM

Many different conditions can cause an excess secretion of thyroid hormone. Sometimes a nodular goiter or a solitary thyroid adenoma may produce excess hormone and cause hyperthyroidism. A few other uncommon conditions may also increase hormone output. However, usually the hyperthyroidism is caused by an autoimmune disease in which various autoantibodies target thyroid cells. This condition is usually called either **Graves disease** after the Irish physician who described the condition many years ago, or **exophthalmic goiter**, which describes a common eye manifestation of the disease. The most important of the antithyroid autoantibodies in this disease is the one that mimics the function of TSH and combines with TSH receptors on thyroid cells, which drives the thyroid to secrete excess hormone unresponsive to the inhibitory feedback control mechanism that regulates normal thyroid activity. Indeed, the normal TSH produced by the pituitary gland is suppressed by the excess hormone output, but nevertheless, the autoantibody continues to force the thyroid gland to produce hormone. In most subjects, the thyroid gland is diffusely enlarged, but the degree of enlargement is not marked (FIGURE 25-9).

The eye changes that occur in many subjects with Graves disease are also caused by the autoimmune disease. Activated T lymphocytes infiltrate the fat, connective tissue, and the muscles that move the eyes (extraocular muscles) located in the orbital cavities behind the eyes, which causes inflammation and swelling of the tissues and pushes the eyes forward. The eye protrusion may interfere with the ability of the eyelids to close the eyes and with the function of the extraocular muscles. In severe cases, the eyes may be pushed so far forward that the optic nerves are stretched and may be injured. The eye changes are responsible for the other name exophthalmic goiter (*exo* = out + *ophthalmos* = eye) applied to this disease. Fortunately, although some degree of eye protrusion is present in many affected persons, extreme eye protrusion and its complications are uncommon.

Treatment of Hyperthyroidism

At present, no method is available to block the stimulation of the thyroid gland by the autoantibodies that are causing the unregulated hypersecretion of thyroid hormone. It is possible, however, to control the hyperthyroidism. Three different methods of treatment can be used:

1. Antithyroid drugs can be administered to block the synthesis of hormone by the hyperactive gland.
2. A large portion of the gland can be removed surgically, reducing the source of the hormone.
3. A large dose of radioactive iodine can be administered to be taken up by the thyroid gland. The irradiation destroys part of the gland and reduces its hormone output.

Successful treatment of hyperthyroidism may stop further protrusion of the eyes, but sometimes the protrusion progresses even though the hyperthyroidism has been controlled. Immunosuppressive therapy may be helpful by reducing the swelling of the tissues behind the eyes. As a last resort, when there is no response to more conservative treatment, it may be necessary to enlarge surgically the orbital cavities by removing one or more of its bony walls so that the stretched optic nerves will not be irreparably damaged.

The following case illustrates successful treatment of a diffuse toxic goiter by means of antithyroid drugs and thyroidectomy.

CASE 25-1

A 15-year-old girl was referred to her physician because of recent onset of hyperactivity, rapid speech, and some prominence of the eyes (see FIGURE 25-9). Examination revealed prominent eyes, a fine tremor, and hyperactive reflexes. Thyroid function studies indicated an elevated level of thyroid hormone in her blood, together with an increased uptake of iodine and increased synthesis of hormone as demonstrated by radioactive iodine tracer studies. The patient was considered to have a diffuse toxic goiter. She was treated initially by an antithyroid drug to control the hyperthyroidism, and a thyroidectomy was subsequently performed.

HYPOTHYROIDISM

Hypothyroidism in the Adult

Hypothyroidism in the adult is sometimes called **myxedema** (FIGURE 25-10). It is manifested by a general slowing of the body's metabolic processes. Frequently, there are localized accumulations of mucinous material in the skin, from which the disease received its name (*myx* = mucin + *edema* = swelling). Hypothyroid individuals have low levels of circulating thyroid hormone and high levels of TSH that reflect stimulation of the gland in an unsuccessful attempt to increase hormone output. The condition is treated by supplying the deficient hormone, which results in clinical improvement, return of thyroid hormone level to normal, and a fall in TSH, as illustrated by the following case.

Myxedema
(mix-uh-de'muh)
Hypothyroidism in the adult.

CASE 25-2

A 25-year-old woman visited her physician because of recent weight gain and menstrual irregularities. On examination, she was moderately overweight, and her thyroid gland was slightly enlarged; however, there were no other abnormalities. The level of thyroid hormone in her blood was reduced to 2.1 μg/dl (normal range 4.5–11.0 μg/dl), and the thyroid-stimulating hormone (TSH) level was markedly increased to 310 microunits/ml (normal range 2–10 microunits/ml). She was considered to have hypothyroidism. She was treated with a thyroid hormone preparation. The level of thyroid hormone rose, and the elevated TSH level gradually returned to normal. She felt much better and lost some weight. Her menstrual periods became normal.

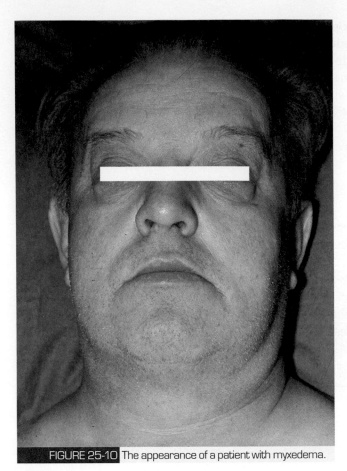

FIGURE 25-10 The appearance of a patient with myxedema.

Neonatal Hypothyroidism

Hypothyroidism in the newborn infant is called congenital hypothyroidism. This condition may be caused by failure of the thyroid gland to develop or may result from a genetically determined deficiency of enzymes necessary for thyroid hormone synthesis. In the latter condition, the gland undergoes hyperplasia caused by excessive TSH stimulation but is unable to produce adequate hormone because of the enzyme deficiency.

Usually the affected infant appears normal at birth because the mother has supplied the fetus with significant amounts of thyroid hormone, which crossed the placenta to make up for the deficient fetal hormone synthesis. However, as the level of passively transferred maternal thyroid hormone in the newborn infant gradually falls, clinical manifestations of hypothyroidism appear within the first few months after birth. Thyroid hormone not only regulates metabolic processes, but is also required for normal growth. The hormone is also essential for the normal development of the nervous system, which continues for several months after birth. If neonatal hypothyroidism is recognized and treated promptly, the affected infant will usually grow and develop normally. If the condition remains undetected, the unfortunate infant will remain permanently stunted in growth and mentally retarded. This condition is called **cretinism** (FIGURE 25-11). Fortunately, we have effective screening tests for neonatal hypothyroidism that are performed routinely on newborn infants. The tests, which require only a few drops of blood, can identify neonatal hypothyroidism by detecting the low levels of thyroid hormone and elevated levels of TSH in newborn infants that are characteristic of this condition. Such screening tests have assured early recognition and prompt treatment of affected infants, thereby preventing cretinism, which is the unfortunate late manifestation of unrecognized and untreated neonatal hypothyroidism.

Cretinism
(krē'tin-izm)
Hypothyroidism in the infant.

CHRONIC THYROIDITIS: HASHIMOTO THYROIDITIS

Acute and chronic inflammation of the thyroid gland caused by a bacterial or viral infection is usually called either acute or chronic thyroiditis depending on its clinical manifestations and the type of inflammatory cells present. Another thyroid disease in which the gland is infiltrated by lymphocytes was described by a Japanese physician named Hashimoto and is called either **chronic thyroiditis** or **Hashimoto thyroiditis**. It is not an infection. It is an autoimmune disease in which antithyroid autoantibodies and activated T lymphocytes directed against thyroid antigens attack and destroy the thyroid gland. It is the most common cause of hypothyroidism in adults, which occurs predominantly in middle-aged women. One of the autoantibodies formed in this disease is directed against TSH receptors on the thyroid cells, which destroys the receptors so that TSH is unable to attach to thyroid cells and stimulate the thyroid gland. Consequently, output of thyroid hormone falls as TSH receptor damage progresses. The normal feedback control system that regulates hormone output (Figure 25-1) responds to the low hormone level, and TSH rises as thyroid hormone falls. The behavior of

Chronic thyroiditis
An autoimmune disease in which an autoantibody directed against thyroid epithelial cells causes progressive destruction of the thyroid gland, leading to hypothyroidism. Also called Hashimoto thyroiditis.

Hashimoto thyroiditis
Another name for chronic thyroiditis.

the autoantibody in chronic thyroiditis (Hashimoto disease) is quite different from that of the autoantibody in hyperthyroidism (Graves disease). In one disease, the antibody destroys the receptors, causing hypothyroidism; in the other, the autoantibody stimulates the receptors, causing hyperthyroidism.

The thyroid gland of a person with Hashimoto thyroiditis is usually enlarged by diffuse infiltration of activated T lymphocytes and plasma cells that are destroying the thyroid gland (FIGURE 25-12). No specific treatment is available to arrest the relentless progression of the disease, but the hypothyroidism can be treated by administration of thyroid hormone. The physician is guided both by the level of thyroid hormone in the blood and the level of TSH when determining how much thyroid hormone to give the patient. The level of thyroid hormone rises and TSH falls in response to therapy. When both thyroid hormone and TSH are within the normal range, the patient's thyroid function is considered to be normal, and the amount of thyroid hormone required to achieve this result is continued.

TUMORS OF THE THYROID

The thyroid gives rise to benign adenomas and several different types of carcinoma. Thyroid adenomas are well-circumscribed tumors composed of mature follicles that often contain large amounts

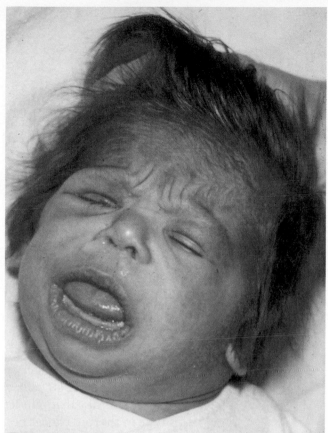

FIGURE 25-11 The characteristic appearance of neonatal hypothyroidism (cretinism) as a result of a congenital absence of thyroid gland. Treatment with thyroid hormone reversed manifestations of hypothyroidism.

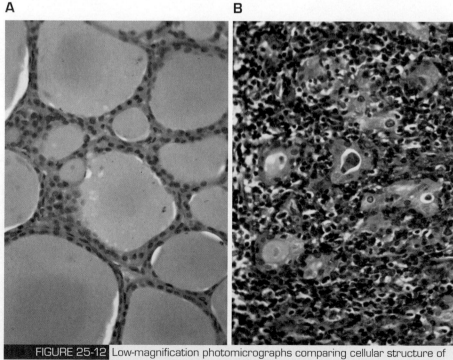

A **B**

FIGURE 25-12 Low-magnification photomicrographs comparing cellular structure of normal thyroid gland (**A**) with that in chronic thyroiditis (**B**). Gland is heavily infiltrated by lymphocytes. Follicles are small and lack colloid (original magnification × 100).

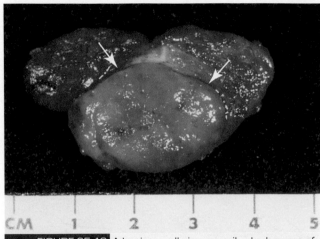

FIGURE 25-13 A benign, well-circumscribed adenoma of the thyroid gland (*arrows*). The surrounding thyroid tissue appears normal.

of colloid (FIGURE 25-13). There are three distinct types of thyroid cancer:

1. Well-differentiated carcinoma
2. Undifferentiated carcinoma
3. Medullary carcinoma

Well-differentiated carcinoma usually occurs in young adults and is of very low-grade malignancy. The most common type, illustrated in FIGURE 25-14, is called a papillary carcinoma because the tumor is composed of well-differentiated papillary processes covered by well-differentiated thyroid epithelial cells. A less common type of tumor is called a follicular carcinoma because the tumor cells form colloid-filled follicles, which resemble normal thyroid tissue. Treatment of both types is by surgical resection of the thyroid gland (thyroidectomy).

Undifferentiated carcinoma develops in older persons, is composed of rapidly growing bizarre tumor cells, and has a poor prognosis. Treatment is by means of surgical resection combined with radiation and chemotherapy.

Medullary carcinoma is an uncommon tumor that is derived from the calcitonin-secreting parafollicular cells of the thyroid. It has a characteristic histologic pattern. Measurement of calcitonin levels in the blood has been used as a diagnostic test for this type of thyroid cancer because the tumor cells often secrete calcitonin. Although the effect of calcitonin is to lower blood calcium, the excess hormone secretion has no significant effect on blood calcium because the effect of the calcitonin is counteracted by an increased secretion of parathyroid hormone, preventing blood calcium from falling. (The physiologic effects of parathyroid hormone are considered in conjunction with diseases of the parathyroid glands.)

Radiation and Thyroid Tumors

The incidence of both benign and malignant tumors of the thyroid has been increasing, and the increase appears related to previous thyroid radiation. In the 1930s and early 1940s, radiation therapy was used to treat enlargement of the thymus gland in infants, hypertrophied tonsils and adenoids, some fungus infections of the scalp,

A   **B**

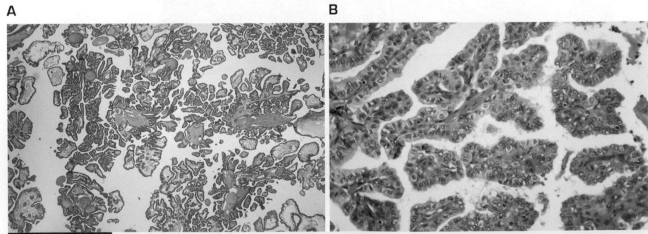

FIGURE 25-14 Well-differentiated papillary carcinoma of thyroid. **A**, A low-magnification view illustrating papillary structure (original magnification × 40). **B**, Higher magnification of papillary processes covered by well-differentiated neoplastic thyroid epithelium (original magnification × 160).

acne, and various other conditions of the head and neck. The treatments also exposed the thyroid gland to radiation. A small percentage of these patients developed various benign and malignant tumors of the thyroid from 5 to 30 years after the radiation exposure. Fortunately, most of the postradiation malignant tumors are well differentiated and of low malignancy. Because persons who have had previous radiation to the head and neck have an increased risk of thyroid tumors, they should have periodic medical examinations to assure that any thyroid tumors that develop subsequent to radiation will be recognized and treated promptly.

The Parathyroid Glands and Calcium Metabolism

The blood calcium is in equilibrium with the calcium salts present in bone. Half the blood calcium is present as calcium ions (Ca^{2+}) and is the active form. The other half is bound to blood proteins and is biologically inactive. An adequate concentration of ionized calcium is required for normal cardiac and skeletal muscle contraction, for transmission of nerve impulses, and for coagulation of the blood. A subnormal level of ionized calcium causes increased excitability of nerve and muscle cells, leading to spasm of skeletal muscles, which is called **tetany**. Conversely, a high level of ionized calcium diminishes neuromuscular excitability and leads to generalized muscular weakness.

Tetany
(tet′an-ē)
Spasm of skeletal muscles caused by subnormal level of ionized calcium in the blood.

The level of ionized calcium in the blood is regulated primarily by parathyroid hormone, which is secreted by four small parathyroid glands located on the posterior surface of the lateral lobes of the thyroid gland. The parathyroid hormone regulates the level of calcium by regulating the release of calcium from bone, the absorption of calcium from the intestine, and the rate of excretion of calcium by the kidneys. The secretion of parathyroid hormone is regulated by the level of ionized calcium in the blood rather than by a tropic hormone elaborated by the pituitary gland. If the level of ionized calcium in the blood decreases, the parathyroids secrete more hormone. If the ionized calcium level rises, parathyroid hormone secretion declines. Any abnormality in the secretion of parathyroid hormone changes the concentration of ionized calcium in the blood and will eventually alter the amount of calcium deposited in bone.

HYPERPARATHYROIDISM

Hyperparathyroidism is a relatively common problem and is usually the result of a hormone-secreting parathyroid adenoma. In response to increased output of hormone, the blood calcium rises (hypercalcemia), and excessive calcium is withdrawn from bone. The bones become excessively fragile and are easily broken.

Excessive amounts of calcium are excreted in the urine (hypercalciuria), sometimes leading to formation of calcium stones within the urinary tract. Occasionally, calcium precipitates out of the blood and becomes deposited in the kidneys, lungs, and other tissues, producing tissue injury and functional impairment. Treatment consists of surgical removal of the tumor.

HYPOPARATHYROIDISM

Hypoparathyroidism usually results from accidental removal of all four parathyroid glands during an operation for a diffuse toxic goiter or a nodular goiter in which most of the thyroid gland is removed. Blood calcium falls precipitously, which leads to increased neuromuscular excitability and tetany. Treatment consists of raising the level of blood calcium by the administration of a high-calcium diet and supplementary vitamin D, which promotes absorption of calcium from the intestinal tract.

The Adrenal Glands

The adrenals are paired glands located above the kidneys. Each adrenal consists of two separate endocrine glands: an inner adrenal medulla surrounded by an outer adrenal cortex. The two glands secrete different hormones.

THE ADRENAL CORTEX

The adrenal cortex secretes three major classes of steroid hormones:

1. Glucocorticoids
2. Mineralocorticoids
3. Sex hormones

Glucocorticoids

Glucocorticoids have three main actions:

1. They raise the blood glucose by decreasing glucose utilization in many tissues, except the brain, and promote fat breakdown with utilization of fatty acids rather than glucose as an energy source.
2. They inhibit protein synthesis and promote breakdown of body proteins, some of which are converted into glucose by the liver. The net effect is to deplete tissue proteins and raise blood glucose. (The adverse effect of glucocorticoids on wound healing and tissue repair is a result in part of their protein-depleting effects.)
3. They act at multiple sites to suppress the inflammatory reaction. (The use of adrenal corticosteroids to treat various types of inflammatory disease is related to the anti-inflammatory property of the glucocorticoids.)

Glucocorticoids are secreted in response to stimulation by adrenocorticotropic hormone (ACTH), and their output is controlled by the same type of negative feedback mechanism that regulates secretion of thyroid hormone. The major glucocorticoid is **cortisol**.

Mineralocorticoids

Mineralocorticoids regulate electrolyte and water balance by promoting absorption of sodium and water and excretion of potassium by the renal tubules. The major mineralocorticoid is **aldosterone**, and its secretion is regulated by more than one mechanism. Although ACTH increases aldosterone secretion to some extent, the most potent stimulus for aldosterone secretion is the renin-angiotensin system (discussion on the urinary system), which responds to a reduction in renal blood flow or blood pressure. One can think of the kidneys as "interpreting" the reduced blood flow and pressure to mean that blood volume is low; aldosterone secretion is then called for to promote retention of sodium and water, thus increasing blood volume.

Sex Hormones

The adrenal cortex also produces weak androgenic (testosteronelike) steroid hormones in response to ACTH stimulation, which are further metabolized into testosterone and into estrogens by both males and females. In men, the estrogens have little effect because of the much greater testicular production of testosterone. In women, the testosterone is responsible for sex drive but otherwise has little physiologic effect because it is overshadowed by estrogen produced by the ovaries. The additional estrogens made from adrenal androgenic hormones do not add much to the large

---

Glucocorticoid
An adrenal cortical hormone that regulates carbohydrate metabolism.

Cortisol (kō r′ti-sol)
The major glucocorticoid.

Mineralocorticoid
(min′ril-ō-kor′tik-oid)
Adrenal cortical hormone that regulates salt and water metabolism.

Aldosterone
A steroid hormone produced by the adrenal cortex that regulates the rate of sodium absorption from the renal tubules.

amount already made by the ovaries. However, in estrogen-deficient postmenopausal women, the estrogens produced from adrenal androgens may be very significant, as described in the discussion on the breast. In some diseases, the output of adrenal androgens is greatly increased, which may exert undesirable masculinizing effects, as illustrated in FIGURE 25-19.

DISTURBANCES OF ADRENAL CORTICAL FUNCTION

Abnormal adrenal cortical function produces abnormalities in the metabolism of carbohydrates and protein as a result of abnormal glucocorticoid secretion, as well as disturbances of salt and water metabolism caused by disturbed mineralocorticoid secretion.

Addison Disease

Adrenal cortical hypofunction is called **Addison disease**. It results from atrophy or destruction of both adrenal glands leading to a deficiency of all of the steroid hormones produced by these glands. In most cases, the disease results from an autoimmune disorder in which destructive autoantibodies directed against adrenal cortical cells and invading cytotoxic lymphocytes destroy the cortex. Less commonly, the adrenal destruction is caused by tuberculosis, histoplasmosis, or metastatic carcinoma involving both adrenal glands.

As a result of a glucocorticoid deficiency, the blood glucose level is subnormal and may decline during fasting to such a low level that symptoms develop. The body's ability to regulate the content of sodium, potassium, and water in body fluids is disturbed as a result of the mineralocorticoid deficiency. Blood volume and blood pressure fall, as does the concentration of sodium in the blood, and blood potassium rises. The blood volume may become so reduced that the circulation can no longer be maintained efficiently.

Persons with Addison disease also frequently exhibit increased pigmentation of the skin that is caused by increased secretion of ACTH along with MSH, which is produced from the same precursor molecule that gives rise to ACTH. The MSH simulates the melanin-producing cells in the skin and is responsible for the increased skin pigmentation characteristic of Addison disease (FIGURE 25-15). ACTH output is

Addison disease
A disease caused by chronic adrenal cortical hypofunction.

A

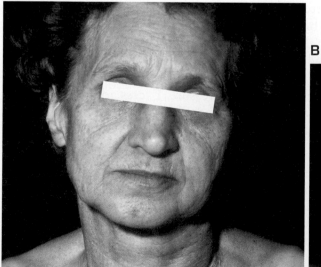

B

FIGURE 25-15 Patient with Addison disease (Case 25-3). **A**, Appearance of face illustrating increased skin pigmentation. **B**, Appearance of hand (*right side* of photograph) compared with hand of normal subject.

regulated by a negative feedback mechanism. In Addison disease, secretion of cortisol is greatly diminished, which causes ACTH to rise in an unsuccessful attempt to increase cortisol output. Treatment of Addison disease consists of administering the deficient corticosteroids, as illustrated by the following case.

CASE 25-3

A 66-year-old woman had noted gradual loss of energy and some weight loss over the previous 2 or 3 years. Her skin had become darker. She was in the habit of working outdoors in the summer and becoming suntanned, but recently, her tan did not fade in the winter. Physical examination was unremarkable except for increased skin pigmentation. Pigmentation was also noted in the oral mucosa and in the skin creases. Laboratory studies revealed normal thyroid function. Plasma corticosteroid hormone level was reduced to 5 μg/dl (normal range 7–28 μg/dl). The plasma adrenocorticotropic hormone (ACTH) level was markedly increased to more than 2,000 pg/ml (normal level is less than 120 pg/ml). A diagnosis of Addison disease was made. The very high ACTH level represented a loss of feedback inhibition with stimulation of the adrenal by the pituitary in an attempt to increase hormone output. The patient was treated with cortisone and responded satisfactorily.

Cushing Disease and Cushing Syndrome

Adrenal cortical hyperfunction causes a rather characteristic clinical syndrome, which results from excess production of adrenal corticosteroids. The glucocorticoid excess causes disturbances of carbohydrate, protein, and fat metabolism. The blood glucose rises. Protein synthesis is impaired, and body proteins are broken down, which leads to loss of muscle fibers and muscle weakness. Bones become weaker and more susceptible to fracture (osteoporosis) as the protein breakdown leads to loss of the connective tissue framework of the bones. The amount and distribution of body fat are altered. Fat tends to accumulate on the trunk, while the extremities appear thin and wasted because of muscle atrophy.

The skin becomes thin and bruises easily. Stretch marks (striae) often appear in the skin as fat deposits accumulate in the subcutaneous tissues of the trunk. The face appears full and rounded, which is sometimes called a "moon face." Salt and water are retained because of the increased output of mineralocorticoids, leading to an increase in blood volume and a rise in blood pressure. Excess adrenal androgens may lead to increased growth of facial and body hair in women.

Four distinct conditions may give rise to this syndrome:

1. An ACTH-producing tumor of the pituitary gland, which stimulates the adrenal glands to enlarge and produce excess hormone.
2. A corticosteroid–hormone-producing tumor of the adrenal cortex.
3. Administration of large amounts of corticosteroid hormone to treat diseases that respond to the hormone, as may be required to help suppress the immune response in recipients of organ transplants or patients with autoimmune diseases, or to help induce remission in patients with leukemia.
4. A malignant tumor, such as a lung tumor, that produces ACTH or a similar protein that resembles the "real" hormone, as described later in this chapter.

The most common cause of a corticosteroid excess is a small ACTH secreting pituitary adenoma (microadenoma), and this condition is called Cushing disease after the physician who described the clinical features of the disease and identified its relationship to a pituitary tumor. When this condition is caused by an adrenal tumor, excess corticosteroid administration, or ACTH production by a non-endocrine tumor, the term Cushing syndrome is used.

The treatment of this condition depends on the cause. If it is Cushing disease caused by a pituitary microadenoma, the usual method of treatment is transsphenoidal resection of the tumor. Cushing syndrome caused by an adrenal cortical tumor is treated by resection of the adrenal tumor.

Successful treatment is followed by regression of the clinical manifestations of the disease (FIGURES 25-16 AND 25-17).

Overproduction of Aldosterone

Aldosterone promotes absorption of salt and water by the kidneys in exchange for potassium which is excreted, and its secretion is regulated primarily by the renin-angiotensin–aldosterone mechanism described in the discussion on the urinary system. However, sometimes the adrenal cortex gives rise to an aldosterone-secreting adenoma called an aldosteronoma. The aldosterone excess produced by the tumor promotes excessive absorption of sodium and excessive excretion of potassium by the kidneys. Because water is absorbed along with the sodium, the blood volume

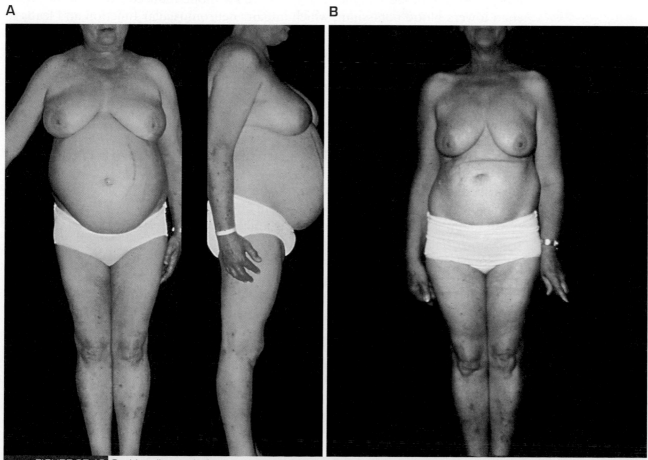

A   B

FIGURE 25-16 Cushing disease before and after treatment. **A**, Before treatment, front and side views of subject illustrating trunk obesity with relatively thin extremities. **B**, After treatment, illustrating normal body configuration.

A   B

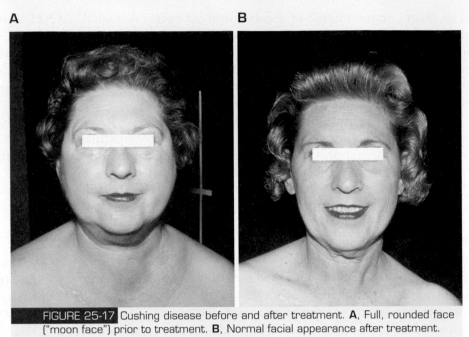

FIGURE 25-17 Cushing disease before and after treatment. **A**, Full, rounded face ("moon face") prior to treatment. **B**, Normal facial appearance after treatment.

increases along with the sodium concentration, and the blood pressure also rises along with the blood volume. The excessive hormone-induced excretion of potassium lowers blood potassium, which impairs neuromuscular function and leads to muscle weakness. The high aldosterone output exerts a negative feedback effect on renin production by the kidneys, and plasma renin falls.

An aldosterone-secreting adenoma is not a common cause of hypertension but may be suspected by the physician when the hypertension is associated with an elevated plasma sodium and a low plasma potassium, and can be confirmed by additional laboratory studies that reveal an elevated plasma aldosterone and low renin. Treatment consists of identification of the adrenal tumor, which can often be accomplished by CT or MRI examinations, followed by removal of the tumor.

Overproduction of Adrenal Sex Hormones

Adrenal gland dysfunction associated with abnormal production of sex hormone is uncommon. This may result from congenital hyperplasia of the adrenal glands or from an adrenal sex-hormone–producing tumor.

Congenital adrenal hyperplasia is the result of a congenital deficiency of certain enzymes required for the synthesis of various steroid hormones. In the normal biosynthesis of hormones by the adrenal cortex, cholesterol is initially converted into an intermediate compound (pregnenolone), which is a precursor of the other steroids produced in the adrenal (FIGURE 25-18). The chief metabolic pathways are concerned with the conversion of the intermediate compound into aldosterone, the major mineralocorticoid (pathway 1) and into the glucocorticoid cortisol (pathway 2). A third minor metabolic pathway leads to the production of adrenal androgens (pathway 3).

Biosynthesis of hormones in the major pathways (1 and 2) requires a series of additions of hydroxyl groups to the steroid molecules, and the enzymes that catalyze these reactions are called hydroxylases. If certain hydroxylases are absent or deficient, synthesis of aldosterone and cortisol will be impaired. This leads to increased ACTH secretion (because the pituitary interprets the low steroid levels

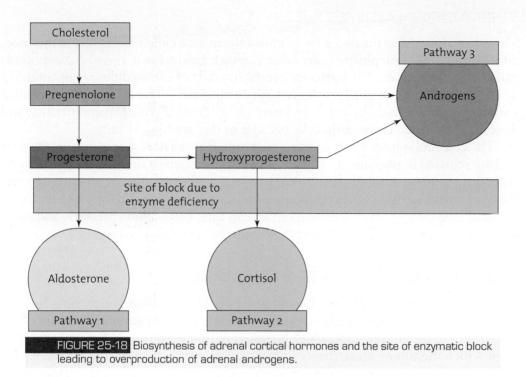

FIGURE 25-18 Biosynthesis of adrenal cortical hormones and the site of enzymatic block leading to overproduction of adrenal androgens.

in the blood as a signal to produce more ACTH). ACTH stimulation produces hyperplasia of the adrenal glands and increased synthesis of precursor compounds. However, because an enzymatic block affects the major pathways of steroid production, biosynthesis is shifted in the direction of androgenic steroids (pathway 3). Consequently, the major steroid output from the adrenals consists of androgenic compounds.

The clinical disorder produced by these enzymatic defects is often called the **adrenogenital syndrome**. This syndrome has several clinical varieties depending on which of the hydroxylase enzymes is deficient and the extent of the deficiency. All have the common feature of producing premature sexual development, called precocious puberty. In the female, sexual development is masculine because of the effect of the androgens. The age at which the hormonal effects become manifest depends on the degree of the enzyme deficiency. Congenital virilization may be noted at birth (FIGURE 25-19). If the deficiency is less severe, symptoms may not appear until the child is older.

Adrenal tumors that elaborate sex hormones are rare. When such a tumor develops, however, either androgen or estrogen may be produced. The clinical features depend on the age of the individual when the tumor becomes manifest and on the sex of the affected person. In a child, the tumor produces precocious puberty, and the character of the sexual development depends on the type of hormone elaborated. In adults, an estrogen-producing neoplasm elicits no hormonal symptoms in women but induces feminization in men. An androgen-secreting tumor masculinizes a woman but causes no hormonal symptoms in a man.

Adrenogenital syndrome
(ad-rēn′ō-jen′i-tul)
Clinical disorder of adrenal function characterized by overproduction of adrenal sex hormones.

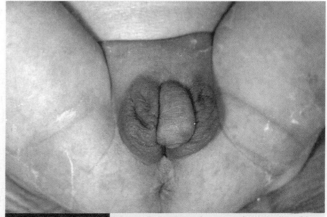

FIGURE 25-19 Masculinization of external genitalia of infant girl. Enlarged clitoris resembles penis. Vulvar labia are wrinkled and resemble scrotum.

THE ADRENAL MEDULLA

Norepinephrine
(nor′ep-in-ef′rin)
One of the compounds
(catecholamines) *secreted
by the adrenal medulla.*

Epinephrine
(ep-in-ef′rin)
One of the compounds
(catecholamines) *secreted
by the adrenal medulla.*

Catecholamines
(kat-eh-kōl′uh-mēnz)
*The adrenal medullary
hormones* epinephrine *and*
norepinephrine.

Pheochromocytoma
(fē′o-krō′mō-sī-tō′muh)
*Catecholamine-secreting
tumor of the adrenal
medulla.*

The adrenal medulla produces two similar hormones called **norepinephrine** (nor-adrenaline) and **epinephrine** (adrenaline), which belong to a class of compounds called **catecholamines**. The hormone-producing cells of the medulla are arranged in small groups surrounded by a rich network of capillaries. The cell cytoplasm is filled with fine granules that become dark brown when treated with chromium salts, and the cells are termed chromaffin cells because of this staining affinity.

The catecholamines produced by the chromaffin cells are stored within the cells and are released in response to nerve impulses transmitted to the medulla by the sympathetic nervous system. Any emotional stress such as anger, fear, or anxiety activates the sympathetic nervous system and causes the adrenal medulla to release its hormones. The liberated catecholamines cause a rapid heart rate, rise in blood pressure, and other effects that prepare the individual to cope with the stress of an emergency.

TUMORS OF THE ADRENAL MEDULLA

Rarely, a benign tumor called a **pheochromocytoma** arises from the chromaffin cells of the medulla. The tumor derives its unusual name from the staining reaction of the tumor cells to chromium salts, which is similar to that of the normal chromaffin cells from which the tumor arose (*pheo* = dark + *chromo* = color + *cyte* = cell + *oma* = tumor). A pheochromocytoma often secretes large amounts of catecholamines and produces severe effects on the heart and vascular system. The tumor may discharge catecholamines intermittently and induce periodic episodes of high blood pressure and increased heart rate. At times, the blood pressure may rise so severely that a cerebral blood vessel ruptures, causing a cerebral hemorrhage. In other cases, the increased output of catecholamines by the tumor is continuous and causes a sustained high blood pressure. Treatment consists of surgical removal of the tumor.

The Pancreatic Islets

In addition to manufacturing digestive enzymes, the pancreas functions as an endocrine gland. Scattered throughout the pancreas are more than a million small clusters of cells called the pancreatic islets or islets of Langerhans, which produce three different hormones: insulin, glucagon, and somatostatin. Diseases of the islets were considered in conjunction with diseases of the pancreas (discussion on the pancreas and diabetes mellitus).

The Gonads

The gonads have two functions: the production of germ cells, either eggs or sperm, and the production of sex hormones responsible for the development of secondary sexual characteristics. (This function is controlled by the gonadotrophic hormones of the pituitary gland.)

Occasionally, sex-hormone–secreting tumors develop in the ovary or testis. They may secrete sex hormone appropriate to the sex of the individual or, paradoxically, sex hormone characteristic of the opposite sex. No endocrine symptoms result from a tumor that produces the "proper" sex hormone; however, elaboration of the inappropriate sex hormone by the tumor causes masculinization in the female or feminization in the male. Sex-hormone–secreting tumors of the gonads are usually benign, and the disorder can be cured by surgical excision.

Hormone Production by Nonendocrine Tumors

Sometimes nonendocrine tumors secrete hormones that produce the same clinical manifestations as those of tumors arising from endocrine glands. Such hormones are called ectopic hormones (*ecto* = outside) because they are formed outside the endocrine glands, which are the normal sites of hormone production. An ectopic hormone is a protein that is either identical with the true hormone produced by the endocrine gland or has such a close resemblance that it mimics the action of the true hormone. Many different ectopic hormones have been identified, including ACTH, TSH, gonadotropins, ADH, parathyroid hormone, and insulin. Most hormone-producing nonendocrine tumors are malignant, and the majority have been elaborated by carcinomas of lung, pancreas, or kidneys or by malignant connective-tissue tumors.

Stress and the Endocrine System

The body is an integrated collection of cells organized into complex organ systems and regulated by a wide variety of control mechanisms, all designed to maintain a stable internal environment in which the cells can function efficiently. The maintenance of a steady state by the body's internal control systems is called homeostasis, and anything that disturbs the body's well-ordered internal environment brings into play regulatory mechanisms that attempt to reestablish the steady state under which the body functions most effectively. In a general sense, stress is any event that disturbs this stable internal environment. The event may be physical trauma, such as an injury or surgical operation, prolonged exposure to cold, vigorous exercise, pain, or a strong emotional stimulus such as anxiety or fear. Any of these events call forth a response that helps the body cope with the stress. There are two distinct but overlapping responses to stress, and the type of response generated depends on both the intensity and the duration of the stress. The acute, short-term response is mediated by the sympathetic nervous system and the adrenal medulla, and the chronic, longer term response includes the participation of several endocrine glands, with the adrenal cortex playing the major role. Both the acute and the chronic responses are initiated in the hypothalamus, which directs both the autonomic nervous system and many endocrine glands, and the hypothalamus in turn receives input from higher cortical centers.

The acute stress response is the well-known fear-fight-flight reaction triggered by the sympathetic nervous system. Norepinephrine released from sympathetic nerve endings, supplemented by norepinephrine and epinephrine released from the adrenal medulla in response to sympathetic nerve impulses, prepares the body to deal with the acute situation. Blood glucose rises as liver glycogen is broken down into glucose and released into the bloodstream. Peripheral vessels constrict, diverting more blood to the brain, heart, and skeletal muscles. The blood pressure rises, and the heart beats more forcefully. All of these systemic effects are of short duration and gradually subside when the stressful event is no longer present.

In contrast, long-term stress of any type, either physical or emotional, initiates a slower but more complex chain of events. Hypothalamic-releasing hormones, acting through the pituitary gland, cause the adrenal cortex to increase its output of cortical hormones; they also increase the output of growth hormone and thyroid hormone while suppressing the output of gonadotropic hormones. Excess cortisol production has pronounced effects on glucose, protein, and fat metabolism, as described earlier in connection with Cushing disease. The cortisol excess also dampens the inflammatory response and reduces the responsiveness of the immune system. In addition, cortisol excess tends to raise blood pressure by making the peripheral arterioles more responsive to the vasoconstrictor effect of norepinephrine released from sympathetic nerve endings. Increased aldosterone output promotes retention of salt and water, which also tends to raise blood pressure by increasing intravascular fluid volume.

The stress-related fall in gonadotropin output impairs gonadal function, which has widespread physiologic effects, and in women may lead to stress-related cessation of menstrual periods. Stress-related amenorrhea has well-defined adverse effects on the skeletal system as described in the discussion on the muskoloskeletal system.

The increased output of thyroid hormone speeds up metabolic processes in order to allow the body to deal more effectively with the stress, as does increased output of growth hormone, which also stimulates the body's metabolic processes.

Unfortunately, chronic stress takes its toll on the body and, over the long term, may predispose to illness. Excessive demands are placed on the cardiovascular system, which may contribute to heart disease, and the chronic corticosteroid excess places undue demand on the vascular system, as well as on other organ systems. Perhaps even more important, the chronic corticosteroid excess may increase our susceptibility to many types of illnesses by reducing our ability to generate an effective inflammatory reaction and by reducing the responsiveness of our immune system.

Stress initiates many physiologic responses that are designed to help protect us from harm, but chronic, unrelieved stress can cause us harm, and stress-relieving activities can help protect us from its long-term injurious effects.

QUESTIONS FOR REVIEW

1. What are the major hormones produced by the pituitary gland? What factors regulate secretion of pituitary hormones?
2. What is the effect of overproduction of growth hormone?
3. What factors regulate the rate of production of thyroid hormone? What are the major effects of an abnormal output of thyroid hormone? What is the difference between cretinism and myxedema?
4. Why does the thyroid gland become enlarged as a result of iodine deficiency?
5. What is the difference between thyrotoxicosis and thyroiditis?
6. What are the main classes of hormones elaborated by the adrenal cortex? What diseases result from adrenal cortical dysfunction?
7. What factors regulate the output of parathyroid hormone? What are the possible effects of parathyroid dysfunction?
8. What factors regulate the release of prolactin? What are the clinical effects of hyperprolactinemia? What are the causes of hyperprolactinemia?
9. What is Addison disease? What is the cause of the skin pigmentation?

SUPPLEMENTARY READINGS

Abboud, C. F. 1986. Laboratory diagnosis of hypopituitarism. *Mayo Clinic Proceedings* 61:35–48.
▶ Reviews the endocrine manifestations of hypopituitarism and useful diagnostic tests.

Amino, N. 1988. Autoimmunity and hypothyroidism. *Clinics in Endocrinology and Metabolism* 2:591–617.
▶ A review.

Greenspan, F. S. 1977. Radiation exposure and thyroid cancer. *Journal of the American Medical Association* 237:2089–91.

► Radiation exposure is carcinogenic.

Melmed, S. 2006. Medical progress: Acromegaly. *New England Journal of Medicine* 355:2558–73.

► Growth hormone is produced by somatotropes under the control of two separate hypothalamic hormones: growth hormone releasing hormone, which stimulates synthesis and secretion of growth hormone, and somatostatin, which inhibits these activities. Growth hormone normally is secreted as about 10 pulses every 24 hours, with the highest hormone levels occurring at night during sleep. Growth hormone secreting pituitary adenomas grow slowly, and the clinical manifestations of acromegaly also appear slowly. Treatment options include surgery, radiotherapy, or medical treatment. Transsphenoidal surgical resection is the preferred initial treatment. Radiotherapy is reserved for treatment of recurrent tumors. Medical treatment employs drugs that suppress growth hormone secretion by stimulating secretion of somatostatin.

Mitchell, M. L., Larsen, P. R., Levy, H. L., et al. 1978. Screening for congenital hypothyroidism. Results in the newborn population of New England. *Journal of the American Medical Association* 239:2348–51.

► Effective screening methods can identify congenital hypothyroidism, permitting effective treatment.

Randall, R. V., Laws, E. R., Jr., Abbound, C. F., et al. 1983. Transsphenoidal microsurgical treatment of prolactin-producing pituitary adenomas. Results in 100 patients. *Mayo Clinic Proceedings* 58:108–21.

► Reviews Mayo Clinic experience.

Samaan, N. A. 1977. Hormone production in non-endocrine tumors. *CA: A Cancer Journal for Clinicians* 27:148–59.

► Describes the various hormones produced by nonendocrine tumors and why this phenomenon occurs.

Vance, M. L., and Thorner, M. O. 1987. Prolactinomas. *Endocrinology and Metabolic Clinics of North America* 16:731–53.

► A relatively common pituitary tumor. Describes diagnostic approaches and treatment methods.

Wass, J. A. H., Laws, E. R., Jr., Randall, R. V., et al. 1986. The treatment of acromegaly. *Clinics in Endocrinology and Metabolism* 15:683–707.

► Describes medical and surgical methods. See also several articles on growth hormone deficiency and excess in the same issue.

OUTLINE SUMMARY

Pituitary Gland

STRUCTURE

Arises from base of brain. Located in pituitary fossa just behind optic chiasm.

Anterior lobe connected to hypothalamus by portal blood vessels.

Posterior lobe connected to hypothalamus by nerve fibers extending down stalk.

PITUITARY HORMONES

Anterior lobe:

Growth hormone: stimulates tissue growth.
Prolactin: stimulates secretion of milk.

TSH: stimulates thyroid.
ACTH: stimulates adrenal cortex.
FSH: gonadotropic hormone.
LH: gonadotropic hormone.

Posterior lobe:

ADH: causes more concentrated urine.
Oxytocin: stimulates uterine contractions and milk secretion.

PHYSIOLOGIC CONTROL OF PITUITARY HORMONE SECRETION

Tropic hormones are regulated by level of hormone produced by target gland.

A self-regulating mechanism to maintain uniform hormone output.

Prolactin secretion differs.

Tonic inhibition by hypothalamic PIF.

TSH stimulates release of prolactin as well as thyroid hormones.

CLINICAL DISTURBANCES OF PITUITARY HORMONE SECRETION

Hypofunction:

Panhypopituitarism: failure of secretion of all hormones. Secondary hypofunction of all target organs.

Pituitary dwarfism: deficiency of growth hormone.

Diabetes insipidus: lack of ADH causes excretion of large volume of extremely dilute urine.

Pituitary tumors.

Overproduction of growth hormone: caused by pituitary adenoma.

Causes gigantism in child.

Causes acromegaly in adult.

May cause visual disturbances caused by tumor encroachment on optic chiasm.

Overproduction of prolactin:

Causes amenorrhea and galactorrhea.

Often the result of small pituitary adenoma.

May be the result of other factors affecting hypothalamic function.

Thyroid Gland

STRUCTURE

Bilobed gland in neck regulated by TSH.

Composed of thyroid follicles which produce and store hormone.

Parafollicular cells produce calcitonin.

ACTIONS OF THYROID HORMONE

Controls metabolic functions.

Abnormal secretion causes hypothyroidism or hyperthyroidism.

GOITER

Nontoxic goiter:

Caused by inadequate hormone output, iodine deficiency, enzyme deficiency, inefficient enzyme function, or increased hormone requirements.

Gland enlarges to increase hormone output.

Treated by supplying hormone: gland decreases in size.

HYPERTHYROIDISM

Caused by autoantibody that stimulates gland.

Treated by antithyroid drugs, thyroidectomy, or radioiodine.

HYPOTHYROIDISM

In adult: causes metabolic slowing. Treated by thyroid hormone.

In infant: causes impaired growth and central nervous system development as well as hypometabolism. Early diagnosis and treatment required to assure normal development.

THYROIDITIS

Autoantibody destroys thyroid tissue and causes hypothyroidism.

Term refers to immunologic reaction, not true infection.

TUMORS OF THYROID

Benign adenomas.

Carcinoma.

Well-differentiated follicular and papillary carcinoma— good prognosis. Treated by surgical resection.

Poorly differentiated carcinoma—rapidly growing with poor prognosis. Treatment by surgery, radiation, and chemotherapy.

Medullary carcinoma—rare. Secretes calcitonin.

Radiation and thyroid tumors.

Radiation increases incidence of benign and malignant thyroid tumors after latent period of 5–30 years.

Most tumors well differentiated and easily treated.

Persons who received head or neck radiation should have periodic follow-up examinations.

Parathyroid Glands and Calcium Metabolism

PHYSIOLOGIC CONCEPTS

Blood calcium in equilibrium with calcium in bone.

Ionized fraction is physiologically active form.

Calcium level regulated by parathyroid glands.

Reduced calcium causes tetany. Elevated level reduces neuromuscular excitability.

HYPERPARATHYROIDISM

Usually the result of parathyroid adenoma.

Hypercalcemia and hypercalcuria.

Formation of renal calculi and calcium deposition in tissues.

Decalcification of bone.

Treated by removal of tumor.

HYPOPARATHYROIDISM

Usually the result of accidental removal of parathyroids during thyroid surgery.

Hypocalcemia causes tetany.

Treated by supplementary oral calcium and vitamin D to raise calcium levels.

Adrenal Glands

HORMONES OF ADRENAL CORTEX

Glucocorticoids: control carbohydrate metabolism.

Mineralocorticoids: control mineral metabolism.

Sex hormones: minor component.

ABNORMALITIES OF ADRENAL CORTICAL FUNCTION

Addison disease:

Glucocorticoid deficiency: hypoglycemia.

Mineralocorticoid deficiency: fall in blood volume and blood pressure.

Hyperpigmentation: caused by increased ACTH (loss of feedback inhibition).

Treated by supplying deficient corticosteroids.

Cushing disease and Cushing syndrome:

Glucocorticoid excess: disturbed carbohydrate, fat, and protein metabolism.

Mineralocorticoid excess: increased blood volume and blood pressure.

Treatment depends on cause: removal of pituitary microadenoma or adrenal adenoma or removal of hyperplastic adrenal glands.

OVERPRODUCTION OF ALDOSTERONE

Caused by aldosterone-secreting adrenal cortical tumor.

Blood sodium, volume, and pressure rise.

Blood potassium falls, leading to neuromuscular manifestations.

Removing the tumor cures the disease.

Overproduction of adrenal sex hormones:

Congenital adrenal hyperplasia: disturbed biosynthesis of hormones caused by enzyme deficiency.

Sex-hormone–producing tumors.

The Adrenal Medulla

Produces catecholamines (epinephrine and norepinephrine), which stimulate sympathetic nervous system.

Adrenal medullary tumors secrete catecholamines.

Produce pronounced cardiovascular effects.

May cause cerebral hemorrhage from high blood pressure.

Treated by removal of tumor.

Pancreatic Islets

See the discussion on the pancreas and diabetes mellitus.

The Gonads

FUNCTION

Production of sex hormones: controlled by FSH and LH.

Production of germ cells.

TUMORS

May secrete sex hormones.

Treated by surgical resection.

Hormone Production by Nonendocrine Tumors

ECTOPIC HORMONES

Identical with or closely resemble normal hormones.

Usually produced by malignant tumors.

Stress and the Endocrine System

Stress is any event that disturbs homeostasis.

Both acute and chronic responses to stress.

Acute response: fear-fight-flight response mediated by sympathetic nervous system and adrenal medulla.

Chronic response: primarily involves adrenal cortex but other endocrines involved.

Chronic stress alters body metabolism, taxes cardiovascular system, impairs inflammatory and immune responses, and predisposes to illness.

CHAPTER 26

The Nervous System

1 Describe the normal structure and basic functions of the brain, meninges, and cerebrospinal fluid as they relate to neurologic disease.

2 Define muscle tone and voluntary motor activity, and relate these concepts to the two forms of muscle paralysis.

3 Explain the pathogenesis and clinical manifestations of closure defects of the central nervous system. Name the techniques used for prenatal diagnosis.

4 Describe the pathogenesis and manifestations of hydrocephalus, and relate them to treatment measures.

5 Name the causes, manifestations, and treatment of transient ischemic attacks.

6 Differentiate between the two principal types of stroke in regard to pathogenesis, prognosis, and treatment.

7 Describe the pathogenesis, manifestations, and treatment of congenital cerebral aneurysms.

8 Name the types of tumors that affect the central nervous system, and explain their origin, pathogenesis, clinical manifestations, and treatment.

9 Explain the pathogenesis, major clinical manifestations, and general principles of treatment of Parkinson's disease, meningitis, multiple sclerosis, and Guillain-Barré syndrome.

Meninges (men-in′jēz)
The membranes covering the brain and spinal cord.

Dura (dū′rä)
The outer covering of the brain and spinal cord.

Structure and Function

The central nervous system (CNS) consists of the brain and spinal cord, surrounded by several membranes called **meninges.** The firm, fibrous outer membrane is called the **dura.** The thin inner membrane, which adheres to the surface of the brain and spinal cord, is called the **pia**. The middle membrane, interposed between the pia and dura, is called the **arachnoid**. The space between the arachnoid and the underlying pia is called the **subarachnoid space**. It contains cerebrospinal fluid (CSF) together with fine strands of arachnoidal connective tissue that extend through the space and attach to the tips of the gyri.

The brain is divided into the cerebrum, brain stem, and cerebellum. The brain is hollow, containing four interconnected cavities called **ventricles**. Arterial blood is supplied to the brain by large blood vessels entering the base of the skull. These arteries join to form a circle of vessels (the circle of Willis) at the base of the brain. Branches from the circle extend outward to supply all parts of the brain. Venous blood is returned from the brain into large venous sinuses in the dura, which eventually drain into the jugular veins.

The brain and spinal cord are surrounded by cerebrospinal fluid and are encased within protective bony structures: the cranium and the vertebral column. The bony case protects the soft and rather fragile nervous tissue, and the cerebrospinal fluid acts as a hydrostatic cushion to insulate the brain from shocks and blows.

The nerve tissue of the brain and spinal cord is composed of nerve cells called **neurons** and supporting cells called **neuroglia** (discussion on cells and tissues: their structure and function of health and disease). Each individual neuron has a central body and one or more long processes extending from the cell body to transmit the impulses. According to traditional concepts, a process that transmits impulses toward the cell body is called a dendrite and one conducting impulses away from the cell body is called an axon. Often, the noncommittal term nerve fiber is used when describing cell processes because the term can be applied to any nerve process without regard to its direction of impulse transmission. Most nerve fibers are covered by a fatty insulating myelin sheath.

Neurons are frequently arranged in chains; the neurons interconnect with other neurons to transmit impulses, but they are not in direct contact with one another. They are separated by minute gaps called synapses. The transmission of a nerve impulse across a synapse is by means of a chemical called a neurotransmitter that is released from the end of an axon and activates receptors on the dendrite or cell body of the adjacent neuron. There are several types of neurotransmitters, and each type of neuron has its own specific type of neurotransmitter. Some of the more important neurotransmitters are acetylcholine, norepinephrine, and dopamine, which is closely related to norepinephrine.

When a nerve fiber leaves the central nervous system, it becomes invested by elongated spindle cells called Schwann cells, which wrap around the fiber. These cells produce the myelin that insulates the fiber. (The myelin surrounding fibers within the central nervous system is produced by **oligodendroglia**.)

A nerve that transmits impulses into the nervous system is called a sensory nerve or afferent nerve (*ad* = to + *ferre* = carry). A motor nerve or efferent nerve (*e* = away) conducts impulses from brain or spinal cord to muscle. The gray matter of the brain and cord is composed primarily of nerve cells and their processes. The white matter consists mostly of bundles of nerve fibers covered by fatty myelin sheaths.

The nervous system may be regarded as a giant switchboard, receiving sensory impulses and relaying this information to brain and spinal cord centers concerned with perception of sensation and with motor activity. The cerebral cortex receives sensory input and initiates voluntary motor activity. In the depths of each cerebral hemisphere are masses of gray matter: the thalami and the basal ganglia (basal nuclei). The paired thalami, which form the lateral walls of the third ventricle, function as relay stations that receive sensory impulses from lower levels and transmit them to the cortex. The basal ganglia in each hemisphere, which consist of the caudate nucleus and lenticular nucleus, are connected to another important group of neurons in the brain stem that are called the substantia nigra (meaning literally black substance),

Pia (pē'yuh)
The innermost of the three membranes covering the brain and spinal cord.

Arachnoid (ar-ak'noyd)
The middle of the three meninges that cover the brain.

Subarachnoid space
(sub-är-ak'noyd)
The space between the arachnoid and the pia, containing large blood vessels supplying the brain.

Ventricle (ven'tri-kul)
A small cavity, especially one in the brain or heart. Ventricles of brain: *The hollow cavities in the brain.* Ventricles of heart: *The muscular chambers that receive blood from the atria and pump the blood into the aorta (left ventricle) or pulmonary artery (right ventricle).*

Neuron (nū'ron)
A nerve cell, including the nerve cell body and its processes.

Neuroglia
(noo-rog'-lē-ah)
Supporting cells of tissue of the nervous system.

Oligodendroglia
(ol'ig-o⁻-den-drog'li-ah)
One type of neuroglia that surrounds nerve fibers within the central nervous system.

so named because the neuron cell bodies contain melanin pigment and the neuron collections appear gray-black in color. Passing between the basal ganglia and the thalamus in each hemisphere is a large compact bundle of nerve fibers called the internal capsule, which carries impulses to and from the cortex.

The brain stem contains neurons that are involved in multiple functions not under direct cortical control; it also carries the bundles of nerve fibers that pass to higher and lower levels within the central nervous system. The cerebellum regulates muscle tone, coordination, posture, and balance.

The spinal cord is the continuation of the brain stem. Its central gray matter receives sensory input from spinal nerves entering the cord, and motor neurons exit from the cord to innervate muscles. Spinal sensory and motor neurons are involved in many reflex functions not under cortical control, but spinal motor neurons are also activated by motor impulses originating from cortical neurons. The spinal motor neurons in turn discharge impulses to the skeletal muscles that they supply, causing them to contract.

The fiber tracts conveying sensory impulses to the cortex and those conveying motor impulses from the cortex cross within the brain stem to the opposite side as they transmit impulses to their destination. Consequently, the right hemisphere registers sensation from the left half of the body and innervates the muscles on the left side. Conversely, the left hemisphere receives sensation from the right side of the body and activates muscles on the right side.

Development of the Nervous System

In the embryo, the central nervous system first appears as a thickened band of surface cells (ectoderm) called the neural plate. Its lateral margins become elevated to form neural folds, and the two folds then fuse to form a hollow tube called the **neural tube.** Fusion begins in the middle of the developing tube and progresses toward both ends until a completely closed tube is formed by the end of the fourth week of embryonic development. Three expansions, called the forebrain, midbrain, and hindbrain, develop from one end of the neural tube (FIGURE 26-1A). The other end remains narrow and becomes the spinal cord.

The cerebral hemispheres develop as lateral outgrowths from the forebrain and soon overgrow the remaining parts of the brain. The remainder of the forebrain becomes the diencephalon, which is located between the cerebral hemispheres (*dia* = between + *encephalon* = brain). The midbrain persists as a small area connecting forebrain and hindbrain. The hindbrain gives rise to parts of the brain called the pons, medulla, and cerebellum. The diencephalon, midbrain, pons, and medulla together form the brain stem. The central cavity within the neural tube develops into the ventricular system of the adult brain (FIGURE 26-1B). Each ventricle contains a choroid plexus, which secretes cerebrospinal fluid (CSF) that flows through the ventricles and into the subarachnoid space through a midline and two lateral openings in the fourth ventricle. The CSF flows around the brain and spinal cord and is absorbed into the large veins located in the dense fibrous covering of the brain called the cerebral dura. The embryonic cells (mesoderm) surrounding the developing neural tube give rise to the cranial cavity, vertebral bodies, and adjacent tissues.

Muscle Tone and Voluntary Muscle Contraction

A skeletal muscle contracts in response to impulses discharged from motor neurons in the spinal cord or from corresponding neurons of the cranial nerves in the brain stem. These neurons are often called the lower motor neurons. Voluntary motor

Neural tube
The ectodermal tube formed in the embryo that gives rise to the brain and spinal cord.

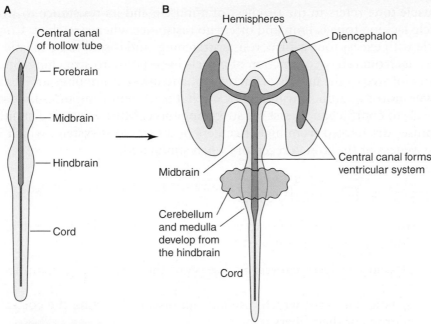

FIGURE 26-1 Early development of the nervous system. **A**, Formation of neural tube, which normally closes at both ends. Central canal in tube is the precursor of the ventricular system. **B**, Cerebral hemispheres grow from the forebrain and the central region becomes the diencephalon. The midbrain undergoes little change. The hindbrain gives rise to the pons and medulla, and the neural tube develops into the ventricular system. The two lateral ventricles follow the contours of the developing hemispheres, which communicate with the third ventricle in the diencephalon by channels called interventricular foramina. The channel in the midbrain becomes the cerebral aqueduct, which expands into the fourth ventricle in the medulla. Each ventricle develops a choroid plexus to make the cerebrospinal fluid that flows through the ventricular system, exits through openings in the fourth ventricle, and circulates around the brain and spinal cord.

activity is controlled by nerve impulses originating in motor neurons in the cerebral cortex, sometimes called upper motor neurons. Voluntary motor activity is controlled by two separate motor systems. One system, called the pyramidal system, controls voluntary motor functions, and the other system, called the extrapyramidal system, regulates muscle groups concerned primarily with balance, posture, and coordination.

The axons of the pyramidal system motor neurons descend in fiber tracts called the pyramidal tracts or corticospinal tracts. The corticospinal tracts cross in the brain stem, and their axons synapse with lower motor neurons in the brain stem and spinal cord, activating the lower motor neurons and causing them to discharge an impulse. Acetylcholine is the neurotransmitter released by the axon terminals of both the corticospinal tract neurons and the motor neurons in the brain stem and spinal cord with which they synapse.

The nerve fibers of the extrapyramidal tract neurons also cross and descend to synapse with the same lower motor neurons that receive impulses from the pyramidal tract neurons, but the extrapyramidal system is a much more complex multineuron pathway. It has multiple connections with neurons in the cerebellum, basal ganglia, substantia nigra, and other groups of brain stem neurons.

The pyramidal system and the extrapyramidal system function together as a single system under cortical control to produce the smooth integrated functions of muscle groups involved in voluntary motor activity. Malfunction of the extrapyramidal system leads to loss of coordinated motor functions. The muscles do not function smoothly, and the malfunction also gives rise to abnormal uncontrollable muscular movements.

Muscle tone
The slight contractility (tension) present in resting muscles.

Muscle tone refers to the firmness of a muscle and its resistance to stretching. A muscle lacking tone is limp and offers no resistance when stretched. Conversely, a muscle with excess tone is firm, resists stretching, and is said to be spastic. Muscle tone results from reflex contraction of muscle in response to stretching. Specialized receptors located in the muscle are activated, and afferent impulses are conveyed to the lower motor neuron, causing reflex discharge of motor impulses that stimulate the muscle to contract and resist the stretching force. Muscle tone is also influenced by impulses discharged from higher centers in the nervous system, which vary the responsiveness of the stretch receptors when stimulated.

Muscle Paralysis

A muscle that is no longer subject to voluntary control is said to be paralyzed. There are two different types of paralysis:

1. Flaccid paralysis, caused by disease of the lower motor neurons or their fibers
2. Spastic paralysis, which results from disease affecting the cortical motor neurons or their fibers

Spastic paralysis occurs more frequently than flaccid paralysis because cortical neurons are more often damaged by disease than are spinal motor neurons.

FLACCID PARALYSIS

If the lower motor neuron in the spinal cord is destroyed by a disease such as poliomyelitis or if the peripheral nerve supplying the muscle (which contains the nerve fibers of the spinal neurons) is interrupted, the reflex arc responsible for muscle tone is interrupted. Muscle tone is abolished because the muscle is deprived of its innervation. The muscle becomes limp and undergoes severe atrophy.

SPASTIC PARALYSIS

If cortical motor neurons or their fibers that travel in the motor pathways are interrupted, as in a stroke, voluntary control of the muscles supplied by the affected neurons is lost because the pyramidal tract pathway is interrupted. However, because the reflex arc that maintains muscle tone is not disturbed and the muscle retains its innervation, significant atrophy of the muscle does not occur. Generally, muscle tone is in fact increased because extrapyramidal motor impulses descending from the cortex tend to inhibit muscle tone, and this inhibitory effect is lost after an upper motor neuron injury.

Cerebral Injury

Concussion
A temporary loss of consciousness caused by a head injury without any memory of the events that occurred shortly before or after the head injury.

The brain is well protected from moderate trauma but may be injured by a blow to the head that jars the brain with its protective cranial cavity. The mildest form of head injury is called a **concussion**, which may be caused by an auto accident or contact sports injury such as football or boxing. A concussion usually is characterized by temporary loss of consciousness without any memory of the events that occurred shortly before and after the head injury (amnesia). The concussion may be associated with a headache, temporary disorientation, and confusion. Usually there are no long-term complications related to a single concussion, but repeated head injuries related to football, boxing, or other contact sports may lead to permanently impared cerebral function. However, a severe blow may injure the brain, and sometimes, the skull also is

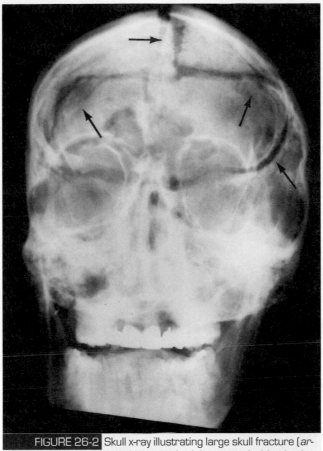

FIGURE 26-2 Skull x-ray illustrating large skull fracture (*arrows*) associated with extensive injury to underlying brain.

fractured (FIGURE 26-2). Injury to the brain may be manifested by loss of consciousness and various neurologic disturbances. The injured brain becomes swollen and often shows evidence of pinpoint hemorrhages caused by disruption of small intracerebral blood vessels. Usually the brain injury is located immediately adjacent to the site of the blow, but sometimes the brain injury is caused by violent contact of the displaced brain against the cranial cavity on the side opposite the injury. For example, the force of a blow to the back of the head may displace the brain forward, injuring the front of the brain where it strikes against the front of the bony cranial cavity (FIGURE 26-3).

Sometimes, a head injury tears blood vessels located between the cranial bones and the dura or under the dura. The escaping blood may accumulate in any of several locations, depending on which vessels have been damaged:

1. Between the outer layer of dura and the cranial bones (epidural hemorrhage)
2. Between the dura and the arachnoid (subdural hemorrhage)
3. Between the arachnoid and the pia (subarachnoid hemorrhage)

A localized epidural or subdural collection of blood (a hematoma) may compress the brain and impair its function. In a subarachnoid hemorrhage, the blood often mixes with the cerebrospinal fluid and spreads diffusely through the subarachnoid space.

Unfortunately, the rigid cranial cavity, which normally serves a protective function, is a disadvantage if the brain is seriously injured. The brain often swells at the site of injury, and the unyielding cranial cavity restricts the swelling and compresses the swollen brain, leading to high intracranial pressure. The elevated pressure adversely affects cerebral function and may also interfere with the blood supply to the brain by compressing cerebral blood vessels.

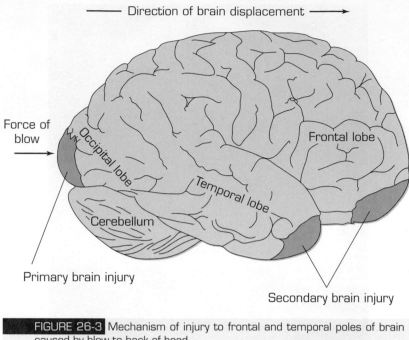

← Direction of brain displacement →

Force of blow →

Occipital lobe

Frontal lobe

Temporal lobe

Cerebellum

Primary brain injury

Secondary brain injury

FIGURE 26-3 Mechanism of injury to frontal and temporal poles of brain caused by blow to back of head.

Neural Tube Defects

Failure of either end of the neural tube to close properly leads to serious congenital malformations called neural tube defects, which involve not only the nervous system but the surrounding tissues as well. A closure defect involving the end of the tube destined to form the cerebral hemispheres (called the cephalic end) leads to a condition called **anencephaly** (*ana* = without + *encephalon* = brain). If the opposite end of the tube (the caudal end) is involved, **spina bifida** results. These are the two most common congenital malformations of the nervous system. The combined incidence of these malformations is about 2 per 1,000 births in the United States and even higher in some other countries. The malformations follow a multifactorial pattern of inheritance (discussion on congenital and hereditary diseases) and tend to recur in subsequent pregnancies. If parents have already given birth to an offspring with a neural tube defect, the risk of recurrence in a subsequent pregnancy is approximately 1 in 20. The risk is 1 in 10 when the parents have had two affected infants.

A deficiency of folic acid during the early part of pregnancy when the neural tube is forming plays an important role in causing neural tube defects. Intake of 0.4 mg (400 μg) of folic acid daily beginning before conception and during the early part of pregnancy can reduce by one-half the frequency of neural tube defects. However, these defects follow a multifactorial inheritance pattern, and the folic acid deficiency functions along with genetic factors to cause the neural tube defect. Consumption of folic acid will reduce the frequency of neural tube defects but will not eliminate the problem, and a woman who has previously given birth to an infant with a neural tube defect still has a greater than normal risk of having an infant with a neural tube defect in a subsequent pregnancy.

ANENCEPHALY

Anencephaly occurs most commonly in female infants and is incompatible with postnatal life.

Because the cephalic end of the neural tube fails to close, the exposed neural tissue undergoes secondary degenerative changes that convert it into a mass of vascular

Anencephaly
(an-en-seff'uh-lē)
A congenital malformation: absence of brain, cranial vault, and scalp as a result of defective closure of the neural tube.

Spina bifida
(spī'-nuh bif'fid-duh)
Incomplete closure of vertebral arches over the spinal cord, sometimes associated with protrusion of meninges and neural tissue through the defect (cystic spina bifida).

A   B

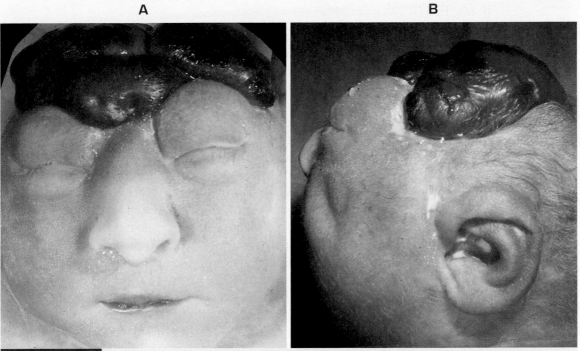

FIGURE 26-4 Characteristic appearance of anencephalic infant. Most of brain, top of skull, and scalp are absent. Maldevelopment of skull causes protrusion of eyes. **A**, Frontal view. **B**, Lateral view.

connective tissue intermixed with masses of degenerated brain and choroid plexus. The anencephalic infant has a striking appearance (FIGURE 26-4). The brain is absent, as are the soft tissues of the scalp and the bones making up the vertex of the skull. The exposed base of the skull is covered only by a vascular membrane. The base of the cranial cavity is abnormally formed, and the orbits are shallow, causing the eyes to bulge outward. The trunk is short, the shoulders are broad, and the neck is not normal; the head arises directly from the trunk and cannot be flexed.

Sometimes the closure defect affects not only the brain, but also the part of the neural tube that forms the upper part of the spinal cord. When this occurs, the vertebral arches are absent, as well as the vertex of the skull, and the unclosed spinal cord lies exposed within the wide-open spinal canal.

The following case illustrates some of the obstetric problems associated with anencephaly.

CASE 26-1

A female anencephalic infant was born to a 28-year-old woman who was pregnant for the first time. The fetal heartbeat could be heard by the obstetrician throughout the last part of the pregnancy. When the patient's abdomen was examined near term, the obstetrician became concerned about the possibility of anencephaly because of the inability to feel the fetal head. An x-ray film taken of the patient's abdomen confirmed the clinical impression because only the base of the fetal skull could be seen in the x-ray film. The bones of the cranial vault were absent. The rest of the fetal skeleton appeared normally formed. The patient was delivered at term with some difficulty because the anencephalic head was unable to flex normally as it passed through the mother's pelvis, and the infant was delivered face first. The infant survived for several hours after delivery. The autopsy revealed complete absence of the cerebral hemispheres, the cerebellum, and most of the brain stem.

SPINA BIFIDA

Malformations of the opposite (caudal) end of the neural tube and related vertebral arches are generally considered together under the term spina bifida. This term means literally split spine and refers to the characteristic failure of fusion of the vertebral arches common to all types of spina bifida (FIGURE 26-5). Failure of fusion of vertebral arches in the lower lumbar region occurring as an isolated abnormality is called occult spina bifida (FIGURE 26-5A); this type produces no clinical symptoms. The more severe types of spina bifida, sometimes called collectively cystic spina bifida, are characterized by a saclike protrusion of meninges or meninges and nerve tissue through the defect in the vertebral arches. The malformation is called a **meningocele** if the protrusion consists only of meninges (FIGURE 26-5B) and is called a **meningomyelocele** (*myelo* = cord) if parts of the spinal cord or nerve roots also are included in the sac (FIGURE 26-5C).

In meningomyelocele, there is often a severe neurologic deficit below the level of the sac because the nerve tissue is actually incorporated into the wall of the sac and is disorganized so that the conduction of nerve impulses is impaired or completely interrupted. In the most severe (and fortunately rare) form of spina bifida, the caudal end of the neural tube completely fails to close. The distal end of the spinal cord is represented by a flattened mass of nerve tissue that is continuous with the adjacent skin (FIGURE 26-5D). The larger meningomyelocele sacs often are covered not by skin but merely by a thin, easily ruptured membrane composed only of meninges (FIGURE 26-6).

Treatment of Spina Bifida

Occult spina bifida is asymptomatic, and no treatment is required. A meningocele usually can be repaired without difficulty by excising the sac and closing the spinal dura,

Meningocele
(men-in′go-sēl)
 A protrusion of meninges through a defect in the spinal vertebral arches.

....

Meningomyelocele
(men-ing-gō-mī′el-ō-sēl)
A type of spina bifida characterized by protrusion of meninges and cord through the defect in the vertebral arches.

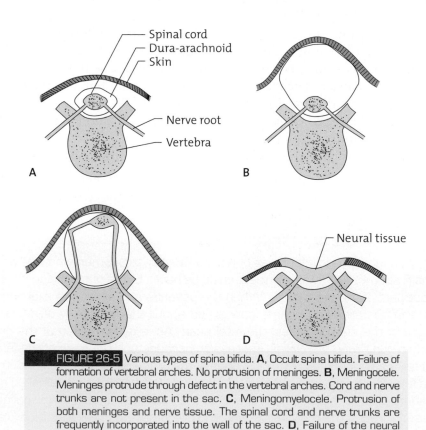

FIGURE 26-5 Various types of spina bifida. **A**, Occult spina bifida. Failure of formation of vertebral arches. No protrusion of meninges. **B**, Meningocele. Meninges protrude through defect in the vertebral arches. Cord and nerve trunks are not present in the sac. **C**, Meningomyelocele. Protrusion of both meninges and nerve tissue. The spinal cord and nerve trunks are frequently incorporated into the wall of the sac. **D**, Failure of the neural tube to form and separate from the surface ectoderm. The neural tissue is continuous with the adjacent skin.

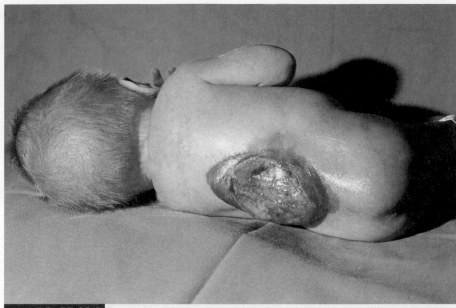

FIGURE 26-6 Large thoracic meningomyelocele covered only by a thin membrane. This condition is associated with neurologic disturbances resulting from incorporation of neural tissue into the wall of the sac.

and the results are usually very satisfactory. Unfortunately, a large meningomyelocele is much more difficult to treat, and results are much less satisfactory. Because spinal cord and nerve roots are often incorporated in the sac, there is frequently some loss of sensation and motor power in the lower extremities. Bowel and bladder function also may be impaired, leading to stasis of urine in the bladder and predisposing to urinary tract infections. These unfortunate individuals are managed best by a team of specialists in a medical center specializing in the care of patients with severe disabilities of this type. Many patients can be treated successfully and are able to lead happy and productive lives despite their disability. Unfortunately, the most common type of cystic spinal bifida is a meninogomyelocele, which has a frequency of 3.4 per 10,000 live births despite widespread use of preconception folic acid. A meninogomyelocele in which nerve tissue is incorporated in the sac is a more complex treatment problem because the condition may be complicated by hydrocephalus. This subject will be considered later along with other causes of hydrocephalus.

The following case illustrates some of the problems encountered by the physician in the care of infants and children with large meningomyeloceles.

CASE 26-2

A female infant was born with a very large meningomyelocele associated with complete loss of sensation and motor power below the level of the protruding sac (FIGURE 26-7). Because of the severe neurologic deficit, she was not considered a suitable candidate for surgical treatment, and she was discharged to a boarding home for care. She was returned to the hospital 6 months later because the surface of the sac had become eroded, permitting the cerebrospinal fluid to leak from the sac. The hole in the sac had also allowed bacteria to gain access to the spinal canal, causing a meningitis that proved fatal despite supportive treatment and antibiotics.

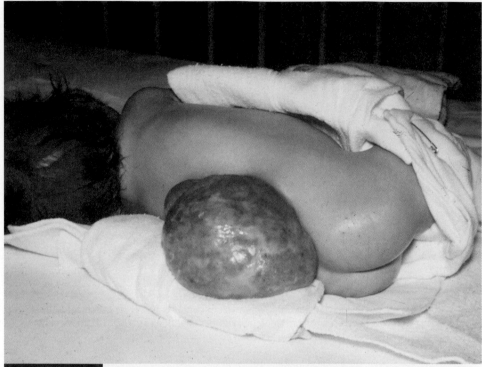

FIGURE 26-7 Very large meningomyelocele that was associated with severe neurologic deficit. Perforation of the sac was followed by meningitis.

PRENATAL DETECTION OF NEURAL TUBE DEFECTS

It is usually possible to identify a fetus with a neural tube defect prior to birth. An elevated concentration of alpha-fetoprotein (AFP) detected on a routine screening test of maternal blood may suggest the possibility of a neural tube defect, and the defect can be confirmed by an ultrasound examination of the fetus performed at about 16-weeks gestation, as described in the discussion on congenital and hereditary diseases. An increased concentration of AFP can also be detected in amnionic fluid if an amniocentesis is performed.

Alpha-fetoprotein is produced in the fetal liver beginning early in pregnancy and can be readily detected in the fetal blood. The concentration in fetal blood is highest at about 13 weeks and then gradually declines. A small amount of AFP normally diffuses from the fetal blood into the amnionic fluid and also into the mother's blood. High-amnionic fluid AFP levels are encountered when the fetus is anencephalic or has a cystic spina bifida in which the defect is covered only by a thin membrane because AFP can more easily diffuse from the fetal blood and cerebrospinal fluid through the defect directly into the amnionic fluid. Consequently, AFP levels are much higher than in a normal pregnancy.

Hydrocephalus

Cerebrospinal fluid serves as a protective cushion around the brain and spinal cord. The fluid is secreted by the choroid plexuses of the ventricles. It flows from the lateral ventricles into the third ventricle, through the cerebral aqueduct (aqueduct of Sylvius) into the fourth ventricle and then out into the subarachnoid space through three small openings in the roof of the fourth ventricle. The fluid circulates around the cord and over the convexity of the brain and is resorbed into the large venous sinuses in the dura. Secretion of cerebrospinal fluid continues even if the flow of fluid through the ventricular system is blocked. Obstruction to the normal circulation of spinal fluid distends the ventricles proximal to the site of obstruction, with associated compression atrophy of brain tissue around the dilated ventricles (FIGURE 26-8). This condition, which is called **hydrocephalus,** may be either congenital or acquired.

Congenital Hydrocephalus

Congenital hydrocephalus is usually caused by a congenital abnormality in the ventricular system, either a congenital obstruction or abnormal formation of the cerebral aqueduct, a narrow channel connecting the third and fourth ventricles, or failure of the openings in the roof and lateral walls of the fourth ventricle to form normally, which blocks escape of cerebrospinal fluid into the subarachnoid space. An aqueduct obstruction leads to distention of the lateral and third ventricles. An obstruction of the outlet channels in the fourth ventricle leads to distention of all four ventricles. Because the distention develops before the skull bones have fused, the head enlarges greatly and the brain undergoes pronounced atrophy secondary to compression by the dilated ventricles. Hydrocephalus may occur in the fetus prior to birth, and the head may become so large that it is unable to enter the maternal pelvis during labor. More often, the hydrocephalus develops insidiously after birth.

Hydrocephalus
Dilatation of the ventricular system caused by pressure arising from accumulation of cerebrospinal fluid within the ventricles.

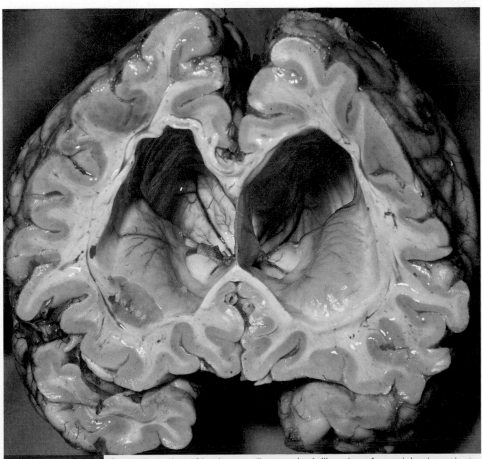

FIGURE 26-8 | Coronal section of brain revealing marked dilatation of ventricles in patient with congenital hydrocephalus.

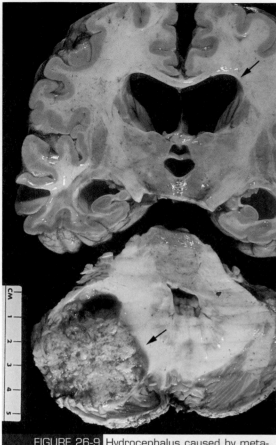

FIGURE 26-9 Hydrocephalus caused by metastatic carcinoma in cerebellum. The upper section of the brain illustrates dilation of the ventricular system, best seen in the lateral ventricles (*upper arrow*). The lower section illustrates a tumor in the cerebellar hemisphere (*lower arrow*), which has compressed fourth ventricle, impeding outflow of cerebrospinal fluid.

Acquired Hydrocephalus

Acquired hydrocephalus is most commonly caused by obstruction of the circulation of the cerebrospinal fluid in the region of the fourth ventricle by fibrous adhesions, which sometimes form after a bacterial infection of the meninges (**meningitis**) and block the outflow of fluid from the fourth ventricle, or by blockage of the ventricular system secondary to a brain tumor (FIGURE 26-9). Acquired hydrocephalus develops after the skull bones fuse, and the skull cannot enlarge as in the congenital form of hydrocephalus.

Treatment of Hydrocephalus

Hydrocephalus can often be treated successfully by inserting a plastic tube into one of the dilated ventricles and rerouting (shunting) the fluid into another part of the body where it can be absorbed. The fluid can be shunted into the right atrium (ventriculoatrial shunt) or into the peritoneal cavity (ventriculoperitoneal shunt). A small opening is made in the skull to allow insertion of a plastic drainage tube through cerebral hemisphere into one of the dilated lateral ventricles. The other end of the tube is passed through the subcutaneous tissues behind the ear. In a ventriculoatrial shunt, the tube is inserted into the jugular vein and threaded down the vein so that the tip is positioned in the right atrium. In the more commonly used ventriculoperitoneal shunt, the tube is passed through the subcutaneous tissues of the neck, chest, and upper abdomen and introduced into the abdominal cavity through a small incision in the peritoneum. Whatever type of shunt is used, a one-way valve is incorporated in the tube to prevent any reflux of blood or peritoneal fluid into the ventricles (FIGURE 26-10).

Meningitis

(men-in-jī'tis)
Inflammation of the meninges.

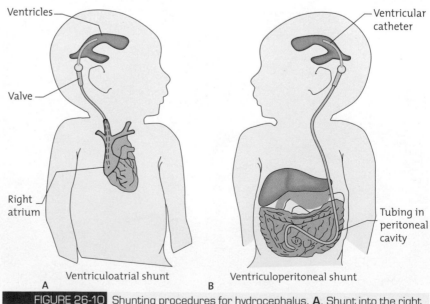

FIGURE 26-10 Shunting procedures for hydrocephalus. **A,** Shunt into the right atrium. **B,** Shunt into the peritoneal cavity.

Hydrocephalus Associated with a Meningomyelocele

An infant born with a meningomyelocele not only has a neurologic defect but also is likely to develop hydrocephalus. Normally, during fetal development, the spine grows faster than the spinal cord, and the end of the spinal cord occupies a progressively higher position in the spinal canal as the fetus grows. Unfortunately, in a fetus with MM, often the end of the spinal cord is fixed within the MM sac and is unable to rise in the spinal canal as the fetus grows; instead, the fixed end of the spinal cord pulls the medulla and part of the cerebellum through the foramen magnum into the spinal canal as the spine grows, which disrupts the normal circulation of cerebrospinal fluid and leads to hydrocephalus.

Prenatal Correction of Hydrocephalus Associated with Meningomyelocele

Although a fetus with a meningomyelocele can be identified relatively early in a pregnancy, usually delivery is delayed until close to term to avoid fetal problems related to premature delivery. Moreover, the displaced hindbrain of the affected fetus disrupts the circulation and absorption of CSF, and the longer the hindbrain displacement persists, the more marked is the damage to the nervous system. Perhaps earlier repair of the meningomyelocele while the fetus is still in the uterus would produce a better long-term result. A recent study reported in the *New England Journal of Medicine* compared the results of prenatal intrauterine repair as early as 30 weeks of gestation with postnatal repair in a comparable group of women with affected fetuses. Prenatal surgery reduced the need to insert a shunt to control hydrocephalus and improved the outcomes of affected infants when evaluated 30 months after prenatal surgery when compared with postnatal surgery results in a control group. However, there were significant maternal complications including a weak uterine scar, which would require delivery by cesarean section in a subsequent pregnancy, as well as fetal complications related to prematurity. An accompanying editorial suggested that the gains were less than optimal when compared with the maternal and fetal risks associated with the prenatal surgery.

Case 26-3 illustrates some of the obstetric and pediatric problems encountered when hydrocephalus occurs in the fetus before delivery.

CASE 26-3

A 24-year-old woman who was pregnant for the first time noted marked enlargement of her abdomen during the last part of pregnancy. X-ray examination of the abdomen revealed a hydrocephalic infant having a head diameter that was larger than the diameter of the mother's pelvis, indicating that delivery could not be accomplished vaginally. At term, an elective cesarean section was performed, and the infant was evaluated soon after delivery by a neurosurgeon. A shunt was performed in order to control the progressing hydrocephalus. The shunt prevented further enlargement of the head, and the infant did reasonably well after this operation.

Stroke

The term **stroke**, also called a **cerebrovascular accident** or simply **CVA**, is used to designate any injury to brain tissue resulting from disturbance of blood supply to the brain and encompasses three conditions: (1) cerebral thrombosis, (2) cerebral embolism, and (3) cerebral hemorrhage.

Stroke
Any injury to the brain caused by disturbance of its blood supply.

Cerebrovascular accident (CVA)
An injury to the brain resulting in a disturbance of cerebral blood flow caused by a cerebral thrombosis, cerebral embolism, or cerebral hemorrhage.

Cerebral thrombosis
A stroke caused by thrombosis of an arteriosclerotic cerebral artery.

Cerebral embolus
A stroke caused by blockage of a cerebral artery by a blood clot that had formed elsewhere in the circulatory system and was transported in the bloodstream to the brain.

Cerebral hemorrhage
A stroke caused by rupture of a cerebral artery, usually in a person with hypertension, which allows blood to escape under high pressure into the brain.

Encephalomalacia
(en-seff'uh-lō-mu-lā'shuh)
Cystic lesion of degenerated brain tissue as a result of obstruction of cerebral blood supply. Same as cerebral infarct.

A **cerebral thrombosis**, as indicated by the name, results from thrombosis of a cerebral artery narrowed by arteriosclerosis and is the cause of most strokes.

A **cerebral embolus**, which occurs less frequently than a cerebral thrombosis, is caused by blockage of a cerebral artery by a fragment of a blood clot dislodged from the surface of an ulcerated arteriosclerotic plaque in the carotid artery and carried to the brain or from a blood clot that formed within the heart. Three cardiac conditions predispose to cerebral emboli: (1) a mural thrombus that formed on the wall of the left ventricle adjacent to a healing myocardial infarct, (2) a thrombus that formed on the rough surface of a diseased mitral or aortic valve, and (3) a small thrombus in the left atrial appendage (auricle) of a person with atrial fibrillation. Atrial thrombi tend to develop because the atria are not contracting normally. Consequently, the blood pools in the atrial appendages instead of being ejected normally, which predisposes to formation of blood clots in the stagnant atrial appendage blood.

A **cerebral hemorrhage** is the most serious type of stroke. It is caused by rupture of a cerebral artery in a person with hypertension. Blood under high pressure escapes from the ruptured vessel and causes marked damage to the brain.

CEREBRAL THROMBI AND EMBOLI

When a cerebral artery is blocked by either a thrombus on an embolus, the brain tissue in the distribution of the blocked vessel becomes necrotic and degenerates, which is called a cerebral infarct (FIGURES 26-11 AND 26-12). The myelin sheath material breaks down, and the debris resulting from the necrosis of brain tissue is eventually cleaned up by phagocytes, leaving a cystic cavity. Because the end stage of a brain infarct is cystic, in contrast to the appearance of infarcts in other tissues, the term **encephalomalacia** (*encephalon* = brain + *malacia* = softening) is sometimes used to describe this kind of lesion (FIGURE 26-13).

In most cerebral infarcts, no blood leaks into the degenerated brain tissue, and this type of infarct is often called an ischemic infarct (pronounced is-key-mik), which means literally that blood is held back (*ischo* = hold back + *heme* = blood).

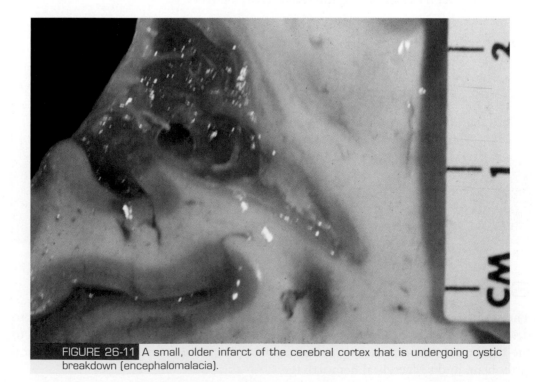

FIGURE 26-11 A small, older infarct of the cerebral cortex that is undergoing cystic breakdown (encephalomalacia).

A   **B**

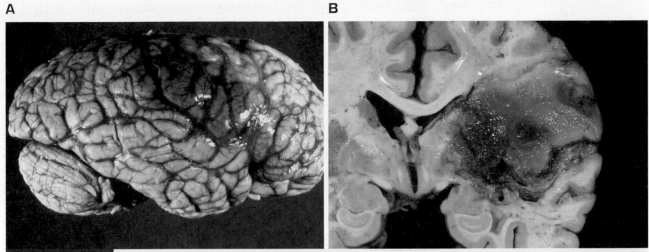

FIGURE 26-12 Large recent infarct of right cerebral hemisphere caused by thrombosis of middle cerebral artery. **A**, External surface of brain illustrating the swollen, dark, infarcted area in the right hemisphere. **B**, Coronal section through hemispheres at level of basal ganglia. Cerebral tissue is necrotic and discolored and involves a large part of the hemisphere.

However, sometimes a relatively small amount of blood leaks into the degenerated brain tissue from adjacent damaged cerebral blood vessels, as illustrated in FIGURE 26-12. This type of infarct may be called a hemorrhagic infarct, but the term should not be confused with a cerebral hemorrhage, which is large hemorrhage within the brain resulting from ruptured cerebral artery, a very different and much more serious condition.

Some patients who have had a cerebral thrombosis may benefit from the same type of thrombolytic drugs used to dissolve blood clots in coronary arteries (discussion on the cardiovascular system). Unfortunately, there is very little time available to restore flow through a blocked cerebral artery before permanent brain damage occurs, and sometimes the thrombolytic drug treatment may be complicated by hemorrhage within the damaged brain tissue.

B

A

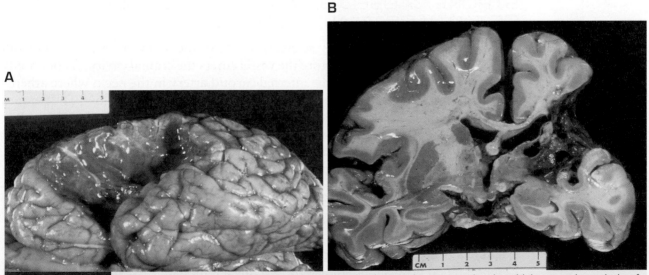

FIGURE 26-13 A large old infarct in the left hemisphere sustained several years previously, which caused paralysis of right side of body and loss of speech. **A**, External surface of the brain, illustrating the large defect in the left hemisphere at the site of the old infarct. **B**, Coronal section through the hemisphere revealing complete loss of cerebral tissue at the site of the old infarct, leaving only a few strands of glial tissue.

STROKE CAUSED BY A PARADOXICAL EMBOLUS

A paradox is an event that seems unbelievable but is actually true. A paradoxical embolus is a blood clot detached from a leg vein that does not cause a pulmonary embolism. Instead, the clot enters the systemic circulation where it blocks a cerebral artery and causes a stroke, which is not the expected behavior of an embolism coming from a detached leg vein thrombus.

Occasionally a young, apparently healthy person has a stroke, even though the affected person has no evidence of cardiovascular disease or other risk factors that predispose to strokes. Although an uncommon cause of strokes, the condition may result from a patent foramen ovale, the opening in the atrial septum guarded by a flap-type valve that allows one-way blood flow from right to left atrium in the fetus, bypassing blood flow to the nonfunctional fetal lungs, as described in the discussion on the cardiovascular system. After birth, the left atrial pressure rises, which presses the flap valve against the atrial septum, where it fuses to the atrial septum and closes the communication.

In about 25% of adults, the flap valve does not fuse completely, but the foramen ovale remains nonfunctional as long as the left atrial pressure remains higher than the right atrial pressure. However, if the foramen ovale is not completely sealed shut, any action involving attempted forced expiration with the glottis closed raises the pressure within the thoracic cavity and also raises right atrial pressure. Actions such as vigorous coughing, straining to expel bowel contents during defecation, or "pushing" to deliver a baby during childbirth may raise right atrial pressure high enough to force some blood from the right atrium into the left atrium. If a small embolus from a leg vein happens to be in the right atrium when right atrial pressure rises, the clot may be carried into the left atrium and from there into the systemic circulation to block a cerebral artery and cause a stroke. A paradoxical embolus is considered to be the usual cause of a stroke in an otherwise normal young adult. Further studies can be performed to document that the foramen ovale is patent in the stroke patient, and also can determine how much blood flows across the patent foramen ovale when the right atrial pressure rises. Based on the results of these studies, it may be advisable in some patients to seal shut the patent foramen ovale in order to prevent another embolus-related stroke.

STROKE CAUSED BY ARTERIOSCLEROSIS OF EXTRACRANIAL ARTERIES

A stroke may also be caused by sclerosis of one of the major arteries arising from the aorta to supply the brain before the vessel enters the cranial cavity. A commonly affected site is at the origin of the internal carotid artery in the neck, where atheromatous plaques may narrow the lumen and reduce cerebral blood flow. The plaques may also become ulcerated, and thrombi may form on the roughened surfaces. Bits of arteriosclerotic debris or thrombus material may break loose from the plaque and be carried into the intracerebral circulation, where they may block small cerebral arteries. Rarely, the internal carotid artery may become completely blocked by a thrombus that has formed on the roughened surface of the artery, leading to a large cerebral infarction. FIGURE 26-14 illustrates the possible effects of arteriosclerosis of the internal carotid artery in the neck.

Diagnosis of Extracranial Vascular Disease

Cerebral blood flow can be studied by injecting a radiopaque dye into the carotid and vertebral arteries that arise from the arch of the aorta to supply the brain. In this procedure, called a cerebral angiogram, the course of the dye is followed by serial x-ray studies, using methods similar to those used to visualize the coronary arteries (FIGURE 26-15).

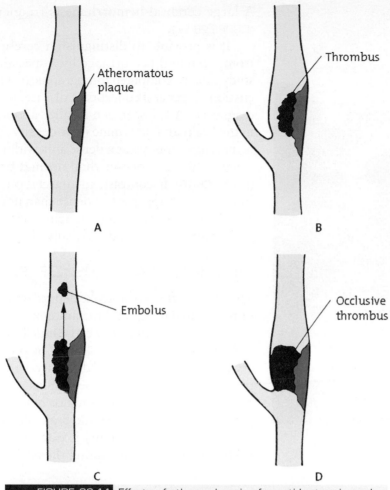

FIGURE 26-14 Effects of atherosclerosis of carotid artery in neck. **A**, Atherosclerotic plaque narrows lumen, and surface frequently becomes ulcerated. **B**, Formation of thrombus on ulcerated surface of plaque, further narrowing vessel. **C**, Thrombus material dislodged from plaque to form emboli, which are carried to brain. **D**, Complete occlusion of artery by thrombus. (Escourolle, R., and Poirier, J. 1977. *Manuel élémentaire de neuropathology.* Paris: Masson S. A. English translation: Philadelphia: W. B. Saunders, 1978.)

Arteriosclerotic plaques that occlude the carotid artery and impede cerebral blood flow can be removed surgically by making an incision in the carotid artery and dissecting out the arteriosclerotic lining and plaque, thereby opening up the artery (FIGURE 26-16). The procedure is called a carotid endarterectomy (*endo* = within + artery + *tome* = incision). Other less invasive methods are also being investigated in selected patients, including the same type of balloon angioplasty and stent insertion procedures that are used to treat coronary artery plaques (discussed in the section on the cardiovascular system). Studies on large groups of patients comparing the two treatment methods favor endarterectomy over angioplasty with stenting of the carotid artery, which is associated with more stroke-related complications than is endarterectomy.

CEREBRAL HEMORRHAGE

A cerebral hemorrhage is a much more serious type of stroke to which persons who have high blood pressure are prone. Blood from the ruptured vessel escapes into the brain under high pressure and causes extensive damage to brain tissue.

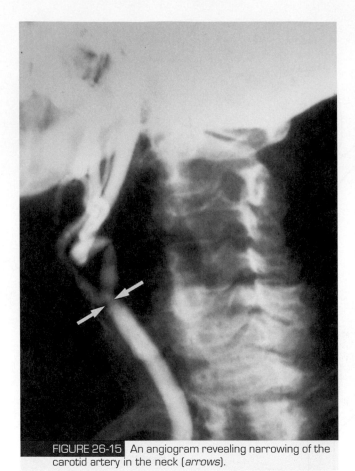

FIGURE 26-15 An angiogram revealing narrowing of the carotid artery in the neck (*arrows*).

A large cerebral hemorrhage is frequently fatal (FIGURE 26-17).

It is possible to distinguish a cerebral infarct from a cerebral hemorrhage by a specialized x-ray study called a computed tomographic (CT) scan (discussion on general concepts of disease: principles of diagnosis). A CT scan can localize abnormal areas in the brain and determine their density. A cerebral hemorrhage appears as a dense area within the brain because blood is denser than normal brain tissue (FIGURE 26-18). In contrast, an infarct is often swollen by edema and appears less dense than normal brain tissue. Magnetic resonance imaging (MRI) provides similar information and is equally effective.

MANIFESTATIONS OF STROKE

The clinical effects of a stroke depend on the location of the brain damage and the amount of brain tissue injured. Small infarcts may cause little functional disturbance and are usually followed by prompt recovery with little or no residual disability. Unfortunately, many strokes result from occlusions of the middle cerebral artery or one of its major branches or from a hemorrhage in a part of the brain supplied by the artery. Frequently the injury is extensive and causes partial paralysis by disrupting the nerve fibers that

A   **B**

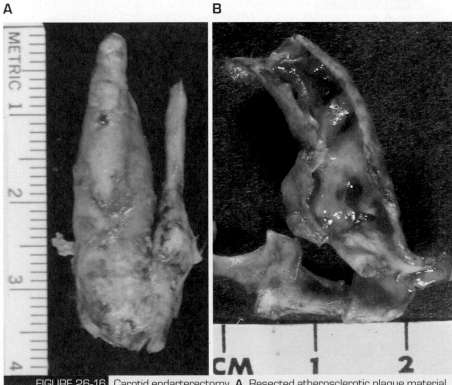

FIGURE 26-16 Carotid endarterectomy. **A**, Resected atherosclerotic plaque material has the contour of the common carotid artery and its two major branches, where it formed. **B**, An opened endarterectomy specimen revealing rough internal surface with areas of ulceration and hemorrhage in the atheromatous plaque.

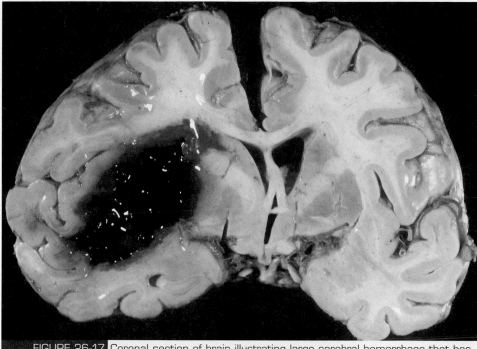

FIGURE 26-17 Coronal section of brain illustrating large cerebral hemorrhage that has compressed and displaced the cerebral ventricles.

carry impulses to the spinal motor neurons and motor neurons of the cranial nerves (lower motor neurons). Nerve fibers carrying sensory impulses to the cortex are often damaged as well, leading to various sensory disturbances.

As mentioned earlier, sensory and motor fiber tracts cross in the brain stem as they ascend or descend; so the motor neurons from the right cerebral hemisphere supply the left side of the body, and sensory impulses received by this hemisphere come from the left side of the body. Conversely, the left hemisphere controls the right half of the body and receives sensory input from the right side. Consequently, a stroke involving one cerebral hemisphere often leads to weakness or paralysis on the opposite side, called **hemiplegia** (*hemi* = half + *plege* = stroke) or hemiparesis (*paresis* = weakness) and often to some sensory impairment on the paralyzed side as well. Speech also may be affected, but usually the affected individual does not lose consciousness.

Hemiplegia
(hem-ē-plē′-jē-uh)
Paralysis of one side of the body.

REHABILITATION OF THE STROKE PATIENT

Many patients who suffer a major stroke are partially paralyzed, and some may have speech impairment as well. Rehabilitation, which is begun as soon as possible, helps the patient achieve several goals:

1. To regain the ability to walk
2. To relearn self-care activities, such as washing, combing the hair, and eating, that may have been impaired by the stroke

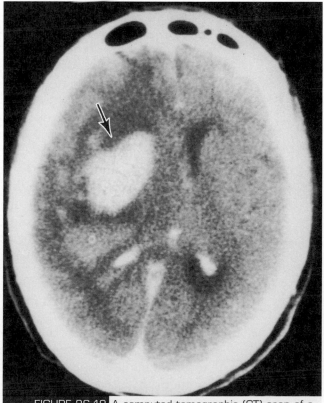

FIGURE 26-18 A computed tomographic (CT) scan of a patient with cerebral hemorrhage (*arrow*), which appears white because blood is denser than brain tissue.

3. To prevent stiffness and limitation of motion in the joints of the paralyzed limbs
4. To make an emotional adjustment to the disability

These goals are achieved primarily by a program of exercises and relearning. If speech is impaired, speech therapy also is started. Many patients can learn to walk again, although in some cases, a leg brace and cane may be required. It is more difficult to regain useful function in a paralyzed upper limb.

Transient Ischemic Attack

Transient ischemic attack (TIA)
(isskē′mik)
Temporary cerebral dysfunction as a result of transient obstruction of a cerebral vessel by a bit of atheromatous debris or blood clot usually embolized from an arteriosclerotic plaque in the carotid artery.

The term **transient ischemic attack**, often abbreviated to TIA, refers to brief episodes of neurologic dysfunction such as temporary paralysis of an arm or leg, loss of speech, or disturbances of vision. The episodes, which tend to occur in older persons, last from a few minutes to a few hours and clear completely. They are usually caused by bits of thrombus or arteriosclerotic debris that break loose from an ulcerated plaque in the internal carotid artery and obstruct a small cerebral artery. The episodes are brief because the obstructing debris or small clot becomes fragmented and dissolved, and the circulation through the blocked vessel is restored before permanent damage to brain tissue occurs.

About one-third of patients with transient ischemic attacks eventually suffer a major stroke, but the majority experience no further difficulties. Treatment consists either of surgical resection of the ulcerated plaque in the carotid artery by means of a carotid endarterectomy or administration of drugs that decrease the likelihood that thrombi will form on the ulcerated plaques, thereby reducing the risk of embolization. A narrowing of the carotid artery is significant if the lumen of the artery is reduced by 50%. This degree of narrowing corresponds to a 75% reduction in the cross-section area of the lumen and is associated with a large reduction in flow rate through the artery.

Vascular Dementia

Not all cerebral infarcts result in paralysis. In persons with vascular disease caused by hypertension, diabetes, or abnormal blood lipids, the smaller cerebral blood vessels are affected as well as the large cerebral arteries. These affected persons may have repeated small strokes caused by blockage of smaller cerebral blood vessels that damage brain tissue but may not affect motor neurons or lead to muscle paralysis. Each additional small stroke further compromises cerebral function. Eventually the cumulative brain damage causes manifestations of dementia similar to those seen in Alzheimer disease. The condition is called vascular dementia or multi-infarct dementia. Diagnosis of vascular dementia is made by computed tomography (CT) or magnetic resonance imaging (MRI) studies that reveal the marked brain damage caused by multiple small strokes. Progression of the vascular dementia can be slowed or even prevented by treating the conditions that predispose to the cerebral vascular disease.

Cerebral Aneurysm

Aneurysm (an′ūr-izm)
A dilatation of a structure, such as the aorta, a cerebral artery, or a part of the ventricular wall. See ventricular aneurysm.

Occasionally, **aneurysms** occur in the large cerebral arteries at the base of the brain. The most common type, a congenital cerebral aneurysm, results from a congenital defect in the elastic and muscular tissue of the vessel wall, usually at the point where the artery branches. Because of the congenital weakness, the lining of the arterial wall (intima) eventually protrudes through the defect at the point of branching, leading to the formation of a saclike outpouching (FIGURE 26-19).

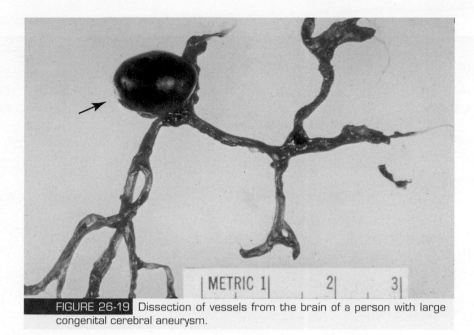

FIGURE 26-19 Dissection of vessels from the brain of a person with large congenital cerebral aneurysm.

Although the weakness of the vessel wall is congenital, the actual aneurysm does not develop until young adulthood or middle age. Persons with congenital polycystic kidney disease (discussion on the urinary system) are prone to develop aneurysms of this type. Congenital aneurysms are hazardous because they may rupture, producing severe and sometimes fatal hemorrhage within the cranial cavity (FIGURE 26-20). Persons with high blood pressure are especially prone to this complication. The initial symptoms of a ruptured aneurysm are severe headache and a stiff neck. The headache results from the increased intracranial pressure caused by the sudden escape of blood into the subarachnoid space. The stiff neck occurs because the escaping blood irritates the meninges, setting off reflex contraction of the neck muscles.

The location of the aneurysm can be determined by a cerebral angiogram. Radiopaque material (contrast medium) is injected into the arteries supplying the brain and fills the aneurysm sac, defining both its size and position (FIGURE 26-21). Treatment usually consists of occluding (closing off) the aneurysm by applying a small metal clip to the narrow neck of the sac at its attachment to the arterial wall. Another approach involves filling the aneurysm sac with coils of material in order to stop blood from filling the aneurysm. To perform the coiling procedure, a catheter is inserted into the femoral artery, advanced through the aorta into the carotid artery, and then advanced to the base of the aneurysm. Then, multiple coils of material are passed through the catheter into the aneurysm to completely fill the aneurysm sac. Various types of coils with specific advantages are being developed continually, including coils that expand within the aneurysm sac to fill it more completely. Many neurosurgeons believe that the coiling technique is safer and has fewer complications than clipping, especially

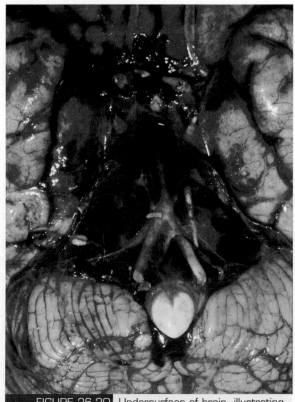

FIGURE 26-20 Undersurface of brain, illustrating subarachnoid hemorrhage secondary to ruptured cerebral aneurysm.

A   B

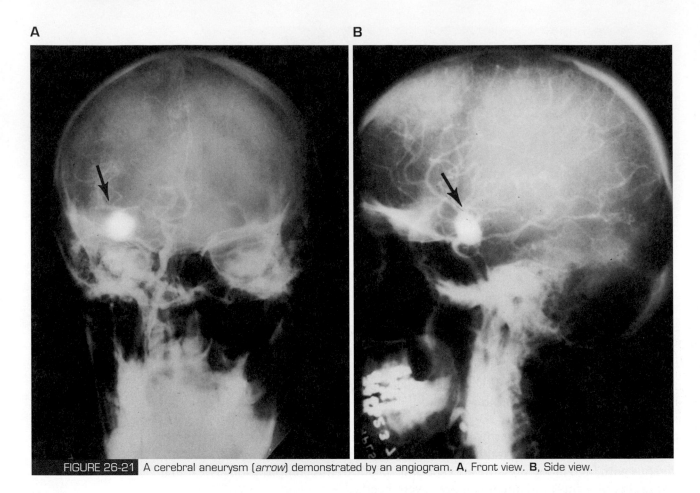

FIGURE 26-21   A cerebral aneurysm (*arrow*) demonstrated by an angiogram. **A**, Front view. **B**, Side view.

when dealing with a ruptured aneurysm. Another procedure can be used to treat an aneurysm that has such a wide opening that it cannot be closed by clipping and is also less suitable for filling with coils. This type of aneurysm sometimes can be treated successfully by injecting into the sac a viscous material that hardens into a solid mass as it fills the sac. Consequently, blood is no longer able to flow into the aneurysm, which reduces the risk of rupture.

Rarely, one of the large cerebral arteries undergoes aneurysmal dilation as a result of arteriosclerosis. This is termed an arteriosclerotic aneurysm. The aneurysm may compress the adjacent brain tissue but usually does not rupture (FIGURE 26-22).

Infections of the Nervous System

Meninges (men-in′jēz)
The membranes covering the brain and spinal cord.

Meningitis
Inflammation of the meninges.

Encephalitis
(en-sef-ăl-ī′tis)
An inflammation of the brain.

Myelitis (mī-el-ī′tis)
An inflammation of the spinal cord.

Many different organisms can infect the nervous system, including bacteria, viruses, and fungi. An infection that predominantly affects the **meninges** surrounding the brain and spinal cord is called a **meningitis**. An infection of the brain tissue is called an **encephalitis**. If both brain and meninges are affected, the term meningoencephalitis is often used. An infection of the spinal cord is called a **myelitis**.

The manifestations of an infection of the central nervous system are those of any systemic infection: elevated temperature and other nonspecific symptoms. In addition, there are manifestations of meningeal irritation, consisting of a headache and a stiff neck. Involvement of brain tissue is associated with alteration of consciousness and neurologic symptoms resulting from dysfunction of localized areas within the brain.

Diagnosis of a central nervous system infection is established by examination of the spinal fluid, which contains a large number of leukocytes and an elevated protein concentration if infection is present. In bacterial infections, the leukocytes are primarily neutrophils, whereas lymphocytes predominate in viral infections. In bacterial and fungus infections, the organism responsible for the infection can often be identified in stained smears prepared from the spinal fluid and by culture of the spinal fluid.

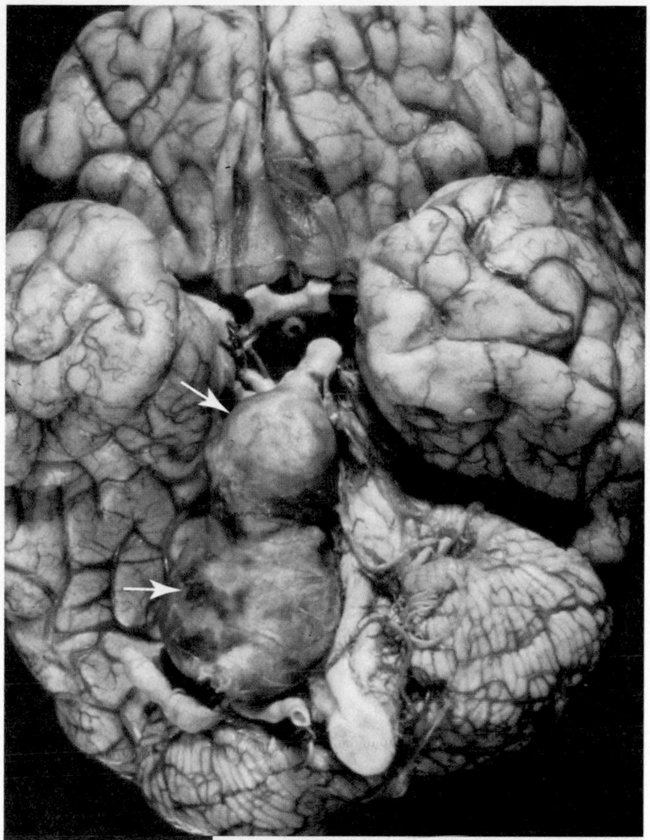

MENINGITIS CAUSED BY BACTERIA AND FUNGI

Two organisms are responsible for most cases of bacterial meningitis: the meningococcus (*Neisseria meningiditis*) and the pneumococcus (*Streptococcus pneumoniae*). Until recently, a third organism, *Haemophilus influenzae*, was a common cause of meningitis in children. Now infants and children are routinely immunized against this organism, and *Haemophilus influenzae* meningitis, as well as other infections caused by this organism, occur much less frequently than in the past.

Meningococcal infections occur primarily in young adults and often become epidemic where people live in close quarters, such as college dormitories and army camps. If an individual develops meningococcal meningitis, persons who have had

FIGURE 26-22 A large arteriosclerotic aneurysm (*arrows*) that compressed and distorted the brain stem.

close contact with the infected individual are treated with prophylactic antibiotics. If several cases occur in a community, college dormitory, or army camp, mass immunizations are undertaken to prevent an epidemic of meningococcal meningitis. In contrast, pneumococcal meningitis occurs sporadically in older adults, but it is not transmitted from person-to-person as is meningococcal meningitis. Consequently, persons who have had contact with an individual who develops pneumococcal meningitis do not require antibiotic prophylaxis, and communitywide immunizations are not required. Other bacteria may occasionally cause meningitis, especially in persons whose immunologic defenses have been weakened by disease or immunosuppressive therapy or under conditions in which bacteria are introduced directly into the nervous system.

Bacterial meningitis is often preceded by a mild upper-respiratory infection, during which small numbers of bacteria gain access to the bloodstream. They are carried to the meninges, where they localize and initiate an acute infection (FIGURE 26-23). Occasionally, the pathogens may spread directly to the meninges from a sinus or middle-ear infection, or they may be introduced into the nervous system directly from a serious head injury such as a gunshot wound or severe skull fracture.

Meningitides caused by the tubercle bacillus or pathogenic fungi are uncommon and tend to be chronic rather than acute. Tuberculous meningitis results from spread of bacteria from a primary infection in the lung (discussion on the respiratory system). Fungus meningitis also is usually secondary to a fungal infection of the lung, and many of the cases develop in immunocompromised persons. The most common type of fungal meningitis is that caused by the *Cryptococcus neoformans* (discussion on pathogenic microorganisms).

Bacterial and fungal infections are treated with appropriate antibiotics.

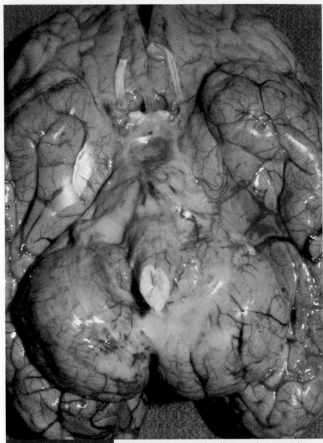

FIGURE 26-23 Bacterial meningitis, illustrating purulent exudate in the meninges. Exudate is most noticeable over the pons (*middle* of photograph) and cerebellum.

VIRAL INFECTIONS

Many viruses can infect the nervous system, including the measles and mumps viruses, various intestinal and respiratory viruses, the herpes simplex virus, cytomegalovirus, poliomyelitis virus, and an important group of viruses called arboviruses.

MANIFESTATIONS OF NERVOUS SYSTEM VIRUS INFECTION

A viral infection may affect either the meninges (meningitis) or the brain tissue (encephalitis). A viral infection restricted to the meninges is often called aseptic meningitis to distinguish it from suppurative (pus-producing) meningitis caused by pathogenic bacteria. The affected individual has an elevated temperature, headache, and a stiff neck but does not usually appear seriously ill and recovers completely. Viral encephalitis is a much more serious infection. Affected patients are often very sick and exhibit various neurologic disturbances, such as confusion, disorientation, coma, cranial nerve dysfunction, weakness, and paralysis. Some cases are fatal, and patients who recover may be left with some permanent neurologic disability. Unfortunately, there is no specific treatment for most cases of viral encephalitis. However, some antiviral drugs may be effective in herpes simplex encephalitis if administered early in the course of the disease (antiviral drugs were considered in the pathogenic microorganisms discussion).

ARBOVIRUS INFECTIONS

This important group of viruses is responsible for many cases of meningitis and encephalitis. The viruses infect birds and animals as well as humans and are transmitted by mosquitoes. The term arbovirus is a contraction of the term **arthropod-borne virus**. Several different types of arboviral encephalitis are recognized. In the United States, western equine encephalitis occurs primarily in the West, and eastern equine encephalitis in the eastern part of the county. As the names imply, the viruses also cause encephalitis in horses (*equus* = horse). Two other types of encephalitis, called St. Louis encephalitis and California encephalitis, are not limited to the area implied by their names but are quite widely distributed. Encephalitis caused by various other arboviruses occur in other countries, but until recently, "foreign" arbovirus infections were uncommon in the United States and Canada. Unfortunately, this situation changed recently with the arrival of the **West Nile virus** in the United States in 1999, where the first case was identified in a person living in the New York City area. The virus also became established in many wild birds at about the same time, where the virus infected and killed many birds in this same area.

West Nile Virus Infections

The West Nile virus was first identified in 1937 in an infected woman living in the West Nile province of Uganda in Africa. From there, the virus soon spread to

Arthropod-borne virus
An infectious nucleic acid particle (virus) transmitted by mosquitoes.

West Nile virus
An arbovirus that infects birds, animals, and humans.

Europe, where it became established and eventually spread to the United States. Since the first case was identified in 1999, the virus has spread rapidly through the United States, as well as into Canada and Mexico. The virus has caused the largest outbreak of arbovirus infections ever recorded in the Western Hemisphere. The West Nile virus infects many species of wild birds, horses, and other animals, as well as people, and many species of mosquitoes can transmit the virus. The virus has also been transmitted by transfusion of blood from blood donors infected with the virus and by organ transplants. Now these routes of transmission are no longer possible because all blood collected for transfusion and all organ transplants are screened to exclude West Nile virus infections. The virus can also be transmitted across the placenta from a pregnant virus-infected mother to her infant and in breast milk from an infected mother to a nursing infant.

Most persons infected with West Nile virus have no symptoms of infection, but about 20% of infected persons develop a fever and neurologic manifestations that can vary from mild aseptic meningitis to severe and sometimes fatal encephalitis. Some affected persons have developed a poliomyelitislike flaccid paralysis. No vaccine is available to immunize against the virus, and no antiviral therapy is available to treat the disease.

Poliomyelitis

Poliomyelitis was formerly a very important and serious disease that caused much disability and many deaths. The virus enters the body through the gastrointestinal tract, localizing in the gray matter of the spinal cord and sometimes also in the cell bodies of cranial nerves in the brain stem. Destruction of motor neurons leads to paralysis of the muscles supplied by the affected neurons. The name of the disease refers to the affinity of the virus for the gray matter of the spinal cord (*polios* = gray). Fortunately, widespread immunization has eliminated this disease in the developed countries of the world, and an extensive immunization effort directed toward persons at risk in third world countries may soon lead to worldwide elimination of poliomyelitis. Hopefully, poliomyelitis will soon join smallpox as another disease that has been completely eradicated by an effective immunization program.

The Postpolio Syndrome

About half the persons who survived paralytic poliomyelitis have begun to experience slowly progressive muscular atrophy, weakness, and muscle fatigue, and the onset of these manifestations began many years after the original episode of acute poliomyelitis from which they had recovered. This late-onset muscle weakness and muscle atrophy have been called the postpolio syndrome. The weakness usually involves muscles or muscle groups that had been affected during the original bout of poliomyelitis and from which the individual had made a partial or apparent complete recovery.

The exact cause of the postpolio syndrome is unknown. One likely explanation is that the surviving spinal motor neurons that were not damaged by poliomyelitis took over the function of the spinal neurons destroyed by poliomyelitis. These neurons established new axon connections with the muscle fibers that had lost their nerve supply, thereby reestablishing function in the previously paralyzed muscles. Overuse of the reinnervated muscles for many years eventually caused the overworked neurons to fail, which led to weakness and atrophy of the involved muscles as they gradually lost their nerve supply. Unfortunately, there is no specific treatment that can restore function to the muscles that have become weak and atrophic. A program of mild exercise that does not overstress the muscles may be helpful, and measures to improve pulmonary function may be required if respiratory muscles are affected.

Creutzfeldt-Jakob Disease

Named after the physicians who described it, Creutzfeldt-Jakob disease is a very unusual disease caused by a very unusual infectious agent. The disease occurs sporadically but can also be transmitted like an infectious disease, from contact with the infected tissues of a person with the disease.

The infectious agent is unusually resistant to inactivation by heat, by many disinfectants, and by ultraviolet light, but it can be destroyed by autoclaving or by household bleach. Creutzfeldt-Jakob disease was originally considered to be a virus infection caused by an unusual virus, but we know now that the disease is caused by an abnormal form of a specific protein called a **prion**, which is a contracted term for proteinaceous infectious particle. The normal form of the protein (the "good prion" designated PrP^C) is found in the cell membranes of neurons and in some other tissues. The abnormal form of the protein (the "bad prion" designated PrP^{SC}) is identical except for the way the protein is folded, which causes the protein to have a different configuration (conformation) when viewed in three dimensions. The abnormal prion is able to function as an infectious agent because of its ability to convert normal prions into abnormal forms. As progressively more prion proteins are converted into abnormal forms, a self-perpetuating chain reaction follows as the newly formed abnormal prions convert more normal prions. As the abnormal prion proteins continue to accumulate, they disrupt the functions of the brain cells, which leads to the characteristic clinical and histologic manifestations of Creutzfeldt-Jakob disease.

The sporadic cases of Creutzfeldt-Jakob disease, which occur in older adults (as does Alzheimer disease), are caused by a spontaneous mutation of a normal gene (called *PRNP*) located on the short arm of chromosome 20. Although we do not yet know the function of the protein coded by the normal gene, we know that a mutation of the gene codes for the abnormal prion protein that is responsible for Creutzfeldt-Jakob disease.

Clinically, Creutzfeldt-Jakob disease is characterized by rapidly progressive mental deterioration (dementia) associated with neurologic disturbances. The disease is usually fatal within 6 months after the onset of symptoms. Histologically, the brains of affected persons contain a large number of vacuoles within the neurons, which causes the affected brain tissue to have a spongy appearance. The affected neurons degenerate, and astrocytes proliferate in response to the neuron loss; however, there is no inflammatory reaction (FIGURE 26-24). Unfortunately, no treatment is available for this devastating disease.

The cases of Creutzfeldt-Jakob disease caused by contact with infected tissues have been traced to biologic products or tissue contaminated with abnormal prions. Human growth hormone, formerly prepared from pituitary glands obtained at autopsy, was sometimes contaminated with abnormal prions. This is no longer a potential source of infection because growth hormone is now produced by recombinant DNA technology. Other infections have followed corneal, tissue, or organ transplants obtained from persons with unsuspected Creutzfeldt-Jakob disease.

Prion (prī′-on)
A protein infectious particle responsible for Creutzfeldt-Jakob disease and some other degenerative diseases of the nervous system.

Mad Cow Disease

Somewhat similar prion diseases occur in animals, which can be transmitted between animals of the same or different species by feeding animal tissues from infected to healthy animals. One such disease occurs in cattle and has raised concerns that it may cause Creutzfeldt-Jakob disease in humans.

In 1985, several dairy cows in the United Kingdom developed bovine spongiform encephalopathy, a prion disease that is usually called by the more familiar

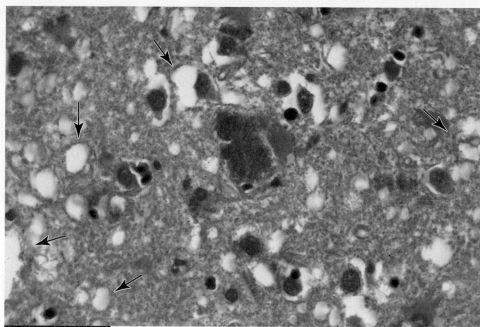

FIGURE 26-24 A photomicrograph of cerebral tissue from patient with Creutzfeldt-Jakob disease, illustrating multiple small vacuoles throughout the cortex (*arrows*) with loss of neurons and proliferation of astrocytes but no inflammatory reaction. The clump of eosinophilic material in the center of the photomicrograph is an aggregate of abnormal prion protein (original magnification × 400).

term mad cow disease because of the bizarre behavior of infected animals. During subsequent years, the number of infected cows increased to over 170,000. This epidemic was traced to cattle feed that had been mixed with protein-rich tissues obtained from sheep that had been infected with another prion disease called scrapie. This feeding practice was discontinued, and the frequency of the cattle disease declined. Now use of animal tissues in animal feed is banned in both Britain and the United States.

The disease in cattle was followed several years later by cases of Creutzfeldt-Jakob disease, which had clinical features that were somewhat different from the usual manifestations of Creutzfeldt-Jakob disease, and has been called new variant Creutzfeldt-Jakob disease. This variant disease was contacted from eating meat from infected cows, and many people were concerned that more cases would occur since there was a lag time between consumption of infected beef and onset of clinical manifestations, but a great increase in new cases has not materialized.

Alzheimer Disease

Alzheimer disease is a chronic progressive disease that affects primarily middle-aged persons older than 65 years, and its frequency increases with advancing age. Approximately 10% of people older than 65 years have the disease, which increases to almost 50% in people older than age 85. The disease is characterized by progressive failure of recent memory followed by difficulties in thinking, reasoning, and judgment; it is often associated with emotional disturbances such as depression, anxiety, and irritability. Alzheimer disease is the most common cause of dementia in elderly people. The disease is preceded by about 6 years of declining cerebral function before Alzheimer disease is diagnosed. The course of the disease differs among individuals but usually is fatal within about 6–8 years, although some affected persons survive more than 10 years.

The brains of affected patients exhibit progressive loss of neurons with atrophy of cerebral cortex and two rather characteristic histologic changes: neurofibrillary tangles and neuritic plaques. Neurofibrillary tangles result from degenerative changes affecting the thin, delicate, wirelike neurofilaments, which are located within the cytoplasm of the neurons. They become converted into thick, tangled, ropy masses encircling or displacing the nuclei of nerve cells and are demonstrated by special stains containing silver compounds (FIGURE 26-25A). Neuritic plaques are masses of broken, thickened nerve filaments that stain intensely with silver-containing stains and that surround a core of acellular protein material, called amyloid protein, with distinct staining properties (FIGURE 26-25B). In general, there is a correlation between the degree of intellectual deterioration and the severity of the histopathologic changes. The brains of patients with advanced Alzheimer disease contain large numbers of neuritic plaques and neurofibrillary tangles, whereas those with mild disease have less striking changes.

A number of biochemical abnormalities also have been described in the brains of patients with Alzheimer disease. One of the more important is a decrease in the concentration of acetylcholine and an acetylcholine-synthesizing enzyme (choline acetyl transferase) in the brain.

Unfortunately, we do not yet understand the basic cause of Alzheimer disease, even though we can recognize the associated anatomic and biochemical changes. Undoubtedly, these changes are the result of some underlying disturbance in brain metabolism. Further research in this field should help us understand the pathogenesis of the disease and perhaps point the way to effective treatment.

The diagnosis of Alzheimer disease is made by excluding other conditions that can impair brain function, such as chronic infections of the nervous system or multiple strokes. Unfortunately, there is no specific treatment that can arrest the relentless progression of the disease, although some drugs may be useful to improve cerebral function temporarily. One group of drugs (cholinesterase inhibitors) prolongs the activity of the acetylcholine in the brain by inhibiting the enzyme (cholinesterase) that breaks down acetylcholine, and other drugs may be helpful to improve the affected person's quality of life. More drugs are being investigated, but no prevention or cure is yet available despite intensive research efforts.

A

B

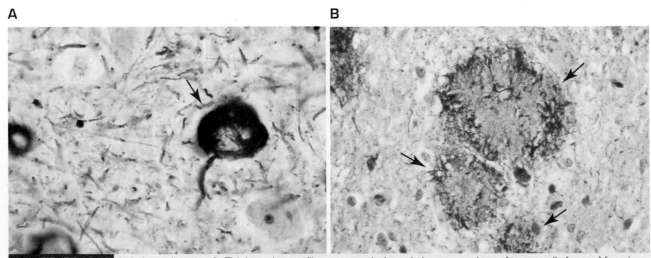

FIGURE 26-25 Alzheimer disease. **A,** Thickened neurofilaments encircle and obscure nucleus of nerve cells (*arrow*) forming neurofibrillary tangle (silver stain, original magnification × 400). **B,** Three neuritic plaques (*arrows*), composed of broken masses of thickened neurofilaments (silver stain, original magnification × 100).

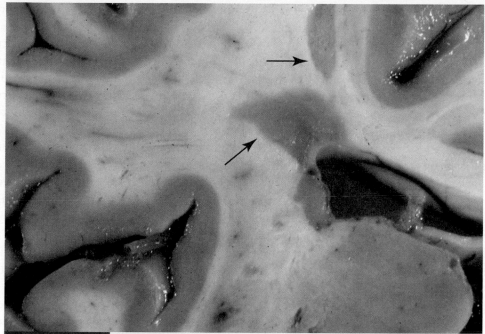

FIGURE 26-26 Coronal section of brain illustrating areas of glial scarring (*arrows*) adjacent to ventricle in multiple sclerosis. The demyelinated areas appear much darker than the adjacent normal white matter because of loss of myelin.

Multiple sclerosis
Chronic disease characterized by focal areas of demyelination in the central nervous system, followed by glial scarring.

Astrocyte
A large stellate cell having highly branched processes. Forms the structural framework of the nervous system. One of the neuroglial cells.

Multiple Sclerosis

Multiple sclerosis is a chronic disease of unknown etiology characterized by the development of focal areas of degeneration of the myelin sheaths of the nerve fibers in the brain and spinal cord. The lesions develop in a random manner throughout the brain and spinal cord. The areas of demyelination eventually heal by forming masses of glial scar tissue (FIGURE 26-26). The name of the disease is derived from the characteristic multiple areas of involvement that heal by sclerosis (another name for scarring). The glial scarring in this disease is produced by a type of neuroglial cell called an **astrocyte** and differs somewhat from the usual fibrous scar produced by connective tissue cells. The discrete areas of myelin loss with glial scarring are called multiple sclerosis plaques. They are readily demonstrated within the nervous systems of affected persons by means of magnetic resonance imaging (MRI, described in the discussion on general concepts of disease: principles of diagnosis). This diagnostic procedure is extremely useful for evaluating patients with neurologic disease in whom multiple sclerosis is suspected (FIGURE 26-27).

Multiple sclerosis is a disease of young adults. The onset of symptoms before the age of 15 or after the age of 40 is rare. Clinically, the disease is characterized by periodic episodes of acute neurologic disturbances, the nature depending on the location of the demyelination.

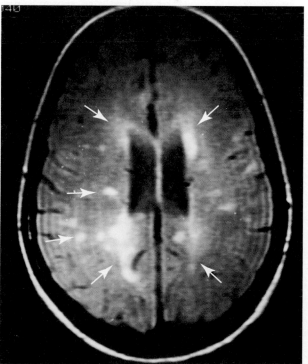

FIGURE 26-27 Multiple sclerosis demonstrated by MRI. The ventricular system is well demonstrated in the *center* of the photograph. Dense white areas adjacent to posterior horns of the ventricles and scattered throughout the brain lateral to the ventricles (*arrows*) are multiple sclerosis plaques.

Each episode is followed by a period of recovery and remission. The course of the disease is prolonged and quite unpredictable, with repeated acute episodes followed by remissions extending over many years. Eventually, the neurologic disabilities become permanent as a consequence of multiple areas of glial scarring, which impair conduction of nerve impulses in the brain and spinal cord. There is no specific treatment that can arrest the progression of the disease. A number of measures, however, are available to relieve symptoms and minimize the neurologic disabilities. Corticosteroids may shorten the recovery from an acute episode. In persons with progressive disease, beta interferon may reduce the frequency of relapses, and immunosuppressive therapy may also be useful in selected patients.

Much evidence indicates that multiple sclerosis is an autoimmune disease, possibly initiated by a viral infection in a genetically predisposed person, that stimulates an abnormal immune response. Activated T lymphocytes and monocytes target myelin proteins and destroy the myelin insulation.

The striking geographic variation in its prevalence suggests that the disease is infectious. The incidence is quite low in tropical areas, ranging from 5 to 10 cases per 100,000 population. It is 10 times as high in temperate zones. Moreover, exposure to the presumed infectious agent that predisposes to the development of multiple sclerosis occurs at an early age, which would be consistent with some type of viral infection having a long incubation period. There is also a genetic susceptibility to multiple sclerosis that appears to be related to multiple genes, including genes that code for the individual's HLA antigens. (The relationship of HLA antigens to disease susceptibility is considered in the chromosomes, genes, and cell division discussion). As an example, a specific HLA antigen designated HLA-DR2 is present in 60% of patients with multiple sclerosis but in only about 25% of control subjects, which is a highly significant difference. The incidence of multiple sclerosis is higher than usual in persons with a family history of the disease, probably because some of the family members may have inherited some of the same HLA and other susceptibility genes as those possessed by the affected individual. Apparently, persons having specific HLA types react to a viral infection by an abnormal immune response that is manifested by focal demyelination of nerve tissue.

Parkinson Disease

Parkinson disease
A chronic disease of the central nervous system characterized by rigidity and tremor, caused by deceased concentration of dopamine in the central nervous system.

Parkinson disease is a chronic disabling disease characterized by rigidity of voluntary muscles and tremor of fingers and extremities. The disease results from a progressive loss of neurons in the substantia nigra of the midbrain. The axons of these neurons synapse with neurons in the basal ganglia, where they release the neurotransmitter dopamine, and this is one of the important connections of the extrapyramidal motor system. As a result of the progressive neuron loss in the substantia nigra, fewer fibers are available to release dopamine in the basal ganglia, and the concentration of dopamine in the basal ganglia falls. The muscular rigidity, increased muscle tone, and abnormal repetitive involuntary movements, which are common manifestations of the disease, result from the deranged function of the extrapyramidal system.

In most cases, the cause of Parkinson disease is unknown. Some cases develop subsequent to viral infections of the nervous system (encephalitis) that damage the dopamine-producing extrapyramidal circuits or to the use of illicit or toxic drugs that damage these neurons. Parkinsonlike extrapyramidal symptoms may also develop after the administration of some of the drugs used to treat mental and emotional illnesses. These drugs inhibit the action of dopamine on brain neurons, and generally, the effects subside when the drugs are discontinued.

The manifestations of the disease can be relieved by a drug called L-dopa, which is converted within the brain into dopamine. The drug therapy alleviates symptoms because it raises the concentration of dopamine in the basal ganglia, thereby supplying the neurotransmitter that is deficient. Various other drugs also have been used successfully to control the manifestations of Parkinson disease. Some surgical procedures also are available to reduce the tremors associated with the disease when they are not controlled adequately by drugs. Treatment, however, does not arrest the progressive neuron loss in the substantia nigra, nor does it stop the progression of the disease.

An experimental approach to treatment is to transplant dopamine-producing cells into the brains of affected patients, using cells from the adrenal medulla or from fetal brain tissue. Some results have been promising. Many research studies on experimental animals are investigating the best way to establish a population of functional dopamine-producing cells within the brain and eventually find a "cure" for Parkinson disease. Many investigators believe that embryonic stem cells are the key to successful treatment. Stem cells are the precursors from which all other cells are derived, and it may be possible to induce stem cells to differentiate into dopamine-producing neurons, which can be used to treat Parkinson disease.

Huntington Disease

This is an uncommon but relatively well-known hereditary autosomal dominant disease that is characterized by progressive mental deterioration associated with abnormal jerky and writhing movements. The first manifestations in affected persons occur between age 30–50 years. The disease progresses slowly and is usually fatal within about 15–20 years. Huntington disease causes progressive atrophy of groups of neurons called basal ganglia that are located deep within the cerebral hemispheres. These structures are part of the extrapyramidal motor system, which regulates smooth and coordinated muscle movements, and damage to the system gives rise to the abnormal movements characteristic of the disease. The cerebral cortex is also affected, which eventually leads to dementia as the disease progresses. CT scans of affected subjects demonstrate the cortical and basal ganglia atrophy characteristic of the disease.

The normal gene (*HD*) located on chromosome 4 contains from 6 to 35 repeating groups of three nucleotides, cytosine, adenine, and guanine, which are called CAG triplet repeating sequences, or simply *repeats*. Persons with Huntington disease have a larger number of repeats, and the greater the number, the earlier the onset of the disease. This is another disease in which an increased number of triplet repeats disrupts gene function and leads to disease, as described in the fragile X syndrome (discussion on congenital and hereditary diseases). As in the fragile X syndrome, the number of repeats increases during gametogenesis, so the number of repeating sequences in the gene transmitted to the child may be greater than the number in the parent's gene, depending on which parent transmits the gene. In Huntington disease, however, the expansion of triplet repeats increases during spermatogenesis rather than during oogenesis, as occurs in the fragile X syndrome, and it is the affected father instead of the mother who passes a gene with expanded repeats to the child.

Unfortunately, there is no way to arrest the progression of the disease, but drugs are available to help control some of its manifestations. Children of persons with Huntington disease should be offered genetic counseling and should be advised that they can be tested to determine whether they carry the abnormal gene. However, not all of the children of affected persons want this information. Some prefer living with an uncertain future rather than being tested and possibly learning that they carry the abnormal gene and are destined to acquire the disease.

Degenerative Diseases of Motor Neurons

A group of diseases of unknown cause affecting middle-aged and older adults is characterized by degeneration of motor neurons in the cortex, of cranial nerve neurons in the brain stem, and of spinal motor neurons. A small proportion of these cases are familial and follow an autosomal dominant inheritance pattern. Most cases, however, occur sporadically, and no hereditary background can be identified. Many of these diseases receive specific names, depending on which neuron groups are affected most severely, and the clinical manifestations of the neuron degeneration depend on what part of the nervous system suffers the greatest degenerative changes. In general, the symptoms are rapidly progressive muscular weakness leading to severe incapacitation and breathing difficulties resulting from weakness or paralysis of respiratory muscles. Death usually results from respiratory failure, often complicated by superimposed pulmonary infections. Unfortunately, there is no way to arrest the relentless progression of these devastating diseases.

One of the best known of these neuronal degenerative diseases is called amyotrophic lateral sclerosis, better known as Lou Gehrig disease. The disease affects not only cortical motor neurons (upper motor neurons) but also cranial nerve and spinal motor neurons (lower motor neurons). The loss of lower motor neuron function leads to weakness and eventual flaccid paralysis of muscles. The degeneration of the cortical neurons is followed by secondary degeneration of the corticospinal tracts that descend to synapse with the lower motor neurons in the spinal cord.

Tumors of the Nervous System

Tumors of the nervous system may arise from three sites:

1. The peripheral nerves
2. The meninges
3. Cells within the brain or spinal cord

TUMORS OF THE PERIPHERAL NERVES

Tumors of peripheral nerves arise from the Schwann cells that invest the nerve fibers. Such tumors may be solitary or multiple, benign or malignant.

Most solitary Schwann cell tumors are benign. They form discrete, well-circumscribed nodules attached to larger nerve trunks and usually can be dissected easily from the adjacent nerve (see discussion on neoplastic disease, FIGURE 10-2). This type of tumor is often called a neuroma, although the terms Schwannoma or neurofibroma also are used.

Sometimes a neuroma arises from one of the cranial nerves at the base of the brain or from one of the spinal nerves within the spinal canal. A tumor in either of these locations is much more difficult to remove. One of the more common locations for an intracerebral neuroma is the vestibulocochlear nerve (cranial nerve VIII), which is often called by its older name of acoustic nerve. The nerve exits the brain at the junction between the pons, medulla, and cerebellum. The tumor arising from this nerve is usually called an acoustic neuroma. Frequently, the tumor compresses the adjacent brain and the nearby cranial nerves as it grows, and it may also erode the adjacent temporal bone. Clinically, the tumor causes ringing in the ear (tinnitus) on the affected side. Compression of the nerve causes partial hearing loss on the affected side, and symptoms related to pressure on the adjacent cranial nerves and the brain stem also may be present. Although the tumor is benign, its inaccessibility makes surgical removal difficult.

Multiple tumors of the peripheral nerves occur in a hereditary disease called multiple neurofibromatosis or von Recklinghausen disease, an uncommon condition transmitted as a Mendelian dominant trait. In this condition, the skin is disfigured by multiple tumors that grow from the cutaneous nerves and appear as variously sized nodules covering the entire body (FIGURE 26-28). The nodules are usually associated with localized light brown patches of hyperpigmented skin. The neoplastic proliferations involve all the components of the nerves, including nerve fibers as well as Schwann cells. Multiple tumors also arise from the more deeply placed nerves supplying the internal organs.

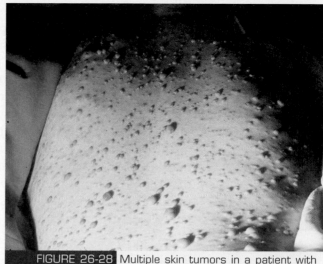

FIGURE 26-28 Multiple skin tumors in a patient with multiple neurofibromatosis (von Recklinghausen disease).

Sometimes, in localized areas, the cellular proliferation extends diffusely through the skin and subcutaneous tissue instead of forming discrete tumors. This causes the skin to become so greatly thickened that it hangs in large, disfiguring folds. In addition to being disfigured, the affected individual is at risk of having one or more of the tumors undergo malignant change. A malignant tumor of this type is called a Schwann cell sarcoma and occurs in about 10–15% of persons with this disease. There is no specific treatment for this disease. Large tumors that encroach on vital organs or are cosmetically disfiguring can be removed surgically. A Schwann cell sarcoma is treated by wide surgical excision, in the same way as is any malignant tumor.

TUMORS OF THE BRAIN

Malignant tumors arising in the breast, colon, lung, or other sites frequently metastasize to the brain. Primary brain tumors are less common than metastatic tumors. They may arise from the meninges, from the glial supporting tissues of the brain, from the cells lining the ventricular system, or rarely from other tissues such as the blood vessels within the brain. Neuromas may also arise from the cranial nerves, as described in the foregoing section. Tumors do not develop from neurons because adult nerve cells are no longer capable of cell division.

A tumor of meninges is called a **meningioma**. This is a well-circumscribed benign tumor arising from arachnoid cells and is firmly adherent to the dura. The tumor causes symptoms as a result of compression of the underlying brain and can be removed successfully if it is located in an accessible location.

Any tumor of neuroglial origin is called a **glioma**. These tumors are further classified according to the type of glial supporting cell from which the neoplasm arises. The most common type arises from astrocytes and is called an astrocytoma. A special name, glioblastoma multiforme, is applied to a highly undifferentiated, rapidly growing astrocytoma. The name describes the primitive appearance of the neoplastic astrocytes (*blast* = primitive cell) and their great variability in shape and appearance (*multiform* = having many shapes). Gliomas arise less frequently from other supporting cells. One arising from oligodendroglia is called an oligodendroglioma. Two other types of tumors are often considered along with the gliomas. One is an uncommon malignant tumor arising from primitive cells in the cerebellum of young children, which is called a medulloblastoma. The other is a tumor arising from the cells lining the ventricular system. These cells are called ependymal cells, and the tumor is called an ependymoma.

Meningioma
(men-in-jē-ō'muh)
A benign tumor arising from the meninges.

Glioma
(glē-ō'muh)
Any brain tumor arising from glial (supporting) cells of the brain.

Lymphomas also may arise within the central nervous system, and they are relatively common tumors in patients with AIDS.

Primary central nervous system tumors do not normally spread outside the nervous system, but many carry a poor prognosis because they often lie deep within the brain. Treatment consists of surgical resection of as much of the tumor as possible. In selected cases, surgery is followed by radiation and sometimes by anticancer chemotherapy as well. Primary lymphomas respond poorly to treatment, although radiotherapy may control the tumor for a time.

The symptoms of a brain tumor depend on the size and location of the neoplasm. Headache is a common initial manifestation because the increased volume within the cranial cavity caused by the tumor raises the intracranial pressure. Growth of the tumor also disrupts nerve cells and fiber tracts within the brain, leading to various neurologic disturbances.

TUMORS OF THE SPINAL CORD

Multiple myeloma
(my-el-ō′muh)
A malignant neoplasm of plasma cells.

The types of tumors that affect the brain may also occur in the spinal cord. Ependymomas may arise from the thin filament of tissue extending from the caudal end of the spinal cord, which is called the filum terminale. In addition, metastatic tumors within the vertebral bodies or **multiple myeloma**, a tumor of plasma cells within the bone marrow (discussion on neoplastic disease), may extend from the vertebrae to compress or invade the adjacent spinal cord. If this occurs, sensation and motor function below the level of cord injury may be partially or completely lost.

Peripheral Nerve Disorders

Polyneuritis
(päl-ē-nū-rī′tis)
An inflammation of multiple nerves.

Peripheral nerves and nerve roots may undergo demyelination and varying degrees of axon degeneration. Clinical manifestations depend on the degree of nerve degeneration and on which nerves are affected. Involvement of a single nerve is usually secondary to injury or external compression. Involvement of multiple nerves, called **polyneuritis** or peripheral neuritis, is usually a manifestation of systemic disease. A special type of autoimmune polyneuritis with characteristic clinical manifestations is called the Guillain-Barré syndrome or idiopathic polyneuritis. Tumors of peripheral nerves were discussed in the foregoing section.

PERIPHERAL NERVE INJURY

Paresthesia
(par-es-thē′ze-ah)
An abnormal sensation, such as burning, prickling, or numbness.

A peripheral nerve may be damaged in association with a deep laceration, a fracture, or a crushing injury. A common cause of a more chronic type of nerve injury is external compression by a fibrous band or ligament. This condition is often called a nerve-entrapment neuropathy. The median nerve that supplies sensory and motor fibers to the hand is often involved. The nerve is usually compressed on the anterior surface of the wrist, within the confined space between the wrist bones and the overlying ligaments that cross the wrist joint and stabilize the positions of the flexor tendons. The nerve compression causes pain and **paresthesias** (abnormal sensations such as burning, numbness, and tingling) in the index and middle fingers, together with decreased sensation in the part of the hand supplied by the nerve. The small muscles of the hand at the base of the thumb, which are supplied by the nerve, may also undergo atrophy. Sometimes symptoms can be relieved by conservative measures such as injecting a corticosteroid mixed with a local anesthetic into the confined space (called the carpal tunnel) in which the nerve is compressed. In many cases, however, it is necessary to relieve the compression surgically by resecting the part of the ligament that compresses the nerve.

POLYNEURITIS (PERIPHERAL NEURITIS)

Polyneuritis, also called peripheral neuritis, is characterized by progressive muscular weakness, numbness and tingling, tenderness, and pain in the parts of the body supplied by the peripheral nerves (called the distribution of the nerves). Often, the muscles supplied by the involved nerves also exhibit some degree of atrophy. Usually, the weakness and sensory disturbances affect the distal parts of the limbs, whereas strength and sensation remain relatively normal in the proximal parts of the extremities. This "glove and stocking" pattern of sensory and motor dysfunction is quite characteristic of polyneuritis. Most cases result from systemic diseases such as long-standing diabetes or various collagen diseases or from occupational exposure to toxic drugs, heavy metals, or industrial compounds. Alcoholism is another common cause of peripheral neuritis, which is probably related to a coexisting deficiency of B vitamins. Treatment of the underlying disease may produce some symptomatic improvement.

GUILLAIN-BARRÉ SYNDROME (IDIOPATHIC POLYNEURITIS)

Guillain-Barré syndrome, or idiopathic polyneuritis, is characterized by widespread patchy demyelination of nerves and nerve roots with mild inflammatory changes and sometimes by axon degeneration as well. Onset is usually a few weeks after a mild respiratory infection or after a viral infection such as measles or mumps; some cases have followed immunizations. The illness appears to be a type of autoimmune reaction to myelin that is triggered by a preceding viral infection.

Guillain-Barré syndrome (gil'yän bär rä') *A type of polyneuritis resulting from an autoimmune reaction to myelin.*

Clinically, the disease is characterized by muscular weakness that usually begins in the legs and often spreads rapidly to affect the muscles of the trunk and upper extremities. Sensory disturbances are infrequent. Severe respiratory distress may occur if the nerves supplying the intercostal muscles are involved. Cranial-nerve involvement causes difficulty in swallowing and other neurologic disturbances related to cranial-nerve dysfunction. The muscular weakness generally progresses for 1–2 weeks, remains stationary for a time, and then gradually improves. The patient usually recovers rapidly if the nerve injury is limited to demyelination. Recovery may take several months, however, if the nerve axons are damaged, and some weakness may persist. The spinal fluid characteristically contains an increased concentration of protein without an increase in white cells, a valuable diagnostic test. The high protein concentration is apparently secondary to the inflammatory and degenerative changes within the spinal nerve roots in the subarachnoid space. There is no specific treatment, although corticosteroids are frequently used because of the apparent immunologic nature of the disease. A mechanical ventilator may be necessary temporarily if respiration is impaired.

Neurologic Manifestations of Human Immunodeficiency Virus Infections

The nervous system is often involved in persons infected with the human immunodeficiency virus (HIV, described in the discussion on communicable diseases). Neurologic manifestations fall into three large categories:

1. Infections of the nervous system directly caused by the virus
2. Infections of the nervous system caused by opportunistic pathogens
3. AIDS-related tumors of the nervous system

HIV INFECTIONS OF THE NERVOUS SYSTEM

Although HIV causes its major damage by infecting and destroying helper T lymphocytes, the virus also infects monocytes that can transport the virus into the brain, where it can injure the nervous system. In some patients, the infection may be manifested as an acute viral meningitis occurring soon after the initial infection with the AIDS virus. In others, the infection causes a more chronic progressive degeneration of the brain with symptoms similar to those of Alzheimer disease, which is called AIDS-related dementia or AIDS encephalopathy (*encephalon* = brain + *pathy* = disease). Polyneuritis involving either cranial or spinal nerves also may occur in some patients as a result of infection by the virus.

OPPORTUNISTIC INFECTIONS OF THE NERVOUS SYSTEM

Many of the opportunistic viruses, bacteria, fungi, and parasites that afflict AIDS patients can cause a primary infection of the nervous system. The clinical manifestations depend on the location of the infection within the nervous system and the amount of neurologic damage caused by the pathogen. Some of the more common opportunistic infections of the nervous system are those caused by the herpes virus, cytomegalovirus, the fungus *Cryptococcus neoformans* (discussion on pathogenic microorganisms), and the protozoan parasite *Toxoplasma gondii* (discussion on animal parasites). Some of these infections respond to appropriate antibiotics and chemotherapeutic agents.

AIDS-RELATED TUMORS

Persons with AIDS are at risk for various malignant tumors, especially Kaposi's sarcoma and lymphoma, and these tumors may metastasize to the nervous system as well as to other sites within the body. AIDS patients may also develop primary lymphomas of the nervous system. These tumors carry a very poor prognosis and do not respond well to treatment.

QUESTIONS FOR REVIEW

1. Briefly describe the organization of the central nervous system. Describe the function and circulation of cerebrospinal fluid. What is meant by the following terms: *upper motor neuron lesion*, *lower motor neuron lesion*, *flaccid paralysis*, and *spastic paralysis*?
2. What are some of the possible effects of a severe blow to the head?
3. What is a stroke? What are the common causes of a stroke? What is a congenital aneurysm of the circle of Willis?
4. What are the common causes of hydrocephalus? How does a brain tumor cause hydrocephalus?
5. What is a neural tube defect? How can it be recognized before birth?
6. What is meant by the following terms: *arachnoid*, *subdural hemorrhage*, *anencephaly*, and *meningioma*?
7. What is a transient ischemic attack? How is it treated?
8. Describe the common tumors of the nervous system. What are their clinical manifestations?
9. What is the difference between a polyneuritis (peripheral neuritis) and Guillain Barré syndrome?

10. Compare Creutzfeldt-Jakob disease and Alzheimer disease.
11. Describe the role of magnetic resonance imaging in the diagnosis of multiple sclerosis.
12. Describe the effects of human immunodeficiency virus infections on the nervous system.

SUPPLEMENTARY READINGS

Adzick, N. S., Thom, E. A., Spong, C. Y., et al. 2011. A randomized trial of prenatal versus postnatal repair of myelomeningocele. *New England Journal of Medicine* 364:993–1004.

▶ Prenatal surgery reduced the need to shunting to treat hydrocephalus caused by hindbrain herniation. There were no maternal deaths, but there were more maternal and fetal complications than in the postnatal treatment group. Thirteen percent of infants were delivered before 30 weeks. The prenatal treatment group had better outcomes and better mental and motor function at age 30 months, but the benefits came with an increased maternal and fetal risk.

Barnett, H. J., Gunton, R. W., Eliasziw, M., et al. 2000. Causes and severity of ischemic strokes in patients with internal carotid artery stenosis. *Journal of the American Medical Association* 283:1429–36.

▶ Not all strokes in persons with significant carotid artery stenosis are caused by embolism of thrombi from atheromatous plaques in carotid arteries. Expectation of benefit from endarterectomy in symptomatic patients with moderate carotid atherosclerosis or in asymptomatic patients must consider that a large number of later-developing strokes will be caused by intracerebral vascular disease and will not be related to carotid artery atherosclerosis.

Brisman, J. L., Song, J. K., and Newell, D. W. 2006. Cerebral aneurysms. *New England Journal of Medicine* 355:928–39.

▶ Intracranial aneurysms are common. Most are small, and usually small aneurysms less than 10 mm diameter have a very low risk of rupture. Aneurysms appear to be caused by congenital segmental defects in the muscular walls of cranial arteries at sites where an artery branches, which allows the arterial wall to bulge and form an aneurysm. They are relatively common in persons with autosomal dominant polycystic kidney disease. Normally, an aneurysm is asymptomatic until it ruptures and causes a subarachnoid hemorrhage, which causes a severe headache. Computed tomography (CT) without using contrast material is the initial diagnostic test to identify a subarachnoid hemorrhage resulting from a ruptured aneurysm, and lumbar puncture to examine cerebrospinal fluid is only performed on patients in whom no abnormality is identified. Applications and limitations of the treatment methods are discussed.

Caplan, L. R. 1998. Stroke treatment: Promising but still struggling. *Journal of the American Medical Association* 279:1304–6.

▶ Many technical advances have improved the management of affected patients. Thrombolytic therapy may be helpful in selected cases but carries a risk of causing a brain hemorrhage and must be used within a few hours after the onset of stroke symptoms.

Caplin, L. R. 2008. A 70-year-old man with a transient ischemic attack: Review of internal carotid artery stenosis. *Journal of the American Medical Association* 300:81–90.

▶ An excellent review of the current status of internal carotid artery revascularization procedures: applications, limitations, benefits, and complications of treating internal carotid artery stenosis. Comparable results are obtained with carotid endarterectomy compared with stenting procedures. Treatment must be individualized based on multiple factors.

Clark, W. M., Wissman, S., Albers, G. W., et al. 1999. Recombinant tissue-type plasminogen activator (alteplase) for ischemic stroke 3 to 5 hours after symptom onset. The ATLANTIS study: A randomized controlled trial. Alteplase thrombolysis for acute noninterventional therapy in ischemic stroke. *Journal of the American Medical Association* 282:2019–26.

▶ Alteplase increased the risk of cerebral hemorrhage and was of no benefit when given after 3 hours.

DeAngelis, L. M. 2001. Brain tumors. *New England Journal of Medicine* 344:114–23.

▶ A comprehensive review article dealing with the clinical features, classification, diagnosis, prognosis, and management of the various types of glial and meningeal tumors.

Hogancamp, W. E., Rodriguez, M., and Weinshenker, B. G. 1997. The epidemiology of multiple sclerosis. *Mayo Clinic Proceedings* 72:871–8.

▶ A review of the interaction of environmental influences and genetic susceptibility in the pathogenesis of this disease.

Hollander, H., Schaefer, P. W., and Hedley-Whyte, E. T. 2005. Case records of the Massachusetts General Hospital Case 22-2005: An 81-year-old man with cough, fever, and altered mental status. *New England Journal of Medicine* 353:287–95.

▶ A clinical and pathological case study of an older man with the fatal West Nile virus infection. Autopsy revealed encephalomyelitis with the most marked damage in spinal cord anterior horn cells and in motor nuclei of the brain stem, changes similar to those encountered in poliomyelitis. Less marked changes were also detected in thalamus, cerebellum, and cerebral cortex.

JAMA Patient Page. 1998. How do you know when someone is having a stroke? *Journal of the American Medical Association* 279:1324.

▶ A review for the lay person of risk factors, manifestations, and what to do.

Johnson, R. T., and Gibbs, C. J., Jr. 1998. Creutzfeldt-Jakob disease and related transmissible spongiform encephalopathies. *New England Journal of Medicine* 339:1994–2004.

▶ This review article discusses the relationship of mad cow disease to Creutzfeldt-Jakob disease.

Jubelt, B., and Agre, J. C. 2000. Characteristics and management of postpolio syndrome. *Journal of the American Medical Association* 284:412–4.

▶ A discussion of clinical manifestations and management of postpolio syndrome, which affects about half the persons who developed paralytic poliomyelitis many years previously.

Kizer, J. R., and Devereux, R. B. 2005. Clinical practice. Patent foramen ovale in young adults with unexplained stroke. *New England Journal of Medicine* 353:2361–72.

▶ Strokes in young persons without any known cardiovascular risk factors are often associated with a patent foramen ovale, which allows a small blood clot from leg vein thrombus to travel to the right atrium, enter the left atrium through the patent foramen ovale, and travel in the systemic circulation to plug a cerebral artery. Diagnostic studies to evaluate the degree of blood shunting across the foramen ovale are described, and treatment recommendations are discussed.

Noseworthy, J. H., Lucchinetti, C., Rodriguez, M., and Weinshenker, B. G. 2000. Multiple sclerosis. *New England Journal of Medicine* 343:938–52.

▶ A comprehensive review of clinical manifestations, epidemiologic features, genetic factors, and treatment.

Prusiner, S. B. 2001. Shattuck lecture—neurodegenerative disease and prions. *New England Journal of Medicine* 344:1516–26.

▶ A review of neurodegenerative disorders involving abnormal processing of neuronal proteins, with emphasis on prion diseases.

Sacco, R. L. 2001. Clinical practice. Extracranial carotid stenosis. *New England Journal of Medicine* 345:1113–8.

▶ A review of methods of treatment, risk of strokes and other complications under various conditions, and guidelines for treatment. Patients with symptoms who have severe carotid artery stenosis should be treated surgically.

Sila, C. A., Higashida, R. T., and Clagett, G. P. 2008. Clinical decisions. Management of carotid stenosis. *New England Journal of Medicine* 358:1627–31.

▶ The preferred method for treating a specific patient with caroid artery stenosis, as discussed by three physicians, each with special expertise in a specific approach: medical management, carotid stenting, and carotid endarterectomy. Each physician explains reasons why his or her approach is preferable for the specific patient under discussion.

Simpson, J . L., and Green, M. F. 2011. Fetal surgery for myelomeningocele? *New England Journal of Medicine* 364:1076–7.

▶ The study by Adzick and associates is a major step in the right direction, but the maternal risks and suboptimal fetal outcome of prenatal surgery require caution; less invasive approaches are required if prenatal surgery is to be recommended.

Tyler, K. L. 2003. Creutzfeldt-Jakob disease. *New England Journal of Medicine* 348:681–2.

▶ Current status of new variant Creutzfeldt-Jakob disease and tests available for diagnosis. The number of new cases in the United Kingdom is decreasing.

Vermeer, S. E., Prins, N. D., de Heijer, T. K., et al. 2003. Silent brain infarcts and the risk of dementia and cognitive decline. *New England Journal of Medicine* 348:1215–22.

▶ "Silent" strokes are a risk factor for dementia. Depending on the size and location of the stroke, there may not be any paralysis caused by damage to motor tracts or other easily detectable manifestation in a standard neurologic examination. Repeated small strokes may cause a progressive deterioration of cerebral function without significant loss of motor functions, which resembles Alzheimer disease. The condition is called vascular dementia or multi-infarct dementia.

OUTLINE SUMMARY

Structure and Function of the Brain and Nervous System

THE MENINGES

Dura: fibrous outer covering.
Pia: inner membrane adherent to brain and cord.
Arachnoid: middle membrane interposed between other two. Contains cerebrospinal fluid and blood vessels.

THE BRAIN

Divided into cerebrum, cerebellum, and brain stem.
Surrounded by cerebrospinal fluid secreted by choroid plexus.
Ventricles: hollow interior cavities.
Blood supply from arterial circle (circle of Willis) at base of brain.
Venous blood returns into venous sinuses in dura.

VOLUNTARY MUSCLES

Muscle tone caused by reflex arcs.
Voluntary motor activity controlled by cortical neurons.

Development of the Nervous System

EARLY DEVELOPMENT

Neural plate becomes tube.
Forebrain forms cerebral hemispheres and diencephalon.
Midbrain and hindbrain form remainder of adult brain.
Mesoderm surrounding neural tube forms cranial cavity, vertebral bodies, and surrounding structures.

Muscle Paralysis

FLACCID PARALYSIS

Destruction of motor neurons by disease.
Peripheral-nerve destruction.

SPASTIC PARALYSIS

Injury to cortical neurons stops voluntary control.
Reflex arc unaffected.
Tone increased and atrophy does not develop.

Closure Defects

ANENCEPHALY

Failure of normal development of brain and cranial cavity.
Multifactorial inheritance.

SPINA BIFIDA

Several types: differ in severity.
Most severe type associated with meningomyelocele.

PRENATAL DETERMINATION OF NEURAL TUBE DEFECT

Alpha-fetoprotein leaks from fetal blood into amnionic fluid through open neural tube defect; high levels found in amnionic fluid.
Perform amniocentesis and measure alpha-fetoprotein.

Hydrocephalus

FORMATION AND ABSORPTION OF CEREBROSPINAL FLUID

Secreted by choroid plexuses.
Flows through ventricles and exits through openings in roof of fourth ventricle.
Circulates around brain and spinal cord.
Absorbed into venous sinuses in dura.

CONGENITAL HYDROCEPHALUS

Caused by congenital obstruction of aqueduct or absence of openings in roof of fourth ventricle.
Head enlarges as ventricles dilate because cranial structures have not fused.

ACQUIRED HYDROCEPHALUS

Obstruction of cerebrospinal fluid by tumor or adhesions blocking opening in fourth ventricle.
Ventricles dilate but head does not enlarge because cranial structures are fused.

TREATMENT OF HYDROCEPHALUS

Shunt cerebrospinal fluid into venous system by tube extending from ventricles into jugular vein or peritoneal cavity.
Pressure in ventricles falls and enlargement of ventricles is arrested.

Stroke

ENCEPHALOMALACIA

Thrombus or embolus in vessel leads to breakdown of brain tissue.
Cystic cavity forms.
May be caused by atherosclerosis of internal carotid artery in neck.
Thrombi form on ulcerated plaque.
Atheromatous debris or thrombi from plaque form emboli carried to brain.
Rarely, artery is completely occluded in neck.
Condition of artery in neck can be determined by x-ray studies using radiopaque material.
Treated by carotid endarterectomy.
Stroke caused by a paradoxical embolus.
Uncommon complication in persons with patent foramen ovale.
High right atrial pressure may allow embolus from leg vein thrombus to traverse patent foramen ovale into left atrium.
Systemic circulation carries embolus to brain and obstructs cerebral artery.

HEMORRHAGE

Ruptured artery in brain discharges blood under high pressure.
Hypertension predisposes.
Can be distinguished from encephalomalacia by CT scan.

MANIFESTATIONS OF STROKE

Depend on location and size.
Paralysis or sensory loss or both on opposite side of body.

REHABILITATION OF THE STROKE PATIENT

A program of graduated exercises and relearning.
Most patients can learn to walk; useful function of upper limbs less likely.

Transient Ischemic Attack (TIA)

MANIFESTATIONS AND TREATMENT

Brief episodes of neurologic dysfunction.
Dysfunction usually a result of embolization of material from plaque in carotid artery in neck.
Treated by endarterectomy or medical therapy.

Vascular Dementia

MULTIPLE SMALL INFARCTS CAUSE PROGRESSIVE BRAIN DAMAGE WITH MANIFESTATIONS SIMILAR TO ALZHEIMER DISEASE.

PERSONS WITH HYPERTENSION, DIABETES, ABNORMAL BLOOD LIPIDS AT RISK.

PREVENTION AND SLOWING PROGRESSION REQUIRES MANAGEMENT OF RISK FACTORS.

Cerebral Aneurysm

CONGENITAL ANEURYSM OF CIRCLE OF WILLIS

Congenital weakness in arterial wall allows lining (intima) to protrude.

Weakness is congenital but aneurysm develops in adult life.

Hypertension predisposes.

Rupture causes subarachnoid hemorrhage.

Treated by occluding aneurysm surgically.

ARTERIOSCLEROTIC ANEURYSM

Arteriosclerotic cerebral artery dilates and compresses adjacent brain.

Rupture very uncommon.

Infections of the Nervous System

MANIFESTATIONS

Systemic infection: fever, nonspecific symptoms.

Meningeal irritation: headache, stiff neck.

Infection of brain: alteration of consciousness, focal neurologic symptoms.

Abnormalities of spinal fluid: neutrophil increase in bacterial infection. Lymphocyte increase in virus infection.

BACTERIAL AND FUNGAL MENINGITIS

Usually caused by pneumococcus, meningococcus.

Bacteria carried to meninges in bloodstream. Less commonly spread from sinuses or middle ear or introduced after cerebral injury.

Tuberculous and fungus infections less common.

Usually spread from lung.

VIRAL INFECTIONS

Meningitis: usually mild illness with complete recovery.

Encephalitis: more serious disease with occasional deaths and late complications.

> Many cases caused by arboviruses that infect animals and are transferred to humans by mosquitoes.
>
> Herpes virus may cause severe destructive inflammation.
>
> No specific treatment for most cases. Antiviral chemotherapy may be useful in some cases of herpes infection.

Poliomyelitis:

> Affects gray matter of spinal cord; damages motor neurons, causing paralysis.
>
> Largely eradicated in developed countries by widespread immunization.

Postpolio syndrome:

> Late onset of muscle weakness and atrophy many years after recovery from poliomyelitis.
>
> Results from degeneration of "overworked" neurons that reinnervated muscles affected by poliomyelitis.

Creutzfeldt-Jakob Disease

Caused by small protein particle (prion) produced as a result of gene mutation.

Causes dementia and neurologic dysfunction.

Most cases sporadic, but transmissible by contaminated biologic products or infected transplanted cornea or organs.

Invariably fatal. No treatment available.

MAD COW DISEASE

Prion disease affecting cows.

Cows became infected from animal feed mixed with protein-rich tissue obtained from sheep infected with a prion disease called scrapie.

Cases of atypical (variant) Creutzfeldt-Jakob disease related to eating meat from infected cows.

Alzheimer Disease

CHARACTERISTICS

Affects chiefly middle-aged and elderly.

Progressive mental deterioration and emotional disturbances.

Relentless progression. No treatment available.

ANATOMIC AND BIOCHEMICAL FEATURES

Reflect unknown disturbance in brain metabolism.

Thickening of neuron neurofilaments forming neurofibrillary tangles.

Clusters of thick, broken neurofilaments form neuritic plaques.

Brain enzyme deficiencies.

Multiple Sclerosis

PATHOGENESIS AND MANIFESTATIONS

Probably autoimmune disease in genetically predisposed individual.

Random foci of demyelination followed by glial scarring.

Neurologic symptoms depend on location of plaques.

MRI useful diagnostic test to demonstrate plaques in CNS.

Parkinson Disease

MANIFESTATIONS AND PATHOGENESIS

Rigidity of muscles and tremor.

As a result of decreased concentration of dopamine in central nervous system.

Symptoms relieved by L-dopa, which is converted into dopamine in brain.

Huntington Disease

MANIFESTATIONS AND PATHOGENESIS

Progressive hereditary autosomal dominant disease.

Abnormal gene contains too many CAG triplet repeats.

The greater the number of repeats, the earlier the onset of the disease.

Characterized by brain degeneration and involuntary movements.

Degenerative Diseases of Motor Neurons

Affect both upper and lower motor neurons.

Cause weakness, paralysis, respiratory problems.

Some cases are familial.

No specific treatment.

Tumors of Nervous System

PERIPHERAL NERVE TUMORS

Usually solitary: arise from Schwann cells.

Neuromas of cranial nerves often involve acoustic nerve and are difficult to remove surgically.

Multiple nerve tumors occur in multiple neurofibromatosis.
Transmitted as Mendelian dominant trait.
Disfiguring skin nodules, thickened patches of skin, and focal hyperpigmentation of skin.
Sarcoma arises from preexisting tumors in 10–15% of cases.

BRAIN TUMORS

Metastatic tumors common.

Meningioma: from arachnoid cells. Good prognosis.

Gliomas: including ependymoma and medulloblastoma. Many carry poor prognosis because of deep location in brain. Treatment by surgery, radiation, and chemotherapy.

SPINAL CORD TUMORS

Same types of tumors that arise in brain.

Tumors involving vertebral bodies may invade or compress cord.

Peripheral Nerve Disorders

PERIPHERAL NERVE INJURY

Traumatic injury: associated with lacerations, fractures, crush injury.

Nerve entrapment neuropathy.
External compression by fibrous band.
Median nerve commonly involved.
May require surgical release if no response to conservative treatment.

POLYNEURITIS (PERIPHERAL NEURITIS)

Sensory and motor dysfunction in "glove and stocking" distribution. Proximal sensation and motor function preserved.

As a result of systemic disease, toxins, alcoholism.

Treatment of underlying disease may lead to improvement.

GUILLAIN-BARRÉ SYNDROME (IDIOPATHIC POLYNEURITIS)

Patchy demyelination of nerves and nerve roots with mild inflammation and sometimes axon degeneration.

An autoimmune reaction to myelin triggered by preceding viral infection.

Progressive weakness usually followed by complete recovery. No specific treatment.

Neurologic Manifestations of Human Immunodeficiency Virus Infection

AS A RESULT OF HIV INFECTION OF NERVOUS SYSTEM

Acute viral meningitis.

AIDS encephalopathy—chronic and progressive.

Polyneuritis.

CAUSED BY OPPORTUNISTIC INFECTIONS OF NERVOUS SYSTEM

Many pathogenic organisms can infect nervous system directly.

Manifestations depend on location of infection and extent of damage to nervous system.

Herpes, cytomegalovirus, *Cryptococcus neoformans*, and *Toxoplasma gondii* are commonly implicated organisms.

AIDS-RELATED TUMORS

Kaposi sarcoma, lymphoma, or other malignant tumors may metastasize to nervous system.

Primary lymphoma of brain may occur.

Tumors respond poorly to treatment.

CHAPTER 27

The Musculoskeletal System

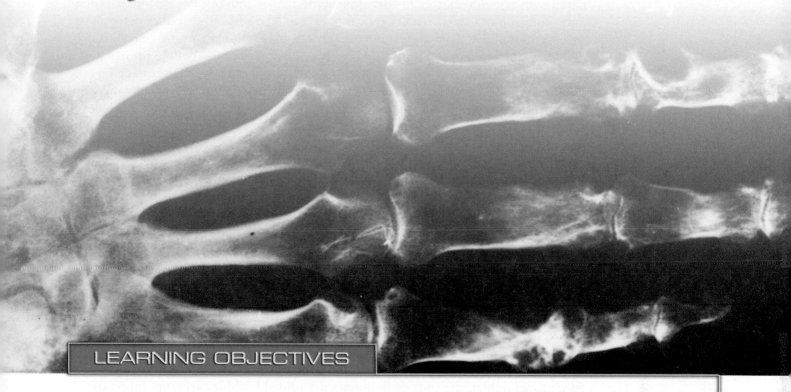

LEARNING OBJECTIVES

1 Name the common congenital abnormalities of the skeletal system.

2 List the three major types of arthritis. Describe their pathogenesis and clinical manifestations, and explain the methods of treatment.

3 Describe the causes and effects of osteoporosis, and name the methods of treatment.

4 Describe the structure of the intervertebral disks, and explain their function. Describe the clinical manifestations of a herniated disk.

5 Compare the pathogenesis and clinical manifestations of muscular atrophy and muscular dystrophy. Name and describe the common types of each.

6 Describe the pathogenesis, manifestations, and treatment of myasthenia gravis.

7 Describe the manifestations, complications, and treatment of scoliosis.

Structure and Function of the Skeletal System

The skeleton is the rigid supporting structure of the body. All bones have the same basic structure. They are composed of an outer layer of compact bone, the cortex, and an inner, spongy layer in which the bone is arranged in a loose meshed latticework of thin strands called bone trabeculae. The spaces between the trabeculae contain the bone marrow, which consists of fat and blood-forming tissue.

Individual bones vary in size and appearance. They may be long, short, flat, or irregular in shape. The typical long bone, such as is found in the upper and lower limbs, has a tubular shape with expanded ends. The shaft is the long cylindrical part, and the expanded ends of the shaft are called the epiphyses. The center of the shaft is hollowed out to form the marrow cavity, which is filled with fat and bone marrow. This type of construction provides considerable strength without excessive weight.

Bone is a specialized type of connective tissue. It is composed of a dense connective-tissue framework (called osteoid before it is calcified), which soon becomes impregnated with calcium phosphate salts along with smaller amounts of calcium carbonate and other minerals. Three different types of cells are found in bone: osteoblasts, osteocytes, and osteoclasts. Osteoblasts are the active bone-forming cells that produce the collagenous bone matrix. They secrete an enzyme, alkaline phosphatase, that promotes deposition of calcium phosphate salts in the bone matrix to calcify the bone. As the bone matrix is formed and calcified, the osteoblasts become incorporated within the bone and become transformed into relatively inactive mature bone cells called osteocytes. Osteoclasts are multinucleated cells concerned with bone resorption. They remove the bone matrix by phagocytosis, dissolve the bone salts, and release the calcium and phosphate ions into the circulation. Bone is not a static structure. It is continually being broken down and reformed, and calcium salts in bone and calcium ions in the blood and body fluid are continuously interchanged.

In general, the strength and thickness of the bones depend on the activities of the individual. A person accustomed to strenuous physical labor has thicker, heavier bones than one who is normally engaged in light, sedentary activities. If an extremity is immobilized and is not allowed to bear weight, as after a fracture, the immobilized bone undergoes significant thinning and decalcification, called disuse atrophy.

The bones of the skeleton are connected by joints. There are three types: fibrous joints, cartilaginous joints, and synovial joints. In a fibrous joint, such as occurs between the bones of the skull, the bones are firmly joined by fibrous tissue to form a firm union called a suture line. In a cartilaginous joint, such as occurs between adjacent vertebral bodies in the spine and between the pubic bones of the pelvis (symphysis pubis), the ends of the bones are joined by fibrocartilage. Joints of this type have very little mobility. A synovial joint is a movable joint. The ends of the bones that move against one another are covered by smooth hyaline cartilage, which is called the articular cartilage (*articulare* = to connect). The ends of the bones are held together by dense fibrous bands (ligaments). The joint capsule is lined by a thin synovial membrane (the synovium), which secretes a small amount of mucinous fluid to lubricate the joint. FIGURE 27-1 illustrates the structure of a typical movable joint. FIGURE 27-2 illustrates the histologic appearance of the articular cartilage and

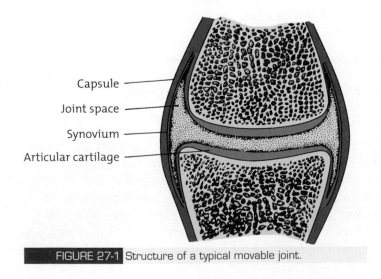

Capsule
Joint space
Synovium
Articular cartilage

FIGURE 27-1 Structure of a typical movable joint.

A

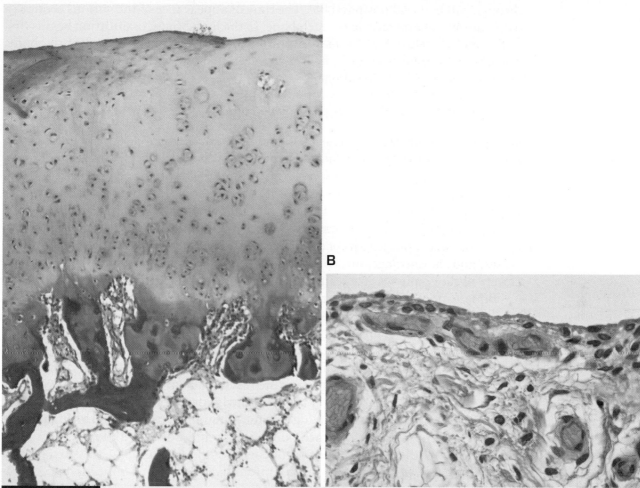

FIGURE 27-2 **A**, A low-magnification photomicrograph of cellular structure of normal articular surface, illustrating articular cartilage at *top* of photograph, junction of bone and cartilage in *middle* of photograph, and normal bone with fatty bone marrow at *bottom* of photograph (original magnification × 40). **B**, Normal synovium composed of synovial cells (*top* of photograph) covering loose connective tissue.

underlying bone and the appearance of a normal synovium. In joint disease, the structures are altered by inflammation and degeneration, leading to derangement in the functions of the joints.

BONE FORMATION

There are two types of bone formation, and they are fundamentally similar. In one type, called **intramembranous bone formation**, the embryonic connective-tissue cells (mesodermal cells) are transformed directly into bone-forming cells (osteoblasts). The osteoblasts secrete a collagenous material called osteoid, which then becomes calcified to form bone. The bones of the vertex of the skull, the facial bones, and a few other bones are formed in this manner. Most of the skeletal system, however, is formed by a process called **endochondral bone formation** (*endo* = within + *chondral* = cartilage). In endochondral bone formation, the mesodermal cells differentiate first into cartilage cells, and the bones are formed initially as cartilage models. The cartilage is then absorbed and replaced by bone. Conversion of cartilage into bone is accomplished by vascular bone-forming mesoderm, which invades the cartilage. The areas of active bone formation are termed centers of ossification.

Intramembranous bone formation
Direct formation of bone by osteoblasts without prior formation of a cartilage model.

Endochondral bone formation
(en-dō-kon′drul)
Formation of bone as, first, a cartilage model that is then reabsorbed and converted into bone.

Bones that have been preformed in cartilage undergo ossification at specific times throughout fetal and postnatal life. The time of appearance of the various centers of ossification is characteristic for each bone. In the long bones, ossification begins first in the shaft; later, centers of ossification form at the ends (epiphyses) of the bone. The actively growing zone of cartilage between the shaft and the epiphysis of a long bone is called the epiphyseal plate.

BONE GROWTH AND REMODELING

Periosteum
The tough, fibrous membrane that covers a bone, except for its articular surfaces.

Bone grows in both length and thickness and is continually remodeled as it grows by absorption of bone in some areas and formation of new bone in others. Bone grows thicker by adding to its external surface newly formed bone that is produced by the **periosteum**, a layer of specialized connective-tissue cells surrounding the bone. The periosteal cells differentiate into osteoblasts, which in turn produce bone. Growth in the length of bone is the result of proliferation of cartilage at the epiphyseal plate, which is converted into bone. Growth in bone length continues into adolescence. Eventually, epiphyseal growth ceases, and the cartilagenous epiphyseal plate becomes converted into bone—called closure of the epiphyses. Thereafter, no further growth in length of bone is possible.

Bone is not a stable unchanging tissue. Bone breakdown and replacement by newly formed bone occurs continuously. The process is called **bone remodeling**. It occurs during bone growth in childhood and adolescence, during repair of bone fractures, when required to increase bone strength in response to greater weight-bearing requirements, and even in association with normal weight bearing. Often, microscopic breaks occur in bone structure resulting from the stresses of daily weight bearing, which are repaired or replaced by newly formed bone. Many other factors influence bone remodeling, including calcium, vitamin D, parathyroid hormone, and steroid hormones, which influence bone growth and bone breakdown. Normally, bone breakdown and replacement occur concurrently so, normally, the strength and density of the skeletal system are not compromised. However, if bone loss exceeds replacement, the bone density falls and the bones become more susceptible to fractures.

Normal bone growth and maturation require a normal amount of vitamin D, which can be obtained by exposure of the skin to sunlight, or obtained from the diet in vitamin D–fortified milk and other foods. Normal amounts of calcium and phosphate are also needed to calcify the bone as it is formed, and the parathyroid glands that regulate the level of blood calcium must function normally (as described in the discussion on the endocrine glands).

BONE GROWTH DISTURBANCES CAUSED BY VITAMIN D DEFICIENCY: RICKETS AND OSTEOMALACIA

Rickets
Impaired calcification of bone in a growing child caused by vitamin D deficiency, which leads to bowing of leg bones when weight bearing is attempted.

Children lacking adequate vitamin D develop **rickets**, which is an uncommon disease because most children receive vitamin D supplements. However, if vitamin D is insufficient, calcium is not absorbed normally from the intestinal tract, and the blood calcium tends to fall. The parathyroid glands respond to the low calcium by increasing the secretion of parathyroid hormone, which raises blood calcium but also causes the level of phosphate in the blood to fall. As a result, the deposition of calcium phosphate in the bone matrix is impaired because there is not enough phosphate available to combine with calcium, and the bone matrix is not adequately calcified. Osteoid is formed in excess at the epiphyseal ends of the growing bones, but it lacks strength because it is so poorly calcified. Consequently, the weakened bones tend to become bowed when weight bearing is attempted. Treatment consists of supplying vitamin D along with additional calcium and phosphate.

A similar condition caused by vitamin D deficiency in adults is called **osteomalacia,** a term that means softening of bone. The condition occurs in middle-aged and elderly adults, and the deficiency is caused by several factors: (1) inadequate exposure to sunlight, which is required to produce vitamin D; (2) reduced intake of vitamin D–fortified foods; and (3) increased vitamin D requirements associated with aging. The poorly calcified bone formed in persons with osteomalacia may contribute to the loss of bone strength and bone density associated with aging, which is called osteoporosis.

In addition to the role of vitamin D and calcium on bone growth, many other less well-documented functions also have been attributed to vitamin D, such as regulation of the immune system and regulating cell division. In addition, many physicians and scientists in health-related fields believe that intake of both calcium and vitamin D are inadequate. To clarify the functions and requirements of vitamin D and calcium, the United States and Canadian governments asked for an evaluation by an independent organization not affiliated with either government called the Institute of Medicine. The conclusions of the study were (1) the only well-established function of vitamin D is related to the skeletal system; (2) most persons have an adequate intake of both vitamin D and calcium; (3) large doses of vitamin D may be harmful; and (4) a high-calcium intake may lead to calcium kidney stones. The Institute of Medicine also recommended further research studies to evaluate some of the currently unsupported claims attributed to vitamin D.

Osteomalacia
(ä′stē-ō-măh-lāy′see-yăh) *Impaired calcification of bone in an adult caused by vitamin D deficiency, which also contributes to bone loss caused by osteoporosis.*

Achondroplasia
(a-kon-dro-pla′zi-yuh) *A congenital disturbance of endochondral bone formation that causes a type of dwarfism.*

Osteogenesis imperfecta
A congenital disturbance of bone formation characterized by excessively thin and delicate bones that are easily broken.

Congenital Malformations

ABNORMAL BONE FORMATION

The two most important genetically determined diseases of the skeletal system that result from abnormal bone formation are achondroplasia and osteogenesis imperfecta.

In **achondroplasia,** endochondral bone formation is faulty. The abnormality, which is transmitted as a Mendelian dominant trait, is characterized by disturbed endochondral bone formation at the epiphyseal lines of the long bones. The disturbance impairs growth of the extremities, causing a type of dwarfism in which the limbs are disproportionately short in relation to the trunk (achondroplastic dwarfism). The head is also abnormally formed because of disturbed endochondral ossification of the bones forming the base of the skull, and there is usually also an exaggerated curvature (lordosis) of the lumbar spine (FIGURE 27-3).

Osteogenesis imperfecta (meaning literally "imperfect bone formation") is characterized by the formation of very thin and delicate bones that are easily broken under very minimal stress. In the most severe cases, the infant is born with multiple fractures. Some fractures occur before birth, having been sustained as a result of the very minor stresses resulting from the movements of the fetus within the uterus; other fractures occur during delivery. The intrauterine fractures of the extremities usually heal in poor alignment, causing the limbs to appear bent and disproportionately short (FIGURE 27-4). In milder forms of the disease, the abnormal fragility of the bone may not become apparent until childhood or adolescence.

There are several different types of osteogenesis imperfecta that differ in their severity and method of transmission. The disease results from a mutation of a gene concerned with producing the type of connective tissue protein (called type 1 collagen) that

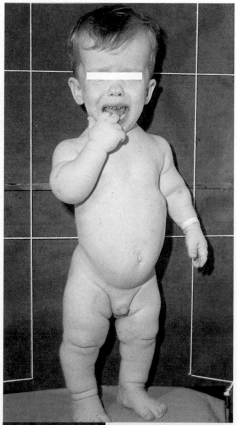

FIGURE 27-3 Characteristic appearance of child with achondroplasia, illustrating the relatively large head and disproportionate shortening of the extremities.

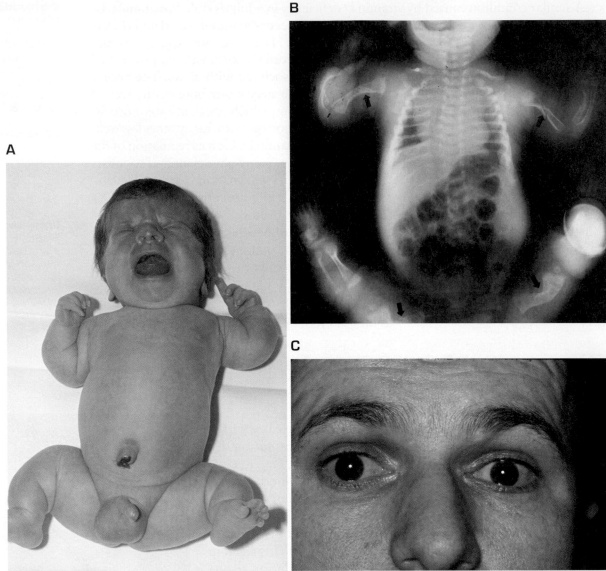

FIGURE 27-4 Severe form of osteogenesis imperfecta. **A**, Shortening and bowing of the limbs resulting from multiple intrauterine fractures that have healed in poor alignment. **B**, X-ray film showing multiple fractures of ribs and limb bones, some showing poor alignment and evidence of healing. *Arrows* indicate the location of four fractures. **C**, Blue sclerae of subject with osteogenesis imperfecta. The thin sclerae allow the black choroid layers to show through the sclerae, which changes the scleral color from white to blue or blue-grey.

forms the structural framework of the skeletal system, which later calcifies to form bone. Unfortunately, the newly formed bone is easily broken under very minimal stress in persons who do not make enough type 1 collagen or who make such poor quality collagen that the bones cannot withstand normal stress. Other connective tissues containing type 1 collagen such as ligaments and tendons are not as strong as they should be, which leads to excessive joint mobility. Even the connective tissue in the sclerae (the white outer layers of the eyes posterior to the corneas) are affected. Because the sclerae are thinner than normal, the black pigmented choroid layers in the eyes under the sclerae show through the thin sclerae. As a result, the sclerae of persons appear blue or blue-grey instead of white (FIGURE 27-4C).

The characteristic features of osteogenesis imperfecta vary greatly from person to person even within the same family. There is no cure for the condition. The diagnosis of the disease is based on the clinical features and family history of the disease;

genetic testing is also available to identify the mutation responsible for the disease in the affected person and family members. Affected persons are encouraged to lead as normal a life as possible. Exercise to maintain muscle strength is best achieved by swimming and other in-water activities to minimize the risk of exercise-induced fractures. Affected persons may obtain limited benefit from some of the same drugs that are used to treat older adults with thinning bones caused by a condition called osteoporosis, as described later in this chapter.

MALFORMATION OF FINGERS AND TOES

Abnormalities of the fingers and toes are relatively common and, generally, can be corrected surgically. The fingers and toes may fail to separate normally during development (syndactyly) leading to the formation of spadelike hands and feet (FIGURE 27-5A). In other instances, extra digits are formed (polydactyly, FIGURE 27-5B).

CONGENITAL CLUBFOOT (TALIPES)

Clubfoot is a relatively common congenital abnormality, having an incidence of about 1 in 1,000 infants. The malformation is characterized by an abnormal position of the foot that prevents normal weight-bearing, the affected individual tending to walk on the ankle rather than on the sole of the foot (*talus* = ankle + *pes* = foot). FIGURE 27-6 illustrates the most common type of clubfoot deformity called talipes equinovarus, in which the foot is turned inward at the ankle (varus position) and fixed in tiptoe (equinus) position. Less commonly, the foot is rotated outward (valgus position) and fixed so that the weight is born on the heel (calcaneus position). Talipes follows a multifactorial pattern of inheritance (discussion on congenital and hereditary diseases). Any intrauterine fetal position that causes the foot to assume an abnormal position may cause the foot to develop abnormally if the fetus is genetically predisposed to this malformation. Talipes is treated by manipulating the foot into a normal position and maintaining the corrected position with casts or splints.

CONGENITAL DISLOCATION OF THE HIP

Congenital dislocation of the hip has an incidence of about 1 in 1,500 infants, and it occurs most commonly in females. In this malformation, the hip-joint socket (acetabulum) on the affected side is shallow, its upper rim is less well developed

A   **B**

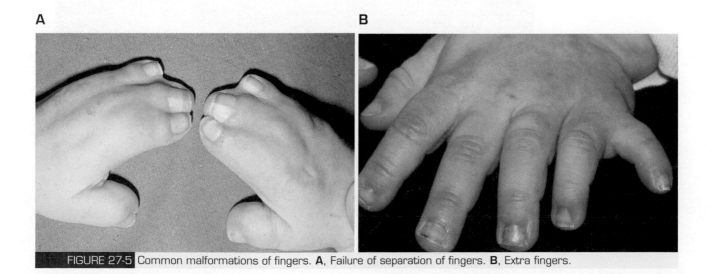

FIGURE 27-5 Common malformations of fingers. **A**, Failure of separation of fingers. **B**, Extra fingers.

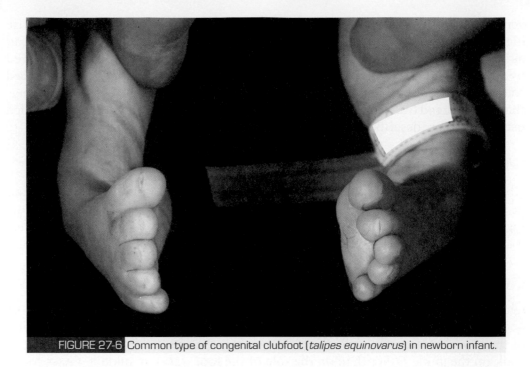

FIGURE 27-6 Common type of congenital clubfoot (*talipes equinovarus*) in newborn infant.

than normal, and the ligaments holding the head of the femur in the socket are relatively lax. As a consequence, the head of the femur fails to maintain its normal position and becomes displaced upward and backward out of the shallow socket (FIGURE 27-7). Like clubfoot, congenital hip dislocation results from the interaction of genetic factors in conjunction with an abnormal intrauterine fetal position. The

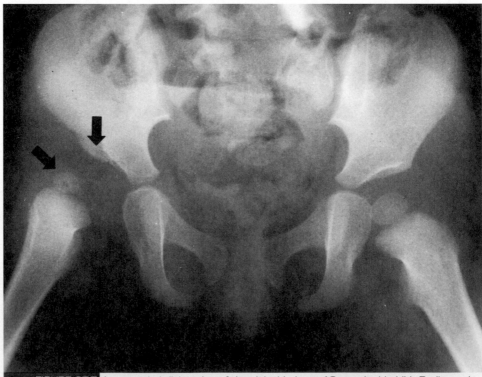

FIGURE 27-7 A congenital dislocation of the right hip in an 18-month-old child. Radiograph shows that right hip socket (*left*) is shallow, and its upper end (*upper arrow*) is less well developed than normal, permitting the head of the femur (*lower arrow*) to be displaced upward out of the hip-joint socket. The dislocated head is also less well developed than normal.

depth of the hip socket and the laxity of the ligaments are genetically determined. Ligamentous laxity is also related to the sex of the infant, being greater in female infants (which accounts for the more frequent occurrence of congenital hip dislocation in females). If, in addition, the fetus assumes a position that causes the foot and leg to be rotated externally, the thigh also is rotated externally, which tends to displace the head of the femur out of its socket. Some types of breech positions (fetal buttocks rather than head in the lower part of the uterus and the lower extremities with knees extended pressed against the fetal abdomen and chest) predispose to hip dislocation in a genetically susceptible infant.

Congenital dislocation of the hip can frequently be treated effectively by manipulating the displaced femoral head into the acetabulum and maintaining the head within the socket by means of some device that maintains the leg and thigh in proper position, such as a splint or plaster cast.

Arthritis

Arthritis is one of the most common and disabling diseases of the skeletal system. Although there are many different kinds of arthritis, the three most common are

1. Rheumatoid arthritis
2. Osteoarthritis
3. Gout

TABLE 27-1 compares the major features of these conditions.

TABLE 27-1

Comparison of major features of common types of arthritis

	Rheumatoid arthritis	Osteoarthritis	Gout
Age and sex of usual patient	Young and middle-aged, female	Adult, older persons, both sexes	Middle-aged, male
Major characteristic	Systemic disease with major effects in joints; causes chronic synovitis	"Wear and tear" degeneration of articular cartilage	Disturbance of purine metabolism; acute episodes caused by crystals of uric acid in joints
Secondary effects of disease	Ingrowth of inflammatory tissue over cartilage destroys cartilage, leads to destruction of joint space; deformities common	Overgrowth of bone; thickening of periarticular soft tissues	Deposits of uric acid in joints with damage to joints (gouty arthritis); soft tissue tophi
Joints usually affected	Small joints of hands and feet	Major weight-bearing joints	Small joints; joint at base of great toe often affected
Special features	Autoantibody against gamma globulin (rheumatoid factor)	No systemic symptoms or biochemical abnormalities	High blood level of uric acid

RHEUMATOID ARTHRITIS

Rheumatoid arthritis
(rōōm′uh-toyd)
A systemic disease primarily affecting the synovium with major manifestations in the small joints.

Rheumatoid arthritis is a systemic disease affecting the connective tissues throughout the body, but the most pronounced clinical manifestations are in the joints. Clinically, the disease is seen as a chronic, disabling, and often deforming arthritis affecting several joints. Rheumatoid arthritis is encountered most frequently in young and middle-aged women; it usually affects the small joints of the hands and feet. In the joints, the arthritis produces a chronic inflammation and thickening of the synovial membrane. The inflammatory tissue extends over the surface of the articular cartilage, destroying the cartilage (FIGURE 27-8). The severe damage to the articular surfaces makes the joint unstable; this in turn leads to deviation or displacement of the bones owing to the pull of the surrounding ligaments and tendons (FIGURE 27-9). Fibrous adhesions often develop within the joint, and the ends of the adjacent bones may become completely fused. The end result of these various structural derangements is often severe disability and conspicuous deformity of the affected joints (FIGURE 27-10).

The blood and synovial tissues of patients with rheumatoid arthritis often contains a substance called rheumatoid factor, which is an autoantibody produced by B lymphocytes that is directed against the individual's own gamma globulin. Immune complexes composed of gamma globulin and autoantibody form within the joints, which activates complement and attracts inflammatory cells that damage the joints. The lymphocytes and macrophages (activated monocytes) in the synovial tissues also contribute to joint damage by secreting various injurious cytokines, including **tumor necrosis factor** and interleukin-1 (discussion on immunity, hypersensitivity, allergy, and autoimmune diseases). Much of the joint damage characteristic of rheumatoid arthritis appears to be caused by tumor necrosis factor, which is a very destructive cytokine. Because of the systemic nature of the disease and the presence of auto-antibodies, rheumatoid arthritis is often classified as one of the autoimmune diseases (discussion on immunity, hypersensitivity, allergy, and autoimmune diseases).

Tumor necrosis factor
A cytokine that can destroy foreign or abnormal cells.

As with some other autoimmune diseases, there is a genetic susceptibility to rheumatoid arthritis that is related to the individual's HLA antigens. About half the persons with rheumatoid arthritis have the HLA antigen designated HLA-DR4, which is present in only about 20% of control subjects, and this is considered a highly significant difference.

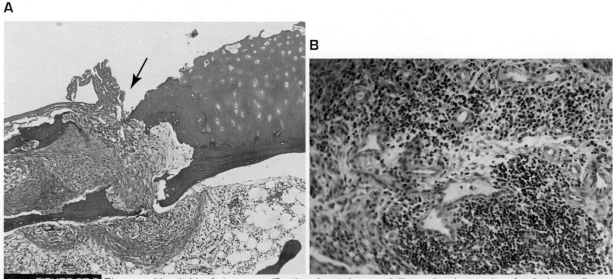

FIGURE 27-8 Rheumatoid arthritis. **A,** Low-magnification photomicrograph illustrating destruction of articular cartilage by inflammatory reaction (*arrow*) extending from synovial surface (original magnification × 25). **B,** Photomicrograph of chronic inflammatory reaction in synovium (original magnification × 100).

Rheumatoid arthritis tends to fluctuate in severity. Periods in which the disease is active may alternate with periods in which it is inactive. Although there is no cure for rheumatoid arthritis, a number of measures can be used to control the disease and minimize its attending disability and deformity.

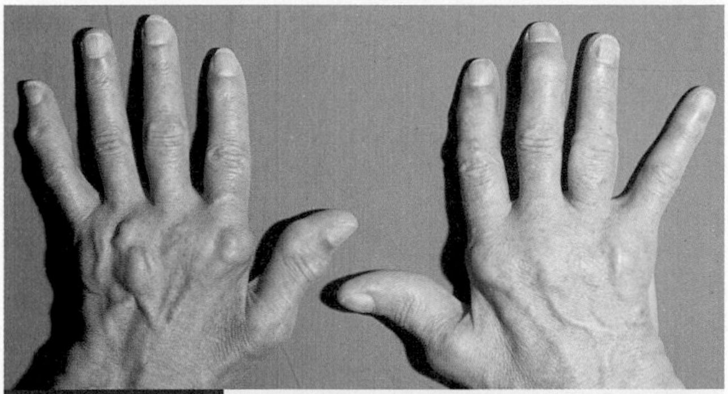

TREATMENT OF RHEUMATOID ARTHRITIS

The primary objectives of treatment are reduction of joint inflammation and pain, maximal preservation of joint function, and prevention of joint deformity (if possible). Treatment consists of rest periods for several hours every day while the disease is active,

FIGURE 27-9 Rheumatoid arthritis. Early manifestations, illustrating swelling of knuckle joints (metacarpophalangeal joints) as a result of inflammation and ulnar deviation of fingers.

use of splints to support inflamed joints and reduce deformities caused by muscle spasm, and use of crutches and braces to aid weight bearing. The affected joints are exercised gently in order to preserve joint mobility and muscle strength. Anti-inflammatory drugs such as aspirin are prescribed to reduce inflammation within the joints. In selected cases, corticosteroids are administered orally or injected into the affected joints. Often, other measures are used to slow the progression of the disease, which are grouped under the general term of disease-modifying anti-rheumatic drugs. Many take several weeks or months to exert an effect, and all have some toxicity. Methotrexate (a cytotoxic immunosuppressive drug) is often used, and many patients are treated with methotrexate combined with other drugs. Newer agents called tumor necrosis factor inhibitors also have been useful for controlling the disease in patients who do not respond adequately to immunosuppressive therapy. The drugs act by blocking the effect of tumor necrosis factor, which is the destructive cytokine responsible for much of the joint damage. However, tumor necrosis factor also plays a role in protecting us from infections, and blocking its effect increases the infection risk, which can lead to potentially serious complications. For example, in patients who had been previously infected with the

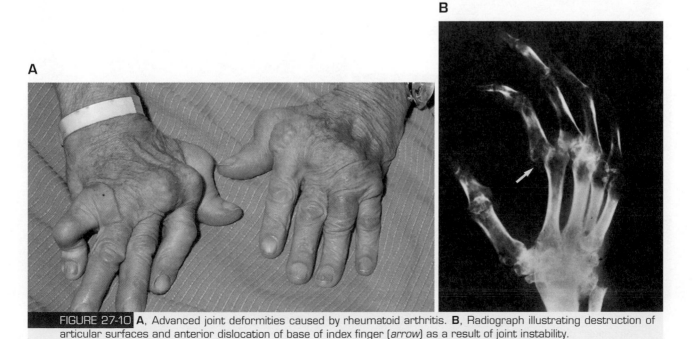

FIGURE 27-10 **A**, Advanced joint deformities caused by rheumatoid arthritis. **B**, Radiograph illustrating destruction of articular surfaces and anterior dislocation of base of index finger (*arrow*) as a result of joint instability.

tubercle bacillus and have latent inactive infections, blocking the tumor necrosis factor inhibitor also blocks a control mechanism that was holding the tubercle bacilli in check, and some patients developed active pulmonary tuberculosis. Drugs have also been developed that block the effect of interleukin-1, another important cytokine that contributes to joint inflammation. However, interleukin-1 also helps protect us from infection. Blocking this cytokine also increases the risk of infection and may lead to the same complications that occur when the tumor necrosis factor is inhibited. Often a combination of drugs may be required to control the disease. If severe joint deformities develop, surgical procedures can be performed to improve joint function. These measures include excision of thickened inflamed synovium, surgical correction of joint dislocations, or even complete reconstruction of damaged joints.

OSTEOARTHRITIS

Osteoarthritis (ä'stē-ō)
A "wear and tear" degeneration of the major weight-bearing joints.

In contrast to rheumatoid arthritis, which is a systemic disease, **osteoarthritis** is a result of "wear and tear" degeneration of one or more of the major weight-bearing joints (*osteo* = bone + *arthro* = joint + *itis* = inflammation). The disease is seen in older adults and may be considered a manifestation of the normal aging process. The primary change in osteoarthritis is degeneration of the articular cartilage, leading to roughening of the articular surfaces of the bones (FIGURE 27-11). As a consequence,

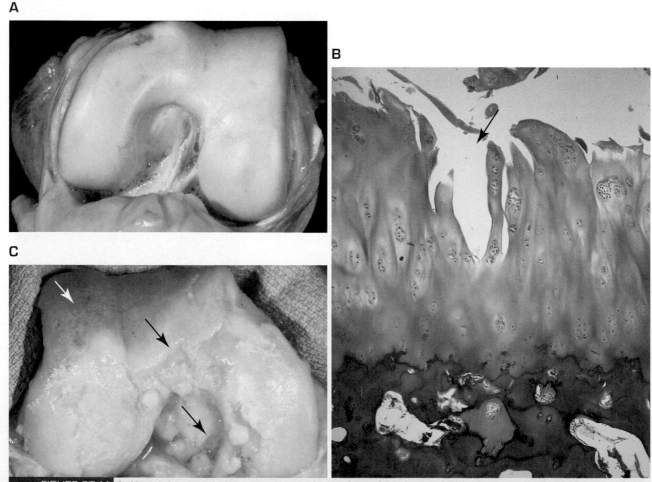

FIGURE 27-11 **A**, Knee joint, illustrating smooth articular surface of femoral condyles. **B**, Early histologic changes of osteoarthritis, illustrating splitting and fragmentation of articular cartilage (*arrow*) (original magnification × 160). Compare with normal articular cartilage in Figure 27-2A. **C**, Advanced osteoarthritis, illustrating loss of articular cartilage (*left arrow*) and nodular overgrowth of bone (*right arrows*).

the bones grate against one another when the joint moves, instead of gliding smoothly. Degeneration of the cartilage sometimes leaves large areas of underlying bone exposed. Secondary overgrowth of bone frequently occurs in response to the trauma of weight-bearing (FIGURE 27-12), and some thickening of the synovium and adjacent soft tissues is also common.

Clinically, persons with osteoarthritis experience stiffness, creaking, and some pain on motion of the joints, but disability is usually not severe, and the joints are not destroyed. However, occasional patients may experience considerable pain and disability from advanced arthritis affecting one or both hip joints. In such cases, it is possible to remove the affected femoral head and articular surface of the hip bone surgically and to replace them with an artificial hip joint. The procedure is called a total hip joint replacement (FIGURE 27-13). Similar types of joint replacement procedures have been performed on the knee joint and some other joints as well. Joint replacement operations can provide excellent pain relief and greatly improved joint function in many patients.

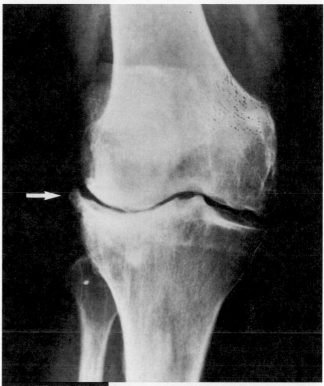

FIGURE 27-12 Osteoarthritis. Radiograph illustrates increased bone density of femoral condyle (*left side* of photograph) and adjacent tibia, with overgrowth of bone at margin of tibia (*arrow*).

GOUT

Gout is a clinical syndrome associated with an elevated level of uric acid in the blood and body fluids (hyperuricemia), leading to precipitation of uric acid as sodium urate crystals in joints and other tissues. In most patients, the condition is caused by a metabolic disorder of purine metabolism, which leads to an overproduction of uric

A   B

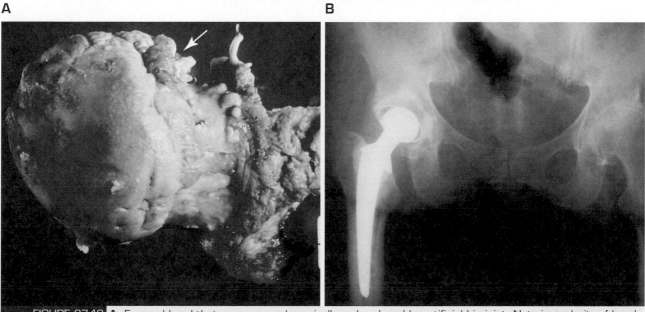

FIGURE 27-13 **A**, Femoral head that was removed surgically and replaced by artificial hip joint. Note irregularity of head and overgrowth of bone at margin of femoral head (*arrow*). **B**, X-ray illustrating total hip replacement.

acid, an inadequate excretion of uric acid, or a combination of both. This condition is sometimes called **primary gout** to distinguish it from the much less common **secondary gout** in which the elevated uric acid is secondary to some other disease or condition.

Primary Gout

Purines are double-ring nitrogen compounds that are used to form the nucleotides adenine and guanine. Along with the pyrimidine nucleotides, they make up the large DNA molecules within the nuclei of our cells. Although our body can produce purines from nonpurine precursor substances, most of the purines that we use to make nucleoproteins for new cells are salvaged (recycled) from our own worn-out cells when the cells are broken down. The purines that are not salvaged and recycled are converted into the end-product uric acid, which is excreted in the urine. Because uric acid is not very soluble in body fluids, any significant elevation may lead to precipitation of the uric acid in joints and other tissues.

Clinically, the person afflicted with gout experiences periodic episodes of extremely painful acute arthritis usually involving initially only a single joint, often the joint at the base of the great toe (FIGURE 27-14A). The acute episodes are caused by crystallization of uric acid within the joint, which incites an intense inflammatory reaction. Gradually the symptoms of an acute attack subside, and joint function returns to normal until the next attack. If the disease is not treated, however, the attacks last longer, occur more frequently, and may involve several joints. Eventually, lumpy masses called gouty tophi are deposited in the soft tissues around the joints (FIGURE 27-14B) and in other locations. The tophi consist of large masses of urate surrounded by macrophages, multinucleated giant cells, and fibrous tissue. When viewed under polarized light, the needlelike urate crystals have a characteristic appearance diagnostic of gout (FIGURE 27-15). In untreated patients, masses of urate crystals deposited in and around the articular surfaces of the joints damage the joint surfaces and adjacent bone; this is called gouty arthritis (FIGURE 27-16).

In many persons with gout, the disease also targets the kidneys and urinary tract. Many develop uric acid kidney stones. The uric acid also may precipitate from the tubular filtrate within the kidney tubules, which blocks the tubules, damages the kidneys, and impairs renal function. This condition is called urate nephropathy, as described in the discussion on the urinary system.

B

A

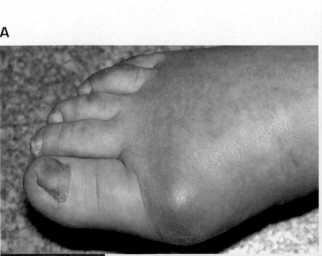
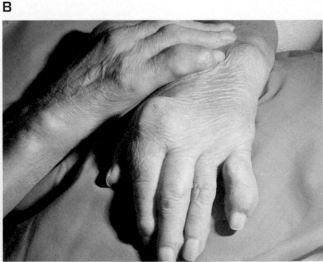

FIGURE 27-14 **A**, Acute gout affecting right great toe (© Dr. Allan Harris/Phototake). **B**, Deformities of hands caused by accumulation of uric acid crystals (tophi) in and around finger joints.

A B

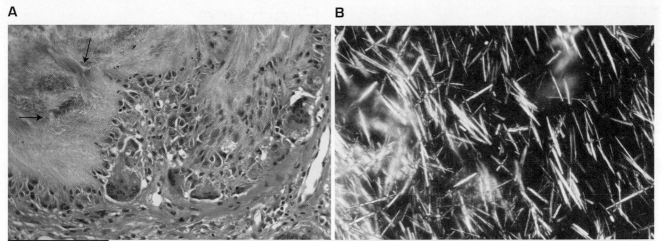

FIGURE 27-15 **A,** Margin of tophus illustrating mass of urate crystals (*arrows*) and adjacent zone of macrophages, multinucleated giant cells, and fibrous tissue formed in response to crystal deposits (original magnification × 250). **B,** Characteristic histologic appearance of needlelike sodium urate crystals from tophus viewed under polarized light (original magnification × 400).

Gout is treated by administering drugs that reduce the concentration of uric acid in the blood by interfering with the formation of uric acid within the body, or by promoting the excretion of uric acid by the kidneys. Patients are usually advised to avoid foods rich in nucleoproteins, such as liver, kidney, and pancreas, because they tend to raise uric acid levels. Heavy intake of alcohol also should be avoided because alcohol indirectly impairs excretion of uric acid by the renal tubules, causing the blood uric acid level to rise.

Patients also are advised to drink lots of fluids in order to maintain a high urine volume so that the urine is less concentrated, in order to reduce the likelihood of forming kidney stones or developing urate nephropathy.

Secondary Gout

Other conditions also may raise blood uric acid, and at times, the level may be so high that the uric acid precipitates from the blood and produces the same manifestations as gout caused by the metabolic disorder of purine metabolism. The hyperuricemia results either from inadequate renal excretion of uric acid or from excessive nucleoprotein breakdown. This condition is often called secondary gout because the elevated uric acid is secondary to some other disease. Patients with kidney failure may have high blood uric acid because the diseased kidneys are unable to excrete the uric acid efficiently, and some diuretics also may impair renal uric acid excretion. Hyperuricemia may be a problem in **leukemia** when patients have a greatly increased number of white blood cells, especially after treatment with drugs that destroy the leukemic cells and release large amounts of nucleoprotein from the disrupted cells. The breakdown of the nucleoprotein yields a large amount of uric acid derived from the purine-containing nucleotides in the nucleoprotein. In these conditions, there is no underlying metabolic defect in purine metabolism.

Leukemia
(lōō-kē′mē-yuh)
A neoplastic proliferation of leukocytes.

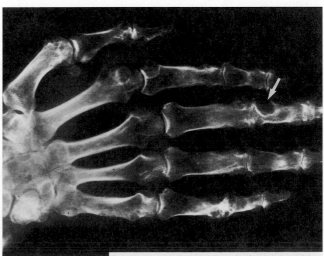

FIGURE 27-16 Radiograph of right hand of patient with gouty arthritis illustrating area of bone destruction (*arrow*) caused by masses of uric acid crystals.

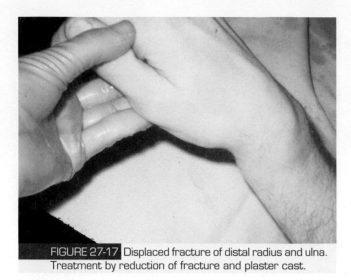

FIGURE 27-17 Displaced fracture of distal radius and ulna. Treatment by reduction of fracture and plaster cast.

Fracture

A fracture is a break in bone. In a simple fracture, the bone is broken into only two pieces. The term comminuted fracture is used when the bone is shattered into several pieces. A compound fracture is one in which the overlying skin has been broken. A compound fracture is more serious than the other types because of the possibility that bacteria may invade the fracture site and cause secondary infection of bone (osteomyelitis).

After a fracture, the ends of the broken bone may remain aligned, or they may be displaced out of position (FIGURE 27-17). The term reduction of a fracture refers to realigning the ends of the broken bone so that the bone will heal in its normal anatomic position. Sometimes, this can be accomplished by manipulating the injured extremity to realign the ends of the bone and then immobilizing it in a plaster cast. However, a surgical operation must sometimes be performed to reduce the fracture and hold it in position by means of a metal plate and screws or a similar device. This procedure is called an open reduction. Sometimes, a bone may become so weakened by disease, such as metastatic tumor, that it breaks after minimal stress (for example, coughing or sneezing). A fracture of this type through a diseased area in bone is called a pathologic fracture.

Osteomyelitis

Osteomyelitis
(ä′stē-ō-mī-el-ī′tis)
An inflammation of bone.

Osteomyelitis is an infection of bone and adjacent marrow cavity (*osteo* = bone + *myelos* = marrow + *itis* = inflammation) that is usually the result of staphylococci or various gram-negative bacteria. The infecting organisms gain access to bone in two ways:

1. They may be transported to bone from a distant site by way of the bloodstream, which is called hematogenous osteomyelitis.
2. Bacteria may be implanted directly in the bone from various causes.

HEMATOGENOUS OSTEOMYELITIS

Hematogenous osteomyelitis is more common in children than in adults. The bacteria are usually carried to the bone from a skin infection, such as a boil, from a kidney infection, or from some other distant site. In children, the organisms tend to lodge in the growing end of the bone on the diaphyseal side of the epiphyseal plate, where they proliferate and incite an acute inflammation. Local injury to bone near its very vascular growing end seems to favor localization of bacteria in the bone, probably because a small hemorrhage forms secondary to the injury, and the collection of blood provides conditions favorable for the growth of bacteria.

Once the infection is established, it tends to spread through the bone. In children, the epiphyseal plate cartilage generally prevents the infection from spreading into the adjacent joint. The infection may spread through the cortex, however, and pus may accumulate under the periosteum, stripping the periosteum away from the underlying cortex. Because much of the blood supply to the cortex comes from the periosteum, the part of the cortex deprived of its blood supply may undergo necrosis. Spread of the infection within the bone may also compress blood vessels that nourish bone, thereby further compromising the blood supply to the infected bone. In adults, in whom hematogenous osteomyelitis is less frequent, the periosteum is more firmly applied to the cortex than it is in children, tending to prevent pus from accumulating under the periosteum. However, the infection may instead spread to the end of the bone and break into the joint, causing a secondary infection in the adjacent joint. This condition is called septic arthritis.

New bone formation proceeds concurrently with the inflammatory process, as the body attempts to repair the damage and localize the infection. Initial x-rays taken soon after the onset of the infection may show only swelling of the soft tissues surrounding the bone but no radiologic abnormalities in the affected bone at the site of infection. After the infection has been present for a time, however, evidence of bone destruction and new bone formation can be seen in the x-ray films.

Hematogenous osteomyelitis sometimes occurs in adults. Intravenous drug abusers are at risk because they often inject drugs with unclean needles and syringes that are contaminated with bacteria. Although hematogenous osteomyelitis may affect any bone, the infection frequently localizes in the vertebral bodies rather than in the long bones. Probably, the stresses and trauma associated with weight-bearing predispose to localization in the spine.

OSTEOMYELITIS AS A RESULT OF DIRECT IMPLANTATION OF BACTERIA

Various conditions may expose bone to direct infection, including compound fractures, gunshot wounds, or other severe injuries affecting bone. Various surgical procedures performed on bone, such as open reduction and internal fixation of fractures or total joint replacement, may also be complicated by osteomyelitis. Chronic ulcers of the feet, which sometimes develop in diabetic patients, may expose the small bones of the feet to chronic infection.

CLINICAL MANIFESTATIONS AND TREATMENT

Usually, osteomyelitis is manifested as an acute febrile illness associated with localized pain, tenderness, and swelling over the affected bone. Sometimes, however, the manifestations are less acute, and the inflammation is manifested only as chronic pain and localized tenderness over the affected bone. X-rays taken after the inflammation is well established show characteristic changes.

Osteomyelitis is treated by a prolonged course of antibiotic therapy. In some patients, the infection may become chronic and may recur periodically. Chronic osteomyelitis is much more difficult to treat. In addition to intensive antibiotic treatment, surgical procedures may be required to remove infected degenerated bone and drain collections of pus in the bone.

Pathogenic fungi, tubercle bacilli, and various unusual opportunistic organisms may at times cause osteomyelitis, especially in immunocompromised adults. The infections are treated by appropriate antibiotics supplemented by various surgical procedures, if needed.

Tumors of Bone

Bone is often affected by metastatic tumors. Carcinoma of breast or prostate, as well as many other tumors, frequently metastasize to bone (FIGURE 27-18).

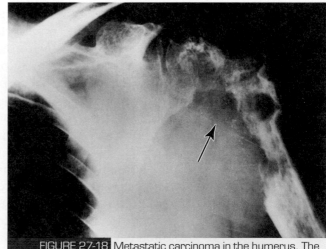

FIGURE 27-18 Metastatic carcinoma in the humerus. The primary tumor was in the kidney. Bone destruction by metastatic carcinoma is indicated by marked irregularity in the contour of the head and neck of the humerus (*arrow*).

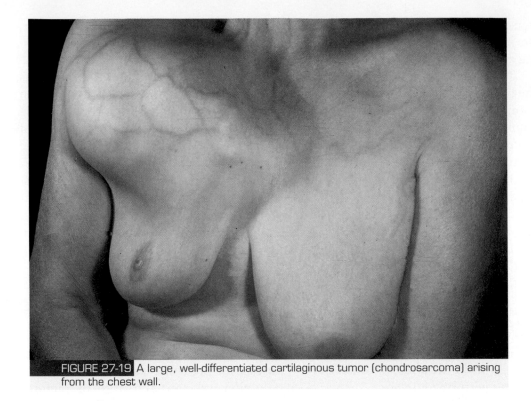

FIGURE 27-19 A large, well-differentiated cartilaginous tumor (chondrosarcoma) arising from the chest wall.

Occasionally, the skeletal system may be so heavily infiltrated by tumor that hematopoietic cells within the marrow are crowded out, leading to anemia, leukopenia, and thrombocytopenia (discussion on the hematopoietic and lymphatic systems). Nodular deposits of neoplastic plasma cells are frequently present throughout the skeletal system in **multiple myeloma** (discussion on neoplastic disease). Benign cysts and benign tumors of bone are encountered occasionally, but primary malignant tumors of bone are unusual. A malignant tumor of cartilage is called a chondrosarcoma (FIGURE 27-19). One arising from bone-forming cells is called an osteosarcoma.

Multiple myeloma
(my-el-ō′muh)
A malignant neoplasm of plasma cells.

Osteoporosis

Osteoporosis
(ä′stē-ō-por-ō′sis)
Generalized thinning and demineralization of bone that tends to occur in post-menopausal women.

Osteoporosis, literally meaning "porous bones," is a generalized thinning and demineralization of the entire skeletal system. Most cases are found in postmenopausal women, beginning in their 50s, and a significant degree of osteoporosis is said to be present in approximately one-fourth of all women in their 60s. Osteoporosis develops whenever bone resorption exceeds bone production. The incidence is high in postmenopausal women because the loss of ovarian function results in estrogen deficiency. Estrogen inhibits bone resorption, and loss of estrogen accelerates the rate of bone resorption, which results in slowly progressive thinning of the bones. Osteoporosis also develops in older men, but it occurs at a much later age and is usually less severe than in women.

The osteoporotic bones are quite fragile and susceptible to fracture. Fractures of vertebral bodies are frequent, either from the stress of weight-bearing or after minor exertion (FIGURE 27-20). Such fractures produce back pain and tenderness and are often characterized by collapse of the anterior portions of the vertebral bodies (compression fractures). Collapse of vertebral bodies may compress the spinal nerve roots passing through the intervertebral foramina, causing pain to radiate along the course of the compressed nerve.

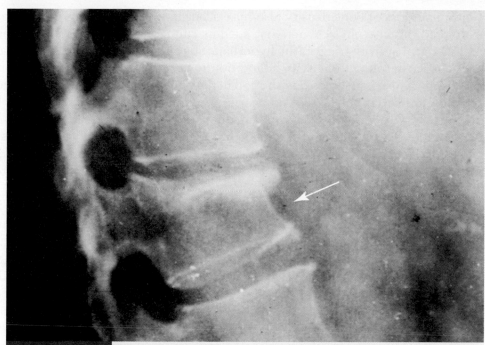

FIGURE 27-20 Osteoporosis with a compression fracture of vertebral body. Vertebral bodies are less dense than normal, and the front of one vertebral body has collapsed (*arrow*). Compare the compression fracture in this vertebral body with the vertebra above in which the anterior and posterior surfaces are the same height.

Maximum bone density is attained in young adults, and then it slowly but steadily declines as they get older. The greater the bone density one has as a young adult, the longer it will take before there is enough bone loss to increase the risk of fractures. To use an analogy, bone density is like a savings account at a bank where money is deposited for retirement. The more money one has accumulated, the longer it takes before the savings account is depleted.

Bone loss can be retarded by regular weight-bearing exercises, which help maintain bone density, by a high-calcium diet and calcium supplements if necessary to assure an adequate calcium intake, and by an adequate intake of vitamin D, which is required to promote calcium absorption from the intestine and incorporation into bone. Estrogens are no longer recommended to retard bone loss in postmenopausal women because of the long-term risks associated with estrogen use.

Once marked osteoporosis has developed and fractures occur, it is difficult to restore bone density. The following groups of drugs are available to restore bone density. Each has advantages and disadvantages:

1. Bisphosphonate drugs, which are usually taken orally, are the most popular drugs to treat osteoporosis. They act primarily by inhibiting bone resorption by osteoclasts, but also may inhibit bone formation to such a degree that the skeleton has insufficient bone density to maintain skeletal strength.

2. Selective estrogen receptor modulators, which are estrogenlike drugs taken orally that inhibit bone resorption like estrogens but do not have the adverse effects of estrogen on the breast and uterus.

3. Calcitonin, a nasal spray containing a hormone produced by thyroid cells that inhibits the osteoclasts that break down bone.

4. Parathyroid hormonelike drugs, daily injections that increase bone density by stimulating osteoblasts, but the amount used is not enough to stimulate osteoclasts.

Significant loss of bone density also may occur in women athletes who engage in prolonged, intense physical activity, such as runners and gymnasts. The high level of physical activity triggers the hypothalamus and pituitary gland to increase adrenal corticosteroid output as an adaptation to the exercise-induced stress. This event, however, also is associated with a fall in the pituitary gonadotropic hormones that stimulate ovarian function. The ovaries, no longer adequately stimulated by pituitary gonadotropins, fail to produce adequate estrogen, which leads to cessation of menses called exercise-induced amenorrhea. In addition, the estrogen-deficient athlete is also at risk of the same type of estrogen-deficiency osteoporosis that develops in postmenopausal women and is subject to the same osteoporosis-related complications.

Osteoporosis related to exercise-induced amenorrhea can be prevented by reducing the level of physical activity enough to reestablish normal menstrual cycles. Alternatively, the athlete who elects to continue the same level of exercise can reduce her risk of osteoporosis by taking supplementary estrogen and progesterone hormones to replace the missing ovarian hormones and by taking calcium supplements.

New x-ray and radioisotope methods are now available that make a quantitative assessment of a patient's bone density and compare the results with normal ranges established for persons of the same age and sex. Those patients whose bones are losing mineral content to a greater extent or more rapidly than normal are at high risk of fractures and other complications related to osteoporosis. They should be treated vigorously in an attempt to retard further bone demineralization.

Avascular necrosis
(ā-vas′kēw-lär
nek-rō′sis)
Bone necrosis caused by interruption of its blood supply.

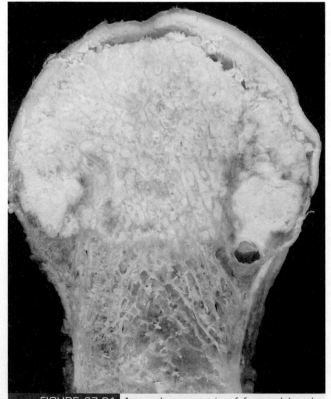

FIGURE 27-21 Avascular necrosis of femoral head. Articular cartilage has separated from underlying bone, which appears dense and lacks normal structural pattern. In contrast, bone of femoral neck (*lower part* of photograph) appears normal. Treated by removal of femoral head and replacement with artificial hip joint.

Avascular Necrosis

Occasionally, the growing cartilaginous ends of bone (epiphyses) in children and adolescents undergo necrosis and degeneration, owing to interference with the blood supply to the epiphysis. This condition is termed **avascular necrosis**. Sometimes it follows an injury, but in most cases, the reason for the vascular disturbance is unknown. Common sites of avascular necrosis are the femoral head (FIGURE 27-21), the tibial tubercle, the articular surface of the femoral condyle, and occasionally the small bones of the ankle and foot. Symptoms consist of pain and disability related to motion of the affected joint. Avascular necrosis may also occur in adults if the blood supply to a bone is interrupted for any reason, as, for example, if the circulation to the femoral head is disrupted as a result of a hip fracture or dislocation.

Structure and Function of the Spine

The vertebral column forms the central axis of the body. It consists of a series of vertebrae joined by intervertebral disks and fibrous ligaments. The vertebral column has four curves. The cervical and lumbar curves arch forward. Those in the thoracic and sacral regions bend in the opposite direction (FIGURE 27-22A).

A typical vertebra has a large cylindrical body and a bony arch that encloses the spinal canal and protects the spinal cord. The parts of the arch that extend posteriorly from the body are called the pedicles, and the parts that roof the spinal canal are called the laminae (singular, lamina). A single midline spinous process projects posteriorly from the bony arch, and paired transverse processes extend laterally. Each vertebra also has two superior articular processes and two inferior articular processes. The superior processes articulate with the inferior processes of the vertebra above, and the inferior processes articulate with the superior processes of the vertebra below. The articulations form synovial joints that contribute to the mobility of the spine. (FIGURE 27-22B).

When the vertebrae are viewed from the side, the superior and inferior margins of the vertebral pedicles appear concave. The spaces between the concave surfaces of the pedicles of adjacent vertebrae form oval openings called intervertebral foramina (singular, foramen), through which the spinal nerves leave the spinal canal (FIGURE 27-22C).

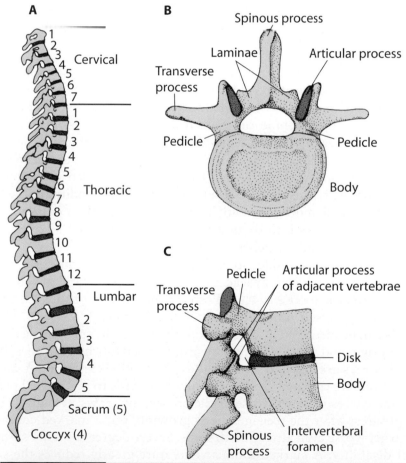

FIGURE 27-22 **A**, Side view of vertebral column illustrating normal curves. Vertebrae are numbered. **B**, Structure of typical vertebra viewed from above. The vertebral arch extends posteriorly from the vertebral body. The spinous process projects posteriorly from the arch, and the transverse processes project laterally. The articular processes of adjacent vertebrae articulate with each other by means of small synovial joints. **C**, Side view of two vertebrae, illustrating the intervertebral disk, articular processes, and intervertebral foramen.

intervertebral disk
A fibrocartilaginous joint between adjacent vertebral bodies.

Annulus fibrosus
(an′ū-lus)
The dense peripheral ring of fibrocartilage making up the intervertebral disk.

Nucleus pulposus
(nū′klē-us)
The soft elastic center of the intervertebral disk.

The **intervertebral disks**, interposed between adjacent vertebral bodies, consist of a peripheral fibrous ring, the annulus fibrosus, and a soft central nucleus pulposus. The **annulus fibrosus** ("fibrous ring") is structured as a ring of interlacing connective-tissue bundles firmly adherent to adjacent vertebral bodies. Longitudinal bands of connective tissue called the anterior and posterior longitudinal ligaments run the entire length of the vertebral column to reinforce the annulus. The **nucleus pulposus** ("pulpy nucleus") consists of a gelatinous material containing a carbohydrate substance called a mucopolysaccharide and about 80% water. Because of its very high water content, it is relatively incompressible.

The position of the nucleus pulposus within the disk changes slightly during flexion and extension of the spine. During flexion, as when one bends forward to pick up an object on the ground, compression forces are concentrated on the anterior parts of the vertebral bodies and cause the nucleus to shift slightly posteriorly, moving away from the compressing force. Conversely, when compression forces are concentrated on the posterior part of the vertebral bodies during extension, the nucleus pulposus tends to shift anteriorly. Slight lateral movements of the nucleus also occur during lateral flexion of the spine. The intervertebral disks function somewhat like shock absorbers. Pressure applied to the disks is distributed evenly around the annulus by the soft nucleus pulposus, absorbing the forces of compression to some extent and preventing direct impact between adjacent vertebral bodies.

SCOLIOSIS

Scoliosis is an abnormal lateral curvature of the spine and is a common abnormality which is estimated to occur in about 4% of people. A small percentage of cases result from a congenital abnormality of a spinal vertebra that disturbs the normal vertical alignment of the spinal vertebrae, or results from a neurologic problem that disturbs the innervation of the muscles that maintain the spinal vertebrae in proper position. The vast majority of cases, however, occur during adolescence as the teenager is growing, and we do not know why this occurs. This condition is called **idiopathic scoliosis**. (The term idiopathic means that we don't know why this condition develops.) The condition occurs much more frequently in adolescent girls than in boys.

Idiopathic scoliosis
(id′-ē-opath′-ik skō-lē-ō′-sis)
Lateral curvature of the spine. Idiopathic means cause of condition is unknown.

The spinal curvatures lead to an asymmetry of the trunk, so one shoulder is higher than the other, and the pelvis is tilted so that one iliac crest is higher than its counterpart on the opposite side. Some degree of rotation of the vertebrae accompanies the curvatures, which may lead to some asymmetry of the ribs that attach to the thoracic vertebrae (FIGURE 27-23A). Posterior protrusion of the ribs on one side of the thorax may cause a noticeable humplike deformity.

Scoliosis can be identified by careful examination of the spine while the teenager is standing upright and while bending forward, as when touching the toes. If scoliosis is identified, x-rays are taken to measure the extent of the curvature. A small curvature may not require treatment, but the adolescent needs to be checked periodically because some curves may get worse as the adolescent grows. Usually, a curvature does not progress after the teenager stops growing, but a marked curvature may continue to get worse even after growth stops. Severe degrees of scoliosis may cause significant disability. A marked thoracic curvature greatly reduces the size of the thorax, which interferes with lung function (FIGURE 27-23B).

Treatment depends on the degree of curvature. Slight curves may not require treatment but should be watched because the curve may get worse. A growing teenager with a curvature that is getting worse is treated by means of a spinal brace to help maintain the normal position of the spine and stop the progression of the curvature. A marked scoliosis may require surgical treatment, and various surgical procedures are used to stabilize the spine and correct the curvature.

A

B

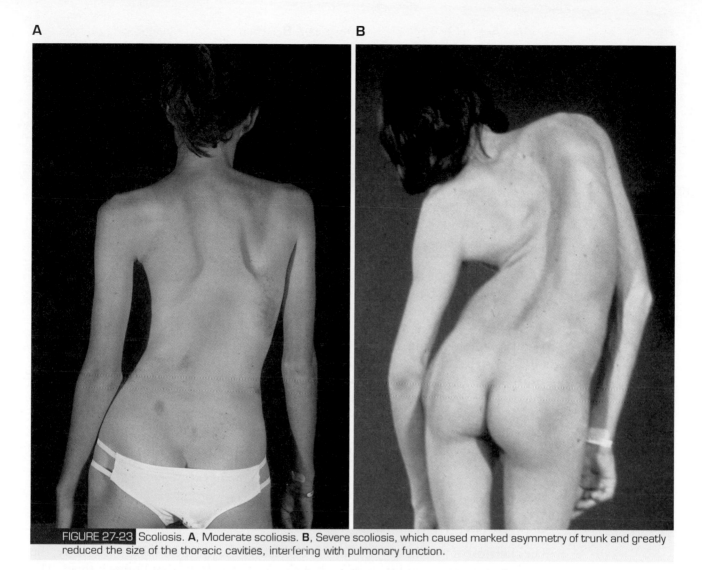

FIGURE 27-23 Scoliosis. **A**, Moderate scoliosis. **B**, Severe scoliosis, which caused marked asymmetry of trunk and greatly reduced the size of the thoracic cavities, interfering with pulmonary function.

Intervertebral Disk Disease

With age, the intervertebral disks undergo a progressive wear-and-tear degeneration of both the nucleus and the annulus. The nucleus becomes more dense because its water content is reduced, and the annulus becomes weakened and thinned. When marked compression force is applied to the anterior part of the disk during flexion of the spine, the nucleus is forced posteriorly against the weakened annulus, and part of the nucleus may be forced into the spinal canal through a weak area or tear in the annulus (FIGURE 27-24). Generally, a disk protrusion occurs in the lumbosacral region because this is the part of the vertebral column where the disks are subject to the greatest mechanical compression during lifting. The disk usually protrudes in a posterolateral direction because the dense posterior longitudinal ligament reinforces the annulus in the midline, preventing a direct posterior protrusion.

Symptoms of disk protrusion, sometimes called a "slipped disk," consist of sudden onset of acute back pain after an episode of lifting. Frequently, the pain is also felt in the leg and thigh on the side of the protrusion. This occurs because the extruded disk material often impinges on lumbosacral nerve roots, causing pain to radiate along the course of the nerve compressed by the protruded nucleus pulposus. Treatment consists of bed rest and measures to minimize pain and disability, such as administration of aspirin or other pain-relieving medications, local application of heat, and

A   **B**

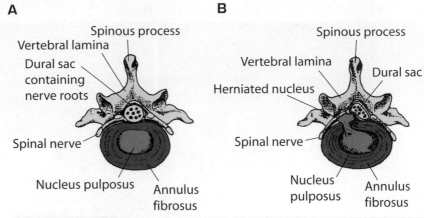

FIGURE 27-24 Cross-section through the lumbar spine at the level of the intervertebral disk. **A**, Normal relationships of intervertebral disk to spinal canal, dura, and spinal nerves. **B**, Posterior protrusion of nucleus pulposus, impinging on dural sac and spinal nerve exiting through intervertebral foramen.

use of muscle-relaxing drugs to relieve spasm of the back muscles that occurs after a disk protrusion and contributes to the disability. Protruded disk material may be resorbed, and the tear in the annulus may be repaired by fibrous tissue. Sometimes, however, surgical removal of the protruded disk material may be required.

The protrusion of the disk material into the spinal canal can be demonstrated by CT and MRI scans, noninvasive radiologic examinations described in the discussion on general concepts of disease: principles of diagnosis (FIGURE 27-25).

Structure and Function of the Thorax

The skeleton of the chest wall (thorax) consists of the thoracic spine posteriorly, the sternum anteriorly, and the ribs with their costal cartilages that connect them. The upper part of the sternum is called the manubrium, to which the first ribs attach by

A   **B**

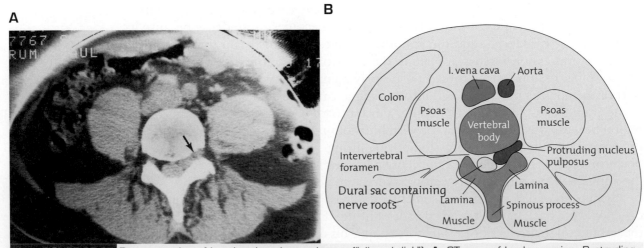

FIGURE 27-25 Demonstration of herniated nucleus pulposus ("slipped disk"). **A**, CT scan of lumbar region. Protruding nucleus pulposus (*arrow*) is located adjacent to dural sac and fills intervertebral foramen (*arrow*). Compare with appearance of normal intervertebral foramen on opposite side. **B**, Schematic of anatomic structures and lesion as demonstrated on CT scan.

their costal cartilages. The body of the sternum is attached to the manubrium by a movable joint that acts as a hinge, allowing the sternal body to angle forward and the attached ribs to become more horizontal as the diaphragm descends during inspiration. The ribs articulate posteriorly with the thoracic vertebrae, and all except ribs 11 and 12 also attach to the sternum anteriorly by their costal cartilages. Below the sternal body is the small attached xiphoid process, which moves with the sternal body. The costal cartilages of ribs 3 through 5 attach to the body of the sternum so that the anterior surfaces of the costal cartilages and the body of the sternum form a uniform, relatively flat surface that is characteristic of the anterior surface of the chest wall. Ribs 6 and 7 attach to the lower part of the sternal body and xiphoid process.

The ribs protect the lungs, and the sternum protects the heart, which is located in the mediastinum (the region between the lungs). However, the space available to the heart in the mediastinum is limited anteriorly by the sternum, and posteriorly by the vertebral bodies of the thoracic spine. Consequently, part of the left ventricle must project into the left pleural cavity to obtain additional space, which reduces slightly the space for expansion of the left lung during inspiration when compared to the size of the right pleural cavity.

Chest Wall Abnormalities

Chest wall abnormalities result from abnormal growth and attachment of the rib cartilages to the body of the sternum, which changes the position of the sternum. In the most common and important condition, the lower part of the sternum is displaced posteriorly, which is called **pectus excavatum** (*pectus* = chest + *excavatum* = hollowed out), sometimes called a "funnel chest." An anterior sternal protrusion is called **pectus carinatum** (*carina* = prow of a ship), which is sometimes called a "pigeon breast" because it resembles the anterior protrusion of the sternum in a bird.

PECTUS EXCAVATUM

In this condition, the lower two-thirds of the sternum is displaced posteriorly along with the lower costal cartilages, which curve inward to form a broad midline chest depression with the deepest depression in the lowest part of the sternum just above the xiphoid process. The posterior displacement of the sternum appears to be caused by excessive unbalanced growth of the lower costal cartilages 3 through 5, which pushes the sternum posteriorly (FIGURE 27-26A). The sternal displacement also affects the position of the ribs, which may lead to some asymmetry of the thorax manifested as slight scoliosis. The manubrium and the attached first and second costal cartilages are unaffected. The abnormality usually becomes apparent soon after birth, progresses during childhood, and becomes even more pronounced during the rapid skeletal growth phase associated with adolescence.

Pectus excavatum (PE) is a relatively common abnormality, which occurs in about 1 in 300 to 400 white males, and less often in white females and other ethnic groups. About 40% of affected persons also have family members with PE, but the genetic basis has not yet been established. The condition usually is recognized soon after birth and often progresses slowly during childhood. Usually, the abnormality becomes more pronounced during the accelerated growth phase associated with adolescence, but does not progress after skeletal growth ceases.

Clinical Effects of Pectus Excavatum

A relatively minor posterior sternal depression may not encroach to a significant extent on the heart or the adjacent pleural cavities, but can be a psychological

Pectus excavatum
Posterior displacement of the sternum caused by excessive growth of costal cartilages, which reduce the size of the retrosternal space available for the heart within the mediastinum.

Pectus carinatum
Ridgelike projection of the sternum anteriorly.

A

B

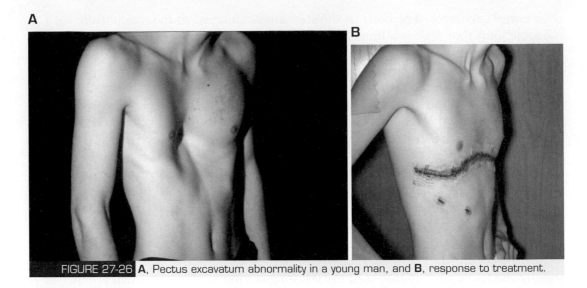

FIGURE 27-26 **A**, Pectus excavatum abnormality in a young man, and **B**, response to treatment.

problem to a teenager concerned about his or her body image. However, a marked posterior sternal depression can compromise both cardiac and pulmonary function. The reduced space available to the heart between the posterior surface of the sternum and the thoracic spine compresses and displaces the heart laterally, which reduces cardiac output, especially during exercise when the heart rate and cardiac output increase. In addition, the laterally displaced heart projects further into the left pleural cavity, leaving less space available for full expansion of the left lung during exercise; and pulmonary ventilation becomes less efficient. The impaired exercise-related marked as the person ages.

Treatment of Pectus Excavatum

Only a major degree of sternal depression is treated surgically so it is important to document the severity of the deformity. X-ray or CT examinations can be used to determine the extent of the posterior sternal displacement and other studies can assess its effects on cardiac and pulmonary function. Only marked posterior sternal displacement is considered for surgical repair, especially if cardiac and pulmonary function studies are abnormal. A severe posterior sternal displacement can be treated surgically in children, but surgery is usually deferred until adolescence if possible.

Surgical treatment involves moving the sternum into a more normal position to enlarge the space available for the heart located in the mediastinum between the sternum and the spine. There are two ways to do this. The first, described in 1949, surgically exposes the pectus deformity and "reshapes" the chest wall by elevating the sternum and adjusting the length of the costal cartilages (FIGURE 27-26B). A strutlike device holds the repositioned sternum in proper position until the surgical repair heals. The strut is left in place for about 6 months and then removed as an outpatient procedure.

A more recent procedure introduced in 1998 is less invasive but forces the chest wall structures abruptly into a new position. A long curved metal bar is inserted through a small lateral chest incision with the concave surface of the bar positioned anteriorly. Then the bar is passed through the chest behind the sternum. When properly positioned, the bar is turned ("flipped') so that the convex surface of the bar is directed anteriorly, which pushes the sternum anteriorly along with the attached ribs. The bar is left in place for 2–4 years and then removed. The goal is to maintain the chest bar in place until the bones and joints reshape to the new chest position, and the chest muscles are able to help maintain the new chest position.

PECTUS CARINATUM

This less common chest wall abnormality (FIGURE 27-27) is called pectus carinatum because of the anterior ridgelike projection of the sternum that has been compared to the prow of a ship (*carina* = ship's prow). Another commonly used term is "pigeon breast" from its resemblance to a bird's sternum. Although the abnormality may be a concern to the subject, usually there are no associated disturbances of cardiac or pulmonary function. Braces worn by the patient have been used to push the sternum back into a more normal position, but are not very effective. Surgical reconstruction of the chest wall can be performed if desired.

MARFAN SYNDROME: A CONNECTIVE TISSUE DISEASE

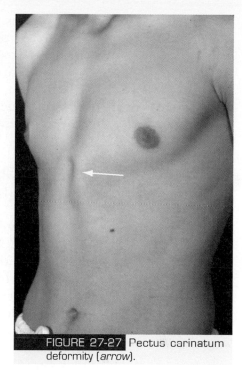

FIGURE 27-27 Pectus carinatum deformity (*arrow*).

The two important types of connective tissue are the widely distributed collagen fibers that provide strength but lack flexibility, and elastic tissue fibers that can stretch and return to their former shape when the stretching force ceases. Elastic fibers are abundant in blood vessels where their elasticity permits the aorta and its branches to stretch and recoil in response to the blood pumped into the vessels during ventricular systole. Elastic fibers are present in many other tissues along with collagen fibers, where they perform various "stretchability" functions in the skin and subcutaneous tissues, and in the eyes where they attach the lens to the ciliary body in the correct position required for normal vision. Connective tissue fibers are constructed from a precursor protein called *fibrillin*, and a mutation of the gene coding for fibrillin (*FBN1*) gives rise to a group of abnormalities grouped together as a relatively common disease called **Marfan syndrome**. Its incidence is about 1 in 5,000 persons and usually the condition is transmitted as a dominant trait. Less often, the disease is not transmitted from a parent, but instead results from a new spontaneous *FBN1* gene mutation in the affected person. When the mutation is transmitted from a parent, its severity may differ among affected individuals in the same family. The gene mutation leads to excessive growth in height; excessively long, thin fingers and toes with excessive joint flexibility; and various chest wall abnormalities, usually pectus excavatum. The fibers that hold the lens in correct position behind the iris may not be able to maintain the lens in proper position, which leads to visual disturbances. However, the most serious complications of Marfan syndrome involve the cardiovascular system, which is caused by defective elastic fibers in the aorta. As a result, the aorta gradually dilates because the defective elastic fibers in the aortic wall are unable to maintain the normal shape of the aorta. Excessive dilation of the aorta may lead to a dissecting aneurysm of the aorta and its complications, as described in the discussion on the cardiovascular system. If the excessive dilation occurs in the ascending aorta, the cusps of the aortic valve, which are attached to the dilated aorta, are unable to fit closely together in diastole to close the aortic valve, which leads to aortic valve insufficiency. Mitral valve function is also compromised because the mitral valve leaflets do not fit together as well in diastole as the aorta dilates. There is no specific nonsurgical treatment of the disease, although some drugs may retard the rate of aortic dilation and reduce the risk of a dissecting aneurysm. Surgical procedures are also available to treat the complications caused by dilation of the aorta and disturbed

Marfan syndrome
A hereditary connective tissue disease characterized by excessive joint flexibility along with various skeletal and cardiovascular abnormalities.

valve functions. Annual ultrasound examinations are recommended to monitor the progression of the aortic dilation, which may require eventual surgical repair in order to reduce the risk of a dissecting aneurysm or rupture of the aorta.

Since pectus excavatum and Marfan syndrome both are associated with pectus excavatum, it has been suggested that they may be related to connective tissue diseases. In one series of cases, one-third of a group of patients treated for pectus excavatum were later considered to have Marfan syndrome.

Structure and Function of Skeletal Muscle

Muscle cells are highly specialized contractile cells. Three different types of muscle are recognized: smooth muscle, skeletal muscle, and cardiac muscle. Smooth muscle is found in the walls of the gastrointestinal tract, biliary tract, urogenital system, respiratory tract, and blood vessels. Skeletal muscle is attached to the skeleton by tendons and ligaments; it functions in voluntary muscular activity. Cardiac muscle closely resembles skeletal muscle but has certain special features related to its function of producing rhythmic contractions of the heart. Lesions of smooth muscles are rare, and disorders of cardiac muscle are considered in the discussion on the cardiovascular system. A discussion of skeletal muscle, the great bulk of muscle within the body, follows.

CONTRACTION OF SKELETAL MUSCLE

Skeletal muscles are long, straplike fibers that measure as much as 30 cm in length. The cytoplasm (sarcoplasm) contains multiple nuclei located just beneath the cell membrane (sarcolemma). Filling the cytoplasm are long threadlike myofibrils composed of the contractile myofilaments actin and myosin. The cytoplasm also contains many energy-rich organic compounds, ions, and enzymes required for the metabolic activity of the muscle cell.

Muscle cells contract in response to motor nerve impulses conveyed to the muscle. The area of communication between the nerve endings and the muscle cell is called the myoneural junction. The actual stimulation of the muscle cell is the result of a chemical called **acetylcholine**, which is released from the nerve endings at the myoneural junction and interacts with acetylcholine receptors on the surface of the muscle fibers. The chemical mediator acetylcholine initiates the biochemical chain of events that causes the actin and myosin filaments to slide together, which leads to shortening of the muscle fiber. The duration of the chemical mediator is quite brief because this substance is rapidly broken down by the enzyme cholinesterase, which is present at the myoneural junction.

Acetylcholine
(as-et-il-kō′lēn)
A chemical secreted by nerve endings that activates neurons or muscle cells.

FACTORS AFFECTING MUSCULAR STRUCTURE AND FUNCTION

The normal structural and functional integrity of skeletal muscle depends on an intact nerve supply, normal transmission of impulses across the myoneural junction, and normal metabolic processes within the muscle cell.

As considered in the discussion on the nervous system, skeletal muscles that are not used or muscles deprived of their nerve supply undergo marked atrophy. Conversely, when additional work is required of the muscles, they undergo hypertrophy in response to the increased demands.

Muscle cells contain a highly complex metabolic machinery capable of translating nerve impulses into muscle contractions. Any disturbance in the metabolism of the muscle cell leads to a disturbance in the function of the cell. The intracellular metabolic processes are also influenced by the endocrine glands that regulate the rate of metabolism within the muscle cell and affect the concentration of the various ions required for normal muscle contraction.

Diseases of skeletal muscle are uncommon. The principal disorders consist of inflammatory lesions, muscular atrophy, degeneration (dystrophy) of muscle, and disturbance of impulse conduction at the myoneural junction.

Inflammation of Muscle (Myositis)

LOCALIZED MYOSITIS

Small areas of inflammation in skeletal muscle are encountered in many systemic diseases and have no major clinical significance. Inflammation of muscle may also follow injury or muscular overexertion. The inflammation is secondary to necrosis and disruption of muscle cells and is associated with swelling and tenderness of the affected muscle. The inflammation gradually subsides as the muscle injury heals.

GENERALIZED MYOSITIS

Generalized inflammation of skeletal muscle (polymyositis) is an uncommon but serious systemic disease of unknown etiology, characterized by widespread degeneration and inflammation of skeletal muscle. One type of polymyositis, associated with swelling and inflammation of the skin, is called dermatomyositis. These disorders are often classified as connective tissue (collagen) diseases (discussion on immunity, hypersensitivity, allergy, and autoimmune diseases) because of the necrosis of connective tissue fibers in the affected muscles and because these diseases are presumed to have an immunologic basis.

Muscular Atrophy and Muscular Dystrophy

A group of relatively rare diseases is characterized by progressive atrophy or degeneration of skeletal muscle. Many are hereditary. Various clinical syndromes are recognized, depending on the muscle groups affected, the patterns of inheritance, and the rate of progression of the disease. In general, the diseases are characterized by progressive muscular weakness and gradually increasing disability, eventually terminating in death from paralysis of the respiratory muscles or superimposed respiratory infection.

It is customary to classify these diseases into two large categories: the muscular atrophy group and the muscular dystrophy group.

In the progressive muscular atrophy group of diseases, the muscular weakness and atrophy are secondary to progressive degeneration of motor nerve cells in the cerebral cortex, brain stem, and spinal cord, described in the discussion on the nervous system (degenerative disease of motor neurons). The clinical manifestations are related to the location of the degenerating nerve cells within the central nervous system and the rate at which the neuronal degeneration progresses.

In the muscular dystrophy group, the nerve supply to the muscles is unaffected. The basic disturbance is an abnormality in the muscle fibers that causes them to degenerate. The most common and severe type is called Duchenne muscular dystrophy, and a milder form of muscular dystrophy is called Becker muscular dystrophy. Both forms result from the mutation of a large gene on the X chromosome, and the disease is transmitted as an X-linked trait to male children of women who carry the defective gene. The normal gene codes for a muscle protein called dystropin, which is located on the inner surface of the sarcolemma, where it plays a role in maintaining the structure and functions of the muscle fibers.

As a result of the gene mutation, dystropin is absent in the muscle fibers of persons afflicted with Duchenne muscular dystrophy and is apparently responsible for the manifestations of the disease, which appear first during early childhood and progress rapidly, leading to death in late adolescence or early adulthood. The muscles primarily affected are those of the lower extremities, trunk, hips, and shoulder girdle. Often, the extent of atrophy is masked because the muscles are infiltrated by fat and fibrous tissue as they atrophy. The fat infiltration may at times be so extreme that the affected muscles appear hypertrophied, leading to the paradox of profound muscular weakness in an individual whose muscles appear very well developed. The apparent hypertrophy is an illusion, which is why the term pseudohypertrophic is applied to this type of muscular dystrophy.

The less-severe Becker muscular dystrophy also is caused by a mutation of the same dystropin-producing gene that causes Duchenne muscular dystrophy. Dystropin is produced by the mutated gene but is either abnormal or produced in insufficient amounts. In both diseases, the muscle enzyme creatine kinase (CK) leaks from the abnormal muscle fibers, and very high enzyme levels can be detected in the blood of affected persons. (This is the same enzyme that leaks from heart muscle when the muscle is damaged, as described in the discussion on the cardiovascular system.) The diagnosis of muscular dystrophy is made on the basis of the clinical features together with the very high CK blood concentration. Genetic testing reveals the gene mutation, and muscle biopsies reveal absence of dystropin in Duchenne dystrophy and an abnormal or reduced amount of dystropin in Becker dystrophy.

Although the various types of muscular atrophy and muscular dystrophy are uncommon, they are of major concern not only to the patient, but to the family because of the hereditary nature of many of these illnesses. Unfortunately, there is no way at present to arrest the relentless progression of the disease. Gene therapy to eventually allow insertion of replacement genes in muscle fibers to code for the synthesis of the missing or defective dystropin is being actively investigated but has not yet been successful.

Myasthenia Gravis

Myasthenia gravis
An autoimmune disease characterized by abnormal fatigability of muscle and caused by an autoantibody that damages the acetylcholine receptors at the myoneural junction.

Myasthenia gravis is a chronic disease characterized by abnormal fatigability of the voluntary muscles as a result of an abnormality at the myoneural junction. Fatigue develops rapidly when the muscles are used and subsides when they are rested. Often, the dysfunction is most conspicuous in the small muscles of the face and in the muscles concerned with eye movement (extraocular muscles). Myasthenia gravis appears to be an autoimmune disease. The blood of affected patients contains an autoantibody directed against acetylcholine receptors on the surface of the muscle fibers at the myoneural junction. The manifestations of the disease occur because the antibody damages and greatly reduces the number of receptors available to interact with the acetylcholine liberated from motor nerve endings.

Symptoms can be relieved by drugs that inhibit the action of the enzyme cholinesterase. This prolongs the action of the chemical mediator acetylcholine so that it can continue to stimulate the reduced numbers of receptors for a longer time. Many patients with myasthenia gravis have either a tumor or a benign hyperplasia of the thymus gland, which is probably also related to a disturbance of the immune system. Patients with hyperplasia or a tumor of the thymus gland sometimes are improved by removal of the thymus.

QUESTIONS FOR REVIEW

1. Describe the structure of the typical movable joint (see Figure 27-1).
2. What are the three most common types of arthritis? What are their distinguishing features (see Table 27-1)?
3. What is the difference between a simple fracture and a compound fracture? What are the complications of a compound fracture? What is a comminuted fracture? A pathologic fracture?
4. What is osteoporosis? Why does it develop? What symptoms and complications result from osteoporosis?
5. What is a "slipped disk"? Why does it occur? Why does it sometimes produce pain radiating down the leg? How is it treated?
6. What is meant by the following terms: *osteoporosis, multiple myeloma, nucleus pulposus,* and *rheumatoid factor*?
7. What are the types of muscle cells?
8. What is meant by the following terms: *myoneural junction, acetylcholine,* and *myositis*?
9. What is the difference between muscular atrophy and muscular dystrophy? What are the most common types of atrophic disease of the muscles? Of dystrophic disease?
10. What is myasthenia gravis? What is its relationship to the immune system? How is it treated?

SUPPLEMENTARY READINGS

Arn, P. H., Scherer, L. R., Haller, J. A. Jr., et al. 1989. Outcome of pectus excavatum in patients with Marfan syndrome and in the general population. *The Journal of Pediatrics* 115:954–58.

▶ Records of 28 patients with Marfan syndrome were compared with 30 age-matched control patients with presumed pectus excavatum. Isolated pectus excavatum may indicate an underlying connective tissue disorder such as Marfan syndrome.

Bitton, A., Yialamas, M., Levy, B. D., et al. 2009. Clinical problem-solving. A fragile balance. *The New England Journal of Medicine* 361:74–79.

▶ Osteogenesis imperfecta is a genetic disorder of collagen production leading to thin and insufficiently mineralized bone. There are several variants which differ in their severity. The abnormal collagen production may also involve the sclerae of the eyes, ear drums, skin, and other collagen-containing tissues. Early diagnosis and treatment may reduce the risk of fractures. Bisphosphonate drugs (used to treat patients with osteoporosis) may also be helpful, along with additional calcium and vitamin D.

Brender, E., Burke, A., and Glass, R. M. 2005. JAMA patient pages Vitamin D. *Journal of the American Medical Association* 294:2386.

▶ A short 1-page article designed for patient education describing the amount of sunlight exposure required to ensure adequate vitamin D (10–15 minutes twice per week), the diseases resulting from the deficiency (rickets and osteomalacia), and the persons at risk of deficiency (breast-fed infants receiving less than 2 cups a day of vitamin D–fortified formula or milk, people with dark pigmented skin, people with very limited sun exposure, people with fat malabsorption diseases, people with liver or kidney disease, people in the northern hemisphere during winter).

Cauley, J. A., Lui, L. Y., Ensrud, K. E., et al. 2005. Bone mineral density and the risk of incident nonspinal fractures in black and white women. *Journal of the American Medical Association* 293:2102–08.

▶ Age, female sex, slender body configuration, and white race are well-known risk factors for osteoporosis. Although many factors affect bone mineral density (BMD), middle-aged and older black men and women have higher BMD and lower fracture rates than whites. Decreased total hip and femoral neck BMD is associated with increased fracture risk in both black and white women. At any level of BMD, fracture rates in black women were 30–40% lower than in white women. Separate race-specific databases may be appropriate to define osteoporosis and fracture risk in black and white women.

Drinkwater, B. L., Nilson, K., Ott, S., et al. 1986. Bone mineral density after resumption of menses in amenorrheic athletes. *Journal of the American Medical Association* 256:380–82.

▶ Bone mass may not be completely restored.

Felson, D. T. 2006. Clinical practice. Osteoarthritis of the knee. *The New England Journal of Medicine* 354:841–48.

▶ Describes risk factors, manifestations, and principle of treatment.

Fonkalsrud, E. W. 2000. Surgical management of pectus excavatum. *Operative Techniques in Thoracic and Cardiovascular Surgery* 5:94–102.

▶ A comprehensive description and illustration of the standard open surgical technique.

Holick, M. F. 2007. Vitamin D deficiency. *The New England Journal of Medicine* 357: 266–81.

▶ Vitamin D deficiency is still a problem despite fortification of foods with supplements. In adults, the deficiency may increase the risk of bone fractures by contributing to the development of osteoporosis, and also may cause osteomalacia. Without vitamin D only about 10–15% of dietary calcium and about 60% of phosphorous is absorbed. Most cells and tissues in the body have vitamin D receptors, and the vitamin has many effects unrelated to the skeletal system. Vitamin D inhibits cell proliferation of both normal cells and cancer cells, and promotes normal differentiation of cells. Vitamin D is required for normal immune system function, which may explain why black Americans, who are often vitamin D deficient, are more prone to tuberculosis than are whites, and tend to have more aggressive disease. People living at higher or lower latitudes (farther away from the equator, where sunlight is most intense and prolonged) have a greater risk of a number of diseases than persons living closer to the equator.

▶ Current recommendations for vitamin D supplements are too low, and many persons are vitamin D deficient. There are two forms of vitamin D (vitamin D_2 and vitamin D_3) and recommended supplement is 1,000 international units (IU) of vitamin D_3 or 3,000 IU of vitamin D_2.

Jaroszewski, D., Notrica, D., McMahon, L., et al. 2010. Current management of pectus excavatum: A review and update of therapy and treatment recommendations. *Journal of the American Board of Family Medicine* 23:230–39.

▶ A review article dealing with the current management and clinical manifestations of pectus excavatum.

Johnson, R. J., and Rideout, B. A. 2004. Uric acid and diet—Insights into the epidemic of cardiovascular disease. *The New England Journal of Medicine* 350:1071–73.

▶ Neither the total protein intake nor the intake of purine-rich vegetables was correlated with the development of gout. Gout is most common among people whose diet is high in meat and low in dairy products. Genetic and other factors also modulate the uric acid levels. Many patients with chronic gout and persisting high uric acid develop urate nephropathy. Diets that contain abundant fruits, vegetables, and low-fat dairy foods not only reduce the frequency of hypertension but also the frequency of gout.

LeBoff, M. S., Kohlmeier, L., Hurwitz, S., et al. 1999. Occult vitamin D deficiency in postmenopausal US women with acute hip fracture. *Journal of the American Medical Association* 281:1505–11.

▶ Postmenopausal women with hip fractures had occult vitamin D deficiency, which impairs absorption of calcium and mineralization of bone and also stimulates compensatory increase in parathyroid hormone secretion. These factors predispose to fractures. Older people need 600 IU of vitamin D daily, which should be increased to 800 IU in winter.

Loucks, A. B., Mortola, J. F., Girton, L., et al. 1989. Alterations in the hypothalamic-pituitary-ovarian and the hypothalamic-pituitary-adrenal axes in athletic women. *The Journal of Clinical Endocrinology and Metabolism* 68:402–11.

▶ Describes pathophysiology of exercise-induced amenorrhea.

O'Dell, J. R. 2004. Therapeutic strategies for rheumatoid arthritis. *The New England Journal of Medicine* 350:2591–602.

▶ Irreversible joint damage occurs early in rheumatoid arthritis. Early diagnosis and prompt treatment with disease-modifying antirheumatic drugs (DMARD) are essential to minimize joint damage. Nonsteroidal anti-inflammatory drugs improve symptoms but do not slow the progression of the disease. Corticosteroid drugs suppress inflammation and slow disease progression but have significant side effects. DMARD vary in effectiveness and toxicity. Methotrexate is the most widely used, and many patients are treated with methotrexate combined with two other DMARD agents. Tumor necrosis factor inhibitor drugs are generally reserved for patients whose disease cannot be controlled by a combined therapy with DMARD.

Raisz, L. G. 2005. Clinical practice. Screening for osteoporosis. *The New England Journal of Medicine* 353:164–71.

▶ Measurement of bone mineral density in the lumbar spine and proximal femur is a reliable and safe way to assess the risk of fracture. Screening should provide an estimate of fracture risk during the subsequent 5 or 20 years.

Rott, K. T., and Agudelo, C. A. 2003. Gout. *Journal of the American Medical Association* 289:2857–60.

▶ Current concepts on pathogenesis, factors raising uric acid, clinical manifestations, drugs available for treating gout, and new treatment methods being investigated.

Shahinian, V. B., Kuo, Y. F., Freeman, J. L., et al. 2005. Risk of fracture after androgen deprivation for prostate cancer. *The New England Journal of Medicine* 352:154–64.

▶ Orchiectomy or drug-induced suppression of testicular function in men with prostate cancer significantly increases their risk of fractures by promoting more rapid decline in bone density resulting from loss of androgens.

Sellmeyer, D. E. 2010. Atypical fractures as a potential complication of long-term bisphosphonate therapy. *Journal of the American Medical Association* 304:1480–84.

▶ Bisphosphonates reduce risk of spine, hip, and other site fractures in postmenopausal women, but prolonged therapy may suppress bone remodeling (proliferation) to such an extent that normal bone remodeling is impaired, which results in increased fracture risk. Such fractures are considered "atypical" because they usually affect the shaft of the femur instead of the femoral neck or the upper femur just below the femoral neck (intertrochanteric fracture). The fractures are not associated with an injury, have a radiologic appearance that differs from the usual femoral fracture, and clinically are characterized by thigh pain and subsequently by inability to bear weight on the affected limb. Apparently, prolonged bisphosphonate treatment can suppress bone remodeling to such a degree that the skeleton has insufficient bone turnover to maintain skeletal strength. Management consists of treating the fracture, a 12-month interruption of bisphosphonate therapy every 5 years, and administering a parathyroid hormonelike drug to help restore bone density.

OUTLINE SUMMARY

Skeletal System

STRUCTURE AND FUNCTION

Rigid supporting framework.
Impregnated with calcium salts.
Bone continually being broken down and reformed.
Density of bones depends on activity.
Bones connected by joints.
Movable joints are covered by articular cartilage, lubricated by synovial fluid.
Ligamentous joint capsule lined by synovium.

BONE FORMATION

Intramembranous bone formation: mesoderm converted directly into bone.
Endochondral bone formation: cartilage model becomes converted into bone.

BONE GROWTH

Growth in length from epiphysis.
Growth in thickness from periosteum.

FACTORS REQUIRED FOR NORMAL BONE GROWTH

Vitamin D.
Normal amounts of calcium and phosphate.
Normal parathyroid function.

INADEQUATE VITAMIN D CAUSES RICKETS IN CHILDREN AND OSTEOMALACIA IN ADULTS

CONGENITAL ABNORMALITIES

Achondroplasia:
Faulty endochondral bone formation impairs growth of extremities and disturbs formation of skull bones.
Causes dwarfism with disproportionately short limbs.
Osteogenesis imperfecta:
Thin and delicate bones, easily broken.
Infant may be born with multiple fractures.
Malformations of digits:
Extra digits (polydactyly): easily removed.
Fused digits: more difficult to correct.
Congenital clubfoot (talipes):
Multifactorial inheritance.
Talipes equinovarus most common type.
Treated by casts and splints.
Congenital dislocation of hip:
Multifactorial inheritance: more common in females.

Shallow acetabulum causes femoral head to be displaced out of socket.
Breech position favors development.
Treated by manipulation and casts.

RHEUMATOID ARTHRITIS

A systemic disease of chiefly small joints.
More common in women.
Inflammatory tissue from synovium destroys joint.
Dislocation occurs owing to joint instability.
Autoantibodies to gamma globulin demonstrated in many patients.

OSTEOARTHRITIS

"Wear and tear" degeneration of joints.
Affects major weight-bearing joints.
Usually little disability.
Severe disability can be treated by joint replacement.

GOUT

Disorder of purine metabolism.
Deposition of uric acid in and around joints.
Frequent acute episodes caused by precipitation of uric acid crystals in joint fluid.
Diet and drugs control disease by lowering uric acid.

FRACTURES

Simple: bone broken into two pieces.
Comminuted: bone shattered.
Compound: overlying skin broken with potential for infection.
Pathologic: secondary to disease such as metastatic carcinoma.
Treatment by reduction and casts or internal fixation.

OSTEOMYELITIS

Hematogenous: predominantly in children.
Occurs at ends of bone.
Spread of infection may strip periosteum from cortex and devitalize bone.
Infection may spread into joint in adults.
Infection in drug abusers tends to localize in vertebral bodies.
As a result of direct implantation: after trauma or surgical procedures.
Manifestations and treatment:
Febrile illness with localizing manifestations.
X-rays reveal changes in bone.
Treatment by antibiotics supplemented by surgical procedures if needed.

BONE TUMORS
Metastatic tumors: relatively common.
Multiple myeloma: plasma cell neoplasm.
Benign cysts and tumors: occur occasionally.
Primary malignant bone tumors: relatively rare.

OSTEOPOROSIS
Generalized thinning of bone.
Most common in postmenopausal women.
Treatment by high-calcium diet.

AVASCULAR NECROSIS
Necrosis and degeneration at ends of bone.
Probably caused by disturbance in blood supply as a result of injury.
Causes local pain and disability.

Structure and Function of the Spine

STRUCTURE
Fibrocartilaginous cushions interposed between adjacent vertebral bodies.

FUNCTION
Spine forms central axis of body
Disks function as shock absorbers.

SCOLIOSIS
An abnormal lateral curvature of the spine.
Most cases are idiopathic and occur during adolescence.
Large curves cause pronounced disability and reduce size of thoracic cavities.
Treatment depends on extent of curvature.

STRUCTURE AND FUNCTION OF THORAX
Sternum and ribs function as a unit.

ABNORMAL STERNUM–SPINE RELATIONSHIP MAY DISTURB CARDIOPULMONARY FUNCTION
Posterior displacement of sternum (pectus excavatum) restricts space available to heart located between spine and sternum that may compromise cardiopulmonary function.
Marked posterior sternal displacement may require correction. Treatment methods available.

Anterior sternal protrusion (pectus carinatum) is primarily a cosmetic defect.
Usually, surgical correction is not required.

Intervertebral Disk Disease

PATHOGENESIS
Disk wears out with age.
Nucleus pulposus may be extruded through tear in annulus fibrosus and impinge on nerve roots.
Sudden onset of back pain radiating down leg.

DIAGNOSIS AND TREATMENT
Protrusion can be demonstrated by myelogram or CT scan.
Disk material may be absorbed but often must be removed surgically.

Skeletal Muscle

CONTRACTION OF SKELETAL MUSCLE
Myofilaments slide together.
Communication between nerve and muscle at myoneural junction.
Nerve stimulation liberates acetylcholine, which interacts with receptors on muscle fibers and initiates contraction.

INFLAMMATION OF MUSCLE
Localized myositis follows injury or overexertion.
Generalized myositis: a systemic disease.

HEREDITARY DISEASES CHARACTERIZED BY MUSCLE ATROPHY AND DEGENERATION
Progressive muscular atrophy: nerve cell degeneration with secondary muscle atrophy.
Muscular dystrophy: primary degeneration of muscle.

MYASTHENIA GRAVIS
Abnormal fatigability of voluntary muscles.
Autoantibodies formed against acetylcholine receptors at myoneural junction.
Symptoms relieved by drugs that prolong action of acetylcholine.

General References

ANATOMY AND PHYSIOLOGY

Ganong, W. F. 2004. *Review of medical physiology.* 21st ed. New York: Lange Medical Books/McGraw-Hill.

Guyton, A. C., and Hall, J. E. 1997. *Human physiology and mechanisms of disease.* 6th ed. Philadelphia: W. B. Saunders Company.

Martini, F. H. 2006. *Fundamentals of anatomy and physiology.* 7th ed. San Francisco: Pearson/Benjamin Cummings.

Martini, F. H., Timmons, M. J., and Tallitsch, R. B. 2009. *Human anatomy.* 6th ed. San Francisco: Pearson/Benjamin Cummings.

MEDICINE

Andrioli, T. E., Carpenter, C. C. J., Griggs, R. C., et al. 2006. *Cecil essentials of medicine.* 6th ed. Philadelphia: W. B. Saunders Company.

Beers, M. H., Fletcher, A. J., and Berkow, R. 2003. *The Merck manual of medical information: Home edition.* 2nd ed. New York: Pocket Books/Simon and Schuster, Inc.

Gardner, D. G., Shoback, D. M., and Greenspan F. S. eds. 2010. *Greenspan's basic and clinical endocrinology.* 8th ed. New York: Lange Medical Books/McGraw-Hill.

McPhee, S. J., Papadakis, M. A., and Rabow, M. W. eds. 2011. *Current medical diagnosis and treatment.* 50th ed. New York: Lange Medical Books/McGraw-Hill.

MICROBIOLOGY

Murray, P. R., Rosenthal, K. S., and Pfaller, M. A. 2005. *Medical microbiology.* 5th ed. Philadelphia: Mosby.

OBSTETRICS AND GYNECOLOGY

Boston Women's Health Book. 2005. *Our bodies, ourselves for the new century: A book for and by women.* New York: Simon and Schuster, Inc.

Decherney, A. H., Nathan, L., and Goodwin, T. M. 2007. *Current obstetric & gynecologic diagnosis and treatment.* 10th ed. New York: Lange Medical Books/McGraw-Hill.

PATHOLOGY

Kumar, V., Abbas, A. K., Fausto, N., et al. 2009. *Robbins and Cotran pathologic basis of disease.* 8th ed. Philadelphia: Elsevier Saunders.

PEDIATRICS

Hay, W. W., Levin, M. J., Sondheimer J. M., et al. 2005. *Current pediatric diagnosis and treatment.* 17th ed. New York: Lange Medical Books/McGraw-Hill.

SURGERY

Doherty, G. M. 2006. *Current surgical diagnosis and treatment.* 12th ed. New York: Lange Medical Books/McGraw-Hill.

Sabiston, D. C., and Lyerly, H. K. 2008. *Textbook of surgery: The biological basis of modern surgical practice.* 18th ed. Philadelphia: W. B. Saunders Company.

UROLOGY

Schrier, R. W. 2003. *Renal and electrolyte disorders.* 6th ed. Baltimore: Lippincott Williams & Wilkins.

Glossary

COMMON PREFIXES AND SUFFIXES

Prefixes

a, an—without
ab—from, away from
ad—toward
ante—before
bi—twice, two
circum—around
co—together
contra—against, opposed
de—down, from, away
dis—apart
dys—abnormal, difficult

endo—within
epi—upon
exo—outside
extra—outside
hemi—half
hetero—different
homo—same
hyper—above, beyond, excessive
hypo—below, under, deficient
infra—beneath
inter—between

intra—within
meta—after, beyond
para—beside
peri—around
post—behind, after
pre—before
pro—before
sub—beneath
supra—above
syn—together

Suffixes

—**blast**, applied to formative cells (e.g., osteoblast)
—**cyte**, applied to adult cells (e.g., osteocyte)

—**itis**, inflammation of
—**oid**, like

—**ology**, study of
—**oma**, a swelling or tumor

An Approximate Guide to Pronunciation

a: as in lad
ā: as in late
ä: as in calm
e: as in met
ē: as in meet

i: as in pill
ī: as in pile
o: as in rob
ō: as in robe
u: as in shut

ū: as in chute
oi: as in joy
ōō: as in fool
ou: as in loud

A

ABO hemolytic disease A mild hemolytic disease in group A or B infants or group O mothers, as a result of maternal anti-A and anti-B antibodies.

abscess (ab′sess) A localized accumulation of pus in tissues.

acetone (as′e-tōn) An organic compound (ketone) derived from the ketone bodies acetoacetic acid and beta-hydroxybutyric acid.

acetylcholine (as-et-il-kō′lēn) A chemical secreted by nerve endings that activates neurons or muscle cells.

ac′etyl coen′zyme A (acetyl CoA) A combination of a two-carbon acetate fragment with a complex organic compound called coenzyme A.

achondroplasia (a-kon-dro-pla′zi-yuh) A congenital disturbance of endochondral bone formation that causes a type of dwarfism.

acido′sis A disturbance in the acid–base balance of the body in which body fluids have a lower pH than normal.

acinus (as′in-us) A functional unit of the lung consisting of a cluster of respiratory bronchioles, alveolar ducts, and alveoli derived from a single terminal bronchiole.

acquired immune deficiency syndrome (AIDS) An infection caused by the human immunodeficiency virus. The virus attacks and destroys helper T lymphocytes, which compromises cell-mediated immunity, leading to increased susceptibility to infection and some tumors.

acromegaly (ak′ro-meg′al-ē) A condition resulting from excessive secretion of growth hormone in the adult.

ACTH See *adrenocorticotropic hormone.*

actinic keratosis (ak-ti′-nik ke-rä-tō′sis) A precancerous warty proliferation of squamous epithelial cells in sun-damaged skin of older persons.

acute coronary syndrome A general term for the three most serious manifestations of coronary artery disease: unstable angina, non–ST-segment elevation myocardial infarction, and ST-segment elevation myocardial infarction.

Addison disease A disease caused by chronic adrenal cortical hypofunction.

adenoma (ad-en-ō′muh) A benign tumor arising from glands.

adenperoxisone′osine triphos′phate (ATP) A high-energy phosphate compound that liberates energy to power numerous cellular metabolic processes.

ADH See *antidiuretic hormone.*

adhesions (ad-hē′shuns) Bands of fibrous tissue that form subsequent to an inflammation, and bind adjacent tissues together.

adjustable gastric banding A method for treating obesity by applying an adjustable gastric band to the stomach in order to reduce its capacity, thereby promoting weight loss.

adjuvant chemotherapy (ad′joo-vent) Anticancer chemotherapy administered after surgical resection of a tumor in an attempt to destroy any small undetected foci of metastatic tumor before they become clinically detectable.

adrenaline (ad-ren′a-lin) Another name for epinephrine, one of the hormones of the adrenal medulla.

adrenocorticotropic hormone (ACTH) (ad-rēn′o-cor′tico-trō′pik) A hormone secreted by the anterior lobe of the pituitary that stimulates the adrenal cortex to manufacture and secrete adrenal cortical hormones.

adrenogenital syndrome (ad-rēn′ō-jen′i-tul) Clinical disorder of adrenal function characterized by overproduction of adrenal sex hormones.

agonist (ag′-on-ist) A drug that can combine with a specific cell receptor and cause an effect characteristic of the receptor. See *dopamine receptor.*

aldos′terone A steroid hormone produced by the adrenal cortex that regulates the rate of sodium absorption from the renal tubules.

alkalo′sis A disturbance in the body's acid–base balance in which the pH of the extracellular fluids is shifted toward the alkaline side of normal. See also *acidosis.*

alkylating agent (al′kil-ā-ting) An anticancer drug that disrupts cell function by binding DNA chains together so that they cannot separate.

allele (äh′lēl) One of several related genes that may occupy the same locus on a homologous chromosome.

allergen (al′ler-jen) A substance capable of inducing an allergic reaction in a predisposed individual.

allergy A tendency to form specific IgE antibody to antigens that do not affect most persons.

alpha cells (al′fuh) Glucagon-secreting cells of the pancreatic islets.

alpha fetoprotein (al′fuh fē′tō-prō′tēn) Protein produced by fetal liver early in gestation. Sometimes produced by tumor cells. Level is elevated in amnionic fluid when fetus has neural tube defect.

alveolus (alvē′olus) One of the terminal air sacs of the lung.

Alzheimer disease (ahls′-hīm-er) A degenerative disease of the nervous system with characteristic structural abnormalities within neurons.

amenorrhea (äh-men-ō-rē′äh) Absence of menses.

amniocentesis (am′ni-ō-sen-tē′sis) Removal of amnionic fluid, usually accomplished by inserting a needle through the mother's abdominal and uterine walls into the amnionic cavity.

amnionic fluid (am-nē-on′ik) Fluid within the amnionic cavity surrounding the developing organism.

amnionic sac (am-nē-on′ik) The fluid-filled sac surrounding the embryo. One of the fetal membranes.

anaerobic (an-air-o′bik) Not requiring oxygen for growth.

anaphylactoid reaction (a-na-fil-ack′-toyd) A hypersensitivity reaction resembling anaphylaxis but not caused by IgE antibodies.

anaphylaxis (a-nä-fil-aks′is) A severe generalized IgE-mediated hypersensitivity reaction characterized by marked respiratory distress and fall in blood pressure.

anastomosis (ä-nas-ta-mō′sis) A communication between two blood vessels or other tubular structures. Also refers to a surgical connection of two hollow tubular structures, such as the divided ends of the intestine or a blood vessel (*surgical anastomosis*).

anemia (an-ē′mē-uh) A decrease in hemoglobin or red cells or both.

anencephaly (an-en-seff′uh-lē) A congenital malformation: absence of brain, cranial vault, and scalp as a result of defective closure of the neural tube.

aneurysm (an′ūr-izm) A dilatation of a structure, such as the aorta, a cerebral artery, or a part of the ventricular wall. See *ventricular aneurysm*.

angina pectoris (an-jī′nuh pek′tōr-is) Precordial pain experienced on exertion owing to inadequate blood supply to the heart muscle.

angiogram (an′jē-ō-gram) Same as *arteriogram*.

angiotensin (an-jē-o-ten′sin) A component of the renin-angiotensin-aldosterone system, formed from interaction of renin with a blood protein (*angiotensinogen*). The first product formed, called angiotensin I, is converted rapidly to a second product called angiotensin II by angiotensin converting enzyme (ACE). Angiotensin II raises blood pressure and stimulates the adrenal gland to secrete aldosterone.

angiotensin converting enzyme An enzyme that converts angiotensin I to angiotensin II.

angiotensinogen (an-jee-o-ten-sin′-o-gen) A blood protein converted to angiotensin I by renin secreted by the kidneys. Part of the renin-angiotensin-aldosterone system.

anion (an′ī-on) An ion carrying a negative charge.

annulus fibrosus (an′ū-lus) The dense peripheral ring of fibrocartilage making up the intervertebral disk.

anorexia nervosa Excessive self-induced weight loss because of a false perception of being fat.

antibiotic sensitivity test A laboratory test to determine the ability of antibiotics to inhibit bacterial growth.

antibody A globulin manufactured by plasma cells in response to contact with a foreign antigen.

anticoagulant drugs Drugs that inhibit the process of blood coagulation.

antidiuretic hormone (ADH) (an-ti-dī-u-ret′tik) Posterior lobe pituitary hormone that regulates urine concentration by altering the permeability of the renal collecting tubules.

antimetabolite (an-ti-met-ab′o-līte) A substance that competes with or replaces another substance (metabolite) required for cell growth or multiplication.

aplastic anemia (ā-plas′tik) An anemia caused by bone marrow failure.

apoptosis (ah-pop-toe′-sis, or ah-po-toe′-sis) Programmed cell death that occurs after a cell has lived its normal life span.

arachnoid (ar-ak′noyd) The middle of the three meninges that cover the brain.

areola (a-rē′o-la) The pigmented area surrounding the nipple.

aromatase inhibitor (air-ō′-muh-tase) A drug that inhibits the conversion of adrenal androgenic steroids to estrogens, used as postresection adjuvant therapy to treat postmenopausal women with estrogen-positive breast carcinoma.

arrhythmia (a-rith′mi-uh) An irregularity of the heartbeat.

arteriogram (är-tēr′ē-ō-gram) An x-ray technique for studying the caliber of blood vessels by injection of radiopaque material into the vessel.

arteriolosclerosis (är-tēr-ē-ólo-skler-ō′-sis) One type of arteriosclerosis characterized by thickening and degeneration of small arterioles.

arteriosclerosis (är-tēr′ē-ō-skler-ō′sis) A general term for degenerative change in the wall of an artery, often associated with narrowing of its lumen.

arteriosclerotic aneurysm (an′ūr-izm) A ballooning of the aorta or a large artery as a result of weakening of the wall secondary to atherosclerosis.

arthritis (ärth-rī′tis) An inflammation of a joint. Term is also used to refer to a degenerative process in joints, as in osteoarthritis.

arthropod (är′thrō-pod) Invertebrate animal with jointed limbs and segmented body, such as insect and spider. Important arthropods that parasitize humans include the crab louse and the organism causing scabies.

arthropod-borne virus An infectious nucleic acid particle (virus) transmitted by mosquitoes.

articular Pertaining to a joint.

asbestos body (as-bes′tus) An asbestos fiber coated with protein and iron that is found in lungs and sputum of patients with asbestosis.

asbestosis (as-bes-tō′sis) A type of pneumoconiosis caused by inhalation of asbestos fibers.

Ascaris (as′kar-is) A large parasitic roundworm that infests humans.

ascites (a-si′tēz) Accumulation of fluid in the abdominal cavity.

as′trocyte A large stellate cell having highly branched processes. Forms the structural framework of the nervous system. One of the neuroglial cells.

atelectasis (ah-tel-ek′tuh-sis) Collapse of the lung, either caused by bronchial obstruction (*obstructive atelectasis*) or external compression (*compression atelectasis*).

atheroma (ah-ther-ō′muh) A mass of lipids and debris that accumulates in the intima lining of an artery and narrows its lumen.

ath′erosclero′sis A thickening of the lining (*intima*) of blood vessels caused by accumulation of lipids, with secondary scarring and calcification.

athyreotic (ā-thī-rē′äh′tik) Lacking a thyroid gland, as in one type of cretinism caused by failure of gland development.

atopic (ā-top′ik) Having a genetic predisposition to certain allergic conditions such as hay fever and asthma.

atrioventricular (AV) valve (a′trē-o-ven-trik′ū-lar) The flaplike heart valve located between the atrium and ventricle.

atrophy (ah′trō′fē) A reduction in size of a structure caused by decreased function, inadequate hormonal stimulation, or reduced blood supply.

autoantibody (aw′tō-an′ti-bod-ē) An antibody formed against one's own cells or tissue components.

autoimmune disease A disease associated with formation of cell-mediated or humoral immunity against the subject's own cells or tissue components.

autosome (aw′tō-sōm) A chromosome other than a sex chromosome.

avascular necrosis (ā-vas′kew̄-lär nek-rō′sis) Bone necrosis caused by interruption of its blood supply.

Babesia (bă-bē′-zē-ă) A tick-borne malarialike parasite that multiplies within the red cells of infected persons and animals.

bacterial endocarditis An inflammation of the endocardium. Term usually refers to an inflammation of the heart valves.

Barr body The inactivated X chromosome that is applied to the nuclear membrane in the female. Sex chromatin body.

Barrett esophagus A condition in which the epithelial lining of the esophagus changes from squamous to columnar type, usually as a result of reflux esophagitis.

base A solution containing an excess of hydroxyl ions and having a pH greater than 7.0.

basement membrane A thin layer of acellular material upon which epithelium rests.

bas′ophil A cell that contains numerous variable-sized granules that stain intensely purple with basic dyes. See also *eosinophil*.

beta cells (bā′tuh) Insulin-secreting cells of the pancreatic islets.

bile A secretion of the liver containing bile salts, cholesterol, and other substances.

bile canaliculus (kan-al-ik′u-lus) Small terminal bile channel located between liver cords.

bile salts Derivatives of bile acids present in bile that act as emulsifiers to promote fat digestion and absorption.

biliary cirrhosis Diffuse liver cell damage and scarring with distortion of liver cell structure and function (cirrhosis) caused by obstruction of bile ducts.

bil′iary colic Abdominal pain that results when a gallstone enters the biliary duct system.

bilirubin (bil-i-rū′bin) One of the bile pigments derived from breakdown of hemoglobin.

biopsy (bī′op-sē) Removal of a small sample of tissue for examination and diagnosis by a pathologist.

blas′tocyst A stage of development of the fertilized ovum (*zygote*) in which a central cavity accumulates within the cluster of developing cells.

blastomycosis (blast-ō-mī-kō′sis) A systemic fungus infection caused by the fungus *Blastomyces dermatitidis*.

blighted twin A twin that fails to develop normally.

B lymphocyte A lymphocyte that differentiates into plasma cells and is associated with humoral immunity.

body stalk The structure connecting the embryo to the chorion. Eventually develops into the umbilical cord.

bone remodeling Normal physiologic bone breakdown and replacement by an equivalent amount of newly formed bone without any loss of normal bone density.

botulism (bo′-chôô-lizm) Food poisoning caused by ingestion of a neurotoxin produced by an anaerobic spore-forming bacillus *Clostridium botulinum* growing in improperly canned or preserved food.

Bowman's capsule The cuplike expanded end of the nephron that surrounds the tuft of glomerular capillaries.

bradykinin (brā-dē-kī′nin) A chemical mediator of inflammation derived from components in the blood plasma.

bronchiectasis (bron-kē-ek′tuh-sis) Dilatation of bronchi caused by weakening of their walls as a result of infection.

bronchiole (bron′ke-ōl) One of the small terminal subdivisions of the branched bronchial tree.

bronchus One of the large subdivisions of the trachea.

buffer A substance that minimizes change in pH of a solution when an acid or base is added.

bulimia nervosa Weight control by compulsive overeating followed by self-induced vomiting and other methods in order to prevent weight gain.

caged-ball valve An artificial heart valve consisting of a small ball in a metal cage in which the position of the ball in the cage determines the blood flow through the valve.

calcito′nin A hormone that lowers blood calcium, produced by the interfollicular cells of the thyroid gland.

cal′culus A stone formed within the body, as in the kidney or gallbladder.

capsid (kap′sid) The protein covering the central nucleic acid core of a virus.

capsomere (kap′sō-mēr) One of the subunits that make up the protein shell (*capsid*) of a virus.

carcinoembryonic antigen (CEA) (kär′sin-ō-em-bry-on′ik) A tumor-associated antigen that resembles the antigen secreted by the cells of the fetal gastrointestinal tract.

carcinoma (kär-sin-ō′-mah) A malignant tumor derived from epithelial cells.

cardiac arrest Complete cessation of cardiac activity.

cardiac catheterization A specialized technique to determine the blood flow through the chambers of the heart and to detect abnormal communications between cardiac chambers.

cardiac cycle The sequence of events during a single contraction and relaxation of the atria and ventricles.

cardiomyopathy (kar-dē-o-my-op′-a′thē) A general term for any noninflammatory disease of heart muscle.

cardiospasm (kär′-dē-o-spazm) Spasm of the lower gastroesophageal (cardiac) sphincter.

caries (ka′rēz) Tooth decay.

catecholamines (kat-eh-kōl′uh-mēnz) The adrenal medullary hormones *epinephrine* and *norepinephrine*.

cation (kat′ī-on) An ion that carries a positive charge.

cavity (dental) A loss of tooth structure caused by the combined action of mouth bacteria and organic acids derived from bacterial fermentation of retained food particles.

cell-mediated defense mechanism The defense against foreign antigens provided by a population of T lymphocytes that can attach and destroy the foreign antigens.

cell-mediated immunity Immunity associated with population of sensitized lymphocytes.

cellulitis (sell-ū-lī′tis) An acute spreading inflammation affecting the skin or deeper tissues.

cen′trioles Short cylindrical structures located adjacent to the nucleus that participate in the formation of spindle fibers during cell division.

cen′tromere The structure that joins each pair of chromatids formed by chromosome duplication.

cerebral embolus A stroke caused by blockage of a cerebral artery by a blood clot that had formed elsewhere in the circulatory system and was transported in the bloodstream to the brain.

cerebral hemorrhage A stroke caused by rupture of a cerebral artery, usually in a person with hypertension, which allows blood to escape under high pressure into the brain.

cerebral thrombosis A stroke caused by thrombosis of an arteriosclerotic cerebral artery.

cerebrovascular accident (CVA) An injury to the brain resulting in a disturbance of cerebral blood flow caused by a cerebral thrombosis, cerebral embolism, or cerebral hemorrhage.

chenodeoxycholic acid (kēn′-ō-dē-ox′i-ko′lik) A bile salt that is administered orally to promote dissolution of cholesterol gallstones by reducing the saturation of the bile with cholesterol.

Chlamydia (klä-mi′dē-uh) Small gram-negative organisms that are deficient in certain enzymes and must function as intracellular parasites.

cholecystitis (ko′lē-sis-tī′-tis) An inflammation of the gallbladder.

cholelithiasis (kō′lē-lith-ī′uh-sis) Formation of gallstones.

cholesterol (kō-les′ter-ol) A complex compound (*sterol*) containing several ring structures.

chordae tendineae (kor′dā ten-din′ē-ā) Fibrous cords that extend from the free margins of the atrioventricular valves to attach to the papillary muscles.

choriocarcinoma (kōr′rē-ō-kär-sin-ō′muh) A malignant proliferation of trophoblastic tissue.

chorion (kō′ri-on) The layer of trophoblast and associated mesoderm that surrounds the developing embryo.

chorionic vesicle The chorion with its villi and enclosed amnion, yolk sac, and developing embryo.

chorionic villi Fingerlike columns of cells extending from the chorion that anchor the chorionic vesicle in the endometrium.

chromatid (krō′mä-tid) One of two newly formed chromosomes held together by the centromere.

chromophobe cells (krō′-mo-fōb) Anterior lobe pituitary epithelial cells containing sparse poorly stained granules. See also *eosinophil* and *basophil*.

chronic thyroiditis An autoimmune disease in which an autoantibody directed against thyroid epithelial cells causes progressive destruction of the thyroid gland, leading to hypothyroidism. Also called *Hashimoto thyroiditis*.

cirrhosis of the liver (si-rō′sis) A disease characterized by diffuse intrahepatic scarring and liver cell degeneration.

clearance test (klēr′ans) A test of renal function that measures the ability of kidneys to remove (clear) a substance from the blood and excrete it in the urine.

cleft lip Defect in the upper lip of variable degree, as a result of a developmental disturbance.

cleft palate Defect in hard palate allowing communication between oral cavity and nasal cavity, as a result by a developmental disturbance.

clone (klōn) A group of identical cells produced from a single precursor cell.

Clostridium (klä-strid′ē-yum) Anaerobic gram-positive spore-forming rod-shaped bacterium.

clubfoot Congenital malposition of foot. In most common type, foot is turned inward at ankle and heel is elevated.

Coccidioides immitis (kok-sid-ē-oy′dēz im′mi-tis) A highly pathogenic fungus causing the disease coccidioidomycosis.

coccidioidomycosis (kok-sid-ē-oy′dō-mī-kō′sis) A disease caused by the pathogenic fungus *Coccidioides immitis*.

colitis (kō-lī′tis) Inflammation of the colon, such as chronic ulcerative colitis.

collateral circulation An accessory circulation capable of delivering blood to a tissue when the main circulation is blocked, as by a thrombus or embolus.

colloid An eosinophilic protein material present within the thyroid follicles.

colposcope (kol′pos-kōp) A binocular magnifying instrument used to view the cervix and endocervical canal.

coma Loss of consciousness, resulting from various causes.

communicable disease A disease transmitted from person to person.

computed tomographic (CT) scan (tō-mo-graf′ik) An x-ray technique producing detailed cross-sectional images of the body by means of x-ray tube and detectors connected to a computer. Sometimes called a CAT scan.

concussion A temporary loss of consciousness caused by a head injury without any memory of the events that occurred shortly before or after the head injury.

condyloma (kon-di-lō′ma) A warty tumorlike overgrowth in the squamous epithelium of the anorectal or genital tract, caused by a virus that is spread by sexual contact.

congen′ital Present at birth.

congenital cerebral aneurysm (an′ū-rizm) A saclike protrusion of the inner layer (*intima*) of a cerebral artery through a congenital defect in its muscular wall.

congenital polycystic kidney disease A hereditary condition characterized by formation of multiple, progressively enlarging cysts throughout both kidneys, which gradually destroy renal function.

conjoined twins Identical twins that are joined to one another and often share organs in common. Siamese twins.

conjugated bilirubin A more soluble form of bilirubin produced by the addition of two molecules of glucuronic acid to the bilirubin molecule.

consumption coagulopathy See *disseminated intravascular coagulation syndrome*.

cortex The outer layer of an organ. See also *medulla*.

corticotropin (kōr-tik-kō-trō′pin) Another name for adrenocorticotropic hormone (ACTH).

cortisol (kōr′ti-sol) The major glucocorticoid.

Corynebacterium (kōr-rī′nē-bak-te′rī-yum) An aerobic nonspore-forming gram-positive rod-shaped bacterium.

cotyledon (co-ti-lē′don) A unit of the placenta visible grossly on the maternal surface as an irregularly shaped lobe circumscribed by a depressed area.

crab louse A parasite of the pubic area; causes intense itching.

cranial fossa One of the depressions in the base of the skull, which is terraced to receive the undersurface of the brain.

creatinine (krē-at′in-ēn) A waste product derived from the breakdown of a compound present in muscle (phosphocreatine) that is excreted in the urine.

cretinism (krē′tin-izm) Hypothyroidism in the infant.

Crohn disease (krō′-nz) A chronic autoimmune disease characterized by segmental areas of inflammation and scarring within the intestine, often involving primarily the distal ileum. Also called *regional enteritis*.

crossover Interchange of genetic material between homologous chromosomes during synapse and meiosis.

cul-de-sac (kul′de-sak) A blind pouch or cavity. The term is commonly applied to the rectouterine pouch, a peritoneum-covered recess located between the posterior fornix of the vagina and the rectum.

cystic fibrosis Hereditary disease characterized by glandular dysfunction, eventually leading to serious disturbances of pancreatic, hepatic, and pulmonary function.

cystitis (sis-ti′tis) Inflammation of the bladder.

cytokine A general term for any protein secreted by cells that functions as an intercellular messenger and influences cells of the immune system. Cytokines are secreted by macrophages and monocytes (monokines), lymphocytes (lymphokines), and other cells.

cytomegalovirus (sī-tō-meg′u-lō-vī-rus) One of the herpes viruses. Causes an infectious mononucleosislike syndrome in adults; may cause congenital malformation in fetus.

cytopathogenic (sī-tō-path-ō-jen′ik) Pertaining to cell necrosis and degeneration.

cytoskeleton (sigh′-toe-skeleton) Protein tubules and filaments that form the structural framework of cells.

cytotoxic (sī-tō-tok′sik) Producing cell necrosis or destruction.

D & C Dilatation and curettage of the uterus. A scraping out of the uterine lining, often performed as a diagnostic or therapeutic procedure.

daughter cell A cell resulting from division of a single cell (called the *parent cell*).

decidua (de-sid′ū-ah) The endometrium of pregnancy.

deciduous (de-sid′ū-us) Pertaining to anything that is cast off at maturity, as for example the first set of teeth.

delta cells (del′tuh) Somatostatin-secreting cells of the pancreatic islets.

delta hepatitis A type of hepatitis caused by a defective virus that can infect only persons already infected with the hepatitis B virus.

dental plaque Masses of bacteria, bacterial products, and salivary proteins adherent to teeth, which predisposes to tooth decay.

dentine (den′tēn) Bony structure of the tooth.

deoxyribonucleic acid (DNA) The nucleic acid present in the chromosomes of the nuclei of cells that carries genetic information.

dermatomyositis (der-ma′to-mī-ō-sī′tis) A systemic disease characterized by inflammation and scarring of both skin and muscle.

dermatophyte (der-mat′o-fīt) A fungus that causes a superficial infection of the skin.

dermoid cyst (derm′oyd) A common type of benign cystic teratoma that commonly arises in the ovary.

DES See *diethylstilbestrol*.

desensitization A method of inducing a diminished response to allergens by inducing the formation of specific IgG and IgA antibodies.

diabetes insipidus (dī-u-bē′tēz in-sip′id-us) A condition resulting from a deficiency of antidiuretic hormone, characterized by excretion of a large volume of very dilute urine.

diabetes mellitus (dī-u-bē′tēz mel′lit-is) A metabolic disease characterized by hyperglycemia and caused by insufficient insulin secretion or inefficient utilization of insulin.

diabetic ketosis A disturbance of the body's acid–base balance (acidosis) caused by an inability to utilize glucose, which requires the body to use fat as an energy source. Fat metabolism generates excessive amounts of acid ketone bodies, which disrupts the normal alkalinity of body fluids.

diagno′sis The determination of the nature and cause of a patient's illness.

dial′ysis The diffusion of dissolved substances and water across a semipermeable membrane.

diaphragm (di′ä-fram) A partition separating one thing from another, applied to the dome-shaped partition between the thoracic and abdominal cavities. The term is also applied to a contraceptive device placed over the cervix prior to intercourse.

diastolic heart failure Heart failure caused by inadequate filling of the ventricles during diastole, in contrast to systolic heart failure in which ejection of blood from the ventricles during systole is inadequate.

diethylstilbestrol (DES) (dī-ethyl-stil-bes′trol) A nonsteroidal estrogen capable of inducing abnormalities in the genital tract of women whose mothers took the drug in pregnancy.

diffusion The process whereby particles of liquid, gas, or solids spread from a region of higher concentration to a region of lower concentration.

disease Any disturbance of the structure or function of the body.

dissecting aneurysm of the aorta (an′ūr-izm) A dissection of blood into the wall of the aorta secondary to degeneration of the arterial wall with an associated tear of the lining (*intima*) of the artery.

disseminated intravascular coagulation syndrome A disturbance of blood coagulation as a result of activation of the coagulation mechanism and simultaneous clot lysis.

diverticulitis (dī-vur-tik-u-lī′tis) An inflammation of a diverticulum.

diverticulosis (dī-vur-tik-u-lō′sis) A condition characterized by an outpouching of the colonic mucosa through weak areas in the muscular wall.

diverticulum (dī-vur-tik′u-lum) An outpouching from an organ, as from the mucosa of the colon, which projects through the muscular wall.

DNA repair genes Genes that monitor and correct errors in DNA replication during cell division.

dominant gene A gene that expresses a trait in the heterozygous state.

dopamine (dō′puh-mēn) Chemical mediator released by hypothalamic neurons.

dopamine agonist (do′-pă-mēn ag′-on-ist) A drug such as bromocriptine that combines with cell dopamine receptors and causes the same cell response that would be produced by dopamine, such as inhibition of prolactin secretion.

dopamine receptor (do′-pă-mēn rē-sep′ tōr) A protein molecule on the cell surface that binds to dopamine, which is a precursor of epinephrine and norepinephrine.

Down syndrome A congenital syndrome caused by an extra chromosome 21.

ductus arteriosus A fetal artery connecting the pulmonary artery with the aorta that permits pressure determined blood flow from pulmonary artery into the aorta, bypassing blood flow to the nonfunctional fetal lungs.

dura (dū′rä) The outer covering of the brain and spinal cord.

dysfunctional uterine bleeding (DUB) Irregular uterine bleeding caused by disturbance of the normal cyclic interaction of estrogen and progesterone on the endometrium.

dysmenorrhea (dis-men-ō-rhē′uh) Painful menstruation.

dysplasia (dis-plă′sē-yuh) Abnormal maturation of cells.

dyspnea (disp′nē-uh) Difficult or labored breathing.

E

ecchymosis (ek-im-ō′sis) A black-and-blue spot caused by extravasation of blood into the skin.

echocardiogram (eko′-kar-dē-o-gram′) A record obtained from an ultrasound examination of the heart and related blood vessels, used to assist in the diagnosis of cardiovascular disease.

eclampsia (ek-lamp′-sē-ă) One or more convulsions in a pregnant woman with preeclampsia.

ectoderm (ek′tō-derm) The outer germ layer in the embryo that gives rise to specific organs and tissues.

ectopic pregnancy A pregnancy outside the endometrial cavity.

edema (e-dē′muh) Accumulation of an excess of fluid in the interstitial tissues.

effector T cells Cytotoxic and delayed hypersensitivity T cells that protect the body by attacking and destroying body cells infected with bacteria or viruses.

electrocardiogram (ē lek-trō-kär′dē-ō-gram) A technique for measuring the serial changes in the electrical activity of the heart during the various phases of the cardiac cycle. (Often called ECG or EKG.)

electrolyte (ē-lek′trō-līt) A compound that in solution dissociates into positive and negative ions.

embolism (em′bō-lizm) A condition in which a plug composed of a detached clot, mass of bacteria, or other foreign material (*embolus*) occludes a blood vessel.

embryo (em′brē-ō) The developing human organism from the third through the seventh weeks of gestation.

embryonal carcinoma A malignant testicular tumor in which the malignant cells have features resembling rapidly growing trophoblastic tissue.

emphysema (em-fuh-sē′muh) A disease characterized by enlargement and distention of the pulmonary air spaces distal to the terminal bronchioles.

enamel Dense outer covering of the exposed surface of the tooth.

encephalitis (en-sef-äl-ī′tis) An inflammation of the brain.

encephalomalacia (en-seff′uh-lō-mu-lā′shuh) Cystic lesion of degenerated brain tissue as a result of obstruction of cerebral blood supply. Same as cerebral infarct.

endarterectomy (end-är-ter-ek′tō-mē) Surgical resection of arteriosclerotic lining of an artery to increase its caliber and improve blood flow through the vessel.

endemic disease (en-dem′ik) A communicable disease in which small numbers of cases are continually present in a population.

endochondral bone formation (en-dō-kon′drul) Formation of bone as, first, a cartilage model that is then reabsorbed and converted into bone.

endocrine glands A gland that discharges its secretions directly into the bloodstream, in contrast to an exocrine gland that discharges its secretion through a duct onto a mucosal surface.

endometrial cyst (en-dō-mē′trē-ul) An ovarian cyst lined by endometrium and filled with old blood and debris. A manifestation of endometriosis.

endometriosis (en-dō-mē trē-ō′sis) Presence of endometrial tissue in abnormal locations, such as in the ovary or pelvis.

endoplas′mic reticulum A mass of hollow tubular channels within the cytoplasm of the cell, frequently bordered by ribosomes.

endoscopy (en-däs′kō-pē) An examination of the interior of the body by means of various lighted tubular instruments.

endothelium (en-dō-thē′lē-um) The internal lining of blood vessels and interior of heart.

endovascular aneurysm repair A nonsurgical treatment of an abdominal aortic aneurysm in which the aneurysm graft is inserted through the femoral arteries, positioned within the aneurysm, and anchored within the aorta above and below the aneurysm.

Entamoeba histolytica (en-tuh-mē′buh his-tō-lit′ti-kä) A protozoan parasite causing amebiasis.

enteritis (en-ter-ī′tis) Inflammation of the intestine.

entoderm (en′tō-derm) The inner germ layer of the embryo that gives rise to specific organs and tissues.

eosinophil (ē-ō-sin′o-fil) A cell whose cytoplasm is filled with large, uniform granules that stain intensely red with acid dyes. See also *basophil.*

epidemic disease (ep-i-dem′ik) A communicable disease affecting concurrently large numbers of persons in a population.

epidural space (ep-i-dū′rul) Potential space between the dura and overlying cranial bones.

epinephrine (ep-in-ef′rin) One of the compounds (catecholamines) secreted by the adrenal medulla.

Epstein-Barr virus A virus that causes infectious mononucleosis.

erythroblast (e-rith′rō-blast) A precursor cell in the bone marrow that gives rise to red blood cells.

erythropoiesis (er-ith′rō-poy-ē′sis) Production of red blood cells.

erythropoietin (er-ith-rō-poy′e-tin) A humoral substance made by the kidneys that regulates hematopoiesis.

esophageal varices (var′i-sēz) Dilated (varicose) veins of the esophagus, which are often present in patients with cirrhosis of the liver.

etiology (ē-tē-ol′ō-jē) The cause, especially the cause of a disease.

exchange transfusion Partial replacement of blood of infant with hemolytic disease by blood lacking the antigen responsible for hemolytic disease, as when transfusing Rh-negative blood to an Rh-positive infant. Performed to reduce intensity of hemolytic jaundice.

exocrine gland A gland that discharges its secretions through a duct onto a mucosal surface, in contrast to an endocrine gland that delivers its secretions directly into the bloodstream.

exon The part of a chromosomal DNA chain that codes for a specific protein or enzyme.

exophthalmic goiter (ex-āf-thal′-mik) Another term for Graves disease, named for the protrusion of the eyes seen in many patients with this disease.

exudate (ex′yū-dāt) The fluid, leukocytes, and debris that accumulate as a result of an inflammation.

F

fatty acid A long, straight-chain carbon compound that contains a terminal carboxyl group, which enters into the formation of a triglyceride.

feedback mechanism A mechanism whereby the output of a hormone by a target gland controls the release of the regulatory hormone that stimulates the target gland.

fetal hemoglobin A type of hemoglobin containing two alpha and two gamma chains, which is able to take up and release oxygen at much lower PO_2 (oxygen partial pressure) than in adult hemoglobin.

fe′tus The unborn offspring after 8 weeks' gestation.

fibrillation (fi-bril-lā′shun) Uncoordinated quivering of cardiac muscle that prevents normal contraction of the heart muscle.

fibrin The meshwork of protein threads that form during the clotting of the blood.

fibrin monomer (mä′nō-mer) A derivative of fibrinogen that polymerizes to form the fibrin clot during blood coagulation.

fibrinogen (fī-brin′ō-jen) A precursor in plasma converted into fibrin by thrombin during blood coagulation.

fibrinolysin (fī-brin-o-lī′-sin) A component of blood plasma capable of dissolving fibrin clots.

filtration membrane The thin membrane covering the filtration slit between pedicels of the podocytes that cover the glomerular capillaries of the kidneys.

filtration slits The narrow spaces between the pedicels of the podocytes that cover the glomerular capillaries of the kidneys.

flagellum (fla-jel′um) A whiplike process that propels an organism or sperm.

follicle-stimulating hormone (FSH) One of the gonadotropic hormones secreted by the anterior lobe of the pituitary, which regulates growth and function of the gonads (ovary and testis).

foot processes The highly branched cytoplasmic processes of the podocytes covering the glomerular capillaries of the kidneys.

foramen ovale An opening in the atrial septum covered by a one-way flap valve regulated by pressure differences between the atria, permitting blood flow from right to left atrium but not in the opposite direction, thereby bypassing blood flow from right cardiac chambers to the nonfunctional fetal lungs.

fracture (frak-tūr) A broken bone.

frozen section A method of rapid diagnosis of tumors used by the pathologist; tissue is frozen solid, cut into thin sections, stained, and examined microscopically.

FSH See *follicle-stimulating hormone.*

functional disease A disease that is not associated with any recognizable structural changes in the body.

G

galactorrhea (gā-lak-tō-rē′yuh) Secretion of milk by breast not associated with pregnancy or normal lactation.

gametes Reproductive cells, eggs, and sperm, each containing 23 chromosomes, which unite during fertilization to form a zygote containing 46 chromosomes.

gam′ēto gen′esis The development of mature eggs and sperm from precursor cells.

gamma globulin (gam′ah glob′ū-lin) A protein antibody found in the blood.

gangrene (gang-grēn′) Term has two different meanings. Refers to (1) infection caused by gas-forming anaerobic bacteria (*gas gangrene*) or (2) necrosis of an extremity caused by interruption of its blood supply (*ischemic gangrene*).

gastric bypass An operation to treat massive obesity in which the capacity of the stomach is reduced.

gene (jēn) A unit of heredity located at a definite position (*locus*) on a chromosome.

gene mutation A change in the structure of a gene, which may alter its functions.

gene product A protein or enzyme specified (coded) by a gene.

gene splicing Same as recombinant DNA technology.

gene therapy Treating cells by inserting a gene into the cell to accomplish a specific purpose, such as supplying a missing enzyme in a subject with a genetic disease.

genetic code (jen-et′ik kōd) The information carried by the codons of DNA molecules in chromosomes.

genetic engineering Same as recombinant DNA technology.

genome (jee′ nōm) The total of all the genes contained in a cell's chromosomes.

genomics (jen ōm′ iks) The study of the genome, with special reference to the effect of genetic variations on the expression of a gene, such as susceptibility or resistance to a disease.

germ disk A three-layered cluster of cells that will eventually give rise to an embryo.

germ layers The three layers of cells derived from the inner cell mass, each layer destined to form specific organs and tissues in the embryo.

gestational diabetes Elevated blood glucose caused by insulin resistance resulting from elevated hormones related to the pregnancy. Blood glucose returns to normal postpartum, but woman has increased risk of diabetes later in life.

gestational trophoblast disease (jes-tay′-shun-ul tro′-fo-blast) A general term for all diseases characterized by abnormal trophoblast proliferation. Includes both hydatidiform mole and choriocarcinoma.

Giardia (jē-är′-dē-uh) A small pear-shaped parasite that causes an acute inflammation of the small intestine.

glioma (glē-ō′muh) Any brain tumor arising from glial (supporting) cells of the brain.

glomerulonephritis (glo-mär′ū-lō-nef-rī′tis) An inflammation of the glomeruli caused by either antigen–antibody complexes trapped in the glomeruli or by antiglomerular basement membrane antibodies.

glomerulosclerosis (glo-mēr′ū-lō-skler-rō′sis) Diffuse and nodular thickening of glomerular basement membranes, a common occurrence in patients with long-standing diabetes mellitus.

gluten enteropathy Damage to intestinal villi caused by ingesting gluten-containing foods by persons sensitive to a protein in gluten; characterized by passage of large bulky stools containing a large amount of poorly absorbed fat.

glu′cocorticoid An adrenal cortical hormone that regulates carbohydrate metabolism.

α-glucosidase (glu-kō-si-dās) **inhibitor** Inhibitor of an enzyme required to break down a glucose-containing disaccharide so glucose can be absorbed from the small intestine.

glycated hemoglobin (gli-ko′-sil-ay-ted) Hemoglobin to which glucose molecules have become permanently attached. Concentration is related to concentration of glucose in the blood.

glycated hemoglobin test A test that measures the amount of glucose permanently attached to hemoglobin, which is higher than normal in many persons with diabetes.

glycogen (glī′kō-jen) A storage form of glucose present chiefly in liver and muscle.

goiter (goy′ter) Any enlargement of the thyroid gland.

Golgi apparatus (gol′jē) A group of membrane-lined sacs found in the cytoplasm of the cell near the nucleus.

gonad (gō′nad) A general term referring to either the ovary or the testis.

gonadotrop′in A hormone produced by the anterior lobe of the pituitary gland that controls the function of the gonads.

gout A disorder of nucleoprotein metabolism characterized by elevated uric acid and deposition of uric acid in and around joints.

granulosa cells (gran-u-lō′suh) Cells lining the ovarian follicles.

granulosa cell tumor (gran-u-lō′suh) A tumor arising from granulosa cells, usually associated with excess production of estrogen.

granulosa-theca cell tumor An estrogen-producing, ovarian tumor arising from the estrogen-producing granulosa cell of an ovarian follicle.

Graves disease An autoimmune thyroid disease in which autoantibodies resembling thyroid-stimulating hormone stimulate an excessive output of thyroid hormone, causing hyperthyroidism.

growth factor A soluble growth promoting substance produced by cells that attaches to receptors on the cell membrane of other cells, which activates the receptors and initiates events leading to growth or division of the target cells.

growth hormone An anterior lobe pituitary hormone that stimulates growth of bone and other body tissues.

gubernaculum (goo′-ber-nak′-ū-lum) A band of fibrous tissue extending from the fetal testis into the scrotum that promotes descent of the testis.

Guillain Barré syndrome (gil′yän bär rā′) A type of polyneuritis resulting from an autoimmune reaction to myelin.

gynecomastia (gī-ne-ko-mas′ti-uh) Excessive development of the male breast.

H

haplotype (hap′lō-tīp) A set of HLA genes on one chromosome that is transmitted as a set.

Hashimoto thyroiditis Another name for chronic thyroiditis.

heart block Delay or complete interruption of impulse transmission from the atria to the ventricles.

hematoma (hēm-uh-tō′muh) A large collection of blood in the tissues, such as might occur if coagulation factors are deficient.

heme (hēm) An iron porphyrin complex. Part of the hemoglobin molecule.

hemiplegia (hem-ē-plē′-jē-uh) Paralysis of one side of the body.

hemizy′gous A term applied to genes located on the X chromosome in the male.

hemochromatosis (hemo-crow-mah-toe′-sis) A genetic disease characterized by excessive iron absorption, leading to accumulation of excessive amounts of iron in the body, causing organ damage.

hemodialysis (hēm-ō-dī-al′i-sis) A dialysis procedure by which waste products are removed from the blood of patients in chronic renal failure, usually by means of an artificial kidney machine.

hemoglobin An oxygen transport protein within red cells composed of an iron-porphyrin complex (heme) combined with a protein chain (globin).

hemolysis (hēm-ol′i-sis) Destruction of red blood cells with escape of hemoglobin into the surrounding medium.

hemolytic anemia An anemia caused by increased blood destruction.

hemolytic disease of the newborn A hemolytic anemia resulting from maternal sensitization and antibody formation to fetal blood group antigens, leading to destruction of fetal cells.

hemophilia (hē-mō-fil′ē-yuh) A sex-linked coagulation disturbance characterized by a deficiency of antihemophilic globulin.

hemorrhoids (hem′or-oyds) Varicosities of anal and rectal veins.

he′mo sid′erin One of the storage forms of iron.

heparin An anticoagulant obtained from the liver.

hepatitis (hep-ah-tī′tis) Inflammation of the liver.

hepatitis B core antigen The antigen contained in the core of the hepatitis B virus.

hepatitis Be antigen One of the antigens associated with the hepatitis B virus.

hepatitis B surface antigen The coating of the hepatitis B virus that is also found in great excess in the blood of infected patients.

hernia (her′nē-yuh) A protrusion of a loop of bowel through a narrow opening, usually in the abdominal wall.

herniated intervertebral disk (interver′tē-bral) Protrusion of the nucleus pulposus through a tear in the annulus.

heterophile antibody (het′er-o-fīle) A type of antibody, capable of agglutinating sheep red cells, that is formed in patients with infectious mononucleosis.

heterozygous (het′er-o-zī′gus) Having two different alleles at given gene loci on the homologous pair of chromosomes.

high-density lipoprotein (HDL) cholesterol (li-pō-prō′tēn kō-les′ter-ol) The fraction of cholesterol carried by high-density lipoprotein, which is correlated with protection against atherosclerosis.

histocompatibility complex A cluster of genes on chromosome 6 that determines antigens on the surface of cells.

Histoplasma capsulatum (his′tō-plas′-muh kap-sōō-lā′tum) A highly pathogenic fungus causing the disease histoplasmosis.

histoplasmosis (his′tō-plas-mō′sis) An infection caused by the fungus *Histoplasma capsulatum.*

HLA A shortened form for *human leukocyte antigens.* Antigens on the surface of cells determined by genes of the major histocompatibility complex.

HLA system The genes of the histocompatibility complex and the antigens that they determine on the surface of cells.

Hodgkin's disease One type of lymphoma.

homol′ogous chromosomes A matched pair of chromosomes, one derived from each parent.

homozygous (hō-mo-zī′gus) Possessing identical alleles at a given locus on each of a pair of homologous chromosomes.

host Individual infected with a disease-producing organism.

human chorionic gonadotropin (HCG) (kōr-ē-on′ik gō-na-dō-trō′pin) A hormone made by the placenta in pregnancy having actions similar to pituitary gonadotropins. Same hormone is made by neoplastic cells in some types of malignant testicular tumors.

Human Genome Project (jee′-nōm) An international collaboration of scientists who mapped the nucleotide sequence of the entire human genome.

human leukocyte antigens Unique histocompatibility antigens (self-antigens) on the surface of cells. Also called major histocompatibility complex (MHC) antigens.

human papillomavirus (HPV) (pap-i-lō′ma-vī-rus) A virus that stimulates epithelial cell proliferation. Causes warts and genital tract condylomas.

human placental lactogen (HPL) (lak′tō-jen) One of the hormones produced by the placenta that has properties similar to pituitary growth hormone.

humoral immunity Immunity associated with formation of antibodies produced by plasma cells.

Huntington disease A hereditary autosomal dominant disease characterized by degeneration of basal brain nuclei concerned with regulation of automatic motor functions, leading to abnormal uncoordinated spasmodic involuntary movements, and degeneration of cortical neurons leading to dementia.

hydatidiform mole (hī-da-tid′i-form mōl) A neoplastic proliferation of trophoblast associated with formation of large cystic villi.

hydrocele (hī′-drō-cēl) An accumulation of excess fluid within the tunica vaginalis of the testis.

hydrocephalus Dilatation of the ventricular system caused by pressure arising from accumulation of cerebrospinal fluid within the ventricles.

hydronephrosis (hydro-nef-rō′sis) A dilatation of the urinary drainage tract proximal to the site of an obstruction.

hydrostat′ic pressure Pressure that filters fluid from the blood through the capillary endothelium.

hydrothorax (hī-drō-thor′ax) Accumulation of fluid in the pleural cavity.

hydroureter A dilatation of the ureter secondary to obstruction of the urinary drainage system, often associated with coexisting dilatation of the renal pelvis and calyces (*hydronephrosis*).

hypercholesterolemia (hī′per-ko-les′ter-ol-ē′mi-uh) Excessive concentration of cholesterol in the blood.

hyperglycemia (hī-per-glī-sē′mi-uh) Excessively high blood glucose concentration.

hyperglyceridemia (hī-per-glis′er-id-ē′mi-uh) An elevated concentration of triglycerides in the blood.

hyperosmolar coma (hī-per-oz-mō′lär) Coma resulting from neurologic dysfunction caused by hyperosmolarity of body fluids as a consequence of severe hyperglycemia.

hyperplasia (hī-per-plā′sēē-uh) An increase in the number of cells.

hypersensitivity A state of abnormal reactivity to a foreign material.

hypertension High blood pressure.

hyperton′ic Having an osmotic pressure (*osmolarity*) greater than that of body fluids.

hypertonic solution A solution having a greater osmolarity than body fluids, which causes cells to shrink in such a solution because water moves by osmosis from the cells into the hypertonic solution.

hyper′trophy An enlargement or overgrowth of an organ caused by an increase in size of its constituent cells.

hyphae (hī′fāy) Filamentous branching structures formed by fungi.

hypoglycemia (hī-pō-glī-sē′mē-ah) Lower than normal concentration of glucose in the blood.

hy′pothal′amus A portion of the brain stem that forms the floor of the third ventricle. It contains clusters of nerve cells that regulate various body functions.

hypotonic solution A solution having a lower osmolarity than body fluids, causing cells in the solution to swell because water moves by osmosis from the hypotonic solution into the cells.

I

idiopathic scoliosis (id′-ē-opath′-ik skō-lē-ō′-sis) Lateral curvature of the spine. Idiopathic means cause of condition is unknown.

ileal bypass A surgical procedure performed on the small intestine to promote weight loss.

immune response genes Genes on chromosome 6 that control the immune response to specific antigens.

immunity Resistance to disease.

immunoglobulin (im′mū-nō-glob′u-lin) An antibody protein.

immunotherapy (im′mū-nō-ther′uh-pē) Treatment given to retard growth of a disseminated malignant tumor by stimulating to body's own immune defenses.

imperforate anus (im-per′for-āt) Congenital absence of anal opening, often associated with absence of distal rectum as well.

inclusion bodies Spherical structures in the nucleus or cytoplasm of virus-infected cells.

infarct (in′färkt) Necrosis of tissue caused by interruption of its blood supply.

infection Inflammation caused by a disease-producing organism.

inflamma′tion A reaction produced by an irritant or infectious agent, characterized by swelling of the affected tissue as a result of vascular congestion and exudation of fluid and white blood cells.

inguinal canal (in′gwin-ul) An oblique tunnel in the muscles of the abdominal wall through which the testes and spermatic cords descend into the scrotum.

inner cell mass A group of cells that are derived from the fertilized ovum and are destined to form the embryo.

in situ carcinoma (in-sī′tū kär-sin-ō′muh) A malignant epithelial tumor that is still confined to the surface epithelium and has not yet invaded deeper tissues.

insulin (in′su-lin) A hormone that lowers blood glucose, produced by the beta cells of the pancreas.

interferon (in-tur-fēr′on) A broad-spectrum antiviral agent manufactured by various cells in the body.

interleukin-2 (inter-loō′kin) A lymphokine that stimulates growth of lymphocytes.

interstitial (in-tur-stish′al) Pertaining to the spaces between the cells.

interver′tebral disk A fibrocartilaginous joint between adjacent vertebral bodies.

intramem′branous bone formation Direct formation of bone by osteoblasts without prior formation of a cartilage model.

intrauterine device (IUD) A small plastic device inserted in the uterus to prevent pregnancy.

intron A noncoding part of a chromosomal DNA chain.

intussusception (in′tus-us-cep′shun) A telescoping of one segment of bowel into an adjacent segment.

invasive mole An aggressive hydatidiform mole that invades the uterine wall.

ischemia (iss-kē′mē-uh) Reduced blood flow to a tissue or organ.

ischemic heart disease (iss-kē′mik) Used synonymously with coronary heart disease. Designates heart disease as a result of inadequate blood flow through the coronary arteries.

islets of Langerhans (län′ger-hänz) Cluster of endocrine cells in the pancreas.

isoton′ic Having an osmotic pressure (*osmolarity*) equal to that of body fluids.

isotonic solution A solution having essentially the same osmolarity as body fluids so that cells neither shrink nor swell when exposed to the solution.

isotope (ī′sō-tōp) A substance that emits a characteristic radiation; used in medicine to label various substances as a means of determining their uptake and excretion.

J

jaundice (jawn′dis) Yellow color of the skin that results from accumulation of bile pigment within the blood.

juxtaglomerular apparatus (jux′tu-glo-mär′ū-lär) A specialized group of cells at the vascular pole of the glomerulus that regulates blood flow through the glomerulus of the kidneys.

K

karyotype (kar-ē-ō-type) An arrangement of chromosomes from a single cell arrangement in pairs in descending order according to size of the chromosomes and the positions of the centromeres.

ker′atin An insoluble sulfur-containing protein that is the principal constituent of the hair and nails.

keratinocyte (ker-u-tin′ō-cyte) A keratin-forming cell in the epidermis.

ketone bodies Various derivatives of acetyl-CoA, resulting from excessive mobilization of fat as an energy source.

ketosis (kē-tō′sis) An excess of ketone bodies (acetoacetic acid, beta-hydroxybutyric acid, and acetone) in the blood resulting from utilization of fat as the primary source of energy.

kinin (kī′nin) A chemical mediator of inflammation formed from components in plasma; same as *bradykinin.*

Klinefelter syndrome (klīn′felt-er) A congenital syndrome caused by an extra X chromosome in the male. Characterized by testicular atrophy, sterility, feminine body configuration, and subnormal intelligence.

L

laparoscope (lap′-ă-rō-skōp) A long tubular telescopelike instrument passed through the abdominal wall to examine structures within the peritoneal cavity.

latent infection An infection without clinical symptoms.

lecithin (les′ith-in) A phosphorus-containing lipid (*phospholipid*) having detergent properties similar to bile salts.

Legionnaires' disease A type of pneumonia caused by an airborne bacterium called *Legionella pneumophila.*

lentigo maligna A precancerous, pigmented skin lesion arising from proliferation of atypical melanin-producing epithelial cells (melanocytes).

lesion (lē′shun) Any structural abnormality or pathologic change.

leukemia (loō-kē′mē-yuh) A neoplastic proliferation of leukocytes.

leukocyte (loō′kō-sīt) A general term for a white blood cell.

leukopenia (loō-kō-pē′ni-uh) An abnormally small number of leukocytes in the peripheral blood.

leukoplakia A white patch of hyperplastic and usually atypical squamous epithelium on the oral mucosa or genital tract mucosa.

leukotriene (loō-kō-try′-ēn) A prostaglandinlike mediator of inflammation.

LH See *luteinizing hormone.*

lipoprotein (li-pō-prō′tēn) A protein that carries cholesterol and other lipids in the blood.

liver lobule A histologic subdivision of the liver in which columns of liver cells converge toward a central vein and portal tracts are located at the periphery.

locus The position of a gene on a chromosome. Different forms (*alleles*) of the same gene are always found at the same locus on a chromosome.

low-density lipoprotein (LDL) cholesterol (li-pō-prō′tēn kō-les′ter-all) The fraction of cholesterol carried by low-density lipoproteins, which is correlated with atherosclerosis.

lung acinus (ä-sīn′us) A cluster of respiratory bronchioles and their subdivisions derived from a single terminal bronchiole. Same as *respiratory unit.*

lung lobule A small group of terminal bronchioles and their subdivisions.

lupus erythematosus (loō′pus er-i-thē-muh-tō′sis) A type of autoimmune connective tissue disease.

luteinizing hormone (LH) One of the gonadotropic hormones secreted by the anterior lobe of the pituitary that regulates growth and function of the gonads (ovary and testis).

Lyme disease (lī'm) A tick-borne systemic infection caused by a spiral organism, *Borrelia burgdorferi*, characterized by neurologic, joint, and cardiac manifestations.

lymphadenitis (limf-a-den-ī'tis) An inflammation of lymph nodes draining a site of infection.

lymphangitis (limf'an-jī'tis) An inflammation of lymph vessels draining a site of infection.

lymphocyte (limf'ō-sīt) A mononuclear blood cell produced in lymphoid tissue that takes part in cell-mediated and humoral immunity.

lymphokine (limf'ō-kīn) A soluble substance liberated by lymphocytes.

lymphoma (limf-ō'muh) A neoplasm of lymphoid cells.

Lyon hypothesis Concept of random inactivation of one X chromosome in cells of females, so that the number of functioning X chromosomes in males and females is equivalent.

ly'sosome A small cytoplasmic vacuole containing digestive enzymes.

M

macroglobulin One type of immunoglobulin of high molecular weight.

macrophage (mak'ro-f āj) A wandering phagocytic cell found in the blood and tissues.

magnetic resonance imaging (MRI) A diagnostic procedure that yields computer-generated images based on the movement of hydrogen atoms in tissues subjected to a strong magnetic field.

major histocompatibility complex (his-tō'com-pat-i-bil'i-tē) A group of genes on chromosome 6 that determine the antigens on the surface of cells.

Mallory body An irregular red-staining structure in the cytoplasm of injured liver cells, usually resulting from alcohol-induced liver injury.

mammogram (mam'ō-gram) An x-ray of the breast, used to detect tumors and other abnormalities within the breast.

Marfan (mahr-fahn') **syndrome** A connective tissue disease characterized by skeletal and cardiovascular abnormalities.

mast cell A specialized connective tissue cell containing granules filled with histamine and other chemical mediators.

matrix (mā'trix) Material in which connective tissue cells are embedded.

Meckel diverticulum (dī-vur-tik'kū-lum) A tubular outpouching from the distal ileum; remnant of the vitelline duct.

mediastinum (mē-de-as-tī'num) The central partition that separates the pleural cavities. It contains the heart, major blood vessels, and other midline structures.

mediators of inflammation Chemical agents released from mast cells and certain blood proteins (kinins and complement) in response to tissue injury.

medulla (med-ul'ah) The innermost part of an organ. See also *cortex*.

megaloblast (meg'al-ō-blast) An abnormal red cell precursor resulting from vitamin B_{12} or folic acid deficiency.

meiosis (mī-o'sis) A special type of cell division occurring in *gametes* (ova and sperm), in which the number of chromosomes is reduced by one-half in the ovum and sperm.

mel'anin Dark pigment found in the skin, in the middle coat of the eye, and in some other regions.

melanin-stimulating hormone (MSH) One of the hormones produced by the pituitary. Causes darkening of the skin.

melanocyte (me-lan'o-cyte) Melanin-producing cell in the epidermis.

melanoma (mel-uh-nō'muh) A malignant tumor of pigment-producing cells.

meninges (men-in'jēz) The membranes covering the brain and spinal cord.

meningioma (men-in-jē-ō'muh) A benign tumor arising from the meninges.

meningitis (men-in-jī'tis) Inflammation of the meninges.

meningocele (men-in'go-sēl) A protrusion of meninges through a defect in the spinal vertebral arches.

meningomyelocele (men-ing-gō-mī'el-ō-sēl) A type of spina bifida characterized by protrusion of meninges and cord through the defect in the vertebral arches.

mesangial cell (mes-an'jē-yul) Modified connective tissue cells at the vascular pole of the glomerulus that hold the capillary tuft together.

mesoderm (me'zō-derm) The middle germ layer of the embryo, which gives rise to specific organs and tissues.

mesothelium (me-sō-thē'li-um) A layer of flat squamous epithelial cells that covers the surfaces of the pleural, pericardial, and peritoneal cavities.

metabolic syndrome A group of conditions consisting of obesity, hypertension, elevated blood glucose, and blood lipids, which predisposes to cardiovascular disease and diabetes.

metaplasia (met-uh-plā'sē-yuh) A change from one type of cell to a more resistant cell type.

metas'tasis The spread of cancer cells from the primary site of origin to a distant site within the body.

metastasize (me-tas'tuh-sīz) To spread to distant sites, as applied to the spread of a malignant tumor.

metazoa (me'tuh-zō-uh) Complex multicelled animal parasites, such as worms and flukes.

micelle (mi-sell') An aggregate of bile salt and lecithin molecules by which cholesterol is brought into solution in bile.

microcytic hypochromic anemia (mīk-ro-sit'ik hī-pō-krō'mik) An anemia characterized by red cells that are smaller than normal and have a reduced concentration of hemoglobin, usually because of chronic iron deficiency.

microglia (mī-krog'-lē-ă) Phagocytic cells of the nervous system comparable to macrophages in other tissues.

microRNA A unique RNA that regulates the activity of individual genes.

miliary tuberculosis (mi'lē-air-ē) Multiple foci of tuberculosis throughout the body as a result of bloodstream dissemination of tubercle bacilli from a primary focus in the lung or peribronchial lymph nodes.

milliosmol (mOsm) (mil ī-oz'mol) A unit of osmotic activity that depends upon the number of dissolved particles in a solution.

mineralocorticoid (min'ril-ō-kor'tik-oid) Adrenal cortical hormone that regulates salt and water metabolism.

mitochondria (mīt-o-kon′drē-uh) Rod-shaped structures in the cell capable of converting foods into energy to power the cell.

mito′sis The type of cell division of most cells in which chromosomes are duplicated in the daughter cells and are identical with those in the parent cell. The characteristic cell division found in all cells in the body except for the gametes.

monocyte (mon′ō-sīt) A leukocyte having a kidney-shaped nucleus and light blue cytoplasm; a phagocytic cell that forms part of the reticuloendothelial system.

monokine A cytokine secreted by monocytes and macrophages.

monoso′my A condition of a cell in which one chromosome of a homologous pair is missing.

morphology (mor-fähl′ō-jē) Structure or architecture of a tissue or organ.

mor′ula A mulberry-shaped solid cluster of cells formed by division of the fertilized ovum.

motor neuron A neuron that carries nerve impulses from the brain and spinal cord to muscles and glands.

MRI See *magnetic resonance imaging.*

MSH See *melanin-stimulating hormone.*

multifactorial inheritance Inheritance of a trait or condition related to the combined effect of multiple genes rather than a single gene, as in Mendelian inheritance.

multiple myeloma (my-el-ō′muh) A malignant neoplasm of plasma cells.

multiple sclerosis Chronic disease characterized by focal areas of demyelination in the central nervous system, followed by glial scarring.

muscle tone The slight contractility (tension) present in resting muscles.

muscular dystrophy (dis′trō-fē) A hereditary disturbance of a skeletal muscle leading to necrosis and degeneration of muscle.

mutation (mū-tā′shun) An alteration in a base sequence in DNA; may alter cell function. Transmitted from parents to offspring only if mutation is in gametes.

mutator gene A gene that monitors and corrects errors in DNA duplication during cell division. Same as *DNA repair gene.*

myasthenia gravis (mī-as-thē′nē-uh grä′vis) An autoimmune disease characterized by abnormal fatigability of muscle and caused by an autoantibody that damages the acetylcholine receptors at the myoneural junction.

mycelium (mī-sē′lē-yum) Matted mass of hyphae forming a fluffy colony characteristic of fungi.

mycoplasma (mī-kō-plas′muh) Small bacteria lacking a cell wall.

myelin (my′e-lin) The fatty insulating material surrounding nerve fibers.

myelitis (mī-el-ī′tis) An inflammation of the spinal cord.

myelodysplastic syndrome (my′elo-dis-plas′tik) A disturbance of bone marrow function that is characterized by anemia, leukopenia, and thrombocytopenia and that may be a precursor to leukemia in some patients.

myelogram (mī′el-′o-gram) A procedure for visualizing the contour of the dural sac surrounding the spinal cord and nerve roots by injection of a radiopaque material into the dural sac.

myocardial infarction (mī-o-kar′dī-ul in-färk′shun) Necrosis of heart muscle as a result of interruption of its blood supply.

May affect full thickness of muscle wall (*transmural infarct*) or only part of the wall (*subendocardial infarct*).

myoma (mī-ō′muh) A benign smooth muscle tumor such as commonly develops in the uterus.

myoneural junction (mī-o-nū′ral) The specialized communication between motor nerve endings and muscle cells.

myositis (mī-ō-sī′tis) Inflammation of muscle.

myxedema (mix-uh-de′muh) Hypothyroidism in the adult.

N

natural killer cells Lymphocytes capable of destroying foreign or abnormal cells, although they have not had any prior antigenic contact with the cells.

necrosis (nek-rō′sis) Structural changes associated with cell death.

Neisseria (nī-sēr′ē-uh) Gram-negative diplococci, some species of which cause meningitis and gonorrhea.

neoplasia (nē-ō-plā′se-yuh) The pathologic process that results in the formation and growth of a tumor.

nephron (nef′rän) The glomerulus and renal tubule.

nephrosclero′sis Thickening and narrowing of the afferent glomerular arterioles as a result of disease.

nephrotic syndrome (nef-rä′tik sin′drōm) A generalized edema resulting from excessive protein loss in the urine, caused by various types of renal disease.

neural tube The ectodermal tube formed in the embryo that gives rise to the brain and spinal cord.

neuroglia (noo-rog′-lē-ah) Supporting cells of tissue of the nervous system.

neuron (nū′ron) A nerve cell, including the nerve cell body and its processes.

neutrophil (nū′trō-fil) A leukocyte having a multilobed nucleus whose cytoplasm is filled with fine granules.

nevus (nē′vus) A benign tumor of pigment-producing cells.

NK cells An abbreviation for natural killer cells.

Nonalcoholic fatty liver Fatty liver without significant inflammation or scarring within the liver, which usually occurs in insulin-resistant obese subjects with lipid abnormalities.

Nonalcoholic steatohepatitis Fat-associated liver damage associated with inflammation and scarring similar to the features seen in alcohol-related liver disease.

non nucleoside reverse transcriptase inhibitors Drugs used to treat HIV infections that bind to reverse transcriptase, blocking DNA polymerase that converts RNA to DNA.

nontoxic goiter Thyroid enlargement not associated with overproduction of thyroid hormone.

noradrenaline (nor-ad-ren′a-lin) Another name for *norepinephrine,* one of the hormones of the adrenal medulla.

norepinephrine (nor′ep-in-ef′rin) One of the compounds (*catecholamines*) secreted by the adrenal medulla.

normocytic anemia (nor-mō-sit′ik) An anemia characterized by red cells having normal size and hemoglobin concentrations.

nucleoside analogs "Look alike compounds" that resemble normal nucleosides required for viral DNA synthesis, and which disrupt DNA synthesis when used by a virus instead of the required normal nucleosides.

nucleoside reverse transcriptase inhibitors Nucleoside analogs ("look alike compounds") that resemble the normal nucleosides that a virus uses to construct DNA. Synthesis is disrupted when the analog substitutes for the required nucleoside.

nucleus pulposus (nū′klē-us) The soft elastic center of the intervertebral disk.

O

oligodendroglia (ol′ig-ō-den-drog′li-ah) One type of neuroglia that surrounds nerve fibers within the central nervous system.

oligohydramnios (ol-ig-ō-hī-dram′nē-yus) An insufficient quantity of amnionic fluid.

oncogene (on′-koh-jēn) An abnormally functioning gene that causes unrestrained cell growth leading to formation of a tumor. Results from mutation or translocation of a proto-oncogene.

one-second forced expiratory volume (FEV₁) The maximum volume of air that can be expelled from the lungs in 1 second.

oocyte (ō-ō-sīt) A developing ovum contained within a follicle in the ovary.

oogenesis (ō-ō-jen′es-is) Formation and development of the mature ovum from the oocyte.

open surgical aneurysm repair A surgical procedure in which an aortic aneurysm is opened; a graft is placed within the aneurysm sac and sutured to the aorta above and below the aneurysm so that the blood flows through the graft rather than through the aneurysm.

opportunistic infection (op-por-too-nis′tik) An infection in an immunocompromised person caused by an organism that is normally nonpathogenic or of limited pathogenicity.

optic chiasm (kī′asm) The point where the fibers of the optic nerves of each eye cross.

organ A group of different tissues organized to perform a specific function.

organ systems A group of organs that function together as a unit, such as the various organs of the gastrointestinal tract.

organelle A small structure present in the cytoplasm of the cell, such as a mitochondrion.

organic disease A disease associated with structural changes in the affected tissue or organ.

osmol The standard unit of osmotic pressure. See also *milliosmol.*

osmolar′ity A measure of the osmotic pressure exerted by a solution.

osmo′sis Passage of a solvent, such as water, through a semipermeable membrane from a solution of lesser to one of greater solute concentration.

ossifica′tion The process of forming bone.

osteoarthritis (ä′stē-ō) A "wear and tear" degeneration of the major weight-bearing joints.

osteogen′esis imperfec′ta A congenital disturbance of bone formation characterized by excessively thin and delicate bones that are easily broken.

osteomalacia (ä′stē-ō-măh-lāy′see-yăh) Impaired calcification of bone in an adult caused by vitamin D deficiency, which also contributes to bone loss caused by osteoporosis.

osteomyelitis (ä′stē-ō-mī-el-ī′tis) An inflammation of bone.

osteoporosis (ä′stē-ō-por-ō′sis) Generalized thinning and demineralization of bone that tends to occur in postmenopausal women.

oxyhemoglobin (ox-ē-hēm′ō-glō-bin) Compound formed by combination of hemoglobin with two atoms of oxygen.

oxytocin (ox-i-to′sin) A hormone that is stored in the posterior lobe of the pituitary gland that causes uterine contractions during labor and ejection of milk from the breast lobules into the larger ducts.

P

panhy′popitu′itarism Failure of secretion of all anterior lobe pituitary hormones.

papilloma (pap-pil-ō′muh) A descriptive term for a benign tumor projecting from an epithelial surface.

Pap smear A study of cells from various sources, commonly used as a screening test for cancer.

parenchyma (par-en′ki-muh) The functional cells of an organ, as contrasted with the connective and supporting tissue that forms its framework.

parenchymal cell (par en′ki-mul) The functional cell of an organ or tissue.

paresthesia (par-es-thē′ze-ah) An abnormal sensation, such as burning, prickling, or numbness.

Parkinson disease A chronic disease of the central nervous system characterized by rigidity and tremor, caused by deceased concentration of dopamine in the central nervous system.

partial pressure The pressure exerted by a single gas in a mixture of gases, designated by the letter "P" preceding the chemical symbol for the gas (as in PCO₂).

partial thromboplastin time (PTT) test (throm-bō-plas′tin) A test that measures the overall efficiency of the blood coagulation process.

pathogenesis (path-ō-jen′e-sis) Manner in which a disease develops.

pathogenic (path-ō-jen′ik) Capable of producing disease.

pathology The study of the structural and functional changes in the body caused by disease.

PCI See *percutaneous coronary intervention.*

pectus carinatum Ridgelike projection of the sternum anteriorly.

pectus excavatum Posterior displacement of the sternum caused by excessive growth of costal cartilages, which reduce the size of the retrosternal space available for the heart within the mediastinum.

pedicel (ped′i-cel) One of the small terminal processes of the podocytes that cover the glomerular capillaries.

pelvic inflammatory disease (PID) A general term for an infection affecting the fallopian tubes and adjacent pelvic organs.

peptic ulcer A chronic ulcer of the stomach or duodenum related to hypersecretion of gastric juice.

percutaneous coronary intervention (PCI) (per cue tāy′ne yus) An angioplasty procedure in which a balloon catheter covered by a stent is inserted into the site of a severely narrowed or blocked coronary artery, followed by expansion of the balloon, which enlarges the lumen of the artery and simultaneously expands the stent to keep the artery open.

periodontal disease (per-i-ō-don′tal) An inflammation of the gums around the roots of the teeth.

perios′teum The tough, fibrous membrane that covers a bone, except for its articular surfaces.

peristal′sis The wavelike contractions of the wall of the alimentary tract that propel contents through the bowel.

peritoneal dialysis A type of hemodialysis used to treat patients with chronic renal failure, in which dialysate is instilled into the patient's peritoneal cavity and the peritoneum functions as the dialyzing membrane.

peritoneum (per-i-to-nē′um) The membrane that lines the abdominal cavity and also invests the external surfaces of the abdominal organs.

pernicious anemia (per-ni′shus) A macrocytic anemia caused by inability to absorb vitamin B_{12} as a result of inadequate secretion of intrinsic factor by gastric mucosa.

peroxisome (per-ok′-si-sōm) A cytoplasmic organelle containing various enzymes, including those that decompose potentially toxic hydrogen peroxide.

petechia (pe-tē′kēy-uh) A small pinpoint hemorrhage caused by decreased platelets, abnormal platelet function, or capillary defect.

pH Symbol for the negative logarithm of the hydrogen ion concentration—pH 7.0 is neutral; pH less than 7.0 is acid; pH greater than 7.0 is alkaline.

phagocytosis (fag-o-sī-tō′sis) Ingestion of particulate of foreign material by cells.

pheochromocytoma (fē′o-krō′mō-sī-tō′muh) Catecholamine-secreting tumor of the adrenal medulla.

Philadelphia chromosome A chromosomal abnormality found in patients with chronic granulocytic leukemia; abnormality is characterized by a reciprocal translocation of broken end pieces between chromosomes 9 and 22.

phototherapy Fluorescent light treatment of jaundiced babies to reduce the concentration of unconjugated bilirubin in their blood.

pia (pē′yuh) The innermost of the three membranes covering the brain and spinal cord.

pinocytosis (pīn′o-sī-tō′sis) Liquid absorption by cells in which a segment of cell membrane forms small pockets and engulfs the liquid. Similar to *phagocytosis*, except that liquids rather than particulate material are ingested.

pinworm A small parasitic worm infecting humans. Lives in lower bowel and causes perianal pruritus.

placenta Flat disk-shaped structure that maintains the developing organism within the uterus.

placenta previa (prē′vē-yuh) Attachment of the placenta in the uterus such that it partially or completely covers the cervix.

plasma The fluid part of the blood.

plasmid (plas′-mid) A small, circular DNA molecule separate from the main bacterial chromosome.

platelet A component of the blood; a roughly circular or oval disk concerned with blood coagulation.

pleura (plōōr′äh) The mesothelial covering of the lung (*visceral pleura*) and chest wall (*parietal pleura*).

pneumoconiosis (nōō′mō-kō-nēēiō′sis) An occupational lung disease caused by inhalation of injurious substances such as rock dust.

Pneumocystis jiroveci (new-mō-cis′tis •••) A protozoan parasite that causes severe pulmonary infections in immunocompromised persons.

pneumonia (nōō-mōn′yuh) Inflammation of the lung.

pneumothorax (nōō-mō-thor′ax) Accumulation of air in the pleural cavity.

polar body Structure extruded during the meiosis of the oocyte. Contains discarded chromosomes and a small amount of cytoplasm.

poliomyelitis (pō′lē-yo-mī-e-lī′tis) An inflammation of the gray matter of the spinal cord, caused by a virus.

polycythemia (pål-ē-sī-thē′mē-yuh) Increased number of red cells. May be caused by some types of chronic heart or lung disease (*secondary polycythemia*) or by marrow erythroid hyperplasia of unknown causes (*primary polycythemia*).

polyhydramnios (pä-ē-hī-dram′nē-yus) An excess of amnionic fluid.

polyneuritis (pål-ē-nū-rī′tis) An inflammation of multiple nerves.

polyp A descriptive term for a benign tumor projecting from an epithelial surface.

portacaval shunt (por′tuh-kay′vul) Surgically created anastomosis between the portal vein and the vena cava, performed to lower portal pressure in the treatment of esophageal varices.

portal hypertension Elevated pressure in the portal vein and its branches; usually caused by obstruction of blood flow through the liver resulting from cirrhosis.

portal tract Branch of hepatic artery, portal vein, and bile duct located at periphery of liver lobule.

portosystemic shunt (por′-toe-sis-tem′-ik) A surgical or radiologic procedure that connects the portal vein or one of its branches with a systemic vein, performed to lower elevated pressure in the portal vein and its tributaries.

prediabetes Higher than normal blood glucose but high enough to establish diagnosis of diabetes.

preeclampsia (prē-e`k-lamp′-sē-ă) A pregnancy-related complication characterized by hypertension and proteinuria, which usually occurs after the 20th week of gestation, thought to be caused by placental dysfunction.

pregnancy test A test performed on blood or urine to detect the presence of human chorionic gonadotropin (HCG) characteristic of pregnancy.

premyeloma An early stage of multiple myeloma in which plasma cell proliferation in the bone marrow is only slightly increased and only minor blood protein abnormalities are present.

primary gout A metabolic disease caused by overproduction of uric acid, reduced excretion of uric acid, or a combination of both factors. Clinical manifestations are related to precipitation of uric acid in joints, kidneys, and other sites.

prion (prī′-on) A protein infectious particle responsible for Creutzfeldt-Jakob disease and some other degenerative diseases of the nervous system.

proges′terone A steroid hormone that is secreted by the corpus luteum that functions to prepare the endometrium for reception and development of the fertilized ovum.

progno′sis The probable outcome of a disease or a disorder; the outlook for recovery.

progressive inflammatory neuropathy An autoimmune neurologic caused by inhalation of pig brain tissue.

prolac′tin Hormone produced by the anterior lobe of the pituitary gland that stimulates milk secretion.

prolactin inhibitory factor (PIF) Hypothalamic hormone that suppresses release of prolactin from the anterior lobe of the pituitary.

prostaglandin (pros-ta-glan′din) A complex derivative of a fatty acid (prostanoic acid) that has widespread physiologic effects.

prostate-specific antigen An antigen produced by prostatic epithelial cells that is often found in higher than normal concentrations in the blood of patients with prostatic cancer and other diseases of the prostate.

protease inhibitors Drugs used to treat HIV infection that block the enzyme that cuts the viral protein into segments and assembles them around the viral RNA to form the infectious virus particle. As a result, the virus particle is improperly constructed and is not infectious.

prothrombin time test A test that measures the phase of the coagulation mechanism after the formation of thromboplastin.

pro′ton A positively charged particle in the nucleus around which electrons rotate.

proto-oncogene (pro-to-on′-koh-jēn) A normal gene that regulates some aspect of cell growth, maturation, or division.

protozoa (prō-tō-zō′uh) Simple one-celled animal parasites, such as the plasmodium causing malaria.

pulp cavity Central cavity in tooth containing nerves, blood vessels, and lymphatics.

purpura (pur′pura) A condition characterized by hemorrhage in the skin and mucous membranes (petechiae and ecchymoses).

pyelogram (pī′el-o-gram) A means for studying the contour of the urinary tract by intravenous injection of radiopaque material or by direct injection of the material into both ureters.

pyelonephritis (pī′el-ō-nef-rī′tis) A bacterial infection of the kidney and renal pelvis.

R

receptor (rē-sep′-tōr) A protein molecule on the cell surface or within the cytoplasm that binds to a specific factor, such as a drug, hormone, antigen, or neurotransmitter.

recessive gene A gene that expresses a trait only when present in the homozygous state.

recombinant DNA technology Methods for combining a gene from one organism, such as a gene specifying insulin synthesis, with genes from another organism, such as a bacterium.

Reed-Sternberg cell The characteristic cell of Hodgkin's disease, containing two "mirror image" nuclei with prominent nucleoli.

reflex An automatic action, such as a knee jerk, not under voluntary control.

reflux esophagitis Inflammation of the lining of the esophagus caused by reflux of acidic gastric secretions through an incompetent lower gastroesophageal sphincter.

regional enteritis Another name for Crohn disease.

regulator T cells T4 (CD4+) helper T cells that secrete various cytokines to regulate the intensity of the immune response.

rejection An immunologic process characterized by destruction of a transplanted organ.

releasing hormone Hypothalamic hormone that causes release of hormone from the anterior lobe of pituitary.

renal colic Intense flank pain radiating into the groin, resulting from passage of a renal calculus into the ureter.

renin (ren′in) A humoral substance secreted by the kidneys in response to fall in blood pressure, blood volume, or sodium concentration.

resolution A regression of an inflammatory process without significant tissue destruction and with return of the tissues to normal.

respiratory bronchiole A small bronchiole containing alveoli in its walls.

respiratory unit A functional unit of the lung consisting of a cluster of respiratory bronchioles, alveolar ducts, and alveoli derived from a single terminal bronchiole. Another term for *acinus*.

reticulocyte (rē-tik′ū-lō-sīt) A young red cell that can be identified by special staining procedures.

reticuloendothelial system (rē-tik-ū-lō-en-dō-thē′lē-yul) A system of phagocytic cells distributed throughout the body.

Reye syndrome (Rīz) A disease characterized by a fatty liver and neurologic disturbances, probably related to aspirin administration in association with a viral infection.

rheumatic fever A disease caused by hypersensitivity to antigens of the beta streptococcus, characterized by fever, joint pains, and inflammation of heart valves and muscle.

rheumatoid arthritis (rōōm′uh-toyd) A systemic disease primarily affecting the synovium with major manifestations in the small joints.

Rh immune globulin A gamma globulin containing a high concentration of anti-D (Rh$_o$) antibody; used to prevent Rh sensitization of Rh-negative mothers.

ribonucleic acid (RNA) A type of nucleic acid contained in the nucleoli of cells. A component of messenger, transfer, and ribosomal RNA.

ribosome A small cytoplasmic organelle that serves as the site of protein synthesis. Ribosomes are usually attached to the endoplasmic reticulum but may be free in the cytoplasm.

rickets Impaired calcification of bone in a growing child, caused by vitamin D deficiency, which leads to bowing of leg bones when weight bearing is attempted.

Rickettsiae (rik-ket′sē-yuh) Small bacterialike intracellular parasites that parasitize endothelial cells.

roentgenogram (rent′gen-ō-gram) A photograph taken with x-rays.

rubella (rū-bel′luh) German measles.

S

salpingitis Inflammation of the fallopian tubes.

sarcoma (sar-kō′muh) A malignant tumor arising from connective and supporting tissues.

scabies (skā′bēz) An infestation caused by the small parasite *Sarcoptes scabiei*.

Schwann cell (shwän) An elongated cell that surrounds a peripheral nerve fiber and produces the myelin that insulates the fiber.

sclerotherapy (skler′-o-ther′-a-pē) Treatment of varicose veins in esophagus or elsewhere by injecting them with a solution that scars and obliterates the veins.

scoliosis (sko-lee-oh′-sis) An abnormal lateral curvature of the spine.

secondary gout Elevated uric acid and clinical manifestations of gout not caused by the metabolic disease, primary gout, but instead caused by some other disease that raises the blood uric acid excessively, such as kidney failure or excessive breakdown of white blood cells in patients with leukemia.

sella turcica (sel-la tur′sik-uh) Depression in sphenoid bone at base of skull in which pituitary is located. Also called the *pituitary fossa.*

semilunar valve The cup-shaped valve located between the ventricles and the aorta or pulmonary artery.

seminoma (sem-in-ō′ma) One type of malignant tumor of testis.

sen′sory neuron An afferent neuron that carries impulses into the central nervous system.

sentinel lymph node The lymph node in a group of lymph nodes that is located closest to a malignant tumor, which is examined to determine whether the tumor has spread to the node. If the sentinel node is not involved, additional lymph node dissection is not required.

septic embolus (sep-tik em′bo-lus) Infected infarct resulting from embolization of blood clot containing pathogenic bacteria.

septicemia (sep-ti-sē′mē-yuh) An infection in which large numbers of pathogenic bacteria are present in the bloodstream.

serotonin (sēr-o-tō′-nin) A vasoconstrictor mediator of inflammation released from platelets.

serum The fluid expressed from clotted blood. It differs from plasma chiefly in the absence of fibrinogen and some other plasma proteins that are consumed in the process of clotting.

sex chromosomes The X and Y chromosomes that determine genetic sex.

sex-linked gene Gene present on the X chromosome.

shingles Another term for herpes zoster.

shock A general term for any condition leading to such a marked fall of blood pressure that body tissues do not receive an adequate amount of oxygen, most often caused by acute blood loss or severe infection (sepsis).

shock wave lithotripsy (lith-o-trip′sē) A method for removing stones from the urinary tract by breaking them into small bits that can be excreted in the urine.

sickle hemoglobin An abnormal hemoglobin that crystallizes under reduced oxygen tension.

silicosis (sil-ik-ō′sis) A type of occupational lung disease caused by inhalation of rock dust.

sinusoid (sī′nus-oyd) A special type of capillary with a wide lumen of irregular caliber.

slow viral infection An infection of the nervous system caused by an unusual virus with a very long latent period.

somatotropin (so-ma-to-tro′pin) Another name for growth hormone.

spermatids Germ cells in a late stage of sperm development just before complete maturation to form mature sperm.

spina bifida (spī′-nuh bif′fid-duh) Incomplete closure of vertebral arches over the spinal cord, sometimes associated with protrusion of meninges and neural tissue through the defect (*cystic spina bifida*).

splenorenal shunt (splē′no-rē′nul) Surgically created anastomosis between splenic vein and renal vein, performed to lower portal pressure in the treatment of esophageal varices.

spontaneous pneumothorax (nōō-mō-thor′ax) Pneumothorax occurring without apparent cause in healthy young persons.

spores Spherical structures formed within some bacteria that are extremely resistant to heat, disinfectants, and other agents that destroy bacteria. Spores form when conditions are unfavorable for the bacteria, and they can germinate to form actively growing bacteria when conditions are more favorable.

staghorn calculus (kal′kū-lus) A large renal calculus that has adopted the configuration of the renal pelvis and calyces where it formed.

stent An expandable metal hollow tubular device placed within the lumen of a structure such as a blood vessel, often used to expand the lumen of the vessel, where it functions as a support to prevent narrowing of the dilated vessel.

steroid A complex lipid composed of carbon atoms arranged in a four-ring structure.

stomatitis (stō-mäh-tī′tis) Inflammation of the oral cavity.

stricture (strik′tūre) A narrowing of a tubular channel, usually a result of scarring, such as an esophageal stricture.

stroke Any injury to the brain caused by disturbance of its blood supply.

stroma (strō′muh) The tissue that forms the framework of an organ.

subarachnoid space (sub-är-ak′noyd) The space between the arachnoid and the pia, containing large blood vessels supplying the brain.

subdural space (sub-dōōr′rul) The potential space between the dura and the arachnoid.

surfactant (sur-fak′tant) A lipid material secreted by alveolar lining cells that facilitates respiration by decreasing the surface tension of the fluid lining the pulmonary alveoli.

synapse (sin′aps) Pairing of homologous chromosomes in meiosis.

synovium (si-nō′vē-um) The lining of joint cavities, bursae, and tendon sheaths.

systolic heart failure Heart failure caused by inadequate ejection of blood from the ventricles during systole, in contrast to diastolic heart failure in which filling of the ventricles in diastole is inadequate.

T

tension pneumothorax (nōō-mō-thor′ax) Accumulation of air under pressure in the pleural cavity, with displacement of mediastinum away from the side of the pneumothorax.

teratoma (tār-uh-tō′muh) A tumor of mixed cell components.

tetany (tet′an-ē) Spasm of skeletal muscles caused by subnormal level of ionized calcium in the blood.

thrombin A coagulation factor formed by activation of prothrombin in the process of blood coagulation.

thrombin time A laboratory test measurement that determines the concentration of fibrinogen in the blood by determining the clotting time of the blood plasma after addition of thrombin.

thrombocytopenia (throm′bō-sī-tō-pē′ny-yuh) A deficiency of platelets.

thromboplastin (throm-bō-plas′tin) A component formed during blood coagulation from interaction of platelets and plasma components (*intrinsic system*) or liberated from injured tissues (*extrinsic system*).

thrombosis A blood clot formed within the vascular system.

thyroglobulin A protein within the colloid of the thyroid follicles to which the thyroid hormone is attached.

thyroiditis (thī-roy-dī′tis) Inflammation of the thyroid gland. Term often refers to infiltration of gland by lymphocytes and plasma cells as a manifestation of an autoimmune process.

thyroid-stimulating hormone (TSH) Hormone secreted by the anterior lobe of the pituitary; regulates thyroid function.

thyrotropin (thī-ro-tro′pin) Another name for thyroid-stimulating hormone (TSH).

thyroxine (T_4) (thī-rox′sin) One of the thyroid hormones.

tissue A group of similar cells joined to perform a specific function.

tilting disk valve An artificial heart valve in which the flow through the valve is determined by the position of a flat circular disk within the valve.

T lymphocyte A type of lymphocyte associated with cell-mediated immunity.

tone The slight continuous contraction of muscles, which aids in the maintenance of posture.

toxic shock syndrome (TSS) A symptom complex in menstruating women who use high-absorbency tampons, caused by a toxin produced by a staphylococcus that grows in the vagina.

Toxoplasma gondii (tähk′sō-plas′muh gän′dē-ī) A small intracellular parasite of birds, animals, and humans. Causes the disease *toxoplasmosis.*

transient ischemic attack (TIA) (isskē′mik) Temporary cerebral dysfunction as a result of transient obstruction of a cerebral vessel by a bit of atheromatous debris or blood clot usually embolized from an arteriosclerotic plaque in the carotid artery.

transjugular intrahepatic portosystemic shunt A nonsurgical method used to lower portal vein pressure in a person with cirrhosis by connecting an intrahepatic branch of the portal vein to a hepatic vein branch.

translocation A transfer of a piece of one chromosome to a nonhomologous chromosome.

transurethral resection of prostate (TUR) (trans-yūr-ēth′rul) Removal of prostatic tissue by means of a specially designed instrument inserted into the penis.

Treponema pallidum (trep-pō-nē′muh pal′lid-dum) The spiral organism causing syphilis.

Trichinella spiralis (trik-in-el′luh spī-rā′lis) A parasitic worm that infects humans, causing the disease *trichinosis.*

trichomonad (trik-kō-mō′nad) A small motile parasite of the genus *Trichomonas,* one of which causes vaginitis.

triglyceride (trī-glis′er-īd) A compound composed of three molecules of fatty acid combined with one molecule of glycerol.

tri-iodothyronine (T_3) (trī′ī-ō-dō-thi′rō-nēn) One of the thyroid hormones.

tri′somy The presence of an extra chromosome within a cell; having three of a given chromosome instead of the usual pair.

tro′phoblast Cell derived from the fertilized ovum that gives rise to the fetal membranes and contributes to the formation of the placenta.

TSH See *thyroid-stimulating hormone.*

tumor A benign or malignant overgrowth of tissues that serves no normal function.

tumor-associated antigen An antigen associated with growing tumor cells, which serves as an indicator of tumor growth in the body.

tumor necrosis factor A cytokine that can destroy foreign or abnormal cells.

tumor suppressor gene A gene that suppresses cell proliferation.

Turner syndrome A congenital syndrome usually caused by absence of one X chromosome in the female.

two leaflet valve An artificial heart valve in which the flow through the valve is determined by two flat "half moon" leaflets that pivot to open and close the valve.

tyrosine kinase (tī′-rō-sēn kī′-nās) An enzyme that transfers phosphate groups from adenosine triphosphate to the amino acid tyrosine in various cell proteins. Plays an important role in many cell functions concerned with cell growth and cell division. A hyperactive unregulated form of this enzyme is responsible for leukemia in Philadelphia chromosome positive individuals.

ulcer Lesion caused by loss of a portion of a cutaneous or mucous surface, such as a peptic ulcer of the stomach or duodenum.

urate nephropathy (něf-rop′-uh-thē) Kidney damage caused by precipitation of urate crystals within the kidney tubules of a person with gout.

urea (ū-rē′yuh) The nitrogen waste product derived from protein metabolism and excreted in the urine.

uremia (ur-ē′mi-yuh) An excess of urea and other waste products in the blood, resulting from renal failure.

urinalysis (ur-in-al′i-sis) A commonly performed chemical and microscopic analysis of the urine.

valve stenosis (sten-ō′sis) Impaired flow of blood through a heart valve that does not open properly.

valvular regurgitation (rē-gurg-i-tā′shun) Reflux flow of blood through a heart valve that does not close properly.

varices (var′i-sēz) Dilated veins (singular term *varix*).

varicocele (var′-ik-kō-sēl) Varicose veins within the spermatic cord that drain blood from the testis.

vasodilatation Increase in the caliber of a blood vessel.

vasodilator A substance that dilates blood vessels.

velamentous insertion of umbilical cord (vel′uh-men-tus) Attachment of the umbilical cord to the fetal membranes rather than to the placenta.

ventricle (ven′tri-kul) A small cavity, especially one in the brain or heart. *Ventricles of brain:* The hollow cavities in the brain. *Ventricles of heart:* The muscular chambers that receive blood from the atria and pump the blood into the aorta (*left ventricle*) or pulmonary artery (*right ventricle*).

ventricular aneurysm (ven-trik′ū-lär an′ūr-izm) A localized ballooning out of a scar of the ventricle resulting from a previous myocardial infarction.

vertical banded gastroplasty A surgical procedures to promote weight loss in obese subjects by reducing the capacity of the stomach.

vesicoureteral reflux (ves′i-kō-ūr-ēt′er-al) Retrograde flow of urine from the bladder into the ureter during voiding.

virulence (vir′u-lenz) The ability of an organism to cause disease.

virus A small infectious particle. An obligate intracellular parasite.

vital capacity The maximum volume of air that can be forcefully expelled after a maximum inspiration.

volvulus (vol′vū-lus) A rotary twisting of the intestine on its mesentery, with obstruction of the blood supply to the twisted segment.

vulvar dystrophy (vul′vär dis′trō-fē) An abnormality of the vulvar epithelium characterized by hyperkeratosis and epithelial maturation disturbances.

W

West Nile virus An arbovirus that infects birds, animals, and humans.

Wilms tumor A malignant renal tumor of infants and children.

Y

yolk sac A sac that is formed adjacent to the germ disk and that will form the gastrointestinal tract and other important structures in the embryo.

Z

zona pellu′cida A layer of acellular material surrounding the ovum.

zy′gote (zī′gōt) The fertilized ovum.

Index